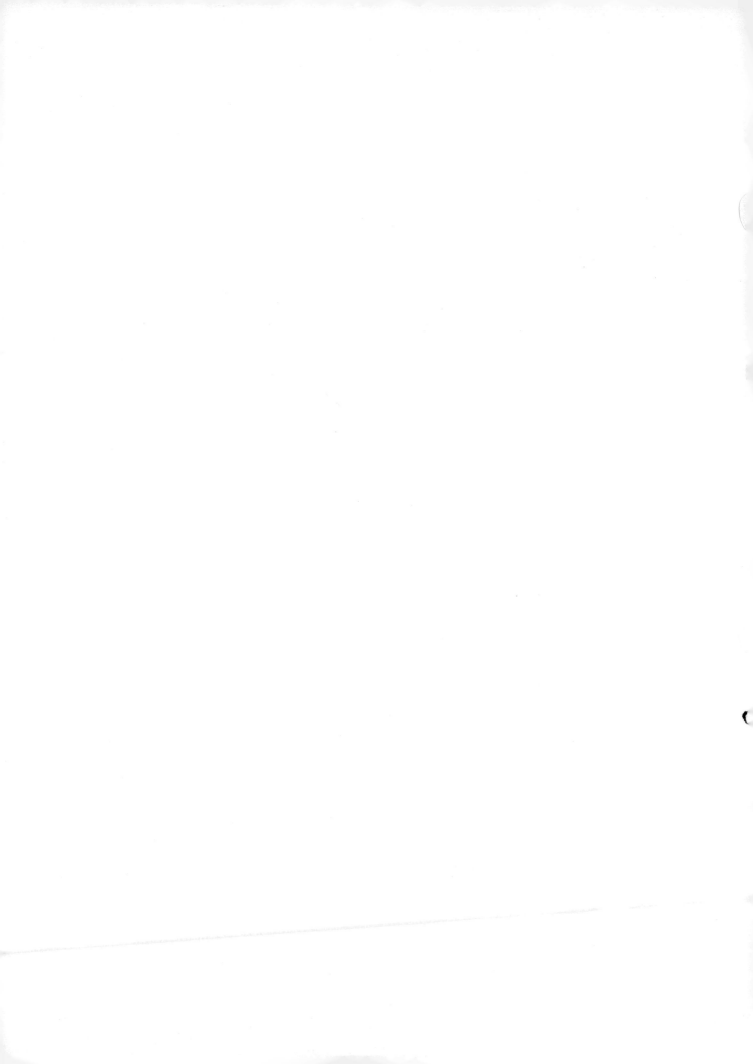

Principles and Practice in Ophthalmic Assisting

A Comprehensive Textbook

PRINCIPLES AND PRACTICE
IN OPHTHALMIC ASSISTING

A COMPREHENSIVE TEXTBOOK

Editors

Janice K. Ledford, AS, COMT
Editor
EyeWrite Productions
Franklin, North Carolina

Al Lens, COMT
Associate Editor and Illustration Manager
Merritt, British Columbia, Canada

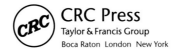

CRC Press
Taylor & Francis Group
Boca Raton London New York

CRC Press is an imprint of the
Taylor & Francis Group, an **informa** business

First published 2018 by SLACK Incorporated

Published 2024 by CRC Press
2385 NW Executive Center Drive, Suite 320, Boca Raton FL 33431

and by CRC Press
4 Park Square, Milton Park, Abingdon, Oxon, OX14 4RN

CRC Press is an imprint of Taylor & Francis Group, LLC

© 2018 Taylor & Francis Group, LLC

Cover photo credits: Cheryl Pelham, Jan Ledford, Wendy M. Ford, Colleen Schreiber

Library of Congress Cataloging-in-Publication Data

Names: Ledford, Janice K., editor. | Lens, Al, editor.
Title: Principles and practice in ophthalmic assisting : a comprehensive
  textbook / edited by Janice K. Ledford, Al Lens.
Description: Thorofare, NJ : Slack Incorporated, [2018] | Includes
  bibliographical references and index. |
Identifiers: LCCN 2017044370 (print) | ISBN 9781617119330 (hardback : alk. paper)
Subjects: | MESH: Eye Diseases | Vision Disorders | Diagnostic Techniques,
  Ophthalmological | Ophthalmic Assistants
Classification: LCC RE46 (print) | NLM WW 140 | DDC

  617.7--dc23
  LC record available at https://lccn.loc.gov/2017044370

ISBN: 9781617119330 (hbk)
ISBN: 9781003525899 (ebk)

DOI: 10.1201/9781003525899

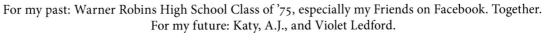

DEDICATION

For my past: Warner Robins High School Class of '75, especially my Friends on Facebook. Together.
For my future: Katy, A.J., and Violet Ledford.
—*Jan Ledford, COMT*

To my wife, Sheila, for her incredible patience as I spent countless hours working on this book.
—*Al Lens, COMT*

CONTENTS

Dedication .... *v*
Acknowledgments .... *xi*
About the Editors .... *xiii*
Contributing Authors .... *xv*
Introduction .... *xvii*

Section I   **General Ophthalmic Knowledge** 1
Chapter 1   Introduction to the Field of Eye Care 3
Jan Ledford, COMT

Chapter 2   Ocular Anatomy 11
Charles A. Beck, DO, FAAO

Chapter 3   Ocular Physiology 27
Al Lens, COMT

Chapter 4   Optics 39
Al Lens, COMT

Section II   **Ophthalmic Skills** 55
Chapter 5   Ophthalmic Equipment 57
Al Lens, COMT

Chapter 6   Scribing and Chair-Side Assisting 69
Jane T. Shuman, MSM, COT, COE, OCS, CMSS, OSC

Chapter 7   History Taking 77
Ellie Bessarab, COT, NCLEC, OSC, and Duanna VanCamp, COT

Chapter 8   Vision Testing 93
Jan Ledford, COMT

Chapter 9   Basic Eye Exam 117
Suzanne Hansen, MEd, COMT, and Anna Kiss, BS, COMT

Chapter 10   Ocular Motility, Strabismus, and Amblyopia 137
Colleen Schreiber, OC(C), COMT, CCRP

Chapter 11   Retinoscopy and Refractometry 179
Aaron V. Shukla, PhD, COMT

Chapter 12   Slit Lamp Microscopy 213
Sergina M. Flaherty, COMT, OSC

Chapter 13   Tonometry 233
Gayle Roberts, COMT, BHS

Chapter 14   Visual Fields 253
Gayle Roberts, COMT, BHS

Chapter 15   Ophthalmic Photography 275
Sarah M. Armstrong, CRA, OCT-C, FOPS

Chapter 16   Diagnostic Imaging 297
Al Lens, COMT

Chapter 17   Ophthalmic Ultrasound 307
Monique Rinke, COMT, and Laura Barry, BSc, COMT

Chapter 18   Electrophysical Testing 335
Jacob P. McGinnis, BA, COT

Section III   Optical Skills **345**
Chapter 19   Optical Procedures 347
                Sumáya "Sumi" Rodríguez, COT, OSC, ABO-AC, FNAO, USN (Ret)

Chapter 20   Eyewear: Spectacles and Lenses 363
                Anne West-Ellmers, COT, OSC, LDO, NCLEC, AAS

Chapter 21   Contact Lenses 379
                Wendy M. Ford, BS, COMT, FCLSA, NCLEM

Section IV   Ophthalmic Medical Sciences **417**
Chapter 22   Pharmacology 419
                Peter D. Anderson, Pharm D, BCPP, CMI-IV, and Gyula Bokor, MD

Chapter 23   Microbiology 439
                Catherine Horan, BA, COMT

Chapter 24   Genetics 459
                James Walsh, MD, PhD, and Sandra Johnson, MD

Chapter 25   Neuro-Ophthalmology 473
                Beth Koch, COT, ROUB, and Lisa Lystad, MD

Chapter 26   Ocular Disorders and Conditions: External and Anterior Segment 485
                Jessica M. Barr, COMT, ROUB

Chapter 27   Ocular Disorders and Conditions: Posterior Segment 499
                Jessica M. Barr, COMT, ROUB

Chapter 28   Cataract 511
                Roxanna Martin, BSc, OSC

Chapter 29   Glaucoma 523
                Sandra Johnson, MD, and Eric Areiter, MD

Chapter 30   Diabetes 537
                Christine McDonald, COE, COA, ROUB, OSC

Chapter 31   Other Systemic Disorders/Conditions Affecting the Eyes 549
                Al Lens, COMT

Chapter 32   Ocular Trauma 557
                Adel Ebraheem, MD, MS

Chapter 33   Nontraumatic Ocular Emergent and Urgent Situations 573
                Gayle Roberts, COMT, BHS

Chapter 34   Subspecialties in Ophthalmology and Optometry 593
                Donna Bong, COMT

Chapter 35   Low Vision 611
                Beth Koch, COT, ROUB

Section V   Surgical Services and Skills **621**
Chapter 36   Overview of Ophthalmic Surgery 623
                Cynthia Matossian, MD, FACS, Henry Lee, MD, and Sebastian Lesniak, MD

Chapter 37   In-Office Minor Surgery 631
                Kesha Hyde, COT, and Jan Ledford, COMT

Chapter 38   Refractive Surgery 645
                Paul M. Larson, MBA, MMSc, COMT, COE, CPC, CPMA

Chapter 39   Ophthalmic Laser Surgery 655
                Adeline Stone, COT, CRA, CDOS

Chapter 40   Surgical Assisting 665
                Robert M. Kershner, MD, MS, FACS, and Jacob P. McGinnis, BA, COT

Section VI   Administrative Skills **681**

Chapter 41   Around the Office 683
Jane T. Shuman, MSM, COT, COE, OCS, CMSS, OSC

Chapter 42   Record Keeping and Electronic Medical Records 689
Jane T. Shuman, MSM, COT, COE, OCS, CMSS, OSC, and Amanda J. Shuman, Esq

Chapter 43   The Basics of Coding in an Outpatient Setting 695
Jane T. Shuman, MSM, COT, COE, OCS, CMSS, OSC

Chapter 44   Health Care Compliance and Regulatory Issues 705
Gloria Garcia-Garza, COA, CMC, and Cheryl Pelham

Appendices **715**

Appendix A   *Review of Sciences and Applications* 717
Jan Ledford, COMT

Appendix B   *In-Office Training* 733
Savory Turman, COMT, OCS

Appendix C   *Medical Terminology* 773
John P. Rowan, COMT

Appendix D   *Commonly Used Ophthalmic Medications* 779
Jan Ledford, COMT

Glossary 785
Financial Disclosures 797
Index 799

ACKNOWLEDGMENTS

Ella Rosamont-Morgan was the original author on the Visual Fields chapter, but passed away before she could complete the work. Her legacy to those of us in the field, including her devoted work with the Association of Technical Personnel in Ophthalmology (ATPO), will never be forgotten.

Every author in this text unselfishly gave time and expertise because he/she believes that eye sight is important… and interesting. Many endured very long wait periods between submission and feedback on their manuscripts. Many also endured seemingly innumerable emails from me, as well as my eternal comments and changes to their work. The goal that united us all was and is to provide readers with the tools and information they need to "help others see better, one person at a time." Thank you, each and every one.

From SLACK Incorporated, I would like to thank Tony Schiavo, Jennifer Kilpatrick, Julia Dolinger, Nathan Quinn, John Bond, April Billick, Katherine Rola, Erika Gonzalez, and Danielle Yentz. You've all been very patient and professional. But my biggest thanks must go to Jennifer Cahill, Senior Project Editor. Her many roles have included cheerleader, permissions watchdog, and sometimes mess-cleaner-upper, not to mention putter-upper with this sometimes testy book editor. Fortunately, she and I never hyperventilated at the same time! She's been a great sounding board, and has worked very hard to make this book happen. And she let me stubbornly cling to my Oxford commas.

I can never pay my debt of gratitude to Al Lens for handling the photos and illustrations. In the 4+ years it has taken to bring this project to fruition, he has never complained. He has worked his Al Magic on countless photos, created numerous drawings, and made every requested figure alteration (no matter how subtle). He's often been the calm in the editorial storm, and endured countless emails from me. Our profession owes him a great deal; so do I.

Others who helped me personally by posing, donating, and providing photo sites include Kelly Ledford, Katy Ledford, AJ Ledford, Violet Ledford, and Heather Ledford; Val Sanders and Johnny Gayton of Eyesight Associates of Middle Georgia; Debbie McCall and Charles Shaller of Franklin Eye Center; Courtney McGaha; Eric Meinecke (Georgia Eye Bank); and Todd Cranmore (Erickson Labs Northwest).

For helping in other ways: Julie Iverson, COT; Frank Wenger, Product Manager General Diagnostics; and Stephanie McMillan, MHA, COT.

For being in my corner always: Cheera Roadarmel (Mom) and Cheryl Pelham.

—*Jan Ledford, COMT*

Dr. Michael Boyd, Dr. Suren Sanmugasunderam, and Dr. Perry Maerov were kind enough to lend their expertise in reviewing some of the material. Without them, it would have taken much longer to verify statements.

The creators of Photoshop have my gratitude for enabling someone like me, with virtually no artistic talent, to create graphics that are respectable. (I was never really good at coloring between the lines without a computer!)

Not all clinics have all the "toys" that we talk about in this book. That meant I relied on a few photographers to come up with images, mostly on short notice. Those who contributed a high number of photos are Kimberly McQuaid, Sergina Flaherty, and Adeline Stone.

Jan Ledford is a very knowledgeable person, and an incredibly understanding editor. I have had the pleasure of working with her on numerous books over the years and she always maintains her professionalism. During the long journey this book was, I had taken 4 months off of work and left the continent. Jan limited her contact with me as much as possible to allow me to enjoy my leave of absence. And to top it all off, she was able to find all the authors for this book!

—*Al Lens, COMT*

ABOUT THE EDITORS

Author, editor, and speaker *Jan Ledford, COMT*, began her ocular adventure as a job-trained assistant. Three certifications, 20+ books, and thousands of eye exams later, she is still very happy in an exam room with a patient, doing refractometry and other fun things.

She is currently owned by only one cat (Nadia Narci), but hopes to one day retire (although no time soon) and become a crazy cat lady. Jan lives in the mountains of western North Carolina where she enjoys singing, reading, spending time with her grandkids and other family, and watching *Judge Judy* and *NCIS*. Oh, and bleeding red ink on other people's manuscripts.

Al Lens, COMT, began his career in ophthalmology in 1986 and has enjoyed teaching new ophthalmic medical personnel how to evaluate and care for patients in the best way possible. He is a firm believer that you should never stop learning. When students face a new scenario, Al encourages them to gain knowledge from the experience, possibly undertaking further study to fill in the blanks. Continuous study makes the job more enjoyable and better serves the patients.

CONTRIBUTING AUTHORS

Peter D. Anderson, Pharm D, BCPP, CMI-IV (Chapter 22)
Clinical Pharmacist
Inpatient and Emergency Department
Boston Medical Center
Boston, Massachusetts

Eric Areiter, MD (Chapter 29)
Department of Ophthalmology
Hendrick Medical Center
Abilene, Texas

Sarah M. Armstrong, CRA, OCT-C, FOPS (Chapter 15)
University of North Carolina
Chapel Hill, North Carolina

Jessica M. Barr, COMT, ROUB (Chapters 26 and 27)
Camden County College
Blackwood, New Jersey
Quidel Corporation
San Diego, California

Laura Barry, BSc, COMT (Chapter 17)
Technical Supervisor
Rockyview Eye Clinic
Calgary, Canada

Charles A. Beck, DO, FAAO (Chapter 2)
Osteopathic Vision
Indianapolis, Indiana

Ellie Bessarab, COT, NCLEC, OSC (Chapter 7)
Portland Community College
Portland, Oregon
Vancouver Eye Care
Vancouver, Washington

Gyula Bokor, MD (Chapter 22)
Independent Practice of Psychiatry
Taunton, Massachusetts

Donna Bong, COMT (Chapter 34)
Outpatient Eye Clinic
Eye Institute of Alberta
Edmonton, Alberta, Canada

Adel Ebraheem, MD, MS (Chapter 32)
Doheny Eye Institute
University of California
Los Angeles, California

Sergina M. Flaherty, COMT, OSC (Chapter 12)
Ophthalmic Technologist
Stone Oak Ophthalmology
Principal
Ophthalmic Seminars of San Antonio
San Antonio, Texas

Wendy M. Ford, BS, COMT, FCLSA, NCLEM (Chapter 21)
President—Contact Lens Society of America
Clinical Administrator/Contact Lens Specialist
Eye Consultants of Northern Virginia, PC
Springfield, Virginia

Gloria Garcia-Garza, COA, CMC (Chapter 44)

Suzanne Hansen, MEd, COMT (Chapter 9)
Ophthalmic Medical Technology Program
University of Arkansas for Medical Sciences
Little Rock, Arkansas

Catherine Horan, BA, COMT (Chapter 23)

Kesha Hyde, COT (Chapter 37)
Kesha Hyde Eye Consulting, Inc
Lindenhurst, New York

Sandra Johnson, MD (Chapters 24 and 29)
Associate Professor
Department of Ophthalmology
University of Virginia
Charlottesville, Virginia

Robert M. Kershner, MD, MS, FACS (Chapter 40)
Eye Physician and Surgeon
Refractive and Cataract Surgery
President and CEO, Eye Laser Consulting
Consultant Specialist-Biomedical, BioPhotonics,
Pharmaceutical, and Ophthalmic Medical and
Laser Devices
Professor and Chairman
Department of Ophthalmic Medical Technology
Palm Beach State College
Palm Beach Gardens, Florida

Anna Kiss, BS, COMT (Chapter 9)
Ophthalmic Medical Personnel Training Program
Georgetown University
Washington, DC

Beth Koch, COT, ROUB (Chapters 25 and 35)
Cole Eye Institute
Cleveland Clinic
Cleveland, Ohio

*Paul M. Larson, MBA, MMSc, COMT, COE, CPC, CPMA
(Chapter 38)*
Senior Consultant
Corcoran Consulting Group
Atlanta, Georgia

Henry Lee, MD (Chapter 36)
Lee Aesthetic Center
Warren, New Jersey

Sebastian Lesniak, MD (Chapter 36)
Matossian Eye Associates
Hopewell, Pennsylvania

Lisa Lystad, MD (Chapter 25)
Cole Eye Institute
Cleveland Clinic Foundation
Cleveland, Ohio

Roxanna Martin, BSc, OSC (Chapter 28)
Akler Eye Center
Dearborn, Michigan

Cynthia Matossian, MD, FACS (Chapter 36)
Clinical Assistant Professor of Ophthalmology (Adjunct)
Temple University School of Medicine
Philadelphia, Pennsylvania

Christine McDonald, COE, COA, ROUB, OSC (Chapter 30)
Association of Technical Personnel in Ophthalmology
President 2015-2016
The Retina Institute
St. Louis, Missouri

Jacob P. McGinnis, BA, COT (Chapters 18 and 40)
Dartmouth Hitchcock Ophthalmology
Lebanon, New Hampshire

Cheryl Pelham (Chapter 44)
Franklin, North Carolina

Monique Rinke, COMT (Chapter 17)
Rockyview Eye Clinic
Calgary, Canada

Gayle Roberts, COMT, BHS (Chapters 13, 14, and 33)
iScreen Vision
Cordova, Tennessee

Sumáya "Sumi" Rodríguez, COT, OSC, ABO-AC, FNAO, USN (Ret) (Chapter 19)
Virginia Eye Institute
Richmond, Virginia
Fellow of the National Academy of Opticianry

John P. Rowan, COMT (Appendix C)
National Eye Institute, National Institutes of Health
Bethesda, Maryland
Mr. Rowan contributed to this work in his personal capacity. The views expressed are his own and do not necessarily represent the views of the National Institutes of Health or the US Government.

Colleen Schreiber, OC(C), COMT, CCRP (Chapter 10)
Alberta Health Services
Alberta, Canada

Aaron V. Shukla, PhD, COMT (Chapter 11)
Professor and Program Director
Ophthalmic Technician Program
St. Catherine University
Eye Care Associates, PA
Minneapolis, Minnesota

Amanda J. Shuman, Esq (Chapter 42)
Danger Law
Newton, Massachusetts

Jane T. Shuman, MSM, COT, COE, OCS, CMSS, OSC (Chapters 6, 41, 42, and 43)
President
Eyetechs, Inc
Needham, Massachusetts

Adeline Stone, COT, CRA, CDOS (Chapter 39)
Ophthalmic Medical Technology Program Director and Faculty Chair
Portland Community College
Portland, Oregon

Savory Turman, COMT, OCS (Appendix B)
Eye Center of Northern Colorado, PC
Fort Collins, Colorado

Duanna VanCamp, COT (Chapter 7)
Ophthalmic Medical Technology Program
Portland Community College
Portland, Oregon

James Walsh, MD, PhD (Chapter 24)
University of Virginia School of Medicine
Charlottesville, Virginia

Anne West-Ellmers, COT, OSC, LDO, NCLEC, AAS (Chapter 20)
Cleveland Sight Center
Cleveland, Ohio

Note: Some of the authors and illustrators are affiliated with the armed forces or governmental agencies of the United States. The opinions and information in this text are the authors' own, and should not be construed as that of the government agencies with which they are associated. Some of the authors and illustrators are affiliated with universities, colleges, and technical schools. The opinions and information in this text are the authors' own, and should not be construed as that of the institutions with which they are associated.

INTRODUCTION

It took more than 40 professionals more than 4 years to put together the volume you now hold in your hands. Whether you are new to ophthalmology or optometry (or opticianry, ocular surgery, etc) or you've been around a long time, this book is for you.

From "A" measurement to zygoma, we have endeavored to include everything you need to know in order to do your job, assist your patients, and advance your career. The authors include professionals in ophthalmology, optometry, osteopathy, pharmacy, opticianry, surgery, and more. The tone is friendly, as if we're sitting next to you in your living room at home. The information is practical, usable, and forward-looking. (And even now we're contemplating the next edition!) Color photos, drawings, diagrams, tables, case studies, and sidebars all contribute to your experience.

I'm still convinced, even (especially!) after 30+ years, that working in the field of eye care is the best career ever. I hope you will learn, explore, and agree.

—*Jan Ledford, COMT*

I

GENERAL OPHTHALMIC KNOWLEDGE

1

Introduction to the Field of Eye Care

Jan Ledford, COMT

Of the many different fields of medicine, eye care has to be one of the most fascinating and rewarding. Advances in instrumentation now let us measure, photograph, scan, and evaluate virtually every part of the eye's complex structure. The continuing study of how we see allows vision correction in both traditional and innovative ways.

Yet it all boils down to patient care. We are helping others "see better," one person at a time. Whether it is a simple matter of greeting the patient or the detailed task of assisting in surgery, we contribute by belonging to a preventing, restoring, preserving, and healing team of professionals.

Regardless of a person's clinical role, there are specific parameters within which one must work. This is known as *scope of practice*. Scope of practice can be identified via legal methods, such as laws that govern whether or not a practitioner can perform surgery, and what type. It can also be delineated by a professional body (organization) or even local clinic protocol, as long as these do not conflict with the law. For example, a local practice might allow competent technicians to remove corneal foreign bodies as long as this is not legally regarded as "practicing medicine." Yet another clinic might require all unlicensed assistive personnel to take and pass a course before they are permitted to instill eye drops.

The text that follows gives an overview of the various types of professionals involved in eye care, each with its own specific scope of practice. If you want to know more after reading this, there is a list of websites at the end of the chapter (Sidebar 1-1) where you can get more information.

Licensed Practitioners

Ophthalmologist

Ophthalmologists are medical doctors (MD) who have specialized in care and treatment of the eye. After obtaining a 4-year college degree, they attend 4 years of medical school, then spend 1 year as an intern. Next is a minimum of 3 years as a resident in ophthalmology. Some go on to an additional 1 or 2 years of specialty training in specific areas of eye care. (See Chapter 34 for subspecialties.)

An ophthalmologist may set up a practice of his/her own, work as part of a group, or be part of a hospital staff. An ophthalmologist is licensed to diagnose and treat disorders of the eye. Treatment may include prescribing glasses, contact lenses, and medications, as well as performing eye surgery of all types.

Ledford JK, Lens A, eds.
Principles and Practice in Ophthalmic Assisting:
A Comprehensive Textbook (pp 3-10).
© 2018 Taylor & Francis Group.

Doctor of Osteopathy

The *doctor of osteopathy's* (DO) schooling and training closely parallels that of an MD. Following a 4-year college degree, he/she attends 4 years of osteopathic medical school followed by 3 to 8 years of specialty training in ophthalmology. A licensed DO may set up a private practice or work in a clinic or hospital, diagnosing and treating eye problems via medication and/or surgery.

The osteopathic method of medicine tends to be more focused on the body as a cohesive unit, vs just the system (visual) or part (the eye) under consideration. Prevention of problems and maintenance of wellness are emphasized.

Optometrist

Like MDs and DOs, an *optometrist* (OD) starts off with a 4-year college degree. The optometrist follows that with a 4-year degree from an optometry school, and must be licensed to practice. An OD may work in his/her own private practice or as part of a group or clinic, and may choose to specialize in a specific area of vision/eye care.

The scope of services that an OD may provide is regulated by national as well as state legislation, and thus may vary from state to state. The general practice of optometry includes diagnosing ocular disease, as well as prescribing glasses and contact lenses. Then, depending on location, licensure, and specialized training, an OD may also prescribe medications to treat specific ocular disorders. Some states also allow ODs to perform certain laser procedures.

Mid-Level Practitioners

Physician Assistant

A *physician assistant* (PA) generally has an undergraduate degree prior to undergoing a rigorous 2- to 3-year training program in medicine and surgery, taking many of the same courses as the MD/DO students. At the end of the academic and practical training, the graduate is awarded a bachelor's or master's degree. This qualifies the candidate to sit for a board examination leading to licensure.

PAs generally must work under a medical doctor and thus cannot set up their own practices, but the scope of their abilities is wide. Depending on state law, a PA in ophthalmology may diagnose and treat eye disease, prescribe glasses and contact lenses, order and interpret tests, and perform certain surgical procedures.

Nurse Practitioner

The hallmark of the licensed nursing profession is patient care, but a *nurse practitioner* (NP) moves into the realm of practicing medicine. The typical NP program accepts registered nurses with a 4-year degree, and results in a master's degree. An NP may work in any branch of medicine, and in some states may set up his/her own practice.

Assistive Personnel

In contrast to the previously mentioned eye care professionals, who must be licensed in order to practice, it does not take a license or even certification to be an ophthalmic or optometric assistant. It is an important distinction that none of these paraprofessionals (also sometimes referred to as *ocular care techs*) practice medicine, which includes prescribing (medications, glasses, or contacts), although they routinely perform measurements and tests used by the practitioner who then prescribes. Persons attaining certification must usually maintain their status with approved continuing education, as well as sponsorship by a licensed practitioner in the field. Where there is more than one level in a particular field, each advancing level builds on the one before it and adds more advanced knowledge and skills in each category.

Regardless of certification or lack of it, eye care techs may work in a variety of settings performing an interesting array of tasks as indicated by the broad subject matter of this book. One study indicated that the top five skills performed by ophthalmic techs are the following:
1. History taking (patient interview)
2. Patient education
3. Checking vision
4. Handling ocular medications
5. Applanation tonometry[1]

Ophthalmic

The generic term for those assisting an ophthalmologist is *allied ophthalmic personnel* (AOP), but they are also commonly called ophthalmic assistants, technicians, or techs. (Note: Until recently the generic term was ophthalmic medical personnel [OMP].) This profession does not require certification and is not a licensed position, but certification does indicate that certain standards have been met and maintained. Certified or not, all AOP must work under the supervision of a licensed practitioner.

The International Joint Commission on Allied Health Personnel in Ophthalmology (IJCAHPO®) is the certifying body for ophthalmic techs. There are three levels of general certification, as well as several specialties. However, just because a person may be certified at the entry level does not mean he/she is limited to specific duties, and may carry out tasks that those certified at higher levels also perform.

AOP usually provide direct patient care (Figure 1-1). Duties include taking the patient history, which is interviewing the patient about his/her eye and vision problems and history, general medical background and conditions, medications and allergies, and other areas. Verifying glasses/contact lens prescriptions, measuring vision, checking pupils and eye muscles, applying eye medications, providing patient education, and performing special tests and measurements are considered basic tasks. Some AOP assist in minor and major surgery, research, or eye banking. Yet others may specialize in specific techniques (such as photography) or specific patient populations (such as pediatrics).

A *certified ophthalmic assistant* (COA®) is the entry-level certification, requiring either completion of an approved school or a combination of work experience, an independent study course, and sponsorship of an ophthalmologist. Once these requirements are met, one may apply to take the certification exam.

The *certified ophthalmic technician* (COT®) is the mid-level certification. Again, the candidate may be either a graduate of an accredited program or a COA with further work experience and education credits. This level requires passing both a written and a practical examination.

The highest level of AOP is the *certified ophthalmic medical technologist* (COMT®). One can qualify to take the written and practical exams by completing a formal program or by being a COT with extended work experience and continuing education.

Optometric

Like their ophthalmic counterparts, optometric assistants are generally involved in direct patient care. While certification is not mandatory, passing the exams signifies a standardized level of knowledge. The certifications were developed by the American Optometric Association (AOA), and the tests are developed and administered by the Commission on Paraoptometric Certification (CPC). Much of the content is the same as for ophthalmic techs, with a greater emphasis on optical skills (eg, ordering, handling, and fitting glasses).

Certified paraoptometric (CPO) is the entry-level designation. In order to sit for the exam, the candidate must have a high school diploma or equivalent, as well as 6 months' experience working in the field of eye care. Basic knowledge of ophthalmic terms, anatomy, and disorders is required, as well as patient examination techniques. There is a marked emphasis on understanding spectacle and lens features and dispensing. Practice management and business skills are also stressed.

Certified paraoptometric assistant (CPOA) is the second level in optometric assisting. One may become eligible to take the exam either by being a CPO and gaining another 6 months' experience or by graduating from

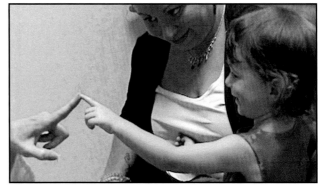

Figure 1-1. Working with children is often a part of the eye care profession.

an approved assistant program. (There may be additional options; see the AOA website.) The content areas include office operations; prescriptions, lenses, frames, adjusting and dispensing; a more advanced level of patient testing (including testing peripheral vision); contact lenses (types, patient education, dispensing); and advanced knowledge of anatomy and physiology; and pharmacology.

Certified paraoptometric technician (CPOT) is the highest level. A CPOA may apply for this certification after another 6 months' work experience. Graduates from an approved technician program may also apply. At this level, less emphasis is placed on office management and more on patient evaluation, including sophisticated testing and instrumentation. Advanced skills in contact lenses and spectacles are required, as well as vision therapy and rehabilitation. Knowledge of ocular anatomy and physiology, disorders of the eye, optics, and pharmacology is likewise more complex.

Medical Assistant

The term *medical assistant* is often used to refer to any nonphysician who works in a medical setting. However, this is a specific profession with certifications of its own (although certification is not required in order to work). Training (often on-the-job or through vocational school) is geared toward a general medical knowledge and skill set, both clinical and administrative. In eye care, a clinical medical assistant will perform many of the same skills as an ophthalmic or optometric tech.

Certification is offered by the American Association of Medical Assistants (AAMA). The *certified medical assistant* (CMA) candidate must have graduated from an approved program for medical assistants before applying to take the exam.

Licensed Nursing Staff

Nursing is a very complex profession when one starts trying to assign classifications. The tasks that a nurse at

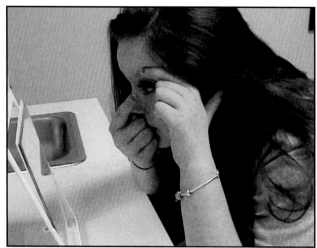

Figure 1-2. Contact lens technicians assist patients in learning how to handle their lenses.

any level may perform vary widely from state to state. In eye care, duties may range from in-office testing and patient counseling to assisting in surgery (laser, minor, and major).

The *licensed practical nurse* (LPN) or *licensed vocation nurse* (LVN) is generally involved in direct patient care and while licensed must still practice under the supervision and direction of a registered nurse or physician. The LPN/LVN must graduate from an approved program, and then pass a licensing exam. In eye care, his/her duties might include basic testing, monitoring, patient education, administering medication, and assisting in surgery. Some states allow them to start intravenous lines and perform other tasks as directed by a registered nurse or practitioner.

A *registered nurse* (RN) must graduate from an approved nursing program or obtain an associate's (2-year) or bachelor's (4-year) degree in nursing, then pass exams in order to become licensed. A master's degree is also available, as well as nurse practitioner (see Licensed Practitioners). In addition to direct patient care, the RN may function in a supervisory role and perform other duties that vary from state to state.

If desired, an RN may become a *certified registered nurse of ophthalmology* (CRNO) through the National Certifying Board for Ophthalmic Registered Nurses (NCBORN). In order to sit for the exam, an RN in good standing must log 2 years' experience in the field of eye care. Exam content areas include ocular conditions, pharmacology, and patient assessment and education.

Clinical Specialties

Contact Lenses

The fitting and (especially) dispensing of contact lenses often falls to an ophthalmic or optometric tech (Figure 1-2). Fitting is more complex, requiring not only special measurements, but some clinical judgment as various lenses are placed on the patient and evaluated for vision and fit. This must be done under the supervision of a licensed practitioner. (For more information, see Chapter 21, Contact Lenses.) Dispensing involves patient education as to lens handling, care, and hygiene.

While certification is not required to work with contact lenses, the National Contact Lens Examiners (NCLE) offers three levels of certification:
1. Basic (NCLE)
2. Advanced (NCLE-AC)
3. Master's (NCLE-M)

These certifications are often sought by opticians as well. Each has specific prerequirements for education, experience, and testing. And while not a certification per se, IJCAHPO has a contact lens home-study course that offers a "certificate of completion" once the program is successfully finished.

Photography and Imaging

Ophthalmic imaging is one area of eye care that has experienced a technological explosion. In fact, the term *imaging* no longer refers only to conventional ophthalmic photography with a camera, but includes other sophisticated methods of capturing images of the eye. Techniques include conventional external photos, photos of the surface and front portion of the eye using the slit lamp microscope, photographing the interior part of the eye (including the optic nerve and retina), as well as specialized techniques utilizing special filters, video, ultrasound, and laser interferometry.

Certification is not required in order to take ocular photos, but there are several types. The Ophthalmic Photographers' Society (OPS) Board of Certification offers the *certified retinal angiographer* (CRA) credential for those proficient in photography (both single-frame and stereoscopic) and angiography (a technique where dye is injected into a vein and rapid-sequence photos are taken as the dye enters and exits the eye's vasculature). Eligibility requirements to take the exam include experience and submission of a portfolio.

OPS also offers an *optical coherence tomographer-certified* (OCT-C) credential for techs specializing in optical coherence tomography. This sophisticated technology involves imaging the layers of the retina as well as other ocular structures (see Chapter 16). In order to take the exam, a candidate must have sponsor-verified work experience and a portfolio.

Low Vision

The field of low vision (for definitions, see Chapter 35) is populated by eye care professionals who must have an extra dose of empathy. There are certifying exams for ophthalmic and optometric techs at every level, but certification is not required in order to work with patients. IJCAHPO does offer technicians a certificate of completion for a self-study course in low vision. Tasks that may be needed for patients with low vision include special vision testing and measuring, training patients to use optical and other low vision aids, patient education, documentation of disabilities, and referral to assistive agencies.

There are other professionals who work with low vision patients (outside of the eye care office or clinic) who must be certified. The Academy for Certification of Vision Rehabilitative and Education Professionals (ACVREP) oversees three areas that provide direct patient assistance. The *certified orientation and mobility specialist* (COMS) helps the patient learn to utilize any remaining vision, as well as other senses, in order to negotiate such skills as maneuvering in traffic areas and using public transportation. A *certified vision rehabilitation therapist* (CVRT) works with the patient to use assistive technology and other skills for independent living and vocational pursuits. A *certified low vision therapist* (CLVT) helps the patient learn to handle activities of daily living (ADLs), which include coping with the impact of low vision on educational, vocational, and social areas.

Surgical Assisting/Surgical Technologist

Ophthalmic surgery is an exciting field that can involve procedures of many kinds, from cosmetic to sight-saving. An ophthalmic surgical assistant is not required to be licensed or certified, but this role is often filled by licensed nurses. The National Board of Surgical Technology and Surgical Assisting (NBSTSA) also certifies graduates of accredited surgical assisting programs (or other pathways) who pass their exams as a *certified surgical technologist* (CST) or *certified surgical first assistant* (CSFA). IJCAHPO offers a specialized credential as an *ophthalmic surgical assistant* (OSA), but one must first be IJCAHPO certified as an assistant, technician, or technologist prior to taking the exam.

Tasks performed by any OSA might include preoperative patient education and consent; instrument and operating room set-up; scrubbing, gloving, and gowning (self and others); directly assisting the surgeon; circulating; set-up and troubleshooting of specialized equipment; postoperative care of instruments and equipment; and postoperative patient care and education.

Ultrasound/Sonography

Ophthalmic Biometry

The generic term *biometry* refers to measuring something; in eye care, this usually refers to ultrasonically measuring the length of the eye, but can also refer to measuring tissue thicknesses as well as tumors. While any appropriately trained tech might perform this task, one can become a *registered ophthalmic ultrasound biometrist*

(ROUB) through IJCAHPO. There are three ways to qualify to take the exam. A person who is already certified in ophthalmic assisting may either complete a special training program or log a specific number of work hours in the field. The third option is for a noncertified tech, who must attain specific educational credits in biometry as well as log hours of biometry experience.

The most common form of biometry uses an A-scan ultrasound, which gives a one-dimensional (linear) image as well as dimensions. A measurement of the eye's length (called axial length) is used in selecting the power of the intraocular lens (IOL), a plastic lens that is implanted into the eye during cataract surgery.

Ophthalmic Sonography

Sonography is often associated with obstetrics and cardiology, but it plays a significant role in eye care as well. B-scan ultrasonography can be used to provide a real-time two-dimensional image of the eye and its structures, as detailed in Chapter 17. It is more complex than A-scan biometry, and is used to evaluate the eye's interior structures, especially when these structures are not visible for any reason. (For example, if a cataract is so dense to the point that the practitioner cannot view the retina, a B-scan might be done to make sure that there is not a retinal detachment prior to performing cataract surgery.) Dimensional measurements may be obtained as well. These tasks might be done by any trained tech or medical sonographer, but IJCAHPO does offer designation as a *certified diagnostic ophthalmic sonographer* (CDOS). In order to qualify for the exam, one must have work experience or certification, plus a portfolio and case log of appropriate scans.

Orthoptics and Vision Therapy

Orthoptics is the branch of eye care that deals with the alignment of the eyes and related subjects, such as the eye muscles and nerves that control movement. While most ophthalmic and optometric techs perform some basic testing of alignment, a *certified orthoptist* (CO) is specially trained and certified (by the American Orthoptic Council) to test for, diagnose, and nonsurgically treat disorders of alignment (eg, "crossed eyes" or strabismus) and vision (eg, "lazy eye" or amblyopia). Because of the importance of early detection and therapy, many orthoptists work with children (Figure 1-3). A prospective orthoptist must hold a 4-year college degree and then attend an approved 24-month fellowship program and pass an exam in order to be certified.

Vision therapy involves training the eyes to work together and may benefit patients with focusing problems, perceptual problems (including learning disabilities), and acquired brain injuries. Certification is not required, but the College of Optometrists in Vision Development (COVD) does offer a credential as a *certified optometric vision therapist* (COVT). First, candidates

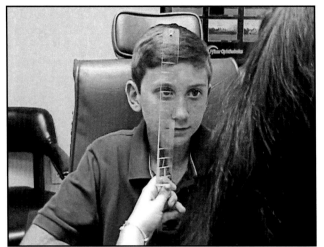

Figure 1-3. Orthoptics involves taking detailed measurements.

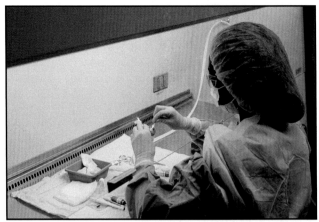

Figure 1-4. Eye banking tech evaluating donor tissue. (Photo is courtesy of Georgia Eye Bank, Inc.)

must be employed by an optometrist who has a fellowship in vision therapy. Then requirements for guided study, experience, and passing both written exams and oral interviews must be completed.

Corporate Certified Ophthalmic Assistant

As ophthalmic technology has expanded, there is a greater need for a knowledgeable task force who can represent companies directly to eye care clinics and offices. These specialists might work for a pharmaceutical company or be more involved in technology. Not only must they know their own products, they must be familiar with the language and needs of those involved in direct patient care. IJCAHPO offers credentialing as a *corporate certified ophthalmic assistant* (CCOA) to these professionals, who must fulfill specific study and work requirements before passing a written exam that covers much the same content as that of a COA.

Eye Bank Technician

Eye banking involves the recovery ("harvest"), preservation, evaluation, and use of ocular tissues retrieved from deceased donors (Figure 1-4). This tissue might be used for research or transplantation. The Eye Bank Association of America (EBAA) administers the examinations (both written and practical) for the *certified eye bank technician* (CEBT). To be eligible, a candidate must have at least a high school diploma or equivalent, as well as on-the-job experience and training in eye banking. Tasks include donor screening, obtaining consent, knowledge of legal and regulatory issues, evaluating tissue, and removing the ocular tissue from the deceased donor.

OPTICAL PERSONNEL

Optician

Simply put, the *optician* is a professional who "fits glasses." In actuality, this is a complex occupation that involves handling, interpreting, manipulating, and filling prescriptions for eyeglasses (and often contact lenses). From assisting and advising the patient in selection of frames and lenses (including material, style, shape, tints, and other features) to adjustment, repair, and patient instruction, these professionals are an essential part of the eye care team (Figure 1-5). An optician may have his/her own private shop or work in a clinic or eye care office. Services offered vary, but might include specialties in fitting children or in dispensing low vision aids. Spectacle lenses might be cut and tinted on the premises or ordered from an outside lab.

Opticianry skills are generally learned on the job. About half the states require opticians to be licensed and/or registered. The American Board of Opticianry (ABO) offers 3 levels of certification:
1. ABOC (basic)
2. ABOC-AC (advanced)
3. ABOM (master's)

Each level requires specific amounts of experience and training/education, as well as passing written and practical exams. Those who also handle contact lenses can seek specific certifications (as outlined under Contact Lenses), and may be required to obtain an additional permit.

Ocularist/Prosthetist

Making and fitting prosthetic eyes (or ocularism) is an art involving fabricating, sculpting, painting, and dispensing of artificial eyes (Figure 1-6). This is the purview of the *ocularist* or *prosthetist*. There is no specific school

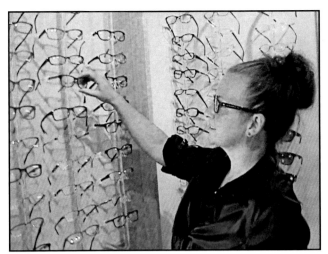

Figure 1-5. Opticians assist patients with every aspect of frame and lens selection.

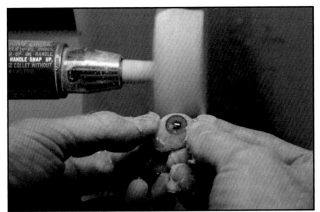

Figure 1-6. Polishing a custom ocular prosthesis. (Photo by: Erickson Labs Northwest, LLC. Todd Cranmore BCO/BADO.)

to learn ocularistry; those wishing to enter the profession must find someone willing to take them on as an apprentice. After a number of years in the field, one may apply to become a Diplomat of the American Society of Ocularists. Additionally, the National Examining Board of Ocularists (NEBO) offers credentialing as a *board certified ocularist* (BCO) to those meeting its criteria and passing both written and practical exams. Some states may require registration with the state labor board in order for a prosthetist to advertise as a registered ocularist.[2] With the advent of three-dimensional printers, ocular prosthetics is a field that continues to evolve.

Ophthalmic Laboratory Technician

The *ophthalmic laboratory technician* (also called *manufacturing optician*) works in an optical lab and fabricates lenses for prescription spectacles and contact lenses. Once cut to prescription, spectacle lenses are shaped, polished, inserted into frames, and checked for accuracy. A high school diploma or the equivalent is usually required, and training is on the job. While there is no official certification for the profession, some vocational schools offer a certificate of completion once the candidate has completed the course work. Although this job does not generally provide face-to-face contact with patients, the lenses that are made affect patients' welfare and quality of life.

ADMINISTRATIVE

Certified Ophthalmic Executive

For those managing an ophthalmic practice, the American Society of Ophthalmic Administrators (ASOA) offers credentialing as a *certified ophthalmic executive* (COE). In order to qualify for the exam, the candidate must have experience in medical management, some of which must be specifically in ophthalmology. The exam covers basic knowledge about the eye, as well as management skills, including human resources, accounting and finances, marketing, risk management, regulatory issues, and information systems.

Certified Patient Service Specialist

While the main emphasis of this book involves working directly with patients, nonclinical personnel also play a big role in providing eye care. The ASOA established the *certified patient service specialist* (CPSS) credential for those involved in the administrative side of practice. The practice itself must make a commitment to the program in order for its employees to be eligible. The candidate him-/herself must complete a distance-learning program and then pass an exam in order to become credentialed. Not only must he/she have knowledge of regulatory issues, customer service, coding/billing, and human resources, but he/she must also have an understanding of ophthalmic equipment and services, common ocular disorders, and triage.

Coding Certifications

Coding involves properly designating the diagnostic and procedure codes for a patient's ophthalmic or optometric visit and/or services (including optical) required for billing and reimbursement. Mistakes can result in delays and denials of reimbursement and even fines to the practice.

While certification is not required, the American Academy of Professional Coders (AAPC) offers the *paraoptometric coding certification* (CPOC). To sit for this exam one must have a high school diploma or equivalent, as well as 2 years' experience in medical coding and billing. The exam covers knowledge of the eye and its pathology, ocular procedures, medical terminology, medical records, and details regarding coding.

SIDEBAR 1-1
CERTIFICATION WEBSITES

▶ Academy for Certification of Vision Rehabilitation and Education Professionals (ACVREP): www.acvrep.org

▶ American Board of Opticianry (ABO): www.abo-ncle.org/

▶ College of Optometrists in Vision Development (COVD): www.covd.org/

▶ Contact lenses: www.abo-ncle.org

▶ Corporate ophthalmic assistant: www.jcahpo.org/certification-recertification/

▶ Diagnostic ophthalmic sonography: www.jcahpo.org/certification-recertification/

▶ Medical assisting: www.aama-ntl.org

▶ National Board of Surgical Technology and Surgical Assisting (NBSTSA): www.nbstsa.org/index.asp

▶ National Examining Board of Ocularists (NEBO): www.neboboard.org/

▶ Ophthalmic assisting: www.jcahpo.org/certification-recertification/

▶ Ophthalmic coding: www.aao.org/aaoe/coding/ocs-exam.cfm

▶ Ophthalmic photography: www.opsweb.org/

▶ Ophthalmic registered nurse: www.asorn.org/certification/

▶ Ophthalmic surgical assisting: www.jcahpo.org/certification-recertification/

▶ Ophthalmic ultrasound biometry: www.jcahpo.org/certification-recertification/

▶ Opticianry: www.abo-ncle.org

▶ Optometric assisting (paraoptometry): www.aoa.org/paraoptometrics/certification

▶ Orthoptics: www.orthoptics.org

▶ Paraoptometric Coding Certification (CPOC): www.aoa.org/paraoptometrics/certification/paraoptometric-coding-certification-%28cpoc%29

For those working in an ophthalmic practice, the American Academy of Ophthalmic Executives (AAOE) and IJCAHPO offer the *ophthalmic coding specialist* (OCS) credential, awarded after passing an open-book test with content areas similar to that of a CPOC.

REFERENCES

1. Woodworth KE, Campbell RC, Dean CA, DuBois LG, Ledford JK. Analysis of tasks performed by certified ophthalmic medical personnel. *Ophthalmology*. 1995;102(12):1973-1986.

2. House Bill 4392. www.legislature.mi.gov/documents/2013-2014/billanalysis/house/htm/2013-HLA-4374-C368A7DB.HTM. Accessed April 23, 2016.

BIBLIOGRAPHY

Bureau of Labor Statistics. Healthcare occupations. US Department of Labor website. www.bls.gov/ooh/healthcare/home.htm. Published December 17, 2015. Accessed April 23, 2016.

Unless otherwise noted, the figures in this chapter were contributed by the following, who are associated with this book as authors:
Jan Ledford: Figures 1-2, 1-3, 1-5
Cheryl Pelham: Figure 1-1

2

OCULAR ANATOMY

Charles A. Beck, DO, FAAO

In order to talk scientifically about the eye and its surrounding structures, we need an agreed-upon language that will help orient us as we explore (Sidebar 2-1).

We also need to define specific areas of the eyeball (*globe*, Figure 2-1). The different structures mentioned here will be covered in detail later.

The eye has three *chambers*. The *anterior chamber* is the fluid-filled space between the cornea's innermost surface and the iris. The *posterior chamber* occupies the space behind the iris and in front of the lens. The *vitreous chamber* is the jelly-filled space that extends from behind the lens to the retina and makes up the majority (two-thirds) of the eye.

The globe has two *segments*. The *anterior segment* is made up of the anterior chamber, posterior chamber, cornea, iris, lens, ciliary body, and the anterior portion of the sclera. The *posterior segment* is bound anteriorly by the back of the lens; this is the largest portion and contains the vitreous body, retina, and optic disc.

THE SKULL

The bones of the head (skull) are joined together by specialized joints called *sutures*. These sutures allow some slight movement of the bones as well as adaptation to external forces (ie, trauma) placed on the skull (Sidebar 2-2). The motion of the sutures has been measured in the range of 380 microns to 1 mm.[1] This fluctuation, or its lack, has been suggested to have an impact on vision.

The Bony Orbit

There are seven bones that make up the bony housing (*orbit*, Figure 2-2) of the eye. Together these bones shape the globe, offer protection, and provide the origins of the ocular muscles. They create a space that is filled by the globe of the eye and its accompanying structures. The bones can also contribute to visual disturbances. We will explore variations in the orbit as we progress through the chapter.

The *frontal bone* makes up the superior portion, or roof, of the orbit and is the largest of the orbital bones. Embryologically, this bone starts as a left and right portion that come together in the midline. In most people the two halves fuse by adulthood into a single bone, but in 7% of the population the halves do not close completely. Such a suture could impact a spectacle prescription or the way eyeglasses fit because different forces on one-half of the frontal bone could physically create a different pressure and shape of the orbit. This change could be nearly instantaneous if caused by a car accident, for example, or happen over a longer time if caused by less powerful forces.

Ledford JK, Lens A, eds.
Principles and Practice in Ophthalmic Assisting:
A Comprehensive Textbook (pp 11-26).
© 2018 Taylor & Francis Group.

SIDEBAR 2-1

ANATOMICAL TERMS

▸ Midline: The center of the body—Usually an imaginary line that divides the forehead, nose, mouth, etc, into left and right parts

▸ Superior, supra-: Above, referring to the top

▸ Inferior, infero-: Below, referring to the bottom

▸ Medial: Toward the middle (of the body)

▸ Lateral: Toward the outside (of the body)

▸ Ipsi-: Prefix meaning "same"

▸ Contra-: Prefix meaning "opposite"

▸ Suture: The interlocking joint between two bones of the head

▸ Origin (of a muscle): The place where a muscle attaches to the body part that does not move when the muscle contracts

▸ Insertion (of a muscle): The place where a muscle attaches to the body part that moves when a muscle contracts

▸ Embryology: The study of the development of the body from conception through birth

▸ Afferent nerve: Primary direction of conduction is toward the brain (sensory)

▸ Efferent nerve: Primary direction of conduction is away from the brain (motor/movement)

SIDEBAR 2-2

THE OSTEOPATHIC VIEW

The field of osteopathy (see Chapter 1) offers a unique perspective to all branches of medicine. Founded by A. T. Still in the late 1800s, osteopathy set out to improve the (then) practice of medicine and surgery by incorporating physical manipulation as a part of medical treatment. Solidly based in anatomy, osteopathy believes that the body can heal itself in most cases if unhealthy anatomy is restored to health by correcting its altered motion. Today, this philosophy is what distinguishes osteopaths from traditional medical doctors.

Historically, only the Italian anatomists wrote of the movement (bony motion) and nonfusion of the bones of the skull. Most medical professionals trained in the United States and Britain are taught that these bones fuse and do not move at all once we reach adulthood. This has lead to many medical professionals having reservations about bony motion and its implications. The Osteopathic Cranial Academy (www.cranialacademy.org) is a good place to explore this phenomenon.

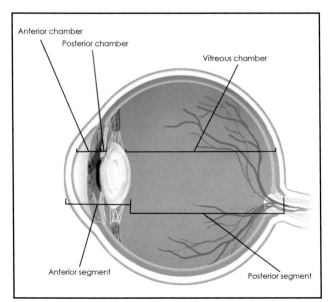

Figure 2-1. Chambers and segments of the globe.

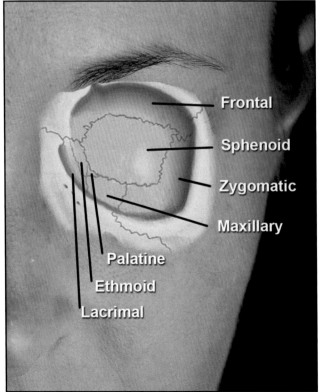

Figure 2-2. The seven bones of the orbit.

Moving clockwise around the left orbit, the next bone is the *zygoma*, or *cheekbone*. The zygoma is a paired bone and joins the frontal bone to make up the continuation of the lateral border of the orbit. The zygoma forms the lateral, inferolateral, and much of the inferior border of the orbit. It also abuts the maxilla. Because of its prominence, the zygoma is the receiver of many of life's facial impacts. This kind of trauma can jam the bone into its neighbors and cause or contribute to visual disturbances.

Continuing clockwise we come to the *maxilla*, a paired bone that forms the remainder of the inferior border of the orbit and the majority of the medial border. Because it holds the upper teeth, the maxilla also falls into the realm of dentistry. From an osteopath's and facial surgeon's perspectives, aberrations here can impact vision. Theoretically, this means that something as common as having the teeth cleaned might alter the inherent movement of the maxilla, slightly altering its position. Orthodontia and facial surgery may affect vision as well.

Directly posterior to the medial border of the maxilla we reach the *lacrimal* bone. It is also a paired bone. It shares a suture with the maxilla (maxillary/ethmoid suture), as well as the frontal (frontal/lacrimal) and ethmoid (lacrimal/ethmoid) bones. The lacrimal bone also houses the lacrimal (or tear) gland (covered later).

Continuing to move into the deeper parts of the orbit, we come next to the *ethmoid* bone. The ethmoid is the only bone of the face that cannot be palpated directly from the outside. The ethmoid is a midline bone. It is mostly hollow and incredibly delicate.

The smallest component of the orbit is the *palatine* bone. This bone also makes up the posterior portion of the palate. It is a paired bone and, along with the maxilla, makes up two arches (the arch of the teeth and the arch of the palate). Because of its location at the posterior part of the orbit (and thus its closeness to the retina), alterations in the palatine bone may affect vision.

The last bone of the orbit is the *sphenoid*, which is located on the midline. Since most of the ocular muscles attach here and because it makes up the retinal portion of the orbit, it is the most important bone for ocular function.

NERVE SUPPLY

Cranial Nerves Affecting the Eye

Cranial nerves (CNs) come directly from the brain. There are 12, usually designated by Roman numerals. There are four CNs that principally involve vision or the eye: CNs II, III, IV, and VI.

CN II, the *optic nerve*, is the key nerve for vision. Its primary functions are detection of light and vision. Compromise to this nerve can affect vision in one or both eyes causing blindness, visual field defects, blurring,

blind spots, and double vision (diplopia). It enters the eye at the optic disc, making the eye actually an extension of the brain.

CN III, the *oculomotor nerve*, primarily moves four of the six ocular muscles. (This is discussed in more detail later, as well as in Chapter 10.) Problems with this nerve can cause outward and downward deviation of the eye, drooping of the eyelid, and (in a complete palsy) pupillary dilation on the affected (*ipsilateral*) side. Primary functions are eye movement (upward, downward, and inward), raising the eyelids, and constricting/dilating the pupil in response to light changes.

CN IV, the *trochlear nerve*, moves the superior oblique muscle. Disorders of this nerve can cause vertical diplopia upon looking downward. Its primary function is eye movement downward and inward.

CN VI, the *abducens* nerve, stimulates the lateral rectus muscle to pull the eye laterally (toward the ear). Malfunctions of this nerve can affect medial deviation of the eye (ie, toward the midline, or inward). In a complete nerve injury, the eye is turned in. If the injury is only partial, the eye may be straight when looking forward, but cannot move laterally from the midline.

The eye is also innervated by segments of CN V, the *trigeminal nerve*. The *maxillary division* of CN V supplies the lower lid. The *ophthalmic division* of CN V has three branches that affect the eye. The *lacrimal nerve* goes to the lacrimal gland and has subdivisions that go to the skin of the superior eyelid and the conjunctiva. The *frontal nerve* provides sensory input to the scalp, forehead, and superior eyelid. The *nasociliary nerve* provides sensory input to the eyeball. This nerve further subdivides to the *infratrochlear nerve*, which innervates the eyelids, conjunctiva, and lacrimal sac.

Finally, there is a bundle of nerve cell bodies called the *ciliary ganglion,* which supplies parasympathetic fibers that support the oculomotor nerve and ophthalmic nerve. (The nervous system is divided into voluntary and involuntary branches. The voluntary we can control [eg, movement] and the involuntary we cannot [eg, heartbeat, breathing]. The involuntary branch is further broken into the sympathetic and parasympathetic. Sympathetic ["fight or flight"] is controlled by adrenaline and the parasympathetic by noradrenaline [the body relaxed]. In the eye, the parasympathetic division constricts the pupil and causes accommodation. See also Appendix A.)

BLOOD SUPPLY

We will begin our discussion of the eye's blood supply (Figure 2-3) with the blood vessels (arteries) leaving the heart via the aorta. The left and right common carotids branch off from the aorta. Each common carotid travels up the side of the neck to the level of the thyroid cartilage, where it splits into the external and internal carotid artery.

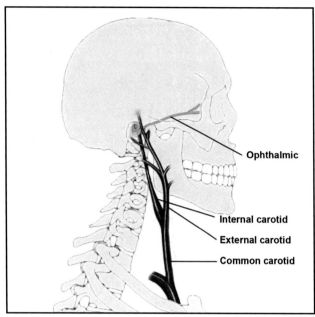

Ophthalmic

Internal carotid

External carotid

Common carotid

Figure 2-3. Arterial blood supply to the eye.

The internal carotid artery travels up and enters the head via the carotid canal. (This canal extends through an opening [foramen] in the temporal bone). After passing through the cavernous sinus, the internal carotid becomes the ophthalmic artery. It supplies all of the structures of the orbit as well as some parts of the meninges (three-layered protective covering over the brain and spinal cord), face, and nose. The branches of the ophthalmic artery are listed in Table 2-1.

The ophthalmic artery and vein branch to form the central artery and vein of the retina. These run next to the anterior part of the optic nerve and cross through the subarachnoid space around it. Pulsation of the retinal artery is usually visible through an ophthalmoscope.

Any increase in the fluid around the brain and in the spine (cerebrospinal fluid) can cause pressure that slows the drainage of blood from the veins, causing fluid accumulation and edema in the eye. Edema of the retina can be observed through an ophthalmoscope as swelling of the optic disc. This is called *papilledema*. Inspection of the optic fundus is thus an essential part of a neurologic examination.

	TABLE 2-1	
OCULAR BLOOD SUPPLY (BRANCHES OF THE OPHTHALMIC ARTERY)		
Artery	**Location**	**Function**
Central retinal artery	Briefly runs under the optic nerve, then penetrates into the nerve sheath	Supplies blood to inner retinal layers and optic nerve
Lacrimal artery	Arises just as the ophthalmic artery enters the orbit and runs along the lateral rectus muscle	Supplies blood to eyelids, lacrimal gland, and conjunctiva
Posterior ciliary arteries	There are one to five of these; they enter the sclera posteriorly near the optic nerve	Supply blood to posterior uveal tract (the iris, ciliary body, and choroid)
Muscular branches	There are superior and inferior muscular branches	Supply blood to extraocular muscles
Supraorbital artery	Passes anteriorly along the medial border of the superior rectus and levator palpebrae muscles and through the supraorbital foramen	Supplies blood to muscles of skin and forehead
Anterior ethmoidal artery	Enters nose through anterior ethmoidal canal	Supplies blood to anterior and middle ethmoidal sinuses, frontal sinus, and meninges
Posterior ethmoidal artery	Enters nose via posterior ethmoidal canal	Supplies blood to posterior ethmoidal sinuses and meninges
Medial palpebral arteries	Anterior to the trochlea (ear); there is a superior and inferior artery	Supply blood to eyelids
Terminal branches	Supratrochlear (frontal bone) artery and dorsal nasal artery	Supply blood to forehead and scalp

EXTRAOCULAR MUSCLES

There are six extraocular muscles (EOMs) that move the eye (Figure 2-4). When these ocular muscles work well together, smooth and balanced eye motion is the result. Ultimately, we are then able to process a three-dimensional image in the brain derived from the input of both eyes. This is covered in great detail in Chapter 10.

Each EOM has two designations, and is usually further identified by indicating which eye (ie, right or left). The *recti* (from the Latin meaning "straight") attach to the eye at the anatomical "compass directions"—superior, inferior, medial, and lateral. The *obliques* (from the Latin meaning "situated at an angle") attach to the globe at an angle, one upper (superior) and one lower (inferior). The actions and nerve supply of the EOMs are listed in Table 2-2.

The four rectus muscles arise from the Annulus of Zinn, a tendinous sheath surrounding the optic canal (Table 2-3). The superior oblique arises from the sphenoid bone close to the tendinous ring. The inferior oblique originates on the orbital surface of the maxilla.

Contraction of the oblique muscles when the eye is rotated laterally is accompanied by some slight protrusion of the eyeball. The rectus muscles have the opposite effect.

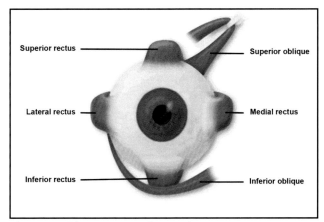

Figure 2-4. The six extraocular muscles.

EYELIDS AND LASHES

The eyelids are a thin layer of skin that protects and helps spread lubrication for the eye. The levator palpebrae superioris muscle can voluntarily or involuntarily open the eyelid. The eyelashes are added protection against sweat dripping into the eye and help to keep dust and other foreign objects out of the eye (Figure 2-5).

TABLE 2-2
EXTRAOCULAR MUSCLES

Muscle	Action	Cranial Nerve Supply
Inferior oblique	Rotates laterally (excyclotorsion), turns up (when looking toward nose), and turns laterally	CN III
Inferior rectus	Turns down, rotates laterally (excyclotorsion), and turns medially	CN III
Lateral rectus	Turns laterally (abduction)	CN VI
Medial rectus	Turns medially (adduction)	CN III
Superior oblique	Rotates medially (incyclotorsion), turns down (when looking toward nose), and turns laterally	CN IV
Superior rectus	Turns up, rotates medially (incyclotorsion), and turns medially	CN III

TABLE 2-3
ORIGINS AND INSERTIONS OF THE EXTRAOCULAR MUSCLES

Muscle	Origin	Insertion
Superior rectus	Annulus of Zinn	Anterior, superior surface of the globe
Inferior rectus	Annulus of Zinn	Anterior, inferior surface of the globe
Lateral rectus	Annulus of Zinn	Anterior, lateral surface of the globe
Medial rectus	Annulus of Zinn	Anterior, medial surface of the globe
Superior oblique	Sphenoid	Posterior, superior, lateral surface of the globe
Inferior oblique	Maxilla	Posterior, inferior, lateral surface of the globe

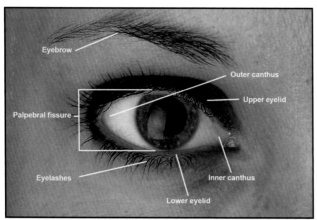

Figure 2-5. The external eye.

Sensory input for the upper eyelid comes via divisions of the ophthalmic branch of CN V (the *infratrochlear*, *supratrochlear*, *supraorbital*, and *lacrimal* nerves). The medial portion of the lower eyelid is supplied by the infratrochlear nerve. The rest of the lower lid is supplied by the *infraorbital nerve* (maxillary branch of CN V).

If CN III is damaged, the upper eyelid cannot be voluntarily raised due to the impact on the levator palpebrae superioris muscle. However, if CN VII is damaged, the orbicularis oculi muscle is affected and the eyelids cannot close. In this case, protective blinking is lost and tears cannot be swabbed across the cornea. This may result in excessive tearing as the body tries to lubricate the eye.

The eyelids keep the cornea moist and protect it from injury and excessive light. The lids are covered externally by thin skin and lined internally by the highly vascularized *conjunctiva*. The conjunctiva is a mucous membrane that covers both the inner lid (*palpebral* conjunctiva) and the eyeball (*bulbar* conjunctiva). Where they merge, deep pockets known as the conjunctival *fornices* (Latin for "vault" or "arch") occur. The fornices (also called the *cul de sac*) can trap dust or other foreign objects, which may cause severe pain until the object is removed. Because the palpebral and bulbar conjunctiva are continuous, it is impossible for an object to "get lost behind the eye."

Internally, each eyelid has a tough, dense connective tissue band known as the *tarsal plate* or *tarsus*. This gives the lids their shape. The orbicularis oris muscle lies between the skin and this connective tissue band. The tarsal plates contain a number of tarsal glands, which produce fatty secretions to lubricate the edges of the eyelids. These secretions prevent the eyelids from sticking together when closed as well as compose part of the tear film (discussed later).

The margins of the eyelids are further protected by *cilia*, or *eyelashes*. These are arranged in two or three irregular rows. Between the hairs are modified sweat glands, as well as sebaceous glands (*ciliary* glands). The ciliary glands secrete oil to the superficial layer of tears that helps to retard evaporation. The *gray line* (also known as the *muscle of Riolan*) represents the division between the anterior and posterior part of the lid. The gray line is often used as a landmark during eyelid surgery as a point where the lid can be split. It is actually the superficial portion of the orbicularis muscle. This muscle, along with the outer skin, make up the *anterior lamella*. (The *posterior lamella* consists of the conjunctiva and the tarsus.)

The "corner" where the eyelids meet is known as the *canthus*. Each eye has a medial (toward the midline or nose) and lateral (toward the outside or ear) canthus. Some persons or races may have an extra skin fold at the nasal canthus, called the *epicanthal fold*.

The space between the upper and lower eyelids is called the *palpebral fissure*. In most races the fissure is nearly horizontal; however, in some races (such as Asian) it slants up at the lateral edge.

LACRIMAL SYSTEM

The *lacrimal gland* is a small, almond-shaped gland that secretes watery tears (lacrimal fluid). It contains 3 to 90 excretory ducts that open into the superior fornix. There are also accessory lacrimal glands. Those found in the lacrimal caruncle are called *Ciaccio's glands*. The ones found underneath the eyelid and where the upper and lower conjunctiva meet are *Krause's glands*. The function of these accessory glands is to produce tears. The physiology of the tears and tear film is discussed in Chapter 3.

As tears drain from the lacrimal gland, they moisten the corneal surface. When the cornea becomes dry, the eye blinks and lacrimal fluid is carried in a thin film over the surface of the cornea. Excess fluid (and any debris that may be carried with it) is moved toward the medial canthus.

If you evert the medial lower eyelid, you will notice a small elevation called the *lacrimal papilla* in the center of which is a tiny pit call the *lacrimal punctum*. (There is a similar punctum and papilla on the upper eyelid.) The lacrimal punctum is the exterior opening of the canal called *lacrimal canaliculus*. This canal channels tears into the *lacrimal sac* (Figure 2-6).

Some fibers from the orbicularis oris muscle run to the lacrimal sac and insert into the crest of the lacrimal bone. When these muscle fibers contract, the lacrimal sac is squeezed, forcing tears through the *nasolacrimal duct* and into the nasal cavity. From there, tears drain into the throat.

During embryonic formation, there is a membrane between the lacrimal sac and nasolacrimal duct. This membrane normally disappears before birth. Sometimes, however, it remains and causes tearing and infection in infants. In such a case the membrane must be mechanically broken through so that the tears can drain properly.

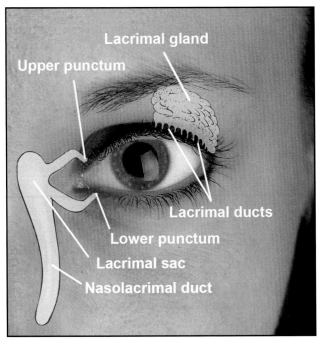

Figure 2-6. The nasolacrimal system.

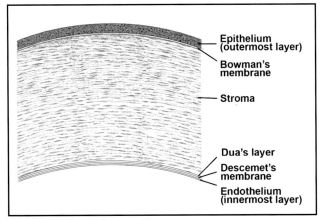

Figure 2-7. The six layers of the cornea.

Any of the glands or ducts of the lacrimal system can become infected and/or blocked. Swelling is usually the result. If an eyelash follicle becomes obstructed or infected, a painful red swelling known as a *sty* develops on the eyelid. *Chalazia* are cysts of the sebaceous glands of the eyelids. A tarsal chalazion is an obstruction of a tarsal gland, and protrudes toward the eyeball. Usually chalazia are more painful than sties.

THE ANTERIOR SEGMENT

The External Globe

Sclera

The visible white portion of the eye is known as the *sclera*. It is continuous with the dural sheath of the optic nerve and the dura (membranous covering) of the brain. If we think of the eyes as an extension of the brain (because they share the same covering membranes) it is easy to see why eye infections can become life-threatening and why ocular trauma can be debilitating. The sclera is tough and opaque. It can appear bluish in children and yellowish in older people.

The clear covering of the front of the eye is the *cornea* (described momentarily), and its margins are continuous with the sclera, meeting at a junction known as the *corneoscleral limbus* (usually shortened to just *limbus*). Interestingly, the cornea and sclera are made of the same type of collagen fibers, but with some important differences. The fibers in the cornea are arranged at right angles to each other, and thus are transparent. The scleral

fibers are haphazardly arranged. In addition, the innermost layer of the cornea keeps the entire tissue dehydrated. The sclera is opaque in part because it is hydrated.

Conjunctiva

As discussed previously, the external eyeball/sclera is covered by a thin, moist mucous membrane called the bulbar conjunctiva. This conjunctiva continues from the sclera to line the inside of the eyelids, where it becomes the palpebral conjunctiva (which is continuous with the skin of the eyelid). The palpebral conjunctiva has lots of blood vessels. These become visible when dilated and congested, commonly called bloodshot eyes (or more formally, *hyperemia*). An infection that causes the conjunctiva to become red and inflamed is known as *conjunctivitis* (see Chapter 26).

Sensory innervation of the conjunctiva comes from the trigeminal nerve through its maxillary, lacrimal, and infratrochlear branches.

The Anterior Chamber

Cornea

The cornea is circular, transparent, and dome shaped. It makes up the anterior part of the outer fibrous coat of the eyeball. It is a specialized, dense connective tissue that is responsible for nearly two-thirds of the eye's focusing power (40 to 43 diopters). It contains no blood vessels and must get its nutrients from the tear fluid, environmental air, aqueous (discussed in a moment), and blood vessels at the limbus. Because the central portion of the cornea receives its oxygen from the air, any contact lens that is worn on the eye for a long period of time must be permeable.

The cornea has more nerve endings than almost any other tissue in the body, so any irritation here can cause severe pain. The cornea is continuous with the sclera of the eye, with which it merges at the limbus.

The cornea is 0.5 mm thick and made up of six layers (Figure 2-7 and Table 2-4).

Corneal Layer	Function
Epithelium	Five to six cells thick, this layer is an important barrier to infection
Bowman's membrane	Tough layer protecting the eye from injury
Stroma	Made up of collagen, this layer is principal in the cornea's transparency
Dua's layer	Only 15 microns thick, it has only recently been discovered, and its purpose is not yet known; some consider it part of the stroma
Descemet's membrane	Tough but thin layer that protects the underlying endothelium from injury and infection
Endothelium	A single cell layer thick, it pumps water from the cornea, keeping it from becoming swollen with excess fluid (excess fluid will cause the cornea to become hazy)

TABLE 2-4

CORNEAL LAYERS

The exterior layer is the *epithelium*. It is a fast-growing layer, continually shed and replenished. It has the most significant refractive power of the eye and is continuous with the conjunctival epithelium. Because it is exposed to the environment, it is most susceptible to injury.

Just beneath the epithelium is *Bowman's membrane*. It serves as a protective layer for the underlying stroma, and is composed mainly of tightly woven, randomly organized collagen fibers.

The *stroma* is the middle layer and provides the majority of the bulk of the cornea. It is composed of regularly arranged collagen and has sparsely interconnected keratocytes, cells that are activated in injury to repair the layer. Unfortunately, this repair consists of scarring, which decreases the clarity of the tissue.

Dua's layer, identified in 2013, is a thin and very strong layer between the stroma and *Descemet's membrane*. Some researchers regard it as part of the stroma and not a separate layer. Descemet's membrane serves as the basement layer for the corneal endothelium.

The *endothelium* is the innermost layer of the cornea, bathed interiorly by the aqueous. This layer is only one cell thick and is responsible for regulating the balance between fluids and dissolved compounds in the cornea. The cells of the endothelium cannot regenerate, so cells lost to aging and injury are not replaced. If enough cells are compromised, the cornea's fluid balance is upset and the tissue becomes hydrated and opaque.

Any injury to the cornea can result in permanent damage and scars. If only the outer epithelium is injured, an abrasion will generally heal completely within 24 hours (making the epithelium the fastest-healing tissue in the body). However, if the deeper layers are also injured, then scarring will result. The closer a scar is to the center of the cornea, the more impact it will have on vision. In severe cases a corneal transplant may be needed, a surgery where the scarred tissue is removed then replaced with clear donor tissue. (Ocular surgery is covered in Chapter 36 and other places; see the Index.)

Aqueous Humor

The *aqueous humor* is a clear, watery fluid that fills both the anterior and posterior chambers of the eye. It is produced continually by the *ciliary processes* (finger-like projections at the base of and behind the iris), and is made up of 98% water plus immunoglobulins, electrolytes, ascorbic acid, amino acids, and glutathione (an antioxidant).

The aqueous circulates constantly. After passing from the posterior to the anterior chamber, this nutrient-rich fluid drains off through an area at the base of the iris called the *iridocorneal angle*. In the angle are a tangle of openings called the *trabecular meshwork* (or *trabeculum*). These spaces open into a circular venous canal, called the *canal of Schlemm*. This drains into the *scleral venous plexus* (Figure 2-8).

If any part of this drainage system is partially or totally blocked, or if the ciliary process makes too much aqueous, the pressure in the eye (*intraocular pressure*) increases. If the excess pressure causes damage to the optic nerve, glaucoma develops (see Chapter 29).

Iris and Pupil

The *iris* (the "colored part of the eye") is made up of two muscles that control the size of the pupil, the round opening in its center. The *dilator* muscle (*dilator papillae*) acts to enlarge the pupil, and the *sphincter* muscle (*sphincter papillae*) makes it smaller. The purpose of these muscles is to act like the diaphragm of a camera, controlling the amount of light that enters the eye.

The iris has four layers. The outer layer contains pigment cells that give the iris its color. The stroma is made up of blood vessels, nerves, and connective tissue. The

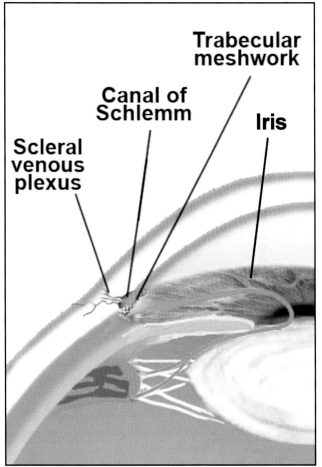

Figure 2-8. Flow and drainage of the aqueous humor.

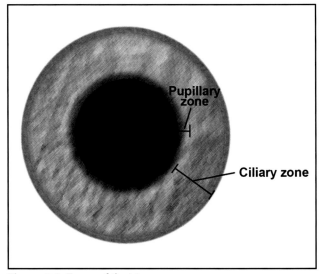

Figure 2-9. Zones of the iris.

The sphincter muscle, with its opposite action to make the pupil smaller, is under the influence of the parasympathetic division of the ANS. Thus, pupil constriction is controlled by the "rest and digest" system. Pupillary constriction is triggered by increased light, looking at near objects, and being in a relaxed state.

The iris is rich with blood vessels, and is part of the so-called vascular tunic of the eye, or *uveal tract* (covered next).

The Posterior Chamber

Crystalline Lens

The crystalline lens is a flexible, transparent, biconvex structure of approximately 15 to 20 diopters that is enclosed in a capsule. It is located behind the iris and in front of the vitreous humor. It is encircled by the *ciliary muscle* and, like the cornea, is both transparent and avascular. The lens is held in position by a series of highly elastic, radially arranged fibers called *zonules*. Collectively, these are known as the *suspensory ligament* of the lens (Figure 2-10).

The zonules are attached to the capsule of the lens and to the ciliary muscle. When the eye must focus on something close, the ciliary muscle is stimulated to contract. This releases the zonules and allows the lens to attain its maximum focal length by thickening, thus increasing its magnifying power. This process is part of *accommodation* (discussed more in Chapter 3).

Traditionally, as a person ages, the lens becomes harder, thicker, more flattened, and more resistant to movement. These changes gradually reduce a person's focusing power and result in a condition known as *presbyopia*. In some elderly people, there is also a yellowing of the lens and a loss in transparency, which is known as a *cataract*. Cataracts (covered in great detail in Chapter 28) can also

dilator muscle is a ring-like muscle within the stroma, near the pupil's edge. Beneath the stroma is the sphincter muscle (resembling a washer), which runs from the base of the iris to the point where the dilator muscle lies in the stroma. Beneath the sphincter muscle lies the heavily pigmented posterior epithelium. The dark pigment of this inner-most layer prevents light from passing through the iris itself. If this pigment is minimal or missing (eg, as in albinism), then light is transmitted through the iris as well as the pupil, usually causing light sensitivity that can be quite intense.

The iris also has two zones (Figure 2-9). The inner central region at the edge of the iris's opening is the *pupillary zone*. The *ciliary zone* extends from the pupillary zone to the ciliary body.

The nerves to the muscles of the iris are controlled by the autonomic nervous system (ANS), which can be thought of as handling the "automatic" functions of our body (heart beat, digestion, etc). The dilator muscle is controlled by the sympathetic branch of the ANS. That means that pupil dilation occurs as part of the "flight or fight" response. Dilation can be instigated by decreased light, pain/fear, arousal, and looking from near to distance.

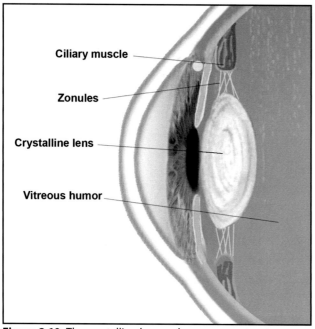

Figure 2-10. The crystalline lens and suspensory structures.

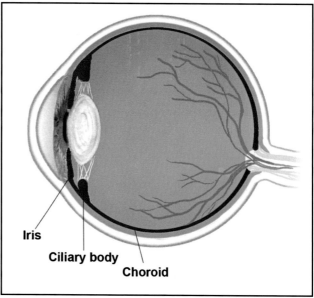

Figure 2-11. The three structures of the uveal tract.

be the result of diseases (such as diabetes), trauma, or prolonged exposure to sunlight. They can also occur as a birth defect in children. Surgery to remove cataracts is the most common of all eye surgeries.

From an osteopathic viewpoint, preventing the zonular fibers from experiencing chronic, abnormal tension is the best way to keep the lens healthy for the longest duration. Reducing abnormal tension allows the lens to contract and relax, and maintains a healthy flow of nutrients.

UVEAL TRACT

The vascular "tunic" of the eye is called the *uveal tract*. Not only does it bring nourishment to the ocular structures, it also contains the pigment *melanin*. The amount of melanin in a person's eye is a product of genetics. The uveal tract consists of three parts: the iris, ciliary body, and choroid (Figure 2-11). It thus contains elements in both the anterior and posterior segments.

The *ciliary body* has several components. First, it contains the ciliary processes mentioned earlier. At its base is the ciliary muscle (discussed in a moment because of its relationship with the crystalline lens). The ciliary body stretches to the edge of the retina; the point where these meet is the *ora serrata*.

The *choroid* is a dense network of blood vessels that begins at the optic nerve and runs under the retinal layers to the ora serrata. Bruch's membrane overlies the choroid on the eye's interior. Exteriorly, the sclera covers the choroid.

POSTERIOR SEGMENT

The posterior segment begins behind the crystalline lens and extends to the retina.

Vitreous Body

The vitreous chamber occupies the space from the lens to the retina. It is filled with a jelly-like, transparent gel known as the *vitreous humor* (or simply *vitreous*), which is formed during the embryonic period. It is a meshwork of collagen fibers that holds the retina in place and provides support for the lens. The gel is normally clear and not visible during an exam. But its front surface, the *vitreous face*, is just behind the lens and can be evaluated with the slit lamp microscope. The clarity of the vitreous allows light to pass through it.

Unlike the aqueous, the vitreous is not continuously replaced. The vitreous is almost 100% water and forms about four-fifths of the eyeball. It has a consistency like egg whites and is actually very sticky. If the vitreous comes forward during eye surgery (cataract extraction being the most common example), it can be very difficult to handle and must actually be cut with a special instrument. If lost or removed, the vitreous is replaced with a synthetic substitute.

With age, the vitreous can liquefy to the point where the collagen fibers and clumps of protein can move around inside the eye. These cast shadows on the retina, causing *floaters* to appear, which patients often describe as a spider web or bugs. Other patients claim to see something moving rapidly across the floor (*scoots*), but when they look, nothing is there.

	TABLE 2-5
	RETINAL LAYERS
Layer Name	**Function**
Inner limiting membrane	Basement membrane; contacts the vitreous
Nerve fiber layer	Contains axons of the ganglion cell nuclei
Ganglion cell layer	Contains nuclei of the ganglion cells
Inner plexiform layer (amacrine cells)	Contains the synapse layer between the dendrites of the ganglion cells and the bipolar cell axons
Inner nuclear layer (bipolar cells)	Contains the nuclei of the bipolar cells
Outer plexiform layer (horizontal cells)	Contains the synapse layer between the bipolar cells and the rods and cones
Outer nuclear layer (Müller cells)	Contains the cell bodies of the rods and cones
Outer/external limiting membrane	Separates the photoreceptors from their cell nuclei
Photoreceptor layer	Contains the rods and cones
Retinal pigment epithelium	Contains a single layer of pigmented epithelium; overlies the choroid

If the vitreous tugs on the retina, the patient will experience *light flashes*, little jagged lightning bolts that are more prominent in the dark. These occur because when stimulated (by something sensory [ie, light] or mechanical) the only way the retina can respond is by generating light.

A patient complaining of flashes, floaters, and/or scoots is considered an urgent case to be seen within 24 hours. That is because these phenomena can indicate a retinal detachment, which can result in blindness. More commonly, however, only the vitreous has pulled loose. This can be annoying, but is not sight threatening. However, the only way to determine whether the detachment is vitreous or retinal is to perform a dilated exam.

Retina

The retina lines the inside of the eye. It is very thin (0.5 mm) and delicate, and can be divided into the pigmented portions (the *pigment epithelium*, which abuts the vitreous) and the underlying neural portion (which overlies the blood-rich choroid). Most references agree that taken together, these comprise 10 layers (Table 2-5 and Figure 2-12), nine of which are neural. The retina ends at the ciliary body in a wavy border called the *ora serrata*. A thin segment that is not sensitive to light continues anterior into the iris and ciliary body.

Because the retina gathers light impulses to form an image, it has much the same function as the film in a camera. The nine neural layers contain millions of *photoreceptors* that capture light rays and convert them into electrical impulses. These photoreceptors come in two varieties: *rods* and *cones*. There are about 125 million rods. They function best in dim lighting and are located in the peripheral retina. The rods are responsible for night and peripheral vision. The cones are contained

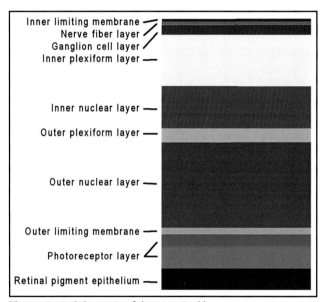

Figure 2-12. Schematic of the 10 retinal layers.

in the macula and are responsible for central and color vision. There are about 6 million of them, and they are most densely packed at the fovea. These function best in bright light.

When an image strikes the retina, the first reaction is a chemical one as the light activates pigments in the rods and cones. These are converted to electrical impulses that pass along the visual pathway, eventually to be interpreted in the visual cortex of the brain.

The optic *fundus* is a collective term for the posterior portion of the eye's interior (Figure 2-13). In general, it refers to the anatomy that is visible using an ophthalmoscope. One landmark of the fundus is a small, oval, yellowish spot called the *macula lutea* (usually called the *macula*; Latin for yellow spot). This lies just lateral

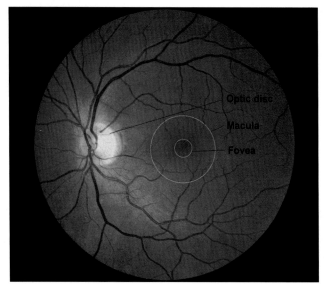

Figure 2-13. The normal fundus.

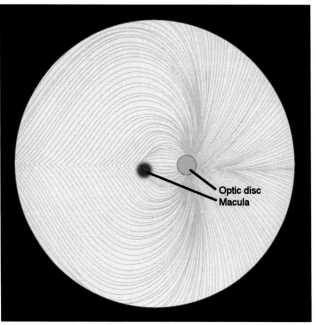

Figure 2-14. Schematic showing the arrangement of the retinal nerve fibers.

to the optic disc (discussed in a moment). The center of the macula is a tiny pit known as the *fovea centralis* (or simply, the *fovea*). This is the area where most of the cone cells are concentrated, making it the area of most acute vision. The fovea is surrounded by an area that is free from blood vessels, called the *foveal avascular zone.* Blood vessels in this area, such as those that can form in diabetic retinopathy and wet macular degeneration, can cause visual impairment.

It is important to understand that an object on the viewer's right stimulates the retina on the left, and vice versa. An object from below will be imaged on the upper part of the retina. This concept is key when it comes to interpreting a patient's side (peripheral) vision during visual field testing. Evaluation of the visual field is covered in Chapters 9 and 14.

The blood supply to the retina comes from the central artery of the retina, which is a branch of the ophthalmic artery, and enters the eyeball with the optic nerve. The blood drains via the retinal veins, which unite to form the central vein of the retina. The arteries and veins run in conjunction with one another.

Optic Nerve

One of the most prominent features of the fundus is the *optic papilla* (more commonly, *optic disc*). This is a circular indentation where the optic nerve enters the eyeball. Because this area contains no photoreceptors, it does not process light. It is sometimes referred to as the *blind spot* for this reason.

From the optic disc, retinal nerve fibers fan out like the lines of a magnetic field to join the photoreceptor cells of the retina (Figure 2-14). This unique arrangement can help us identify where in the pathway a visual field

defect is occurring. Certain disorders (notably glaucoma, Chapter 29) tend to destroy nerve fibers in a specific pattern. This translates to a unique pattern of change and loss on visual field testing.

The *optic nerve*, or CN II, is the messenger of the visual pathway. It carries the visual input gathered from the rods and cones and carries it to the brain via a complex network known as the *visual pathway.*

The Visual Pathway

CN II begins at the optic disc. The fibers that make up the optic nerve are largely afferent (sensory) and are derived from ganglion cells in the retina. Behind the optic disc, the optic nerve is surrounded by the EOMs. The nerve exits the globe via an opening in the sclera called the *lamina cribrosa.* The lamina is a mesh-like structure believed to help regulate the pressure gradient between the eye and its surrounding structures. The nerve then courses back and toward the center, then exits the bony orbit by way of the optic canal at the back wall of the orbit.

Once exiting the optic canal, the optic nerve continues to the *optic chiasm.* The optic chiasm is an X-shaped structure where the optic nerves of both eyes meet. It is located just anterior to the pituitary gland in the chiasmatic groove of the sphenoid bone.

At the chiasm, the nerve fibers from the nasal side of the retina (which receive stimuli from the viewer's temporal field of vision) divide out and cross over to travel on the opposite side. The lateral fibers remain on the original (ipsilateral) side. This has important implications in the study of peripheral vision, or visual fields (Table 2-6).

TABLE 2-6
CORRELATION OF OCULAR ANATOMY WITH VISUAL FIELDS

Characteristic of Visual Field Defect	Ocular Structure Likely Involved
One eye only	Retina
Temporal defect both eyes	Chiasm
Curtain coming over eye	Retinal detachment (retina)
Looking through a half pulled down window shade in one eye	Arterial occlusion, inferior retinal detachment, branch retinal vein thrombosis
Superior quadrant of (left) side of both eyes	(Right) temporal lobe of brain lesion
Entire (left) side of both eyes	(Right) optic radiation or visual cortex
Central vision loss on (left) side of both eyes	Lesion at tip of (right) occipital lobe
Partial deficits in one eye	Glaucoma, macular degeneration or macular edema

After it crosses the chiasm, the optic nerve becomes the *optic tract*. The optic tract continues its course posteriorly and goes around the midbrain toward a structure called the *lateral geniculate nuclei* (or *lateral geniculate body*) located on the *thalamus* (a part of the brain that relays nerve signals and also manages consciousness). From this point, the majority of the optic tract becomes *optic radiations*, and the visual information is transferred to the brain. (A small portion of fibers from the optic tract go to the *superior colliculus*. This is a part of the brain that directs eye movements.) The upper optic radiations project directly posterior via the medial occipital lobe to the superior of the calcarine fissure (the central area of visual processing).

The optic radiations course anterior and inferior into the temporal lobe of the brain, then laterally into the inferior horn of the lateral ventricle of the brain, then posterior toward the inferior lip of the calcarine fissure (a fissure between the two parts of the occipital lobe). This curved pathway is called *Meyer's loop*. The occipital lobe is the final point in the visual pathway; it is the main site for visual interpretation. A blow to the back of the head can thus cause visual disturbance.

EMBRYOLOGY

Now that we have established the basics of ocular anatomy, it is pertinent to look at how it all begins (Figure 2-15 and Table 2-7).

The retina and the optic nerve develop from an outgrowth in the embryonic forebrain, known as the optic vesicle. This vesicle pulls the covering of the brain (meninges) with it as it grows, forming the optic stalk. Thus, the meningeal layers and the subarachnoid space (space between the inner part of the skull and the brain) extend from the brain to also surround the optic nerve and the eyeball.

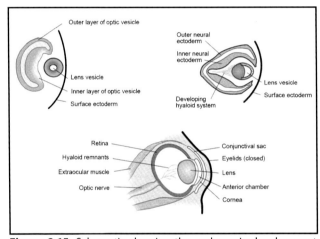

Figure 2-15. Schematic showing the embryonic development of the eye.

Embryologically, the outer layer of the optic cup becomes the pigment epithelium of the retina. The inner layer of the optic cup becomes the neural layer. These two layers are separate in the embryo and fuse during the early fetal period. The pigment layer becomes firmly attached to the choroid, but the attachment to the neural layer is not as tight. This is why a blow to the eye can potentially separate, or detach, areas of the retina. The retina is more tightly adhered to the choroid at the optic disc and the ora serrata than anywhere else.

As the human body forms, embryonic structures give rise to the more mature structures needed to make an organ. The embryonic structure is then no longer needed and will usually disappear by the time the child is born. Sometimes, however, the embryonic form remains and can be observed in the adult eye (Table 2-8). An example of this would be the place where the hyaloid artery attached to the crystalline lens; if a remnant remains it may be visible as a tiny round opacity (Mittendorf's dot) on the posterior surface of the lens.

TABLE 2-7
EMBRYOLOGICAL DEVELOPMENT OF THE EYE

Ocular Structure	Gestational Period
Optic groove forms in forebrain Optic groove becomes optic vesicle Optic stalk connects forebrain to optic vesicle; this will become the optic nerve	Day 22
Optic vesicle interacts with ectoderm to form the lens vesicle	Day 28
Optic vesicle invaginates (turns in on itself) to form optic cup Hyaloid artery and vein form	Day 32
Retinal pigment layer begins to form in optic cup	Days 35 through 37
Eyelid groove forms	Day 37
Mesenchyme (undifferentiated cells) on outer surface of optic cup develop into choroid and sclera Iris, ciliary body, and ciliary processes form from the rim of the optic cup Vitreous body forms	Weeks 6 and 7
Eyelids and conjunctiva begin to form (lids are sealed) Extraocular muscles form from mesenchyme in three areas close to the ear; each area is separately innervated by CN III, IV, or VII	Week 6
Eyelids separate	Week 27
Hyaloid artery and vein disintegrate All layers of retina present (but will further mature after birth)	8 months

TABLE 2-8
CONGENITAL OCULAR FINDINGS

Ocular Finding	Affected Structure	Notes
Persistent pupillary membrane	Pupil	Remnants of fetal membrane crossing the pupil
Mittendorf's dot	Crystalline lens	Remnant of anterior hyaloid artery
Bergmeister's papilla	Anterior to the optic disc	Remnant of posterior portion of the hyaloid artery
Vitreous cyst	Vitreous	Abnormal regression of the anterior or posterior hyaloid vascular system
Anterior persistent fetal vasculature syndrome	Vitreous	Persistent capillary network around lens, usually dissolves soon after birth
Posterior persistent fetal vasculature syndrome	Vitreous	Persistent posterior hyaloid artery
Cataract	Crystalline lens	
Glaucoma	Cornea, optic nerve	
Retinopathy of prematurity	Retina	
Coloboma	Lids, iris, choroid, retina, optic nerve	Failure of tissues with right and left halves to fuse
Nasolacrimal sac obstruction	Tear drainage mechanism	Failure of membrane over nasolacrimal sac to dissolve

Fetal development often requires the fusing of the left and right parts an organ, structure, or tissue. If fusion does not take place or is incomplete, a cleft remains. (Think of a cleft lip.) This can also occur with ocular structures as well, notably with the optic nerve, choroid, retina, iris, and eyelids (see Table 2-8). Such a defect is known as a *coloboma*.

Some ocular disorders may be present at birth, such as congenital cataracts and glaucoma (see Table 2-8). Still other problems may be associated with birth itself, such as retinopathy of prematurity or physical trauma.

Chapter Quiz

1. Which bone of the orbit is most likely to be the contributor to visual disturbance following trauma to the face?
    a. maxilla
    b. nasal
    c. zygoma
    d. frontal

2. Having teeth extracted can sometimes cause visual problems. Which bone is most commonly the cause of this phenomenon?
    a. palatine
    b. maxilla
    c. mandible
    d. premaxilla

3. A thrombus (debris or a clot) that lodges in an artery would cause complete loss of vision if located in the:
    a. anterior ciliary artery
    b. temporal lobe of the brain
    c. retinal artery
    d. posterior ciliary artery

4. The ocular muscle that responds to impulses from CN IV is:
    a. superior rectus
    b. medial rectus
    c. inferior oblique
    d. superior oblique

5. Damage to CN III will cause what kind of change?
    a. unconsciousness
    b. the eyelid on the affected side cannot be raised
    c. no change will be noted
    d. sweating

6. The final step of visual processing occurs in:
    a. occipital lobe of the brain
    b. optic chiasm
    c. optic nerve
    d. Edinger-Westphal nucleus

7. When looking at the eye through an ophthalmoscope, the part that is visible is commonly called the:
    a. macula
    b. retina
    c. fundus
    d. chiasm

8. A patient comes into your office to let you have a look at his eye. Using the slit lamp microscope, you notice a foreign object that appears to be a sliver of metal protruding from the cornea. The clear fluid coming out from around the sliver is likely:
    a. sweat
    b. tears
    c. aqueous humor
    d. vitreous humor

9. A patient presents to your office with dry eyes. You suspect faulty blinking. Which cranial nerve(s) could be involved?
    a. CN II
    b. CNs III and VII
    c. CNs IV and VI
    d. CN V

10. The crystalline lens of the eye is located between which two structures?
    a. cornea, iris
    b. iris, vitreous humor
    c. cornea, vitreous humor
    d. ciliary body, choroid

Answers

1. c
2. a
3. c
4. d
5. b
6. a
7. c
8. c
9. b
10. b

REFERENCE

1.   King HH. The inherent rhythmic motion of the cranial bones. www.cranialfoundation.org/pdf/CranialBoneMotion.pdf. Accessed April 24, 2016.

BIBLIOGRAPHY

Ort V, Howard D. Development of the eye. http://education.med. nyu.edu/courses/macrostructure/lectures/lec_images/eye.html. Accessed April 23, 2016.

The figures in this chapter were contributed by the following, who are associated with this book as authors:
Sarah M. Armstrong: Figure 2-13
Al Lens: Figures 2-1 through 2-12, 2-14, 2-15

3

OCULAR PHYSIOLOGY

Al Lens, COMT

In simple terms, physiology is the science of how things work. The eye, however, is a complex structure with complex interactions. A review of ocular anatomy (Chapter 2) is essential to understanding how the parts function together to result in vision. Ocular physiology helps us understand why the eye behaves as it does. This further aids us in performing the tests and diagnostics that lead to an identification of what's different or wrong (Sidebar 3-1).

BLINKING: EYELIDS AND LASHES

Even though the muscles that close the eyelid are only about 1 mm thick, anyone who has had to pry an eye open can tell you how strong those muscles are. This thin layer of muscle and skin allows a person to blink the eyes, spreading tears across the surface and keeping the tissues moist. The eyelid muscles work at such a high speed, the interruption to vision is virtually imperceptible when we blink. The typical blink lasts about one-tenth of a second. We can also wink by selectively closing just one eye. (Interestingly, a lot of people are not able to wink with their dominant eye.)

The majority of the tear film (discussed momentarily) is produced in the lacrimal gland (located above the eye and temporally), so the blink needs to spread the tears across the entire eye. This is done with a zipper-like motion from the lateral to nasal side, even though it looks like the eyelids move straight up and down.

The normal blink rate is roughly 15 times per minute. This decreases to less than half that during visually demanding tasks or intense concentration, which can lead to dryness. However, when someone is anxious, stressed, or engaged in conversation, the blink rate increases to 20 or more times per minute. This type of blinking is involuntary (although one can voluntarily prolong the time between blinks) and spontaneous (ie, no physical stimulus is required to cause the blink).

A *reflex blink* occurs in response to some sort of stimulus, such as an object heading toward the eye (like a dropper bottle), something brushing against the eyelashes, an irritant in the eye, or a loud noise. This response helps protect the eye from injury, pollen, etc. A flash of light, as from a camera, will also cause a reflex blink. Prolonged bright lights can cause squinting in an effort to limit the amount of light entering the eye.

When a person tries to close the eyes against resistance, there is a tendency for the eyes to roll upward and outward. This is known as *Bell's phenomenon*. The degree of this eye movement is in direct relation to how much effort is being applied to close the eyes. Bell's phenomenon occurs in almost all younger people (about 90%), but tends to be less noticeable in senior years.

Ledford JK, Lens A, eds.
Principles and Practice in Ophthalmic Assisting:
A Comprehensive Textbook (pp 27-37).
© 2018 Taylor & Francis Group.

TEAR FILM

Tears are composed of the secretions of several glands, mainly the lacrimal gland, as discussed previously. The zipper-like motion of blinking pushes the tears toward the nose. There is a tiny opening in each eyelid called punctum (one each in the upper and lower eyelids) that provides access to the small tube called the canaliculus, which channels the tears to the nasolacrimal sac. The tears continue their journey into the nasal cavity, which is why the nose tends to run when the eyes are watering.

If the nasolacrimal duct becomes obstructed, *epiphora* (tears rolling down the cheeks) can occur. In most cases, the blockage can be opened with irrigation. Other causes of epiphora include malposition of the eyelid (entropion, ectropion), inward turning of the eyelashes (*trichiasis*), or irritants that cause tearing.

There are two types of tears—normal, lubricating tears and reflex tears.

Lubricating tears, also known as *basal tears,* provide moisture, nutrition, defense against microorganisms, and a smooth optical interface for best vision. This tear form has three layers. The watery layer, called aqueous, is produced by the lacrimal gland and accessory glands of Krause and Wolfring. About 98% of the tear volume consists of aqueous. Dry eye can result from a decreased production of aqueous and/or either of the other two tear layers.

The *mucin layer,* produced primarily by the goblet cells in the conjunctiva, allows the tear film to adhere to the cornea. The mucin coats the corneal epithelium and "fills in" any tiny irregularities. Without this layer, the cornea is like a waxed car where the water just beads up on the surface. The eye then dries easily, and its optical quality is compromised.

The third, remaining portion of the tear film is the outermost *oil* or *lipid layer,* which is produced mainly by the meibomian glands with a minor contribution from the glands of Zeis in the eyelids. The oil inhibits the evaporation of the tears, helping to keep the tear film on the eye.

Basal tears are very important in maintaining the health of the eye and clear, stable vision. The electrolytes and proteins in the tears provide nutrition and a defense against microorganisms. This makes it understandable that a dry eye is more prone to infection. If the tear film is not confluent across the surface of the cornea, the optical quality of the eye suffers. Patients with dry eyes will often complain of decreased or fluctuating vision, usually made clearer by blinking.

Reflex tears occur as a result of some stimulus, such as emotions or physical irritants. It is composed mainly of water and actually does little to keep the ocular tissues moist.

Dry Eye

Patients are often confused when they tell the doctor that they have excessive tearing and are subsequently informed they have dry eyes. However, if the lubricating tears are not adequate, tiny dry spots develop on the eye. This causes the eyes to feel "gritty" or "sandy" with every blink. There is then enough irritation to initiate reflex tears because the brain believes something needs to be flushed out.

Dry eye compromises all of the benefits of the lubricating tear film. It is more common among postmenopausal women and the elderly, but can be a problem for anyone (Table 3-1). Other common causes of dry eye include autoimmune diseases, some medications (such as antihistamines, antidepressants, and birth control pills), eyelid surgery, and laser refractive surgery. The eyes of people with Graves' disease (hyperthyroidism) can protrude from the orbit more than usual (Figure 3-1). This can lead to dry eye because the lids may have difficulty completely covering the globe.

Sometimes the volume of lubricating tears is adequate but the quality of the tears is poor. Many patients complaining of dry eye have a compromised oil layer, often due to clogged meibomian gland orifices (Figure 3-2).

If it is an inadequate volume of tears that is causing the dry eye, the punctum can be occluded (usually just the lower punctum) with temporary or permanent punctal plugs. It can also be useful to increase room humidity, make an effort to increase blinking, and/or use artificial tear drops.

TABLE 3-1	
CAUSES OF DRY EYE	
Problem/Entity	**Mechanism**
Antihistamines	Dry up the sinuses but also dry up the tear film
Aging	Tissue breakdown, decreased function, increased evaporation of tear film, thinner lipid layer
Moving air	Physically dries the eye's surface
Ocular decongestant drops	Chemicals that decrease redness also dry the surface
Autoimmune disease	Disease targets ocular surface
Menopause	Hormone change alters tear composition
Low environmental humidity	Dry air causes more rapid tear film evaporation
Incomplete lid closure	Prolonged exposure causes evaporation of tears
Incomplete blinking	Lids inadequately spread tears across the eye

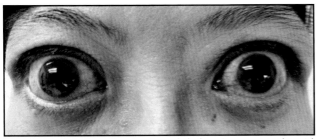

Figure 3-1. Ocular protrusion (exophthalmos) as seen in thyroid disorder.

BONY ORBIT

Only about one-sixth of the eyeball is visible. The rest of the globe is hidden behind eyelids and within the bony orbit. While it is a safe place for the eyeball, the orbit would not be a very hospitable environment without the orbital fat to provide a cushion for the eye.

It is not uncommon for frail, elderly people to lose some of their orbital fat volume. This causes the eye to sink into the orbit more than normal.

Also within the orbit are the extraocular muscles (EOMs) that allow precise eye movements (six muscles for each eye). Each muscle attaches to a unique place in the orbit, making specific movements possible (discussed next).

Blunt trauma can cause bones of the orbit to fracture, most often the orbital floor (see Chapter 32). If an EOM is trapped in the fracture (Figure 3-3), the movement of the eye will be restricted and cause double vision. Surgery may be required to release the entrapped muscle.

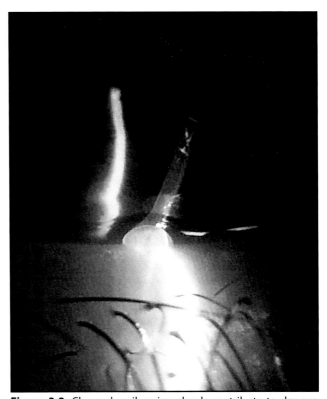

Figure 3-2. Clogged meibomian glands contribute to dry eye disease.

EXTRAOCULAR MUSCLES

The primary reason we have two eyeballs is for a higher degree of depth perception (stereopsis) than what is possible with just one eye. This is a great feature to have, but requires that the eyes move in unison. Failure to do so will usually result in double vision. To move the eyes together requires the cooperation of at least four EOMs— One in each eye will contract and the opposing muscle

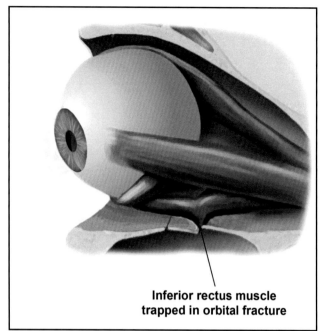

**Inferior rectus muscle
trapped in orbital fracture**

Figure 3-3. Herniation of a muscle through a fractured orbital floor.

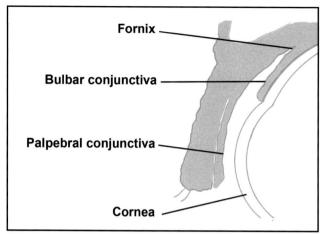

Figure 3-4. The conjunctiva.

of the same eye needs to relax a proportionate amount. Other benefits of having two eyes are a wider field of view and having a back-up in case vision is lost in one eye.

Physiology of the EOMs is complex and is further discussed in Chapter 10.

There are four types of eye movements: saccades, smooth pursuit, vergence, and vestibulo-ocular. *Saccades* are rapid eye movements to quickly change the point of fixation. This happens when we want to look at a different object (or in the case of reading, a different word). *Smooth pursuits* are slower movements to follow a moving object. *Vergence* is moving both eyes either inward (convergence) or outward (divergence) for looking at a closer or farther object, respectively. The *vestibulo-ocular reflex* causes the eyes to move in the opposite direction of head movement. This includes tilting the head—the top of the eye rotates in the opposite direction of head tilt. Emergency response personnel use the involuntary vestibulo-ocular reflex to determine the function of the brainstem in an unconscious person; the head is moved rapidly side to side (assuming no spinal injury), if the eyes move in the opposite direction of the head, then the reflex is intact and the brainstem is also intact.

Conjunctiva

The smooth, transparent tissue that covers the visible part of the sclera and the inside of the eyelids is the conjunctiva. It secretes mucus, water, and electrolytes into the tear film. The *bulbar conjunctiva* is the portion that covers the sclera and provides nutrients to the peripheral cornea. Veins that underlie the conjunctiva transport aqueous that has drained out of the anterior chamber.

The *palpebral conjunctiva* lines the inside of the eyelids and is continuous with the bulbar conjunctiva (Figure 3-4). This seamless attribute of the conjunctiva prevents foreign bodies (including contact lenses) from "disappearing behind the eye" where they would be able to fester and cause infection.

The conjunctiva can be host to bacterial or viral infections. It can also suffer from allergic reactions. Because the conjunctiva is highly vascular, when the blood vessels dilate as a result of any of these conditions, the eye becomes quite red.

Cornea

The multilayered cornea has two roles: as a powerful lens to focus incoming light and to protect the contents of the eyeball. The average cornea has about 40 to 43 diopters of focusing power. The refractive index of the cornea is 1.376. The high density of nerves makes the cornea one of the most sensitive parts of the human body. This helps to keep the eye safe from foreign bodies. (We know how irritating something as minor as an eyelash can be on the surface of the cornea.)

To uphold its clarity, the cornea must maintain a somewhat dehydrated state. When too much water is in the corneal structure, it swells and loses some of its transparency. The *endothelium* (innermost layer of the cornea) is responsible for keeping the proper amount of hydration by pumping out excess fluid, while allowing nutrients in the aqueous to enter the cornea. Endothelial cells cannot reproduce, so with the natural death of cells throughout a person's life, the remaining endothelial cells enlarge to close any gaps left by dead cells. At birth, the average cornea has about 3500 cells/mm². The cell density decreases to about 2000 cells/mm² in a person's 80s. The ability of the endothelium to maintain corneal clarity is compromised when the cell density falls below 1000 cells/mm². When the density falls to 500 cells/mm², corneal edema is probable, and a corneal transplant of some sort is indicated.

The cornea and sclera (white of the eye) are made of essentially the same type of collagen. It is, in part, the organization of those fibers in the cornea that results in its clarity. The sclera appears white because the cells are more hydrated and lack the structural uniformity of the cornea. If the endothelium fails, the cornea can become as opaque as the sclera.

Next to the endothelium is the posterior basement membrane called *Descemet's membrane*, which thickens with age from about 3 to 10 microns. This layer does not adhere very strongly to the stroma, which makes it possible to surgically separate it for procedures where the endothelium needs to be replaced.

The recently proposed *Dua's layer* is located between Descemet's and the stroma. (Whether or not it is actually a layer in and of itself or instead just a part of the stroma is controversial.) Its physiological significance is not fully understood, but it is impervious to air. This has an impact on corneal surgery, especially deep anterior lamellar keratoplasty (DALK), which is discussed in Chapter 36.

The *stroma* overlies Descemet's and makes up 90% of the cornea's thickness. Damage to the stromal layer will result in a permanent scar.

Bowman's layer is the anterior basement membrane of the cornea, just above the stroma. Bowman's membrane tends to get thinner throughout life. This layer is resistant to injury and infections. However, once this layer is damaged, it does not regenerate. When photorefractive keratectomy (PRK) laser eye surgery is done, this layer is obliterated, yet seemingly with no ill effects. In fact, a pseudomembrane eventually develops to replace Bowman's, usually with an even greater adhesion to the overlying epithelium. Because of this feature, phototherapeutic keratectomy (PTK) is performed on eyes with a defective Bowman's membrane.

The *epithelium* (outermost layer) is about 50 microns (0.05 mm) thick. The epithelial cells regenerate very quickly, being totally replaced about every 7 days. An epithelial defect (an area of the cornea that is missing the epithelium) may be due to surgery or injury. The epithelium will regenerate across the defect from remaining cells at a rate of 1 to 3 mm per day. In the case of PRK, an 8- to 9-mm circle of epithelium is removed and takes 3 to 5 days to regenerate. Since most of the cornea's nerve endings are in the epithelium, it can be very painful while this layer is damaged and the nerve endings are exposed.

AQUEOUS HUMOR

The *aqueous humor* is the fluid that fills the anterior and posterior chambers of the eye. It is a source of nutrients to the cornea and the crystalline lens. Aqueous has a refractive index of 1.336. Since the aqueous is providing nourishment, it must be continually produced so fresh fluid replaces the exhausted fluid (ie, that in which the nutrients have been used up). It is very similar to blood plasma in composition.

The aqueous is produced by the ciliary processes at the base of the ciliary muscle (which surrounds the crystalline lens). The fluid then flows through the pupil into the anterior chamber, where it finally escapes the eye through the trabecular meshwork, then to Schlemm's canal, and into the bloodstream via episcleral veins beneath the conjunctiva.

As long as the rate at which the aqueous drains from the eye matches the rate that it is being produced, equilibrium is maintained. If the pathway from where aqueous is produced (behind the iris) to where it drains (through the trabecular meshwork at the corneal limbus) is obstructed, or if aqueous is produced faster than it can drain, the intraocular pressure (IOP) rises, which can lead to glaucoma (discussed momentarily under Optic Nerve and also in Chapter 29).

UVEAL TRACT

Uvea is Latin for grape. The eye would look like a purple grape if the outer coat (sclera) were not there. The uveal tract is rich with blood vessels and consists of the iris, ciliary body, and choroid.

The iris is what gives the eye its color. Whether the eye is blue, green, hazel, or brown depends on the amount of pigment within the iris. (Regardless of the eye color, the pigment is brown.) If there is not much pigment, the eye will be blue; add a little more pigment and you get a green eye, and so on, up to dark brown. The two eyes are usually the same color, but a small number of people have eyes of different colors (Figure 3-5)—either between the two eyes or different colors in the same eye. This is called *heterochromia iridis*, sometimes referred to as simply *heterochromia*. Some people are born this way, but the condition can be acquired. Most acquired cases of heterochromia are related to disease or trauma and should be investigated.

The iris is made up of two muscles: the dilator and the sphincter. These control the amount of light entering the eye by adjusting the size of the pupil. The pupil also constricts as part of the accommodative response, discussed later.

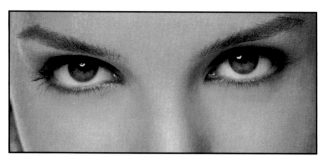

Figure 3-5. Heterochromia: Irises of different colors.

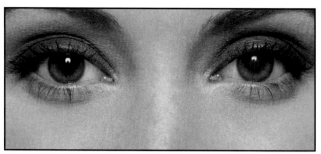

Figure 3-6. Left eye lacking red reflex.

When the *dilator muscle* contracts, it expands the pupil's diameter. It is a radial muscle that is innervated by *sympathetic* nerves (the fight-or-flight response is activated by the sympathetic system) and is stimulated by the release of the sympathetic hormone norepinephrine. The dilator muscle is the target when using phenylephrine drops to dilate the pupil. The iris *sphincter* constricts the pupil and is stimulated by the parasympathetic system (which has the opposite effect on the body as the sympathetic system). Cycloplegic drops, such as tropicamide or Cyclogyl (cyclopentolate), block the nerve pathway of the iris sphincter and cause pupil dilation, as well as inhibit accommodation.

The pupil appears black under normal circumstances because the inside of the eye is very dark. However, if a light is shone into the eye close to the observer's visual axis, a red reflection can be seen. ("Red eye" on photographs is an example.) Known as the *red reflex*, the color is caused by the blood vessels in the retina. The absence of a red reflex (Figure 3-6) indicates there is something blocking light from getting to/from the retina. This may be due to a dense cataract, a vitreous hemorrhage, or an intraocular tumor, to name a few.

The *ciliary body* has two purposes. One is to produce the aqueous humor as detailed previously. The second is to change the eye's focusing power by providing *accommodation*. Accommodation is made possible by the ciliary muscle contracting around the lens. The muscle is not directly connected to the lens itself. Rather, it releases tension on the fine fibers (known as *zonules*) that connect the crystalline lens to the ciliary muscle. This allows the lens to thicken.

Underneath the retina is a rich bank of blood vessels in the *choroid*. These vessels provide nutrition to the retinal pigment epithelium and outer layers of the sensory retina.

CRYSTALLINE LENS

Like the cornea, the crystalline lens is avascular. It gets nutrition from the aqueous humor. The lens accounts for about one-third of the eye's focusing power (15 to 20 diopters).

Unlike the cornea, the crystalline lens is able to adjust its focus to nearby objects (*accommodation*), and then refocus for the distance. When an object is perceived to be close, the *near triad* is initiated: the eyes converge (to maintain singular vision), the pupil constricts (to increase the eye's depth of focus), and the ciliary muscle contracts (releasing tension on the zonules). Without the zonules pulling on the lens, it bulges a bit, making it more convex. This effectively adds "plus power" to the eye, bringing the object into focus.

The crystalline lens changes throughout life. At birth, the lens material is very pliable, like putty. This means that there is a high range of accommodation. However, the lens lays down layers as it progresses through life. Like a tree, it gets thicker with age and the center becomes compacted and rigid. This means that it does not have the large range of focus that it did earlier in life. For most people, *presbyopia* (a natural aging process caused by the decrease in accommodation, discussed in Chapter 4) becomes apparent around the age of 45 when reading becomes more difficult. The eye's accommodative ability continues to diminish until it has lost all of its faculty and the eye can no longer adjust its focus at all. This usually occurs by age 65 to 70 years.

The next step in the life of the crystalline lens is a decrease in clarity, often first yellowing and then becoming brownish. At some point, there will be enough opacification to be considered a *cataract* (discussed in detail in Chapter 28). Age-related cataracts are usually caused by a build-up of protein in the lens.

VITREOUS

The vitreous humor, the "jelly" that fills the posterior segment of the eye, is adherent to the underlying retinal tissue. It is static; that is, it forms completely during gestation and, under normal circumstances, never exits the eye. It is sticky, has a consistency similar to egg whites, and is composed almost entirely of water, along with a small amount of salt, protein, and polysaccharides.

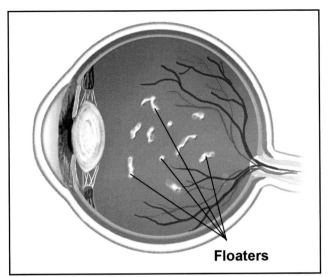

Figure 3-7. Vitreous floaters cast a shadow on the retina, giving patients the impression that "bugs" or "spider webs" are in front of them.

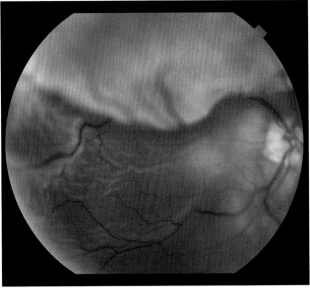

Figure 3-8. Retinal detachment. (Reprinted with permission from Retina Gallery.)

The vitreous is normally clear, which is vital to good vision. The majority of eyes will develop floaters in the vitreous (Figure 3-7) at some time in a person's life. While these are annoying, they tend to settle with time and usually do not interfere with vision unless they are large and in the central visual field. In some cases, large vitreous floaters (mostly those caused by a posterior vitreous detachment) may be treated with an Nd:YAG (neodymium-doped yttrium aluminum garnet) laser. Floaters that are close to the retina are not treatable due to the danger of damaging the retina with the laser.

A hemorrhage in the vitreous will obscure vision, sometimes almost completely. If the retina cannot be viewed, an ultrasound can be performed to determine if there was a retinal detachment; if that is the case, the vitreous would be removed (*vitrectomy*) to allow treatment of the retina. If the retina is attached, the hemorrhage is not treated and usually resolves spontaneously. Persistent blood in the vitreous may also require a vitrectomy.

Unfortunately, the vitreous is an ideal environment for bacterial growth. If the vitreous is exposed to the external environment, it can become a conduit for infection to enter the eye. When the vitreous prolapses (enters the anterior chamber, which is most likely to occur during cataract surgery), it may adhere to the corneal endothelium and/or the surgical wound. An anterior vitrectomy is done to remove any drifting vitreous.

Over time the vitreous tends to shrink and liquefy a bit, and may develop some impurities. These changes can cause floaters to appear. If it pulls away from the retina, a posterior vitreous detachment can occur, generating multiple floaters and/or flashes of light (also called *photopsia*). The flashes are caused by the vitreous tugging on the retina. As long as the vitreous detachment does

not cause a hole or tear in the retina, it is of little concern despite being bothersome to the patient due to the temporary visual effects. Because the visual symptoms of vitreous and retinal detachments are basically the same, any patient with these symptoms is classified as urgent and brought in for a dilated exam.

RETINA

The retina contains all the photoreceptors that are stimulated by incoming light. The signals from these receptors are converted into nerve impulses and sent to the brain for interpretation. So, while the retina is a key element in vision, it does not actually do the seeing, per se.

In order for vision to occur, each of the 10 layers of the retina must be in proper contact with each other. If the layers of the retina separate, it is called a *retinal detachment* (Figure 3-8). This causes the receptor layer to be separated from its nutritional supply, so time is of the essence for repair to prevent permanent loss of vision. Like a plant pulled out of the soil, if the retina is starved of nutrition for more than a couple of days, the prognosis for recovery is poor. Retinal detachments are more common among myopic eyes because the eyeball is longer than average; the retina is essentially a one-size-fits-all structure and must stretch over a larger area when the eye is elongated.

Photoreceptor Layer

The photoreceptor cells are divided into rods and cones.

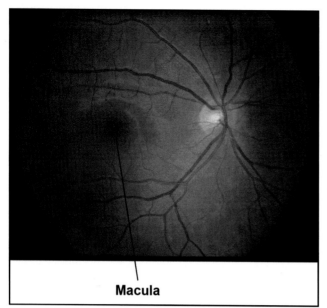

Macula

Figure 3-9. The macula, showing darker pigment in the macular area.

The *rods* are responsible for dim light and night vision, but do not have the capacity to discern color. (Hence, it is not wise to choose what to wear when it is dark!) The retina contains about 125 million rods, mostly in the periphery. Light bleaches the photosensitive pigment *rhodopsin* from the rods, rendering them pretty much useless. This is why it is difficult to see when entering a dark room from a bright environment until rhodopsin has time to build up in the rods again. While the human eye can begin to see in darkness in less than 1 minute, it takes around 30 minutes for full dark adaptation to occur.

Most of the *cone* cells are concentrated in the macula (discussed momentarily), making them responsible for our fine, central vision. Their ability to function, however, decreases as available light decreases. This means that the central vision does not work in the dark. You may have noticed this on a dark night when a star seems to disappear when you look directly at it. That is because the image is falling on the macula. If you look a little to the side of the star, it reappears. That is because the image has moved off the macula and into the periphery where the rod cells can pick it up. There are far fewer cones than rods—only about 6 million.

Color Vision

The cones also provide us with *color vision*. There are three types of cones, each most sensitive to a particular color: red, green, or blue. If one or more sets of the photoreceptors is either deficient or absent, the patient's color vision will be compromised. Congenital color defects are bilateral and originate on the X chromosome; acquired defects can be unilateral or bilateral. (See Chapter 9 for information on color vision testing.)

The layperson's term for color vision deficiency is *color blindness*. This is not really an accurate term, though. It is actually very rare for someone to have a total lack of color vision. Up to 10% of males have congenital color vision deficiencies, but less than 1% of females are born with color vision problems.

We use color vision tests to differentiate between color vision problems by finding out the colors the patient has trouble identifying correctly and then determining which photoreceptors are responsible for the misidentified colors.

An *anomalous trichromat* has all three photoreceptors present, but one is deficient. *Protanomaly* is caused by deficient red photoreceptors, *deuteranomaly* (the most common congenital color vision deficiency) represents green, and *tritanomaly* is for blue. Patients with protanomaly and deuteranomaly see the color spectrum in a similar manner because there is a fair bit of crossover of colors in this range; tritanomaly is a blue/yellow deficiency. Some color vision tests can differentiate between the three.

If the photoreceptors for a color are absent (vs deficient), then we change the suffix to –opia: *protanopia*, *deuteranopia*, and *tritanopia*. (Note that some references will use the suffix –opsia in place of -opia.) The colors affected are the same as above, but more profound.

The *rod monochromat* is someone with no cones (ie, has rod cells only) and is totally color blind and legally blind as well, because there are no cones in the macula where detailed visual acuity originates. This condition is also accompanied by nystagmus (involuntary eye movements) and light sensitivity (because rods are meant for night vision, not daylight).

A *cone monochromat* is very rare, resulting from having just one type of cone. While they perceive everything in one color spectrum (totally color blind), cone monochromats have normal visual acuity and are not abnormally sensitive to light.

Macula

The *macula* is a small spot in the retina, about 5 mm in diameter, which is responsible for fine detailed vision. In the center of the macula is the *fovea* (*fovea centralis*), which measures about 2 mm in diameter. Smaller yet is the *foveola* (about 0.25 mm). The density of photoreceptors is the greatest in the foveola. When the eye is in proper alignment, the image of an object being looked at falls on the foveola.

When observing the eye's interior, the macula normally appears darker than the rest of the retina (Figure 3-9). This is due in part because there is a difference in pigmentation. In addition, the retinal tissue is thinner here, which allows the dark choroid color to show through more.

It is also obvious from fundus photographs that the retinal blood vessels stop short of the macula, yet it appears redder than the rest of the retina. This is because the macula gets its blood supply from the posterior ciliary arteries in the choroid rather than the retinal arteries like the rest of the retina.

Macular degeneration is a common condition where the tissues of the macula break down, affecting the patient's central vision. This is covered in more detail in Chapter 27.

Optic Nerve Head

Laypersons often assume that the image of what they are looking at falls directly on the optic nerve. This might seem to make sense, but the *optic nerve head* (or *disc*), where the optic nerve enters the eye, is devoid of any photoreceptors. That makes it a blind spot. Each eye has a blind spot located about 15 degrees temporal to fixation.

Thankfully, the blind spot is unnoticeable. Even if we close one eye, we cannot detect the blind spot. However, the brain's ability to adapt to any blind spot can mask abnormalities until they become very obvious. Thus, the patient is unaware of a problem, often until it is too late. This is one of the reasons that routine eye exams are highly recommended.

An average disc measures about 1.5 mm by 1.8 mm. This is where all the nerve axons leave the eye and the blood vessels enter/exit the eye. There is a depression in the middle of the disc that is referred to as the *cup*. The size of the cup compared to the disc diameter is called the *cup-to-disc ratio*. Some discs are quite small, but have the same number of axons and vessels crammed into them, so the cup is expected to be quite small. The cup of an average disc usually covers about one-third of the visible disc, or a 0.3 cup-to-disc ratio. A larger cup-to-disc ratio can raise some concern about the presence of glaucoma, especially if there is asymmetry between the eyes. However, some eyes simply have large *physiologic* cups (ie, a variation that is normal for that eye) without being glaucomatous. Glaucoma is discussed in detail in Chapter 29.

Sometimes the optic nerve head will exhibit the first signs of a disease, such as multiple sclerosis. It can also exhibit signs of inflammation or infection. In many cases, the patient has visual or systemic symptoms to correlate with the findings, but sometimes the patient is asymptomatic.

LIGHT AND VISUAL PATHWAYS

Light entering the eye will go through the tear film, cornea, and anterior chamber (and its aqueous). After entering the pupil, light continues its journey into the posterior chamber, crystalline lens, and the vitreous

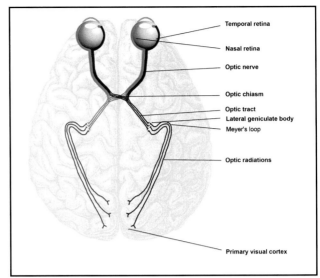

Figure 3-10. The visual pathway.

humor. This is known as the *pathway of light*. An opacity anywhere in this pathway will compromise the vision.

Light that comes from the temporal side will fall on the nasal retina. Light from below will shine on the superior retina. The actual image displayed on the retina will be upside down and backward. (The brain makes the necessary adjustments so we see the image as it really is.)

Once light has stimulated the photoreceptors, the cells send a nerve impulse to the nerve fibers (*axons*). The nerve fibers follow a pattern very similar to the blood vessels, creating a superior and inferior arch, meeting at the horizontal midline. This explains why conditions that affect the nerve fibers, such as glaucoma, will have visual field defects that "respect" (eg, do not cross) the horizontal midline. All the nerve axons exit the eye at the optic nerve of that eye.

The nerve fibers from the temporal half of each eye continue toward the brain, staying on the same side. The nasal fibers of each retina, however, cross over at the *optic chiasm* to join the temporal fibers of the fellow eye. These merged fibers form the *optic tract* that leads to the *lateral geniculate body*, which is like a relay station. The *optic radiations* leave the lateral geniculate body, with the fibers from the inferior retinas (corresponding to the superior visual field) going through *Meyer's loop*. The final destination is the *visual cortex* in the *occipital lobe*, where the brain forms the image. Taken together, this "journey to vision" is the *visual pathway* (Figure 3-10).

Lesions in the visual pathway may affect vision in one or both eyes. If the lesion is in the retina or optic nerve, it will only affect the vision in that eye. The optic chiasm, however, contains nerve fibers from both eyes. Remember that the nasal fibers switch sides here, so are responsible for the temporal visual field. A lesion at the center of the optic chiasm will thus affect the temporal visual field of both eyes. Anything posterior to the optic chiasm will affect the visual field of both eyes on the opposite side (eg, if the lesion is in the right optic tract, it will show up as a visual field defect on the left side of both eyes). The farther back the lesion is in the visual pathway, the more similar (*congruous*) it tends to be in each eye. Thus, the characteristics of the visual field can help pinpoint just where a lesion is in the pathway. Testing the visual field is covered in Chapter 14.

BLOOD AND BLOOD CELLS

Blood contains three types of cells: erythrocytes, leukocytes, and platelets. Erythrocytes are red blood cells that carry oxygen and nutrients to cells. Leukocytes are white blood cells that fight infection and disease. Platelets keep blood loss to a minimum by clumping or plugging up holes when there is a laceration or compromise in a blood vessel.

The liquid component of blood is plasma, which is ultimately the transport system for the erythrocytes, leukocytes, and platelets. It also carries waste away from the body's cells. Oxygen is brought from the lungs to the cells, and then carbon dioxide from the cells is released back into the lungs. The nutrients from the gastrointestinal tract are carried to the cells and cell waste is sent back to the kidneys. Hormones are also transported from various glands to the cells via the bloodstream.

Sometimes the blood vessels can become clogged. If an artery leading into the retina becomes obstructed, the tissue that is "fed" by this vessel will die if blood flow is not restored quickly enough. The extent of tissue death thus depends on how large an area is served by the blocked vessel. A central retinal artery occlusion will affect the entire retina, while a branch retinal artery occlusion causes the death of only a section of the retina. Since veins take blood from the eye to the heart, if a vein is obstructed, retinal hemorrhages occur because the blood cannot leave the eye.

When the eye senses that it is not getting adequate nutrition, it may form new blood vessels (*neovascularization*) in an attempt to be "fed." This commonly occurs in the cornea (which is usually *avascular*, or lacks blood vessels) of patients who wear contact lenses because there is an inadequate supply of nutrients (notably oxygen) through the contact lens. If this situation continues, over time blood vessels start to develop and migrate inward from the periphery of the cornea. Scarring, hemorrhaging, and lipid deposits can occur in advanced cases.

Neovascularization can also occur in the retina of diabetic patients and those with high blood pressure. Treatment is usually initiated in the form of intravitreal injections or laser therapy. If left untreated, the fragile new blood vessels in the retina tend to leak, causing vitreous hemorrhages that result in floaters or loss of vision. If the hemorrhage does not resolve on its own, a vitrectomy (removal of vitreous) may be performed.

RESPONSE TO INSULT
Mechanisms of Infection

An eye that has not been compromised is quite resistant to infection. Mucous membranes of the body, including the conjunctiva, are more prone to infection. The conjunctiva is protected by the tears that contain an enzyme, called lysozyme, which kills bacteria. If the barriers to infection fail, microorganisms can invade the eye. The number of neutrophils and monocytes (types of white blood cells) is increased to destroy microorganisms that penetrate the physical barriers. Other types of white blood cells may also get involved, such as killer T-cells. (See also Chapter 23, Microbiology.)

Mechanisms of Injury and Inflammation

Injuries can be the result of energy from an outside source (blunt trauma or something sharp), thermal (hot or cold), or chemical. When a patient presents with an injury, determining the mechanism of injury can greatly aid the physician in the examination and treatment plan.

Inflammation is a reaction to any trauma to tissue in the body. Blood flow is increased as part of the process to aid the immune system in protecting the eye. The white blood cells ingest or absorb pathogens or toxins that may be present, and platelets will aid in the blood clotting process to keep bleeding to a minimum. Inflammation can also cause swelling and pain, and if excessive, can result in tissue damage.

When inflammation occurs in the uveal tract (uveitis, or more commonly, iritis), white blood cells and protein appear at the site in response. In the aqueous, this is noted as "cells and flare." The cells are actually white blood cells. When viewed with the slit lamp, they appear similar to dust as when seen in a beam of sunlight. Protein is the flare and looks like a haze through the slit lamp. Except in high degrees of inflammation, the cells can be seen circulating in the anterior chamber. Since heat rises, cells close to the iris (which is warmer than the cornea) will be seen to floating upward, while the cells close to the cornea will be sinking downward.

Mechanisms of Allergy

An allergy is a reaction to a substance that the body has previously been exposed to and identified as an allergen. That means that future exposures will result in an allergic reaction. The body produces antibodies that are attached to mast cells (a type of white blood cell that releases histamine and other substances, which lead to allergic and inflammatory responses), waiting to bind to the invader the next time. Substances like histamine and prostaglandins are released, causing redness, swelling, itching, and inflammation. Antihistamines are commonly used to treat the symptoms of allergies by preventing the release of the reaction-causing histamine.

CHAPTER QUIZ

1. The normal blink rate is approximately how many times per minute?
   a. 5
   b. 10
   c. 15
   d. 20

2. What photoreceptors are responsible for color vision?
   a. rhodopsin
   b. rods
   c. cones
   d. all of the above

3. All of the following are types of blood cells *except*:
   a. plasma
   b. erythrocytes
   c. leukocytes
   d. platelets

4. Which of the following is *true* about the optic chiasm?
   a. the temporal nerve fibers from each eye cross over
   b. the nasal nerve fibers from each eye cross over
   c. it contains temporal fibers from one eye and nasal fibers from the other eye
   d. it is where the highest density of cones can be found

5. The primary purpose of the corneal endothelium is to:
   a. provide structural strength
   b. pump fluid from the cornea
   c. provide protection from pathogens
   d. all of the above

6. What substance do the meibomian glands secrete?
   a. aqueous
   b. mucus
   c. lipid/oil
   d. vitreous

7. What is responsible for the eye's physiologic blind spot?
   a. macula
   b. fovea
   c. rhodopsin
   d. optic nerve head

Answers

1. c
2. c
3. a
4. b
5. b
6. c
7. d

Unless otherwise noted, the figures in this chapter were contributed by the following, who are associated with this book as authors:
Al Lens: Figures 3-1, 3-3 through 3-7, 3-9, 3-10
Sergina M. Flaherty: Figure 3-2

4

OPTICS

Al Lens, COMT

BASIC SCIENCES

Physical Optics

Physical optics is the division of optics that relates to the origin and movement of light. In a vacuum (or on a practical level, in air), light travels at 186,282 miles (or 299,792 km) per second. Light slows down a bit when it enters a transparent medium (eg, water or glass). We use this feature to our advantage when we want to alter the direction that light travels, most notably by using lenses.

Two theories of how light travels exist: corpuscular and wave. Sir Isaac Newton came to the conclusion that light is a group of particles (*corpuscles*). Later on, other scientists showed that light must travel in *waves*. Since the corpuscular theory could not explain diffraction (when light changes direction after passing across an edge, such as the ridges on a multifocal intraocular lens [IOL] implant, or through a small aperture) and interference (the new shape that results when two waves meet), the wave theory caught on. However, the wave theory does not explain things like the photoelectric effect (where metal can eject photoelectrons). The wave theory is the one that this chapter will concentrate on mostly, but that does not mean the particle theory does not exist.

A *wavelength* is the distance between the peaks of two adjacent waves. The electromagnetic spectrum covers all light energy (Figure 4-1), ranging from cosmic gamma rays (shortest) to radio waves (longest). In clinical optics, we are referring to light from the ultraviolet to infrared wavelengths, and its interaction with optical media. What most people call "light" is visible light (all the colors of the rainbow; Sidebar 4-1).

Different colors have different wavelengths. Despite the variation in wavelengths (be it in the visible or invisible spectrums), all light travels at the same speed in any given medium. That is, the speed of light in air, for example, is the same regardless of its wavelength. Red light travels just as fast as blue light.

When light is emitted, the waves can be oriented vertically (think of a wave of water), horizontally (like a snake slithering on the ground), and anywhere in between. Light that is reflected is *polarized* (at least to some degree), meaning the light waves are parallel to one another. A polarizing filter allows only light waves that are polarized in the same direction to pass through (Figure 4-2). Placing two polarizers perpendicular to each other prevents any light from getting through.

Light reflected off a horizontal surface, such as a body of water or the road, has light waves that are partially polarized horizontally. Using a polarized filter

Ledford JK, Lens A, eds.
Principles and Practice in Ophthalmic Assisting:
A Comprehensive Textbook (pp 39-53).
© 2018 Taylor & Francis Group.

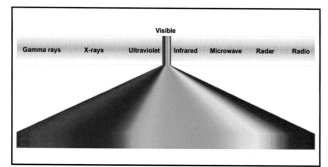

Figure 4-1. The electromagnetic spectrum.

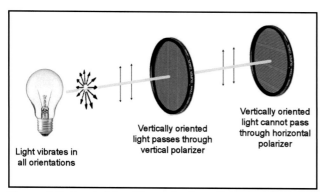

Figure 4-2. A polarizing filter only allows light rays through if they are polarized in the same direction as the filter.

oriented to allow vertically polarized light will drastically reduce the glare from these surfaces; this is the basis of polarized sunglasses. Many camera display screens also have a polarizer to cut down reflections, making it easier to see. If a person wearing polarized sunglasses tries to take a picture with the camera's polarizer perpendicular to that of the sunglasses' polarizer, the screen will turn dark. (On most cameras, this is when the camera is held in the "portrait" orientation, or vertical.) This problem can be remedied by removing the sunglasses or rotating the head in order to view the screen.

Light also has what is referred to as *color temperature*, which is measured in Kelvin (K) degrees. The color temperature, however, has nothing to do with actual temperature (heat). Cameras that have a "white balance" control will show common scenarios depicting differing color temperatures, such as sunny, cloudy, fluorescent lighting, incandescent lighting, and flash photography. The sun is about 5780 K on a sunny day, about 6500 K on an overcast day, and 5000 K when it is close to the horizon (sunrise/sunset). Incandescent light is around 3000 K. Take note that the Kelvin temperature contradicts the way we normally think about temperature; we think of red as "hot," and thus a higher temperature, but red light actually has a lower Kelvin rating than "ice cold" blue. (One way to think of this is "less is more.")

Light intensity or brightness can be measured in *candelas* (cd), *lumens* (lm), *foot candles* (fc), or *lux* (lx).

We use candelas or lumens to measure light at its source (*radiance*), and foot candles or lux to measure light at a given distance from the source (*illuminance*).

Candela (cd) is the unit of measurement of the International System of Units (SI) and quantifies light at its source. Candelas can be calculated by squaring the distance (in feet) from the light source, multiplied by the foot candle (fc) value at that distance (distance^2 x fc = cd). Let's say you are measuring the light intensity 5 feet away from the light source, and the photometer reads 10 foot candles. Thus, 5^2 x 10 = 250 candelas. If we had 10 foot candles measured 8 feet from the source, it would be 8^2 x 10 = 640 candelas. We can tell from this that a much brighter light would be required to keep the intensity the same if the distance is greater. The formula is useful if you want to determine how bright a light needs to be to illuminate an object a particular amount at a given distance. For example, your visual acuity chart specifications may suggest the background illumination for the chart as 2 foot candles and you measure the light source to be 6 feet away. Instead of trying a bunch of different light bulbs, we can calculate how bright it needs to be: 6^2 x 2 = cd, 36 x 2 = 72 candelas. We need to multiply the candelas by 12.6 to get lumens, so the light source would need to emit 907 lumens.

Lumens are used to talk about the total amount of visible light emitted by an object. It is similar to candela in that it measures light output, but candela is more specific because it relates to directional intensity. In the "old days," we used to think of light bulbs in relation to watts—the more watts, the brighter the light. In reality, watts relate to energy consumption, but since pretty much all bulbs were created equal back then, we knew a 100-watt bulb was brighter than a 60-watt bulb. Bulbs are much more efficient now, some more than others, so the wattage rating is not useful with respect to how much light the bulb puts out. Instead, we now consider how many lumens the light emits.

Candela and lumen are great units of measurement for how much light output is provided, but it does not really help when we want to measure how much light reaches a surface, such as a desk, color vision plates, etc. The farther the light source is from the surface, the less light there is. In the United States, we typically use foot

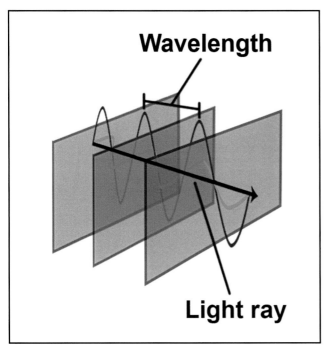

Figure 4-3. Geometric optics is involved with light rays.

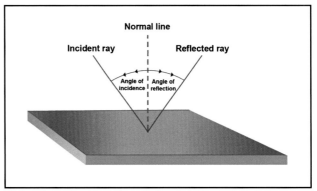

Figure 4-4. The principles of reflection.

candles as the unit of measurement to determine the light level, while most other countries use the metric version of lux. If a typical candle is lit, the amount of light falling on a surface 1 foot away is termed 1 foot candle. Lux would measure the light at 1 meter. One foot candle is about 10.764 lux.

Geometric Optics

We use *geometric optics* a lot in ophthalmology. This part of optics relates to reflection and refraction of light, and the use of lenses, prisms, and mirrors. While physical optics deals with light waves, geometric optics works with light rays, which are lines of light going in a particular direction that are perpendicular to a group of wave fronts (Figure 4-3).

Reflection

In addition to formulas, optics has its fair share of laws to contend with. One of those laws is the *law of reflection*, which stipulates that the *angle of incidence* equals the *angle of reflection*. (In between these two angles is a "normal" line, which is an imaginary line perpendicular to the surface of the mirror at the point where the incoming ray strikes the surface.) A real-life example could be demonstrated by trying to view an object in a mirror. Assuming the mirror is not directly in front of the object, you would have to stand at an equal angle on the other side of the mirror in order to see the object reflected in the mirror (Figure 4-4). The light rays from the object are the *incident* rays, and the image you see is a result of

reflected rays. If we assume the mirror is flat (*plane*), the normal line would extend perpendicular to the mirror's surface and would be an equal angle from the object and you.

The *law of reflection* is valid on curved surfaces as well as plane, the difference being the perceived size of the image. A *concave* mirror (such as a makeup or shaving mirror) will make images appear larger because there are multiple points that will match the angle of incidence (Figure 4-5A). Conversely, a *convex* mirror (like those seen on the passenger side of cars or in stores and buildings) makes things look smaller than they really are because multiple points of incidence will match the angle of reflection (Figure 4-5B).

Refraction

Light rays travel in a straight line until their path is altered by a lens, prism, or mirror. When light enters a transparent optical medium, the speed of that light will be altered. (In this sense, *medium* refers to any material that light can pass through.) The medium will cause a light ray to be bent (*refracted*), unless the ray strikes the medium exactly perpendicular to its surface at its *optical center* (Figure 4-6).

How much the light will be refracted depends on the *index of refraction*, or optical density, of the medium. The index of refraction is calculated by dividing the speed of light in a vacuum (300,000 m/sec) by the speed of light in the specific medium (n = v/c, where n is the refractive index, v is the speed of light in a vacuum, and c is the speed of light in the medium). The slower that light travels in the medium, the higher the index of refraction and the more that the lens will alter the direction of light. Various materials used for lenses are discussed in Chapter 20.

Total Internal Reflection

When light moves from one medium to another, the resulting possibilities are refraction, reflection, or (most commonly) a combination of the two. *Internal reflection* occurs when light is traveling from a dense medium (such as water) into a less dense medium (such as air).

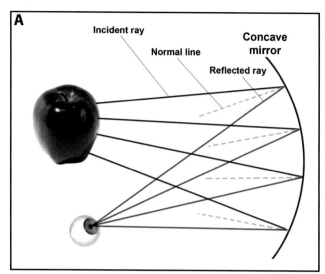

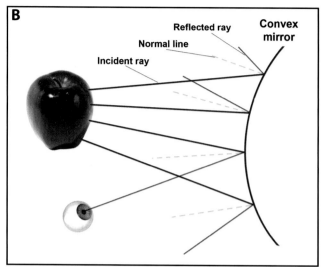

Figure 4-5. (A) A concave mirror makes images appear larger. (B) A convex mirror makes objects appear smaller.

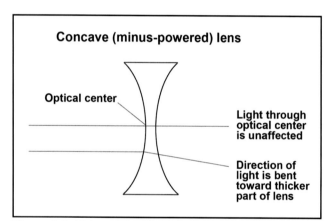

Figure 4-6. Light passing through the center of a lens is not refracted (ie, does not change direction).

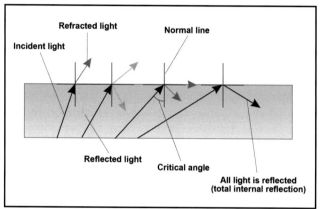

Figure 4-7. The principle of total internal reflection.

As an example, let's think of a laser pointer under water. If the light is pointed straight up, at 0 degrees (°), then there is no refraction or reflection; the beam simply passes straight through the interface between the two media. As soon as you begin to tilt the pointer slowly clockwise, its light will be 100% refracted as it leaves the water and enters the air. At some point, however, if you keep tilting, you will reach an angle where not all of the light enters the air; the beam will hit the interface between the water and the air and some of it will begin to be reflected back into the water. The point where this internal reflection first begins is the *critical angle*. If you continue to tilt the beam beyond the critical angle, the amount of refraction decreases and the amount of internal reflection increases until you reach a point where no light passes through the water-air interface and 100% of the light is bounced back, reflected back into the water. At this point *total internal reflection* (TIR) occurs (Figure 4-7).

In the eye, TIR means that the anterior chamber angle cannot be viewed with the slit lamp alone because light from the structures in the anterior chamber angle is reflected back into the eye. Fortunately, by placing a lens on the surface of the eye (ie, a goniolens), light leaving the eye goes into the lens (which has a higher refractive index than air) allowing a view of the anterior chamber angle. Fiber optics, used in ophthalmic laser, lighting, and imaging, is another technology that uses TIR.

Snell's law is a formula that can be used to determine the angle of refraction, or the index of refraction of the incident or refractive medium. As long as you have three of the four values, the missing value can be determined. Snell's law can also be used to calculate the critical angle of a medium where total internal reflection would occur.

Diffraction

Diffraction is when light bends around the corner of an "obstacle." In the case of the eye, that obstacle is the iris and diffraction is not a desired effect because it creates an

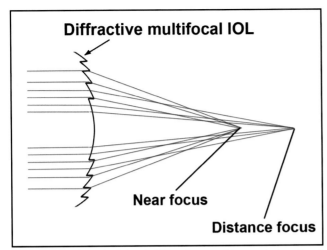

Figure 4-8. The principle of diffraction used to create two focal points in an intraocular lens.

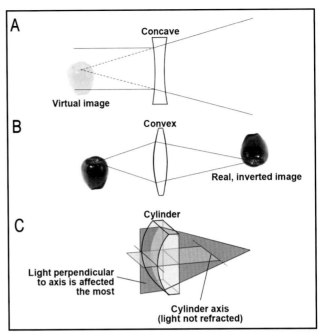

Figure 4-9. (A) A spherical concave (minus) lens diverges light and has a virtual image. (B) A spherical convex (plus) lens converges light and forms a real image. (C) A cylindrical lens focuses light in only one meridian.

aberration (where light going through an optical medium has more than one focal point due to an irregularity in the media). However, some multifocal IOLs use diffraction to an advantage. These IOLs have concentric rings. Light bends around the edge of each ring while the rest of the light is refracted by the optical power of the lens. This creates two focal points: one for distance, one for near (Figure 4-8).

Lenses

The purpose of corrective lenses is to bend peripheral light rays to a focus. Light that goes through the optical center of a lens is not affected by the focusing power of the lens; it continues in a straight line.

A plus-powered lens is convex in shape and will cause parallel light rays to converge (be bent inward) and come to a focus behind the lens. Minus-powered lenses are concave in shape and will cause parallel light rays to diverge (spread apart). Diverging light cannot come to a real focus, but the focal point would be considered to be a *virtual* focus in front of the lens.

The degree that light will bend depends on the power of the lens, measured in units called *diopters* (D). The dioptric power is equal to 1/focal length of the lens (or D = 1/F), measured in meters. For example, if the focal length of the lens (the distance from the lens to where light comes to a focus) is 0.5 meter, D = 1/0.5 or 2 D.

Lenses are used to affect the vergence (direction) of light. A spherical lens affects light the same amount throughout its 360°. Spherical lenses can be concave or convex in shape. A *concave* lens is thinnest at its optical center and gets thicker in the periphery. Since there is more substance or thickness in the periphery, light passing through this part of the lens will slow down more, thus bending in the direction of the thicker part of the lens. This ultimately causes light to *diverge* (spread apart). If the light entering the lens had parallel light

rays (from a distant source), the light would not come to a real focal point (where light comes to a focus). Instead, there would be a *virtual* focal point (not visible) in front of the lens (Figure 4-9A). Concave lenses are "minus-powered" and have the property of *minification* (ie, objects viewed through a minus lens appear smaller). A common use of concave lenses is to correct myopia (nearsightedness).

Convex lenses are thickest at their optical center and thinnest in the periphery. Parallel light rays entering a convex lens will *converge* or be bent toward the thicker center of the lens and come to a focus behind the lens (Figure 4-9B). Convex lenses are "plus-powered" and *magnify* images. They are used to correct hyperopia (farsightedness), as well as in magnifying glasses, cameras, projectors, and telescopes.

Sometimes we do not want to focus light equally in all directions. To correct astigmatism (a refractive error where an image is not focused to a single point, discussed momentarily), we need to focus light selectively—maximally in one meridian, and not at all 90° away from that meridian (Figure 4-9C). *Cylinder* lenses are used in these cases. A cylinder can be convex or concave (plus or minus cylinder), but spectacles and contact lenses are manufactured in the minus cylinder format. Light entering parallel to the axis is not refracted. Thus, the maximum power of a cylinder is 90° perpendicular to its axis, with the power diminishing progressively as it approaches the axis. Cylinders can be combined with spherical lenses to correct refractive errors with astigmatism combined with myopia or hyperopia.

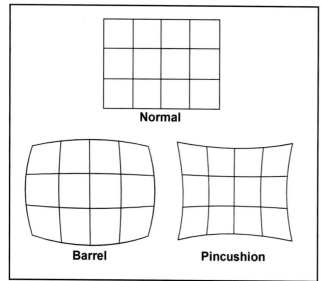

Figure 4-10. Types of distortion.

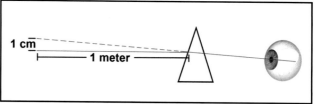

Figure 4-11. A prism displaces an image, bending light rays toward its base so that the image seems moved toward the apex.

Aberrations and Distortion

An *aberration* means that light does not come to a sharp focus. This can occur any time the path of light is altered. *Spherical aberration* occurs when light traveling through a spherical lens comes to a focus at different points. This happens because light entering near the edge of the lens is bent more than at the center of the lens (where it is not bent at all). The power of the human cornea lessens toward the periphery (ie, is *aspherical*) to counteract spherical aberration.

Chromatic aberration is similar, except now it is different colors that are focused differently. Blue light tends to be refracted more than other colors, and red is refracted the least. An *achromatic lens* can help reduce this aberration. The human eye's optical system is not achromatic, but there is yellow pigment in the fovea that helps reduce chromatic aberration (because yellow filters out blue).

Distortion (where straight lines appear bent) is caused from light entering the periphery of a lens. A person wearing low power lenses (say, < 3 D) likely does not notice this. However, as the power of a lens increases, so does the distortion. Minus-powered lenses (concave) cause *barrel distortion,* where the center is stretched out, and plus-powered lenses (convex) produce *pincushion distortion,* where the center is pinched inward. You may note that the distortion is the *opposite* of the shape of the lens—if you look at a minus-powered lens, you would see it is pinched inward (thinnest) in the middle, and a plus-powered lens is kind of barrel-shaped (thicker in the middle; Figure 4-10).

For those who wear glasses, distortion can be bothersome, especially if they switch back and forth between glasses and contact lenses. Because the edges of a contact lens are out beyond the field of vision, contacts do not cause the same distortion as glasses. The brain will adjust

to a constant distortion, but switching between glasses and contacts interrupts this adaptation and may cause headaches, dizziness, and/or eye fatigue.

Prisms

There are times when it is needful to alter the direction of light, but not its focus. That is where prisms come in. Prisms are triangular in shape, with the *base* being the thick end and the *apex* being the pointed end. Light is bent toward the base (thickest part) of a prism, but the image is displaced toward the apex (thinnest part; Figure 4-11). Like other lenses, prisms are measured in diopters, but the power relates to how much *displacement* occurs rather than where a focal point is. One prism diopter will displace light 1 cm when measured at a distance of 1 meter. Two prism diopters displaces light 2 cm at 1 meter, etc. The formula is PD = d/f (PD is prism diopters, d is displacement measured in centimeters, and f is the distance measured from the lens in meters). In ophthalmology, the most common use for prisms is correcting strabismus (misalignment of the eyes). When prescribing prism in glasses, we must always indicate the prism power and the direction of the base (ie, base-in, -out, -up, or -down).

In essence, a minus-powered (concave) lens is prisms placed apex to apex, while a plus-powered (convex) lens is prisms placed base to base. Ideally, the wearer looks through the optical center. But if the alignment is off, there is a prismatic effect. *Induced prism* occurs when looking through a part of the lens other than the optical center. This means that the object appears to have moved; the eyes will have to move in order to "pick up" the image. This can cause discomfort and/or double vision. The problem may be compounded when there is a significant difference between the power of one eye vs the other.

Sometimes, however, lenses are purposely placed into the frames so they *will* be off center (called *decentration*). This is done to correct strabismus and alleviate double vision (see Chapter 10).

Induced prism can be calculated using *Prentice's rule,* discussed in the Clinical Skills section of this chapter.

A high plus-powered lens can induce what is referred to as the *Jack-in-the-box phenomenon*—the prismatic effect of the lenses will displace the object's image outside the edge of the lens. This creates a blind spot that

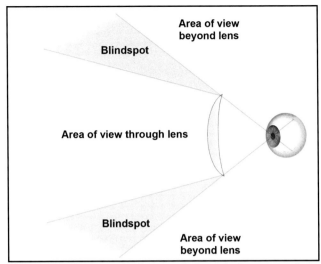

Figure 4-12. A strong plus lens can induce displacement where an object seems to appear out of nowhere.

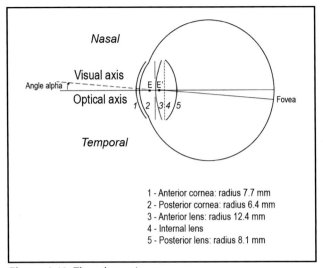

1 - Anterior cornea: radius 7.7 mm
2 - Posterior cornea: radius 6.4 mm
3 - Anterior lens: radius 12.4 mm
4 - Internal lens
5 - Posterior lens: radius 8.1 mm

Figure 4-13. The schematic eye.

surrounds the lens (Figure 4-12). Objects hidden within that blind spot can seem to appear "out of nowhere" when the head is turned a bit, or the object itself moves from the blind spot into the visible area.

Another popular use of prisms in the ophthalmology practice is in the applanation tonometer, used for measuring intraocular pressure. (See Chapter 13.) The tonometer head has a bi-prism (two prisms with the bases pointed in opposite directions) that splits a circle into two half-circles. When properly aligned, the images indicate the endpoint of the measurement.

CLINICAL KNOWLEDGE

Physiologic Optics

This division of optics relates to the eye itself. It might be advantageous to review Chapters 2 and 3 regarding ocular anatomy and physiology prior to studying this section.

In order to provide a basis for theoretical studies of the human eye, a *schematic eye* is used. The schematic eye is a virtual model providing dimensions of the "average" eye (Figure 4-13). The concept has been around a long time. In the early 1900s, Allvar Gullstrand (a Swedish ophthalmologist) improved on earlier, simpler schematic eyes. Others have tried to enhance the design since, taking into account the asphericity (gradual decrease in curvature of the cornea toward the periphery) and aberrations (irregularities in how light focuses) of the real eye. Still, no perfect schematic eye exists. However, what we do have is used as a framework for calculating retinal image size, magnifications, and position/diameter of the pupil, as well as designing optical instruments and analyzing IOLs.

There are two primary "lenses" in the eye's optical system: the cornea and crystalline lens. The cornea is responsible for about two-thirds of the eye's focusing ability, or about 40 D to 43 D in the average cornea. The other one-third of focusing power comes from the crystalline lens (about 15 D to 20 D, in a relaxed state).

The cornea, by itself, really does not have much impact on the direction of light. If you were to remove a cornea, preserve its shape, and look through it, there is virtually no affect on focus. It is the aqueous (and to a certain extent, the tear film) that provides the focusing power; the cornea merely provides the shape. (Similarly, an empty glass has little refractive effect, but fill it with water and it becomes a strong plus-powered lens.) The cornea thus represents a *fixed-focus* lens. From minute to minute, its refractive power does not change.

The crystalline lens is different, at least in our younger years. This biconvex lens can change its focusing power (with the help of the ciliary muscle) when we need to alter our focusing distance. (A common example would be looking at a book, then up at the television, and then back to reading again.) This process (called *accommodation*) is discussed momentarily.

The eye produces four optical reflections known as *Purkinje images* (*Purkinje-Sanson images* or *Purkinje reflexes*). The first reflection is off the front surface of the cornea. (Interestingly, this reflection is that of the observer, so it looks like there is a little person inside the dark pupil. The term *pupil* is actually Latin for "little doll.") The second reflection is from the rear surface of the cornea, the third from the front surface of the crystalline lens, and the fourth and final reflection is from the posterior surface of the crystalline lens. This fourth reflection is the only inverted image. Some instruments use the Purkinje images to track eye movements.

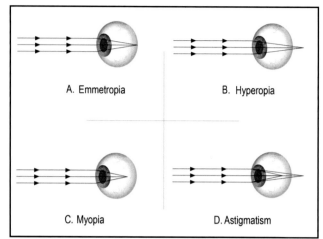

Figure 4-14. (A) Emmetropia, where the image falls properly on the retina. (B) Hyperopia ("farsighted"), where the image focus is behind the retina. (C) Myopia ("nearsighted"), where the image focus is in front of the retina. (D) Astigmatism, where light is broken into two different focal points.

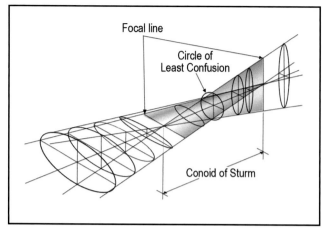

Figure 4-15. The conoid of Sturm.

Refractive Errors

Emmetropia is when light from a distant object (20 feet or more away) comes to a focus on the retina (technically, the macula) due to the eye's natural refractive power (Figure 4-14A). Unfortunately, *refractive errors* exist, moving the focal point off the macula. These can be caused by an anomaly in the eye's focusing power (cornea/crystalline lens), an eye that is longer/shorter than normal (termed *axial*), or both.

Most newborns are hyperopic (farsighted), but undergo a process called emmetropization that is usually complete by the teen years. *Emmetropization* is a phenomenon occurring in the cornea, the lens, and with eyeball size that works to eliminate refractive errors. However, there are no guarantees. Some eyes remain hyperopic, some develop myopia (nearsightedness), and some also have (or develop) astigmatism. Genetics and/or environmental conditions can contribute to the success or failure of emmetropization.

A *hyperopic* eye lacks enough focusing power. It may be that the eye is shorter than average and/or the focusing power is less than average. Parallel light rays entering the eye fail to come to a focus before reaching the retina (Figure 4-14B), virtually falling somewhere beyond the retina instead. If the amount of hyperopia is not excessive, it may go undetected until later in life when the eye can no longer accommodate enough to overcome the hyperopia. Plus-powered lenses are used to correct hyperopia.

Myopic eyes have too much focusing power. In the majority of cases, it is because the eye is longer than average, but it could also be that the eye's focusing power is higher than average. Light from a distant source comes to a focus in front of the retina (Figure 4-14C) instead of on

it (see Figure 4-14A). Myopes can see clearly up close, but distant objects are blurry. A minus-powered lens is used to correct this refractive error.

Astigmatism is a refractive error that is not equal in all meridians (Figure 4-14D). This means there is not a single focal point regardless of whether the eye is looking at near or far. Astigmatism is the result of the cornea and/or lens not being spherically shaped; rather, one meridian is more curved than the other. (Think of a football or the back of a spoon, where the curve is greater in one direction vs the other.) The majority of eyes have at least a small amount of astigmatism, but nominal amounts are negligible to visual acuity and tend to go unnoticed in the absence of any other refractive error. Cylindrical (or toric) lenses are used to correct astigmatism.

In *regular astigmatism*, there are two focal lines positioned perpendicular to each other. The interval between the two lines is called the *conoid of Sturm* (Figure 4-15). In the middle of the conoid is the *circle of least confusion*, where the best vision can be achieved without correcting the astigmatism.

Irregular astigmatism occurs when there are irregularities in the optical media causing multiple focal points, and is not correctable by the typical cylindrical (toric) lens because the axes are not 90° from each other. Irregular astigmatism can be caused by corneal injury or pathology (eg, keratoconus) or irregularities in the crystalline lens (eg, cataract).

Refractive Conditions

There are several situations that are refractive conditions as opposed to refractive errors. By far the most common is *presbyopia*, which involves the elasticity of the crystalline lens.

When a person is born, the consistency of the lens is soft like putty. As we age, the lens laminates (rather like a tree putting down layers). Eventually the center of the lens hardens, which means it is less flexible.

When accommodation occurs (ie, focusing at near), the ciliary muscle contracts, which causes the lens to thicken, adding "plus power" for focusing. A young child, with a soft lens, has a tremendous ability to accommodate. But as the lens's center gets less flexible, the ability to accommodate decreases.

Usually by age 40 years, enough focusing power is gone for a person to notice it. At first, near vision is improved by holding reading material farther away from the eye. But the loss gradually continues and finally you cannot hold your newspaper far enough away and still see it. Eventually the lens cannot accommodate at all. This usually occurs by age 65 to 70 years.

The optical response to presbyopia is to restore the plus power that the crystalline lens can no longer supply via reading glasses or a bifocal (if the patient also needs correction at a distance).

Aphakia is another refractive condition. This means that the crystalline lens is absent from the pathway of light. It may have been surgically removed, or trauma may have torn it away from its usual position and it is no longer aligned. If one were to provide glasses to compensate, you would expect the necessary power to be around +12.00 for distance. A contact lens would need to be a bit stronger (+14.00). The ideal way to correct aphakia is by inserting an IOL as we do when removing a cataract; the power for this might be around +22.00.

If an IOL is inserted, then *pseudophakia* ("false lens") exists. Glasses may still be needed to fine-tune the patient's vision, but not the thick +12.00's you would need in aphakia.

Irregular astigmatism occurs when the curvature of the cornea does not refract light equally. In regular astigmatism, the opposing axes are 90° away and we use a cylinder (or spherocylinder) lens to correct it. But irregular astigmatism may have multiple focal points, and they are not 90° away from each other. There may be ways to improve vision somewhat, but it is unlikely to be perfect. Keratoconus and scarring are two examples of corneal problems that can cause irregular astigmatism.

Accommodation

The physiology of the lens is discussed in Chapter 3. Briefly, the crystalline lens of the eye is very pliable in childhood and can significantly increase its focusing power. The lens thickens and becomes less flexible with each passing year, eventually losing all of its ability to adjust its focus as discussed above.

In order to maintain focus at near for any length of time, we need twice as much accommodative amplitude (focusing power) than the focusing power required at the desired distance. For example, reading at 16 inches (40 cm) requires 2.5 D of focus, so twice that amount, or 5.0 D, of accommodative amplitude would be needed. With each passing year, accommodative amplitude

Age	Amplitude	Age	Amplitude
10	14.00	45	3.50
15	12.00	50	2.50
20	10.00	55	1.75
25	8.50	60	1.00
30	7.00	65	0.50
35	5.50	70	0.25
40	4.50	75	0

Figure 4-16. Donder's table.

decreases. For most people, the decrease in accommodation becomes noticeable around the age of 45 years when the amplitude has dropped to about 3.5 D. If 5 D is required to comfortably maintain focus at 16 inches, and only 3.5 is available, then 5 − 3.5 = 1.50. Hence, a +1.50 D pair of reading glasses is needed (or a +1.50 add in the glasses prescription for bifocal or progressive lenses).

Donder's table (Figure 4-16) shows typical accommodative amplitude at various ages. The amplitude can also be calculated using the formula of 18.5 − (age x 0.3), although the results are slightly different. Bear in mind, like gray hair and wrinkles, the eye's aging process does not occur at the same rate for everyone, so the table and formula are just guidelines.

In between the cornea and lens is the pupil. Technically, the pupil is the opening in the iris. The size of this opening is controlled by the two iris muscles: the sphincter and the dilator. While pupil size controls the amount of light entering the eye, it also affects depth of field (the range that objects are in focus). A smaller pupil has a larger depth of field than a large pupil. A camera lens works the same way—a small aperture will allow the background of an image to be in focus as well as the object of interest. A large aperture will blur the background and foreground (while the object itself is clear) because of the shallow depth of focus. This helps explain why someone with a mild refractive error will say the vision in bright light is better than in dim light; the larger depth of focus created by the small pupil can mask the small refractive error.

When the eyes are looking at a near target, three things should happen (known as the *accommodative triad*): accommodation of the lens, convergence of the eyes (inward turning), and pupil constriction. If there is a problem with any one of these, then near vision will be compromised and/or uncomfortable. The pupil constriction occurs to help increase the depth of field and decrease the amount of accommodation required.

The "ideal pupil size" that provides best vision at any distance is around 3 to 4 mm. Smaller than that and *diffraction* (bending of light around sharp edges; the iris in this case) becomes noticeable, causing a decrease in image quality.

Retinal Image Size

The size of the image on the retina varies from eye to eye, and is also dependent on corrective lenses in higher grades of refractive error (more than 3 D usually makes a noticeable change in image size). To determine if there will be an alteration in image size (usually only a concern if there is a large difference in refractive error between the two eyes), we first need to determine if a refractive error is strictly due to axial length (axial myopia/axial hyperopia), or at least in part to optical issues of the cornea and/or lens (refractive myopia/hyperopia). The image size is not affected as much if the axial length is at fault because an eye that is myopic due to axial length will have a 1.5% increase in image size for each diopter of myopia, which offsets the 1.5% minification per diopter of the typical optical lens (and vice versa for hyperopia). Measuring the corneal curvature and axial length and comparing these to normal values will help calculate the cause (the axial length of the average eye is 23.5 mm, and the average cornea is 43 D).

Next is deciding on the corrective lenses to be used. Spectacle lenses will minify (minus-powered lenses) or magnify (plus-powered lenses). The farther the lens sits from the eye, the more noticeable this effect becomes. If the anisometropia is caused by a difference in axial length between the two eyes, then spectacle lenses will not cause a difference in image size and would be the correction of choice.

Contact lenses do not alter image size to any appreciable amount since they sit directly on the eye. If contact lenses are used to correct eyes with refractive errors caused by axial length, the myopic eye will have a larger retinal image than the hyperopic eye. A "refractive" myope or hyperope (where the refractive error is mostly due to an over- or underpowered optical system) will have an image similar in size to an emmetrope. Putting a spectacle lens in front of eyes with refractive myopia or hyperopia will induce the minification or magnification factors of the minus- or plus-powered lenses, respectively. If a significant amount of *anisometropia* exists (a difference in refractive error between the two eyes of 2 D or more), a disparity of retinal image size (*aniseikonia*) can result. Aniseikonia can be a problem because it can cause double vision, with each image being a different size. This lack of single binocular vision is especially of concern in children because the brain may choose to suppress one image and lead to amblyopia. Aniseikonia is more of an issue for refractive myopes and hyperopes (ie, less noticeable for axial myopes/hyperopes). These cases are often better suited to contact lenses than

spectacle lenses. *Antimetropia* exists when one eye is hyperopic and the other is myopic.

CLINICAL SKILLS

Lens Power

The power of a lens, which is a description of the refracting ability of the lens, is measured in *diopters*. A 1 D lens will bend light rays to a focus (*focal point*) at 1 meter from the lens. The distance from the lens to the focal point is the *focal distance* (or *focal length*). If we know the power of a lens, we can determine where its focal point is. We can also calculate the power of a lens if we know its focal distance. If we know the focal length and are solving for lens power, the formula is D = 1/F (D is the diopter power, F is the focal length in meters). If we know the lens power and want to calculate the focal length, the formula is F = 1/D.

Example 1: Determine the focal length of a lens with a power of +4.00. We know what D is (+4.00), so F = 1/4 meter (or 25 cm).

Example 2: The focal point is 2 meters in front of the lens; what is the lens power? D = 1/2. Because we've been told that the focal point is in *front* of the lens (and thus is a virtual image) we know that this is a minus-powered lens, or -0.50 D.

Optical Cross

An *optical cross* is a visual representation of the power of a lens, most especially of the two primary meridians in a spherocylindrical lens. For example, if the lens measures +2.00 -3.50 x 095, the optical cross would indicate the power is +2.00 at 095 degrees, and -1.50 at 005 degrees (Figure 4-17). This might sound a bit confusing, so let's break it down.

A cylinder's *meridian of power* is 90° *away* from its axis, so the sphere is actually the refractive power that exists along the cylinder axis. The cylinder itself has *no power* along its axis. Thus, the first primary meridian is represented as +2.00 x 095 degrees. Now, where did the -1.50 come from at the 005 meridian? The *difference* between +2.00 and -1.50 is -3.50 (ie, 2.00 − 3.50 = -1.50), which is the cylinder power (90° away from its axis). The optical cross can be used to figure lens power in both plus and minus cylinder format (Sidebar 4-2).

The main use of the optical cross in the exam room is retinoscopy when trial lenses are used to estimate a patient's refractive error, mainly children (see Chapter 11). And while the optical cross may not be something we use daily, it is important to understand the concept. In addition, manipulating the optical cross is likely to show up on some certification exams.

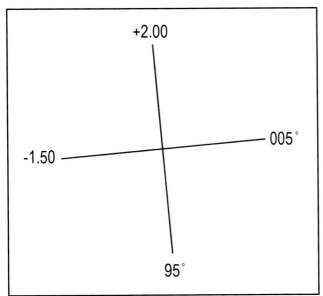

Figure 4-17. An optical cross showing a lens's power at the two principal meridians.

Vertex Distance

Vertex distance (VD) is measured from the back surface of the corrective lens to the front surface of the eye. Most refractors have a vertex scale built into them; using this is covered in Chapter 11. To measure the vertex distance of the patient's glasses, a vertexometer can be used (details in Chapter 19). A conversion chart then determines the lens power required at the new vertex distance. The *effective power* (the adjusted focusing power) of a lens changes as the position of the lens changes. If a lens is moved farther away from the eye, the focal length is moved as well; the actual power of the lens itself does not change, of course, but the focusing effect it has does change. Moving a plus-powered lens away from the eye increases the effective power of the lens. Moving a minus-powered lens toward the eye increases its effective power (Figure 4-18). This phenomenon comes into play when translating a higher refractive measurement to contact lenses or with certain frames that fit a lot closer to or farther from the face than does the phoropter.

For example, when we measure a refractive error, we employ lenses at a certain distance from the cornea (standard is 12 to 14 mm). If the refractive error is less than 4 D, the change in vertex distance from spectacles to contact lenses would have a minimal impact on the effective power, so we can ignore it. However, for anything over 4 D (plus or minus), the change in effective power must be taken into account. A vertex compensation table can be used for this purpose. Alternately, the computation can be done by using the vertex compensation formula: $Dc = D/(1 - vD)$, where Dc is the power (in diopters) corrected for vertex distance, v is the change in vertex distance (in meters), and D is the original lens power (in diopters).

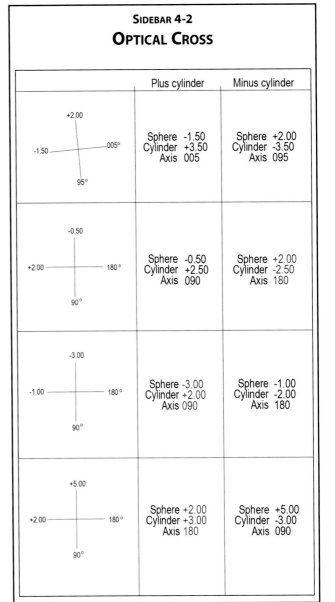

Example 1: You have measured the vertex distance to be 14 mm. The patient's refractive error is -6.00 sphere. He wants a pair of soft contact lenses, so we need to convert the refractive measurement to the corneal plane (0 mm). (Remember school math—*multiply* before adding or subtracting, and if we *subtract* a negative number we actually *add* it [ie, two negatives make a positive]. For more on mathematical operations, see Appendix A.)

$Dc = D/(1 - vD)$ where $D = -6.00$ D and $v = 0.014$ meter (Note: 14 mm must be converted to meters in order to fit the formula.)

$Dc = -6.00/(1 - 0.014 \times -6.00) = -6.00/1 - (-0.084) = -6.00/1.084 = -5.54$ D

Thus, the corrected power for a contact lens would be -5.54 D (or rounded off to -5.50 D).

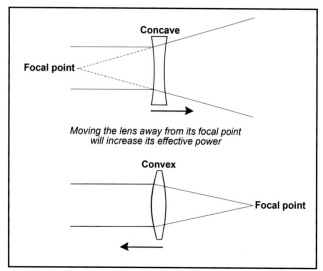

Figure 4-18. The effect of lens position on the effective power of the lens.

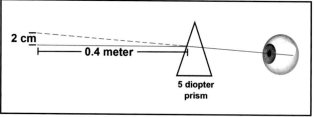

Figure 4-19. Calculating the displacement of an object using prism.

Example 2: Let's use a +6.00 and keep the vertex at 14 mm.

Dc = D/(1 – vD) where D = +6.00 D and v = 0.014 m

Dc = 6.00/(1 – 0.014 x 6.00) = 6.00/(1 – 0.084) = 6.00/0.916 = +6.55 D

Thus, the corrected power for this contact lens would be +6.55 D (or rounded off to +6.50 D).

Example 3: The patient has a pair of glasses with -7.50 lenses that sit at a vertex of 10 mm, but the new frames will have a vertex of 15 mm. That is an *increase* of 5 mm (0.005 m), so we will change the sign in our formula to a plus sign.

Dc = D/(1 + vD) where D = -7.50 D and v = 0.005 m

Dc = -7.50/(1 + 0.005 x -7.50) = -7.50/1 – 0.0375 = -7.50/0.963 = -7.79

What about cylinder? If the cylinder power is *more than 4 D*, the same formula is used. However, if there is sphere and cylinder combined, totalling more than 4 D, then they are calculated a bit differently (see Example 4).

Example 4: If there is more than 1 D of cylinder in addition to the sphere power being *over 4 D*, or vice versa, we need to use the optical cross (previously discussed). Let's say the prescription is -10.00 -2.00 x 010. This means part of the lens is -10.00, while the meridian 90° away is -12.00. We'll apply the formula to this prescription twice: once for the -10.00, and again for -12.00. In this example, we'll use a decrease in vertex (so we will use a minus sign in the formula) of 7 mm.

Dc = -10.00/(1 – 0.007 x 10.00)

Dc = -10.00/1.07 = -9.35

Then for the other meridian, Dc = 12.00/(1 – 0.007 x -12.00)

Dc = -12.00/1.084 = 11.07

The difference between -9.35 and -11.07 is -1.72, which would be the new cylinder power

So, rounding to the nearest eighth of a diopter (because standard prescriptions are in increments of one-eighth of a diopter), our new prescription would read -9.37 -1.75 x 010.

Calculating Prism Power

The formula for calculating prism diopters is: P = C/D (P is prism power in diopters, where C is the displacement of image in centimeters, and D is distance from the prism in meters). For example, we can determine how much the prism will displace the image at a given distance.

Example 1: Let's say we have a 5 diopter prism with an object 1 meter away.

P = C/D where P = 5 D and D = 1 meter

5 = C/1 = 5 cm

Thus a 5 diopter prism would displace the object 5 cm when measured at 1 meter.

Example 2: Let's use the same prism power, but measure at 40 cm (or 0.4 m).

P = C/D where P = 5 D and D = 0.4 m

5 = C/0.4, or C = 5 x 0.4, and C = 2 cm

Thus a 5 diopter prism would displace the object 2 cm when measured at 0.4 meter (Figure 4-19).

The usefulness of this formula in day-to-day eye clinic work may be minimal, but the question could possibly appear on some certification exams.

Prentice's Rule—Induced Prism

Sometimes induced prism can be used (on purpose!) instead of ground-in prism to correct small amounts of strabismus. To calculate the amount of induced prism, we use Prentice's rule: prism power = F x C where F is the diopter power of the lens and C is decentration in centimeters. Keep in mind that cylinders have to be considered and that their maximum power is 90° from their axis. One could use a complicated formula (involving trigonometry) to calculate the exact power at any axis, but for the purpose of Prentice's rule, an estimation is adequate. Three-quarters of the cylinder power is added to the sphere when the axis is 55° to 75° from the direction of decentration, one-half if decentration is 35° to 55° from the axis, and one-quarter of the cylinder is added when the axis is 15° to 35° away.

Example: Let's say we want to induce 3.5 D of base-out prism in a -7.00 lens.

Prism power = F x C where prism power = 3.5 and F = -7.00 D.

3.5 = -7 x C, then C = 3.5/-7.00, then C = -0.50 cm (or 5 mm)

Now we know that we need to decenter the lens by 5 mm, but which way (whether it be in/out or up/down)? Minus-powered lenses will induce prism with the base in the opposite direction as the decentration (Figure 4-20). Our example was a -7.00 (*minus*) lens and we wanted to induce base-*out* prism, so we need to decenter the lens 5 mm *inward*. For plus lenses, the base is in the *same* direction.

Alternately, suppose a patient complains that the new glasses are causing double vision. A common reason for this is that the optical centers are not in line with the patient's visual axis. In this case, you measure the inter-pupillary distance (the distance between the visual axis of the eyes; how-to's covered in Chapter 19) and find it matches the optical centers of the glasses. One physical feature that is often overlooked is that the two eyes are not always at the same height. The pupillometer does a great job at measuring interpupillary distance, but pays no attention to anomalies in the position of the eyes vertically. You notice that one of the patient's eyes is 5 mm below the optical center. The prescription was -8.00 -2.00 x 040 (and the glasses were made to the correct power). Because the cylinder axis is 50° from the direction of decentration (the decentration is vertical [90°] and the axis is at 40°, 90 – 40 = 50), one-half of the cylinder power will be added to the sphere (using the estimation technique mentioned previously). That gives us a power of -9.00 (-8.00 + -1.00). Then 9 x 0.5 = 4.5 D of prism. The lens is minus-powered, so the base is in the opposite direction of decentration (the optical center in this case is UP above the visual axis), so the result is 4.5 D of base-down prism.

Transposition

Prescriptions for spectacles are written in the following format: sphere cylinder x axis. For example, -2.00 -1.00 x 090 means there is a -2.00 sphere combined with a -1.00 cylinder at 90°.

Transposition is required when we want to convert from a plus-cylinder format to minus-cylinder, or vice versa. This is probably one of the most commonly performed mathematical functions used in opticianry, which works almost exclusively in minus cylinder. It is also important to understand transposition when a patient

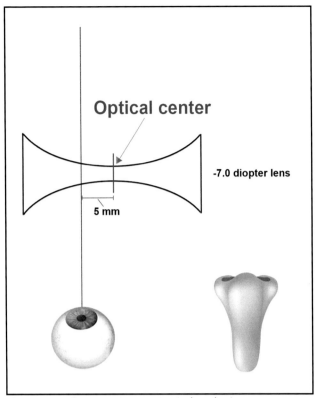

Figure 4-20. Decentration causing induced prism.

comes in comparing your prescription to that of another office and asking, "Which one of these is correct? See how different the numbers are!" One glance and you see that the prescriptions are actually the same: one written in minus cylinder and the other in plus.

To change from one cylinder form to the other, first algebraically add the cylinder to the sphere. If the power of the sphere and cylinder are the same (ie, both positive or both negative), add them together and keep the same sign (ie, + or -). If one is plus and one is minus, then subtract the smaller from the larger number and keep the sign of the larger number. Next, change the sign of the cylinder only. Finally, rotate the axis by 90°. (If the original axis is 90° or less *add* 90; if the original axis is over 90° then *subtract* 90. Remember, the axis cannot exceed 180.)

Example 1: Convert -2.00 +3.50 x 095 to minus cylinder format.

Add +3.50 to -2.00 = +1.50, the sphere power (the signs are opposite, so we subtract the smaller number from the larger and keep the sign of the larger number).

Change the cylinder sign to minus: -3.50, the cylinder power.

Since the axis is over 90, subtract 90 from the 95 = 5, the cylinder axis.

The minus cylinder version of this prescription would be: +1.50 -3.50 x 005.

Example 2: Convert -2.00 -1.25 x 012 to plus cylinder.

The signs are the same, so we add them together an get -3.25 for the sphere. The cylinder sign is changed to plus, and 90 is added to the cylinder axis (since it is <90) to get 102. The plus cylinder format is -3.25 +1.25 x 102.

Example 3: Convert plano +1.50 x 145 to minus cylinder.

Plano is the same as zero. +1.50 added to zero is +1.50 for the sphere. Change the cylinder sign to minus and subtract 90 from the axis (because it is >90). That gives us +1.50 -1.50 x 055.

Spherical Equivalent

Sometimes we need to use only spherical power to provide best vision in someone with astigmatism. This might be the case in fitting contact lenses, determining if the refractive outcome after cataract surgery was on target, or calculating a trial lens for visual field testing. In these situations, we want the "average" of the spherocylindrical prescription, known as the *spherical equivalent* (SE).

To calculate the spherical equivalent, algebraically add 1/2 of the cylinder power to the sphere power. The cylinder power and axis are then deleted from the equation. Thus, the spherical equivalent is the same whether we use the plus or minus cylinder format.

Example 1: Find the spherical equivalent of -2.00 +3.50 x 095.

Half of the cylinder power (+3.50) = +1.75. Add that to the sphere: -2.00 + 1.75 = -0.25. The original cylinder power and axis are removed from the mix; SE = -0.25.

In minus cylinder, the same prescription is +1.50 -3.50 x 005. Half of the cylinder power (-3.50) = -1.75. Add that to the sphere: -1.75 + 1.50 = -0.25. The original cylinder power and axis are removed from the mix; SE = -0.25.

Example 2: -8.00 -2.00 x 180.
Half the cylinder power = -1.00.
-8.00 + (-1.00) = SE -9.00

Example 3: +1.00 +1.00 x 090.
Half the cylinder power = 0.50.
+1.00 + 0.50 = SE +1.50

CHAPTER QUIZ

1. Which color's wavelength travels the fastest?
   a. red
   b. violet
   c. green
   d. none of the above

2. The "Law of Reflection" says:
   a. the angle of reflection increases with the index of refraction
   b. the angle of incidence is equal to the angle of reflection
   c. light is reflected proportionate to the power of the lens
   d. none of the above

3. Regarding light traveling through a prism, the following is *true*:
   a. light is bent toward the apex and the image is displaced toward the base
   b. light is bent toward the base and the image is displaced toward the apex
   c. light is bent toward the apex and the image is displaced toward the apex
   d. light is bent toward the base and the image is displaced toward the base

4. Where is the focal point(s) in a myopic eye?
   a. behind the retina
   b. one focal point is on the retina, the other is behind the retina
   c. one focal point is on the retina, the other is in front of the retina
   d. in front of the retina

5. Which of the following is *not* true about convex lenses?
   a. they are thickest at the optical center
   b. they can induce prism if the optical center is not aligned with the visual axis
   c. they correct astigmatism
   d. they correct hyperopia

6. Which of the following is *not* part of the accommodative triad?
   a. accommodation
   b. convergence of the eyes
   c. pupil constriction
   d. increased blinking

7. What is vertex distance?
    a. the distance from the back surface of a lens to the front of the eye
    b. the distance between the peak of wavelengths
    c. the distance between the visual axis of each eye
    d. none of the above

8. The minus cylinder version of +1.00 +2.00 x 180 is:
    a. +1.00 -2.00 x 090
    b. +2.00 -1.00 x 180
    c. +3.00 -2.00 x 090
    d. +3.00 -2.00 x 180

9. The spherical equivalent of +1.00 -2.50 x 075 is:
    a. +1.00
    b. -1.50
    c. +0.75
    d. -0.25

Answers

1. d, All wavelengths (colors) travel at the same speed.
2. b
3. b
4. d
5. c
6. d
7. a
8. c
9. d

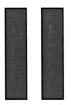

OPHTHALMIC SKILLS

5

OPHTHALMIC EQUIPMENT

Al Lens, COMT

There is a wide variety of equipment available for ophthalmic medical personnel to use. Certainly, select specialties will use some instruments more than others. Anyone new to the field might be overwhelmed with all of the "toys" that exist. This chapter is an overview of the various tools at our disposal. To find "how-to's," check the Contents or Index. For a review on the ocular structures mentioned, see Chapter 2, Anatomy.

INSTRUMENTS USED IN TESTING VISION

Devices used to evaluate vision include projectors, charts (wall charts and hand-held versions), occluders, and pinhole disks, which every office will have (Table 5-1). Other instruments might include desk-top vision machines (like the ones used at the driver's license office), as well as those that evaluate specific elements of vision, such as contrast sensitivity, potential acuity, and glare disability.

INSTRUMENTS USED IN EVALUATING REFRACTIVE ERRORS (TABLE 5-2)

Phoropter

The *phoropter*, or *refractor*, is an instrument used to measure a patient's refractive error. The word Phoroptor is a trademarked name (note the uppercase P and the "-tor" rather than "-ter" at the end) and is used to describe the phoropter made by Reichert Technologies.

This instrument is essentially a series of lenses placed inside a compact case with knobs to exchange the lenses in front of the apertures. It was designed to virtually eliminate the need for loose trial lenses that accomplish the same task, but are much more time-consuming. Most ophthalmic exam rooms will have a phoropter (Figure 5-1) or similar instrument.

Semiautomatic Refractor/Phoropter

The digital, or semiautomatic, refractor takes the phoropter into the digital era. These instruments still require responses from the patient, but the user can

Ledford JK, Lens A, eds.
Principles and Practice in Ophthalmic Assisting:
A Comprehensive Textbook (pp 57-68).
© 2018 Taylor & Francis Group.

	TABLE 5-1	
	INSTRUMENTS USED IN VISION TESTING	
Instrument	**Maintenance**	**Troubleshooting/Repairs**
Projector	▸ Cover when not in use ▸ Keep lens clean • Use lens cleaner and lens cloth with circular motion working from center to edge	▸ Projector will not illuminate • Ensure power cord is affixed • Replace bulb • If operated by remote control, check battery ▸ Chart is dimly illuminated • If projector uses tungsten bulb, it may need to be replaced • Bulb reflector may be out of position
Front-surface mirror	▸ Keep clean • First, use soft brush to clear dust • If there are fingerprints/smudges that need to be removed, use lens cleaner and a cotton ball; gently wipe in one direction only; use fresh cotton ball for each swipe until dry	▸ If mirror surface is significantly scratched or has peeled, the mirror needs to be replaced
Reflecting screen	▸ Keep clean • Use dampened cotton and use light pressure (the reflective surface scratches easily)	▸ Replace the screen if it is blemished or excessively scratched

follow the unit's program to step through the process of refracting. This shortens the learning curve to obtain an accurate refractometry result. Also, instead of having knobs on the phoropter, the user utilizes a separate control panel, making it more comfortable to operate. (Some models allow the use of a computer tablet instead of the control panel). At the end of the test, the results can be electronically submitted to electronic medical records (EMR), eliminating inaccurate input into EMR and making the process more efficient. The EPIC by Marco and the CV-5000 by Topcon Medical Systems, Inc are examples of this technology.

Autorefractor

Autorefractors provide an objective measurement (ie, requires no input from the patient) of an eye's refractive error. In an eye that has no accommodation (due to age or pharmaceutically induced), the results of an autorefractor are typically very close to subjective refractometry (requiring responses from the patient), assuming there are no optical irregularities in the eye (eg, post eye surgery or cloudy media). The basic autorefractor has a target for the patient to view, an infrared light, and a lens. Most current autorefractors analyze the focus of two LEDs (light-emitting diodes). Many clinicians will use the autorefractor results as a starting point for subjective refractometry. This means that the "computer read-out" must still be refined "by hand" with the phoropter.

Trial Lenses and Frames

The phoropter has replaced trial frames and lenses for most situations. However, there are times when having loose lenses in a frame that the patient can wear is the better method. Small children sometimes do not want to have that big phoropter pushed against the face, but will wear a pair of glasses (trial frames). When glasses are prescribed for large refractive errors (hyperopia or myopia), the vertex distance (the distance between the back of the lens and the front of the eye) is important and more easily measured with trial lenses. Also, when determining the power for reading glasses or bifocals, some patients will benefit by assuming any usual reading posture that cannot be accomplished with the phoropter. Lastly, there are some accessory lenses available in a trial lens set that are not in a phoropter.

Retinoscope

The retinoscope (Figure 5-2) is a hand-held device used to objectively measure a refractive error, just as an autorefractor does. There are advantages and disadvantages to using a retinoscope instead of an autorefractor. The retinoscope allows the examiner to view the clarity of the optical media and see irregularities in how light is focusing in the eye, giving some idea if the visual acuity could be less than 20/20. Retinoscopy can be done in conjunction with a phoropter or loose lenses, and does not require the patient to hold still like the autorefractor does.

	TABLE 5-2	
	INSTRUMENTS USED IN EVALUATING REFRACTIVE ERRORS	
Instrument	**Maintenance**	**Troubleshooting/Repairs**
Phoropter (including semiautomatic versions)	▸ Cover when not in use ▸ Sanitize points of patient contact ▸ To spot clean a lens or two, use lens cleaning solution sprayed onto a cotton swab (not directly on the lens) and wipe the lens in a circular pattern starting in the center and working outward	▸ Must be cleaned and serviced by a professional
Autorefractor	▸ Cover when not in use ▸ Sanitize points of patient contact ▸ Replace printer paper when needed ▸ Clean viewing screen with a lens cloth	▸ Replace fuse(s) as needed (if a fuse blows shortly after being replaced, the cause must be investigated) ▸ Difficulties obtaining measurements may be due to media opacities in the eye, a dirty window on the patient side, or ambient light that is too bright
Trial lenses	▸ Clean lenses with lens cleaning solution and a lens tissue or cloth ▸ Put lenses in proper position in the lens tray	
Trial frames	▸ Sanitize patient contact areas (nosepiece and arms) ▸ Tighten any loose screws	
Retinoscope	▸ Clean eyepiece with cotton swab sprayed with lens cleaning solution (do not spray the solution directly on the instrument) ▸ Keep the battery charged	▸ Replace rechargeable battery when it no longer maintains a charge ▸ When replacing a burnt-out bulb, do not touch the glass surface ▸ When the retinoscope will not illuminate, it may be easiest to put the retinoscope head on another battery unit, if available. If the unit still does not work, the bulb is the likely problem. If it does work, the battery needs to be charged or replaced.

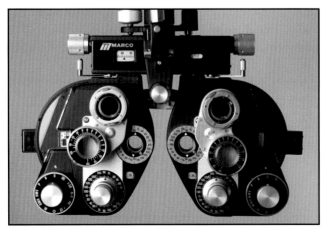

Figure 5-1. Standard refractor/phoropter (Marco).

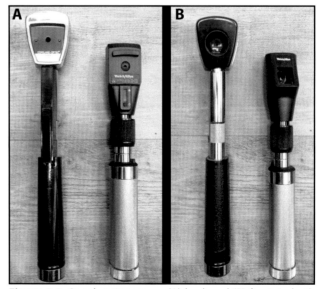

Figure 5-2. Streak retinoscopes (A) back and (B) front. In both pictures, the Copeland Optec 360 (Stereo Optical Co) is on the left, and the Welch Allyn is on the right.

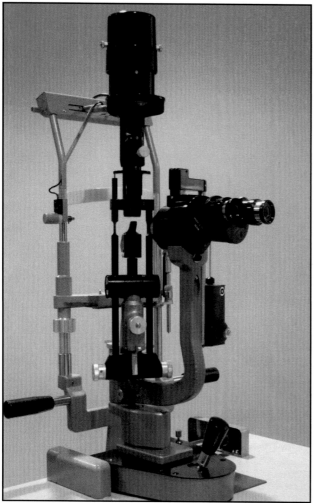

Figure 5-3. Slit lamp.

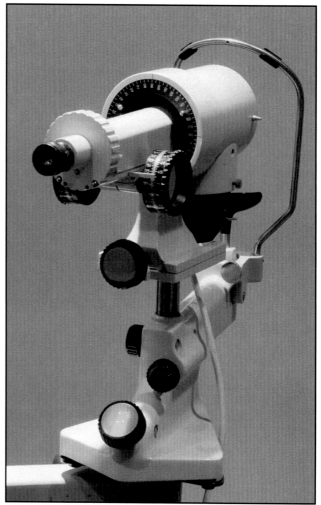

Figure 5-4. Manual keratometer.

However, the retinoscope requires a skilled examiner in order to get accurate results, and is probably equal parts art as science in less-than-perfect cases.

INSTRUMENTS USED TO EVALUATE THE CORNEA

Slit Lamp Biomicroscope

The *slit lamp biomicroscope* (Figure 5-3) is the mainstay of the eye exam. It provides three-dimensional real-time views at a variety of magnifications with adjustable lighting and filters. The use and care of the slit lamp is covered in Chapter 12.

Keratometer

The *manual keratometer* is used to measure the curvature of the cornea. This is important information for contact lens fitting, as well as for planning refractive or cataract surgeries. Certain corneal diseases are monitored by repeating readings (called K readings) over a period of time. The manual unit (Figure 5-4) might look intimidating, with numerous knobs plus a barrel that turns. An automated keratometer (Figure 5-5) takes the measurements with incredible ease and is reproducible. Many automated instruments are combined with autorefractors, but some are stand-alone units.

Pachymeter

A *pachymeter* (or *pachometer*) is used to measure the thickness of the cornea. This is commonly done before corneal refractive surgery, for glaucoma evaluation, to aid in diagnosing keratoconus, and to monitor corneal

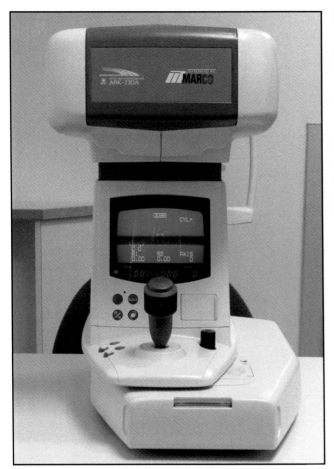

Figure 5-5. Automated keratometer (Nidek Co, Ltd). (Reprinted with permission from Kim McQuaid, COMT.)

edema. Pachymetry can be done using ultrasound or optical methods. Some instruments measure an isolated spot, while others provide a map of the corneal thickness. The most common type is a small hand-held ultrasound unit that provides a spot measurement (Figure 5-6). For corneal specialists or refractive surgery, the industry standard is to map the corneal thickness using corneal topography units that are capable of measuring the front and back surfaces of the cornea.

Corneal Topographer

The *corneal topographer* is an advanced version of the keratometer that is used to measure the shape of the cornea. The topography of the cornea is an important measurement when certain types of corneal pathology are suspected (eg, keratoconus) and for specialty contact lens fitting. Some surgeons prefer to use the corneal topographer instead of a keratometer when calculating intraocular lens (IOL) powers. There are many versions of the corneal topographer available. (See Chapter 16, Diagnostic Imaging, for more information.)

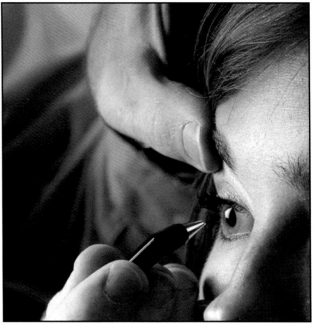

Figure 5-6. Pachymeter probe.

Specular Microscope

A magnified view of the cornea is provided by the *specular microscope*, but is used almost exclusively for analyzing the endothelium (innermost layer). This allows the examiner to look at the cell structure in great detail, determining if the cell sizes/shapes differ significantly from one cell to another. An endothelial cell count is also possible (cells per square millimeter) since the tissue is only one cell thick. A low cell count (< 500/mm²) will lead to corneal swelling and clouding, and may require corneal transplant. Specular microscopes come in contact and noncontact versions.

Confocal Microscope

The *confocal microscope* is used to view optical sections of the cornea to study its structure. The common uses in ophthalmology are for identifying dystrophies, evaluating infections, and inspecting the stroma, as well as analyzing the corneal nerves.

A *confocal scanning microscope* is used for analysis of corneal cellular structure, allowing for better diagnosis and treatment of corneal pathology. All the layers of the cornea are visible and identifiable with this technology. The high resolution provides corneal pachymetry, which can be used to measure flap thickness after laser refractive surgery. It is also useful for differentiating between various corneal dystrophies.

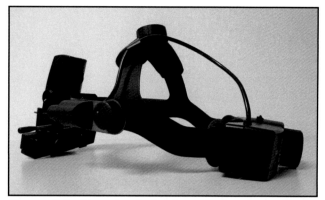

Figure 5-7. Binocular indirect ophthalmoscope (Keeler Ophthalmic Instruments). (Reprinted with permission from Kim McQuaid, COMT.)

INSTRUMENTS USED TO EVALUATE THE RETINA

Binocular Indirect Ophthalmoscope

When the periphery of the retina needs to be seen, the *indirect ophthalmoscope* (Figure 5-7) is the common tool of choice. The examiner also needs a hand-held lens (ranging from 14 to 40 diopters in power, with 20 or 30 diopters being the most commonly used) to position in front of the eye. Without the lens, the indirect ophthalmoscope is virtually useless. With the lens, there is a fairly broad binocular view of the retina (up to 240 degrees of the retina can be seen by scanning around the eye from different positions), enabling the examiner to look for retinal lesions. The three-dimensional view allows an appreciation for any elevated areas of tissue. The view, however, is upside-down and backward. (When drawing what they see, some examiners will turn their page upside down to be able to draw it exactly the way it was viewed.) Higher powered lenses provide a wider field of view (usually between 30 to 40 degrees), but a lower magnification. (A quick calculation can be made to determine the magnification: divide the refractive power of the eye by the power of the lens. For example, if the lens power is 20 and the refractive power of the eye is 60, the magnification is 60/20 = 3. A lens power of 30 nets a magnification of 60/30 = 2.)

Direct Ophthalmoscope

The *direct ophthalmoscope* (Figure 5-8) is a monocular, hand-held instrument that provides a 15x magnified view of the retina. Unlike the indirect ophthalmoscope, this instrument does not invert the image, but it also does not give a three-dimensional view. There is a dial on the instrument to compensate for the refractive error(s) of the patient and examiner. The examiner must be positioned very close to the patient and will use the right eye to view the patient's right eye, and left eye for left eye.

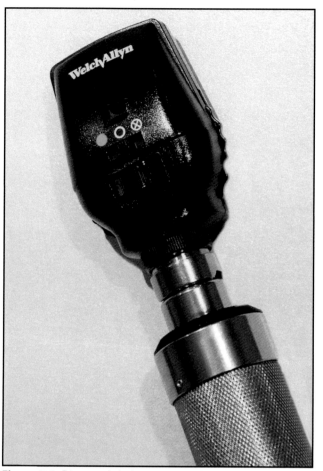

Figure 5-8. Direct ophthalmoscope (Welch Allyn).

INSTRUMENTS USED TO IMAGE THE EYE

Anterior Segment Imaging and Analysis

While the anterior segment can be viewed with a slit lamp biomicroscope, sometimes more detail is required. The *ultrasound biomicroscope* (UBM) and *anterior segment optical coherence tomography* (AS-OCT) are used for viewing details of the conjunctiva, sclera, cornea, iris, and crystalline lens. Looking behind the iris (specifically at the ciliary body) is better done with the UBM as the near-infrared light from the OCT has difficulty penetrating the iris. UBM is a high-frequency ultrasound that, while giving greater detail than typical diagnostic ultrasound, is limited to about 5 mm of penetration. As with diagnostic ultrasound, UBM is a contact method whereas OCT is noncontact and gives a wider field of view.

The common uses for anterior segment imaging is for determining open angles vs angle closure in glaucoma, and determining if an iridotomy (a hole created in the iris by surgery) is open or not. In the cornea, anterior segment imaging may be used to determine corneal thickness, assess corneal opacity depth/cause, and evaluate flap

TABLE 5-3
DIGITAL RETINAL CAMERA MAINTENANCE

Instrument	Maintenance	Troubleshooting/Repairs
Digital retinal camera	► Keep lens cap on when not in use ► Cover unit when not in use for extended periods of time (eg, overnight) ► Sanitize points of patient contact ► Use air blower or soft brush to clear dust from lens and eyepiece ► Clean persistent debris, possibly fingerprints, with lens cleaning paper and lens cleaner solution (fingerprints should not be left on the lens for long periods of time as the oil can cause permanent damage to the lens coatings)	► Refer to user's manual for instructions on replacing illumination and flash bulb ► Must be serviced by a professional for most other problems

thickness and continuity after laser refractive surgery. Other uses include post-cataract IOL position, as well as cyst and tumor size and tissue involvement of growths in the anterior segment.

Digital Retinal Camera

Digital *retinal cameras* are often used to capture an image of an anomaly in the retina. This creates a visual record to compare with at subsequent visits. A nonmydriatic retinal camera can capture images through a nondilated pupil down to about 3 mm. A mydriatic version will require a pupil diameter of 5 mm or more. Some cameras are hybrids and have both nonmydriatic and mydriatic features.

In most cases, a nonmydriatic version is used when documenting the retina for reference or telemedicine. Mydriatic cameras may be equipped with exciter and barrier filters for use in fluorescein angiography. Most digital retinal cameras have options to capture a stereo pair (usually for viewing the optic disc or diabetic retinopathy in three dimensions). Other common features are automatic conversion of standard photos into red-free (increasing the contrast of the blood vessels on the retina), cobalt (useful for assessing the retinal nerve fiber layer, the optic disc, and optic disc drusen), and mosaic (to automatically stitch a series of images together to display a large field of view). Some can also capture fundus autofluorescence, providing a view of the fluorescent pigment lipofuscin. This technique is useful for detecting or monitoring conditions like macular degeneration.

General care and maintenance for a digital retinal camera is shown in Table 5-3.

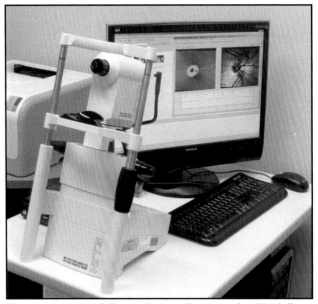

Figure 5-9. Heidelberg Retina Tomograph (Heidelberg Engineering).

Heidelberg Retina Tomograph

The *Heidelberg Retina Tomograph* (HRT; Heidelberg Engineering; Figure 5-9) is used primarily for three-dimensional imaging of the optic disc and is a great tool for documenting and monitoring glaucoma patients. HRT uses a laser to do multiple scans at varying depths to create the image. After the scan of the nerve fiber layer and optic disc are completed, the built-in software analyzes for glaucoma probability by comparing the results to normals for people of similar ethnicity. Consecutive scans can be compared to determine if any change is occurring. The unit can also scan the retina.

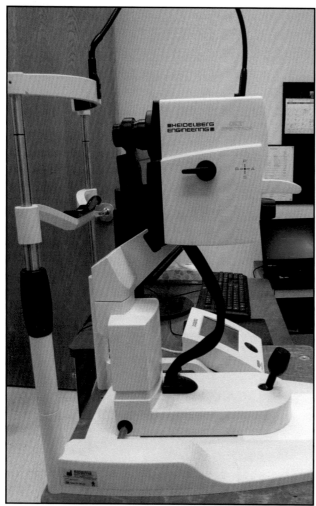

Figure 5-10. Optical coherence tomographer (Heidelberg Engineering). (Reprinted with permission from Kim McQuaid, COMT.)

Optical Coherence Tomography

OCT (Figure 5-10) is similar to ultrasound in that it uses echo time delay to scan the eye; however, it employs light instead of sound. This technology uses near-infrared light, or low coherence interferometry, to create a cross-section image of the tissue, displaying its thickness across multiple scans. These scans can identify differences in thickness down to a micron, revealing anomalies that may not be detectable with conventional methods. OCT is used to better diagnose and treat many retinal conditions. Some units are designed to analyze the cornea and anterior segment.

There are two forms of OCT: time domain and spectral domain. These formats collect the same information, but the mechanism is slightly different. The time domain uses a photodetector to collect the information and measures the time for light to be reflected; the spectral domain uses a spectrometer and collects signals from multiple wavelengths of light simultaneously. This

feature allows the spectral domain OCT to collect more information in a shorter period of time, making it the preferred choice.

Diagnostic Ultrasound

B-scan ultrasound is used mainly to view the contents of the posterior pole of the eye in cases where the media (cornea, lens, or vitreous) is opaque, making it difficult or impossible to view with the ophthalmoscope. Commonly, this is done before considering surgery (cataract or corneal), or if there has been a vitreous hemorrhage to verify that the retina is intact. It can also be used to assess vitreous adhesion and to look for pathology in the soft tissue surrounding the eye. Since it uses sound echoes, it can image through dense opacities, which OCT cannot. B-scans can be performed through the eyelid (using coupling gel), but this can limit the detail seen. The best images are obtained when the probe is placed directly on the anesthetized cornea.

INSTRUMENTS USED TO EVALUATE INTRAOCULAR PRESSURE

Intraocular pressure (IOP) is tested with a device called a *tonometer*. (Patients often refer to this as "the glaucoma test," although that is somewhat of a misnomer.)

There are various makes and models. The Goldmann applanation tonometer (Figure 5-11) is the "gold standard" for checking IOP. It is discussed in Chapter 13, which also explains its care and maintenance.

A second and very common method to quickly check the IOP is with *noncontact tonometry* (NCT, or *air puff tonometry*; Figure 5-12). Since, as the name implies, there is no contact with the eye, these instruments can obtain readings faster than methods that require the instillation of a drop. (Readings with the NCT are often obtained in the amount of time it takes to instill drops for contact versions of tonometry.) Sensors in the instrument detect when the jet of air has flattened the cornea a specific amount. An eye with a higher IOP is more resistant to flattening, and the time required to flatten the cornea will be longer. The instrument calculates the IOP and displays it in millimeters of mercury (mm Hg).

The results from the NCT are typically very close to applanation tonometry, but only when the pressure is within the normal range. Inaccuracy is more prevalent when the pressure is outside normal, with higher pressures often reading higher than and lower pressures appearing lower than the true value. Thus, the NCT is not generally used to follow patients with glaucoma.

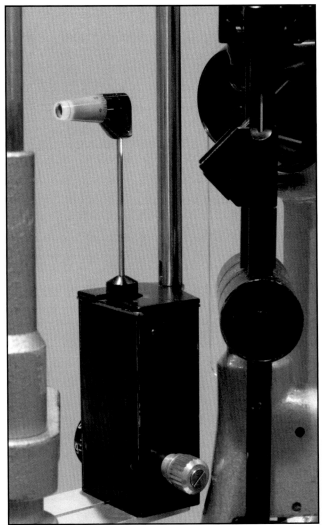

Figure 5-11. Goldmann applanation tonometer.

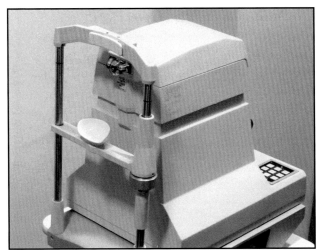

Figure 5-12. Noncontact tonometer (Reichert Technologies).

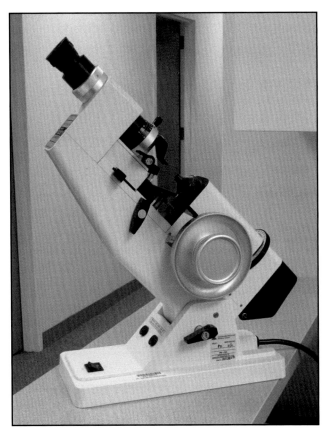

Figure 5-13. Manual lensometer.

OPTICAL INSTRUMENTS

Pupillometer

In the optical division of eye care, the *pupillometer* is used to measure the interpupillary distance (the space between the visual axis of the two eyes) for use in making a pair of spectacles. (Note: A pupillometer can actually be one of two instruments. The other is used to measure pupil diameter, discussed later.)

Lensometer

A *lensometer* (or *lensmeter*) measures the power of a lens, typically mounted in spectacles. This instrument is found in essentially every eye care office, clinic, and lab, as well as optical shops.

There are manual and automated versions of the lensometer. Manual instruments (Figure 5-13) require more user skill than automated editions and some simple mathematics need to be performed. If the spectacle pupillary distance needs to be measured, built-in markers are pressed against the lens. A ruler is then used to measure the distance between the optical centers of the lenses. Prism is calculated by observing a cross-hatch image inside the instrument and either calculating the displacement or else by turning a prism compensation device until the image is aligned.

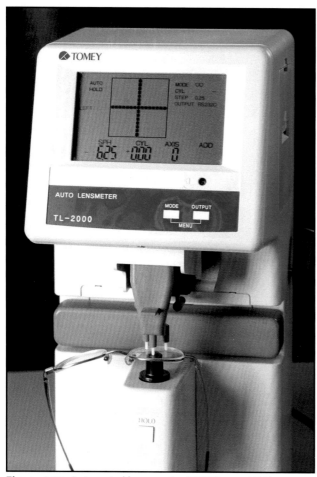

Figure 5-14. Automated lensometer (CBD/Tomey USA).

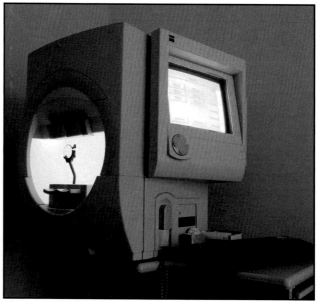

Figure 5-15. Automated perimeter/visual field analyzer (Carl Zeiss Meditec). (Reprinted with permission from Kim McQuaid, COMT.)

The automated lensometer (Figure 5-14) measures lens power simply by aligning the lens on the lens table. Most units can recognize when a "no line trifocal" (progressive add lens [PAL]) is being measured and guides the user to properly position the lens. Some instruments can measure the spectacle pupillary distance. If prism is present, and the lens is positioned on the lens table to match where the patient looks through the lens, the prism power can be measured. One other feature of some automated lensometers is to measure ultraviolet light transmittance and the corresponding ultraviolet protection in a lens.

Radiuscope

The *radiuscope* is used to measure the radius of curvature of a contact lens, better known as the base curve. The contact lens is placed on a drop of water under the scope, and similar to a lensometer, a knob is turned to focus the mires inside the instrument. The base curve is read off the millimeter scale inside the instrument or on an external dial.

INSTRUMENTS USED TO EVALUATE PERIPHERAL VISION

Perimeters

Also known as a *visual field analyzer*, the *perimeter* is used to test the level of light sensitivity in various areas of the retina. The test itself is called a *visual field*.

Almost all perimeters are automated (Figure 5-15), with a large white dome onto which the instrument projects small lights (targets) of various size and brightness. The patient responds whenever a target is seen. There are numerous testing strategies programmed into the perimeter to suit almost any situation that would require a visual field test. Some are screening tests that simply indicate if the patient can see a specific stimulus or not. More commonly, a threshold test is done to determine the dimmest/smallest stimulus that can be seen at any given location of the visual field.

Tangent Screen

A *tangent screen* (see Figure 14-18) is basically a black piece of felt with radial lines sewn into it. The examiner uses the lines as a guide as the target is moved. The targets are various-sized circles attached to the end of a black wand. A popular purpose for using the tangent screen is to test for functional vision loss (possibly due to hysteria or malingering). The fabric screen can be cleaned by gently whisking.

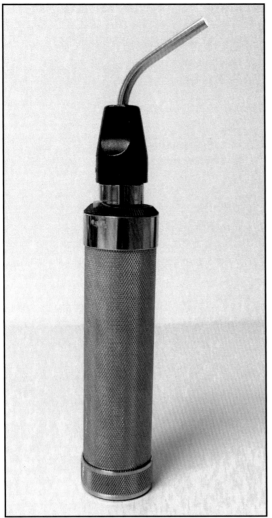

Figure 5-16. Transilluminator (muscle light). (Reprinted with permission from Kim McQuaid, COMT.)

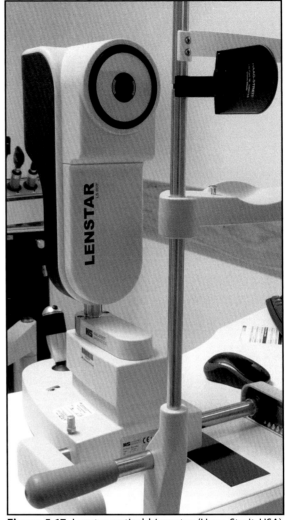

Figure 5-17. Lenstar optical biometer (Haag-Streit USA). (Reprinted with permission from Kim McQuaid, COMT.)

Miscellaneous Instruments

Pupillometer

When the diameter of the pupil is important to know (most notably in neuro-ophthalmology, refractive surgery, and multifocal IOL screening), a *pupillometer* provides an objective value. Static pupillometry is used when a simple pupil diameter is desired. Dynamic pupillometry records the pupil reactions (to light and accommodation) and is the desired method for neuro-ophthalmology. (Note: Another use of the term pupillometer applies to an optical instrument used to measure pupillary distance; see Optical Instruments, this chapter.)

Transilluminator

The *transilluminator* (or *muscle light*; Figure 5-16) is essentially a focused flashlight. It is a useful tool for

viewing the external eye, checking pupillary reactions, and estimating anterior chamber depth. It also serves as a light source for the patient to look at and/or follow when evaluating the alignment of the eyes. A cobalt blue filter can be fit on the unit to view fluorescein patterns on the cornea.

Biometer

The word *biometer* generally refers to an instrument that measures the axial length (front to back) of the eye, usually to be used in calculations for IOL powers.

A biometer can use ultrasound or optical methods. *A-scan* is an ultrasonic unit using either a contact or immersion-type probe. It gives a single (linear) display and calculates the length or depth of ocular structures.

Optical biometers are noncontact and use optical low coherence reflectometry (eg, Lenstar, Haag-Streit USA; Figure 5-17), or partial coherence interferometry (eg,

IOLMaster, Carl Zeiss Meditec). These units have essentially replaced the A-scan in many clinics. In addition to measuring the axial length, they perform keratometry and measure corneal diameter (white to white) and anterior chamber depth. Various IOL calculation formulas are built into the instruments, making it simple to select the appropriate IOL power.

CHAPTER QUIZ

1. A keratometer measures:
   a. refractive error
   b. lenticular astigmatism
   c. corneal curvature
   d. contact lens diameter

2. A pachymeter is used to:
   a. compress the cornea
   b. analyze corneal endothelium
   c. measure pupil diameter
   d. measure corneal thickness

3. What device is currently considered the gold standard for measuring intraocular pressure?
   a. Goldmann applanation tonometer
   b. noncontact tonometer
   c. visual field analyzer
   d. pachymeter

4. What is the tangent screen used to evaluate?
   a. peripheral vision
   b. extraocular muscle function
   c. macular function
   d. astigmatism

5. What is a retinoscope used for?
   a. viewing the retina
   b. measuring retinal thickness
   c. measuring pupil size
   d. estimating refractive error

6. The specular microscope is used for:
   a. measuring epithelial cell density
   b. analyzing the corneal endothelium
   c. viewing an optical section of the cornea
   d. measuring corneal thickness

Answers

1. c
2. d
3. a
4. a
5. d
6. b

Unless otherwise noted, the figures in this chapter were contributed by the following, who are associated with this book as authors:
Al Lens: 5-2
Aaron V. Shukla: 5-1, 5-3, 5-4, 5-6, 5-8, 5-9, 5-11 through 5-14

6

SCRIBING AND CHAIR-SIDE ASSISTING

Jane T. Shuman, MSM, COT, COE, OCS, CMSS, OSC

Medical scribing is an area of ophthalmic assisting that has grown in popularity in the past couple of decades. An increasing number of practices have embraced the use of scribes to document the exam as it occurs; it is multitasking at its finest.

Historically, ophthalmologists have been able to see more patients per session than many other specialists. This volume increased with the introduction of ophthalmic assistants and other allied health personnel to perform the ocular function tests, intraocular pressure (IOP) checks, refractometry, and dilation. With appropriate staffing, patients can be double booked. The job of the doctor then is to assimilate the information, examine the patient, diagnose, and recommend treatment.

The scribe is present in the exam lane recording the dictated findings in the medical chart as the exam is performed. The scribe summarizes the physician's findings and plan as they are discussed, in the words and terms of the physician. In this way, the doctor is able to focus on the patient, communicating directly without having to turn his/her back to record exam findings in the chart. The documentation is often completed by the time the doctor leaves the room. According to Garrett Erskine, President of Emergency Medicine Scribe Systems, a scribe "…frees up the doctor to focus on the patient, which ultimately improves productivity and patient satisfaction levels. Meanwhile, the scribe is capturing all the data for accurate reimbursement."[1] Scribes are viewed as the doctor's agent (some might say right hand).

Changes in the aging population and medicine have created the need for more access to physicians. The Baby Boomers are reaching maturity, the time of life when eye disease is more prevalent. The Affordable Care Act (discussed in Chapter 44) has mandated insurance coverage to a population that previously had none. In many cases, these persons have not had preventative exams that might detect glaucoma, amblyopia, or diabetic retinopathy. Sadly, changing vision due to cataracts has also been neglected because there was no insurance. Now that they are insured, there is an influx of people wanting eye exams and treatment.

Incorporating the use of a scribe has helped high-volume ophthalmologists meet the demands of their increasing patient volume. Once trained, the scribe will be able to complete the charting, requiring only minimal review by the doctor signing the note. Not only will this help the doctor get through the patient volume in a timely fashion, but because charting is not piled up by the end of the day, there is the prospect of getting off on time (or even early!).

Ledford JK, Lens A, eds.
*Principles and Practice in Ophthalmic Assisting:
A Comprehensive Textbook* (pp 69-76).
© 2018 Taylor & Francis Group.

WHO SHOULD BE THE SCRIBE?

There is a lot of discussion as to who is most appropriate as a scribe: the senior technician who is skilled clinically, a new hire, or someone moving from the front desk. There is merit to each scenario.

The technician has an understanding of the tests and the disease process, plus a familiarity with both the patient and the doctor. The learning curve is short, and the documentation probably needs little proofreading. However, this removes an experienced worker from the pool of technicians doing patient work-ups.

When the scribe position is used as an entry position to the clinical jobs, the preliminary learning curve is greater, but it provides the trainee with the knowledge behind the skills that he/she may later perform. Hence, he/she is likely to learn the skills required for work-ups faster and more thoroughly than someone hired initially to get on-the-job training as a tech. He/She will have become comfortable with the patients, who are likely to take pride in watching the progress.

TRAINING THE NEW SCRIBE

Before the scribe is allowed to do the documentation, the trainee must have an understanding of the patient flow in the clinic. By shadowing the current scribe (if there is one), he/she should begin to grasp how the doctor communicates and how the documentation is captured. Provide the trainee with a list of frequently used abbreviations and a breakdown of findings that might pertain to each ocular structure. It is helpful to review a model of the eye so he/she can visualize the inner workings of the globe.

If a scribe is already used in the office, the training is fairly straightforward. He/She should shadow the existing scribe for several days, then write findings on a blank template while the actual scribe is doing the chart documentation. Between patients they should compare notes. When the trainee captures approximately 80% correct, it is time to switch places and alternate between the two scribes for another week.

When the new hire is the first scribe in the practice, he/she should be given the same tools as in the previous example. What is unique in this situation is that the doctor may need training as well, having done his/her own documentation until now.

The order of dictation should remain consistent from one patient to another, beginning with the lids and adnexa, proceeding to the conjunctiva and cornea, and progressing deeper into the anterior segment before moving to the fundus and periphery. When training a new scribe, the doctor should indicate *both* the structure and its findings. In time, dictating the findings alone should

suffice as the experienced scribe will recognize what disorders go with which structure.

Role-playing with other team members is also a means of training the new scribe. The more familiar he/she is with the structures and the disease process, the faster he/she will be able to go solo.

FUNDAMENTALS OF SCRIBING

Principles of Documentation

Whether the record is paper or electronic, the documentation must accurately reflect what transpired during the encounter. The record is a legal document, and as such, it must be legible and complete. There is a key premise in chart documentation: "If it isn't documented, it wasn't done." Every scribe must recognize this as the foundation of the documentation he/she provides.

There are many reasons for strict documentation guidelines. For one thing, accurate documentation provides a review of the patient's condition for future visits. Also, when records are transferred to another provider, the next doctor can have a thorough understanding of the disease progression. Finally, it serves as the substantiation of the code that is billed to the insurance carrier, and stands up to a third-party audit.

Should this patient pursue litigation, or if the record is subpoenaed for any reason, the documentation will summarize the findings, counseling, any recommendations that were made, and subsequent decisions.

A common misconception is that documentation starts with the physical exam, but in actuality, it is when the doctor begins questioning the patient after the initial greeting. The physician often probes more deeply into the patient's history, adding information to what the technician already acquired. It is the scribe's responsibility to add the patient's responses to these questions; pertinent negatives are equally as important as pertinent positives. An example of this is if the doctor asked a patient, who complained of floaters, if flashes were present as well; "+ flashes" (yes) or "– flashes" (no) would be the appropriate addition to the history of present illness (HPI).

All persons involved with a patient's care must indicate their work by signing the record; this includes the technician(s), the scribe, and the physician. When diagnostic tests are performed, the name or initials of the person who did them is included on the test results or on the visit note. When the visit is recorded in an electronic record, the method of signing is dependent on the software (eg, a sign pad or a password/code). The tech usually signs the record at the end of the preliminary work-up. The scribe traditionally uses the same convention as a secretary who transcribed dictation from his/her boss. This is indicated by the provider's initials in capitals followed by the initials of the scribe in lowercase (eg, ABC/def).

Whether electronic or on paper, the physician's signature indicates the validity of the documentation. He/She should review the notes for accuracy prior to finalizing the record. Any new or changed information after the finalization of the chart note should be done in the form of an addendum; this too must be signed. Signature stamps are not to be used on paper charts; most electronic records have a mechanism for capturing the physician's signature once the note is finalized.

Just as when the chief complaint and history of present illness is expressed in the patient's words, the scribe must write the doctor's findings verbatim. The best physician-scribe teams develop a rhythm of the sequence in which the findings are dictated. This often follows the order of the ocular structures beginning with the lids, lacrimal system, and the remainder of the adnexa. Progressing to the anterior segment, findings are dictated regarding the conjunctiva, tear film, cornea, anterior chamber, iris, and lens. In most cases, the posterior segment is examined: the optic nerve (often expressed as the cup-to-disc ratio), macula, and vessels. If the patient is dilated, the periphery is examined using the ophthalmoscope. It should not be taken for granted that the findings are as they were at the previous visit, but rather, the status of each structure must be indicated verbally during every exam so it can be recorded by the scribe.

Legibility is not an issue when the chart is an electronic record. However, neat handwriting is a must when the documentation is on paper.

In order to survive an audit, the chart must be read by up to three reviewers who may not be familiar with ophthalmic terminology. Abbreviations in the record must be used consistently among all staff and doctors. Best practices maintain a list and distribute it to all new employees. Should there be an audit, your manager or doctor will submit this list along with the requested chart notes.

It is only natural, though, that mistakes are sometimes made. There are right and wrong ways to correct the inaccuracies. Consistent with the fact that the record is a legal document, anything entered in the chart (correct or not) must be available for viewing. Therefore, incorrect entries should *never* be scratched out, erased, covered over, or written over; it is also improper to recopy a visit note found to have errors. The approved way to make a correction in a paper chart is to simply draw a single line through the wrong word or phrase, write the word "error," note the correct word or phrase right next to or above it, then date and initial the change.

Spelling, or misspelling, as the case may be, is a source of error for the novice scribe. Some words (like ptosis and phthisis) have a silent p or a silent ph. If the scribe is uncertain of the correct spelling, he/she should

SIDEBAR 6-1
DOCUMENTATION FOR NORMAL EXAM FINDINGS

Anterior Segment
- Lids and lacrimal: No scales, tear film healthy
- Conjunctiva: White and quiet
- Cornea: Clear
- Anterior chamber: Deep and quiet
- Iris: No rubeosis
- Lens: Clear

Posterior Segment
- Vitreous: Clear
- Discs, vessels, macula: Healthy
  - The cup-to-disc ratio is written as a decimal for each eye (eg, 0.3)
- Periphery: Healthy without tears, holes, or detachment

be instructed to leave it blank and check the spelling before completing the chart. It is also a good plan to jot down any unfamiliar terms so they can be looked up later.

Scribing the Examination
Findings

The principle responsibility of the scribe is to document the doctor's findings while he/she is examining the patient.

Abbreviations must be standardized and kept on file in the clinic. There should be consistent phrases when there is no pathology found in each anatomical structure. Keep in mind that the abbreviation *WNL* (within normal limits) is often interpreted by lawyers as "we never looked" and that the best practice is to define the healthy status of each structure. Suggested phrases for normal findings are shown in Sidebar 6-1.

Convention dictates that the right eye is examined first, followed by the left. However, there are times that this is not the case. Keep a periodic eye on the exam (pun intended), making sure you are documenting the findings for the appropriate eye.

Abnormal findings are often graded according to severity, most commonly from 0 (none) to 4 (most). As pathology is detected, it is critical that the scribe annotate the chart with the exact language and grades that are dictated, and that findings are documented under the correct anatomical structure. The anterior segment (from the lens forward) is fairly clear-cut; the retina can be complex and described with terms not frequently heard.

Electronic medical records are often set up with many of the terms already in the user dictionaries and will appear as the typing has begun (much like common phrases in word processors or text messages). Make sure you are selecting the correct phrase. In some systems, the findings from the previous visit are carried forward and need to be selected so they will be relevant to the current exam.

The Assessment

The assessment is a summary of the exam findings that were discussed during the examination and includes the evaluation of the condition(s). The examiner's evaluation is based on:

▶ The patient's subjective report of the symptoms

▶ The course of illness or condition

▶ The examiner's objective findings including data obtained through physical examination

▶ The medical history

▶ Diagnostic tests

▶ Information reported by family and other health care providers

When there are multiple diagnoses, the first one listed must relate to the chief complaint (main reason for the visit). If, for example, the patient arrived for a scheduled glaucoma follow-up and was found to have a visually significant macular pucker that seemed to take precedence over the stable glaucoma, the glaucoma is still listed first, because that is what brought the patient to the office that day.

In addition to listing the diagnoses in the assessment, it is increasingly important to add the *status* of the condition. Examples of this include:

▶ Cataract OS > OD, visually significant

▶ Open angle glaucoma, OU, well-controlled

▶ Wet AMD, OS, responding well to anti-vascular endothelial growth factor treatment

Status of findings is of vital importance as we begin to use the *International Classification of Diseases, 10th Revision* (ICD-10), diagnosis codes. Intrinsic in many of the codes submitted to the carrier is laterality (side of the body affected). Others, such as the diabetic codes, also contain the severity level of the retinopathy and whether there is diabetic macular edema or not. In addition, part of many glaucoma codes is the level of severity for *each* eye. So while the simple notation of "left" or "right" seems minor, it is key. The less time the biller has to spend researching the chart for the information, the faster the claim is billed and paid. Therefore, the information needed should be easily identified in the assessment.

Only diagnoses pertinent to the date of service should be listed in the assessment. However, this does not mean that other conditions have been resolved. One such example might be a person with well-controlled non–insulin-dependent diabetes mellitus (NIDDM) who is seen quarterly for glaucoma; the patient is not dilated during these interval visits, and the diabetes is not pertinent. Only the status of the glaucoma would be listed in the assessment, while the NIDDM remains in the list of active diagnoses in the medical and/or ocular history for reference at a later date.

In the event the symptoms and findings could pertain to a variety of diagnoses (called *differential diagnoses*) and further testing is required to determine which one is accurate, it is acceptable to indicate one condition or another. It is not acceptable to use a "rule out" for billing purposes. This term describes a condition that is to be *excluded* from consideration and is most often used for when testing is performed. When the patient's symptoms combined with the exam findings may lead to several potential diagnoses, the doctor may order diagnostic tests to substantiate his/her thoughts. In this case, the *symptoms* can be billed.

The Plan

The plan is the part of the visit note that can be the most challenging for many scribes. This is where the visit is summarized and the recommendations for future events are detailed. The astute scribe will include the decision-making rationale, as appropriate. This includes tests ordered, prescriptions issued, surgery discussions, and referrals to subspecialists, to name a few.

In order for a test to be billed as a separately identifiable item, there must be an order in the chart for that test, as well as its medical necessity. Without both, the claim will not be paid by the third-party payer and may be the responsibility of the patient (provided that the appropriate form was signed by the patient in advance of the test). These include, but are not limited to, the tests listed in Sidebar 6-2.

Less frequent orders might include a Doppler study or magnetic resonance imaging (MRI). These, too, must be listed as part of the plan. Some insurance carriers require a preauthorization before some of these tests can be performed. It will help expedite the booking process if the scribe is aware of the plans that mandate the prior authorization and communicates this to the appropriate scheduler. In the event that the ophthalmologist returns the patient to the primary care doctor, that should be noted as well, along with any conversations between the two providers, including the recommendation for the tests.

Other important considerations to be included in the record are the intention to review notes from a previous eye care provider when the patient has transferred his/her care. Discussions pertinent to current and future care must also be documented. These include warning signs (ie, explaining flashes and floaters to a patient diagnosed with a vitreous detachment) and the risks and benefits of any proposed procedure. In the case of elective procedures, the documentation should include whether or not the patient chooses to proceed and, when appropriate, the rationale for that decision.

Occasionally, the patient does not meet the state's minimum requirements to maintain a driver's license. This is a difficult conversation for the doctor to have with the patient who equates the car with independence, but one that is necessary. Loss of driving vision is often the justification for cataract surgery, but sometimes there is nothing further that can be done to improve the patient's visual acuity. It is imperative that the scribe document that this conversation took place. If a family member is present in the lane, the documentation should include that this person witnessed the discussion. In the case where surgery will be performed that could possibly restore vision to driving functionality, the documentation should include that the restriction *might* be lifted post surgery (ie, no guarantees are given).

When medications are prescribed or refilled, the chart should reflect the specifics as they are sent to the pharmacy. This includes the name of the medication, the sig (how to label the medication), which eye(s), the dose, and any other special instructions (such as "shake" or "use after warm compresses"). In the event generics are not desired, the prescription must indicate that no substitutions are allowed. The specific number of refills allowed must also be indicated, otherwise none will be issued. The scribe is the person tasked with entering these during the patient encounter.

Meaningful use is a program created by the Centers for Medicare & Medicaid Services that provides incentives for using certified electronic medical records in a "meaningful" way to improve patient care. Of import here are guidelines that specify who is qualified to enter orders and electronic prescriptions in an electronic medical record. In order for documentation to meet this measure, the author of the notes must be a licensed medical professional (including doctors and nurses), or certified

Clinic Name
Clinic Address
Clinic Phone Number
Clinic Fax Number

Name: Aaron Martin

Address: 555 Main Street
My Town, PA

Exam Date: 7/4/2020

Glasses Prescription

	Sphere	Cylinder	Axis	Prism	Base	ADD
OD	+1.25	+2.50	090			1.50
OS	+1.25	+2.25	093			1.50

7/4/2021
Expiration Date

Violet Faux, MD
Provider Signature - Dispense as written

Recommendation:

_x_ Anti-Reflective Coating
___ Polycarbonate
___ High Index Plastic
___ Transitions / Sunglasses

___ Single Vision
___ Bifocal
_x_ Progressive Add Lens
___ Reader / Computer

Comments:

Figure 6-1. Sample eyeglasses prescription.

by a recognized agency other than the employer.[2] This can be a certified medical assistant or a certified ophthalmic or optometric assistant at any level.[3] Certified medical scribes also qualify. (Note: This designation applies to *orders* only. A certification is not required to write *notes* in an electronic record.)

It is often up to the scribe to fill out the prescription for eyeglasses and/or contact lenses as indicated by the doctor. Prescriptions for eyeglasses should be written as shown in Figure 6-1.

Contact lens prescriptions must also include the brand, diameter, and the base curve (Figure 6-2). Contact lens prescriptions expire after 1 year in most states. The life of eyeglass prescriptions also depends on state law.

Assisting the doctor in the lane is an integral part of a scribe's responsibilities as detailed above. But in some practices, the doctor prefers to do his/her own documentation, yet wants a staff member in the room to help as needed. At a minimum, this person will seat the patient and open the electronic record and images (when applicable). Any instruments or materials needed during the exam would be obtained by the assistant. At the end of the exam, the assistant would show the patient the way out and instruct the scheduler about the next visit.

```
                    Clinic Name
                   Clinic Address
                Clinic Phone Number
                 Clinic Fax Number


Name: Kathryn James


Address: 555 First St.
         Anytown, GA
Exam Date: 7/4/20


Contact Lens Prescription
```

Brand Name	B.C.	Sphere	Cylinder	Axis	DM
OD: XYZ Deluxe	8.8	-2.75	-1.25	180	14.5
OS: XYZ Deluxe	8.8	-3.00	-1.50	170	14.5

```
7/4/21
Expiration Date


Paul Taylor, OD
Provider Signature


Comments:
```

Figure 6-2. Sample contact lens prescription.

FOR THE SCRIBE: THE ART OF SCRIBING

Decades ago, children were raised to be seen and not heard, and to speak only when spoken to. This is good advice for the scribe to live by because you are present to help the doctor, not to be a party to the conversation. Often you will be joining the doctor after the exam has begun, coming in late from having helped the previous patient with instructions and remaining questions. In this regard, silence is golden. Silence is also a necessary part of the job when it pertains to patient confidentiality. As someone who is privy to the private nature of the encounter, you are not to share this information with anyone not involved in the patient's care. (Confidentiality and privacy are discussed in more detail in Chapters 7 and 44.)

When entering the room after the doctor is already there, do not slam the door or greet the patient by name. If the patient talks to you, a silent nod is in order, acknowledging the salutation. Quietly take your position. If there are others in the room who are inclined to chat with you, you must let them know that you are there to assist the doctor, perhaps by whispering that you need to pay attention to what the doctor is telling you.

Remember that any noise may be disruptive. This includes shuffling papers, coughs, sneezes, etc. Should you find yourself with a coughing spell, for example, leave the room until it has subsided.

The set-up of the exam room will be unique to each practice, as well as whether the charting is done on paper or in an electronic record. If in a file, it is likely that the doctor will review the previous notes and the work performed by the technician before handing it off to you. If you are working in an electronic medical record, the workflow may differ from doctor to doctor. You may find that you review the record together, either in front of the patient or before entering the room. Alternatively, there might be two computer terminals, one for the doctor to use for review, and one for you.

Anticipation of the doctor's needs during the exam comes after working side by side for many weeks or months, and is akin to the surgeon's relationship with the first assistant in the operating room. Mastering the ability to know what he/she is going to say, prescribe, or need will make you a valuable member of the clinical team. This talent improves efficiency because the time the doctor previously spent providing explanations or looking for a staff person can be better utilized providing direct patient care.

If you have the opportunity to check the patient's chart to read the previous plan or today's reason for the visit, you will know if additional instruments may be needed. For example, a jeweler's forceps or foreign body spud should be available if the patient complains of a foreign body. In addition, perusing the plan recorded at the previous visit and noting that an ordered test was not performed today, you can remind the appropriate technician this test is needed before the physician comes in. This will save the doctor from having to see the patient twice.

Pay attention during the exam for cases where the patient may need to be physically assisted. For example, if he/she has trouble reaching the slit lamp you might step in to support his/her head and back. You may also need to function as a "free hand" for the practitioner, reaching items in the cabinets or drawers.

During the exam, there are some natural breaks that are ideal for asking questions or clarification without interrupting flow. For instance, when the provider is strapping on the indirect ophthalmoscope, you might ask if you should write out the patient's eyeglasses prescription. Or you may need clarification as to which eye the findings pertained to. After working together for a while, you will become familiar with the physician's sequence and can better judge when to ask for additional information.

For invasive procedures done in the office, a consent form must be provided and explained to the patient prior to providing the treatment. Although the assistant may review it with the patient, the *doctor* must discuss the risks and benefits of the procedure and offer the patient the opportunity to ask any remaining questions prior to signing the document. Informed consent is discussed more thoroughly in Chapters 40 and 44.

The frequency of intravitreal injections have increased exponentially since the introduction of new medications for the treatment of macular degeneration.[4] These procedures require that a consent form be signed prior to every injection. However, as long as the same drug is used repeatedly and the risks and benefits of the drug do not change after the first complete consent is signed, subsequent forms only require a signature and date. Some medical malpractice carriers allow one signature for each eye until the pharmacologic agent is changed. If the ophthalmologist changes therapies, a new and complete consent form must be signed. It is up to you to make certain this is in order.

Drug samples might have to be logged prior to giving them to the doctor to issue to the patient. It may be necessary to document how medications are to be used, or to review treatments with the patient, such as the application of hot compresses. These and other topics of patient education are generally done after the doctor has left the exam room. If you are the only chair-side assistant, you will have to do this as quickly as possible, without making the patient feel rushed, before joining the physician in the next room.

Over time, you will know what patient education materials to provide the patient, as you become increasingly familiar with how the findings relate to the plan. For example, scaling and crusting along the lid margin is indicative of blepharitis. Chances are good that you will be providing this patient with written and/or verbal education on lid scrubs. Do not forget to document this instruction in the medical record.

Patient education may be offered in various formats. There are preprinted brochures and information sheets from numerous eye organizations, and others that can be downloaded from your office computer. Videos and animations are other means of communicating this information. Whatever you provide the patient, do not forget to document what materials he/she was given.

Anticipating the physician's needs includes knowing when the exam is over. This is not always clear, if the doctor expects the patient to dismiss him/her. There might be a pregnant pause while each waits for the other. You might break the silence by asking the provider, "When would you like to see Mr. Jones next?" or begin moving toward the closed door.

A key job of the scribe is to remain aware of patient flow. The responsibility of seating the next patient in the doctor's "room on deck" should fall to *all* clinical staff. Because the flow is not always predictable, you should always make sure the doctor will immediately have another patient to examine. This includes calling the patient from the dilating area prior to entering the "active room" with the physician. If there is no one ready and the doctor retreats to his/her office, you must alert the provider when the next patient is ready to be seen.

Just as important as letting him/her know when patients are ready, it falls to the scribe to let the doctor know when things begin to run behind. If the doctor is intent on catching up, he/she will (hopefully) reduce the time spent chatting about nonclinical issues with the next few patients in order to get back on track. You might use some sort of code phrase that will alert the physician (but not the patient) that things are backing up.

Whether the eye care practice is that of a solo practitioner or a large group, the scribe is a valuable member of the ophthalmic team that provides quality care, and is viewed as an agent of the provider.

CHAPTER QUIZ

1. A scribe's responsibility is to:
   a. perform the ocular function tests, intraocular pressure checks, refractometry, and dilation
   b. assimilate the information, examine the patient, diagnose, and recommend treatment
   c. record expected findings in the medical chart before the exam is performed
   d. record dictated findings, then summarize the physician's findings and plan as they are discussed with the patient

2. Provide two reasons for maintaining strict documentation guidelines in the medical record.

3. If the record is changed after it is finalized, the correction should be done by _____ .

4. The severity of a condition is recorded on a scale of _____ .

5. What is the section of the record that lists the diagnoses that pertain to the day's examination?

6. When is a differential diagnosis used in the assessment?

7. True/False: In order to bill for a diagnostic test, there must be an order in the chart.

8. What is meaningful use?

9. In most states, contact lens prescriptions expire after what period of time?
   a. 6 months
   b. 12 months
   c. 18 months
   d. 24 months

10. The responsibility of reviewing risks and benefits for invasive procedures falls to which member of the clinical team?

Answers

1. d

2. Possible answers: Provide a review for future visits. Provide a thorough understanding of the patient's condition should the patient transfer care. Provide risk management in that it substantiates the code billed and helps stand up to an audit.

3. The physician writing an addendum

4. 1 to 4

5. Assessment or impression

6. When the symptoms and findings could pertain to a variety of diagnoses.

7. True

8. Meaningful use is a program created by the Centers for Medicare & Medicaid Services that provides incentives for using certified electronic medical records in a "meaningful" way to improve patient care.

9. b

10. The physician

REFERENCES

1. Erskine G. Medical scribes improve revenue cycle, patient satisfaction. *Healthcare IT News.* www.healthcareitnews.com/press-release/medical-scribes-improve-revenue-cycle-patient-satisfaction. Accessed July 4, 2016.

2. Stage 2 eligible professional meaningful use core measures, measure 1 of 17. Centers for Medicare & Medicaid Services website. www.cms.gov/Regulations-and-Guidance/Legislation/EHRIncentivePrograms/downloads/Stage2_EPCore_1_CPOE_MedicationOrders.pdf. Accessed July 4, 2016.

3. Balasa DA. The CMS order entry rule: what educators need to know. *CMA Today.* 2015;March/April. http://aama-ntl.org/docs/default-source/other/ma15_pa_educators.pdf?sfvrsn=2. Accessed July 4, 2016.

4. Williams GA. IVT injections: health policy implications. *Review of Ophthalmology.* www.reviewofophthalmology.com/content/d/retinal_insider/c/48732/. Accessed July 4, 2016.

The figures in this chapter were contributed by the author, Jane T. Shuman.

7

HISTORY TAKING

Ellie Bessarab, COT, NCLEC, OSC
Duanna VanCamp, COT

BASIC SCIENCES

At its most basic, history taking is recording the patient's story. Yet this is not always (if ever!) a simple task. In order to obtain the information needed, both to guide testing/screening and to assist the practitioner in helping the patient, you need a good understanding of general human anatomy and physiology (see Appendix A), ocular anatomy and physiology (see Chapters 2 and 3), ocular disorders (kindly check the Contents for these), and ocular pharmacology (Chapter 22). This material will provide the background needed for utilizing this chapter.

CLINICAL KNOWLEDGE

To take a good history you must become like a detective, obtaining evidence from the suspects and putting together the clues that will help solve a medical mystery. The mystery is why this patient's vision is not as good as expected, or why the eye is bothering the patient. The clues are the signs and symptoms of the eye condition. The suspects are the systemic and ocular disorders and medications known to cause such signs and symptoms. By carefully questioning the patient, you gather information that narrows down the possible suspects. General and ophthalmic medical knowledge help weave the clues into a case for or against a suspected process.

Privacy Compliance

The Health Insurance Portability and Accountability Act (HIPAA) sets the standard for protecting sensitive patient data. Any company that deals with *protected health information* (PHI) must follow the HIPAA guidelines and make sure that the health information stays protected. The patient history certainly falls under the category of PHI. Measures should be taken by all the employees in the clinical practice to comply with the HIPAA guidelines and handle information accordingly. An overview is provided here; more details are available in Chapter 44.

A patient's record may not be left open on the desk or computer and left unattended; the user must make sure that the work station is secure with information locked up and/or electronic records protected with a password. A computer screen should not be visible to passersby; a filter can be applied to the monitor so that it can only be seen by someone looking directly at it (vs at an angle).

It is also very important to pay attention to the privacy of *personally identifiable information* (PII). PII may include the patient's full name, home address, driver's license number, credit card number, date of birth, phone number, or any other information that may distinguish the patient's identity. If a patient needs help filling out the necessary forms required by the practice and must be asked the questions aloud, this should be done in a

Ledford JK, Lens A, eds.
Principles and Practice in Ophthalmic Assisting:
A Comprehensive Textbook (pp 77-91).
© 2018 Taylor & Francis Group.

private place to avoid sharing PII with anyone else that may be in the area. Also, respect the patient's privacy and ask for any health information behind the closed doors of the exam room.

Patient information may only be shared with those staff members directly involved in the patient's care. The provider will have access to the patient's PHI to examine and treat the patient. The technician will access the patient's PHI to collect a series of diagnostic data and update his/her medical and ocular history. PII may be shared with a diagnostic technician who is to enter the PII into a machine for diagnostic imaging (fundus camera, perimeter, etc). The receptionist will have access to the patient's PII during the registration, check-in, and insurance verification process. The billing office will have access to the PII and the PHI to obtain payment for care.

PHI may also be shared between the clinical staff for consultation purposes. If a provider needs to consult with another provider regarding patient care, he/she may do so. If a technician has questions regarding the patient's care, he/she may consult with another technician or the provider. However, the PHI may not be shared between the office staff for any other reason that does not directly involve caring for the patient. If the PHI has no legitimate reason to be shared (let's say the staff would like to discuss the patient's medical condition to feed their vibe of curiosity), then according to the HIPAA guidelines, this is not ethical and does not protect PHI. Confidentiality is a serious matter of trust, care, and law.

Role of a Technician in Ophthalmic History Taking

The responsibility of collecting an accurate and detailed ophthalmic and medical history that highlights pertinent facts primarily falls on the ophthalmic paraprofessional. Learning to ask the right questions at the right time is an invaluable skill. It is important to be courteous and sensitive to the patient and be respectful of his/her health history. The patient needs to know that he/she can trust you with the personal health information that he/she has shared.

Professionalism defines how you communicate with the patient, how you present yourself to the patient, and how you converse with colleagues during down time. If the patient appreciates your professionalism and your etiquette in the exam room, and then he/she overhears how you were cited for "driving under the influence," his/her impression of you and the image of the clinic will be misleading. Be aware that patients watch your every move, even if you are not communicating with them directly.

With the advancement of technology, more and more patients search for a medical provider based on online reviews. Most of the ratings for providers are based on their customer service skills, bedside manner, and wait time. Even if you work for the greatest doctor in the region, if that doctor does not have good chair-side manners and lacks professional etiquette, the patient will provide a poor review. Patients like to be treated by someone who can blend professionalism, wealth of knowledge, and efficiency, as well as provide a comfortable visit with optimum results. A patient's experience is rated not just on the exam outcome, but on the entire office experience from the time the patient comes in to the time he/she leaves.

Signs and Symptoms

Symptoms of eye problems are what the patient reports experiencing. This is a subjective "story" and requires the patient to express how the eye bothers him/her. These may or may not be related to a specific ocular structure. Gather all the details about any ocular symptoms a patient reports.

The patient may report visual symptoms, visual disturbance, and physical discomfort he/she is experiencing or physical changes he/she is noticing. Visual symptoms may include blurred vision, glare and halos around lights, sensitivity to bright lights, or loss of vision. Visual disturbances may include flashing lights, floaters, curtain or veil shadowing over his/her vision, changes to peripheral vision, double vision, diminished contrast in vision, or diminished color vision. Physical discomfort may include burning sensation, discharge, itching, pain, a dull ache, throbbing sensation, tingling sensation, twitching, numbness, pulling sensation, tenderness, and general eye discomfort. Physical changes may include redness, droopiness, swelling, growths/lesions, and physical changes in size and texture of the area of interest.

Signs of eye problems are abnormalities of the eye that can be directly observed by an eye care professional. Signs are often specific to an ocular structure, but there are times where other anatomical changes may help complete the assessment. Signs of eye problems may be detected by examining the external ocular adnexa, eye muscle alignment, cornea, conjunctiva, sclera, iris, lens, vitreous, and fundus. A variety of ophthalmic diagnostic equipment and measurement tools may also be required.

CLINICAL SKILLS

Communication Skills

Communicating with and understanding the patient is not always cut and dried. There are many variables that come into play that can make or break the communication link that we establish with any patient (Sidebar 7-1).

When the patient is a child, it is important to speak with the parent or guardian regarding the child's medical and ocular health. But it is also critical to speak to the child directly. When a child enters the exam room, provide your undivided attention to the child. You may want to start with "small talk" to put the child at ease. Lead the patient interview by asking a series of direct and closed-ended questions. These types of questions are going to help you obtain the information you need, instead of having to filter out the information a child might provide when asked an open-ended question. It is also important to collect information from the parents about what they have observed, as well as recollect any complaints or struggles the child has been having. At the end of the exam, open up the conversation for any questions or concerns. You may be surprised by things a child may mention that is pertinent to his/her care, once given the opportunity.

Communication with teens may be a delicate issue, and requires compassion and understanding from the technician. After introducing yourself to the teen and the parent or guardian, you may want to "break the ice" with a small conversation about school, hobbies, sports, or whatever else he/she might be interested in. Teens are young adults, treat them with dignity and respect, and take their comments seriously. Use active listening skills and demonstrate interest and concern during the interview process. Gently involve the family in the conversation (as they may have some significant input), but allow the teen to respond first. The teen may volunteer more information when he/she feels more confident and important.

Verbal

It is important to figure out your patient's personality and what kind of communication style he/she uses. Once the communication style is identified, you can apply your response to the patient and figure out the best way to communicate with that patient (Table 7-1).

It may be hard to identify the communication style that any one patient is using. In cases of uncertainty, try to keep neutral ground with the patient and respond with lots of reinforcing interjections to encourage the patient to keep going with what he/she has to say.

Create a smooth transition from a friendly introduction to an ophthalmic history. Keep in mind that you are in control of the history-oriented interview. Avoid too much personal interaction and going into detail about your life, otherwise the patient will feel like he/she is collecting your history, not you taking his/hers.

Nonverbal

Nonverbal cues are used between everyone who communicates. They come from the patient, the person accompanying them, the technician, the provider, and everyone else involved in the encounter.

SIDEBAR 7-1
DO IT BETTER: COMMUNICATION SKILLS

Language barrier: An interpreter must be provided for the exam. Some templates are available that provide questions and answers in two languages so that the patient and personnel can communicate by pointing to text.

Hard of hearing: Speak directly to the patient (including direct eye contact), speak loudly and clearly, but do not scream at the patient. Sitting closer to the patient and speaking in a lower/deeper tone also help. Alternately, provide a tablet and pencil. Gestures may also be helpful (eg, thumbs up for "better," thumbs down for "worse").

Deaf patients: Sign language interpreter might be needed for the visit; alternately, provide a tablet and pencil. Gestures may also be helpful (eg, pantomime taking glasses off). Some deaf people read lips, so look directly at the patient when communicating. Also remember, many are not mute and can give you verbal replies.

Patients with challenges (dementia, Alzheimer's, Down syndrome, etc): Speak directly to the patient as much as possible, including eye contact. If you are unable to collect a complete history from the patient, refer to the family members and/or caregivers accompanying the patient for help.

The technician needs to learn how to interpret the most common nonverbal cues to fully understand what the patient is trying to say. Sometimes the patient might be expressing an emotion like anger or frustration. It is important to understand what the patient is indirectly trying to tell you. You may need to steer your interview to a more comfortable zone for the patient. Body language is also discussed in Chapter 9.

It is likewise important to pay attention to the nonverbal cues that you, as a technician, may be demonstrating. You do not want to appear as someone who is not interested, upset, angry, or sad, by giving off negative nonverbal cues that discourage rapport. This will turn the patient away and give the wrong impression of not only the clinical staff, but the clinic as a whole. Implement positive nonverbal cues that will encourage the patient, such as an affirmative head nod and leaning toward the patient to show interest.

Listening Skills

It is often and rightly said, "If you listen to patients, they'll tell you what's wrong." Yet listening is a skill that needs to be developed. It is easy to "hear" and yet bypass everything that is being said. It takes a lot more effort to

TABLE 7-1
COMMUNICATION STYLES

Communication Style	Positive Aspects	Negative Aspects	How to Use This to Your Advantage as a Clinician
Intuitor	Imaginative Creative Original	Questions everything Sets unrealistic expectations	Ask questions that are more direct and specific to their chief complaint. Set the parameters from the beginning, let patients know what the flow of the exam will be. Don't let patients steer you away from getting your job done.
Thinker	Effective communicator Analytical	Overanalyzes Indecisive	You may get a good history, but be careful and filter out what they say as some of the information may not be relevant to the exam. It may be hard to discern what really needs to be documented.
Feeler	Interpersonal Social	Sentimental Manipulative	While they may be understanding of your time, and very sweet and social, sometimes their emotional state may overcome them. They might try to have you feel sorry them and attempt to manipulate you to a desired response. Be understanding and respectful, but know your boundaries.
Sensor	Objective Confident Determined Action oriented	Arrogant Acts first, then thinks	These people are usually upbeat, and they have their "let's do this" face on. If you steer them in the right direction and put on your game face, you may have a fun time collecting their ophthalmic history. Be confident, don't show them your weaknesses, and power through the exam.

listen with empathy and understanding. When patients describe the symptoms they are experiencing, tune out all the distractions and focus on their story. Get in their shoes and try to visualize what they are going through. Take into account the nonverbal cues they are presenting, their emotional state, and their tone of voice to depict a message they are trying to tell you.

Do not be judgmental of their accent, language barriers, or the way they deliver their information. Everyone has a different delivery method, a unique personality, and a different way of speaking. Not everyone can easily paint a detailed canvas for you that will take your breath away. There are times where you have to dig for the information one clue at a time. Try to ignore any distractions on how the message is presented and focus on what patients are trying to tell you. Your job is to collect the information accurately, bypassing the disturbance in between.

The most important aspect of a good listener is to be patient and affirmative. Listen with empathy and try to understand the patient. Validate the patient's concerns, acknowledge his/her emotional state, and facilitate the interview to encourage the patient and put him/her at ease. The following points and sample comments will serve to illustrate good listening tactics.

▶ Validate patient concerns: Information is summarized and patient's nonverbal cues are taken into account.
 • "Just to make sure I have the facts, your neighbor's kid swung a tree branch that lacerated your child's right lower eyelid this evening. I don't blame you for being upset. I will ask the doctor to see you right away."

▶ Acknowledgment: Acknowledging the patient's positive or negative state of emotion can facilitate the interview.
 • "You appear to be so upbeat, you must have been enjoying the weather outside."
 • "I am sorry about your loss, Mrs. Smith. It must be hard on you. I'm glad you're here today taking care of your eyes."

▶ Facilitative interjections: These are comments and sounds that motivate the patient to go on with the history.
 • "Hmm, uh-huh, interesting, go on, tell me more about that…"

AIDET Model of Patient Satisfaction

AIDET is an acronym for Acknowledge, Introduce, Duration, Explanation, and Thank you.[1] It represents how a patient's clinical experience should progress, and is detailed here along with sample dialogue.

▶ Acknowledge: Welcome your patient with a bright smile and address him/her by name. Escort the patient to the exam room for the visit. Having good chair-side manners will make the patient feel welcome and more open to the health history questions you are about to ask.

- "Hello, Mr. Smith. It is a pleasure to meet you. Welcome to our clinic. Let me escort you to one of our rooms to get started on the exam."

▶ Introduce: Introduce yourself to the patient and whoever is accompanying him/her. Politely let them know who you are and your credentials and what you will be doing. Get permission from the patient to allow any companion (friend or family member) to accompany him/her to the exam room. Give a quick overview of what today's exam entails. Let them know that he/she is in good hands, that you have state-of-the-art equipment (if that applies to your clinic), and that you have an excellent patient care team. Your respect for your team and providers will help lessen any anxiety that your patients may be experiencing and make them feel more comfortable and confident in your care.

- "My name is Ellie, I am a certified ophthalmic technician and I will be asking you some questions and doing some tests before Dr. Johnson sees you. Would you be comfortable having your companion in the exam room with you? It looks like you are here for a complete eye examination. This would include your health history, checking your vision, checking you for glasses, checking your eye pressure, and dilating your pupils. The doctor may request that we do additional testing as we go, but I will let you know of any changes when the time comes. The doctor that will be seeing you is very personable and knowledgeable; I can assure you that you will receive the best care and hope you will be happy with your experience."

▶ Duration: Give patients an overall estimate of the length of their visit. Let them know how long it may take for the pupils to dilate. If your schedule does not go according to plan and your estimated time falls through, let the patient know, and apologize for any delays. If the patient is incapable of waiting to be seen by the provider, you may offer to reschedule the appointment to a different day or time. There are times when the doctor may be caught up with a true ocular emergency, and he/she would not be able to see the patients who were previously put on the schedule. If you explain the reason why the doctor is running behind, your patient may be more understanding, and may accept the delay with a lot more compassion rather than anger and frustration.

- "Your visit today should take about an hour and half. This includes the initial screening with the technician, pupil dilation, and an exam with the doctor. It takes about 20 to 30 minutes for the dilating drops to take effect. Dr. Johnson will see you after your pupils are dilated." If 30 minutes have passed, and Dr. Johnson is still not ready to come in to see the patient…. "I'm sorry, Mr. Smith. Dr. Johnson is running about 20 minutes behind. Are you able to stay a little longer and continue to wait for him?"

▶ Explanation: Explain the importance of collecting a good ophthalmic history. Be patient with any questions he/she may have and answer questions to the best of your ability.

- "I will be asking you some questions regarding your medical history and eye health. All of these components are helpful for the doctor to see the big picture of your general health and how it's related to your overall eye health."

▶ Thank you: Thank patients for their time, recognize their cooperation, and thank them for choosing to come to your clinic. Ask if they have any additional information they would like to address with the doctor.

- "Thank you for coming to the clinic to see Dr. Johnson today. I've enjoyed working with you. Is there anything else you think he needs to know about your eyes or your health?"

Taking the History

Types of Questions

A variety of questioning methods may be used to lead your interview in the right direction by collecting missing clues to the "mystery." This will help your doctor uncover a suitable diagnosis and develop a treatment plan for the patient.

The following is an overview of the types of questions that are commonly used in any type of history taking.

▶ Open-ended questions: These lead the patient to tell you his/her story. More than a few sentences may be expected in response.

- "What brings you in today?"
- "Tell me about the problems you are having with your vision."
- "Tell me about your headaches."

- ▶ Closed-ended questions: These are used to elicit specific information. The patient response should be very minimal (ideally, yes or no).
  - • "Can you see the computer monitor clearly with your current glasses?"
  - • "Do you need a new prescription for your glasses?
  - • "Are you wearing your glasses all the time?
- ▶ Direct questions: These are especially useful for talkative patients to help steer them in the direction to facilitate the interview and stay on topic. These questions may be open-ended or closed-ended, depending on what information you need to gather.
  - • "What kind of activities do you do at work?"
  - • "Are you using the computer a lot?"
  - • "Are you experiencing any glare from headlights of oncoming traffic?"
- ▶ Indirect questions: These questions may be used for patients who seem more sensitive about the exam, and are nervous about the visit. Speaking at an affectionate level and listening with empathy will help relax the patient and put him/her at ease and help you gather more information.
  - • "It looks like you have tried several different glaucoma drops over a short period of time. How are you doing with the current ones that the doctor has given you?"
  - • "I am sorry to hear that your vision is getting worse. How are you handling it?"
  - • "You seem a little nervous. I want to affirm that the doctor is very experienced and will take good care of you."
- ▶ Confronting questions: These are used on difficult patients who are not responding to indirect questions that may be related to drug and alcohol abuse, domestic abuse, etc. You may want to remind the patient that this information will remain confidential and is important for the doctor to know.
  - • "Do you have any history of recreational drug use?"
  - • "Are you currently using tobacco products? How much and/or how often?"
- ▶ Informing questions: These both inform (or remind) the patient and weave in the next question.
  - • "The doctor has noted that you have cataracts. How do you think you are doing with your vision?"
- ▶ Clarifying questions: Summarizing the information that was collected, to ensure the accuracy of the information, and then moving on to the next question.

- • "Your right eye has been red and painful for the last 3 days, then. Have you noticed any changes to your vision?"
- ▶ Laundry list questions: These are helpful if the patient is not sure what you are asking and will help guide him/her. However, be careful not to put words in his/her mouth or tell him/her to choose one of the options you provided. Instead, give the patient an option to decide what to answer on his/her own.
  - • Avoid asking: "How often do you get migraines? Once a week or once a month?" (This gives patient only two options for an answer, both of which are supplied by the interviewer.)
  - • Instead, ask: "How often do you get migraines—every day, once a week, once a month, or at some other interval?" (Indicates that you want a specific answer and makes some suggestions, but leaves an opening for the patient to determine how to respond.)

Some other questioning methods can be counterproductive as well; compound questions and leading question are to be avoided.

- ▶ Compound questions: Compounding more than one question in a sentence should be avoided, as this causes a lot of confusion.
  - • Tech: "Are your eyes red and itchy and blurry?" Patient: "Yes." Tech: "Yes to which one?"
- ▶ Leading questions: These can mislead the patient's response because of the way the questions are formed. These questions should be avoided.
  - • Tech: "You don't have any eye pain, do you?" Patient: "No, of course not..." (See how you just steered them to respond?)

Parts of the History

A general ophthalmic history includes the patient's reason for the visit, characterized by the chief complaint (CC) and explained in detail in the history of present illness (HPI). It also includes the patient's general medical history, ophthalmic history, and his/her family and social history.

If the patient is transferring care and is new to your clinic, it is especially important to request records from his/her previous provider(s). Patients will not always know exactly what kind of medical conditions they have had, or the details of their ocular history. In accordance with HIPAA, a patient must sign a form releasing this information to your clinic; this form is typically known as a *release of information* (ROI) form. This can be accomplished by faxing a signed request to the patient's prior health care practitioners.

Chief Complaint

The CC is the main reason why the patient is coming in for an eye exam. The patient's symptoms or problems may be described in his/her own words. A medical diagnosis or a condition may be used as a CC. If a patient is coming in for a basic eye exam, the CC will be eye or vision related. To get things started, you might ask:

▶ "What brings you to the office today?"

▶ "Are you having any particular problems with your eyes?"

▶ "Are you having any particular problems with your vision?"

▶ Example: CC: "Blurred vision at distance and near for 6 months."

If the patient is coming for a return visit, most likely it would be due to a medical reason. In the CC, include the reason for the visit and the medical condition that it pertains to. Sometimes the patient is scheduled for a follow-up visit, but he/she might be here for an urgent matter that needs to be addressed, unrelated to the original problem requiring the appointment. Make sure you know exactly why the patient is being seen.

▶ Example: CC: "Glaucoma follow-up."

▶ Example: CC: "Iritis follow-up."

▶ Example: CC: "Diabetic follow-up."

▶ Example: CC: "Foreign body sensation in the right eye for 3 days."

▶ Example: CC: "New onset of flashes and floaters in the right eye."

If the patient has more than one CC, list the CCs in the order of importance (which one of these complaints is more vision threatening?) and address the details of the complaints in the HPI. If the complaints are equally important, then list them all.

▶ Example: CC: "Patient is here to evaluate diabetes, glaucoma, and cataracts."

Multiple CCs may all tie together into one diagnosis, as follows:

▶ Example: CC: "Patient complains of a new onset of headaches and a visual disturbance."

If one CC predominates all the rest, and an acute problem presents, this should be recorded as the reason for visit, and the follow-up visit may be rescheduled. For example, if the patient is here for a cataract evaluation, but he/she has a new onset of eye pain, redness, and photophobia, then the acute symptoms should be the primary CC, and a cataract evaluation may be done at his/her next visit when the eye is feeling better and vision is more stable.

History of Present Illness

The HPI is the detailed report of the CC or symptoms that brought the patient to the office. Once the reason for the visit has been determined, the technician needs to find out more. The technician acts like a detective and asks specific questions to get the details about what is bothering the patient. Based on the collected information, the doctor should get a general idea of the patient's perceived problems. A detailed HPI helps the doctor determine if additional diagnostic testing is needed, as well as a diagnosis and treatment plan for the patient.

Document the present illness in terms of the timing, context, onset, location, duration, associated signs and symptoms, modifying factors, severity, and quality. According to the American Academy of Ophthalmology, for a "brief" history, one to three elements must be addressed in the HPI. For an "extended" history, four to eight of these elements must be addressed to properly document the HPI. These descriptive terms are often remembered with the mnemonic FOLDARS:

▶ Frequency: How frequent is the patient experiencing the symptoms? Are the symptoms constant or intermittent? Is the patient experiencing those symptoms once a month, once a week, or at a different interval? Is he/she experiencing these symptoms during any certain activity?

▶ Onset: When did the patient first notice the symptoms? If the patient is not 100% certain, have him/her estimate the initiation of the symptoms.

▶ Location: Be specific with this one. What part of the head? What part of the eye? Eyelid, conjunctiva, sclera? Medial, lateral, upper, lower?

▶ Duration: When the symptom occurs, how long does it last? Days, hours, minutes, seconds? Or do the symptoms come in clusters?

▶ Associated signs and symptoms: Has the patient noticed anything else going on with his/her general health that may be associated with the current signs and symptoms he/she is experiencing? Is there anything else going on in the general health during the time that the symptoms peak?

▶ Relief: What makes these symptoms better? Do artificial tears help? Does the use of ointment help? Do the eyes feel better when they are closed?

▶ Severity: On a scale from 1 to 10, how severe are these symptoms? Is the patient experiencing throbbing pain, a mild ache, or severe sharp pain? Does the problem interfere with activities of daily living (ADLs)?

If the patient has more than one CC, make sure to address the FOLDARS technique in the HPI for each. For example, if a patient complains of both flashing lights and blurred vision, depending on the extent of the history, you must address one to eight of the FOLDARS elements for each complaint.

Past Ophthalmic History

The patient's ophthalmic history includes any disorders/diseases of the eye, any surgeries or treatments, and any eye injuries. These should be noted with approximate dates (although the best you may sometimes get is "back in the 70s"), who performed the surgery/treatment, and any resulting problems.

Past Eye Disease/Disorders

A complete history of the patient's ocular disease/disorders may provide a head start in determining the treatment plan for the patient. For details on any specific eye disorder, check the Index.

Past Eye Injuries

Any previous ophthalmic injury should be noted in the history. Common examples include flash burns (from welding), foreign bodies, and corneal abrasions. Such injuries may explain specific findings (eg, scars) or certain symptoms (eg, early morning eye pain in recurrent erosion syndrome). See Chapter 32, Ocular Trauma, for more detailed information.

Past Ophthalmic Surgeries and Treatments

Some ophthalmic surgeries or treatments may predispose a person to other ophthalmic disorders or affect diagnostic measurements. Some examples are:

▶ LASIK/PRK (laser-assisted in situ keratomileusis/photorefractive keratectomy): May cause dry eye problems, affect intraocular pressure measurements, or cause an error in intraocular lens power selection for cataract surgery.

▶ Radial keratotomy (RK)/corneal transplant: Cornea may be unstable, causing visual distortion and instability.

▶ Cataract surgery: Posterior capsular opacity may develop postoperatively.

▶ Scleral buckle: Usually causes a myopic shift, can extrude over time, can cause double vision.

▶ Blepharoplasty/brow lift: Patient may still have residual ptosis, incomplete lid closure, or dry eye.

▶ Glaucoma filtering surgery: Bleb may scar down, drainage fields/shunts can extrude.

▶ Intraocular and intravitreal injections: May cause a retinal detachment, perforated globe, optic nerve damage, glaucoma, progression of a cataract. Any resulting infection may be as severe as endophthalmitis.

▶ Laser panretinal photocoagulation (PRP): May cause blind spots in vision due to retinal scar tissue.

General Medical History

It is important to collect a complete general medical history because many eye problems are directly related to medical conditions. It is also important to collect a medical history preoperatively (especially prior to anesthesia) for the evaluation of general health.

Review of Systems

A review of systems (ROS) gives a snapshot of the patient's current health. Many systemic diseases and medications can affect the eye. Some ophthalmic medications can have adverse effects in patients with systemic problems. An ROS looks at what the patient is experiencing currently or recently. Many offices have a written intake form asking the patient to provide information on his/her health history, as well as an ROS, which is then used as the starting point for the oral history.

There are 14 recognized body systems (see Appendix A). According to the American Academy of Ophthalmology, how many body systems are reviewed depends on the reason of the visit and the level of the examination to reflect coding compliance. Often, the presenting problem will direct the choice of which systems are reviewed.

Careful documentation of the ROS will help ensure your provider receives full payment for his/her services. There are three levels of documentation for the ROS that coincide with the billable level of service for the examination. The more extensive exams require documentation that more systems were reviewed. The levels of documentation for an ROS include:

▶ *Problem pertinent* is directly related to the problem(s) identified in the HPI. This level is often appropriate for a return check where the patient has no additional problems. Documentation of a review of at least one system (the eye) is needed to bill at this level.

▶ *Extended* includes the problem(s) that was/were identified in the HPI, as well as a limited number of other systems. This level may be appropriate for a return check of a patient experiencing problems or with multiple problems (eg, glaucoma and an adverse reaction to medication, plus diabetic retinopathy, plus Graves' disease). Documentation of a review of two to nine systems must be present to bill at this level.

▶ *Complete* is an evaluation of the patient as a whole, including the problems identified in the HPI. This is often appropriate when a patient is being seen for the first time or returning after an extended time. Documentation of a review of at least 10 of the 14 systems is required to bill at this level.

Ophthalmic personnel responsible for entering the patient information into the medical record should review the systems, listening for clues that could affect the diagnosis and treatment plan. The body systems, examples of questions, and ways each body system may relate to the eye are outlined in Table 7-2. A well-documented, complete ROS reports both the positive (conditions the patient has) and negative (conditions the patient denies having) responses.

TABLE 7-2		
REVIEW OF SYSTEMS		
System	**Possible Questions to Ask: Have You Recently Experienced Any of the Following?**	**Potential Ocular Relevance**
Allergic/ immunologic	Anaphylactic response (difficulty breathing, a choking feeling, swelling of tongue/throat, or hives/itching/flushed or pale skin) after exposure to some trigger. Inhaled: Pollen, dust, animals, molds, or symptoms of runny nose or watery eyes. Ingested: Nuts, eggs, shellfish, or medication. Contact: Latex, paper tape. Poor wound healing. Frequent pneumonia or bronchitis or infections. Fatigue, fever, malaise. Autoimmune disorders or immunodeficiency disorders.	Many allergic conditions and medications affect the eye. Medical exposure to an allergen such as latex or a sulfa drug should be avoided. Many immunodeficiency and autoimmune disorders have ocular effects.
Cardiovascular	Heart attack, heart disease, stroke, swelling of extremities, faintness on standing, loss of consciousness. High blood pressure. Chest pain, shortness of breath, rapid or fluttering heart rate. Intermittent leg pain during exercise or walking relieved by rest.	Heart disease and hypertension can have serious ocular consequences, including retinal artery or vein occlusions, ischemic attacks, and retinal hemorrhage.
Constitutional	Unexplained fever, chills, weight change, sleeping problems, tiredness, falling. Recent trauma or change in environment.	Unexplained constitutional issues may point to disorders such as diabetes or thyroid disease, which have ocular effects.
Ears, nose, throat, mouth, and head	Hearing loss, pain, discharge, or ringing in ears. Runny nose, nosebleeds, sinus infections or pain. Congestion, sneezing. Jaw pain, dental pain, gum disease, or bleeding gums. Dry mouth, mouth sores, sore throat, or pain on swallowing. Facial swelling, neck pain, neck stiffness.	Sinus infection or inflammation can cause eye discomfort. Jaw pain can be a serious symptom of temporal arteritis. Herpes simplex can cause cold sores, as well as affect the eyelids, conjunctiva, and cornea.
Endocrine	Thyroid: Excessively hot or cold. Weight gain and loss of energy or weight loss with increased appetite. Diabetes: Excessive thirst, dizziness, sweating. Frequent urination. Tingling or numbness in hands or feet. Adrenal: High blood pressure resisting treatment. Chronic low blood pressure. Weakness, dizziness, or blurred vision upon standing. Tanning of the skin without sun exposure. Reproductive problems.	Thyroid disease has many effects on the eye. Diabetes can cause vascular changes of the retina and iris. Steroid treatments for adrenal insufficiency may cause cataract and glaucoma.
Eyes	Eye pain. Vision that fluctuates, blurs, or doubles. Flashes, floaters, curtains or veils across vision, halos around lights, light sensitivity, loss of contrast, problems with night vision, or changes in colors. Transient loss of vision or areas of missing vision (blind spots or hemianopia).	Each element of an ocular history gives the physician diagnostic information.

(continued)

	TABLE 7-2 (CONTINUED)
	REVIEW OF SYSTEMS

System	Possible Questions to Ask: Have You Recently Experienced Any of the Following?	Potential Ocular Relevance
Gastrointestinal	Abdominal pain, nausea, vomiting, diarrhea, constipation. Bloating, cramping, excessive gas, anorexia, indigestion, gastro reflux, pain on swallowing (liquids or solids). Bright red blood from rectum or black tarry stools.	Many chronic bowel disorders are treated with steroids, which have several ocular effects. (Episcleritis, scleritis, and uveitis can be ocular manifestations of irritable bowel syndrome.)
Genitourinary	Pain or bleeding on urination or excessive urination. Problems with urinary incontinence, hesitancy, reduced stream, or waking often at night to urinate. Genital pain or discharge. Sexually transmitted diseases. Erectile dysfunction. Menstrual status/menopause. Pregnancy.	Reiter's syndrome presents with arthritis, conjunctivitis, and urethritis. Many sexually transmitted diseases can have ocular manifestations. Post-menopausal women are more likely to have dry eye syndrome. Medications for erectile dysfunction can have effects on vision. Some ophthalmic medications can diminish sexual function.
Hematologic/ lymphatic	Easy or prolonged bleeding. Easy bruising. Anemia, leukemia, sickle cell disease. Red/ purple spots and/or patches. Painless swelling of lymph nodes, fatigue, night sweats, fever, itching.	Many blood disorders have ocular manifestations. Cat scratch disease affects the lymphatic system and the eye.
Integumentary	Itching or burning. Excessive dryness. Rashes, eruptions, scaling, blisters, or hives. Acne. Trauma burns or wounds. New or changing moles. Bruises or bleeding under the skin. Albinism. Birthmarks, brown or tan spots, skin tags. Blueness, redness, jaundice, or white patches. Lumps under the skin or in the breasts. Changes in the shape, appearance, or growth of the fingernails. Thinning, dry, brittle, or coarse hair.	Many diseases affecting the skin have ocular manifestations. Some acne treatments can have serious effects on vision.
Musculoskeletal	Unexplained muscle pain, tremors, wasting, easy fatigability, or weakness. Morning stiffness, arthritis, joint swelling, or pain. Osteoporosis, spinal rigidity, or curving. Limited range of movement, joint dislocations, loss of dexterity.	Many forms of arthritis have ocular manifestations, including uveitis, dry eye syndrome, and conjunctivitis. Treatments for arthritis, including steroids and antimalarial drugs, may have serious ocular effects.
Neurological	Headaches or scalp pain. Lightheadedness. Balance or walking problems. Numbness, weakness, or tingling of the limbs or extremities. Changes of the senses of smell, taste, hearing, or vision. Seizures, tremors, twitching, dizziness, or fainting. Problems with speech, memory, concentration, or thinking.	Neurologic diseases with ocular manifestations include multiple sclerosis, brain tumors, migraine, idiopathic intracranial hypertension, Parkinson's disease, and nerve palsies. Pupil abnormalities and visual field changes are seen in many neurologic diseases. Treatments for seizure disorders can cause vision changes.
Psychiatric	Depression, loss of pleasure, anxiety, or worry. Excitability, irritability, obsessiveness. Changes in mood, performance, or hygiene. Loss of sleep or excessive sleeping. Paranoia, delusions, or hallucinations.	Many antidepressants and antipsychotic agents have ocular side effects. Some ophthalmic medications can have psychoactive effects or cause depression.
Respiratory	Pain on breathing, shortness of breath, choking, labored breathing on exertion, chest tightness. Coughing (dry or producing sputum or blood). Apnea, asthma, emphysema, or wheezing.	Drugs treating asthma may have ocular side effects. Lung cancers may metastasize to the eye. Some glaucoma medications may make breathing problems worse.

Medical Conditions

The patient's medical history, including any current medical diagnoses and any diagnostic testing that he/she has had recently (x-rays, magnetic resonance imaging [MRI], computed tomography [CT] scans, lab work, biopsies, pathology reports) can lead the eye care professional to determine the cause of or the relationship to ophthalmic manifestations. For example, rosacea, hormonal changes (pre- or post-menopausal), and Graves' disease can all cause dry eye syndrome.

Past Surgical History

It is important to know what kind of surgeries the patient has had because that can also impact eye health. For instance, a hysterectomy may cause hormonal changes that directly impact the ocular surface, causing dry eye. If the eye care provider does not know the patient's surgical history, then the ocular manifestations might not make sense and the mystery would not be solved.

Current Medications

A comprehensive list of systemic and ophthalmic prescription medications and over-the-counter medications and supplements should be listed along with the dosage of the medication and the frequency of use. Systemic medications may cause blurred vision, toxicity in the retina or cornea, dryness, redness and irritation, cataracts, or increased intraocular pressure. Over-the-counter medications may cause blurred vision, retinal damage, and cataract progression. An overdose of vitamins and supplements may cause blurred vision, double vision, retinal hemorrhages, or transient vision loss. Topical eye medications may also cause a systemic adverse reaction.

Allergies

Allergies to oral and topical medications, including ophthalmic medications, must be recorded. It is helpful to include what type of reaction occurs (rash, nausea, etc). Allergic reactions may include, but are not limited to, a rash, hives, swelling, itching, difficulty swallowing, difficulty breathing, nausea, vomiting, chest tightness, nasal congestion, diarrhea, and flushing of the face. The most severe allergic reaction is *anaphylaxis*, which is life-threatening. It can be triggered within minutes, and may include swelling of the tongue, lips, and roof of the mouth, causing difficulty breathing, dizziness, a drop in blood pressure, and headache. In many cases, however, the reaction is just sensitivity to the medication or one of its ingredients rather than a true allergy. In other instances, a reaction may be a side effect of the medication itself.

Social History

Sometimes you might feel awkward when you have to ask the patient about his/her social history, especially when it gets as personal as recreational drug use, or if he/she uses tobacco or alcohol. However, this information can have an impact on the patient's ocular health and on the potential outcome of certain disorders and/or treatments.

▶ Smoking and other tobacco products: How often/how much per day? Is there exposure to second-hand smoke? In clinics where providers are required to give cessation counseling, ask the patient if he/she is interested in quitting or has tried to quit before.

- Why ask? Cigarette smoking and using smokeless tobacco products affect the body in the same way. Both may increase the risk of developing age-related macular degeneration (ARMD), cataracts, glaucoma, diabetes, and dry eye syndrome. Dip and chew tobacco products can cause an increase in blood sugar levels, which may predispose the patient to diabetes and diabetic retinopathy.

▶ Alcohol use: How often? How much?

- Why ask? Alcohol may cause double vision, weakening of the eye muscles, blurred vision, optic neuropathy, and liver damage.

▶ Recreational drug use: What kind, and what route of administration? How long has the patient been using? How often? In clinics where providers are required to give cessation counseling, contact information on groups or organizations to help the patient get clean should be provided.

- Why ask? Recreational drug use may cause neurological damage, double vision, pupil irregularities, and strokes.

Family History

While acquiring a thorough family history may be important due to genetic predispositions, you do not need to spend time asking about all of the systemic and ocular conditions the patient's family might have had. Sidebar 7-2 lists some of the most common conditions that you should ask about. However, these may vary depending on the subspecialty of your eye care professional. At the end of the questioning, be sure to ask the patient if anything else should be added to the family history.

Decision-Making— Proceeding With the Exam

As you become familiar with the patient's history, you perform the function of a detective as well as determine your plan of action for the screening part of the exam (if, indeed, you are the one who will conduct said screening). Reviewing the patient's ROS gives a good idea of the patient's general health. Going through the ophthalmic history narrows down the search for how his/her health problems may be eye related and vice versa. Compiling this information navigates the exam to the next level.

When taking a history, use critical thinking to determine which part of the eye the doctor will likely be examining in the most detail. Determine what testing needs to be done in order to provide the practitioner with the most

---

SIDEBAR 7-2
FAMILY HISTORY

Systemic Disease
- ▶ Diabetes
- ▶ Hypertension
- ▶ Cancer
- ▶ Stroke
- ▶ Heart disease
- ▶ Thyroid disease

Ocular Disease
- ▶ Cataracts
- ▶ Glaucoma
- ▶ Macular degeneration
- ▶ Retinal detachment
- ▶ Blindness
- ▶ Strabismus
- ▶ Amblyopia
- ▶ Significant refractive errors

---

vital information. Then consider what is necessary for the doctor to perform a thorough exam, and make your decision whether or not you need to dilate.

The type of visit that the patient is coming in for will reflect how much information you know and how much is to be collected.

▶ New patient: Ask him/her how long it has been since he/she had an eye exam, and where was the last eye exam. Ask if the last practitioner saw anything he/she was concerned about. Ask if he/she is OK with having medical records transferred to this clinic, and then have the new patient sign a release of information form. Be sure to take a complete ophthalmic and medical history. Accurately record the medications that he/she is taking and go over surgical, family, and social history in detail.

▶ Established patient: Look through the patient's last exam notes; ask if he/she has seen any other eye care professional since the last exam. Find out if this is a follow-up visit at the doctor's request or if the patient is coming in with a new problem. Look through the last treatment plan to get a good lead on the exam. If the doctor has previously prescribed an ophthalmic medication, make sure to address the use, compliance, and tolerance of the medication.

▶ Referred patient: Check to see if a referral letter has been sent, or chart notes that have been received from a referring provider. Ask the patient what he/she is being referred for. At the end of the exam, the provider needs to correspond with the referring physician to share the outcome of the visit and the treatment plan.

▶ Follow-up: Be sure to read the treatment plan so that you know what needs to be done at this visit. If the provider has requested the patient to perform warm compresses and eyelid scrubs, or has asked the patient to start a medication, make sure to note if the patient has followed through with the instructions and indicate compliance.

▶ Postoperative: Patients are asked to assess their overall vision and comfort level. Postoperative medications and compliance are documented.

▶ Contact lens wearer: A detailed history about contact lens wear is obtained. Contact lens brand, prescription, and parameters are recorded. The average daily wear time, if the patient sleeps with the contact lenses in (and if so, how frequently), and replacement schedule is noted. Contact lens solutions and rewetting drops are listed. The patient is asked about the comfort of lenses and if he/she is having any problems with vision.

▶ Pediatric history: Congenital disease, growth and development, strabismus, and social issues of being "different" may be addressed. Expand on the history questions depending on the reason for visit:

- Congenital disease: Ask if there is a family history of any significant eye disease: blindness, amblyopia (lazy eye), strabismus (eye misalignments), congenital cataracts or glaucoma, or refractive error.

- Medical conditions: Ask if the patient has any medical conditions or had illnesses or hospitalizations. Some medical conditions may predispose a specific eye condition. Some medical conditions to ask about: arthritis, asthma, bowel issues, cancer, diabetes, ear-nose-throat issues, attention deficit hyperactivity disorder (ADHD), ear infections, headaches, ear issues, neurological problems, skin issues, or thyroid problems.

- Prematurity: Ask about birth history: at how many weeks was the baby born, current age, birth weight, delivery method (vaginal/C-section/forceps), and any complications during pregnancy or delivery. Ask about complications after delivery, if the baby was on oxygen after birth and, if so, for how long.

- Growth and development: Ask if the infant is achieving developmental milestones at an average rate: smiling at about 2 months, rolling over at 4 to 5 months, sitting at 6 months, walking at 12 months, talking between 2 and 3 years of age. Developmental delay may indicate that the patient is having an eye problem. For school-aged children, ask about grades, if there are any struggles with specific subjects, or if there has been a significant change in grades. This may indicate strabismus or a refractive error.

- Strabismus: If there is any concern about strabismus ("crossed eyes") or amblyopia ("lazy eye"), ask the parent which eye crosses/wanders and in what direction (in, out, etc) and is it constant or intermittent? If intermittent, when does it happen (eg, when the child is tired)? Family history is especially important in strabismus cases.

- Amblyopia: Ask if the patient was given a glasses prescription, if it was filled, and if the child wears them. Are the glasses worn full time? Ask if the patient was told to patch one eye, which eye is being patched, and for how many hours a day. Find out if the child is compliant with patching, and what kinds of activities are done during patching.

- Refractive error: Ask if the patient is having problems with distance or near vision, and if the vision in one eye is worse than the other. Ask about family history of refractive errors, as this can be genetic.

A very common CC in pediatric patients is that they have failed a vision screening. They might have failed the screening in school or during their annual pediatric well exam. A failed vision screening may sometimes be due to a lack of cooperation, testing error, or due to refractive error, amblyopia, or an eye disease that limits their visual acuity. In cases like these, family history is important, for it can help to solve some mysteries.

Depending on the child's age and intelligence, try to get as much information directly from the child as possible. If there is something the patient cannot answer, refer to the accompanying parent or guardian. (Note: If the patient is an underage adolescent or young adult and comes into the exam room alone, confidentiality applies. Consult HIPAA guidelines for a review on what information may be shared with the parent or guardian, and what must be excluded under the privacy rule. This depends in part on whether or not the patient is deemed "mature," is emancipated, or is a parent.)

PATIENT SERVICES

Escorting Patients With Special Needs

▶ Wheelchair bound: Ask the patient if he/she is capable of transferring to the exam chair. It is preferred that patients who are wheelchair bound are assisted by a caregiver or a significant other. Offer to assist

the patient if need be ("Need a push?"); however, some patients are very independent, and that should be respected.

▶ Low vision/blind: Offer an elbow to assist them while you walk them to the exam room. It is okay if the patient would like to walk on his/her own, following your voice; some patients are very independent and do not want to feel handicapped by loss of vision. If the patient has a service dog, just escort the dog as you would a sighted patient. Do not grab the dog's halter (or pet the dog, for that matter). As a side note, many clinics require patients to bring a certificate from an accredited program to prove that they are indeed in medical need of the service animal, before they are allowed to be taken back for an exam. There is a difference between a therapy animal and a service animal. Be aware of HIPAA regulations; you may not ask the patient the nature of his/her disability, but you may ask what service the animal provides. Such questioning should still be done in private.

▶ Patient is accompanied: Make sure the patient has verbally consented for the other person to be in the exam room.

CHAPTER QUIZ

1. What is the difference between PHI and PII?

2. Which is *not* an element of PII?
    a. first and last name
    b. date of birth
    c. diagnosis
    d. address

3. According to the HIPAA guidelines, PHI and PII may be accessed for all of the following reasons *except*:
    a. to consult with a physician or a technician about patient care
    b. for transferring information for diagnostic imaging
    c. for registration, check-in, and insurance verification
    d. curiosity about the patient's medical condition

4. What kind of a form needs to be signed by the patient in order to authorize PHI to be released to or from a different clinic?
    a. PHI
    b. ROI
    c. ROS
    d. PII

5. Which of the following is *not* considered a symptom?

    a. lid droop
    b. loss of vision
    c. elevated intraocular pressure
    d. swelling

6. Which of the following is a symptom?

    a. tingling sensation
    b. enlarged blind spot
    c. incomplete blink
    d. corneal scarring

7. What kind of a nonverbal cue are you using when you say the following to a patient: "Hmm, tell me more about your headaches."

    a. acknowledgment
    b. validating patient concerns
    c. leading questions
    d. facilitative interjections

8. Which of the following is *not* part of the AIDET model of patient satisfaction?

    a. introduction
    b. duration
    c. education
    d. thank you

9. Inquiring about the patient's recent systemic health is done in what part of the history?

    a. history of present illness
    b. review of systems
    c. past medical history
    d. past surgical history

10. When dealing with talkative patients, what is the best type of question to use?

    a. confronting questions
    b. direct questions
    c. indirect questions
    d. laundry list

11. When taking an "extended" history of present illness, what is the *minimum* number of questions (as related to FOLDARS) you should ask?

    a. 2
    b. 4
    c. 6
    d. 8

12. In order to bill for an "extended" level of service, how many body systems should be reviewed in the review of systems?

    a. 1
    b. 7
    c. 10
    d. 14

13. Asking the patient if he/she uses tobacco or alcohol is done in what part of the history?

    a. history of present illness
    b. review of systems
    c. past medical history
    d. social history

14. What part of the FOLDARS component covers the following phrase the best: "My vision gets blurred when the blood sugar levels are high"?

    a. frequency
    b. onset
    c. associated signs and symptoms
    d. severity

15. Which of the following is *not* considered an allergy?

    a. hives
    b. swelling
    c. difficulty breathing
    d. upset stomach

16. Do you have to do a separate FOLDARS for each complaint?

    a. yes
    b. no

Answers

1. PHI, Protected health information is any health information in the patient's record. This includes the patient's medical and ocular history, the examination, assessment, and treatment plan. All of this information is protected under the HIPAA guidelines and may not be shared. PII: Personally identifiable information is any information that may distinguish a patient's identity including his/her full name, home address, driver's license number, credit card number, date of birth, and phone number.

2. c, PII does not include any diagnoses (eg, a particular patient could not be identified simply by the word "cataracts").

3. d, Mere curiosity does not meet the "need to know" criteria required for accessing a patient's information.

4. b, ROI, release of information, must be signed before any private patient information may be shared.

5. c, A patient's intraocular pressure is a sign; the rest are symptoms.

6. a, Tingling is a symptom; the rest are signs.

7. d, Facilitative interjections are words or phrases that motivate the patient to keep going with his/her history. (Acknowledgment refers to sensing the patient's emotional state and addressing it. Validating patient concerns will create empathy with the patient. Leading questions are questions that may direct the patient to respond in a specific way; those questions should be avoided.)

8. c, Education is a component that is covered in the patient's chart. For instance, "The patient was educated on how to do eyelid scrubs," or "Information was given to the patient regarding cataracts." This is not part of the AIDET model.

9. b, The review of systems should include recent systemic symptoms the patient is experiencing. (The history of present illness describes the patient's symptoms. Past medical and surgical information is a "history" of what has happened in the past.)

10. b, Direct questions help steer them on topic. Those patients usually like to travel off to a different topic in a short period of time. (Indirect questions are used for patients who are more sensitive about the exam. Confronting questions are used if the patient is not responding well to indirect questions. Laundry list questions help guide the patient if he/she is not sure exactly what you are trying to ask.)

11. b, For an "extended" history, four to eight of these elements must be addressed to properly document the HPI. (For a "brief" history, one to three elements must be addressed in the HPI.)

12. b, For an extended level, two to nine body systems should be reviewed. (For a problem pertinent exam, at least one body system should be reviewed. For a complete evaluation, 10 to 14 systems need to be reviewed.)

13. d, Social history involves tobacco, alcohol, and recreational drug use, as well as social support networks.

14. c, Associated signs and symptoms. There is an association between health changes (blood sugar level spikes) and visual symptoms.

15. d, An upset stomach is intolerance or sensitivity to a medication, not a true allergic/immunologic response.

16. a, For example, if a patient complains of both pain and halos around lights, depending on the extent of the history, you must address 1 to 8 of the FOLDARS elements for each complaint.

REFERENCE

1. Sharp HealthCare. AIDET: five steps to achieving satisfaction. Sharp HealthCare, San Diego Hospitals and Medical Groups website. www.sharp.com/about/the-sharp-experience/aidet.cfm. Accessed June 19, 2017.

BIBLIOGRAPHY

Gallimore G. Dr. Watson's guide to history taking. Eyetec.net website. www.ophthalmictechnician.org/index.php/courses/ophthalmic-assistant-basic-training-course/138-history-taking. Accessed July 4, 2016.

Ledford JK. *The Complete Guide to Ocular History Taking.* Thorofare, NJ: SLACK Incorporated; 1999.

Marks ES, Adamczyk DT, Thomann KH. *Primary Eye Care in Systemic Disease.* Norwalk, CT: Appleton & Lange; 1995.

Moore KJ. Documenting history in compliance with Medicare's guidelines. *Fam Pract Manag.* 2010;17(2):22-27. Family Practice Management website. www.aafp.org/fpm/2010/0300/p22.html. Accessed July 4, 2016.

Ophthalmic Medical Assisting: An Independent Study Course. 5th ed. San Francisco, CA: American Academy of Ophthalmology; 2012.

Review of systems "cheat sheet." Indiana University School of Medicine, Terra Haute campus website. http://terrehaute.medicine.iu.edu/files/8113/4487/0619/Review_of_Systems_Cheat_Sheet.pdf. Accessed July 4, 2016.

Thompson J. A practical guide to clinical medicine. University of California, San Diego website. http://meded.ucsd.edu/clinicalmed/ros.htm. Accessed July 4, 2016.

Trobe JD. *The Physicians Guide to Eye Care.* 2nd ed. San Francisco, CA: The Foundation of the American Academy of Ophthalmology; 1983.

Urban American Indian Tobacco Prevention and Education Network. Diabetes and tobacco use. NARA Northwest website. www.nara-northwest.org/diabetes%20and%20tobacco.pdf. Accessed July 4, 2016.

Wren VQ. Ocular and visual side effects of systemic drugs. *Journal of Behavioral Optometry.* 2000;11(6). www.oepf.org/sites/default/files/journals/jbo-volume-11-issue-6/11-6%20Valeriewren.pdf. Accessed July 4, 2016.

8

VISION TESTING

Jan Ledford, COMT

Testing visual acuity is much more than having the patient read the eye chart. Not only must you accurately record the results, you must properly select the type of test, the test distance, the type of occlusion used, even which eye to test first.

BASIC SCIENCES

Knowledge of ocular anatomy and physiology is important in understanding how we see. Please review Chapters 2 and 3 as needed. Understanding characteristics of light is also helpful (see Chapter 4).

CLINICAL KNOWLEDGE

Fixation

Because the macula is the retinal area responsible for fine, central vision, visual acuity is essentially a test of macular function (ie, as a part of the visual pathway). Ideally, each eye is situated in the head so that the macula is "pointed" at whatever we are looking at (the *object of regard*). For example, if you are looking at the symbol

$$\Delta$$

then the Δ is the object of regard, and you are able to hold your eye steady so its image continues to fall on your macula. This is called *fixation*. (There is more on fixation elsewhere in this text, especially Chapter 10, but it bears mentioning here as well.)

When we check visual acuity, the assumption is that the patient is fixating on the test object with the macula/fovea. In some cases, however, the patient has learned to fixate with a retinal area other than the macula. This is called *eccentric fixation*, and it is likely to develop in a patient whose macula is deficient. Visual acuity in an eye with eccentric fixation is always subnormal because no other area of the retina has the high concentration of cone cells as the macula. Eccentric fixation is common in the later stages of macular degeneration.

Fixation is also very important in testing infants and small children, where the best acuity "measurement" you can get might be whether or not the patient seems to be looking directly at the object of regard (like a fun, noiseless toy) vs consistently looking somewhere else, or if the eyes exhibit "searching" movements as if trying to find something to lock onto. (More on checking young children later.)

The eyes of a patient with nystagmus ("dancing" or jerking eyes) are constantly in motion, so the image of the object of regard is constantly being swept over the macula (or possibly an eccentric fixation point). This will cause blurred vision because fixation is not steady. More later on how to best evaluate vision in these patients.

Ledford JK, Lens A, eds.
Principles and Practice in Ophthalmic Assisting:
A Comprehensive Textbook (pp 93-116).
© 2018 Taylor & Francis Group.

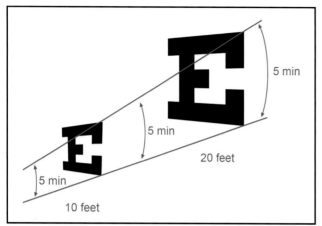

Figure 8-1. Light emanates from an object and converges, creating an angle.

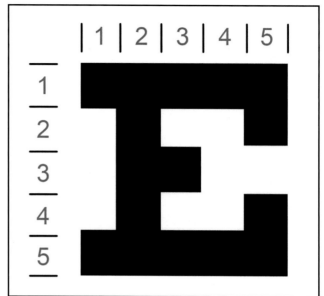

Figure 8-2. Snellen letters are made up of five parts, each subtending 1 minute of arc.

Testing Distance

Light coming from any object is considered to diverge from the object into space. (The physics of light is reviewed in Chapter 4.) Divergent light stimulates the eye to accommodate, which briefly means that the crystalline lens inside the eye tries to focus the incoming light. This changes the refractive power of the eye. When performing refractometry or testing visual acuity, accommodation can get in the way.

Once an object is 20 feet or more away (6 meters, if you are using the metric system), the amount of divergence has become so miniscule that the rays are now considered to be parallel. This means they can be disregarded as a cause of accommodation. For this reason, the standard testing distance for visual acuity is 20 feet (6 meters).

Visual acuity is generally expressed as a fraction, such as 20/20, 20/70, 20/400 (6/6, 6/21, 6/120 in metric), etc. The numerator represents the test distance, which is usually 20 feet. The denominator is the actual measure of the person's vision. We will discuss the eye chart itself in a moment, but for now think about the standard chart with letters that are large on the top and gradually get smaller as you go down. The "20/20" line is considered "normal vision," meaning that from 20 feet away the average and healthy eye can correctly identify this row of letters.

If a person has 20/70 vision, this means that at the 20-foot standard test distance, this person can only identify letters that the normal person can see from 70 feet away. The person with 20/70 vision must move closer, to 20 feet, before being able to correctly identify that line.

So, the larger that bottom number, the worse the patient's vision. Someone who has 20/400 vision must be at the 20-foot test distance before being able to see the "big E," which the normal eye can see from 400 feet away.

Occasionally we must alter the test distance. How to do this, and properly document it, will be covered later.

Angles and Arc

An *angle* is created by the meeting of two rays. The point where they meet is the *vertex*. Angles are measured in degrees. A full circle is 360 degrees. One degree is made up of 60 minutes of arc. To say that an object "subtends XX minutes of arc" means that the rays emanating from an object of a specific size and a specific distance away eventually converge to a specific point, creating a specific angle (Figure 8-1). (In its easiest form, think of the rays coming from the top and bottom [or extremities] of the object.) When we are studying vision, the eye is the "vertex" where the rays converge.

A person with 20/20 vision can just distinguish an object that subtends 5 minutes of arc. So when Snellen developed his eye chart, he designed calibrated letters that were independent of typefaces, so they could be reproduced.[1] His letters are based on 5 minutes of arc and are constructed so that each *part* of the letter subtends 1 minute. Each letter is thus considered to be 5 X 5 (Figure 8-2). One minute of arc is the amount of angle where a normal eye can detect the separation of two points. Not surprisingly, this corresponds to the arrangement and number of cone cells in the macula.[2]

Visual Acuity

Visual acuity is just one component of visual function, and is based on three phenomena: detection, recognition (identification), and resolution.[3] *Detection* is the ability to tell that something is there, which becomes more and more difficult with decreased contrast and size. *Recognition* involves correctly identifying familiar objects/optotypes of decreasing size because small details are visible. (*Optotypes* are simply the symbols, graduated in size, which the patient identifies when we check visual acuity. There are many to choose from; more on this shortly.) Resolution refers to being able to identify smaller and smaller gaps in or orientation of a single optotype or pattern. Tests based on recognition and resolution are generally considered to be interchangeable, but there are differences.

Recognition-Type Tests

The most important factor in selecting an appropriate recognition optotype for a particular patient is that the patient *must* be able to consistently identify the optotype selected.

Letters are the most commonly used optotype. Snellen acuity, developed in 1862, is generally accepted as the clinical standard (Figure 8-3). However, just because a person is illiterate or intellectually impaired does *not* necessarily mean that he/she cannot identify letters…it just means that he/she cannot read. And just because a 4-year-old child "knows his/her A-B-C's" does not mean he/she can recognize them when he/she sees them. If there is any doubt in your mind whether or not a patient will be able to use the letter optotypes, show some of the largest letters on the chart and ask the patient what they are. (No coaching from parents: "Violet, what letter does your name start with?") There are charts that use only the letters HOTV, as these letters are symmetrical (ie, same on left and right) and easy to recognize.

Testing with the standard Snellen chart uses line assignment. But some lines have more letters than others, which is a problem. The 20/100 line often has only two letters. But the 20/20 line probably has five to eight letters. So missing one letter on the 20/100 line has much more bearing than missing one letter on the 20/20 line. Also, many Snellen charts go directly from 20/400 to 20/200. But the patient's vision might actually be 20/300. And finally (for this discussion, anyway), there is the matter of saying that a person has had a "one-line change in visual acuity." There's a lot of difference in the one line between 20/400 and 20/200 and the one line between 20/70 and 20/60. There is no standardization as to what font, which letters, or spacing between letters and rows is used, so charts vary from one manufacturer to another. But, while the system is not perfect, it remains the standard in common clinical use.

Louise Sloan developed a new system in 1952 using the letters C, D, H, K, N, O, R, S, V, and Z.[4] The space between optotypes on any one line is the same size of the optotypes themselves on that particular line. In addition, the space between each line is the same size as the optotypes on the next line down. Thus, the chart looks like an inverted pyramid (Figure 8-4). Sloan letters are more standardized than the Snellen chart.

The Early Treatment Diabetic Retinopathy Study (ETDRS) chart was developed in 1982 by combining the features of several other acuity tests.[1] Notably, each line

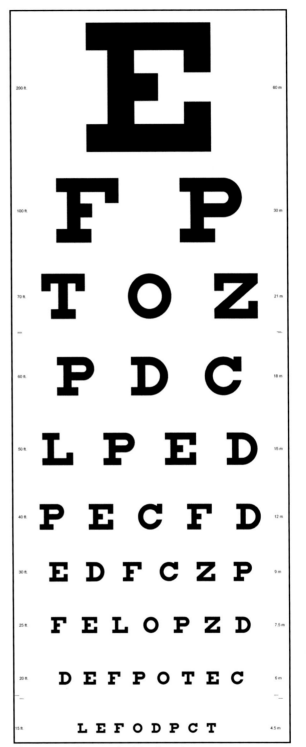

Figure 8-3. The standard Snellen chart.

has the same number of optotypes (5). The chart is set up as an inverted pyramid, similar to the Sloan chart (Figure 8-5). ETDRS has become the preferred system when working with low vision patients, as well as for research, clinical trials, and population studies, because it is more repeatable. For the average clinic, however, many consider the ETDRS chart to be too time-consuming.

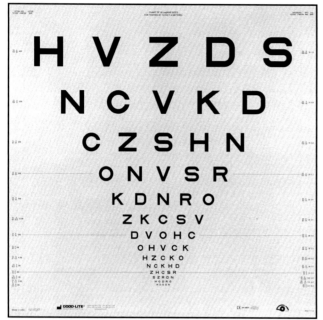

Figure 8-4. Sloan chart (Good-Lite Company).

Numbers are another form of recognition optotype. Many illiterate adults can identify numbers. However, this test is limited to nine possible objects, making it easier to guess; letters are preferred, if the patient is able to name them. *Lea numbers* (using the numbers 5, 6, 8, and 9) blur into nondescript shapes once the patient has passed the limits of his/her recognition ability (Figure 8-6).

Allen pictures use objects that are almost universally recognized, especially by children (Figure 8-7). These can include items such as a hand, truck, horse, etc. Prior to using these, make sure that the patient can consistently identify each picture. It does not matter if he/she calls the horse a "doggy" as long as he/she does it every time. The pictures may be on a wall or hand chart, projector slide, or individual cards. If cards are used, be sure that you know the testing distance for which the cards are calibrated. (More on this later.)

Lea symbols are another set of optotypes useful with children (Figure 8-8). There are only four objects (square, circle, house, and apple), but all four symbols appear to be blurry circles beyond the patient's acuity threshold.

Resolution-Type Tests

Related to the letter chart is *Tumbling E's* or the *E game*. The patient does not have to know that the letter is an "E" in order to tell whether or not the optotype is pointing left, right, up, or down (Figure 8-9). A variation of this test is the Blackbird chart, which uses a stylized "bird" instead of an E.

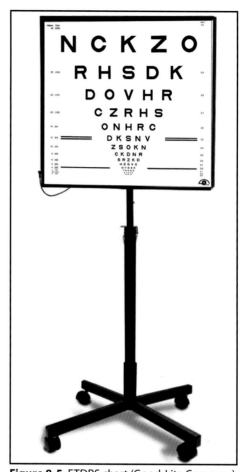

Figure 8-5. ETDRS chart (Good-Lite Company).

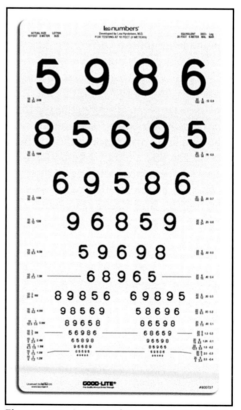

Figure 8-6. Lea numbers chart (Good-Lite Company).

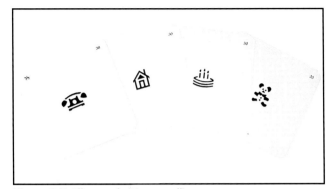

Figure 8-7. Allen cards (Honeywell).

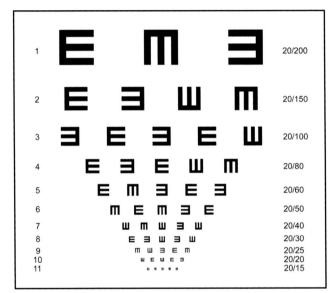

Figure 8-9. Tumbling E chart (Good-Lite Company).

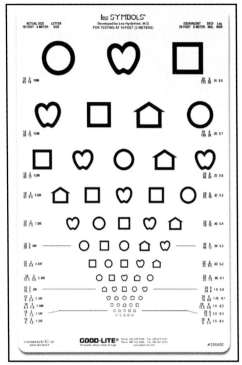

Figure 8-8. Lea symbols chart (Good-Lite Company).

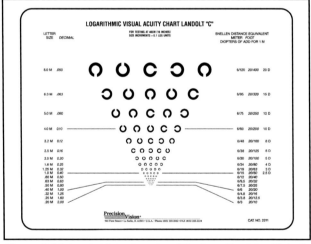

Figure 8-10. Landolt's broken rings/C's chart (Precision Vision).

The optotype in *Landolt's broken rings* or *C's* is a circle with a gap in it. The gap may be positioned right, left, up, or down (Figure 8-10). The rings (and gaps) get progressively smaller.

Testing Systems

Just as there are different optotypes available, there are also numerous systems for displaying them. The how-to's will be covered shortly.

Distance Acuity Systems

For distance acuity, the standard 20-foot test distance must be maintained. If using a poster-style eye chart, you must measure carefully so that the patient's face (not the chair base!) will be 20 feet from the chart. (Note: Low vision evaluation is generally conducted at 10 feet.)

However, not all exam lanes are 20+ feet long. In this case, a projector system or special wall chart (the letters are backward) with mirrors can be used to "bounce" the projected chart back and forth to create an equivalent of 20 feet. (An adjustment of the projector's magnification may also be required to get the optotypes to scale.) For the best optical clarity, the mirrors should be front surface mirrors, which have the silver coating on the front of the glass instead of behind it. A screen is also part of the mirror-system set-up; it has a special nondepolarizing surface that reduces glare.

Manual projectors contain slides that may be changed. Remote-controlled projectors usually have a variety of optotypes built in. Both styles have masks that cover all but a vertical row, or a horizontal row, or a single optotype.

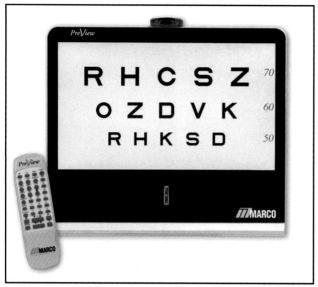

Figure 8-11. Computer-based visual acuity system (Marco).

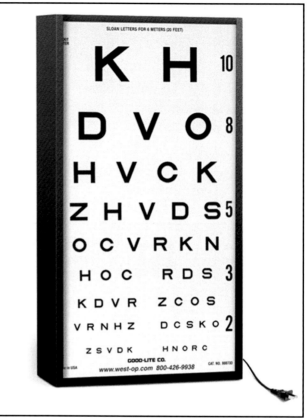

Figure 8-12. Back-lit box chart (Good-Lite Company).

Computer-based systems are now available (Figure 8-11). Features vary from one model to the next, but generally include a wide selection of optotypes and tests. Optotypes can be randomized to prevent memorization, and a moveable pointer means you can indicate a particular figure without isolating it. (Showing single optotypes may not give a true measurement of acuity in amblyopia due to the *crowding phenomenon*; that is, the patient sees smaller letters if he/she is shown one at a time vs a whole [crowded] row.) Video capabilities offer animated fixation loops for evaluating children. Some units have software that provides the ability to adjust to the length of your lane.

Back-lit box-style charts are convenient because they can generally be moved (Figure 8-12). It would probably be helpful to use some type of tape to mark off 5-foot increments on the floor so that you can document the testing distance. (Measure from the patient's position. More later on how to recalculate visual acuity when the testing distance is *not* 20 feet.) The back-lit chart is frequently the ETDRS type used in low vision clinics.

Cards with a single optotype on each can be hand held by the examiner. If the patient is a child and you are using Allen pictures, show the cards up close and make sure that the patient can identify each one. Hold the cards by the edges to avoid soiling. These cards are usually calibrated for a 30-foot test distance, not 20 (it will tell you on the card set). The patient's acuity is the farthest distance from which the pictures can consistently be identified correctly. In addition, the examiner may hold several cards together at once to avoid the crowding phenomenon. Some cards have a row of E's on each card. Be sure to check instructions for use and testing distance.

Another style of card is the single E, which can be used like the Allen cards, changing the orientation of the E (this is a variation of the Tumbling E) as one moves back.

Most everyone is familiar with the "vision machine" used at the driver's license office. There are numerous companies that make these instruments, which simulate a 20-foot testing distance. One disadvantage of checking distance vision with these is that the patient knows that the image is not really 20 feet away and may accommodate.

Near Acuity Systems

Evaluating a patient's vision for near activities is most commonly done with a hand-held card showing optotypes in decreasing size, much like the distance vision chart. An appropriate optotype is selected based on each patient; text, random letters, numbers, E's, pictures, and Landolt C's are available. ETDRS and contrast sensitivity (covered later) charts are also made for near testing.

The Rosenbaum pocket screener is a commonly used near card (Figure 8-13). This reading card offers numbers, tumbling E's, and X's and O's, along with several different result equivalents: point, Jaeger, and distance equivalent.

The *point* system is based on the size of print. It was originally developed to designate the size of the metal "stamp" used to impress a letter onto paper. A 1-inch

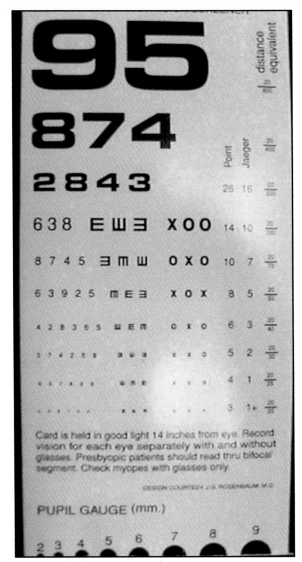

Figure 8-13. Rosenbaum pocket screener.

---

illuminated tablet-style devices, fan-style (where "cards" are joined by a brad in a bottom corner and can be fanned out), and three- or four-sided rotating boxes with different charts on each side.

CLINICAL SKILLS

Standard Visual Acuity Testing

Evaluation of visual acuity is often the first test performed once the history is done. There are some things to be aware of, however, as you plan a particular patient's exam.

If the patient needs detailed extraocular muscle evaluation (especially children), it is important to remember that covering one eye breaks fusion. Thus, stereo testing and other binocular tests should be performed first. This is covered in Chapter 10.

Any test that involves instillation of eye drops (including dilation) and/or physical contact with the eye should be avoided prior to testing vision. An exception to this would be if the patient has had a chemical splash, in which case irrigation should be immediate if it has not already been done in the field.

The first thing to determine prior to performing any test is the purpose of the test. This may seem obvious at first thought, but something as simple as "reading the eye chart" may have important implications (Sidebar 8-1). For example, in testing children, the main purpose may not be to get an exact acuity (although it is ideal if you can do so), but rather to help detect amblyopia (usually defined as a difference of two chart lines in acuity between the eyes, or a distance difference of 5 feet if using Allen cards). So with kids, work rapidly in order to avoid fatigue and loss of interest.

The second step is to select the appropriate optotype and test. This has been discussed previously and is summarized in Table 8-1. (Situations where a child or adult cannot see the optotypes is covered later in the section Beyond Optotypes.)

metallic stamp is designated as 72 point (pt). Note that the printed letter itself is not 1 inch, however, and different fonts in the same point size might not actually be the same size. While that method of printing is going out of use, the point system remains.

The *Jaeger* system was created for near testing. It was originally printed at the State Printing House in Vienna, so it was not reproducible as a standard because different publishers had different typefaces. Even today, the same size print might be labeled as J4, J7, or J10 on different cards.[1]

The *distance equivalent* listed on a near card is merely a conversion of the near acuity to the commonly used "20/20" nomenclature for convenience's sake. (It does *not* indicate a patient's *distance* vision!)

Other near testing modalities include rotating charts (where a wheel is turned to display a specific chart through a "window") and hand-held testers, including

TABLE 8-1
SELECTION OF OPTOTYPE AND VISUAL ACUITY TEST

Patient Characteristic	Suggested Optotype/Test
Infant/preverbal	► Reaction(s) to light, "threatening" stimuli ► Fix ► Follow ► Maintain ► Forced preferential looking ► Optokinetic response
Preschooler/young child	► Letters if possible ► Numbers if possible ► E game/Landolt rings if possible ► Allen pictures ► Stereo fly
Older child/adult	► Letters
Illiterate	► Letters if possible ► Numbers if possible ► E game/Landolt rings

Once the test is selected, make sure that the patient is the appropriate distance from the chart. For distance acuity, this is usually 20 feet (6 meters), as noted earlier. However, some poster-style wall charts are calibrated at 10 feet instead of 20 feet. Projector systems usually come with a template to calibrate the letter size appropriately. This should be checked every so often to make sure that the 20-foot size is maintained. Also, the smallest optotypes on the Allen cards are 20/30, so the *denominator* when using this test is always 30. (That is because the size of the optotypes does not change; you artificially change their "size" by moving closer or farther away. See Sidebar 8-6, later in this chapter.)

Clinic protocol will generally dictate whether you check the patient's vision with or without correction, or both. We usually want to know how well the patient sees with his/her current correction, if worn. If the patient wears multifocals for only one task (reading or driving), check vision both with and without correction. A patient having problems of any kind with new glasses should obviously be tested with the glasses in question. If the patient with a glasses recheck appointment says he/she sees better without the glasses than with, check uncorrected vision as well. Some employers, organizations, and licensing bureaus may require both uncorrected and best-corrected vision on their forms.

If the patient has glasses, make sure you understand what they are for. For example, if a presbyopic patient's single vision glasses are for reading only and you have him/her wear them for checking distance visual acuity, you will get an erroneous measurement. If the lenses do not have a visible segment, you must know if they are

worn for distance, near, or both. If for near, where is the focal point set? If you try to check near acuity at 16 inches, and the glasses are set to focus on a computer screen 24 inches away, your measurement will not be accurate. And remember, a lens that has no visible segment could be a "no-line" (progressive addition) multifocal (see Chapter 20).

Just because a patient is wearing segmented lenses does not mean that the top is set for 20 feet and the bottom for 16 inches. These could be vocational glasses where the top focuses on a workbench at 36 inches and the bottom at 14 inches.

None of these errors is catastrophic. When a patient's corrected acuity is not what you expect and the pinhole vision (discussed in a moment) shows a marked improvement, just take a look at the lens prescription and design, and/or ask the patient.

By convention, we usually check the right eye first. But there are cases where this is not appropriate. If one eye has been injured, check the vision in that eye first, especially on return visits, as long as treatment lasts. In a child who is being treated for amblyopia, always check the amblyopic eye first.

There may be circumstances where neither eye is occluded. This may be especially important in evaluating patients with monovision (one eye for near and one for distance), to give a more accurate idea of what the patient is seeing in "real life." In addition, some practitioners want near vision checked with both eyes together (Figure 8-14). Some driver's license and other forms also require binocular visual acuity.

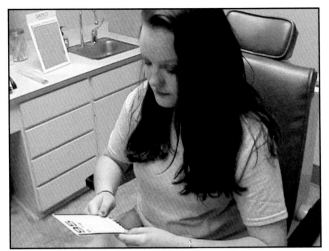

Figure 8-14. Checking vision at near with pocket screener, using both eyes.

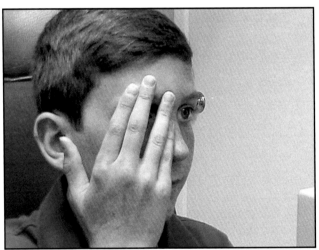

Figure 8-15. If the patient uses his own hand as an occluder, peeking might be too tempting.

Occlusion of the untested eye must be complete and maintained (Sidebar 8-2). It is generally best not to have the patient cover an eye with his/her own hand (Figure 8-15). If the patient's hand must be used, have him/her use the palm. There are several styles of occluders (paddle, mask, etc; Figure 8-16), or patches may be used (pirate patch, adhesive patch, clip-on patch for glasses). If a stick-on occlusion patch is used (especially with children), apply it very lightly. Whatever the method, just make sure that the eye is covered completely and stays that way during the test.

Patients with nystagmus (rhythmic jerking of the eyes) sometimes find that the jerking becomes more intense if one eye is covered.[5] Fog the eye instead of occluding it, by using a strong plus-powered trial lens (+5.00 is fine, held over the patient's glasses if worn). Another option is to have the patient wear the Worth 4 dot glasses (over prescription glasses, if worn), with the

---

SIDEBAR 8-2
DO IT BETTER: OCCLUSION

► If the patient is a child, let him/her see and touch the occluder first. "This looks sort of like an ice cream spoon, doesn't it?"

► If a child is intimidated by the occluder, have him/her cover the eye with his/her own hand, and have the caregiver put his/her palm over the child's hand.

► If the patient is using his/her hand to cover the eye, tell him/her to "cover the eye with your palm." This will help avoid peeking between fingers.

► A patient with a possible infection should probably cover the eye with the palm rather than touching an occluder.

► Sanitize the occluder between every patient.

► Because we cover one eye, checking vision is a dissociative test. Perform extraocular muscle testing first.

► In a patient with nystagmus, use a strong plus sphere trial lens (+5) over the untested eye instead of an opaque occluder.

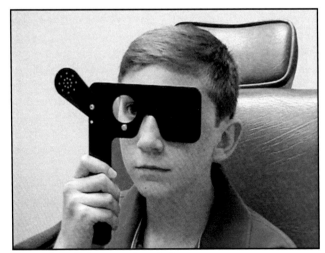

Figure 8-16. Using a mask occluder.

red lens over the eye to be tested. No occlusion is needed. Put up a strip of letters with the red/green duochrome pulled across them and have the patient read the letters. The visual acuity equals the smallest optotype correctly identified *only on the red side* of the chart. (The eye looking through the red lens will see both sides of the chart; the eye with the green lens will see only the green side.) To test the other eye, reverse the Worth 4 dot glasses.

In most cases, you want the patient facing straight ahead (*primary position*) when checking visual acuity, but there are a few exceptions (Sidebar 8-3).

102   Chapter 8

SIDEBAR 8-3
HEAD POSITION WHEN CHECKING VISUAL ACUITY

Normally, the patient should be facing straight ahead when reading the eye chart. There are some exceptions:

▶ The patient has nystagmus and has adopted a head position where the nystagmus is more "quiet" (the null point).

▶ A patient wearing no-line lenses may need to tip the head down a little for distance evaluation, in order to look through the area of the lens that has the maximum distance correction.

▶ A patient wearing no-line lenses may need to tip the head up a little for near evaluation, in order to look through the area of the lens that has the maximum close correction.

▶ A child wearing segmented bifocals must be encouraged to look through the top portion for distant and the bottom segment for near measurements.

SIDEBAR 8-4
VISUAL ACUITY: HELPFUL HINTS

▶ In the case of a painful eye, try to check visual acuity as is. However, if you know that the injury is superficial, recheck the vision after instilling a drop of topical anesthetic. (If in doubt, ask the practitioner or check office protocol before instilling drops.)

▶ Check vision prior to any test that might compromise the tear film or ocular surface (such as applanation, instilling eye drops, etc).

▶ Encourage the patient to blink frequently to avoid dryness of the ocular surface.

▶ Be open to changing your strategy. Some patients respond better if you start with the smallest letters and work your way up. Others require you to "prime the pump" by starting with larger letters and working your way down.

▶ If a patient has eccentric fixation, tell him/her to "look wherever the letters are clearest."

SIDEBAR 8-5
DO IT BETTER: THE E GAME/TUMBLING E'S

▶ The patient is instructed to tell or point in the direction of the E. With children, it may be easier to call the E a table, and ask which way the table legs are pointing.

▶ The patient can be given an E card and instructed to hold it so that it is matching the ones on the chart.

▶ Send the single E card home with parents and let them practice with their child, getting him/her accustomed to having an eye covered and telling which way the E goes, making subsequent exams easier and (hopefully) more accurate.

The patient's visual acuity is the smallest set of optotypes that can be correctly, consistently identified. (For the purposes of this discussion, we will now use the term "letters," but any optotype is indicated.) It is not unusual for a person to miss a few letters here and there as he/she progresses down the chart. These hits (+) and misses (-) are also indicated. For example, if the patient correctly identifies all letters but one on the 20/30 line, this would be documented as 20/30 -1. Or suppose all letters on the 20/60 line are identified, as well as 2 letters on the 20/50 line; this is documented as 20/60 +2.

All sorts of combinations are potentially possible (eg, 20/40 − 1 +3 +1 indicating that one was missed on 20/40, 3 were seen on 20/30, and one was identified on 20/25) but not necessarily useful. In addition, the notation of "-1" does not necessarily mean the same thing for each acuity line. For example, if the 20/100 line only has two letters, then 20/100 -1 indicates that half of the letters were missed. For the 20/40 line, -1 may indicate that only one out of four or five letters were missed. In the case where a patient both identifies and misses letters on most every line, a notation of "misses on all" might be made. Each clinic will have to establish and adhere to its own protocol. More helpful hints are presented in Sidebar 8-4.

It is also important to document any *pattern* the patient has regarding missing letters. For example, the patient consistently does not call out the first two optotypes on every line. Such a pattern may indicate retinal or neurological problems.

Sometimes the patient must read the same chart with each eye, and more than once. If you suspect that the patient is calling out letters from memory, have him/her read backward or ask for specific letters ("Tell me the second letter on that row. Now the last. Now the first."). If you're using a computerized system, it will scramble the optotypes for you.

Some patient education is required if you are going to use the tumbling E's ("E game") or Landolt C's (Sidebar 8-5). This test is scored in the same manner as letters or

---

SIDEBAR 8-6
CONVERSION TO STANDARD OF 20 FEET

▶ Scenario 1: Patient cannot identify the "20/400" E until it is brought closer, to 15 feet.
  - Vision recorded as: 15/400
  - Convert to 20 foot standard: 15/400 = 20/X
  - Cross-multiply: 15X = 20 * 400 = 8000
  - Divide both sides by 15: 15X/15 = 8000/15
  - Result: X = 533.333
  - Converted vision: 20/533

▶ Scenario 2: Child correctly identifies Allen cards at 15 feet but not beyond.
  - Note: The smallest Allen pictures yield 20/30 at 20 feet, so the denominator is always 30 with this test. However, be sure to read any instructions with the cards/test.
  - Vision recorded as: 15/30
  - Convert to 20 foot standard: 15/30 = 20/X
  - Cross-multiply: 15X = 20 * 30 = 600
  - Divide both sides by 15: 15X/15 = 600/15
  - Result: X = 40

SIDEBAR 8-7
DOCUMENTATION OF VISUAL ACUITY

The following should be noted when documenting vision:

▶ Eye tested: OD, OS, OU

▶ With (cc) or without (sc) correction

▶ Distance (DVA) or near (NVA)

▶ Test/optotypes used

▶ If right eye is not tested first, notate "OS checked first"

▶ If standard occlusion is not used, note this (eg, "+5 occlusion used due to nystagmus")

▶ Note if the patient has eccentric fixation

▶ Note any abnormal head position (eg, "right head tilt")

▶ Note any refusal to having an eye occluded (in children, this may indicate amblyopia in the fellow eye)

▶ If near acuity is not tested at the standard 14 or 16 inches, document the distance at which the test is performed

▶ If distant acuity is not tested at the standard 20 feet (6 meters), document the distance at which the test is performed; convert to standard 20 feet if necessary

▶ Note any comments the patient makes about the letters (eg, "There's something in front of my eye, I can't see the top of the chart," "All the letters look like they're slanting to the left")

▶ Make a note if the patient consistently seems to ignore the letters on one side of the chart or the other (eg, "Misses all letters on right side of chart")

---

numbers in that the acuity is the smallest line where the patient gets the majority of the optotypes correct.

When testing distance acuity in young children, it may be helpful to provide a hand-held chart showing the optotypes. The patient is then asked to point to the figure that matches the optotype on the board. Some tests provide a chart for this purpose, or you can make your own. You might also give the guardian a copy to work with the child at home so that the optotypes are more familiar at the next visit. This works especially well with the E game/tumbling E where the guardian can use one E card and the child another. The guardian helps the child practice copying the test E's orientation. (Patching one eye is not necessary, but varying the "test" distance might be beneficial to orient the child to the procedure.)

If the patient is unable to identify the largest optotype at the prescribed distance, there are several alternatives. You may move the patient closer to the chart (or vice versa) until the largest figure is first correctly identified. A situation like this requires you to recalculate the acuity rating, however (Sidebar 8-6).

Another option is to use optotype cards and note the farthest distance at which the patient consistently identifies them. This is helpful in exam rooms that use a mirror system and neither the patient nor the chart can be moved. Again, the acuity will need to be recalculated.

Near vision cards are calibrated for 14 or 16 inches, so be sure to know the requirement for the system you are using. (Note that this distance may *not* be where the letters are the sharpest for the patient.) You may also want to have the patient show you where the letters are the clearest. If you use a different near testing distance than the one your card is calibrated for, be sure to note it in the chart.

The most careful test in the world is useless if it is not documented properly (Sidebar 8-7). Every clinic should have a written protocol that is followed by all.

The patient's visual acuity may be more useful than merely a recording of how well he/she sees on a particular day. You may also get clues to ocular conditions as well (Sidebar 8-8).

SIDEBAR 8-8
CLUES FROM VISUAL ACUITY RESULTS

▶ Poor near vision only
  • Presbyopia
  • Hyperopia
▶ Poor distant vision only
  • Myopia
▶ Poor distant and near vision
  • Hyperopia
  • Astigmatism
  • High myopia
▶ Consistently misses optotypes on one part of the chart
  • Visual field defect
  • Retinal detachment
▶ Central area of chart is blocked out
  • Macular disorder
  • Large floater
  • Posterior subcapsular cataract
▶ Abnormal head posture
  • Astigmatism
  • Extraocular muscle imbalance
  • Nystagmus
▶ In a child, refusal to have one eye occluded
  • Amblyopia
  • Anisometropia
▶ Optotypes are jumbled/distorted/"broken"
  • Astigmatism
  • Macular disorder
▶ Optotypes are moving/dancing
  • Macular disorders
  • Nystagmus
  • Floaters/asteroid hyalosis (deposits in the vitreous jelly)
▶ Optotypes are doubled
  • Extraocular muscle imbalance

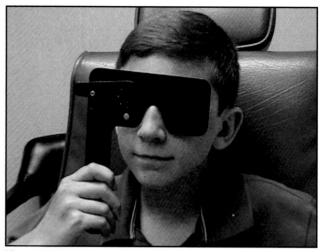

Figure 8-17. Using a multi-pinhole device.

If subnormal distance vision is caused by a refractive error, then acuity should improve through the pinhole. This works because the pinhole cuts out the scattered light rays, and you only get light that is coming straight into the eye. If the pinhole does not improve acuity, then it is assumed that the reduction is due to some type of pathology.

The patient is told to "look straight through one of those little holes" then asked to read the smallest line of letters possible. This is recorded as *pinhole vision*. Theoretically, the patient's refractometric measurement should be at least the pinhole vision or better.

Pinhole vision may usually be done with or without the patient's current glasses. Some patients have difficulty seeing through the pinhole. It may be helpful to isolate the line the patient last read *without* the pinhole as a starting point, as you know he/she should at least be able to see this.

Some clinics have a policy that if a patient's vision is not 20/25 or better (with current glasses, if worn) then a pinhole vision is automatically done. Likewise, if the vision of a returning patient has fallen two lines below his/her last acuity check, a pinhole is done as well. Finally, doing a pinhole on a legally blind patient is key as well, because visual *potential* can be very important when it comes to disability qualifications.

Pinhole

If a patient cannot see 20/20, it is helpful to know if the eye is *capable* of 20/20. This can be determined by using a *pinhole*. Most phoropters and trial lens sets have a pinhole, which is an opaque disk with a tiny hole in the center. It may be easier for the patient, however, to use a pinhole device that has multiple holes in it, making it simpler to "find" a hole to look through (Figure 8-17).

CASE STUDY

A new 75-year-old patient has 20/80 distance vision with and without his current glasses. Pinhole vision is 20/40. Assumption: Refractometry should improve acuity to at least 20/40. In addition, there is probably some type of pathology preventing 20/20 vision.

CASE STUDY

A returning 56-year-old patient has 20/60 distance vision through her current progressive-add glasses. Her vision at the last visit (1 year ago) was 20/20. Pinhole today is 20/20. Refractometry actually shows absolutely no change in the measurement of the current glasses, for 20/20 vision. Assumption: No overt pathology, but what is going on? Think back to the original vision check. In this particular situation, the patient was looking at the chart through a lower part of her progressive addition lenses, and not the uppermost part where the distance correction is located. Lesson: Make sure any patient with progressive addition lenses is looking through the appropriate area of the lens when checking vision at distance and near.

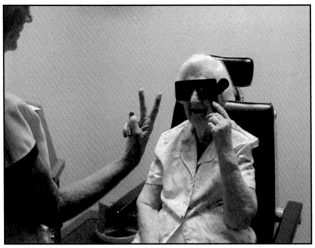

Figure 8-18. Testing vision by counting fingers.

Beyond Optotypes

Even if a patient cannot identify the largest optotype on your chart, you must still evaluate the vision. The next test in the hierarchy is *count fingers*. In this case, the examiner asks the patient to tell how many fingers the examiner is holding up (Figure 8-18). I usually start at about 2 to 3 feet away. If the patient correctly identifies the number of fingers, then gradually back away maybe 2 feet at a time until the patient consistently misses. I may then move gradually closer again just to verify my findings. If the patient cannot correctly identify how many fingers at 2 to 3 feet, I gradually move in closer to see where I first get a response.

The goal is to note the farthest distance at which the patient consistently and correctly identifies the number of fingers presented (Sidebar 8-9). This is documented as "Count Fingers at ____," filling in the blank with the test distance. Some practitioners discourage using this test because standardization is poor, and results are dependent on (among other things) the size of the tester's hand.

If the patient cannot count fingers at about 6 inches, testing must switch to *hand motion*, where the examiner asks the patient to tell if the examiner's hand is moving or still. Again, start at 2 to 3 feet and gradually move closer or farther back to identify the farthest point at which the patient can consistently tell if the hand is moving or not. Make sure that occlusion is complete and encourage the patient to use eccentric fixation, if appropriate. This test is documented as "Hand Motion at ____," again noting the test distance.

Low vision clinics generally do not accept count fingers and hand motion as valid measurements of visual acuity in partially sighted patients. In such a case, it is preferred to do the testing at 10 feet (instead of 20), move the patient/chart closer, or use hand-held cards as outlined earlier.

SIDEBAR 8-9
DO IT BETTER: COUNT FINGERS TEST

▶ Test each eye alone with best correction.

▶ Double-check occlusion! Even when using a plastic occluder, the patient may be seeing around the edge, especially if you are holding your fingers temporally.

▶ You may have to move from one side to the other to find the spot where the patient can see.

▶ The patient may need to use eccentric fixation in order to pick up the target (fingers).

▶ You might need to wave your fingers a little so the patient can locate them. But once you've found the sweet spot, keep your hand still. Moving the fingers effectively makes them larger.

If there is no response to the hand motion test, test the patient's ability to see light. For this test, a hand-held occluder will not work. Ask the patient to cover the other eye with his/her hand making a "seal" around that eye. Hold a strong light several inches away from the eye you are evaluating. (A transilluminator or indirect ophthalmoscope is good for this.) Ask "Can you tell if my light is on?" If yes, then turn it off or move it away and say "Tell me when you notice that the light comes back on." After a brief pause, shine the light into the eye again. (Do not use a light that clicks when you turn it off and on, as this gives an audible clue.)

If the patient can identify if and when the light is shining in the eye, this is called *light perception* (LP). But there is one more level to test. Move the light to various quadrants and ask the patient to identify where the light is coming from (Figure 8-19). If the patient consistently and correctly tells from what direction the light emanates,

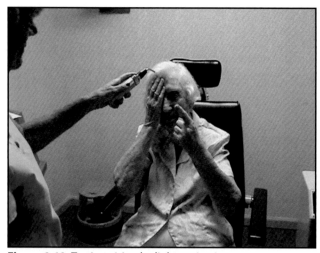
Figure 8-19. Testing vision by light projection.

TABLE 8-2	
VISION IN INFANTS	
Age	**Snellen Equivalent[6]**
Birth	20/120
4 months	20/60
8 months	20/30
	Visual Ability[7]
2 months	Focus on parent's face
3 months	Follow objects
5 months	Depth perception developing
6 months	Color vision is good
9 months	Beginning to refine eye-hand coordination
9 to 12 months	Depth perception refined
24 months	Eye-hand coordination and depth perception well developed

this is noted as *light perception plus projection* (LP+P). Make an additional note indicating where the light is seen (ie, "all four quadrants," "projection in upper quadrants only"). If the patient has light perception but not projection, this is documented as *LP-P* or *LP only*.

If the patient cannot correctly identify that the light is shining in the eye, the eye is considered totally blind with *no light perception* (NLP) and should be noted as such in the patient's record.

The *Purkinje vascular entopic test* is not a measure of acuity per se, but it can give a gross indication of retinal function. Have the patient close both eyes and rotate the eyes downward. Place a strong penlight against the patient's eye through the closed eyelid, just under the brow. Gently move the light. If the retina is functioning at all, the patient may report seeing "tree branches." This is actually a shadow of the retinal vessels, and is called the *Purkinje tree*. Since not everyone can see them, however, it is not a definitive test.

Vision Testing in Infants and Young Children

Parents bringing an infant or very young child to the eye clinic often have specific concerns. Can my baby see? How much can he/she see? Is the vision normal? Answering these questions can be difficult because of the uncertainty in interpreting an infant's responses to testing.

Except perhaps in the very young, it will probably be obvious if the baby has any level of vision prior to any testing. It is generally accepted that a neonate can most easily focus at the distance from the breast to the mother's face, or about 7 to 18 inches. Vision improves (Table 8-2) as the child learns how to control accommodation and the visual pathway in the brain learns to see (more on this later).

Does the Baby See?

Observe how the child responds to visual stimuli. Does the child respond when the room lights are turned off? Turned back on? Is there a response when you shine a penlight in the eyes? What about the brighter (*noxious*) light of an indirect ophthalmoscope? Is there a response if you suddenly wave your hand close to the child's face (a "*visual threat*")?

The *optokinetic tape* or *drum* may be used, although the results are not always conclusive. The drum is held in front of the child and then spun; if there is vision, the patient's eyes will jerk rhythmically as they try to follow the lines. The same result is expected if using the tape, which is held up and moved side to side.

In the *spinning baby test*, the examiner holds the infant at arm's length, spins around several times, and then stops, watching the baby's eyes for prolonged nystagmus (jerking), which *can* indicate poor vision.

Fix and Follow

An infant of 8 weeks can generally fixate on a close object and will follow the object when it moves. The selection of a test object is not important as long as it does not make any noise; even a blind child will turn his/her head toward a set of jangling keys. Babies like to look at faces more than anything else, so you can be the test object yourself. Look directly into the child's face from about 12 inches away, smile, and move from one side to another, up and down. A penlight is also good, or some colorful small toy (Figure 8-20). If the child looks at the object and moves his/her eyes and/or head to follow movement, this is a positive result and documented as *fix and follow*.

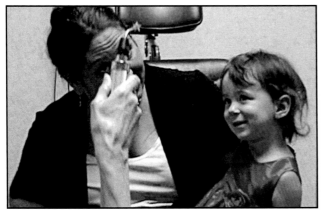

Figure 8-20. Fix and follow test using a transilluminator with a sticker over the light.

Central, Steady, and Maintained

Central, steady, and maintained (CSM) is a simple test based on the examiner's observations. The child is shown a small toy or other object and the following is noted:

▸ Central: Does the patient look at the object? Does he/she seem to be looking at the object using central vision (ie, is the visual axis of the eye(s) aligned with the object)?

▸ Steady: Are the eyes "locked" on the object? Or is there nystagmus?

▸ Maintained: Are both eyes locked on the target? Or does one eye turn in or out? Or do they switch, with one eye sometimes looking at the object and sometimes the other eye?

Forced Preferential Looking

Forced preferential looking (FPL), or *forced choice preferential looking*, is based on the premise that given a choice, a baby will choose to look at something with a pattern vs something that is blank. Using this principle, cards of various types have been developed where one side of the card is blank and the other side has either a picture or grating of varying widths.

The *Teller Acuity Cards* (TAC) use gratings of various frequencies (Figure 8-21). There is a peep hole in the center of each card through which the examiner looks, watching the infant's responses. (That is one of the drawbacks of this type of testing—that it is dependent on the examiner's evaluation of the patient's response.) The examiner is not supposed to know on which side the pattern appears, so as not to bias the results or give the child some unknown clue. Before displaying a card, make sure you have the child's attention. Start with the most obvious grating. Use a test distance of about 15 inches for a child of 6 months or less, and 22 inches for a child over 6 months. A positive result is the finest grating that gets 75% responses. It is helpful and expedient to skip to every

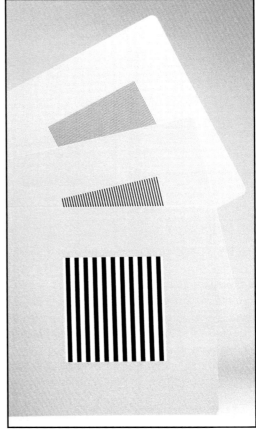

Figure 8-21. Teller Acuity Cards (Bernell).

other card at first until you begin to narrow down the threshold. Then go one by one. More detailed information is supplied with the cards.

Other tests use the same principle. The Cardiff cards (ages 18 to 60 months) have a picture in the upper or lower half of each card. Other versions have the test targets on paddles, such as Lea Gratings (one paddle has grating of varying widths, the other is gray) and Peek-a-Boo Patti (Precision Vision; one paddle is gray and others display a face of fading contrast).

If all else fails, young children who can be persuaded to wear the "neat sunglasses" (Polaroid glasses that come with stereo tests) can be shown the stereo fly. If there is a reaction to the fly (eg, recoils, makes an "ugh" face, refuses to touch it, or tries to touch it and stops above the page), then at least some measure of vision is present in each eye.

Detection of Amblyopia

The progress of vision after birth involves much more than the eye itself. In a way, one must "learn" to see in order for sight to occur. The eyeball is pretty much fully formed at birth, although the retina must still undergo some maturing and accommodation is rather uncontrolled. But the neural pathways for sight in the brain must still develop and mature. If an eye has substandard

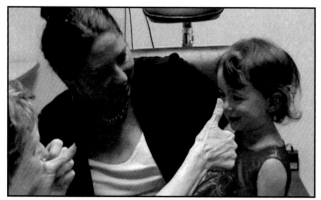

Figure 8-22. Evaluating for amblyopia by surreptitiously blocking an eye.

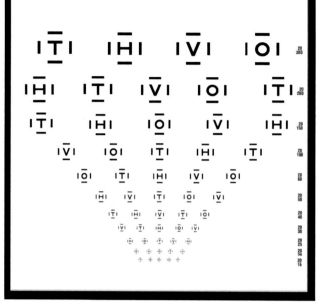

Figure 8-23. Crowding bars (surrounded optotypes; Good-Lite Company).

or occluded vision, then the brain does not receive a proper image from that eye to stimulate this "learning" during the post-natal period. Even if the eyeball is physically healthy, vision will not fully evolve. This is called *amblyopia* (sometimes called *lazy eye*). If not detected and corrected early in life, the poor vision becomes permanent. However, if discovered and treated before the age of 8 to 10 years, the prognosis for improving the vision is usually good. See Chapter 10 for details on amblyopia and its treatment.

When testing visual acuity in infants and children, the main purpose is often the identification of amblyopia. This generally means answering the question, does one eye seem to see better than the other?

Binocular Fixation Preference

The premise of the *binocular fixation preference* test (BFP; sometimes simply called the *fixation preference test*) is that a child will prefer to use a better-seeing eye, and if vision is not equal in both eyes, will object to the good eye being covered.

For infants and very small children, the child is seated on the parent's lap. While talking and smiling at the child, sneak a thumb over one eye (coming up from below) then remove it. Do the same for the other eye (Figure 8-22). If amblyopia is present, the child may move to peek around your thumb, bat your hand away, cry, or lose interest when you cover the good/strong eye. However, if the child has the same reaction with both eyes, then he/she probably sees equally out of either eye. Older children might be shown a small picture or toy. The intensity of the child's reaction when you cover the good eye may give a clue about the *density* (severity) of the amblyopia.

The results of the BFP are documented with such notes as *Seems to see equally OU, No preference OU, Pt will look with either eye, Seems to prefer OD, Prefers OD, Strongly prefers OS,* etc.

Amblyopia and Crowding

Amblyopia also has some important implications in visual acuity testing. The *crowding phenomenon,* where an amblyopic eye is better able to discern optotypes that are presented singly, has already been mentioned. Another option is using optotypes that have bars (*crowding bars*) on all four sides (also known as *surrounded optotypes;* Figure 8-23).

Contrast Sensitivity

Regardless of the fact that "reading the eye chart" is the industry standard for assessing visual acuity, it is not a perfect test. The chart has a high level of contrast: stark, black optotypes against a blank white background. Under such artificial conditions, it is not possible to evaluate what the patient *really* sees. Real life is a mixture of shades and contrasts.

Contrast sensitivity has been defined as the "ability to distinguish between finer and finer increments of light vs dark."[8] Patients with certain ocular conditions (Table 8-3) might have great vision as long as there is high contrast (and thus read 20/20 on the eye chart in the office) but have great difficulty seeing in situations where contrast is diminished. This might occur in foggy weather, night driving, or conditions of glare. They cannot understand why their vision is so good in the clinic when they *know* they "can't see." This can be especially problematic in the case of cataracts, where insurance would normally not pay for surgery on a 20/20 eye. But by measuring the patient's contrast sensitivity, the fact is revealed that the patient really *cannot* see, and surgery might then be approved.

TABLE 8-3
THE EFFECTS OF OCULAR DISORDERS ON VISION TESTING

Conditions That Can Affect Contrast Sensitivity[8]

► Cataracts
► Posterior capsule opacity (following cataract surgery)
► Glaucoma
► Refractive surgery
► Diabetic retinopathy
► Contact lenses

Conditions That Can Affect Glare Disability[9]

► Posterior subcapsular cataract
► Cortical cataract
► Keratoconus
► Corneal dystrophy
► Refractive surgery
► Corneal scarring
► Corneal edema
► Posterior capsule opacity (following cataract surgery)
► Vitreous opacities
► Small pupils (scatter caused by pupillary margins)
► Scratched glasses or contact lenses

Conditions That Can Increase Photostress Recovery Time[10]

► Cystoid macular edema
► Central serous retinopathy
► Age-related maculopathy
► Diabetic maculopathy
► Macular drusen
► Chorioretinitis
► Retinitis pigmentosa
► Toxicity
  • Oxazepam
  • Chloroquine
  • Alcohol
► Advanced age
► Glaucoma (questionable)

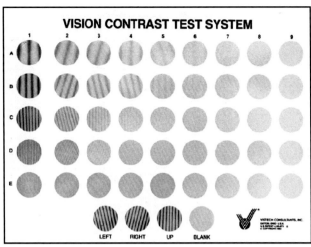

Figure 8-24. Sine-wave gratings of gradient special frequency contrast sensitivity test (Vistech Consultants, Inc).

postoperative refractive surgery, job physicals, etc), then both eyes can be tested together.

First check visual acuity as usual. For the CST, use the patient's own correction or best correction in a trial frame or phoropter. (Note: Some tests recommend a specific reading add; consult the user's guide for your particular test.) Illumination is key to reproducible results, so consult the manufacturer's literature prior to using any test. Light meters are available to help standardize the evaluation. As the test progresses, encourage the patient to try the next row down. Guessing is acceptable. The results are recorded on a special chart and in the patient's record.

Glare Testing

Glare occurs when light is scattered, and may be classified as glare discomfort or as glare disability. *Glare discomfort* would be photophobia (light sensitivity) as seen in iritis or ocular albinism, or reflecting off water on a sunny day. Of interest in this chapter is *glare disability*, or the decrease in vision that occurs when glare causes a reduction in contrast between the background and the object of regard.

Glare disability is generally caused by some sort of media opacity, the most classic of which is posterior subcapsular cataract (PSC). A PSC most commonly occurs directly in the line of vision. As long as the pupil is open wide, the patient can sort of "see around" the cloudy area. But add glare, causing the pupil to constrict, and now the patient is forced to try to look directly through the dense area. This can cause a marked decrease in vision. There are other entities associated with glare disability as well (see Table 8-3).

Glare testing makes it possible to identify and measure glare disability. Being able to document the level of disability may enable the patient to have corrective measures taken sooner rather than later. For example,

There are several different types of *contrast sensitivity tests* (CST; also called *visual contrast sensitivity* [VCS] and *contrast sensitivity function* [CSF]; Figure 8-24 and Table 8-4).

Testing contrast sensitivity is similar to regular visual acuity testing with best correction. If ocular disease is suspected, each eye is tested alone. If only a general idea of the patient's contrast ability is needed (such as in

		TABLE 8-4	
		CONTRAST SENSITIVITY TESTS	
Test	**Description**	**Evaluation Notes**	**Other**
Pelli-Robson	► Fading letter chart: Rows of letters of the same size where each succeeding row is fainter than the one above it	► Lighting: 85 cd/m² ► Testing distance: 40 inches/1 meter ► After first line, each line is worth 0.05 log ► Encourage patient continually to try/guess next line ► Examiner may need key or printed answer sheet	Ages 20 to 50 years: 1.85 log Ages > 50 years: 1.65 log Chart can fade over time; note expiration date and replace
Mars Letter	► Fading letter chart	► Testing distance: 20 inches/50 cm ► Each line is worth 0.04 log	
Low Contrast Chart	► Available in 1.25%, 2.5%, 5%, 10%, and 25% contrast levels ► If only one chart is used, the 2.5% chart is likely to give the most information		
Gradient Spatial Frequency (Figure 8-24)	► Sine-wave gratings: Vary in spatial frequency (bar width), contrast, and direction (straight, left, or right) ► Contrast declines left to right until nearly invisible ► Bar width decreases top to bottom	► For charts with a single row for each spatial frequency: Patient asked to indicate the direction of the bars ► For charts with two rows of disks, only one disk for each contrast level has any gratings: Patient asked to identify whether the top or bottom disk has the lines	Score sheet indicates the number of disks correctly identified at each spatial frequency

a patient with a PSC might have a glare test of 20/40 or worse, making him/her eligible to have insurance pay for cataract surgery.

Glare is most often tested with a Brightness Acuity Tester (BAT; Marco) or a Brightness Acuity Meter (BAM; AMA Optics, Inc). These instruments commonly provide several different levels of glare, simulating room light (the dimmest) to outdoors on a cloudy day (middle setting) to direct sunlight (the most intense). Some autorefractors and other vision analyzers have built-in glare testing.

Glare testing is done prior to dilation. First, the patient's refractive error is measured and this best correction is placed into trial frames. However, if the patient's current glasses also give the best-corrected acuity, they may be used. The BAT should *not* be done through the phoropter, because the phoropter will block some of the light coming from the sides, which is a key part of the test. For the same reason, it is recommended that thin-rimmed trial lenses be used if trial frames are employed.

The smallest acuity line that the patient was able to see with best correction is isolated on the chart (if possible). One eye is occluded, and the patient is directed to

hold the instrument so as to view the eye chart through it (Figure 8-25).

The acuity test light may then be turned on to the desired intensity, and the patient is asked to read the letters. If disabling glare exists, the patient will not be able to see this original, best-corrected line. The next largest acuity line is then presented and the patient asked to read. This is done in rather rapid succession, not giving the patient longer than 30 seconds to work out the letters.

The smallest line that the patient can read with the BAT light turned on is documented. Test results are recorded by noting the visual acuity at each level of lighting. Alternately, a contrast sensitivity chart might be used.

Protocol for performing a glare test varies. If a patient is known to have PSC, a glare test should be done automatically. Likewise, a patient complaining of glare problems (especially a patient of "cataract age"— over 60 years) could have the test done as well. In a patient with cataracts of any type, if the vision is already *not* correctable to 20/50 or better, a glare test will not add much useful information.

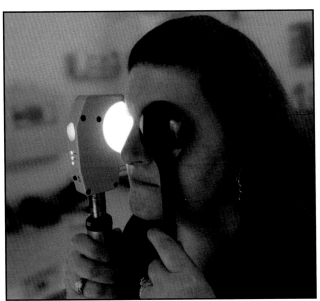

Figure 8-25. Brightness acuity tester in use. (Reprinted with permission from Kim McQuaid, COMT.)

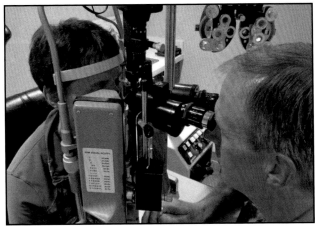

Figure 8-26. Potential acuity meter (Haag-Streit USA) in use.

A simple "glare test" without special equipment can be done by shining a penlight into the patient's eye, either from the side or nearly directly ahead. This can give you a yes/no answer of whether or not glare seems to reduce vision, but does not quantify the disability like BAT or BAM results.

Potential Acuity

Some of the first questions a patient contemplating cataract surgery will ask are, "Will I see better? How much better?" This issue of potential acuity is something that the surgeon is concerned about, too, especially when the patient has more than just cataracts affecting his/her vision. In a case like that, we want to know how much of a vision decrease is due to cataracts or other media opacity and how much is due to something else (macular degeneration being the most common).

Potential acuity can be tested in several ways, but all methods are pretty much based on the same premise: to somehow "bypass" the media opacity and find out what the vision would be if the opacity was not there (sometimes referred to as *retinal vision*). The pupils are first dilated for each of these tests, and each eye is tested individually.

The simplest version of the test, dubbed *super pinhole* or *potential acuity pinhole* (PAP), does not require special equipment. Once dilated, the patient looks through a pinhole at the near acuity card, which must be held at 14 inches in room light. (One reference recommends a +5.00 trial lens as well.[11] Another says to use the patient's glasses.[12] Yet another says use no correction at all.[13]) The muscle light is then used to shine direct, close light on a line of numbers, moving down to the smallest the patient

can identify. The patient is encouraged to make subtle movements of the pinhole and/or head in order to find the position where vision is best. While this method does not use strictly controlled variables, it has been shown to be fairly accurate.[13,14]

A similar test involves having the patient look through a +8.00 sphere at the near card illuminated with the muscle light.[12] There are also *illuminated near card* (INC) charts available on hand-held electronic devices. A variant of this is the *Retinal Acuity Meter* (RAM; Lombart Instrument), which the patient views through a +2.50 trial lens and a pinhole at 16 inches.

The *Super Pinhole Macula* (Richmond Products) is a device that also uses a pinhole, but the target optotypes are displayed on a special cabinet at 5 feet away. This is more controlled than the pinhole tests described previously because the illumination of the cabinet is known. The patient is asked to read the smallest line possible, making adjustments to the pinhole and head position as necessary. The chart may be changed to display letters, numbers, or other figures.

The *potential acuity meter* (PAM) attaches to a slit lamp and projects a tiny eye chart between particles in the lens and directly onto the macula (Figure 8-26). There is a dial that can be set to the spherical equivalent of the patient's refractive error. The examiner manipulates the unit in order to find a spot that might be more clear; this can be done while looking either through or around the slit lamp. The patient reads the smallest line possible. (Note: The acronym PAM seems to have started life as a trademarked item, but has now become a common-use term. The Guyton-Minkowski PAM is manufactured by Mentor.)

The *interferometer* (also called a *retinometer*) creates two beams that are projected onto the retina. There are two types: white light and laser. The patient sees a series of stripes or a grid and is asked to tell the direction of the stripes (vertical, horizontal, slanting left, or slanting

TABLE 8-5

AVERAGE PHOTOSTRESS RECOVERY TEST VALUES

Age (Years)	Approximate/ Average Recovery Time (Seconds)
20 to 30	18 to 70
30 to 40	21 to 74
40 to 50	28 to 76
50 to 60	30 to 80
60 to 70	33 to 84

Test performed using direct ophthalmoscope on brightest setting held as close to eye as possible for 30 seconds.
Adapted from Margrain TH, Thomson D. Sources of variability in the clinical photostress test. *Ophthalmic Physiol Opt.* 2002;22(1):61-67. www.ncbi.nlm.nih.gov/pubmed/11824648/. Accessed July 4, 2016.

right). The finest grid correctly identified is taken as the potential vision as identified on an accompanying chart. It is helpful to test the better eye first, to increase the likelihood that the patient will properly identify the stripes, which may at first look like shooting stars or wiggly lines.

Whatever method is used, the results are documented as "potential acuity" with the type of test used. It is important to explain to the patient that this measurement is not to be taken as a guarantee of a specific postoperative visual result.

Macular Photosensitivity

Normally, the macula is the most sensitive area of the entire retina. This is because the cone cells, rich with visual pigments, are centered here. Some disorders can cause changes in the macula, and some of these can worsen over time.

The *photostress recovery test* (PRT or PSRT) or *macular photostress test* (MPT) evaluates how quickly the pigments in the macular cone cells are regenerated after being "bleached" (ie, depleting the light-sensitive pigments) with a bright light. This regeneration (*photostress recovery time*) is altered in some disorders (see Table 8-3). The test can also help distinguish between central vision loss due to the macula vs the optic nerve, as optic nerve disorders are not associated with prolonged PRT recovery times.[10]

First, the patient's corrected visual acuity is checked. Then, the correction is removed and a bright light (from penlight, muscle light, direct ophthalmoscope, etc) is shone directly into the eye from about 1 to 1.25 inches away for 30 seconds. (Note: Some references give other time lengths for shining the light in the eye, as well as

where to hold the light source; check with your physician to see how he/she wants you to perform the test.) Some brightness acuity instruments have an MPT function. The aperture is blocked with a plug supplied with the instrument, and the patient holds the instrument over the eye to be tested for the prescribed amount of time with the light on full intensity.

The light source is then removed, correction restored, and the examiner clocks the number of seconds it takes before the patient can read one line above (ie, larger than) the previous acuity measurement (Table 8-5). The normal macula takes about 20 to 80 seconds to recover to this level, and younger patients take less.[10] In general, a recovery time of 70 seconds or more (again, depending on age) is considered an abnormal macular response time.[10]

The lack of standardization for this test is obvious: How bright a light, and from what source? How long to shine the light into the eye before testing? If recovery is to one acuity line larger than the patient's best-corrected vision, what happens if there is no intermediate line, as occurs between 20/100 and 20/80 on many charts? Texts differ in their answers to these questions. While the variables will likely never be settled, making it difficult to compare test results from one establishment to another (or, indeed, among examiners in the same practice), one source suggests using the light of the direct ophthalmoscope at full intensity, held as close to the eye as possible, for 30 seconds (the time needed to bleach the macula).[10] At the very least, the tester should document how the test was done.

Functional Vision Loss

When decreased vision is shown to be due to a disease, disorder, trauma, etc, it is known as *organic vision loss.* However, sometimes there is a loss of acuity without known organic cause. These are the cases of *nonorganic* or *functional vision loss,* and it can be a very challenging issue. One source notes, "Neurologists and neuro-ophthalmologists are particularly adept at demonstrating either the organic or nonorganic nature of a symptom or sign because they evaluate an organ system that respects certain anatomical rules that are not intuitively understood by the patient. In addition, the visual system, more than other parts of the sensory system, is closely observable and measurable. Armed with knowledge of neuroanatomy and neurophysiology, a working understanding of basic ophthalmologic tools, and a little sleight of hand, one can demonstrate integrity of the visual system."[15]

There are three types of functional vision loss: malingering, factitious, and hysterical. (Note: These are also sometimes seen as a loss of visual field rather than, or in addition to, central acuity.) Referral to neuro-ophthalmology, neurology, and/or psychiatry may be in order.

Malingering refers to a person who is lying for some type of personal gain, and it knows no age boundaries. Probably the most common scenario is monetary benefit, where a person hopes to become eligible for insurance benefits, legal pay-off, disability payments, etc. The visual acuity test seems "easy" to fake, because it would seem we cannot prove what the patient can or cannot see.

CASE STUDY

A 6-year-old boy was brought in by his mother. The child has been saying he "can't see anything." He walked into the room and took the indicated chair without assistance. But he could not read anything on the eye chart with either eye: not the 20/400 E nor the Allen pictures. He could not count fingers. He could not tell me if the light was shining in his eye or not. By this time, the mother was getting frantic.

I opened the drawer containing the trial lenses. I made a big fuss over choosing one: picked one, said "No...", put that lens back and pulled out another (a +0.12 sphere). "I bet this will work," I said. "Let's see..." I held the lens over his uncovered eye. He now read 20/20. This worked on both eyes.

His best friend got glasses last month.

Factitious vision loss is similar to malingering, but the pay-off is different. In this case, the patient is pretending to have symptoms in order to be regarded as ill. These persons enjoy the role of being sick.

Hysterical vision loss (also called *somatoform loss* or *hysterical amblyopia*) has a psychological root as well. The eye is healthy, and there is no organic reason for the decrease in acuity. However, unlike malingering or factitious loss, the patient has not made a conscious choice "not to see" in order to gain some benefit. Rather, it is generally triggered by some stressful event. Instead of the stress being manifested as something common like a headache or gastrointestinal upset, the mind reacts by impairing the vision.

Because hysterical vision loss is nonorganic, it cannot be conclusively proven. The main goal is to rule out any kind of pathology because there are some organic dysfunctions that can mimic this type of hysteria.

While proof may be lacking, there are still some procedures that can help determine if a patient's vision loss is functional.

▸ Plano sphere trial lens. Hold the lens up over the eye that cannot see (occlude other eye). If vision improves, the loss is functional.

▸ If only one eye is affected, put the patient's prescription, if known, into the phoropter. Leave *both* apertures open, but *fog* the "good" eye with +3.00 sphere

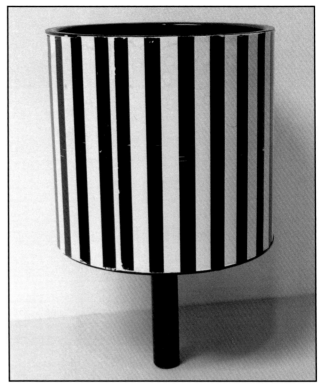

Figure 8-27. Optoknetic drum (Bernell) can be used to evaluate for functional vision loss.

and ask the patient to read the smallest line possible. If the patient now sees more clearly, he/she is doing so with the "bad" eye.

▸ Use the *optokinetic tape* (also called *optokinetic flag*) or *drum* (Figure 8-27). Have the patient cover the "good" eye (if there is one). Do *not* give the patient any explanation of the test. Just hold up the drum and gently spin it, or hold up the tape and move it right to left (not too slowly) and back again. An eye with vision will automatically track the lines/blocks. This corresponds to roughly 20/400 to 20/200 depending on which reference you consult.[15,16]

▸ Perform a stereo test (see Chapter 10). If the patient has stereo vision, then there has to be a degree of decent vision *in both eyes* (Table 8-6). It requires 20/20 vision for the finest degree of arc.

▸ Perform a potential acuity meter test. A substantial improvement is suspicious for functional vision loss.

▸ If the patient claims to have profound vision loss in one eye, check pupils for *afferent pupillary defect*. If there is no afferent pupillary defect, then any vision loss is most likely due to refractive error or media opacity, or else is functional in nature.

▸ Perform an automated visual field with *both* eyes open. If one eye really has a severe vision loss, then it should be possible to plot the blind spot of the "good" eye. If neither blind spot can be plotted, then

TABLE 8-6
RELATIONSHIP OF STEREOPSIS TO VISUAL ACUITY

In Order to Have a Stereo Acuity of:	Patient Must Have Approximate Visual Acuity of:
40	20/20
43	20/25
52	20/30
62	20/40
78	20/50
94	20/70
124	20/100
160	20/200

Adapted from Levy NS, Glick EB. Stereoscopic perception and Snellen visual acuity. *Am J Ophthalmol.* 1974;78(4):722-724. In: Chen JJ, Chen YJ. Functional Visual Loss. University of Iowa Health Care, Ophthalmology and Visual Sciences website. http://webeye.ophth.uiowa.edu/eyeforum/cases/165-functional-visual-loss.htm. March 6, 2013. Accessed July 4, 2016.

it is assumed that each eye has at least some degree of vision.

▶ Have the patient look at an isolated letter on the chart. Hold a 4-diopter prism base-up or base-down in front of the "good" eye. Ask how many images are now seen. If the patient reports seeing two images, then each eye has some degree of vision.

▶ Hold a 10-diopter prism base-out in front of one eye. This should initially cause both eyes to shift toward the prism apex, then one eye will shift back to center. These are movements to restore single vision, and indicate that there is vision in both eyes.

▶ Perform a cross/cover test; an eye that moves to take up fixation sees the target. (Caution: Just because an eye does not move does not mean it does not see.)

▶ Have the patient wear the Worth 4 dot glasses, with the red lens over the "affected" eye. Put up a strip of letters with the duochrome (red/green slide) across them. No occlusion is used. The eye wearing the green lens will see letters *only* on the green side of the chart. If the patient sees both sides, it is because the affected eye is reading the letters on the red side.

▶ Have the patient wear the Worth 4 dot glasses, with the red lens over the affected eye and have him/her look at the Ishihara color plates. The eye with

the green lens will not be able to read the plates. If the patient can read the plates, it is because he/she is using the "affected" eye. This indicates roughly 20/400 vision.[16]

▶ Test visual acuity of the "bad" eye by starting with the smallest letters available (20/10 or 20/15). Encourage the patient to read. Give him/her plenty of time before moving up to the next largest line, which you say is doubling the letter size. Say things like "You should be able to see this." This will sometimes stimulate the patient to see at least 20/25 or 20/30.

▶ Ask the patient to do an arrangement-style color vision test (eg, Farnsworth D-15). You do not really want the color vision results; what you are watching for is enough stereopsis for the patient to pick up the caps without fumbling. Stop the test once you are satisfied with the results.

▶ Visual acuity should double when the testing distance is halved. If this does not occur, then the loss is functional.

▶ Tell the patient you are going to do a coordination test. Say, "I want you to wave your hand," while you do the same. Then say, "Wiggle your fingers," and do the same. Then say, "Do this," and point (or do some other hand motion) *without giving the verbal instructions.* If the patient also points, then he/she can at least see your hand.

▶ A person with vision will usually flinch if you suddenly present a bright light or object.

▶ Without announcing it, put a near card in front of the patient. Watch for convergence and miosis, two indicators that the near image is seen.

▶ Ask the patient to touch his/her two index fingers to each other. This is a test of proprioception that a blind person can pass. A person who cannot do this likely has functional vision loss.

▶ Ask the patient to look at his/her hands. This is another test of proprioception that a blind person can pass. A person who cannot do this is likely to have functional vision loss.

▶ Order electrophysical testing (or at least mention doing so) as a test that can tell whether or not there is vision without any overt response from the patient.

ACKNOWLEDGMENTS

The author would like to thank Sergina M. Flaherty, COMT, OSC; Al Lens, COMT; and Cheryl Pelham for their assistance with this chapter.

CHAPTER QUIZ

For Questions 1 through 8, match the question/scenario to the test that would most appropriately provide the needed information/answer. Each answer is used only once.

   a. contrast sensitivity
   b. glare testing
   c. light projection
   d. macular photostress test
   e. optokinetic drum or tape
   f. pinhole test
   g. potential acuity meter
   h. preferential looking

1. Is this patient's vision loss due to pathology or a refractive error?

2. This patient cannot detect hand motion.

3. This patient has posterior subcapsular cataracts. Does his vision decrease in bright sunlight?

4. This patient has macular degeneration and cataracts. If she has the cataracts removed, how much vision improvement can we expect?

5. This patient has 20/25 vision, yet complains he "can't see."

6. The patient is 12 months old. Her father knows she can see, but is still concerned about her vision.

7. I think the patient is faking her vision loss.

8. Might this patient's vision loss be due to a problem with the macula? Or the optic nerve?

9. In children, the principle objective of visual acuity testing is to detect ____ .

10. True/False: If a patient is malingering, there is no way to prove or disprove it.

11. True/False: A good optotype for an illiterate patient is the number chart.

12. True/False: When checking vision in children, it is especially important to show only one optotype/test object at a time.

13. List at least three types of tests for confirming and evaluating vision in infants.

14. List at least three types of tests for checking visual acuity in children.

15. You are attempting to check near acuity on a 58-year-old patient who is wearing glasses and has just read 20/20 at distance with the right eye. Holding the near card at 14 inches, he can only identify letters of 20/200. What is the possible cause for this unexpected low measurement of near acuity?

Answers

1. f
2. c
3. b
4. g
5. a
6. h
7. e
8. d
9. Amblyopia
10. False
11. True, Most people who are illiterate can recognize numbers.
12. False, To avoid the crowding phenomenon (where a patient with amblyopia has a higher acuity if single optotypes are presented), one must test with an entire line of optotypes if at all possible.
13. Fix-and-follow; central, steady, and maintained; preferential looking test; optokinetic drum/tape; reaction to noxious light; reaction to object coming at face; spinning baby test; Teller Acuity Cards.
14. Allen cards, Lea symbols, E game/tumbling E's, blackbird chart, Landolt C/rings, HOTV chart, number chart.
15. Patient's lenses are for distance only, or with multifocal lenses, patient is not looking through the bifocal/reading portion of the lens.

REFERENCES

1. Colenbrander A. The historical evolution of visual acuity measurement. Presented at the 2001 meeting of the Cogan Society for Ophthalmic History; Stanford, CA. doi:10.1080/13882350802632401.

2. Levi DM. Visual acuity. In: Levin LA, Nilsson SFE, Ver Hoeve J, Wu S, Kaufman PL, Alm A, eds. *Adler's Physiology of the Eye.* 11th ed. Atlanta, GA: Saunders/Elsevier; 2011:633.

3. Newman NJ, Miller NR, Biousse V. *Walsh and Hoyt's Clinical Neuro-Ophthalmology: The Essentials*. Philadelphia, PA: Lippincott Williams & Wilkins; 2008.

4. FAQs: questions that Good-Lite has received. Good-Lite website. www.good-lite.com/faq.cfm. Accessed July 4, 2016.

5. Windsor RL, Windsor LK. Nystagmus: understanding nystagmus. The Internet Low Vision Society website. www.lowvision.org/nystagmus.htm. Accessed July 4, 2016.

6. Hamer RD. What can my baby see? The Smith-Kettlewell Eye Research Institute website. http://www-test.ski.org/Vision/babyvision.html. Accessed July 4, 2016.

7. Infant vision: birth to 24 months of age. American Optometric Association website. www.aoa.org/patients-and-public/good-vision-throughout-life/childrens-vision/infant-vision-birth-to-24-months-of-age?sso=y. Accessed July 4, 2016.

8. Heiting G. Contrast sensitivity testing. All About Vision website. www.allaboutvision.com/eye-exam/contrast-sensitivity.htm. Accessed July 4, 2016.

9. Dhawan S. Glare. www.sdhawan.com/glare.pdf. Accessed July 4, 2016.

10. Margrain TH, Thomson D. Sources of variability in the clinical photostress test. *Ophthalmic Physiol Opt*. 2002;22(1):61-67. www.ncbi.nlm.nih.gov/pubmed/11824648/. Accessed July 4, 2016.

11. Phan T. Super pinhole: when potential acuity meter not available? Optometry Students.com website. www.optometrystudents.com/pearl/super-pinhole-potential-acuity-meter-available/. Accessed July 4, 2016.

12. Koch DD. With coexisting macular disease, how can I tell whether it is worth doing cataract surgery? Healio website. www.healio.com/ophthalmology/curbside-consultation/%7Bef80f54f-0d8a-4207-bdbd-d5f9a9d1159f%7D/with-coexisting-macular-. Accessed July 4, 2016.

13. Melki SA, Safar A, Martin J, et al. Potential acuity pinhole: a simple method to measure potential visual acuity in patients with cataracts, comparison to potential acuity meter. *Ophthalmology*. 1999;106(7):1262-1267. www.ncbi.nlm.nih.gov/pubmed/10406603. Accessed July 4, 2016.

14. Chang MA, Airiani S, Miele D, et al. A comparison of the potential acuity meter (PAM) and the illuminated near card (INC) in patients undergoing phacoemulsification. *Eye*. 2006;20:1345-1351. www.nature.com/eye/journal/v20/n12/full/6702106a.html. Accessed July 4, 2016.

15. Bruce BB, Newman NJ. Functional visual loss. *Neurol Clin*. 2010;28(3):789-802. www.ncbi.nlm.nih.gov/pmc/articles/PMC2907364/. Accessed July 4, 2016.

16. Chen JJ, Chen YJ. Functional visual loss. University of Iowa Health Care, Ophthalmology and Visual Sciences website. http://webeye.ophth.uiowa.edu/eyeforum/cases/165-functional-visual-loss.htm. March 6, 2013. Accessed July 4, 2016.

BIBLIOGRAPHY

Hamrah P, Langston D. Ocular examination techniques and diagnostic tests. In: Langston D. *Manual of Ocular Diagnosis and Therapy*. 6th ed. Philadelphia, PA: Lippincott Williams & Wilkins; 2008.

Levi DM. Visual acuity. In: Goldstein EB, ed. *Encyclopedia of Perception*. Vol 1. Thousand Oaks, CA: Sage Publications; 2009.

Montgomery TM. Visual acuity. www.tedmontgomery.com/the_eye/acuity.html. Accessed March 24, 2015.

Potential acuity meter. American Academy of Optometry website. http://www.aao.org/image/potential-acuity-meter-3. Accessed July 4, 2016.

Rahi JS. Examination of a child with visual loss. *Community Eye Health*. 1998;11(27). www.docs-archive.com/view/92b634ccda60e0cf8d7c7aea1b7aebda/Examination-of-a-Child-with-Visual-Loss-Community.pdf. Accessed July 4, 2016.

Unless otherwise noted, the figures in this chapter were contributed by the following, who are associated with this book as authors:

Jan Ledford: Figures 8-13 through 8-19

Al Lens: Figures 8-1 through 8-12, 8-21, 8-23, 8-24, 8-26, 8-27

Cheryl Pelham: Figures 8-20, 8-22

9

BASIC EYE EXAM

Suzanne Hansen, MEd, COMT
Anna Kiss, BS, COMT

When we first took on this chapter, we chuckled at the title. *Basic Eye Exam.* It seems so simple when stated that way. But, as many of us know (or are on our way to learning) it is often more than just a basic eye exam. Our job as ophthalmic and optometric medical personnel is to be an extra set of eyes, hands, and even brains for the practitioners. The time that a doctor has to spend with a patient is limited, and we play an important role in the eye care office.

Ophthalmic and optometric technicians do not diagnose, plan treatments, or perform surgery. We assist by taking diagnostic measurements and educating patients. It is our ethical and legal responsibility to perform within the scope of our role.

For the many skills we will talk about in this chapter, it is important to keep in mind that doctors and offices may each have a preferred protocol. The methods of performance discussed in this chapter will be presented as suggested best practices. For the knowledgeable eye care technician, you will also use your sound judgment to investigate beyond the preferred protocol in certain circumstances.

Learning basic eye exam techniques and any additional testing required is essential for providing the best care to our patients and assisting our physicians. It is important to prepare and review the order of the exam and make adjustments as needed based on the information obtained in the history. Always consult with your physician if you have any questions about your patient or the results of the diagnostic tests. With continued practice on routine and complex patient work-ups, your technique and efficiency will improve.

BASIC SCIENCES

It may be possible, at least to a limited extent, to perform screening tests and know only how to conduct the evaluation and how to record the results. However, having an understanding of the purpose of a test, its possible variations, and what the results may indicate are imperative for best patient care. Please review, as needed, the following: Chapter 2, Anatomy; Chapter 3, Physiology; Chapter 22, Pharmacology; and others as appropriate.

In addition, some parts of a routine eye exam can be rather complex and have a chapter of their own: Chapter 7, History; Chapter 11, Refractometry; Chapter 12, Slit Lamp; and Chapter 13, Tonometry.

Finally, some topics overlap (eg, lensometry could appear in this chapter as well as Chapter 19, Optical Procedures). In this case, if the information is not presented here, you will be directed to the appropriate text.

Ledford JK, Lens A, eds.
Principles and Practice in Ophthalmic Assisting:
A Comprehensive Textbook (pp 117-135).
© 2018 Taylor & Francis Group.

CLINICAL KNOWLEDGE

Eye care has a screening protocol that is followed for the majority of patients. These ophthalmic vitals include history taking, visual acuity, lensometry, refractometry, tonometry, pupil evaluation, extraocular muscle assessment, and slit lamp examination. The basic eye exam will include these and possibly some additional diagnostic testing performed by the technician, depending on the response or measurements of these ophthalmic vitals. In addition, the required elements for the Centers for Medicare & Medicaid Services exam level relies in part on the screening tests covered here (Sidebar 9-1). See Chapter 43 for information on exam levels.

CLINICAL SKILLS

The order in which some tests are performed can be important. Sidebar 9-2 details some standard protocols.

Simple Observation

In the initial meeting and greeting your patient on the way to the exam chair, it is important to make basic observations as you establish communication and build rapport. These will assist in formulating your screening plan and address some important elements required for thorough history taking.

When you called your patient's name, was he/she able to hear you? You may need to speak louder, slower, deeper, or even obtain an interpreter. Is your patient able

to ambulate to the exam room easily? Is there evidence of stroke from his/her gait? Does your patient require assistance, such as a cane, walker, or wheelchair?

Does your patient seem to have adequate vision to follow you to the exam room, or will he/she need to take your arm to walk there safely? Does he/she appear to see the exam chair and any obstacles in the way? This can begin to give you an idea of the patient's visual acuity.

As your discussion continues into the exam room, is your patient's demeanor and body language appropriate? Your observations should help you determine the patient's cognition or state of awareness (Sidebar 9-3).

SIDEBAR 9-3
COGNITION[2,3]

▶ Cognition: A process: being/becoming aware/ knowing

▶ Orientation: Current state of awareness (X 1, X 2, X 3, X 4)
  • Person
  • Place
  • Time
  • Reason for visit

▶ Dementia: Disorder in which the patient has problems with intellectual functions (memory, judgment, orientation, computation, communication, etc)

SIDEBAR 9-4
MENTAL HEALTH STATUS[2,3]

▶ Overall demeanor

▶ General external appearance: Unkempt, evidence of abuse, malnutrition, poor hygiene, etc

▶ Body language ("normal," crossed arms, leaning away, etc; see Sidebar 9-5)

▶ Affect: Examiner's observations of the patient's emotional response to ideas
  • Appropriate: Patient's emotions seem normal for the circumstances (eg, tears up because of recent death in family, smiles and/or laughs at your jokes, worried about the appearance of a new lesion, etc)
  • Depressive: Withdrawn, sad, self-deprecating, lonely, "dark cloud" without specific cause
  • Labile: Rapidly/suddenly changing affect with no apparent trigger
  • Flat: Little or no emotional response (eg, does not seem appropriately sad at recent death, facial expression never changes, no smiling or laughing at your quips, unresponsive to friendliness, appears unconcerned about anything)
  • Inappropriate: Disharmony between apparent affect and an idea, situation, or what patient is saying (eg, abject laughter while telling you he/she is going blind)

This way you can roughly classify if the patient is aware of self, place, time, and reason for visit. For example, a patient with dementia has problems with intellectual functions such as memory, judgment, orientation, computation, communication, etc, and will have a lower cognition rating.

In some circumstances you may be called upon to estimate the patient's psychological state. The comments in Sidebar 9-4 are not meant to turn us into amateur psychologists, but rather to inform enough to be able to intelligently answer the mental health aspects of the Centers for Medicare & Medicaid Services requirements.

Consider what the patient's body language may be telling you. Also remember that it is essential to put the patient at ease, especially since much of our testing takes place in the personal zone of a person's "space," and some of it even in the intimate zone (Sidebar 9-5).

Once the patient is in the exam chair, continue to evaluate by simply looking (Sidebar 9-6).

History Taking

History taking is one of the first skills that a technician observes, learns, and performs. The goal is to gather data to assist us in our evaluation and the physician in the decision-making process, including diagnosis and treatment planning. See Chapter 7 for details on this vital part of the patient's visit.

It is important to document the patient's symptoms (such as pain, blurry vision, etc) in the history, as well as signs noticed by the patient. *Symptoms* are subjective, meaning something the patient feels or sees, and requires the patient's input for us to know about. For example, we cannot directly observe the patient's floaters; these are a symptom we cannot know about unless the patient tells us.

Signs are objective findings, meaning these are things the technician or practitioner can directly observe or measure, so they are usually noted in the examination portion of the visit's record. Examples of signs would include redness, which we can see, and intraocular pressure (IOP), which we can measure. Signs can be further classified by using a grading scale to indicate severity or quantity. This grading scale is usually from 1 to 4. For example, a patient with an obvious subconjunctival hemorrhage would have +4 redness.

Visual Acuity

Visual acuity is evaluated every time the patient is in the office, with few exceptions. Often it is the first measurement performed. It is important to learn some tricks to speed along visual acuity taking but still get an accurate measurement. Patient encouragement will be necessary at times. Remind the patient to blink, and make sure he/she is not "cheating" by squinting or leaning forward. Visual acuity testing, as well as contrast sensitivity, potential acuity, and glare testing, are discussed in great detail in Chapter 8.

SIDEBAR 9-5
BODY LANGUAGE AND PERSONAL SPACE

► Body language
  • Eyes/face
    ▪ Rapid blinking—Stress
    ▪ Frequently breaking eye contact—Distracted, uncomfortable
    ▪ Pursing lips—Disgust
    ▪ Biting lips—Nervous
    ▪ Covering mouth—Hiding emotion
    ▪ Corners of mouth up—Pleasure, optimistic
    ▪ Corners of mouth down—Dissatisfied, sad
  • Crossed arms—Closed, keeping distance, self-protective (Note: Alternately, the patient could be in pain, or simply cold)
  • Hands on hips—In control, aggressive
  • Clenched fist—Anger
  • Drumming fingers—Impatient, bored
  • Crossed legs—Closed (Note: Could simply be a habit)
  • Leaning forward—Interested, alert
  • Mirrors your body language—In agreement with you
► Personal space
  • 12 to 25 feet—Public
  • 4 to 12 feet—Social
  • 1.5 to 4 feet—Personal
  • 6 to 18 inches—Intimate

SIDEBAR 9-6
EXTERNAL APPEARANCE

► General (unkempt, evidence of abuse, malnutrition, poor hygiene, etc)
► Body position (anything that might preclude patient from reaching slit lamp, phoropter, etc)
► Facial/head evaluation
  • Facial scars
  • Facial lesions
  • Overall facial tone (even color, patches)
  • Facial deformities
  • Drooping of mouth, etc
  • Obvious strabismus
  • Lid abnormalities (ptosis, dermatochalasis, etc)
  • Head tilt
  • Head turn

Lensometry

If the patient brings glasses to the appointment, you need to know the prescription. See Chapter 19 for information on how to read glasses using a lensometer.

Confrontation Visual Fields

Visual acuity is an evaluation of central vision, but it is also necessary to check the patient's peripheral vision (*visual field*). Just a quick screening (as covered here) done properly can pick up visual field defects caused by glaucoma, retinal detachments, and even brain tumors. The physiology of the visual field is covered in Chapter 25. There are several more formal methods of evaluating the visual field, discussed in Chapter 14. These detailed tests are usually ordered by the physician if screening picks up anything suspicious, or if indicated by findings on the fundus exam.

Confrontation visual fields (CVF) can be an excellent estimating tool, and is part of every comprehensive and new patient exam. It will also be performed on an as-needed basis when the patient's history includes complaints of losing side vision or part of the vision being "blocked out." CVF is basically a comparison of the patient's visual field to the examiner's (which is assumed to be normal). The advantages of this test are that it provides important information to the physician, does not require any equipment, and can be done on seated or bedridden patients.

There are several ways to perform the CVF, determined by the doctor's specialty and preference. A suggested best practice includes establishing the outer boundaries of the patient's field by using a moving target (*kinetic* testing), and spot-checking within those boundaries by counting fingers (stationary or *static* testing, as the fingers are not moved).

For testing, the peripheral vision is considered to have four quadrants: lower left, lower right, upper left, and upper right (Figure 9-1).

► Have the patient remove any glasses. With the examination room lights on, sit knee-to-knee to the patient. This will be about 1 meter or 3 feet between patient's and examiner's eyes, and at eye level (may require adjusting chairs of patient and/or the examiner).

► Ask the patient to cover his/her left eye with the palm of the left hand, and to focus on your left eye. While performing the test, always keep watch that the patient is maintaining fixation. Close your own right eye to mirror the patient's visual field.

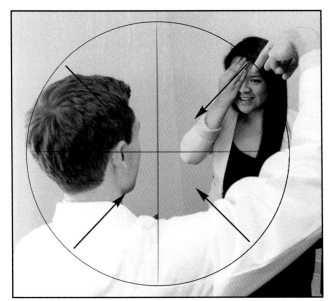

Figure 9-1. Quadrants for confrontation visual field testing.

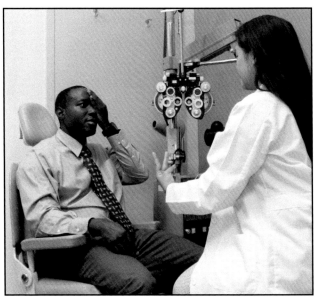

Figure 9-2. Confrontation visual field technique.

▶ For peripheral testing, your purpose is to establish the outer boundaries of the patient's visual field. Instruct the patient, "Tell me when you first notice my finger." Extend one finger in a position where the patient (and you) cannot see it (*nonseeing*). (Note: An object can be used instead of a finger; most common is a red bottle cap.) Then bring your hand slowly inward, toward the center, until the patient responds he/she detects your finger (*seeing*). Think of the field as a clock face. At the very least, check the boundaries at 1:30, 3:30, 7:30, and 10:30. If the screening is for a driver's license or other qualification exam, also test the 3:00 and 9:00 boundaries.

   • It is critical to be aware of patient response time, of the brain seeing the motion of your finger and being able to articulate that it has been seen. If the stimulus is presented too quickly, the field will artificially seem to be smaller than it actually is. Because you are comparing the patient's vision to yours, you should both detect the finger at about the same time. Make a note of any areas where the patient does not see the stimulus when you do. These are areas of *constriction*, where the field boundary has moved inward and is abnormally smaller. If any abnormality is detected, then also check on either side of the horizontal and vertical midlines.

▶ For spot-checking within the boundaries, instruct the patient, "While looking at my eye, guess the number of fingers I'm holding up." Opinions vary regarding presentation: palm in, palm out, and how many fingers to use (1, 2, and 5 seem to be the most common). Present your fingers without moving them in each quadrant (Figure 9-2). (Moving your fingers artificially increases their size.) Make a note of any areas where the patient has difficulty.

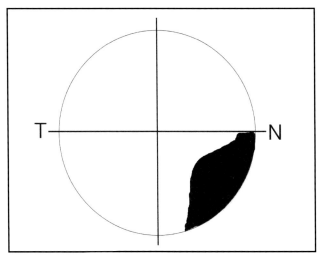

Figure 9-3. Drawing results of confrontation visual field testing, showing an inferior nasal constriction of the right eye (N = nasal, T = temporal) as you look at the patient.

▶ If the patient has repeated difficulty maintaining fixation, you can do the static check by quickly flashing your fingers in the quadrant; keep your hand still, but rapidly put up then retract your fingers, asking the patient, "How many was that?"

Common field defects include constriction, a missing "wedge" (documenting the location of this wedge is very important), and a loss that extends across the vertical or horizontal midline. (Neurological defects, for example, do not cross the vertical meridian.)

When documenting the results, it is important to give enough detail to show what was tested and how. Recording is always done from the *patient's view*. For paper charting, make a quick sketch (Figure 9-3), being sure to insert T (*temporal*) and N (*nasal*) to orient any reader. In electronic medical records, there are a few

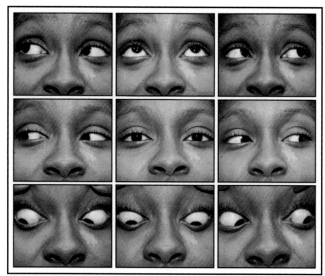

Figure 9-4. Fields of gaze in range of motion testing.

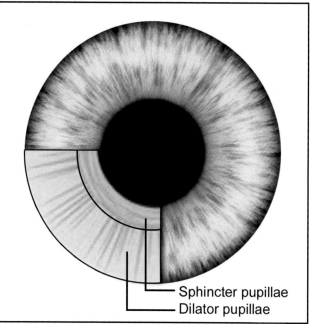

Figure 9-5. Muscles of the iris. (Adapted with permission from Grasycho/Shutterstock.)

different options for recording, depending on the program's set-up. You may just have a check box of normal vs abnormal. However, there should be space to comment on abnormal findings. It is helpful to use the terms *temporal* and *nasal* instead of left and right so that every reader is clear on the location of any defects.

Muscle Balance and Extraocular Muscle Testing

The basic eye exam work-up will include assessment of the six extraocular muscles (EOMs) and how well the eyes work together. The physiology of ocular motility is explained in Chapter 10. Strabismus ("crossed eyes") must be detected then categorized as to direction, whether it is present all the time (tropia) or just some of the time (phoria), and amount (usually measured in prism diopters). For the routine eye exam, the most common muscle balance tests are the cover tests. There are two forms of this test in routine use for screening: the *alternate cover test* and the *cover/uncover* test. This method of EOM evaluation and test interpretation is also discussed in great detail in Chapter 10.

EOM movement (*range of motion*, or ROM) requires watching the patient's eyes move as he/she follows a target (such as a penlight, red cap, a small toy, or the tip of your finger) into the nine positions of gaze (Figure 9-4). These nine positions are primary (straight ahead) up, down, left, right, upper and lower right, and upper and lower left. Determine if the eyes achieve each position together: smoothly, accurately, fast, and equally (shortened to the acronym *SAFE*). Normal results will show equivalent movement of the eyes into each position, which is documented as *full*. If the eyes do not move equally together, further EOM testing is needed. See Chapter 10 for more details of the ROM test.

In addition to watching the movement of the eyes, it is important to note if the patient experiences any pain when moving the eyes. Also observe the lids while moving the target from up to down. Normally, the lids will follow right along with the globe. If, however, there is a time gap where the lids do not automatically and immediately flow with the eyeball from up to down gaze (*lid lag*), there may be thyroid-related problems.

Pupil Assessment

The pupil is the black opening in the center of the iris. The iris controls the amount of light that enters the eye by adjusting the pupil's size. (See also Chapter 2, Anatomy, and Chapter 3, Physiology.)

The iris is composed of two muscles: the iris sphincter and the dilator (Figure 9-5). The *sphincter* muscle is located near the pupil margin and is the stronger of the two muscles. It is regulated by the parasympathetic nervous system and cranial nerve III (oculomotor), and constricts the pupil in bright light. The *dilator* muscle, regulated by the sympathetic system, is located in the periphery of the iris and causes the pupil to enlarge in low-light environments. (For a treatise on the sympathetic and parasympathetic nervous systems, see Appendix A.)

Pupil evaluation gives a glimpse into the operation of the patient's nervous system. Thus, pupil assessment is an essential part of the standard eye exam and should be performed and documented on each patient prior to instillation of any dilation drops. There are numerous categories of pupillary defects.

Performing and Documenting the Test

▶ Direct the patient to look at a distance target with the room lights *on*. Observe and note the size and shape of the pupils, as well as the color of the irides. Each pupil should be round, but there are a number of situations where it might not be (Sidebar 9-7). The pupils should also be the same size (in millimeters) or within 1 mm of each other in both room light and in dim light.

▶ Next, turn the room lights *off* (patient continues to look at a distance target). Again observe and note the size and shape of the pupils.

▶ Now shine a light into the right eye (Figure 9-6). (Best practice uses the transilluminator [muscle light]. If a penlight is used, be sure it has replaceable batteries because this test needs a bright, reliable light.) Note the size of the now-constricted pupils. Use a pupil gauge or millimeter ruler to measure the pupils to 0.5 mm accuracy. You may need a second, dimmer light to shine from the lateral side, to note the pupil size of dark brown irises. The left eye is then similarly evaluated.

A difference in pupil size of greater than 1 mm indicates *anisocoria*. However, 10% of the *normal* population has *physiological* anisocoria (ie, it is normal for them and does not indicate an abnormality of any kind). Anisocoria is usually caused by an efferent pupil defect, where the signal sent from the brain is not getting to the pupil in its entirety. Anisocoria can be further divided as a

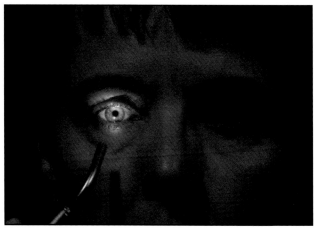

Figure 9-6. Testing the direct pupillary response (ie, in one eye) using a muscle light.

parasympathetic defect (tonic pupil, Argyll-Robertson, or cranial nerve III palsy) or a *sympathetic* defect (Horner's syndrome). Parasympathetic defects are more noticeable in bright light, while sympathetic are more apparent in dim light (Table 9-1.)

▶ After completing the steps of simple observation above, check the pupil's reaction to light. With the room light still off and the patient's focus on a distance target, shine your light into the right eye and observe the right pupil for constriction. Repeat by shining the light into the left pupil and observing the left pupil for constriction. The reaction of each pupil checked individually in this way is called the *direct response*. Best practice would additionally note the size of the patient's pupils (in millimeters) in the dim room light and the size of constriction when illuminated.

The next step involves comparing the light responses of the two eyes to each other, known as the *consensual response*. Because the innervation to the two pupils is linked, if one pupil constricts or dilates, the other will do the same and to the same degree...as long as the connections are normal. If one pupil does not constrict like the other, this indicates that the nerve links to that eye are faulty. This is known as an *afferent pupillary defect* (APD), or *Marcus Gunn pupil*. (Note: APD may be called a *relative afferent pupillary defect* [RAPD] in other texts.)

▶ Begin by shining the light into the right pupil (hold for 3 seconds), quickly move the light to the left pupil, again hold for 3 seconds. It is important to do this switch quickly. Best practice is to take the light straight across from pupil to pupil. This is known as the *swinging flashlight test* (Figure 9-7). Observe the left pupil while simultaneously shining the light into the right pupil. Repeat by shining the light into the left pupil while simultaneously observing the right pupil.

TABLE 9-1				
PUPIL DISORDERS (SIZE AND REACTIONS)‡				
Entity	**Reaction to Light in Affected Eye**	**Reaction to Accommodation**	**Shape/Size**	**Notes**
Normal/PERRLA	Present/normal	Equally brisk in each eye	Round Equal (1 mm or less difference in size)	Hippus may be evident (tiny, readjusting movements of pupil)
Anisocoria (one pupil larger than the other [more than 1 mm difference])	Present/normal	Equally brisk in each eye	Round	Unequal pupil size is a variant of normal in many people Record pupil diameters in room light and dim light Ask practitioner to evaluate prior to dilation as per clinic protocol
Horner's	Dilation lag—Affected pupil takes longer to dilate in dim light	Normal	Anisocoria: Small on affected side	Sympathetic* Efferent† Ptosis and anhidrosis
Argyll-Robertson (syphilitic pupil)	Present/normal	None or very little	May be slightly irregular Pupils are small; possible anisocoria	Tertiary syphilis Light-near dissociation Parasympathetic* Dilate poorly
Tonic pupil (Note: Not all tonic pupils are due to Adie's syndrome)	Little or no reaction to direct light in affected eye; once constricted may remain smaller than other pupil for a while	Slow on affected side; once constricted may remain smaller than other pupil for a while	Anisocoria: Larger on affected side (prior to pupil reaction testing)	Light-near dissociation, may have impaired focus at near Parasympathetic* Efferent† Usually unilateral More common in young women (30s) Some areas of the affected iris may still react to testing Adie's tonic pupil is associated with a specific syndrome that also affects the reflex of tendons (eg, knee-jerk reflex)
Marcus Gunn (afferent pupillary defect, relative afferent pupillary defect)	Present/normal	Affected pupil enlarges or no reaction; nonaffected pupil constricts rapidly	May be oval	Evaluated by the swinging flashlight test Afferent†
CN III palsy (complete)	Poor direct and consensual response	Poor	Anisocoria: Enlarged on affected side	Parasympathetic*
Amaurotic	Absent in affected eye	No direct response; consensual response present		Efferent† Blind eye with severe retinal or optic nerve disease
				(continued)

	TABLE 9-1 (CONTINUED)			
	PUPIL DISORDERS (SIZE AND REACTIONS)‡			
Entity	**Reaction to Light in Affected Eye**	**Reaction to Accommodation**	**Shape/Size**	**Notes**
Iritis	Normal; light may elicit pain	Equal	May be slightly irregular Anisocoria: Smaller in affected eye	Red, painful eye Photophobia May be associated with injury or autoimmune disease
Angle closure glaucoma	Fixed	Fixed	May be oval Mid-dilated	Red, painful eye Blurred vision, hazy cornea Headache, nausea/vomiting Elevated intraocular pressure

‡Pupils are best tested with an appropriate light source (eg, transilluminator or indirect ophthalmoscope) in a room that can be completely darkened.
*The sympathetic nervous system kicks in during a threat (body-wide "fight or flight" response) and is controlled by adrenaline. Parasympathetic is "rest and digest" (confined largely to digestion; body is in non-emergency mode).
†Afferent is an outside stimulus (eg, light) being transmitted to the brain. Efferent is the brain sending a message to part of the body (eg, telling pupil to constrict).

If the pupils are normal, they will pretty much stay constricted throughout this test. (Note: You *may* see a little dilation of the pupil just as you hit it with the light; in this case there will be a corresponding constriction, then maybe a little pulsation of the pupil [known as *hippus*] as the eyes adjust. But these reactions should be roughly the *same* in each eye.)

If the patient does have an APD, instead of constriction you will see a dilation of the affected pupil when the light hits it. This dilation might be from barely discernible (graded as 1+) to blatantly obvious (graded as 4+). Then, when you move the light back to the unaffected eye, you will see constriction (usually rapid), again anywhere from barely there to easily seen.

Neutral-density filters may also be used to quantify the pupil abnormality. These filters are usually arranged in a holder and become increasingly opaque as you go up the holder. The filter (ie, the lightest density or lowest log unit) is placed in front of the normal eye and the swinging flashlight test is continued with each filter setting until equal pupil size and reaction is seen in both eyes. The neutral-density filter that achieves a balanced or equal response between the two eyes indicates the endpoint.

Learning to detect and grade APD is an art (Sidebars 9-8 and 9-9) with several variations.

There are a number of ways to record the test results (Sidebar 9-10). As with any testing you have to record your results so anyone reading the patient's record can visualize what was seen. A common notation is *PERRL*: Pupils equal, round, and reactive to light. Some clinicians also like the notation "w/o APD" (without APD)

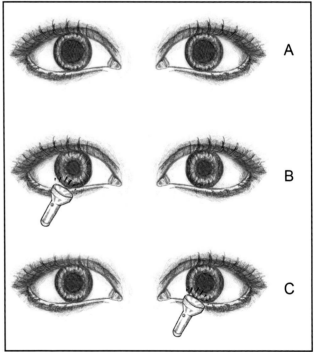

Figure 9-7. Swinging flashlight test. (A) Appearance of pupils in dim light. (B) Direct response to light shining into the right eye, and consensual response in the left eye. (C) Direct response is diminished in the left eye, causing the pupil to dilate when the light is swung from the right to left eye. This indicates an afferent pupillary defect in the left eye. Note that the consensual response of the right eye is similar to the direct response in the left eye.

SIDEBAR 9-8
DO IT BETTER:
PUPIL EVALUATION—
IS IT AN AFFERENT PUPILLARY DEFECT?

▶ Make sure your light is bright. It's been said that the most common "cause" of an APD is a dim flashlight!

▶ Even if your light is bright, if you're still not sure, get an even more intense light. The lamp on the headpiece of the indirect ophthalmoscope turned to high beam is brighter than a muscle light.

▶ Consider the patient's vision in the eye you think may be affected. An eye with an APD will almost always have subnormal vision.

▶ Consider the patient's diagnoses. Any of the following might have an APD:
  • Unilateral optic neuropathy
  • Amaurotic pupil (blind eye)
  • Trauma
  • Unilateral severe glaucoma
  • Optic neuritis
  • Extensive retinal detachment
  • Other neurological disorders

▶ The following diagnoses will not cause APD in and of themselves:
  • Media opacities (including corneal scars and cataracts)
  • Vitreous detachment

▶ Check at the slit lamp. Shine a thin beam at the periphery, just enough so you can see the pupil. (Don't shine it directly on the iris if you can help it.) As you watch that eye through the oculars, shine the muscle light into the other eye. The pupil of the eye you're observing should constrict. Do the same test on the other eye, looking for differences in the way the two pupils react. This is not an "official" technique, but may bail you out on whether or not an APD actually exists.

SIDEBAR 9-9
VARIATIONS OF
AFFERENT PUPILLARY DEFECT

▶ Affected pupil dilates when light shines in that eye.

▶ Unaffected pupil constricts rapidly when light is moved to it.

▶ Affected eye is fixed (does not dilate or constrict); unaffected pupil constricts very rapidly when light is moved to it. This is called detecting APD *by reverse.*

▶ Both pupils constrict with light, but affected eye constricts less than unaffected eye, which may constrict rapidly when the light is moved to it, a variant of detection by reverse.

▶ It is possible to have APD in both eyes. They may react to light equally if the damage is about the same in each eye (in which case you may miss the APDs altogether), or one eye may dilate a little more than the other when the light shines into it; this is the worse eye.

SIDEBAR 9-10
DOCUMENTING PUPIL EVALUATION

Normals
Patient 1:
Rm Lights On: 3.0 mm OU
Rm Lights Off: 6.0 ➡ 3.5 mm, PERRL, brisk OU, no APD

Patient 2:
Rm Lights On: 2.0 mm OD, 3.0 mm OS
Rm Lights Off: 5.5 ➡ 3.0 mm OD, round and brisk, no APD
5.0 ➡ 3.0 mm OS, round and brisk, no APD

Abnormals
Patient 1:
Rm Lights On: 3.0 mm OU
Rm Lights Off: 6.0 ➡ 3.5 mm OD, round, poor light response
5.0 ➡ 2.5 mm OS, round and brisk

Patient 2:
Rm Lights On: 2.0 mm OD, 3.0 mm OS
Rm Lights Off: 5.5 ➡ 2.5 mm OD, round and brisk, +APD
5.0 ➡ 3.0 mm OS, round and brisk, no APD

---

added, because this indicates an awareness on the part of the examiner that an APD is looked for on each patient. If an APD is found, make a note of which eye and grade the defect on a scale from 1 to 4, 4 being the most severe.

The notation *PERRLA* (note the addition of the A) is used if the pupils' reaction to accommodation is also tested and found to be normal. Remember, the pupils should constrict when looking at something close up. This response might be affected in cases of damage to the pupillary fibers, such as Adie's tonic pupil, diabetes mellitus, or chronic alcoholism. To test for accommodation,

observe the pupil size in room light. As you watch, have the patient fixate on a distance object, then switch to looking at a near object. The normal pupil will readily constrict at near then dilate when fixation switches to distance, and vice versa. Make a notation of any sluggishness in the reactions. If the pupils react to near but not to light (or more slowly to light than near), this is a *light-near dissociation*.

Angle Evaluation

The angle of the eye is where the aqueous humor drains out of the anterior chamber. If the angle is not open (either at all or enough), then the aqueous cannot drain properly. In some situations the angle may become blocked completely by the eye's own structures. This is the mechanism of angle closure glaucoma, which is an ocular emergency (see Chapter 29). One precipitating factor can be pupil dilation, which is done routinely in every eye clinic. It is therefore prudent to evaluate the angles for any likelihood of closing prior to instillation of dilating drops.

In the oblique flashlight test, a penlight or transilluminator is used to estimate the anterior chamber. The light is held at the temporal canthus area and the light is projected toward the nasal iris of the eye. If the temporal and nasal iris appear illuminated, this indicates an open angle. However, if the temporal iris illuminates and the nasal iris appears to be dimmer or in a shadow, this indicates a shallow or narrow angle is present (ie, the heaped-up iris casts a shadow across the pupil). At least two-thirds of the nasal iris should be illuminated from the light. A slit lamp evaluation of the angles is preferred (see Chapter 12).

Slit Lamp

The slit lamp or biomicroscope is an essential instrument for examining the external and anterior segments of the eye in greater detail. The physician may also examine the posterior segment with the slit lamp, holding an additional lens in front of the patient's eye. The instrument and various types of illumination are covered in detail in Chapter 12.

The structures of the eye are viewed with the slit lamp in a systematic approach starting with the lashes, eyelids and lacrimal apparatus, conjunctiva (including palpebral and bulbar conjunctiva), sclera, cornea, anterior chamber depth, angles, iris, and lens. Of special note are any media opacities that might explain decreased vision and indicate that refractometry might be compromised.

Conditions to look for prior to dilating the eye are narrow angles, rubeosis (abnormal blood vessel growth in the iris, usually due to diabetes), cells and flare (blood cells and protein particles, respectively), and any transillumination defects (where the red reflex from the retina emits through the iris). It may be difficult to detect any of these once the pupil is fully dilated.

Careful, thorough documentation is imperative. Anyone reading the patient's record should be able to visualize how the eyes appeared on any particular visit.

Tonometry

Tonometry is an indirect measure of the IOP of the eye. This measurement, taken with a *tonometer*, is one of the key factors in diagnosing and treating glaucoma. Tonometry measurements are obtained at annual visits and may be required at certain follow-up appointments. Results are given in millimeters of mercury (mm Hg). Normal tonometry readings are generally considered to be between 10 to 21 mm Hg, and measurements between the two eyes are generally within 3 mm Hg. A reading is recorded for each eye, along with the time of the reading (variations throughout the day can be greater in those with glaucoma) and which instrument or method was used.

There are several types of tonometers. Details of each, including how to perform the measurement, are covered thoroughly in Chapter 13. Because some methods involve the instillation of eye drops and corneal contact, any testing requiring clear media (refractometry, keratometry, corneal scan, etc) should be performed first. In some circumstances, IOP can rise after dilation, so tonometry should also be done prior to dilation to be sure that the patient does not already have high IOPs.

Best practice with tonometry is to perform the slit lamp exam *before* any drops are administered for either tonometry or dilation. The corneal surface should be checked for defects with the cobalt blue light before and after Goldmann applanation. Slit lamp techniques are detailed in Chapter 12.

Dilation

The technician is required to document instillation of any drop(s). Before administration, verify the patient's identity and that the patient is not allergic to dilating drops, and perform any testing that would be contaminated by dilation (Sidebar 9-11). For best practice, note the drop name and concentration, eye(s) instilled, and the time. Chapter 22 covers the pharmacology of dilation and cycloplegia.

You should also be thoroughly familiar with cautions involving pupil dilation. In the case of a new ptosis or new onset of double vision, a careful pupil check and EOM evaluation should be done before dilating. If there are any abnormalities in the pupils (reaction to light, size, shape, etc), this could indicate a specific problem, and the physician should be consulted. In addition, phenylephrine and some other eye drops may change the appearance of the lid droop or the angle of a strabismic deviation. A patient with a red, painful eye should be evaluated carefully for angle closure and not dilated until this diagnosis has been ruled out. Further, if there is any suggestion that there may be intraocular inflammation, the physician may want to check the patient at the slit lamp prior to dilation, as cell and flare in the anterior chamber can be much harder to see once the pupil is dilated.

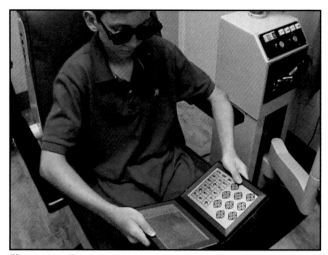

Figure 9-8. Titmus stereo test.

Additional Testing

Based on the results and/or responses from the patient during the history and basic evaluation, it may be necessary to incorporate some of these additional testing elements for a thorough and efficient work-up.

Stereopsis Assessment

Stereopsis testing assesses the ability to use both eyes and the brain's ability to fuse the slightly different image from each eye into one three-dimensional image. (For more details on binocular vision and testing, see Chapter 10.) Often this testing is done during the pediatric screening. Adult patients who present with a history of strabismus, new complaints of diplopia, or self-reported problems with depth perception should also be tested. Stereo acuity is sometimes required for physical exams and licensing forms as well. In order to get the best

measurement of a patient's binocular fusional capability it is best practice to perform stereopsis prior to any monocular testing (ie, testing that covers one eye and disrupts fusion, such as visual acuity).

There are several types of stereo tests. Each has its own instruction manual with which you should be familiar. The Titmus and Randot tests are used for school-aged children and adults (Figure 9-8). The Lang version is preschool age appropriate.

The test is done in good (bright) lighting. If glasses are worn full-time or for reading, they should be used. The test glasses can be worn over regular frames. Hold the stereopsis card/book at the normal reading distance of approximately 14 inches. (The authors recommend that you not let the patient hold the test, adjust the viewing angle, or move his/her head. These give additional, nonstereoscopic clues to the answers.) Ask the patient which of the test objects looks like it is "floating" or "lifting off the page," allowing a few seconds on each item (Sidebar 9-12).

An answer sheet gives the correct responses, which are measured in seconds of arc. The smaller the arc, the finer the patient's stereo vision. The test is stopped after two consecutive wrong answers. The results are recorded by noting what test was used and the finest stereo object that the patient is able to correctly identify.

Amsler Grid

There are several types of Amsler grids (Figure 9-9), and many offices have one that is preferred. This test specifically evaluates the 10 degrees surrounding the center of the visual field. Best practice is to perform and record results of this test when a patient reports a change in his/her central vision including distortion, a stationary dark spot, or a new onset of wavy, broken, or curvy lines. This test should be performed prior to any instillation of drops in the patient's eyes. Also remember this test will not evaluate the blind spot, which is located 15 degrees temporally.

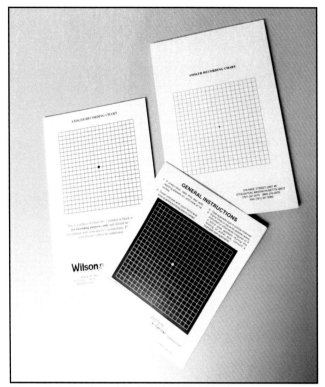

Figure 9-9. Amsler grids. (Reprinted with permission from Kim McQuaid, COMT.)

The grid is placed at a reading distance of 14 inches from the patient. Each eye is tested separately while wearing corrective lenses, if any, for near. Ask the patient to stare at the center dot. While staring at the center dot can the patient see all four corners of the box? Are any of the lines blocked out or wavy? Is any area of the grid blocked out or blurred?

Circle any wavy or distorted areas noted by the patient on the grid. If any parts of the grid are missing, the examiner will shade in those areas. Alternately you may ask the patient to use a pencil to mark the areas that are missing or distorted, but this can be challenging for some. It can be difficult to maintain fixation on the central dot and draw something in the periphery.

The grid should be labeled with the patient's name, date, and which eye was tested. If paper charts are used, the grid can be placed in the record. If an electronic medical record is utilized, then you must document the results by describing them. An example would be "Amsler grid OD, unable to see upper left corner; OS, blurred area in upper right corner with area of distorted lines just inferior to central fixation."

Color Vision

The ability to see the 380 nanometer (violet) to 760 nanometer (red) wavelengths of the electromagnetic spectrum is one of the many great qualities of human vision. Less than 1% of women have a congenital color deficiency. Men have about an 8% chance of being born with a red/green color deficiency. Blue/yellow defects are almost always acquired. There are several subjective methods to assess this particular quality of vision in the eye exam. Color vision testing may be performed on both eyes together (if congenital or job/license testing) or one eye at a time (if it may be an acquired color vision loss). See Chapter 3 for the physiology of color vision and designations for color vision deficiencies.

Testing for color vision is often done during the initial pediatric examination. If the results are normal and you have confidence that the patient understood the test, it need not be repeated at subsequent visits. It is best to perform this test after checking visual acuity and prior to shining lights directly in the patient's eyes or instillation of any eye drops.

For adults, color vision testing plays an important role in the neuro-ophthalmology exam because it can indicate the presence of optic nerve problems. It may also be needed if the patient is taking medication that can affect the retina (eg, hydroxychloroquine [Plaquenil]). Perhaps the most common indication is for job physicals and certain types of driver's licenses. In the typical adult eye exam, it may not be necessary to assess color vision.

The pseudoisochromatic plates, specifically the Ishihara's Tests for Colour Deficiency Test (Figure 9-10, *color* is spelled the British way) or the Hardy-Rand-Ritter

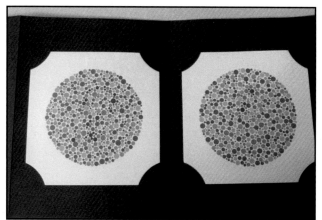

Figure 9-10. Ishihara color vision plates. (Reprinted with permission from Kim McQuaid, COMT.)

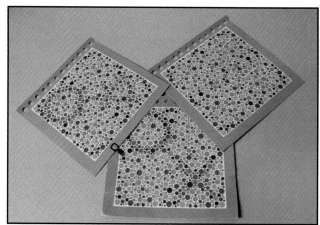

Figure 9-11. Hardy-Rand-Ritter color vision plates (Richmond Products). (Reprinted with permission from Kim McQuaid, COMT.)

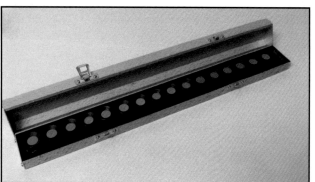

Figure 9-12. Saturated D-15 color vision test (Richmond Products). (Reprinted with permission from Kim McQuaid, COMT.)

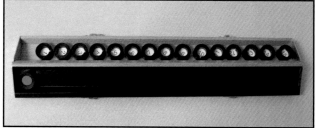

Figure 9-13. D-15 test in box, flipped over showing numbers (Richmond Products). (Reprinted with permission from Kim McQuaid, COMT.)

(HRR) Pseudoisochromatic Plates (Figure 9-11), are frequently used in the clinic to assess the patient's ability to see various colors. There are versions of this test made especially for children.

The plates present a number or symbol that is composed of colored dots embedded in a background field of contrasting dots. (The contrast may be very subtle.) A person with normal color vision will see one number/symbol, and a person with a defect will see a different symbol (or none at all) on the same testing page. The patient's responses are recorded and compared to an answer sheet that interprets the findings.

Ishihara's plates test for red/green deficiencies in a qualitative way, meaning that it gives a yes or no answer as to whether or not one of these problems exists, and which one. It does not tell you how mild or severe the defect is. The HRR plates also test qualitatively for red/green and blue/yellow defects, but give quantitative results as well by indicating if the defect is mild, moderate, or severe.

With the room lights on (additional lighting from the stand lamp may be necessary) and using the patient's glasses if necessary, hold the color book yourself, not letting the patient hold or adjust it. The patient is shown each page and asked to identify the symbol or number

without actually touching the page. With the Ishihara test, the first plate is one that is easily identified by everyone, even someone with a color deficiency. In the HRR test, the first four plates are samples to acquaint the patient with the test. Allow approximately 3 seconds per page. With both tests, the test can be stopped if a specific series of screening plates are identified correctly.

For the Ishihara, record the name of the test along with the correct number of plates identified from the total number of plates shown to the patient: Ishihara 12/14 OD and 14/14 OS. The HRR results are recorded on a special chart that identifies which defect exists as well as its severity.

The *Farnsworth D-15* saturated (Figure 9-12) and desaturated tests are also qualitative color vision tests that can be performed in the office. With the room lights on and additional lighting if necessary, the patient (wearing his/her near correction if used) must arrange caps of various colors in what he/she deems a sequential order between the fixed reference caps in the box. (The cap colors of the *saturated* test are fairly distinct [at least to someone with normal color vision] and the *desaturated* colors are very pale.) Maximum time allowed is 2 minutes. At that point, the examiner closes the box, flips it over, and reopens the box. The flipped caps are now visible, each with a number (Figure 9-13). The order of the

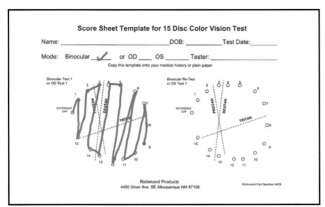

Figure 9-14. Score sheet for D-15 color vision tests (Richmond Products).

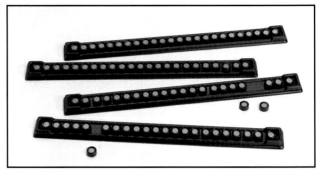

Figure 9-15. Farnsworth-Munsell 100 hue color vision test (Richmond Products).

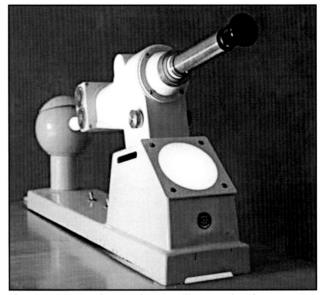

Figure 9-16. Nagal anomaloscope. (Reprinted with permission from Daniel Flück, www.color-blindness.com.)

labeled caps is recorded on special charting paper (Figure 9-14). Difficulty with certain hues/colors will be quickly evident by criss-crosses on the chart based on the patient's arrangement of the caps. Normal results will follow the ordered pattern on the charting paper.

The *Farnsworth-Munsell 100 hue test* (Figure 9-15) is similar to the D-15 color vision tests, but is much more detailed and time-consuming to perform. The patient must arrange 85 colored caps (the "100" is a misnomer) in four boxes in sequential order between the reference caps in each box. The examiner records the order of the numbered caps for each box and calculates the data plot for each cap on the special charting paper. Normal results show a circle of equal depth, whereas abnormal results will show variations or spikes away from the circle pointing to the color areas of confusion for the patient.

The *Nagel anomaloscope* is another color vision test, but is not used as routinely as the popular pseudoisochromatic plates and D-15 (Figure 9-16). This test is able to quantify a red/green color vision defect as mild, moderate, severe, or total. (There is a blue/yellow edition, but these are not found in the basic eye practice.) The patient looks into the instrument and sees a divided circle. The examiner controls the color of one side of the circle. The patient must turn a knob until the other side of the circle seems to match that of the preset side. The results are charted by noting the numbers on the knob as different test colors are presented then matched by the patient.

When performing these color vision tests, be sure to follow the instruction manual for each individual test. In general it will be required to have the patient's near vision corrected and bright, daylight lighting. (Be aware that some lights, such as incandescent bulbs, have a color tinge that can affect the color vision test.) Remind the patient to avoid directly touching the pages of the plates or the top of the colored caps to ensure the natural oils of the fingers do not diminish the colors.

Tear Testing

Adequate tear function is essential for good vision. Blurred vision, a foreign body sensation, and excessive watering are common symptoms of dryness. The physiology of the tear film and the lacrimal system is discussed in Chapter 3.

Fortunately, there are several fairly quick methods to evaluate tear secretion. It is important to determine which test you plan to use and incorporate it into the work-up at the appropriate time. For example, some tear tests do not require anesthetic drops; therefore, it is important to complete this test prior to checking IOP, not after.

The *Schirmer's I* and *basic Schirmer's* tests are tear secretion tests utilizing a small strip of filter paper (Sidebar 9-13 and Figure 9-17). Some brands of tear strips have millimeter markings on them; others do not. The strip is placed in the lower cul-de-sac between the lid and the globe (about one-third the way between the temporal and nasal canthi) for a specified period of time and then removed. At this point the length of the wet portion of the strip is measured.

SIDEBAR 9-13

SCHIRMER'S TEST CONFUSION

Unfortunately, there have been some items of contention where the Schirmer's tear tests are concerned:

▶ Schirmer's I without anesthetic and Schirmer's II with anesthetic

▶ Schirmer's (no Roman numeral designation) with anesthetic and Schirmer's I without

▶ Schirmer's II with anesthetic and irritation of nasal mucosa with a cotton swab

▶ Eyes open vs eyes closed during test

▶ Blink normally vs don't blink during test

▶ Room light vs dim light

▶ Prior to inserting strips wick away excess moisture with a twist of tissue vs more vigorous blotting of palpebral conjunctiva

▶ Look straight vs look up during test

▶ Test time 5 minutes vs half that to make test time faster

The best advice we can offer is to discuss the test(s) preferred by your practitioner and document exactly what was done and how (vs simply recording the name of the test).

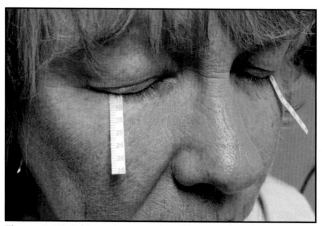

Figure 9-17. Schirmer's tear strips. (Reprinted with permission from Kim McQuaid, COMT.)

Schirmer's I does not require anesthetic; the filter paper is placed in the inferior cul-de-sac for 5 minutes. Evidence of 15 mm wetting essentially indicates adequate reflex (ie, due to irritation) and basal (baseline) tearing combined. The basic Schirmer's test requires an anesthetic drop in the eye prior to insertion of the filter paper in the inferior cul-de-sac. The idea here is to eliminate reflex tearing and measure only basal tearing. A wetting of 10 mm in 5 minutes indicates adequate tearing.

Note: The tear test known as Schirmer's II has not been listed in the American Academy of Ophthalmology's *Basic Clinical Science Course* texts since 2005, although it may still appear in other references. This version also uses the filter strips, but then a cotton-tipped applicator is inserted up the patient's nose to induce reflex tearing.

The *phenol-red thread* (PRT) test measures basal tearing function and can be completed in just 15 seconds. The test utilizes a yellow thread that turns red as it comes into contact with tears. Anesthetic is not used for this test. The upper 3 mm of the thread is placed into the lower cul-de-sac (about one-third of the way from the temporal to the nasal canthus), and then removed after 15 seconds. (Note: To avoid injury, have the patient open the eyes before pulling the thread out.) The length of the red part

of the thread is measured (including the 3 mm). Evidence of greater than 20 mm of wet, red thread indicates normal tear production.

The *tear break-up time* (TBUT or BUT) test is performed at the slit lamp using the cobalt blue filter after instillation of fluorescein in the inferior cul-de-sac. The patient is asked to blink once after the drop is instilled. At that point the patient is told to refrain from blinking, and a timer is started. The tear film will eventually begin to "peel away" from the surface in patches. When this happens, the time is again noted. A normal rate for the tear break-up of the dye is at least 15 seconds.

Finding and treating dry eye syndrome has become increasingly in vogue, particularly since so much of our population uses computers and hand-held electronic devices for a good part of each day. One newer diagnostic tool is called *TearLab* (TearLab Corporation). TearLab measures the osmolarity (in this case the salt content) of the tear film. The test takes a tiny amount of tears from the eyelid. It has been described in literature that increased osmolarity has a negative effect on the tear film.[4]

The TearLab osmolarity test should be performed before any other invasive testing, particularly before anything has touched the tear film. Daily calibration is necessary. Prepare the Pen as indicated by the instruction manual. Seat the patient in an exam chair and have him/her tilt the head back and away from you. Place the TearLab Pen near the lateral canthus to collect the sample. Do *not* pull the lower lid down. The indicator light will go off when sample has been collected. You now have 40 seconds to dock the Pen. Once the Pen is docked properly, push OK. Record the number and repeat the measurement on the other eye.

Margin Reflex Distance

For the external exam it is important to observe the patient's ocular structures for symmetry and note any

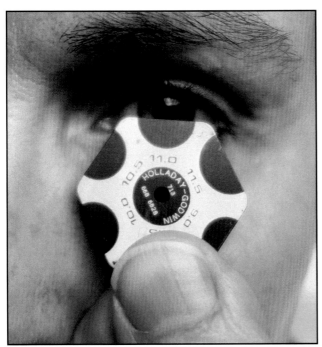

Figure 9-18. Measuring corneal diameter with a gauge (ASICO).

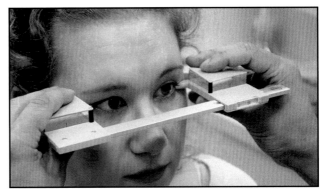

Figure 9-19. Hertel exophthalmometer (Richmond Products).

Exophthalmometry (Hertel)

The protrusion of the globe from the orbit, also known as proptosis, can be measured via *exophthalmometry*. The Hertel *exophthalmometer* (Figure 9-19) is one of the most commonly used instruments for this since it allows the evaluator to measure both eyes and provides a base number for the distance from the lateral orbital margins. This base number is then used for subsequent measurements.

▶ Sit at eye level with the patient about 1 to 1.5 feet away and place the outer edges of the device firmly on the lateral margin of both orbits.

▶ Ensure that the instrument does not rest against either eye/globe and that the patient is looking straight ahead. Note the number indicated on the slide; this is the distance between the right and left orbital rims. The instrument will be set at this base number when measuring this patient from now on. This ensures that future readings can be compared.

▶ View the patient's right cornea (using your left eye) and note the protrusion of the cornea on the scale above the mirror. Repeat the same process for reading the patient's left eye (using your right eye). Ensure that the red lines within the measuring scale are lined up.

▶ The base reading and the measurement for each eye are recorded.

The normal range for this measurement is 12 to 20 mm with a difference of less than 2 mm between the measurements for each eye. Patients who have a history of thyroid-related orbitopathy, trauma, or orbital tumors will need this measurement.

ACKNOWLEDGMENTS

Author Anna Kiss would like to thank the following: Peter Y. Evans, MD; Jay M. Lustbader, MD; Ella Rosamont-Morgan, COMT (deceased); and John P. Rowan, COMT. Editor Jan Ledford would like to thank Mark Lawrence, MD.

abnormalities. The opening of the eyelids, also known as the palpebral fissure height, is on average approximately 11 mm. (The average width is approximately 30 mm.) The *margin reflex distance* (MRD) is a quick set of measurements that provide additional information regarding the palpebral fissure height.

The *MRD-1* measurement is performed using calipers or a simple millimeter ruler to measure the distance from the upper eyelid margin to the pupillary light reflex, while the patient is looking straight ahead. A measurement of 4 mm is average; less than 4 mm is considered ptotic.[5] If the upper lid is below the light reflex, the measurement is a negative number (ie, the number of millimeters the lid must be raised to reach the reflex).

The *MRD-2* measurement is also performed using calipers or a ruler to measure from the center of the pupillary light reflex down to the lower eyelid margin while the patient is staring straight ahead. A measurement up to 6 mm is average; greater than 6 mm might indicate excessive exposure of the globe (and, hence, cornea) related to lid malposition, eye protrusion, etc.[5]

Corneal Diameter

Corneal diameter is often acquired for calculations prior to cataract or other refractive surgeries, and for monitoring corneal abnormalities, such as congenital glaucoma or large or small corneal size. Hand-held calipers, a ruler/gauge (Figure 9-18), or automated instruments are used to measure from the temporal limbus to the nasal limbus (termed *white-to-white*). The average white-to-white measurement is approximately 12 mm.

CHAPTER QUIZ

1. Which of the following is a *sign*?
   a. blurry vision
   b. photophobia OD
   c. redness OD
   d. pain OS

2. The consensual pupil check is:
   a. shining the light in the right eye and observing the left
   b. shining the light in the left eye and observing the left
   c. swinging the flashlight quickly between the eyes
   d. observing pupil size when the patient is looking at a near object

3. Why would an exophthalmometer need to be used?
   a. to measure the corneal thickness
   b. to measure globe protrusion or recession
   c. to measure corneal curvature
   d. to objectively observe the pupils

4. On which adult patient should we use the stereo test?
   a. an adult new patient with a history of strabismus
   b. a patient with complaints of diplopia
   c. patient who is self-reporting problems with depth perception
   d. all of the above

5. True/False: The iris dilator muscle is controlled by the parasympathetic ("rest and digest") nervous system.

6. True/False: The Farnsworth D-15 is a quick screening test for color vision.

7. True/False: The Amsler grid test includes checking the blind spot.

8. True/False: Schirmer's tear testing requires special tear testing paper.

9. True/False: Tonometry should be performed prior to the manifest refraction.

10. _____ visual field testing is a screening test because it does not need any special equipment.

11. One could expect a child to have a congenital color deficiency and adult with optic neuritis to have a(n) _____ color deficiency.

12. The history of present illness (HPI) is required for a comprehensive history and to support the chief complaint provided by the patient. List at least 4 of the 8 HPI elements.

Answers

1. c
2. a
3. b
4. d
5. False
6. True
7. False
8. True
9. False
10. Confrontation
11. Acquired
12. Location, quality, severity, duration, timing, context, modifying factors, and associated signs and symptoms.

REFERENCES

1. Vicchrilli S. E&M documentation requirements, part 4: the exam. American Academy of Ophthalmology website. www.aao.org/young-ophthalmologists/yo-info/article/em-documentation-requirements-part-4-exam. August 19, 2014. Accessed June 19, 2016.

2. Ebert MH, Loosen PT, Nurcombe B, Leckman JF, eds. *Current Diagnosis & Treatment Psychiatry.* 2nd ed. New York, NY: McGraw Hill Lange; 2008.

3. Sadock BJ, Sadock VA. *Kaplan & Sadock's Synopsis of Psychiatry.* 10th ed. Philadelphia, PA: Wolters Kluwer/Lippincott Williams & Wilkins; 2007.

4. Messmer EM, Bulgen M, Kampik A. Hyperosmolarity of the tear film in dry eye syndrome. [abstract taken from *Dev Ophthalmol* 2010;45:129-138]. Pub Med website. www.ncbi.nlm.nih.gov/pubmed/20502033. Accessed June 19, 2016.

5. Kim MM. Margin reflex distance (MRD) 1 and 2. In: Kountakis SE, ed. *Encyclopedia of Otolaryngology, Head and Neck Surgery.* New York, NY: Springer Reference; 2013:1577. doi:10.1007/978-3-642-23499-6.

BIBLIOGRAPHY

American Academy of Ophthalmology (AAO). Basic Clinical Science Course 2013-2014. Section 5: *Neuro-Ophthalmology.* San Francisco, CA: Author; 2013.

American Academy of Ophthalmology. Basic Clinical Science Course 2013-2014. Section 6: *Pediatric Ophthalmology and Strabismus.* San Francisco, CA: Author; 2013.

American Academy of Ophthalmology. Basic Clinical Science Course 2013-2014. Section 7: *Orbit, Eyelids, and Lacrimal System.* San Francisco, CA: Author; 2013.

American Academy of Ophthalmology. Basic Clinical Science Course 2013-2014. Section 10: *Glaucoma*. San Francisco, CA: Author; 2013.

Carlson N, Kurtz D. *Clinical Procedures for Ocular Examination*. 3rd ed. New York, NY: McGraw-Hill; 2004.

Cassin B. *Fundamentals for Ophthalmic Technical Personnel*. Philadelphia, PA: WB Saunders Co; 1995.

Cherry K. Understanding body language. About Health website. http://psychology.about.com/od/nonverbalcommunication/ss/understanding-body-language.htm#step1. Accessed July 4, 2016.

Ledford J. *The Complete Guide to Ocular History Taking*. Thorofare, NJ: SLACK Incorporated; 1999.

Ledford J, Sanders V. *The Slit Lamp Primer*. 2nd ed. Thorofare, NJ: SLACK Incorporated; 2006.

Riordan-Eva P, Witcher J. *Vaughan & Asbury's General Ophthalmology*. 18th ed. New York, NY: McGraw Hill Lange; 2011.

Saleh TA, McDermott B, Bates AK, Ewings P. Phenol red thread test vs Schirmer's test: a comparative study. Eye: The Scientific Journal of the Royal College of Ophthalmologists website. www.nature.com/eye/journal/v20/n8/full/6702052a.html. August 5 2005. Accessed June 19, 2016.

Stein HA, Freeman MI, Stein RM. *The Ophthalmic Assistant: A Text for Allied and Associated Ophthalmic Personnel*. 9th ed. New York, NY: Elsevier; 2013.

Sutphin JE, Verdick RE. The two minute eye exam [video]. EyeRounds.org and MedRounds.org website. http://eyerounds.org/tutorials/Two-Minute-Eye-Exam.htm. Feb 2, 2006. Accessed July 4, 2015.

Van Boemel G. *Special Skills and Techniques*. Thorofare, NJ: SLACK Incorporated; 1999.

10

OCULAR MOTILITY, STRABISMUS, AND AMBLYOPIA

Colleen Schreiber, OC(C), COMT, CCRP

BASIC SCIENCES

Ocular motility refers to the movement of the eyes. Each eye has six extraocular muscles (EOMs): the left (L) and right (R) lateral rectus (LR), medial rectus (MR), inferior rectus (IR), superior rectus (SR), inferior oblique (IO), and superior oblique (SO).

When one eye is out of alignment, the eyes will not be looking at the same object at the same time, and a *strabismus* exists (Figure 10-1). Children can be born with or may develop ocular motility problems. In adults, strabismus may arise due to muscle or nerve dysfunction. The incidence of strabismus in the general population is about 4%.[1]

Orthoptics, the branch of eye care involved with how the eyes move, originates from two Greek words, *ortho* (straight) and *optikas* (eyes). Orthoptists are allied ophthalmic professionals who specialize in evaluating the EOMs (see Chapter 1). However, the typical assistant will also encounter patients with motility problems. While orthoptics can't be learned from just reading this chapter, this material will serve as an introduction to strabismic deviations.

For information regarding the anatomical features of the EOMs, please review Chapter 2. Ocular physiology is covered in Chapter 3 and optics in Chapter 4.

Anatomically, the eyes must be situated in the orbits so that the visual axes of the eyes are aligned. (The *visual axis* is an imaginary straight line from an object to the fovea.) Each muscle must be properly attached and functioning normally with an intact nerve supply. The motor control system must be able to align the eyes so that they can keep the object of regard on each fovea, where vision is sharpest, even as the eyes move to look at various objects.

The six EOMs of each eye control *fixation* (what the eyes lock onto) and coordinate the eyes with one another. Each muscle has its own function(s) (Sidebar 10-1 and Table 10-1) as well as nerve and blood supply, thus there are numerous anatomic locations within the EOM system where abnormalities can occur. Since the brain uniquely controls eye movements, many neurological disorders can affect the EOMs as well as the muscles of the eyelids.

Visual development takes place during childhood, and requires specific anatomical conditions as well as physiological factors such as the *fixation reflex*. This reflex keeps the eyes in position when looking straight, adjusts when looking in another direction, and compensates for movements of the body and head. A *fixing* (or *fixating*) eye is pointed directly at the object of regard.

Fixation reflexes begin to form immediately after birth. By 6 months the reflexes for focusing and

Ledford JK, Lens A, eds.
Principles and Practice in Ophthalmic Assisting:
A Comprehensive Textbook (pp 137-177).
© 2018 Taylor & Francis Group.

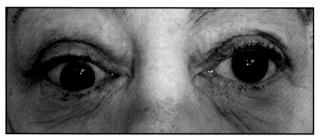

Figure 10-1. Strabismus occurs when the two eyes are not aligned with the same object. In this case, the left eye is looking straight, but the right eye is turned downward.

TABLE 10-1

ACTIONS, NERVE SUPPLY, APPROXIMATE LENGTHS AND WIDTHS OF EXTRAOCULAR MUSCLES[1-4]

	Primary Action	Secondary Action	Tertiary Action	Nerve Supply	Muscle Length	Tendon Length	Muscle Width
Medial rectus	Adduction	None	None	CN III	40 mm	4 mm	10 mm
Lateral rectus	Abduction	None	None	CN VI	40 mm	8 mm	10 mm
Superior rectus	Elevation	Intorsion	Adduction	CN III superior division	42 mm	6 mm	11 mm
Inferior rectus	Depression	Extorsion	Adduction	CN III inferior division	40 mm	5 mm	10 mm
Superior oblique	Intorsion	Depression	Abduction	CN IV	40 mm	20 to 26 mm	11 mm
Inferior oblique	Extorsion	Elevation	Abduction	CN III inferior division	37 mm	1 to 2 mm	9 mm

coordination are also progressing, along with binocular vision. *Fusional reflexes* are conditioned reflexes developed by experience (usually by 6 months of age), and include refixation movements to keep the image on the fovea.

Note: In order to bridge the gap between Basic Sciences and Clinical Knowledge and the Clinical Skills section, refer to Table 10-2, which lists various EOM entities and disorders and the tests used to detect and measure them.

Common Visual Direction and Binocular Single Vision

If the visual axis (also known as the *principle visual axis*) from each fovea intersect (meet) at the fixation point (ie, at the object of regard), it is said that there is *binocular fixation*. Another way of looking at it is if an object stimulates both foveae and the eyes have the same visual direction (*foveal fixation*), then the eyes are said to have a common subjective visual direction of the fovea.

A baby learns to develop *binocular single vision* (BSV) by coordinating the eyes so that a single image is formed by the process of fusion. (In this case the word "single" means one image, as opposed to double images.) If strabismus exists, each eye will be looking in a different direction and double vision (*diplopia*), suppression (where the brain learns to ignore one image), and amblyopia (vision loss due to prolonged suppression in childhood) can occur. These responses to diplopia are discussed shortly.

TABLE 10-2
EXTRAOCULAR MUSCLE ENTITY/FINDINGS PAIRED WITH TESTING

Extraocular Muscle Entity/ Findings	Test(s)*
Versions	Extraocular movements, amblyoscope/synoptophore
Ductions	Monocular range of motion Forced ductions
Stereopsis	Various tests (Lang, Titmus, Random Dot E, Randot) Amblyoscope/synoptophore
Fusion	Worth 4 dot Amblyoscope/synoptophore Red filter test
Fusional amplitudes	Prism vergences Amblyoscope/synoptophore
Convergence	Near point of convergence
Convergence insufficiency	Cover test Near point of convergence Base-out fusional amplitudes
Accommodation	Near point of accommodation Near visual acuity
Accommodative convergence/ accommodation ratio	Heterophoria or gradient method (+3.00/-2.50 lenses)
Tropias	Cover tests Hirschberg/Krimsky Maddox rod Amblyoscope/synoptophore
Phorias	Cover tests Maddox rod Amblyoscope/synoptophore
Paralytic strabismus	Cover tests Extraocular movements Bielschowsky's three-step test Hess/Lees/Lancaster Field of binocular single vision Double Maddox rod Ptosis assessment Pupil assessment
Restrictive strabismus/ traumatic	Cover test Extraocular movements Hess/Lees/Lancaster Field of binocular single vision Forced ductions Pupil evaluation ± Lid lag ± Upper lid retraction Exophthalmometry Color vision
Duane syndrome	Cover test Extraocular movements (assessment of narrowing/widening/retraction of globe)
Brown syndrome	Cover test Extraocular movements

(continued)

TABLE 10-2 (CONTINUED) EXTRAOCULAR MUSCLE ENTITY/FINDINGS PAIRED WITH TESTING	
Extraocular Muscle Entity/ Findings	**Test(s)***
Monofixation syndrome	Cover test Extraocular movements Worth 4 dot Stereopsis 4Δ base-out test Amblyoscope/synoptophore Bagolini After-image
Retinal correspondence	Bagolini After-image
Suppression	Worth 4 dot 4Δ base-out test
Saccades	Two finger versions
Smooth pursuits	Slow versions
Nystagmus	Hirschberg/Krimsky/cover test High plus lens/translucent occluder
Myasthenia gravis	Cover test Extraocular movements Ptosis assessment Ice test Sleep test Tensilon test
Multiple sclerosis	Cover test Extraocular movements Oscillopsia/nystagmus assessment
*Most of these tests are explained in this chapter.	

Common Visual Directions and Corresponding Retinal Elements

If a specific point on the retina of one eye shares a common subjective visual direction with a retinal point of the other eye, then these are said to be *corresponding retinal points* or *elements*. This is referred to as the *Law of sensory correspondence* and is the essence of binocular vision. Any retinal points that do not share a common visual direction are considered *noncorresponding points*. Corresponding retinal points (eg, fovea to fovea) are the essence of binocular vision.

The Eyes as a Sensorimotor Unit

The eyes work as a sensorimotor unit. That is, it involves the sense of vision ("sensory") as well as movement ("motor"). These must work in tandem to create fusion, allowing two images to merge and obtain BSV. The goal of EOM surgery, where muscles may be tightened or loosened, is to straighten the eyes. If this is accomplished and fusion occurs, then ideally the sensory and motor elements will kick in and BSV will result.

What Is Sensory Fusion?

In order to have binocular vision, the eyes must work together. There must be some sensory and motor fusion input for the binocular system to work well, functioning to blend the two similar images into one.

In order for sensory fusion to take place, the image on each fovea must be of similar size, shape, brightness, and clarity. Thus, anything that might affect these qualities can also affect sensory fusion. Other obstacles to sensory fusion can include ptosis, cataract, large uncorrected refractive error, and certain lesions of the retina.

There are many sensory tests (covered later in the Clinical Skills section) used to assess the state of binocularity. Such subjective tests require cooperation, comprehension, verbal response, and/or decision-making from the patient; sometimes results can be misleading.

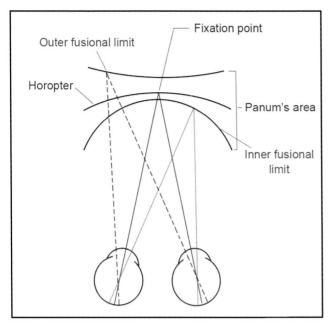

Figure 10-2. Horopter (arc representing corresponding retinal points) and Panum's fusional area (the area in front and behind the horopter that maintains single vision and gives rise to stereopsis).

What Is Motor Fusion?

Motor fusion is the ability of the eyes to hold a position in space so that sensory fusion can take place. Motor fusion is a function of the extrafoveal retinal periphery. When an image is not focused on the fovea, the retinal periphery is stimulated. This in turn signals the brain that movements need to take place in order to shift the image onto the fovea (fusional vergence). Obstacles to motor fusion can include mechanical strabismus, where there is a physical reason that the muscle(s) cannot move, or problems with the nerves that stimulate the muscles.

Testing fusional convergence or divergence amplitudes are examples of motor fusion tests because they measure the ability of the eyes to move inward or outward together until fusion breaks. These tests are explained later in the Clinical Skills section.

Fusion, whether sensory or motor, is always a central process (ie, it takes place in the visual cortex). In children if there are obstacles to fusion, a sensory adaptation to binocular dysfunction such as abnormal retinal correspondence (ARC), suppression, and amblyopia can develop. These are all discussed later. Adults cannot adapt and will present with complaints of double vision.

Retinal Correspondence

Note: Testing retinal correspondence can be done by various methods, discussed later under Clinical Skills.

The Horopter and Diplopia

A *horopter* is an area where fixation occurs when corresponding retinal elements are stimulated. A point seen on the horopter is perceived as single and flat because it projects to corresponding retinal regions.

Panum's fusional area is an area of vision just off the horopter where objects are seen singly and there is a binocular appreciation of an object in depth (three-dimensional vision; Figure 10-2). Disparate retinal elements must be stimulated within Panum's fusional area in order to be perceived as three-dimensional, otherwise known as *stereopsis*.

Points lying off the horopter (in front of and behind the horopter) may stimulate noncorresponding points, thus either double vision or stereopsis (stimulation of Panum's area) may occur. If the points not lying on the horopter are perceived by disparate retinal elements and seen as double, this is called *physiological diplopia* (Sidebar 10-2). This phenomenon occurs even when a person has normal binocular vision.

Pathological diplopia results from the simultaneous stimulation of noncorresponding retinal elements. This means that there are two different subjective visual directions (ie, the two eyes are not looking forward in the same direction). Pathological diplopia is caused by an abnormality in the visual system, such as strabismus or cranial nerve paralysis.

Normal Retinal Correspondence

Objects in the visual field will stimulate the photoreceptors in a certain spot of the retina of each eye, corresponding with where that object is. This retinal correspondence is what lets a person know where an object is located (to the left, right, up, or down). When there is *normal retinal correspondence* (NRC), the fovea of each eye will see the object in the line of fixation. Objects to the left of fixation will have a retinal image in a matching location on the right side of each retina (temporal retina of the right eye and nasal retina of the left eye) and vice versa for objects to the right.

NRC thus occurs when the eyes have a common visual direction. Both foveae and all retinal elements have corresponding retinal elements. If NRC is established and maintained by late childhood, it is there for life.

Abnormal Retinal Correspondence

Abnormal retinal correspondence (ARC) occurs when an image is seen with the fovea of one eye and a nonfoveal point in the fellow eye. Another way of saying this is that the fovea of one eye has a common visual direction with a nonfoveal point of the other eye. Since the fovea has the highest density of photoreceptors, fixating with a different part of the retina results in decreased vision in that eye. Stereopsis requires good visual acuity in *both* eyes, so it can also be affected by ARC. The farther off the fovea that fixation occurs, the greater the loss of stereopsis.

Children with large degrees of anisometropia (marked difference in refractive error between the two eyes) may develop ARC in an attempt to form a compensatory, inferior form of binocularity. The utilization of a nonfoveal point results in a small, constant strabismus that may or may not be detectable by a cover test. (See *monofixation syndrome* [microtropia], later in this chapter. Cover testing is explained in Clinical Skills.)

Because the two foveae are not corresponding, the quality of BSV and visual acuity obtained in ARC will be subpar.

Binocular Vision

There are four advantages to having binocular vision: single vision (ie, not doubled), stereopsis (the most precise kind of depth perception), enlargement of the field of vision (from 150 to 180 degrees [°]), and compensation of the blind spot.

There are three grades of binocular vision, which can be evaluated using an amblyoscope/synoptophore (see Clinical Skills). In *Grade I* there is *simultaneous perception* (the ability to see an object with each eye at the same time). In *Grade II* there is *fusion* (the ability to fuse two images into one). *Grade III* is the finest version of binocular vision where there is stereopsis. Higher levels of stereopsis occur with NRC and are related to visual acuity levels (ie, a person with NRC and 20/40 vision will not have the same stereo level as a person who is 20/20). Stereopsis requires stimulation of disparate retinal elements within Panum's area to produce a three-dimensional effect. If disparate retinal elements are stimulated outside of Panum's area, diplopia is experienced.

Interestingly, *depth perception*, unlike true binocular vision, can be monocular or binocular. For example, a person with only one eye uses monocular clues for spatial orientation (Sidebar 10-3). However, a monocular person does not have stereopsis.

Binocular vision also yields an expanded visual field. The visual field of one eye (monocular) is approximately 150° (90° temporally, 60° nasally). With both eyes open, the binocular visual field extends 180° horizontally (Figure 10-3). This expansion occurs because each eye overlaps a portion of the other eye's monocular field. The field of BSV is an area where both eyes work together and see objects singly. The BSV field extends 120° horizontally because it excludes that little bit of nonoverlapping temporal field. Thus is it smaller than the binocular field. In addition, the overlapping fields mean that the blind spot of one eye is "covered" by the other eye. See Clinical Skills on testing the field of BSV.

Laws of Ocular Motility
Definitions

See Sidebar 10-4 and Table 10-3.

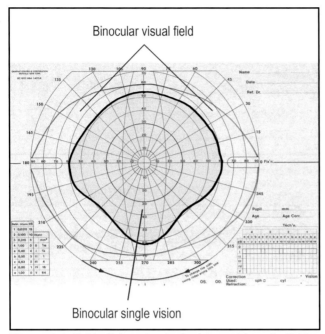

Figure 10-3. Field of binocular single vision vs binocular field.

Hering's Law of Equal Innervation

When a message is sent to an eye muscle to move, the corresponding muscles of each eye receive equal innervations to contract. This is known as *Hering's law of equal innervation*. For example, when the left lateral rectus (LLR) is stimulated to contract and abduct the eye, the right medial rectus (RMR) also receives an equal message to contract. Both actions are required in order to move the eyes into left gaze.

Sherrington's Law of Reciprocal Innervation

Sherrington's law involves the nerve impulse sent to an agonist (or acting) muscle to contract ("draw up") and an inhibitory impulse to its antagonist muscle to relax (lengthen). For example, in order to look right with the right eye, the right lateral rectus (RLR) must contract, and the RMR must relax.

SIDEBAR 10-4
DEFINITIONS

► Agonist—The primary muscle that contracts ("the mover").

► Antagonist—The muscle that opposes the agonist (must relax so that agonist can contract).

► Synergist—Another muscle that contracts (assists the agonist).

► Ipsilateral—A muscle in the same eye. For example, if the RSR elevates, the ipsilateral synergist would be the RIO; the ipsilateral antagonist would be the RIR.

► Contralateral—A muscle in the opposite eye. If it is a contralateral synergist, it helps the agonist keep the eyes parallel. For example, if the RSR is the agonist, then the contralateral synergist would be the LIO.

► Yoke muscles—Muscles that must work together; contralateral synergists. There are six pairs (one from each eye) that produce conjugate ocular movements. For example, the RLR and LMR help move the eyes into right gaze.

Extraocular Muscle Movements

In orthoptics, prism is used to evaluate, measure, and quantify extraocular muscle movements. The strength of a prism is indicated by diopters, designated by a delta sign (Δ) in order to differentiate it from the dioptric strength of a lens. (See also Chapter 4, Optics.) It may also be abbreviated *PD*, but the delta sign will be used in this text.

Saccadic/Smooth Pursuit

Saccadic movements are corrective, fast movements of the eye(s), generally controlled by the frontal lobe of the brain, which help keep a moving image focused on the fovea.

TABLE 10-3
EXTRAOCULAR MUSCLE AGONISTS, SYNERGISTS, AND ANTAGONISTS

Agonist (Right Eye)	Contralateral Synergist/Yoke	Ipsilateral Antagonist	Contralateral Antagonist	Ipsilateral Synergist
Medial rectus (MR)	LLR	RLR	LMR	RSR/RIR
Lateral rectus (LR)	LMR	RMR	LLR	RSO/RIO
Superior rectus (SR)	LIO	RIR	LSO	RIO
Inferior rectus (IR)	LSO	RSR	LIO	RSO
Superior oblique (SO)	LIR	RIO	LSR	RIR
Inferior oblique (IO)	LSR	RSO	LIR	RSR

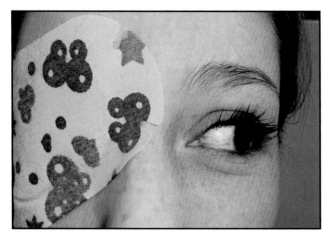

Figure 10-4. Ductions are movements of one eye. In this case, the eye is moving outward, or abducting.

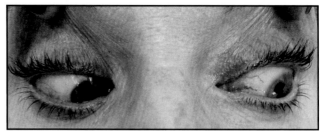

Figure 10-5. Versions are movements of both eyes together, in this case down and left (from the patient's perspective).

Smooth pursuit movements are slow movements of the eyes controlled by an area around the parieto-occipital junction in the brain.

By using a combination of saccades and smooth pursuits, the brain helps maintain the position of the eyes when the head or body moves. A disruption of any of the involved elements may occur with neurological disorders such as Parkinson's.

Ductions

Duction is the movement of one eye alone. *Abduction* is a lateral movement (away from the midline; Figure 10-4), *adduction* is a medial movement (toward the midline), *supraduction* (or *sursumduction*) is upward movement, *infraduction* is downward. Ductions can also include secondary positions such as dextroelevation (up and to the right) or laevoelevation (up and to the left). *Incycloduction* (*intorsion*) is a nasal rotation of the eye, and *excycloduction* (*excyclotorsion*) is a temporal rotation of one eye.

Ductions are tested by occluding one eye and performing the range of motion (ROM) test on the nonoccluded eye. While this test is described in more detail in Clinical Skills, it involves having the patient follow the muscle light while it is moved. The examiner watches the eye move, looking for smooth fluid motion as well as a full movement into each of nine positions (which includes primary [straight ahead] position).

Duction testing is usually done when versions (covered next) are noted to be abnormal. If the eye moves more fully in duction testing vs version testing, there is a strabismus that is likely due to some sort of paralysis. Observing no difference in an abnormal ROM in ductions vs versions may indicate some mechanical reason that the eye muscle(s) cannot act fully.

Versions

Versions are binocular movements of the eyes together in the same direction of gaze. Movement to

the right is *dextroversion, laevoversion* is to the left, *supraversion* is upgaze, and *infraversion* is downgaze of both eyes. Secondary versions may also include dextroelevation (up and to the right), laevoelevation (up and to the left), dextroinfraversion (down and to the right), and laevoinfraversion (down and to the left; Figure 10-5).

Versions are also evaluated by having the patient follow the muscle light as described above, except the examiner is watching *both* eyes to note how they move *together*. In addition to smooth movements, the eyes should be looking at the light together (ie, one eye is not drifting away) and should move together to the full extent of each position. Please see Clinical Skills for more.

There are six cardinal positions of gaze to test EOM function and movement (Figure 10-6). Simply up and right, up and left, down and right, and down and left and lateral and medial movement are included. (Interestingly, up and down are not included as being diagnostic since two muscles are required. All nine positions are considered, however, when checking ductions.) If an abnormality is found, ductions are tested.

Vergence

Vergences are movements of the eyes toward or away from one another (a motor response) to attain and maintain fusion. *Convergence* (both eyes move inward, toward the midline) occurs naturally when one focuses at near, and *divergence* is an outward movement away from the midline as near fixation changes to the distance. The fusional ability to converge the eyes is usually more powerful than divergence.

Fusional convergence takes place when our eyes move inward to avoid double vision. *Proximal convergence* is induced when there is awareness of a near object (such as a bug flying toward your nose). In this case the brain says there's something up close, so the eyes respond by converging. *Tonic convergence* is an inherent reflex that helps reposition our eyes from a divergent position. Under anesthesia, tonic convergence is absent.

Convergence amplitudes are typically between 20Δ to 35Δ, and divergence amplitudes are between 6Δ to 10Δ. Vertical fusion amplitudes are typically only 2Δ to 3Δ, but large amplitudes can exist, particularly in long-standing superior oblique palsies.

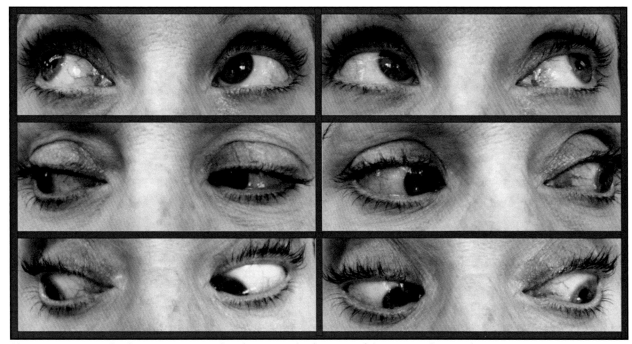

Figure 10-6. Six cardinal positions are used to determine the function of the extraocular muscles.

The range of vergence movements and fusional convergence can be evaluated using prism bars or on the amblyoscope/synoptophore. *Cyclovergence* is not often tested clinically, but it is possible to do so using the amblyoscope/synoptophore. These techniques are discussed in Clinical Skills.

Accommodation and Convergence

Accommodative convergence takes place when both eyes simultaneously accommodate and converge. It is measured at near since accommodation does not take place at a distance of 6 meters and beyond. The *accommodative convergence/accommodation ratio* (AC/A) refers to the amount of convergence needed for each diopter (D) of accommodation.

For example, to see something clearly and singly at 1 meter, 1 meter angle of convergence between the two eyes and 1 D of accommodation are exerted. This is a 1:1 relationship. (A meter angle is the reciprocal of the viewing distance. If an object is 0.5 meters away, the meter angle would be 2, and 2 D of accommodation are exerted. If the object were 2 meters away, the meter angle would be 0.5 [ie, 1/2]. The amount of convergence may also depend on how far apart the eyes are.) A person's AC/A is dependent on the amount of the individual's convergence per diopter of accommodation. A normal AC/A ratio is considered to be 3Δ to 5Δ/1, which means for every 1 D of accommodation, between 3Δ to 5Δ of convergence occurs.

The measurement of the AC/A ratio (see Clinical Skills) can be useful particularly in children who have in-turning strabismus. Some children with high AC/A ratios may respond to a relaxation of accommodation by lenses or other treatment methods.

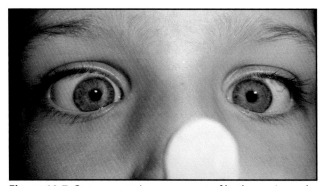

Figure 10-7. Convergence is a movement of both eyes inward.

The *near point of convergence* (NPC) is the closest point a person can converge both eyes while looking at an object (Figure 10-7), thus fusion is required. When convergence breaks, one eye will drift out. Normal NPC is typically 3 to 4 inches (8 to 10 cm). The test itself is covered in Clinical Skills.

A reduced NPC (ie, 10 inches or 25 cm), or *convergence insufficiency*, commonly occurs when one eye turns outward. A reduced NPC may cause eyestrain, headaches, and/or diplopia, and may be treated with exercises (covered in Patient Services).

Patients with a convergence insufficiency usually have a normal *near point of accommodation* (NPA). NPA is a measure of the accommodative ability of the eye, largely of interest during refractometry (Chapter 11). However, NPA may also need to be checked in cases of convergence insufficiency to rule out a combined deficiency.

CLINICAL KNOWLEDGE

Types of Deviations

Definitions

A *heterophoria* (or, more commonly, a *phoria*) is a deviation that is controlled by fusion and is referred to as a *latent strabismus*. It may be discovered by the disruption of fusion (as in covering one eye). A heterophoria may be a horizontal in-turning (*esophoria*, designated as *E*) or out-turning (*exophoria*, or *X*). Less commonly the deviation could be vertical: up-turning (*hyperphoria* of right or left eye, *RH* or *LH*, respectively) or down-turning *(hypophoria* of right or left eye, *R hypo* or *L hypo*, respectively). Generally speaking, if you look at a person who has a phoria you will not be able to see the turn. *Orthophoria* means that the eyes are straight.

A *heterotropia* is a constant deviation that is not controlled. It is often referred to as a *manifest strabismus*. It also may include an in-turning (*esotropia* of right or left eye, *RET* or *LET*, respectively) or out-turning (*exotropia* of the right or left eye, *RXT* or *LXT*, respectively). There is also a vertical heterotropia: up-turning (*hypertropia* of right or left eye, RHT or LHT, respectively) or down-turn (*hypotropia* of the right or left eye, RhypoT or LhypoT, respectively).

Many heterotropias are easily seen when looking at the patient, but some require specialized testing to verify. A tiny heterotropia (ie, 1Δ) would be difficult to pick up with the naked eye.

Rotational (torsional) deviations can also occur. These may take the form of a tropia or phoria, and rotate toward the midline (incyclo-) or laterally (exciclo-). Excyclotorsion is commonly present in fourth nerve palsies.

Intermittent deviation means there is both a phoria (latent) and tropia (manifest) component. In other words, part of the time the deviation is controlled by fusion and other times control breaks down and the turning eye becomes evident. Intermittency is designated by putting parenthesis around the T (for tropia); for example, an intermittent exotropia is written X(T). Fusion might break down due to our testing (ie, covering one eye during vision testing) or if the patient is tired or not feeling well. (The latter case is often noticed by a parent who will then bring the child in for an evaluation.)

An *alternating deviation* (A) is when fixation can be accomplished with either eye. This can be manifest (constant) or intermittent (controlled at times). For example, the patient might switch fixation and sometimes have an RET and at other times an LET, or could be even be intermittent RE(T) or LE(T). There may still be a strong preference to fix with one eye or the other. For example, the documentation AET/RET would mean there is an alternating esotropia, but it is usually the right eye that is turned; this indicates that the patient prefers fixing with the left eye.

Fixation may also swap equally between the eyes (ie, *alternates freely*). Alternating freely is good news. Since both eyes are being used, there is less likelihood that amblyopia will develop.

Deviations of every kind are usually measured in prism diopters and sometimes in *degrees*. One $\Delta = 0.5°$. Thus, if a patient has a 20Δ turn, this means that the eye turns 10°. These measurements are used to manage and monitor strabismus, and for planning strabismus surgery.

Eso Deviations

An *eso* deviation is a misalignment of the eyes where one eye turns in. It may be controlled [*esophoria*, designated by *E*], controlled only at times [*intermittent esotropia, E(T)*], or not controlled [*esotropia, ET*]).

An eso deviation can be refractive (due to uncorrected hyperopia) or nonrefractive in nature. In children this is only determined after a cycloplegic refraction is performed, refraction is prescribed, and strabismus is reassessed.

Eso deviations can also be categorized based on comparing the near and distance measurements. In a *basic* eso deviation, the amount of esotropia is the same at distance as at near. In *convergence excess*, the near eso deviation is larger than the distance deviation. If the distance deviation is larger than the near, then *divergence insufficiency* exists.

Accommodative Esotropia

An accommodative strabismus can produce an eso deviation related to uncorrected hyperopia, accommodative convergence, and/or insufficient fusional divergence. It can occur from infancy to later childhood, but commonly shows up at age 2 to 3 years.

Accommodative esotropia is the most common type of childhood esotropia.[5] Many children with this type of esotropia have high hyperopic refractive errors. Thus, the eyes must work hard to see clearly at a distance, and even harder for objects at near. The more hyperopic a child is, the greater the amount of accommodation required and the more likely he/she is to develop an esotropia. This is because convergence and accommodation are linked together. Some children have high AC/A ratios and tend to overaccommodate/converge, particularly at near.

Accommodative esotropia usually presents with deviations between 20Δ and 30Δ (smaller than a congenital eso that is simply due to a muscle problem), and hyperopic errors are commonly around +4 D.[6,7] It is treated by prescribing plus lenses, which may or may not fully correct the deviation depending on if the eso is fully or only partially linked to accommodation.

A *fully accommodative* esotropia is completely corrected by glasses and does not require surgery. The entire amount of hyperopic correction as determined by cycloplegic retinoscopy is prescribed. A *partially accommodative* esotropia means the deviation is not completely corrected with a hyperopic prescription and there is still a turn even when glasses are prescribed. Surgery may be required to correct the nonaccommodative portion of the strabismus.

Nonaccommodative Esotropia

A *nonaccommodative esotropia* does not have an accommodative component. The deviation is not significantly affected by accommodation or plus lenses. Congenital/infantile esotropia is often nonaccommodative, has a large angle strabismus (ie, 30Δ to 40Δ), and requires surgery.

Exo Deviations

An exo deviation is an out-turning eye. It can be controlled [*latent exophoria*, denoted by an *X*] typically by fusional convergence, controlled only at times [*intermittent exotropia*, *X(T)*], or not controlled [*manifest exotropia*, *XT*]. An exo deviation that is phoric, intermittent, or alternating will not develop amblyopia.

A small exophoria (<10Δ), usually greater at near, is common in the normal population. It is also common for newborns to have a transient exotropia in the first few months.

Intermittent exotropia is the most common type of exo deviation and accounts for about 90% of the out-turning deviations.[8] Unlike a phoria, it breaks down and becomes a manifest deviation, usually due to a lack of fusional convergence. That is, at times the patient cannot converge the eyes enough to fuse, so one eye drifts out. Thus, patients with either exophoria or intermittent exotropia may have complaints of eye fatigue, blurred vision, headaches, photophobia, and decreased depth perception. If the deviation breaks down and becomes manifest, some patients may complain of side-by-side double vision. A child's eye(s) may turn more when tired, if he/she has a cold or the flu, or when daydreaming. An adult may experience the same or notice symptoms after consuming alcoholic beverages or sedatives.

If an exo deviation is larger at near, it may be classified as a *convergence insufficiency* (CI). CI may also be associated with any of the symptoms mentioned above. The NPC and fusional convergence amplitudes should be tested. (See Clinical Skills.) CI may be treated using exercises or prisms in the glasses.

A *sensory exotropia* typically develops after the loss of vision in one eye because the eyes are no longer stimulated to coordinate. The eye with poor or no vision simply drifts out over time.

Exo deviations can also be categorized based on comparing the near and distance measurements. In a *basic* exo deviation, the amount of exotropia is the same at distance as at near. In CI, the near exo deviation is larger than the distance deviation. If the distance deviation is larger than the near, then *divergence excess* exists.

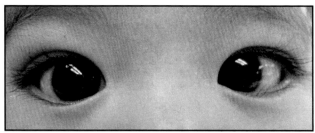

Figure 10-8. Pseudostrabismus is common in children, where the eyes appear to be crossed but aren't.

Vertical and Cyclo Deviations

A *vertical (hyper-* or *hypo-)* deviation or a cyclo (*incyclotorsion* or *excyclotorsion*) deviation can occur alone or in combination with a horizontal deviation.

In adults, a CN (cranial nerve) IV palsy (discussed momentarily) often causes vertical (hyper) and excyclo deviations, and an eso deviation may also be present. Torsion is typical with this palsy.

Vertical deviations also occur as a result of CN III palsies. Often the affected (*paretic*) eye is hypotropic (turns down) as a result of the SR or IO being affected, but can be hypertropic if the IR is affected more. Additionally, torsion may also be present with a CN III palsy but is not as common as with CN IV palsies.

Thyroid eye disease can affect any of the EOMs but most commonly affects the IR, and a hypotropia may be present. This disease can cause a hypertropia as well if the SR is affected, and torsion may also occur particularly when oblique muscles are affected.

Other disorders and diseases, including Brown syndrome, blowout fractures, and myasthenia gravis, can cause vertical deviations as well.

Pseudostrabismus

Pseudostrabismus occurs when the eyes appear to be crossed, but testing reveals that no strabismus exists. A pseudostrabismus can be differentiated from a true strabismus by assessing the corneal light reflexes to see if they are both central. Many babies appear to have an inward-crossed eye (esotropia) due to prominent epicanthal folds (Figure 10-8) that cover the nasal sclera. When shining a penlight in the child's eyes (described in Clinical Skills), the light reflexes are slightly nasal in each eye (normal). Often parents can be reassured that the pseudoturn will disappear as the child grows.

Paralytic Strabismus

Typical strabismus is *comitant*, meaning measurements of the strabismus are similar in different directions of gaze. An *incomitant* strabismus means the measure is different in another direction. For example, in a right CN VI palsy, the esotropia deviation will be worse in right gaze and less in left gaze. Children with strabismus or

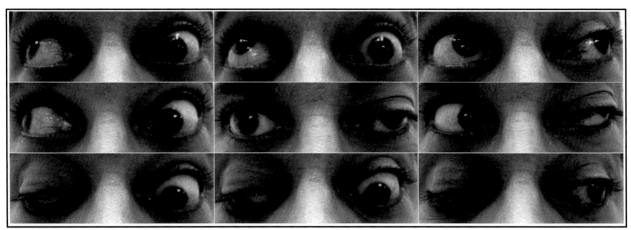

Figure 10-9. CN III palsy (here on the left) can affect all extraocular muscles except lateral rectus and superior oblique.

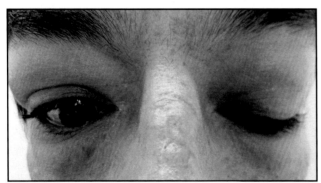

Figure 10-10. Pseudo-Graefe's sign shows a lag of the upper eyelid when looking down with aberrant CN III regeneration.

adults can have incomitant deviations due to syndromes, restrictive anomalies, nerve palsies, etc.

A paralytic strabismus can occur at any age but is more common after the fifth decade. Sometimes the cause of a cranial nerve palsy is idiopathic (unknown), but a neurological or systemic work-up is still necessary to rule out potential causes. Most nerve palsies will recover within 3 to 6 months. In the interim, double vision may be managed with prisms (see Patient Services) or by occluding one eye. If the palsy does not fully resolve, permanent prisms or surgery may be offered, but only after the deviation is stable for a period of time.

When measuring the deviation of a nerve palsy (using prisms and cover test, explained in Clinical Skills), the examiner must be aware that the deviation may be larger if the paralyzed (*paretic*) eye is fixating and the prism is placed over the nonparetic eye. This can be explained via Hering's law (described previously). When the nonparetic eye fixates, this is the *primary deviation*. When the paretic eye fixates, it is referred to as the *secondary deviation*. This difference between the two deviations is commonly seen in new onset palsies. Over time, long-standing palsies tend to have a "spread of comitance" (ie, the "gap" of difference between the two deviations gradually narrows) and eventually there may be no difference.

Third Nerve Palsy

The superior division of the third cranial nerve (CN III, the oculomotor nerve) supplies the SR as well as the levator muscle of the lid. CN III inferior division supplies the IR, IO, and MR. In addition, parasympathetic fibers travel within the CN III and terminate in the ciliary ganglion. These parasympathetic fibers supply the smooth muscle of the ciliary body and the iris sphincter. Thus, the pupil constricts when the iris sphincter is activated.

A total CN III palsy will cause the affected eye to be "down and out" (hypotropia and exotropia) with or without a dilated pupil and/or a drooping lid. A partial third nerve palsy can cause the eye to be misaligned in many different positions depending on which division or muscle is affected. A patient with a CN III palsy (or any palsy; Figure 10-9) must have the pupils checked, as a third nerve palsy with a dilated pupil is suspicious for an aneurysm, which could be serious if left untreated.

Third nerve palsies are typically acquired, but can be present at birth. There are several very serious etiologies including trauma, hypertension, diabetes, aneurysm, and brain tumors, but it can also be idiopathic.

Aberrant Regeneration of Cranial Nerve III

During the recovery of a third nerve paralysis (particularly those due to trauma), as the nerve heals regenerated nerve fibers from one location may sprout to another unexpected location. Aberrant regeneration of CN III inferior rectus nerve fibers may connect to the levator muscle, causing the upper lid to lag behind when the patient looks down (*pseudo-Graefe's sign*; Figure 10-10). If the MR fibers connect to the levator, then the upper lid will be pulled open when the eye is adducted (*lid-gaze dyskinesis*). Sometimes MR fibers or IR fibers get misdirected and end up innervating the iris sphincter; then the pupil will constrict on adduction or downgaze (*pupil-gaze dyskinesis*).

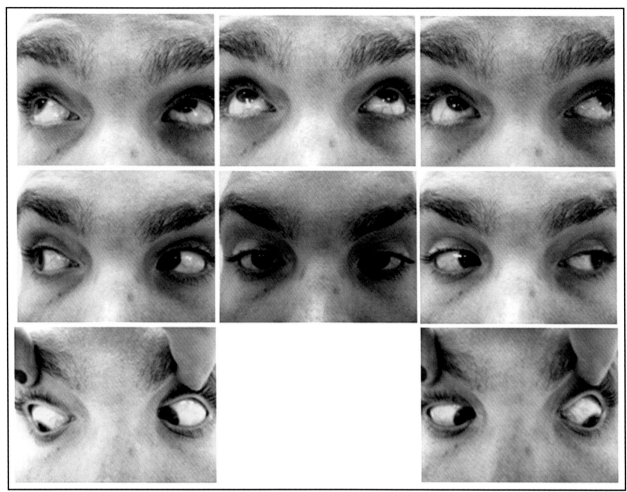

Figure 10-11. Bilateral CN IV palsy limits both superior oblique muscles.

Fourth Nerve Palsy

A CN IV palsy (*trochlear nerve palsy/superior oblique palsy*; Figure 10-11) typically causes a hypertropia with excyclotorsion, often worse in downgaze. Some may have an eso deviation as well. An SO palsy can be unilateral or bilateral. It is not uncommon to see a congenital SO palsy, although the symptoms may appear only later in life. Many people with long-standing SO palsies are able to avoid diplopia by tilting the head to the side opposite the affected eye, and may even demonstrate large vertical fusional amplitudes (an ability to maintain fusion by vertically coordinating the eyes). Fourth nerve palsies can be idiopathic or traumatic. After the age of 50, microvascular disorders may be to blame.

Sixth Nerve Palsy

A CN VI (*abducens*) palsy, which affects the lateral rectus, causes an esotropic deviation typically worse in side gaze (Figure 10-12). It can be congenital but is more often seen in adults, and can be caused by microvascular changes common to hypertension and diabetes, viral infections, trauma, brain tumors, and elevated pressure in the brain.[9] Like all nerve palsies, there are many other causes, and a neurological or systemic work-up may be ordered.

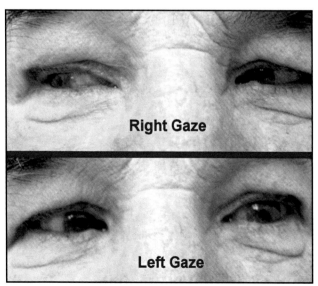

Figure 10-12. CN VI palsy limits the lateral rectus muscle.

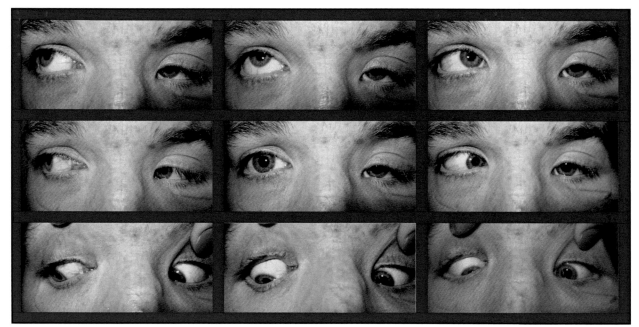

Figure 10-13. Left blowout fracture of all four walls with entrapment of muscles and severe limitation of movement.

Decompensated Strabismus

Latent strabismus can *decompensate* (break down) at any point if the patient does not have adequate fusional reserves. *Fusional* reserves are the strength necessary to keep an image single and fused. For example, a person may have a small esophoria all his/her life and then develop diplopia in the senior years. This is due to a decompensation of the preexisting esophoria. Diminished fusional divergence amplitudes are often seen, and intermittent diplopia and/or blurred vision are common complaints, especially when driving or watching TV.

Secondary Strabismus

Secondary strabismus can result from reduced use or stimulation of the fovea that prevents sensory unification of images. Common causes are anisometropia, trauma, corneal opacities, congenital or traumatic cataract, aphakia, macular lesions, optic nerve anomalies, and any other entity that disrupts fusion.

Another type of secondary strabismus is a *consecutive deviation*, meaning the deviation is now in the opposite direction from what it was previously. This can arise spontaneously or as a result of a surgical overcorrection. For example, an esotropia may be present prior to surgery and an exotropia occurs postoperatively. (If only a small esotropia remained after surgery, it would be called a *residual strabismus*.)

Traumatic

Trauma to the face and head can result in various ocular motility problems. Damage to the brain, nerves, and/or muscles can cause fusional difficulties, nerve palsies, entrapment of EOMs, and various other problems.

For example, a patient may present with diplopia due to lid or EOM swelling. Within a few days to weeks, as the swelling diminishes diplopia usually resolves.

The bones around the eyes help protect the eye from injury. A *blowout fracture* is a break in one or more of the bones in the orbit, usually the floor or medial wall because these bones are very thin.

A patient with a blowout fracture may present with diplopia, pain on eye movement, bruising, tenderness and swelling around the eye, and numbness of the cheek, nose, or teeth. Orbital tissues or muscles can herniate through the break and become caught. This is particularly common in a fracture of the orbital floor, where the IR extrudes through the broken bones of the sinuses. A patient with an IR entrapment may present with a hypotropia worse in upgaze and a limited ability to elevate the eye. MR entrapment would cause an esotropia with a limitation of abduction (Figure 10-13). Surgical repair may be recommended to release trapped tissues and/or muscle and to repair the fracture. Such a repair could include placement of synthetic material over the fracture site to prevent the globe from being displaced and/or to keep a muscle from pushing through the break again.

Special Forms of Childhood Strabismus

Monofixation Syndrome

Monofixation syndrome (MFS) is an abnormality of binocular vision consisting of a foveal suppression scotoma (blind spot), peripheral sensory fusion, and reduced stereopsis. It is a *microstrabismus* (ie, < 10Δ), sometimes referred

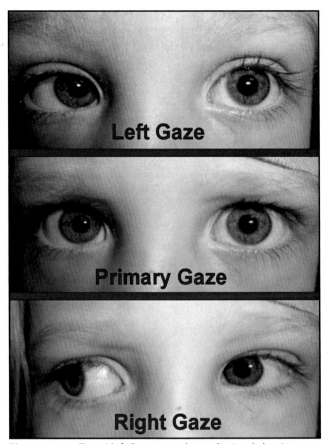

Figure 10-14. Type I left Duane syndrome limits abduction.

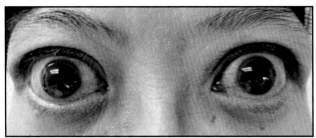

Figure 10-15. Exophthalmos caused by thyroid eye disease.

Brown Syndrome

Brown syndrome is usually a congenital anomaly but can also be acquired due to trauma, surgery, and inflammation. It is also sometimes referred to as *superior oblique tendon sheath syndrome* because the SO tendon is too tight or too short, causing a mechanical limitation. The syndrome is typically unilateral, and the affected eye has difficulty looking up and in. Often a downshoot of the eye is present on adduction.

Strabismus (typically hypo deviations with or without an exo deviation [particularly when looking toward the nose]) and amblyopia may occur. Some children have straight eyes and with impairment only on attempted adduction/elevation. The child may develop a head turn to compensate.[10]

Special Forms of Adulthood Strabismus

Thyroid Eye Disease

Thyroid eye disease (TED) is an autoimmune inflammatory disorder that can cause lymphocytes (immune cells) to infiltrate the EOMs. There is swelling and an expansion of the fat behind the eyeball, causing the eye to bulge forward (exophthalmos; Figure 10-15). A variety of terms are used to refer to thyroid eye disease, such as *Graves' eye disease*, *Graves' orbitopathy* (GO), *dysthyroid/thyroid-associated orbitopathy* (TAO), and *endocrine ophthalmopathy*. The average age on onset for TED is 45 years, and it is three times more common in females.[11,12]

When a patient is suspected of having TED, the practitioner may order orbital imaging (computed tomography/ultrasound) and blood tests to check certain hormone levels or to test for antibodies.

Over time the EOMs become enlarged and fibrotic. The most common muscle affected is the IR (which causes a hypo deviation), followed by the MR (causing an eso), SR (causing a hyper), and the LR (causing an exo). The obliques are less commonly involved.

Over a 2- to 3-year period, symptoms typically progress and then stabilize. Prisms or patching may be used for relief from diplopia. Patients often need reassurance if they are in the active stage, that further medical

to as a microtropia, and is most commonly an eso. This adaptive state usually occurs as a result of anisometropia or a strabismus (corrected or uncorrected). Abnormal retinal correspondence is present.

Monofixation is often detected only by specialized tests. Uniquely a small angle strabismus like this will have a small central scotoma (2° to 5°) with mild (one or two lines) to severe (20/200) amblyopia.

Duane Syndrome

Duane syndrome, also referred to as *Duane retraction syndrome* (DRS), is a congenital condition that involves mis-wiring of cranial nerves: a maldeveloped sixth cranial nerve that supplies the lateral rectus muscle, as well as an irregular innervation of a branch from the third cranial nerve, which controls the MR muscle. There are three types: Type I—abduction deficit (most common; Figure 10-14), Type II—adduction deficit, and Type III—both adduction and abduction deficits. The affected eye may have eyelid narrowing (and possibly an up-shoot or a down-shoot) on adduction. On abduction there may also be eyelid widening. The patient may use a compensatory head posture for BSV (eg, if adduction of the right eye was affected, a head turn left may be used to compensate). Some children have straight eyes in primary gaze and impairment only on adduction and/or abduction.

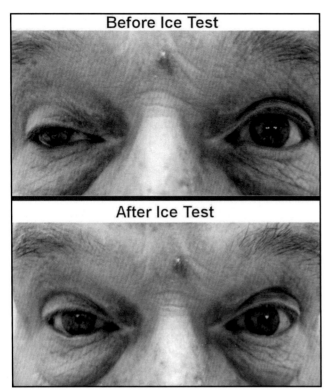

Before Ice Test

After Ice Test

Figure 10-16. Ptosis of the right eye is lessened after ice is applied.

intervention must be delayed until the inflammatory phase is over and the condition is stable.

Those with active disease must be followed closely for potentially sight-threatening compression of the optic nerve. Some cases may require orbital decompression surgery, which involves removal of some of the orbital bone(s) and fat to create more space, eliminate optic nerve compression, and reduce the amount of exophthalmos. Decompression surgery can potentially alter/create strabismus and/or change eyelid position, so it is often performed prior to any strabismus or eyelid procedures.

Neuro-Ophthalmic Disorders

Myasthenia Gravis

Myasthenia gravis (MG) is an autoimmune disease that affects the transmission of impulses between nerves and muscles and results in muscle weakness and/or fatigue.

MG can also occur in association with other autoimmune diseases, such as thyroid eye disease.

About 90% of people with systemic MG have ocular involvement.[13] In many cases, ptosis and/or diplopia are the first signs. Those with MG typically report that diplopia and/or ptosis are worse at the end of the day when they are tired.

The diagnosis of MG can be difficult and may include the ice test (ptosis often improves after ice is applied to the lid for 2 minutes; Figure 10-16); the sleep test (where the

ptosis or diplopia improves briefly after a 30-minute rest with eyes closed); Tensilon test (involves systemic administration of an anticholinesterase agent such as edrophonium chloride [Tensilon/Enlon] or prostigmin); blood tests; and electromyography (an evaluation of electrical activity of the muscle fibers).

If a ptosis extends over the visual axis, the patient may not complain of diplopia. For those who do suffer from diplopia, prisms or occlusion therapy may be needed. Typically strabismus surgery is not performed since this disease is variable in nature; however, it may be done in symptomatically stable patients.

Multiple Sclerosis

Multiple sclerosis (MS) is a chronic immune-mediated disease that attacks the central nervous system (CNS). MS damages myelin, the fatty substance that surrounds and protects the nerve fibers. Consequently, scar tissue (sclerosis) is formed. As a result, nerve impulses traveling to and from the brain, spinal cord, and eye can be interrupted, producing a variety of symptoms, such as sensory disturbances and motor weaknesses. MS affects people differently.

The effects on the eye may include optic neuritis (ON), oscillopsia (a visual disturbance in which objects appear to move), various types of nystagmus, and diplopia. If a patient has diplopia from MS he/she may have eye muscle weaknesses or palsies. Eso deviations and sixth nerve palsies are common.

Nystagmus

Nystagmus is an involuntary to and fro movement of one or both eyes. It can be *manifest,* meaning it is present at all times, or *latent,* which means only present at times. The latent form is often elicited in children with congenital nystagmus when the opposite eye is covered. This can create problems when checking visual acuity, because the increased movement can artificially worsen the vision. (When assessing visual acuity on a patient with nystagmus, a translucent occluder or high plus lens should be used.) Manifest-latent nystagmus is when both types coexist, so it worsens when one eye is covered.

Nystagmus can cause the eyes to move horizontally, vertically, torsionally (rotary), multidirectionally (see-saw), or nonspecifically. If characterized by a slow movement followed by a fast, corrective movement, it is designated as *jerk nystagmus.* The movement can also be pendular (drifting and corrective movements). Downbeating/upbeating nystagmus involves an initial fast phase beating in the downward/upward direction, respectively.

There are other types of nystagmus as well, including congenital or acquired from neurological problems or diseases, including MS and brain tumors.

Children in particular may develop a "null point," which is a head/eye position that may dampen (quiet) the nystagmus and stabilize an image for better acuity. Convergence may also dampen nystagmus. It is not unusual for a person to see 20/200 in the distance and 20/30 at near.

Surgery may be performed in those with nystagmus who have a null position. The idea is to realign the eyes so that the null position is now straight ahead, to lessen the head turn or tilt and hopefully improve cosmetic appearance. Some acquired forms may be medically managed. (The use of botulinum [discussed later] is such an option, although the results are generally temporary.)

Other normal forms of nystagmus are *endpoint nystagmus* (seen when the eyes are moved to extreme gazes) or *optokinetic nystagmus* (OKN), which is induced when objects are passing by. An OKN drum or tape may be used to assess visual status in a baby or in those who may be feigning blindness. (See Chapter 8 for more on malingering and hysterical vision loss.)

Adaptations to Strabismus

Note: *Amblyopia* is a common adaptation in strabismus and other ocular disorders. However, it is a rather extensive topic and is treated under a heading of its own.

Retinal Rivalry, Diplopia, and Suppression

When corresponding retinal points of both eyes are simultaneously excited by dissimilar objects or when noncorresponding retinal areas are stimulated by similar images, fusion becomes difficult. This leads to image confusion, and *retinal rivalry* may occur. In such a case, the retinal points of each eye are competing to be "the" image recognized by the brain.

When a child's eyes are straight but the foveae and other corresponding retinal points do not see an image with equal (or near equal) clarity, the brain will choose to ignore ("turn off" or *suppress*) the blurrier image. The suppressed eye, deprived of proper stimulation, may develop amblyopia and/or strabismus.

When an eye is abnormally turned, then noncorresponding points localized in two different subjective visual directions are stimulated. The disparity causes the object to be seen simultaneously in two directions, appearing doubled. In children, the brain gets rid of the confusion by suppressing one eye, leading to sensory dominance of the other.

If the child continually suppresses, this can eventually lead to a lack of binocularity and the development of strabismus (if not already present) and amblyopia. However, if a child alternately suppresses one eye, then the other, then amblyopia might not occur, since both eyes are receiving visual stimulation.

Adults typically do not have much ability to suppress a sudden-onset strabismus and will have diplopia. If the adult patient does suppress, a long-standing or childhood deviation should be suspected.

Common tests used to assess binocularity can also reveal suppression. These include Worth 4 dot test, Titmus stereopsis test, 4Δ base-out test, Bagolini striated lens test, the synoptophore, and the red filter test. These are covered in the Clinical Skills section.

Eccentric Fixation

Those with long-standing strabismus or deep amblyopia may develop eccentric (nonfoveal) fixation. Eccentric fixation occurs as a result of the inability to fixate centrally and results in the use of a peripheral portion of the retina. Usually vision is poor (ie, worse than 20/400). Often a head turn is noted when testing visual acuity.

Abnormal Retinal Correspondence

As previously discussed (see Retinal Correspondence), ARC is a type of adaptation to strabismus, particularly seen with anisometropia. In those who develop ARC, weaker binocularity is formed and results in subnormal fusion and poor stereopsis. Since there is not fovea-to-fovea correspondence, vision in the strabismic eye can be reduced.

Compensatory Head Postures

A *compensatory head posture* (CHP) may be adopted to fuse images. These can take the form of chin up or down, head turn (right or left), and head tilt (right or left), or in combination. If the position of the head is due to a nonocular problem (eg, a neck problem), it is referred to as an *abnormal head position* (AHP).

CHP is often seen in those with incomitant deviations such as Duane syndrome, V or A patterns, nerve palsies (commonly SO palsies), and thyroid eye disease (chin up head posture to avoid diplopia in upgaze).

Amblyopia

Amblyopia refers to a loss of vision (usually in one eye) during childhood, typically from nonorganic causes. Thus, most types of amblyopia are preventable and/or treatable if detected and treated early. It is seen in 2% to 4% of the population.[8,14,15] It is a sensory adaptation that most commonly occurs as a result of strabismus. (The colloquial term for amblyopia is *lazy eye*, although some patients use that phrase to mean an eye that turns.) Amblyopia is a risk factor for a reduction in visual acuity and binocularity. Timely treatment is imperative for the development of normal vision and binocularity, as the success rate declines with increasing age. Risks factors include positive family history, less than 30 weeks' gestational age at birth, less than 1500 gram birth weight, ptosis, and anisometropia.[15]

The capacity of the visual system to develop amblyopia is limited by its state of maturity.[2] When a baby is born, the visual system is immature because the retino-cortical connections are not firmly established.[2] Babies are estimated to have about 20/400 vision at birth and are often hyperopic. The eyes continue to develop, and vision improves as the baby gradually learns to focus. This is a critical period when any impediment to the development of normal binocular vision (ie, constant strabismus, anisometropia, and deprivation) can cause abnormal visual input frequently resulting in amblyopia.

The vergence control mechanism is not established in newborns. Proper sensory input and maturation of motor fusion must be developed into a well-integrated sensorimotor system to enable good ocular alignment and visual acuity. This occurs in the first 6 months of life and includes a maturation of the central fovea.[2] By the age of 7, the visual system is basically mature and the development of amblyopia would be unusual.[2]

By 6 months of age, children should have straight eyes most of the time. Intermittent strabismus is of less concern than constant a strabismus at age 3 to 6 months, when the visuomotor system is still immature.

Vision impairment from amblyopia is life-long and can be profound if not treated. If amblyopia is detected and treated at an early age, an amblyopic eye may recover vision even up to 20/20. At its most basic level, treatment involves covering or blurring the stronger eye in order to force the weak eye into use. (Treatment is covered more fully in a moment.)

The standard for detecting amblyopia is the visual acuity test, covered in Chapter 8 as well as Clinical Skills in this chapter. The usual definition is a difference of two acuity lines between the two eyes, although sources vary on this interpretation. Amblyopia may also be evaluated with other methods, depending on the age, maturity, and attentiveness (and mood!) of the child.

Types of Amblyopia

There are many different types of amblyopia based on clinical findings.

Strabismic Amblyopia

Strabismic amblyopia is the most common type of amblyopia. If an eye turn develops, a child's brain will often choose to suppress the turned eye rather than have diplopia, which leads to amblyopia from disuse. Children with a phoria, intermittent deviation, or alternating deviation will not develop amblyopia since each eye is fixating at least some of the time. Amblyopia is more common in esotropia than exotropia.[2,15] It is also six times more common in children with developmental delays compared to normal full-term infants.[15]

Refractive Amblyopia

Refractive/ametropic amblyopia is a result of uncorrected refractive error(s) and may occur in combination

with strabismus. It can be unilateral or bilateral. For example, a child could present with a high hyperopic error (eg, +8 D) in each eye. Initially the child may have a corrected visual acuity of 20/50, but over a period of a few months the refractive amblyopia resolves, and the child obtains 20/20 visual acuity in each eye.

Anisometropia with a difference of more than 1.5 D between the eyes can lead to a monofixation syndrome (explained previously) and anisometropic amblyopia.

Meridional amblyopia is a result of uncorrected astigmatism (> 1.5 D) in childhood. Meridional amblyopia is detected on standard visual acuity testing and cycloplegic refraction. A child may be found to have +3 D of uncorrected astigmatism. Once glasses are prescribed, vision may eventually recover to 20/20.

Visual Deprivation Amblyopia

Visual deprivation amblyopia is less common than other types[15] and is caused by visual problems, including congenital/infantile cataracts (most common), ptosis, corneal opacities, retinal disease, retinoblastoma, abnormal optic nerve development, glaucoma, and inflammation. In these cases the abnormality obscures vision in the affected eye, which then does not have the opportunity to "learn" to see. If the cause can be treated, it is imperative that treatment is initiated as soon as possible, as deprivation amblyopia can be the most severe and difficult to treat.[15]

Occlusional amblyopia (also called *reverse amblyopia*) is a form of deprivation amblyopia that occurs as a result of too much patching/penalization of the stronger eye during treatment (discussed later).

Other Types of Amblyopia

Nystagmus causes involuntary movement of the eyes, thus images are constantly swept across the fovea instead of remaining still and focused. If the condition is congenital, vision cannot develop properly, and mild or severe amblyopia of one or both eyes may occur. Congenital nystagmus typically appears between age 6 weeks and 3 months.[16] Some children with nystagmus have a mild reduction in visual acuity (20/50 or better), while in others it is more severe (20/200 or worse).[16] Nystagmus is discussed in more detail in Chapter 25.

So-called *toxic amblyopia* is actually better designated as toxic optic neuropathy. It is caused by substances including medications, tobacco, and alcohol. *Nutritional amblyopia* is in this same category, actually being an optic neuropathy caused by lack of adequate nutrients.

Management of Amblyopia

Amblyopia treatment success depends on the age of onset, cause, severity, and duration of amblyopia, as well as type of treatment prescribed and adherence to therapy.[15] Early detection of childhood amblyopia is crucial as treatment is most successful before the age of 7, although

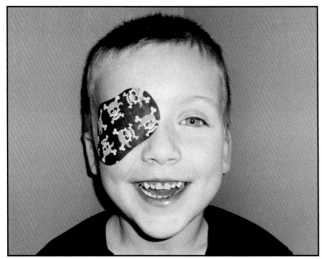

Figure 10-17. Stick-on patch for amblyopia occlusion treatment.

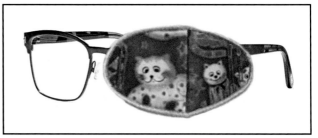

Figure 10-18. Patch on glasses lens for amblyopia occlusion treatment.

some literature supports treatment even into the teenage years.[15,17,18]

The time it takes to see maximum improvement of amblyopia varies from patient to patient and is typically shorter for a younger child.[18] There are several means of treatment, but each focuses on strengthening the amblyopic eye by forcing the patient to use it.

Surgery

Strabismus surgery is performed to align the eyes. Surgery involves loosening and/or tightening muscle(s), sometimes in one eye or sometimes in both. The goal(s) of surgery might include improvement of BSV, stereopsis, and cosmesis, as well as reduction/elimination of diplopia (particularly in adult patients).

In strabismus, amblyopia is treated first so both eyes have best visual acuity before surgery. Then when the eyes are more properly aligned, there is a better chance to gain binocularity (especially if the vision is equal) because the eyes will lock together.

If the cause of a deprivation amblyopia is correctable with surgery, this is usually dealt with first and then followed with amblyopia treatment.

Refractive surgery in children as a treatment for anisometropic amblyopia, bilateral refractive amblyopia, or for those who fail conventional treatment is controversial.[15]

Optical Correction

Untreated anisometropic and strabismic amblyopia is often improved with the correction of refractive errors alone, thus glasses must be prescribed along with other types of amblyopia treatment.[15] Bilateral refractive amblyopia substantially improves with the correction of the refractive error.[15]

Children typically tolerate eyeglasses well due to the improvement in visual acuity. For safety, polycarbonate lenses may be advised. Flexible frames and head straps may be recommended in babies and young children.

Patching

Occlusion involves covering the stronger eye, and can be done on a full- or part-time basis. For example, children with deep amblyopia (ie, 20/400) may need a minimum of 6 hours a day up to all waking hours. Patching is continued until the visual acuity becomes equal in each eye or until there is no improvement after 3 to 6 months. Patching is gradually decreased. If a child has been patched more than 6 hours a day, the chance of recurrence is greater if patching is abruptly discontinued.[15]

There are various types of patches available. Sticky patches are recommended (Figure 10-17). Mild skin irritation often occurs with patching; trying a different patch brand and/or applying skin lotion when the patch is off may help. Cloth patches may be used over glasses (Figure 10-18), but the temptation to peek around it may be too strong. This type of patch is also easy to pull off once the parents disappear around the corner. Arms splints may be used in babies or preverbal children who are not compliant. (This makes them unable to bend their elbows to reach the patch and pull it off.)

Occlusional amblyopia of a patched dominant eye can result during treatment from covering the good eye too much or for too long, but it is almost always reversible. To undo this problem, the formerly amblyopic eye is judiciously patched to improve and restore the originally better-seeing eye. Careful professional monitoring is needed to prevent and resolve this situation.

Children have to be continually evaluated in case the amblyopia returns. Maintenance patching may be needed for some.

Penalization

Penalization involves blurring the good eye through cycloplegic eye drops (*pharmacological penalization*) or lenses/filters (*optical penalization*). It can be a first line of treatment, a second choice (eg, if patching is not working due to noncompliance), or for maintenance. In order for penalization to be effective, the dominant eye must be adequately blurred in order for the amblyopic eye to "want" to work on improvement.

In pharmacological penalization, atropine 1% is instilled into the stronger eye in order to decrease accommodation and the ability to focus. This method is typically used in children over the age of 3.[15] Pharmacological penalization may not work well with deep amblyopia if the fixating eye still maintains better acuity even with the atropine.

Some parents may not be keen on having their child on atropine as there can be side effects, such as photosensitivity due to a dilated pupil (18%) and conjunctival irritation (4%).[15] In addition, other children may comment on the difference between the patient's eyes. Atropine may be given on a daily basis; some physicians may recommend only weekend use.

Optical penalization tends to be recommended less frequently. It involves prescribing glasses with a strong enough plus lens to create a blurred image in the stronger eye. Alternately, a frosted Bangerter filter (a thin translucent paper that resembles waxed paper) might be placed on the lens of the stronger eye.

Amblyopia Follow-Up

Amblyopic children are followed by the ophthalmologist and orthoptist monthly or every few months to monitor therapy results and adjust the treatment plan. Timing varies according to the age of the child and intensity of treatment initiated. Adherence to therapy, side effects, and improvement in visual acuity are noted. A consistent testing environment, using similar charts and a friendly and fun atmosphere, are key. A refraction should be done once yearly to ensure refractive errors are corrected properly.

Maintenance therapy using occlusion, cycloplegia, or optical penalization may be implemented as amblyopia can recur. There is a recurrence rate of 25% within the first year after the conclusion of treatment.[15]

CLINICAL SKILLS

Basic Work-Up

Strabismus testing (especially in children) follows a specific protocol. This is important because some tests should be done before other tests that dissociate the eyes (ie, by occlusion). The correct order of the exam is history, stereo testing, Worth 4 dot testing, prism vergences, and then visual acuity. Before starting, you must gauge the level of cooperation you are likely to get. You may have to alter your strategy and start with the most important test(s) first.

History Taking

Chapter 7 covers taking the ophthalmic history. However, when taking a history on a child or adult with strabismus or diplopia, additional questions should be asked:

▸ Onset (since birth, 2 days ago, etc): Gradual or sudden?

▸ Any precipitating cause (eg, illness, trauma, etc); any prior surgery, treatments, or therapy for strabismus or other eye conditions. Asking about diplopia is very important in patients who have had facial trauma.

▸ Birth history (gestation, delivery, weight, etc), developmental history (milestones—delayed/average).

▸ Family history of strabismus, nystagmus, or other eye diseases/disorders.

▸ General health and medications, recent testing (blood work, magnetic resonance imaging, etc).

▸ Is the diplopia horizontal, vertical, or oblique? Does the diplopia go away if one eye is covered? If the other eye is covered?

▸ Is the turn or diplopia intermittent or constant? Do the symptoms occur at near and/or distance or associated with any specific task?

Vision Testing and Detection of Amblyopia

Chapter 8 discusses visual acuity in great detail, and a review of pediatric acuity testing will be helpful, specifically: fix and follow; fixation steady, central, and maintained (CSM); behavioral response to occlusion; preferential looking; optokinetic drum; Teller Acuity Cards; logMAR charts; and crowding phenomenon and crowding bars.

Strabismic amblyopia is a difference of visual acuity of two lines or more (>0.2 logMAR) between the eyes. The type of tests used to detect amblyopia will depend on the age, maturity, and cooperation of the child. It is ideal if a child can name or match letters on a full chart/line because if optotypes are isolated, amblyopic vision often appears better than it actually is (this is called the *crowding phenomenon*). (See vision testing procedures in Chapter 8).

Preferential looking using Teller Acuity Cards and logMAR charts are often used to test for amblyopia. If the child can match or verbalize, optotypes with 0.1 logMAR decrements should be used, preferably Lea symbols, Sloan, HOTV, or the tumbling E.[15]

In infants and small children, an evaluation for amblyopia may be done by assessing if fixation is CSM. One method is to simply have the child fixate on an accommodative target held at 40 cm. One eye is occluded, which forces the other eye to fixate. Then the other eye is occluded, and the other eye is forced to take up fixation. Once the occluder is removed, if the nonoccluded eye continues to fixate and maintains through a blink or two, then fixation is graded as CSM. If an eye fails to maintain fixation through a blink or spontaneously changes the fixation to the other eye upon removal of the occluder, this is graded as central, steady, and *unmaintained* (CSUM). If fixation is unsteady (ie, uncovered, fixating eye wanders off repeatedly), fixation is called *unsteady* and graded as central, unsteady, and unmaintained (CUSUM). If an eye does not take up fixation at all when the other eye is occluded, this is graded as *uncentral, unsteady, and unmaintained* (UCUSUM) or wandering fixation. An eye that is uncentral, unsteady, and/or unmaintained is more likely to be amblyopic.

The baby's behavioral response to alternate occlusion of each eye may also be assessed. If a child objects to occlusion of one eye in particular, it could mean there is amblyopia of the opposite eye. A child will usually react, sometimes strongly, if the only good eye is covered. If the child objects to occlusion of both eyes, he/she may have bilateral amblyopia or simply does not like to be messed with.

Another method to assess for amblyopia in preverbal children is the 10Δ or induced vertical tropia test. This test uses a 10Δ prism held base-down or base-up to induce a vertical tropia. If the child can hold fixation of either eye, then amblyopia is likely not present. If there is a strong fixation preference, then amblyopia may be present. For example, if the prism is placed over the right eye and the right eye fixates, and then if it is placed over the left eye but the right eye continues to fixate, then amblyopia of the left eye may be present.

If a child is being patched as treatment for amblyopia, check vision in the amblyopic eye first. In all cases, be careful to monitor occlusion. Children frequently peek, so patches are more reliable than hand-held occluders or Mom's hand.

In children or adults with nystagmus, vision should be tested at distance and at near, as convergence often dampens nystagmus, and thus visual acuity is often much better at near. Nystagmus patients should have each eye tested both separately and together at both distances and occluded with a high plus lens (eg, +8) or a translucent occluder, rather than a conventional occluder. Allow testing to be done with any compensatory head posture.

Refractometry

All children with decreased vision or ocular motility problems should have both a nondilated and a cycloplegic refractive exam annually to uncover any latent refractive error. A common mistake is to forgo cycloplegic refractometry. Cycloplegic refractometry helps determine the full amount of hyperopia in patients with accommodative esotropia and prevents overcorrection in myopic patients. (See Chapter 11 for more on accommodation and refractometry.) Cyclopentolate 1% and atropine 1% are commonly used.

Cycloplegic measurements can also be useful in young adults with *asthenopic* ("eyestrain") symptoms who use their accommodation to compensate for a hyperopic refractive error. It can also uncover reasons for blurred vision or headaches (including those due to latent nystagmus) after sustained reading or changing focus from near to far caused by latent hyperopia, or to confirm the diagnosis of accommodative spasm.

Pupil Testing

A pupil assessment is mandatory for any patient with diplopia and/or a strabismus. (See Chapters 9 and 25.) A dilated pupil from a CN III palsy could indicate an aneurysm or other problem that could be a neurological

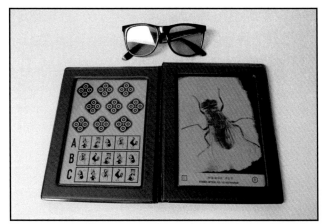

Figure 10-19. Titmus test with polarized glasses (Precision Vision).

emergency. In thyroid eye disease, patients may or may not experience diplopia, but the pupils should be assessed at each visit for a relative afferent pupillary defect (RAPD) in the event of optic nerve involvement.

Fusional Tests

Fusion assessment is essential both for the prognosis and management of strabismus. Fusion must exist for the maintenance and restoration of BSV. Various fusional tests are utilized to determine the presence and extent of fusion.

Stereopsis

In an orthoptic exam, stereopsis is one of the first clinical tests used. It should be performed *before* the Worth 4 dot test, cover test, or even visual acuity, to avoid dissociation of the eyes. If stereopsis exists, it likely indicates the patient has some form of binocularity and is not suppressing. Stereo acuity is maximal at about 0.25° from the fovea, diminishes rapidly from this point outward, and does not exist beyond 15° of the fovea.[19]

Most tests for stereopsis use targets which lie in two planes and stimulate disparate retinal elements in order to give a three-dimensional effect. Common tests include the Titmus test (measures 3000 to 40 seconds of arc), Lang's stereo I and II tests (200 to 1200 seconds of arc), Random dot E, Randot stereo and TNO (The Netherlands Optical Society) tests, and Frisby test. Stereoscopic targets can also be presented on the synoptophore.

With polarization tests such as the Titmus (covered here), Random dot E, and TNO, images are polarized at 90° and are viewed using polarized glasses. Not all children, however, will consent to wear the glasses and other tests can be used, such as the Frisby test or Lang's two-pencil test (covered momentarily).

The commonly used Titmus stereo test (Figure 10-19 and Sidebar 10-5) includes a three-dimensional fly (3000 seconds of arc, or gross/peripheral stereopsis); three rows

---

SIDEBAR 10-5

DO IT BETTER: POLARIZED STEREOPSIS TEST

▶ Put the glasses on yourself. Then ask the child, "Can you wear my fancy sunglasses for a minute?"

▶ If a child is reluctant to put on the glasses, have Mommy try them on first. "Doesn't she look cool? Do you want to try them?"

▶ For the Titmus test, ask the child "Can you pick up the fly's wings? Can you pick out the animal that is popping out in this row? Can you push the circle that is popping out in this box?" For older children, teens, and adults, you can go directly to the circles part of the test (but everyone seems to enjoy picking up that three-dimensional fly!).

▶ If a patient has trouble seeing the circles, jiggle the test booklet a little. (This is more of a vibration, not a wild shaking!) This sometimes makes the dissociated images "pop up."

▶ Be sure that the patient is keeping both eyes open.

▶ If you suspect that the patient has memorized the answers, turn the booklet upside down. The disparate images will now look as if they're sinking.

▶ If you suspect the patient may be suppressing, go back to the fly and ask if he/she sees anything in the circle and square in the lower corners. If he/she is not suppressing, he/she will report seeing the R and L simultaneously (but be aware of alternating suppression!).

▶ The test is concluded once the patient gives two wrong answers in a row. The stereo acuity is then recorded as the last correct response.

▶ If you're not sure if the patient has a phoria or tropia, do a stereo test. Someone who is not using both eyes together will not have fine stereo acuity.

---

of animals, in which one animal in each row is imaged disparately (400, 200, and 100 seconds of arc); and nine sets of four circles, each set arranged in the form of a diamond (800, 400, 200, 140, 100, 80, 60, 50, and 40 seconds of arc). In the circle sequence, one circle in each set is disparate at random. Beneath the fly, there are the letters "R" and "L." If the patient cannot see these two letters at the same time, then he/she is suppressing or diplopic.

If the patient normally wears glasses, put the polarized glasses on over them. The test booklet is held at 16 inches, and the patient is asked to "pinch" the fly's wings. If gross stereopsis exists, the patient will use a scooping motion or stop the fingers just above the page. Some children might refuse to "touch" the fly. (An ugly critter was selected because gross stereopsis makes the fly look very

real and repulsive three-dimensionally.) Patients who respond to the "ugh factor" are likely to have at least some level of stereopsis.

If the child patient responds to the fly, next ask him/her to find which animal is "closer" in each row. "See this row of animals? Which one looks like it's sticking up, closer to you? Can you push it down?" Finer stereopsis is required as you go down the page. If the patient misses any of the animals, then the stereo level of the last correct line is noted.

The set of circles present disparate images from 800 down to 40 seconds of arc, thus overlapping that of the animals. An older child, teen, or adult may be tested with these alone. The patient is asked to identify which circle of each set looks like it's sticking up ("like a door bell you can push, or a nail that needs to be pounded down"). If the patient misses two sets in a row, the last set identified correctly is noted as the result.

Central stereopsis (67 seconds of arc or better) occurs only if the patient has normal acuity in both eyes, thus this can also be a useful test to identify malingers. A person who truly has poor vision or blindness in one eye *cannot* pass the entire circles test.

Although the Titmus test is very useful, it has quite a few monocular clues, meaning that even a person not wearing the polarized glasses can look at the animals or circles and get some right because the "raised" figures look "off."

In the *two-pencil test* the examiner holds one pencil vertically, tip up, 16 inches (40 cm) from the patient. The patient is given the second pencil and asked to hold it vertically tip down, and touch the pencil tips together. If the patient does this accurately, then gross stereopsis (ie, 3000 seconds of arc) is said to exist.

Worth 4 Dot Test

The *Worth 4 dot test* (W4D) is a dissociative test that uses glasses (with one red lens and one green lens) and a special flashlight to evaluate fusion, suppression, and diplopia. The lighted end of the flashlight has four circles (two green, one red, and one white) arranged in a diamond pattern.

The test is performed separately for distance (6 m) and near (33 cm), as deviations can vary. At near, the image falls on about 6° of the central retina. At 6 m it subtends a small angle (1.25°) on the fovea, thus it can uncover a small central scotoma.[8]

The patient is asked to wear the glasses, with Red over the Right eye and green over the left (Figure 10-20). If glasses are normally worn, then put the Worth 4 dot glasses on over the habitual correction. The flashlight is then held so that the two green circles are on either side, the red circle at the top (Red Rises), and the white circle on the bottom. The patient is asked how many lights are seen. (The possibilities are 2, 3, 4, and 5.) The interpretation of this test is shown in Sidebar 10-6.

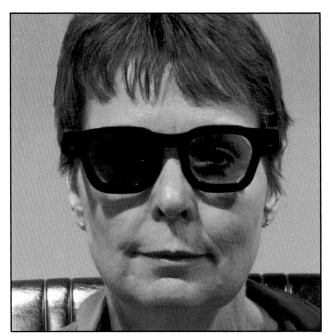

Figure 10-20. Glasses for Worth 4 dot test (note that the red lens is over the right eye).

This test can be done on toddlers, but they may describe the light colors differently, such as reporting red as pink. It is not as important to ensure that their colors are correct as it is to discern the number and position of the lights seen. In a preverbal child, the test can still be done by asking the child to point to the lights (a parent or examiner may help guide his/her hand toward the flashlight to encourage the child to participate). Young children may not want to wear these glasses and may need encouragement. (Make it fun, like a game!)

Remember, patients with ARC may develop an anomalous type of BSV. They may see four lights at near. But if the test is done at 20 feet or even farther, the lights may fall on the fovea and a patient might not see four lights but two or three lights. This demonstrates a central suppression area.

Prism Vergences

Prism vergences are performed to assess the control of a deviation. *Fusional amplitudes* can be evaluated at near or distance. The patient looks at a small target (or a letter two lines above the worst eye to ensure adequate fixation). A prism bar (starting at 1Δ) is placed in front of one eye, gradually increased until the patient reports double vision (fusion is broken). This is denoted as the *break point* or *absolute point*. Some patients may notice a blur point before the break, which may be due to relative fusional convergence (enough to keep the deviation under control).

Once the patient reports diplopia, the prism power is gradually reduced until a single image is again noted (the *recovery point*). This tests the range of vergence

---

SIDEBAR 10-6
INTERPRETATION OF WORTH 4 DOT TEST*

► Seeing four lights means fusion exists from NRC (or even ARC with a manifest strabismus) and is documented as BSV. Neither diplopia or suppression exist. The white light:
  • Is commonly seen as either red or green if one eye is very dominant…
  • …Or a combination of red and green or changing from red to green, in the presence of fusion.

► Seeing five lights indicates diplopia.
  • If the red lights appear to the right of the green lights, there is uncrossed diplopia with esotropia (uncrossed means that from the patient's perspective the red lights are to the right and the green lights are to the left).
  • If the red lights appear to the left of the green lights, then there is crossed diplopia with exotropia.

► Seeing three green lights indicates suppression of right eye.

► Seeing two red lights indicates suppression of left eye.

► If two red then three green lights are alternately seen, this indicates a rapidly alternating suppression. (The patient may state he/she sees five dots but it is important to ask if the lights are seen at the same time or alternately.)

*Assuming the Red lens is over the Right eye and the Red light is Rising (on top).

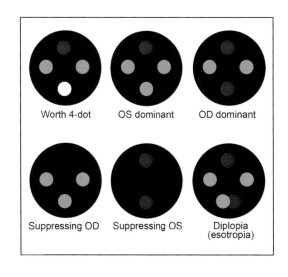

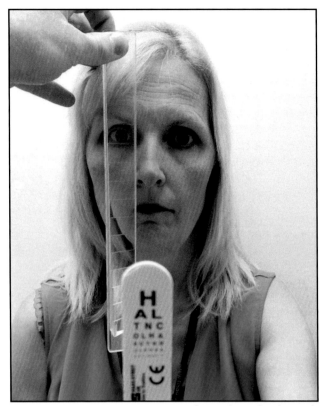

Figure 10-21. Testing convergence fusional amplitudes with base-out prism.

movement (*fusional amplitude*); the amplitude of any vergence movement can be tested.

Convergence fusional amplitudes are tested using base-out prism (Figure 10-21), and *divergence fusional amplitudes* are tested using base-in prism. For example, if a patient has an exophoria with good control, the convergence amplitude might be base-out 35Δ/30Δ at near and base-out 25Δ/20Δ at distance, where the numerator is the break point and the denominator is the recovery point.

Assessing fusion control can be helpful in the management of patients with phoric or intermittent deviations. A person's fusional amplitudes can be compared to normative values (Table 10-4). For example, a patient with a small 6Δ exophoria may have greater than 40Δ of fusional

convergence and have no diplopia because the convergence *reserve* is able to keep the deviation controlled as a phoria.

Vertical amplitudes, which are usually very small, can also be tested using prisms. When performing vertical vergences, base-up and base-down vergences are tested on the same eye. These amplitudes can be particularly useful for vertical deviations, including SO weakness. For example, an RSO palsy (with an intermittent right hypertropia) may have weak base-up vergences (say, 1Δ diplopia is present in the distance) and when the prism is removed fusion is regained. This would be recorded as 1Δ/oΔ.

Cyclovergences may be subnormal (particularly in SO dysfunction) and can be evaluated using the amblyoscope/synoptophore; however, they are not commonly tested (covered later).

Near Point of Convergence

The NPC is measured using a ruler and a small accommodative target. Both eyes are open and correction, if any, is worn. The target is brought from 16 inches (40 cm) toward the bridge of the nose until convergence breaks and you see one eye drift outward. (The patient may report blurring or diplopia, but remember this is an objective test, thus no patient input is required.) The distance at which this break occurs is the NPC.

Cover Testing

A *cover test* is an important orthoptic test that evaluates both the sensory and motor components of the sensorimotor system, because it not only detects and quantifies strabismus but also assesses control. It can be performed on young children (even many infants) up through adults, as long as fixation is adequate.

There are several types of cover tests, discussed in a moment. At its most basic, cover testing involves occluding one eye (Figure 10-22). Then, according to what you are trying to evaluate, you might simply uncover that eye or cover the other. All the while, you are observing the eye(s) for any shifting movements, which indicates the presence of strabismus. Cover testing is performed at near and distance to assess whether an eye turns constantly

TABLE 10-4		
NORMAL FUSIONAL VERGENCE AMPLITUDES[1,2,8]		
	Near Fusional Amplitudes	**Distance Fusional Amplitudes**
Convergence	30Δ to 35Δ	20Δ to 25Δ
Divergence	8Δ to 10Δ	6Δ to 8Δ
Vertical vergence	2Δ to 3Δ	2Δ to 3Δ

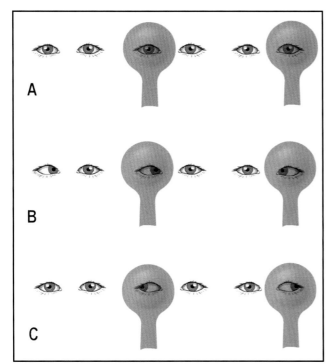

Figure 10-22. Cover testing. (A) Orthophoria—No eye movement detected with cover/uncover, or with cross/cover testing. (B) Right esotropia—No movement is seen when right eye is covered, but right eye moves outward when the left eye is covered (cover/uncover testing). (C) Exophoria—No movement is seen with cover/uncover testing (watching uncovered eye), but an inward movement of each eye is seen with cross/cover testing (watching the eye as it is being uncovered) as they had each wandered outward under the cover.

(tropia), intermittently (intermittent tropia), or only when fusion is disrupted (phoria). In addition, the direction of any strabismus must be determined. Thus a full cover test involves a cover/uncover test, then an alternate cover test, and follow-up with a cover/uncover test.

Any cover test is first performed in primary gaze. For incomitant strabismus, the test may also need to be performed in other diagnostic positions of gaze. However, if the patient has a compensatory head posture (CHP), then cover testing may need to be performed first in the CHP (before fusion is disrupted), then primary gaze and other diagnostic positions of gaze and tilts as required (see also Bielschowsky three-step test).

For distance testing, the patient should fixate on an object at 20 feet (usually two lines above the best-corrected vision of the weaker eye) so accommodation is not a factor.

Near testing is performed in primary position and/or in downgaze, at 33 cm. If downgaze is tested, this should be documented as some disorders can have dissimilar near measurements when evaluated in primary vs downgaze. Appropriate near correction must be used. Sometimes glasses may need to be held up to utilize the near portion and/or to view the eyes.

SIDEBAR 10-7
POSSIBILITIES IN COVER/UNCOVER TEST

1. Cover right eye, left eye does not move (ortho)
2. Cover right eye, left eye moves in (left exo)
3. Cover right eye, left eye moves out (left eso)
4. Cover right eye, left eye moves up or down (left hypo or hyper)

Also:
1. Uncover right eye, left eye does not move (ortho)
2. Uncover right eye, left eye moves out (exo)
3. Uncover right eye, left eye moves in (eso)
4. Uncover right eye, left eye moves down or up (left hyper or hypo)

Finally:
1. Uncover right eye, right eye does not move (ortho)
2. Uncover right eye, right eye moves out (eso)
3. Uncover right eye, right eye moves in (exo)
4. Uncover right eye, right eye moves up or down (hypo or hyper)

A small accommodative target on which both eyes can fixate is used. If either too large of a target or a light is used at near, this may bring out a different deviation. For example, an exophoria that is controlled with fusional convergence on a small accommodative target may become an exotropia if a light is used.

Cover/Uncover

In the *cover/uncover test*, an occluder is placed over the right eye while the examiner watches the left eye for any movement. The cover is then removed while still watching the left eye for any movement. The test is repeated with attention directed this time to the right eye as the left eye is being covered then uncovered. There are several possible results (Sidebar 10-7).

Also observe any movement of the covered eye as the cover is removed. It may move as well, because the test has interrupted fusion and is revealing any latent tendency. In this case, as the cover is removed the eyes are regaining fusion. This situation will be defined more clearly during the alternate cover test (next).

It may seem a little confusing when first learning to determine the direction of a deviation. The question to ask yourself is: In what position is the eye when it's under the cover? That is the correct direction of the strabismus. For example, if a covered eye moves *out* when you remove the cover, then it must have been turned *in* when it was covered: an eso deviation.

TABLE 10-5				
DOCUMENTATION AND PRISM ORIENTATION				
Deviation (Direction Eye Turns)	**Manifest Notations**	**Phoric Notations**	**Intermittent Notations**	**Orientation of Prism Base to Measure This Deviation**
Eso (Inward)	ET	E	E(T)	Base-out
Exo (Outward)	XT	X	X(T)	Base-in
Hyper (Upward)	HT	H	H(T)	Base-down
Hypo (Downward)	HypoT	Hypo	Hypo(T)	Base-up

Alternate Cross/Cover

In the *alternate cross/cover test,* the occluder is moved over the nose bridge from the right eye to the left eye and back six to eight times at a medium rate. (If you go too fast, the uncovered eye may not take up fixation. If you go too slow, the eyes may refixate together while the occluder is in between.) Each eye must also be fully covered to avoid any fusion. This element of the test reveals the phoric part of the deviation. If there is no shift on an alternate cover test, there is no visible strabismus. (But beware, a monofixation/microstrabismus could still exist!)

Repeat Cover/Uncover

Since the alternate cover test disrupted binocularity, repeating the cover/uncover test may reveal that a deviation originally thought to be latent (phoric) is now manifest (tropic). This is an *intermittent deviation*: a deviation that is usually a phoria but can be "broken down" into a tropia. Sometimes you can even watch as, seconds later, the deviated eye once again pulls straight to pick up binocular fixation.

Deviation Measurement: Cover Test With Prism

To measure a deviation using a cover test, a prism is held in front of one eye and the cross/cover test is done, watching for movement of either eye. The apex of the prism is placed in the direction of the strabismus (Table 10-5). Think of the prism as an arrow with the apex as the point. POINT the prism in the direction of the deviation/turn. (Note: Prisms cannot be used to measure torsion.)

The prism should be held over the nonfixing eye in the frontal plane position, meaning that the side of the prism next to the face is parallel to the face. Prisms of similar direction should not be stacked together, as this can induce errors. If a large deviation needs to be measured, use a prism over each eye. In the case of a combined vertical and horizontal deviation, vertical and horizontal prisms can be stacked with no significant error.

Prisms of increasing power are held in front of one eye until there is reversal of movement, and then

decreased until there is no movement (neutralization). It is important to go past what you think is neutral until you see an opposite movement of a deviation, as it may take a few more diopters to see the reversal. Then come back and record the strongest prism that stops the movement just before reversal occurs.

Incomitant strabismus may need to be measured in different diagnostic positions or with and without head tilts (see Bielschowsky's three-step test).

Extraocular Muscle Movement Testing

EOM function can be tested using versions (or ductions, if necessary) in the six diagnostic positions of gaze to include right, left, up and to the right, up and to the left, down and to the right, and down and to the left (see Figure 10-6). (Assessment of straight up and straight down is not typically part of EOM version evaluation.) Spectacles are removed. A muscle light held 33 cm away is used as the target.

When performing version testing (which may also be referred to as ROM testing), the muscle light is moved and the patient is told to follow it (without moving the head) into each of the six positions, always returning to primary position between each one so that each muscle returns to its natural state. It can also be helpful to do EOM testing in primary upgaze and downgaze, as this can evaluate for A and V patterns (discussed next) as well as to assess functionality. Corneal reflexes can also be observed when assessing for restrictions or overactions.

The patient may have to be coached to follow with the eyes alone, without turning his/her head. (For small children and even some adults, you may have to put your hand on the top of their head to hold them still.) Lift the lids when evaluating the downward positions. Finally, be sure to watch the upper lids as you move from upgaze to primary gaze. Thyroid eye disease sometimes causes the upper lids to pause before moving down with the globe (*lid lag*).

When testing versions, one eye should be compared to the other. If versions are *full,* the eyes will move

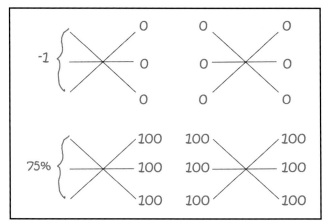

Figure 10-23. Documentation of extraocular muscle under-actions using the number (top) and percentage (bottom) systems.

smoothly together, looking in the same direction at the same angle at the same time. In addition, the patient will not perceive doubling of the light in any gaze.

If versions are full, ductions do not need to be tested. But if a limitation is noted when testing versions, you may see lessening of the restriction on duction testing. For example, an RLR palsy could show 50% restriction on abduction on versions but when the left eye is covered (ie, all the innervation is given to the right eye) only 25% restriction is seen in ductions. In this case, both version and duction findings are documented.

Common childhood strabismus typically does not have restrictions, but can have *overactions*. Other childhood strabismus, such as Duane and Brown syndromes, do have restrictions. Cranial nerve palsies often have restrictions and are often apparent. Finally, sometimes muscles overact to "help" another muscle that is deficient. Horizontal muscles do not commonly have overactions but vertical muscles (especially obliques) often do.

Two different methods may be used to document EOM underactions or overactions in the six diagnostic positions (Figure 10-23).

1. A number scale of overaction (+) or underaction (-) of 0 to 4, with 0 being normal movement. For example, if a -1 RLR is noted, then the RLR muscle is restricted and there is an underaction of 1 out of 4 (Figure 10-23, top).

2. A percentage system. If 25% underaction is noted, the muscle is mildly restricted and is moving only 75% of the expected normal range (Figure 10-23, bottom). If a 25% overaction is seen, this would be noted as >100% or 125%.

A and V Patterns

During EOM testing or measuring, an *A* or *V pattern* may be discovered. This means that there is more or less strabismus (eso or exo) in up- or downgaze than

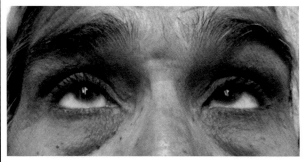
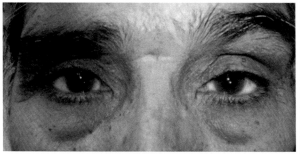
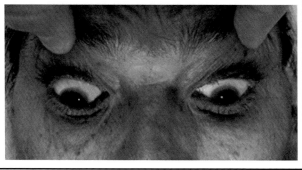

Figure 10-24. This A pattern shows more inward deviation in upgaze (or more straight in downgaze). V patterns are the opposite.

there is in primary gaze. An A pattern is more converged in upgaze (Figure 10-24) and a V in downgaze. The most common scenario is an eso deviation that increases in downgaze, causing a V pattern, but either pattern may be seen in both eso and exo strabismus.

Patterns are commonly seen in childhood strabismus and are most often due to oblique over/underaction. Patterns can also exist with cranial nerve palsies or various syndromes (such as Brown). Patterns must be taken into account when considering surgery so the best functional outcome can occur.

Forced Ductions

The *forced duction test* is typically performed if a mechanical restriction is suspected. It involves attempting to forcibly move the eye in a specific direction using forceps.

The test is mostly performed in patients with suspected blowout fractures where the inferior rectus muscle can become entrapped in the broken orbital floor bones. This causes diplopia in upgaze. However, diplopia could also be due to swelling of the tissues or nerve injury. Forced ductions can help tell the difference.

Forced ductions might also be done on children and adults who have had prior strabismus surgery to assess a restrictive muscle. In this case it is often done under general anesthesia before a subsequent surgery.

The forced duction test can be performed in the office. First, the conjunctiva is anesthetized. The conjunctiva near the limbus is grasped with toothed forceps, and an attempt is made to physically pull the eye in the direction opposite that in which mechanical restriction is suspected. (For example, if an IR entrapment is suspected, then the forceps are positioned at the upper limbus so that the eye can be pulled vertically.) If no resistance is encountered, then the muscle is not entrapped. If resistance is encountered, a mechanical restriction exists.

Measuring AC/A Ratio

The importance of the AC/A ratio in children in particular has been covered earlier. Here we will discuss how to do the measurements and the math. Note: For purposes of this discussion eso deviations are considered to be positive (+) and exo deviations to be negative (-).

The *gradient method* is preferred by most and utilizes ophthalmic lenses (usually plus) to assess the accommodative component of a deviation. The patient wears his/her full distance correction, and the deviation is measured at 33 cm. A lens (+3 is typically used) is placed on top of the full correction and the near deviation is remeasured to see if the added lens affects the deviation. The results are then entered into the following formula:

AC/A = (near deviation with lens) – (near deviation) / power of lens used (in diopters)

Example: The patient requires no correction and has a 25Δ esotropia at near. With a +3.00 lens, the measurement is repeated and results in a 5Δ esotropia.

AC/A = (+5) – (+25)/+3 = 20/3 = approximately 7:1

This is a high AC/A ratio and the child may benefit from the use of plus lenses at near.

Bielschowsky Head Tilt Test

The *Bielschowsky three-step head tilt test* (B3ST, also called simply the *three-step test,* 3ST) is used to give information about a vertical EOM that may not be functioning properly. The process of elimination is used to identify what muscle is most likely dysfunctional.

This test can be especially useful in diagnosing fourth nerve palsies. It can be more of diagnostic use, however, in earlier onset as the spread of comitance has not yet taken place. This innervational test does not work for vertical deviations that are mechanical in nature.

The steps involve implicating four, two, and then finally one muscle as dysfunctional (Sidebar 10-8). The distance deviation is measured in the primary position

using prism and cover. Next, the head is turned to the right to obtain a left gaze measurement (calling upon the RIO, RSO and LSR, LIR), then to the left for a right gaze measurement (calling upon the RSR, RIR and LSO, LIO). The head is next tilted to the right, which causes intorsion of the right eye (calling upon the RSR and RSO) and extorsion of the left eye (calling upon the LIO and LIR), and the measurement is recorded. The last step is to tilt the head left, which causes extorsion of the right eye (calling upon the RIO and RIR) and intorsion of the left eye (calling upon the LSO and LSR).

Saccades and Smooth Pursuit Evaluation

The examiner can test saccades by raising a finger of each hand (about 1 foot apart) and asking the patient to move his/her eyes quickly from one finger to the other (known as *two finger versions*). In normal saccades, the eyes will move in the same direction quickly and smoothly from one object to another, maintaining the image on the fovea. If saccades are impaired, the movements may appear slow, small, or jerky.

Smooth pursuits can be tested by having the patient slowly follow the examiner's light or finger and observing his/her tracking skills.

Light Reflex Tests

Hirschberg and Krimsky tests are methods to detect and estimate or measure manifest strabismus. These tests are especially useful on babies or young children who cannot cooperate with prism cover test measurements or on those who cannot fixate with their strabismic eye (ie, deep amblyopia).

Hirschberg Test

In this test, a light is shone from 33 cm away and the cornea light reflexes are observed (Figure 10-25). The normal, orthophoric (straight) reflex is seen centrally or slightly nasal in each eye. In strabismus, the reflex will be seen in the normal place in the fixating eye and will be displaced in the deviating eye. For example, if the reflex is on the temporal limbus of one eye, then that eye is turning in (esotropic).

The amount of strabismus can be grossly estimated by this method as well. The average cornea is 12 mm in diameter, and a normal pupil is about 4 mm in room light. Each millimeter from the center of the pupil equals approximately 15Δ (7°). If the light reflex falls between the limbus and edge of the pupil nasally (ie, 4 mm from the center), the exotropia is estimated to be about 60Δ.

Krimsky Test

The *Krimsky test* is an approximate measure of strabismus that utilizes a muscle light and prisms to move a deviated light reflex back to the center of the pupil (Figure 10-26). Horizontal prism of increasing power is placed over the deviating eye until both reflexes are central. The

SIDEBAR 10-8
BIELSCHOWSKY THREE-STEP TEST

1. Measure deviation in primary gaze: Identify RHT or LHT.

   - If there is an RHT, then the right depressors aren't working, or if there is an LhypoT, then the left elevators aren't working. RSO, RIR or LSR, LIO are considered.
   - If there is an LHT, then the left depressors aren't working, or if there is an RhypoT, then the right elevators are working. LSO, LIR or RSR, RIO are considered.

2. Measure the deviation in left and right head turns. This identifies whether the vertical hyper deviation increases on right or left gaze, which narrows it down to only two muscles.

   - If there is an RHT or LhypoT and the deviation increases on right gaze, then only the RIR and LIO are considered, or if the deviation increases on left gaze, then only the RSO or LSR are considered.
   - If there is an LHT or RhypoT and the deviation increases on right gaze, then only the RSR and LSO are considered, or if the deviation increases on left gaze, then only the RIO or LIR are considered.

3. Measure the deviation in left and right head tilts. This identifies whether the vertical hyper deviation increases on right or left tilt, isolating the muscle with the problem.

   - That is, the deviation is worse in primary, one side gaze, and one tilt (see example below).
   - If there is an RHT or LhypoT and the deviation increases on right tilt, then only the RSO and LIO are considered, or if the deviation increases on left tilt, then only the RIR or LSR are considered.
   - If there is an LHT or RhypoT and the deviation increases on right tilt, then only the RSR and LIR are considered, or if the deviation increases on left tilt, then only the RIO or LSO are considered.
   - (Step 2 eliminated one of the two options above thus isolating only one muscle which will be circled three times).

Example
Start with worksheet.

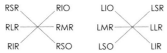

1. Primary position cover test reveals an RHT 6Δ (or L HypoT 6Δ when the right eye is fixating) so RSO, RIR or LSR, LIO are implicated.

2. On left gaze (head turn right) a cover test reveals an RHT 12Δ (increases), and on right gaze (head turn left) the deviation improves to RHT 3Δ. Now only the RSO or LSR are considered.

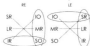

3. On right tilt, a cover test reveals an RHT 14Δ, so the RSO is responsible (as on tilt left the deviation is less RHT 5Δ). The RHT is worse on left gaze and right tilt, thus the RSO is affected in all three steps.

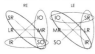

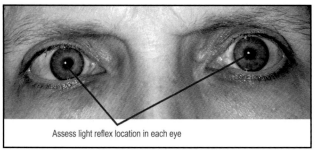

Assess light reflex location in each eye

Figure 10-25. Hirschberg test is a quick visual assessment of eye alignment that compares the position of the corneal reflex of one eye to the other. In this case, the reflex is central in the left eye and decentered temporally in the right, indicating a right esotropia.

prism base is placed in the same direction of the deviating reflex. (For example, if the eye turns out, the reflex will be displaced in, and the prism is positioned base-in.) It is important to measure beyond what you think is a central reflex and record the strongest prism used before it becomes obvious that you have moved beyond central.

A *modified Krimsky test* is when the prism is placed over the straight eye. In this case the prism base is placed in the opposite direction of the displaced reflex in the fellow eye.

Angle Kappa

An *angle kappa* occurs when the visual axis and the pupillary axis do not coincide. An angle kappa may be positive (a slightly *nasal* reflex) or negative (a slightly *temporal* reflex). A positive angle kappa (< 5°) is typically found in the normal population (Figure 10-27).

When performing the Hirschberg or Krimsky tests on orthophoric patients, the examiner must be aware most people have a *physiologic positive* angle kappa. Thus, sometimes a pseudoexotropia may appear with light reflex testing, but when a cover test is performed, no shift is seen. A positive angle kappa can actually hide a small esotropia, or an exotropia can appear larger since the reflex falls nasally.

A negative angle kappa (Figure 10-28) occurs when the reflex falls temporally. It can cause a pseudoesotropia, hide a small exotropia, or make an esotropia appear larger than it actually is. Because of these illusions caused by an angle kappa, it is important to explore any suspected deviation further (eg, cover tests, prism measurements) and not rely simply on appearance.

Red (Bruckner) Reflex Test

The *red reflex* is the red reflection of white light from the eyes. Darken the room and hold a direct ophthalmoscope at arm's length. As the patient fixates on the instrument, look for a symmetric, bright red reflex in each pupil. This is known as the *Bruckner* or *red reflex test*. If the reflex is asymmetrical, absent, irregular, white, or

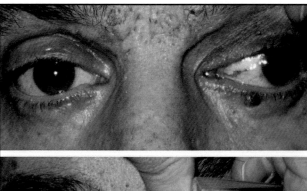

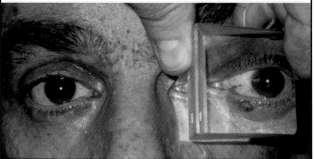

Figure 10-26. Krimsky test uses prisms to align the light reflex in the deviating eye.

there appears to be an opacity within the reflex of a child, this could indicate the presence of potentially amblyogenic factors such as cataract, strabismus, amblyopia, and/or retinoblastoma.

For example, if a patient's left eye is exotropic, then you might see a bright red reflex in the fixating right pupil but a dim or nonexistent reflex in the left. If a superior reflex is seen, it may indicate hyperopia; an inferior reflex may indicate myopia.[20] This test can also help identify other pathologies, such as anisometropia, corneal opacities, and retinal detachments.

Single and Double Maddox Rod Testing

The *Maddox rod* is a transparent "lens" made up of a series of parallel red cylinders. It is available as a single trial lens, on one end of an occluder, or as an auxiliary lens on the phoropter. When a white fixation light is viewed through the rod, it is seen as a red line 90° to the direction of the cylinders.

During testing, the rod is placed over the right eye (by convention) while a fixation light is held at 33 cm with the room lights dimmed. The red line is seen through the right eye, and the left eye sees the white fixation light. Because each eye sees something different, this is a dissociative test and requires the ability to recognize one image from each eye.

To evaluate for a horizontal deviation, the rod is held with the cylinders running horizontally. To test for vertical deviations, the rod is held with the cylinders running vertically. If the eyes are orthophoric, the patient will see the red line going through the white light, or waver a little back and forth through the light. Interpretations of the possible responses are shown in Table 10-6.

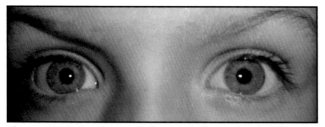

Figure 10-27. Positive angle kappa. Reflexes are slightly nasal in each eye.

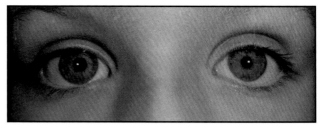

Figure 10-28. Negative angle kappa. Reflexes are slightly temporal in each eye.

TABLE 10-6
SINGLE MADDOX ROD TEST

Rod Orientation (Over the Right Eye)	Patient Observation of Red Line	Patient Response/Interpretation
Horizontal	Vertical	A. Red line is to the right of the white light (uncrossed)—eso deviation
		B. Red line is to the left of the white light (crossed)—exo deviation
		C. Red line is through the white light—no horizontal deviation
Vertical	Horizontal	D. Red line is above the white light—hypo deviation
		E. Red line is below the white light—hyper deviation
		F. Red line is through the white light—no vertical deviation

A. Uncrossed (eso)   B. Crossed (exo)   C. No deviation

D. Right hypo   E. Right hyper   F. No deviation

Prisms can be utilized with the Maddox rod to measure the deviation. With the patient's near prescription in the phoropter or trial frames/clips, the Maddox rod lens is placed in front of one eye and the rotary prism (set at 0) in front of the other. (Detailed instructions are in Sidebar 10-9.)

The *double Maddox rod* test is used to evaluate torsion, most often in those who have an SO palsy. It utilizes a red Maddox rod over the right eye and a white Maddox rod over the left. The rods are set running vertically in a trial frame or clipped onto the patient's glasses (Figure 10-29). The room lights should be dimmed, the target is held at 33 cm in primary position. (Downgaze would also

---

SIDEBAR 10-9
MADDOX ROD AND PRISM MEASUREMENTS (PHOROPTER METHOD)

Note: For purposes of this example, the Maddox rod will be in the RIGHT aperture and a rotary prism will be over the LEFT.

Horizontal Deviations

▶ Patient's near correction in phoropter

▶ Turn MRH (Maddox rod/red/horizontal) in front of OD

▶ Swing rotary prism in front of OS
- Rotate prism so that 0 is at the top
- Turn the thumb screw so the arrow points to 0

▶ Present the muscle light from 33 cm away and verify that the patient sees *both* the red line and the white light, indicating that the eyes are aligned properly. Reconfirm this periodically during the measurement.
- Ask the patient: Do you see the red line? Which way is it going? (If the line is not vertical, you are using the wrong Maddox rod; switch to horizontal.)
- Ask the patient: Do you also see the white light? (If not, adjust the light's position until the patient sees both the red line and the white light.)
- Ask the patient: Does the red line go *through* the white light? (Probably not.)
- Tell the patient: I'm going to move the white light a little.

▶ Rotate the prism just a little bit, either way.
- Ask the patient: Is the white light moving toward or away from the red line?
  - If the images are getting farther apart, rotate the prism in the opposite direction.
  - If the images are getting closer together, you are moving in the correct direction.

▶ Continue to slowly rotate the prism in the appropriate direction.
- Tell the patient: Let me know when the white light has moved onto the red line.

▶ When patient says that the images have intersected, note the prism reading.
- Tell the patient: OK, now I want you to tell me when they just start to split apart again.

▶ Continue slowly rotating the prism in the *same* direction to find the maximum deviation. When the patient says that the images have split apart again you have gone too far: Rotate slowly back in the opposite direction.
- Tell the patient: Let me know when they're back together.

▶ When patient says that the images are together again, note the prism reading.

▶ Note whether the prism base is IN (arrow toward the nose) or OUT (arrow toward the ear).

▶ For example, with the prism set at 0 in front of the left eye, the patient reports that the red line and white light are not together. The patient reports the red line is to the right of the light (uncrossed) so you turn the prism clockwise (base-out), and the line and light are superimposed at 8Δ. You continue to move clockwise and the images move opposite (crossed) and split at 12Δ. Next you turn counterclockwise and the images intersect again at 10Δ. This is your endpoint. If base-out prism has been used, record as an eso deviation (ie, Eso 10Δ); if base-in prism, record as an exo deviation.

Vertical Deviations

▶ Proceed as above, but with the following changes:

▶ Place MRV (red Maddox rod, vertical) in the phoropter. Rotate the prism so the 0 is toward the nose, arrow pointing to 0.

▶ When the endpoint is reached and base-up prism has been used (remember, the prism is over the left eye), record as an L hypo deviation; if base-down prism has been used, record as an L hyper deviation. (By convention we usually indicate the eye that is *higher*, so these would be written R/L and L/R, respectively.)

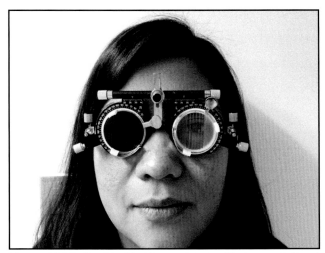

Figure 10-29. Double Maddox rod test will show rotational alignment of the eyes.

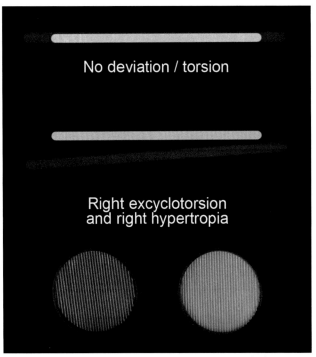

Figure 10-30. Double Maddox rod. (Top) Normal alignment. (Middle) Rotation of the right eye behind the red Maddox rod. (Bottom) Orientation of the red Maddox rod in a 10° right excyclotorsion.

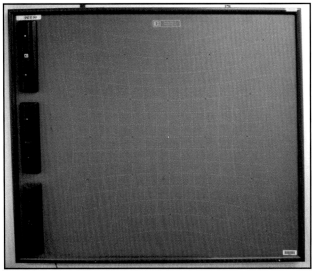

Figure 10-31. Hess screen (Clement Clarke) as seen by the naked eye.

be evaluated for SO palsies as excyclotorsion is often more prevalent when looking down.)

In an orthophoric person the red and white lines will be horizontal and superimposed (Figure 10-30, top). If there is torsion, then at least one of the lines will be tilted. If there is a vertical imbalance, one line will be above the other. Thus, in a patient who has an RSO palsy with excyclotorsion, the red line will be lower than the white line, and tilted (Figure 10-30, middle).

The examiner or patient then turns the Maddox rod of the eye with suspected torsion until the two lines are parallel. The amount of cyclotorsion is measured in degrees using the scale on the trial frame or clip. For example, in an RSO palsy if the red rod must be turned to 100° to be parallel then there are 10° of excyclotorsion (ie, 10° off 90°; Figure 10-30, bottom).

Hess/Lees Testing

This subjective test is commonly performed by an orthoptist to diagnose and monitor muscle imbalances, particularly cranial nerve palsies, thyroid eye disease, and restrictive problems. It assesses the eyes in different diagnostic positions of gaze, similar to EOM testing, to evaluate muscle function and movement in those with NRC.

A *Hess* (or *Lees*) *screen test* uses red/green goggles to dissociate the eyes. Typically this test is done without correction unless the patient cannot fixate without it, but the ROM may be less due to the frame's interference.

For the Hess test, the patient dons the goggles with one red and one green lens, and is seated 50 cm from the screen with chin and forehead stabilized. The red lens fixates the one eye, which sees a red light, while the other eye with the green lens sees a green light. The green and red lights are seen simultaneously; however, the eye being tested is the one wearing the green lens.

The screen is pincushion shaped and divided into squares (Figure 10-31). The examiner uses a remote to move the red light from the center position at 15° fixed increments up, down, left, and right. The patient is given a green flashlight and is asked to place the green light over the red light. The examiner marks on a card the position of the patient's placement of the green light relative to the red dot. The center dot is tested first then eight other points around the center are tested (forming

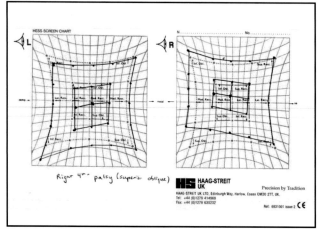

Figure 10-32. Hess test result example (Haag-Streit UK) showing an RSO palsy with a limitation of levodepression of the right eye.

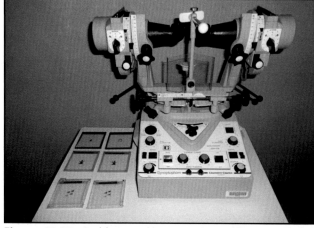

Figure 10-33. Amblyoscope/synoptophore (Clement Clarke) used to assess ocular motility disorders.

an inner square pattern), followed by 16 additional points that form an outer square. After one eye is examined the goggles are flipped over and the other eye is tested.

Each square on the Hess chart represents 5° of strabismus. If the patient places the green light on top of the red light exactly, no deviation is noted.

Once the test has been completed on both eyes, the points are connected and the examiner uses the card to identify muscle underactions and overactions. Typically the smaller "field" is the eye with limited movement (Figure 10-32).

Another, similar test is the Lancaster test. It uses a mirror system to dissociate the eyes, the targets are lines instead of dots, and the screen is a grid of perpendicular lines.

Amblyoscope/Synoptophore

An amblyoscope/synoptophore (Figure 10-33) can be utilized to measure horizontal, vertical, and torsional deviations (in all nine positions of gaze), test fusional vergences (including cyclovergences), stereopsis, and ARC. It is also often used to assess the presence of suppression or fusional ability (with or without the deviation corrected). It is commonly performed by an orthoptist on children but can be performed on adults as well. It can provide an objective as well as subjective measurement of strabismus.

The patient places his/her head and chin forward into the machine. A child's head may have to be held to prevent head movement. There are two movable arms, one for each eye, which move the target sideways. If an object needs to be moved vertically or torsionally, the examiner can move it as directed by the patient. A scale on the examiner's side of the instrument is used to read the angle being measured. The device utilizes +6.50 D lenses in each tube to help eliminate accommodation.

The amblyoscope can identify the three grades of binocular vision.

Grade I: Simultaneous perception. Depending on visual acuity one can use parafoveal, foveal, or macular slides. Separate targets are presented to each eye (eg, a dog and a dog house). The patient is asked to use one of the instrument's arms to move the dog into the house. (The other arm is tightened at zero by the examiner so that the target is maintained straight ahead.) At this point the measurement is noted and recorded. A positive number indicates an eso, and a negative number indicates an exo.

If a patient cannot simultaneously perceive the two dissimilar images even at the corrected angle, then there is a decreased chance that fusion would occur after surgery.

The test can also be done objectively by the examiner centering and observing light reflexes on the eye to assess NRC vs ARC (ie, the patient fuses when the angle of the strabismus is corrected or with ARC at the small partial angle). If this is the same as the objective measurement then there is harmonious ARC; if less, then unharmonious ARC is present.

Grade II: Tests for *true fusion* using similar targets (ie, one eye sees a man holding a pole on one side and the other eye sees a man with a fish on the other side) either at a straight ahead position or at their strabismic angle of anomaly. If fusion exits a single man would appear to be holding both items. If fusion does not exist, either the fish or the pole would be missing. If there are two men, then a diplopia exists. Convergence and divergence amplitudes can be evaluated as well.

Grade III: In well-established binocularity, not only are the images of the two eyes fused, but they perceive *stereoscopic effect.* In this test, images are slightly disparate to create a three-dimensional effect and the patient is asked to state which item appears closer or farther. Slides can be chosen to test gross to fine stereopsis.

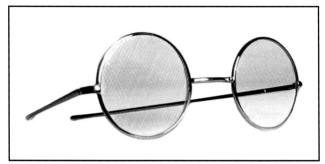

Figure 10-34. Bagolini striated glasses.

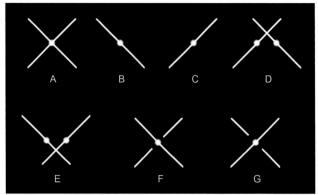

Figure 10-35. Bagolini test results. (A) If the patient has NRC, a perfect cross with no breaks in the lines will be seen. (B, C) If a single line is seen, there is suppression (OD in B and OS in C) and ARC is not present. (D) If the patient has NRC and an exotropia (crossed diplopia), a cross will be seen with the fixation light seen inferiorly. (E) If the patient has NRC and an esotropia (uncrossed diplopia), a cross will be seen with the fixation light seen superiorly. (F, G) If ARC exists, then a cross will been seen but one cross will have a gap (a scotoma OD in F and OS in G).

Retinal Correspondence Tests

Bagolini Test

The *Bagolini test* is a minimally dissociative near test to assess the presence of ARC. Plano striated lenses (Bagolini lenses) are placed either in a trial frame with the patient's prescription or over the patient's glasses (Figure 10-34). The test is usually done on children, but if the patient is an adult, you'd use the near prescription. The right Bagolini lens is obliquely orientated at 45° and the left at 135°. The muscle light is used as a target, and is seen as an elongated streak through the Bagolini lenses. There are several response possibilities (Figure 10-35).

▶ If a complete cross is seen with no breaks in the lines, cover testing reveals no shift, and fixation is central, then the patient has NRC. However, if cover testing reveals a shift, then *harmonious ARC* is present.

▶ If the two streaks are separated and not crossed, this indicates diplopia with NRC. If only one line is seen, there is suppression with NRC.

▶ If a break is seen in the cross, then a *foveal suppression scotoma* (*fixation point scotoma*) is present and peripheral fusion exists (ie, as an adaptation) and ARC exists.

▶ If a single line is seen, there is suppression and ARC is not present.

Bagolini lenses may also be used to assess for torsion if one does not have double Maddox rods.

After-Image Test

The *after-image test* is a highly dissociative test done by stimulating the eyes with a vertical and horizontal line of light to produce an after image. This test is rarely done clinically but may be performed by an orthoptist to confirm if a patient has NRC or ARC. Most people with strabismus have NRC but some children with a small angle strabismus may develop ARC. An amblyoscope/synoptophore can also be used.

The test is performed in a dark room. The target is a 12-inch long, straight filament with a gap in the middle. The light is presented vertically to the right eye (while the

left eye is occluded) and then horizontally into the left eye (while the right eye is occluded). The patient is directed to fixate on the central gap for 10 to 20 seconds each. The patient will then see two images (regardless of if the eyes are open, closed, straight, or crossed).

The interpretation of this test indicates fixation behavior. If the patient has NRC he/she will see a perfect cross irrespective of any deviation (latent or manifest). If the patient has ARC, the vertical and horizontal lines will be displaced (representing the anomalous angle). If there is ARC and right esotropia, the vertical after-image will be displaced to the left. In a case of a right exotropia, the vertical after-image is displaced to the right. These findings are opposite in a left eye strabismus (Figure 10-36).

4Δ Base-Out Test

The *4Δ base-out test* is used to assess whether bifoveal fusion is present or if one fovea is being suppressed, often to evaluate monofixation syndrome. It is used in patients who exhibit reduced stereo acuity and a foveal scotoma where ARC is suspected. If a small (ie, 4Δ) base-out prism is placed over one eye, there will normally be a refixation shift. If no shift is seen, then the image has been moved onto a scotoma and foveal suppression exists.

Red Filter Test

A red filter test may be performed to assess fusion. A red filter is placed over one eye while both eyes fixate on a muscle light. If fusion is present, a pink light may be seen.

If only the white light is seen, the eye looking through the red lens is suppressing and a scotoma is present. If one white then one red light is seen, then alternating suppression is present.

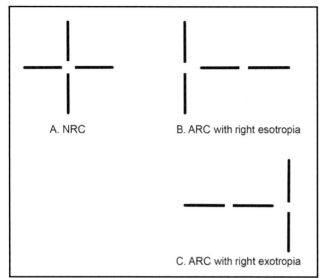

A. NRC   B. ARC with right esotropia

C. ARC with right exotropia

Figure 10-36. After-image test is used to test for normal or abnormal retinal correspondence. (A) NRC. (B) ARC with right esotropia. (C) ARC with right exotropia.

If two lights are seen (one red and one white) simultaneously, then diplopia is present. If the red lens is over the right eye and the red light is seen to the patient's left, then *crossed diplopia* (exotropia) is present. If the red light is seen to the patient's right, then *uncrossed diplopia* (esotropia) is present.

If a patient reports that the red and white images appear to be superimposed, this may indicate an abnormal response in presence of a heterophoria (and possibly ARC).

Field of Binocular Single Vision

A *field of binocular single vision test* uses a Goldmann perimeter to map out and score areas of binocular vision (ie, nondiplopic areas). This test can be utilized in the management of strabismus to assess dysfunction, visual disability, stability, or for driving/legal purposes. For details regarding the Goldmann perimeter, see Chapter 14.

The evaluation is done with both eyes opened. Using a III4e target, areas of diplopia/nondiplopia are mapped out, typically using a kinetic technique. An outline of a normal BSV is used as the test chart. To start, the patient is asked to look straight at the target and report if it is double. The examiner moves the target along the meridians. The patient is told to move the eyes and follow the target, and to report when a single or double target is seen.

A scoring system is used to record the percentage of BSV. Higher scores are given for central BSV, as this is the most important area, and higher scores are also given for downgaze, since functionally we also use this frequently. The scoring template consists of 50 segments ranging from a value of one to three points. A patient with a recent onset total CN VI palsy may only score 50% BSV. As recovery takes place this may increase to 70% then 85% and then 100% if the palsy fully resolves.

Ice Test

The ice test is a relatively sensitive test performed on patients suspected of having a ptosis caused by myasthenia gravis. An ice pack or a glove filled with ice cubes may be used and is applied for 2 minutes. A positive ice test is when a ptosis shows improvement or resolves (see Figure 10-16).

PATIENT SERVICES: EDUCATION, MANAGEMENT, AND TREATMENT

Amblyopia

Early detection and treatment of amblyopia is so important. While guidelines vary, children should generally have an eye exam by the age of 1 year, or sooner if any problems are suspected. It is imperative that parents and the child fully comply with amblyopia treatment. If amblyopia is not treated, it can result in a permanent visual defect or loss of depth perception, which can have far-reaching consequences. For example, if vision in the "good" eye is lost somewhere down the road, one might suddenly be unable to work or drive.

Spectacle Correction

It is so important that children, particularly those with strabismus, have a cycloplegic refraction. Prescribing glasses in children is challenging due to limited cooperation, questionable reliability, and the high-stakes risk of amblyopia. One must take into account the patient's visual needs according to age, accommodative elements, risk of amblyopia, etc. Measuring for glasses is primarily done by objective means until the age of 6.

Many young children with strabismus are hyperopic and require glasses. In the case of a fully accommodative esotropia, parents are often relieved their child does not require surgical correction, but are concerned when the child takes the glasses off and the eye drifts back in.

In partially accommodative esotropia, spectacles are prescribed to lessen the deviation. The patient may still require surgery or further monitoring. Some children with strabismus may be emmetropic or have a minimal refractive error, which is not corrected because there would be little or no improvement in the strabismus or visual acuity. Sometimes children with amblyopia need time to "relax" into the prescription and may take a few months to adjust.

Adults are often prescribed prisms to help control diplopia. Many of these patients are given a trial of Fresnel press-on prisms first, before prism is prescribed in the lenses (discussed momentarily).

SIDEBAR 10-10

CONVERGENCE INSUFFICIENCY TREATMENT, EXAMPLE

Patient Exam Data

▶ 13-year-old with headaches, eyestrain, and double vision associated with near tasks

▶ Deviation at near (intermittent exotropia) X(T) 20Δ

▶ Deviation at distance orthophoric (straight eyes)

▶ NPC fuses up to 20 cm, then convergence is lost and the right eye drifts out

▶ Base-out fusional amplitude 4Δ/2Δ

Pencil push-ups and computer exercises recommended for 3 months.

Post Treatment Exam Data

▶ Headaches, eyestrain, and double vision resolved

▶ Deviation at near X 20Δ (exophoria)

▶ Deviation at distance orthophoric

▶ NPC improved to 10 cm

▶ Base-out fusional amplitude 25Δ/20Δ

Exercises

The most commonly prescribed orthoptic eye exercises are used to treat a *convergence insufficiency* (CI). They are taught in the office and carried out at home. The etiology of CI is not clear, but it is hoped that the exercises will "retrain" the brain, improving convergence, and can be discontinued once that happens. If symptoms reoccur, patients can resume these exercises on their own.

These exercises work to increase convergence ability but are not effective in all patients. Base-in prisms may also be used to help manage the convergence insufficiency in severe cases. Sometimes a combined approach of pencil push-ups, computer exercises, and/or prism may be more effective. Surgery is only offered in rare cases.

Patients given exercises or prisms are often followed by an orthoptist to evaluate any improvement in symptoms. At follow-up visits, the deviation, NPC, and fusional convergence amplitudes are remeasured and used to evaluate the effectiveness of the program (Sidebar 10-10).

Some eye care professionals may offer other forms of vision therapy intended to improve visual processing and visual perception, but this type of therapy is controversial.[21]

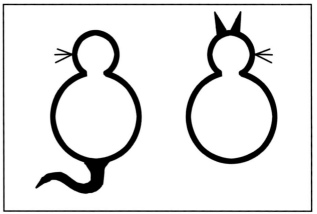

Figure 10-37. Stereogram card (Clement Clarke); each eye sees a slightly different image.

Pencil Push-Ups

For pencil push-ups, a pencil (or small accommodative target) is held at arm's length and brought toward the nose until the patient reports seeing double. The goal is to converge the eyes in order to keep the target clear and single. The patient is instructed to stop the moment the pencil or target becomes double. The patient then tries to refocus the target into a single image. If this can be done, the target is moved closer. This step is repeated over and over until the target touches the nose. If the target becomes double and cannot be merged into one, then the exercise must restart at arm's length. The patient tries to get the pencil closer and closer each day. Exercises may be more difficult if the patient suppresses an image from one eye and cannot recognize when fusion breaks (diplopia or blurred vision). These push-ups are done for a few minutes each day for a minimum of a month. Maintenance therapy may be required.

Stereogram Cards

A stereogram is a card that consists of either two similar or slightly dissimilar images. The card is held at 40 cm, and the patient holds a pen in front of it at 20 cm. The patient then focuses on the pen, converging the eyes to an area in front of the card in order to elicit physiological diplopia. If successful, a third image will appear in the space between the two pictures, forming a combined image.

A cat stereogram card is commonly used (Figure 10-37), where the left and right sides are dissimilar. When the patient converges to focus on the pen he/she should see three cats, the middle one a complete image with whiskers, ears, and tail (Figure 10-38). The cats may appear to be moving as one attempts to converge. If a fourth cat is seen, the patient must expend a little more convergence effort until three cats are seen. It is important that the patient is told to relax the eyes by looking into the

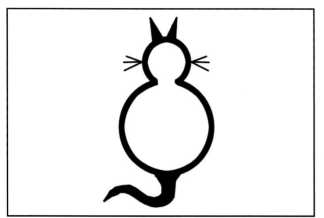

Figure 10-38. Stereogram card with images fused, seen in between the two incomplete images.

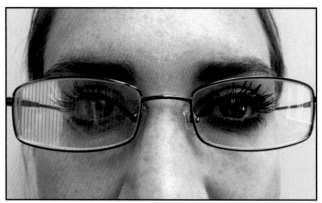

Figure 10-39. Fresnel prism applied to patient's right lens.

distance or closing them briefly after each attempt. When exercises are first started, increased eye strain may occur.

Once this exercise is done easily the patient is asked to practice it without the pen, focusing at an imaginary point in front of the card to see the third, complete cat.

Surgical Correction

The goal of strabismus surgery is to improve ocular alignment to help the eyes gain BSV. In children, amblyopia is always treated before surgery so that there is a better chance of the eyes working together. Adults may have corrective surgery to reduce or eliminate double vision caused by a decompensating strabismus or an acquired strabismus. The surgery may also be done at any age, in whole or in part, to improve cosmesis.

The general principle of strabismus surgery is to weaken or strengthen muscles in order to align the eyes. For example, a child with an esotropia could have bilateral MR recessions to weaken the muscles that pull the eyes inward. Another option might be an MR recession plus an LR resection (which additionally strengthens the muscles that pull the eyes outward) depending on the case and surgeon preference.

Surgery is not performed on small angle strabismus (ie, a horizontal angle of 10∆), as the risk of overcorrection is quite possible even with a tiny amount of correction.

Like every surgical procedure, strabismus surgery has risks. The more common risks are under- or overcorrections of the strabismus and double vision. In children, if double vision occurs after surgery, it is usually temporary. However, in adults persistent double vision is more possible. Other less common risks may include infection, bleeding, retinal detachment, decreased vision, and anesthesia complications.[23]

Children and adults who have strabismus surgery typically have general anesthesia and return home the same day if there are no general health concerns. Some teenagers or adults may be offered local anesthesia.

Adjustable sutures are commonly used in adult strabismus so that modifications can be made postoperatively (by tightening or loosening the suture) for a more desirable outcome.

Some patients experience discomfort for a few days after eye muscle surgery. Most patients can return to their normal activity within a few days to a week. Some ophthalmologists may recommend their patients avoid swimming or heavy physical activity for up to several weeks after surgery.

Botulinum

Botulinum toxin (produced by *Clostridium botulinum*) is a treatment for special strabismus cases and periocular spasms. Botulinum (Botox) is typically administered by strabismus or oculoplastics specialists. Botulinum is injected directly into an EOM to paralyze it to give temporary relief (2 to 4 months) of bothersome diplopia. It has been used in children with strabismus, but is more commonly used in adults. The injection is typically performed in the office under topical anaesthesia.

Botulinum toxin may be used alone or in conjunction with surgery to weaken the opposing muscle. For example, if a patient has a right CN VI palsy, the RMR may be injected to lessen the esotropia, causing the eye to abduct more into a primary position.

Common ocular side effects may include acquired vertical tropias and ptosis.

Prism Treatment in Nerve Palsies

Temporary, plastic stick-on prisms, called Fresnel prisms (Figure 10-39), are typically used for adults with new-onset or decompensating strabismus. They can also be used as a prism adaptation test to assess fusion potential before surgery. Fresnel prisms range from 1∆ to 40∆ and are cut to fit the glasses lens. They can be orientated base-down, base-up, base-out, base-in, or obliquely. They are relatively inexpensive and stick on the inside of the lens (smooth side down) with the application of a little water. A Fresnel prism typically lasts up to 1 year then needs replacement. It can be cleaned with water (not soap) or an alcohol-free lens cleaner and scrubbed lightly with a soft toothbrush, or wiped with a lint-free microfiber cloth.

Unfortunately, the stronger the power of a Fresnel prism, the more distorted and blurred the acuity becomes. Thus, those needing a 40Δ Fresnel often opt for occlusion and/or no prism. Vision should be tested both with and without the Fresnel to determine which will be most tolerable for the patient.

If a patient is using Fresnel prisms for a decompensating deviation or nerve palsy, periodic follow-up is required. Changes in prism power may be needed as the deviation improves or worsens. If a nerve palsy does not fully recover, prism can be permanently incorporated into spectacle lenses once the deviation is stable for at least a few months.

In certain circumstances, a compensatory head turn can be used to help diminish or eliminate diplopia, in which case prism or other treatment is not required. This should be explained to the patient. For example, a person with a mild right CN VI nerve palsy may be able to turn the head to the right (thus moving the eyes left) to avoid the diplopia in right gaze and to achieve BSV.

Follow-Up

A child with a strabismus and/or amblyopia will require close follow-up every few months. Many children are seen by an orthoptist and pediatric ophthalmologist until late childhood when the vision and strabismus is stable and unlikely to change.

Adult patients with paralytic strabismus must be followed for improvement. Typically, paralytic strabismus should show gradual signs of improvement and recovery by 6 months, if there is going to be any recovery at all. Some cases take longer, and some never recover fully, requiring prisms or surgery for relief of symptoms.

CHAPTER QUIZ

1. The medial rectus muscle is innervated by which cranial nerve?
   a. oculomotor
   b. trochlear
   c. abducens
   d. optic

2. Which of the following is *true* of Panum's area?
   a. it is surrounded by the horopter
   b. it is the space within which physiologic diplopia exists
   c. stimulation of slightly disparate retinal points gives rise to stereopsis
   d. stimulation of corresponding retinal points gives rise to stereopsis

3. You cover the patient's right eye and the left eye does not move. You cover the patient's left eye. The right eye moves out. What happens to the left eye under the cover?
   a. moves out
   b. moves in
   c. moves up
   d. does not move

4. In which direction would you orient a prism to measure an esophoria or esotropia?
   a. base-in
   b. base-out
   c. base-up
   d. base-down

5. If vision or refixation is too poor to do an alternate prism cover test, other ways to measure a strabismus would include all the following *except*:
   a. Krimsky
   b. modified Krimsky (prism over fixating eye)
   c. Hirschberg
   d. uncover test alone

6. When measuring a strabismus by the Hirschberg method, a 1-mm decentration of the light reflex in the deviating eye is equivalent to how much of a deviation?
   a. 7Δ
   b. 10Δ
   c. 15Δ
   d. 18Δ

7. What are the signs of a total third nerve palsy?
   a. hypotropia, miotic pupil, and a ptosis
   b. dilated pupil, exotropia, hypotropia, and a ptosis
   c. head tilt, dilated pupil, esotropia, and a ptosis
   d. exotropia, hypertropia, and a dilated pupil

8. When the Maddox rod is placed horizontally over the patient's right eye and the patient states the red streak is on his/her left, which way must the prism be placed over the right eye to correct the deviation?

    a. base-in
    b. base-up
    c. base-out
    d. base-down

9. The following statements are *true* about an accommodative esotropia *except*:

    a. an accommodative esotropia is congenital
    b. an accommodative esotropia usually occurs around age 2 or 3
    c. an accommodative esotropia may improve partially or fully with convex lenses
    d. an accommodative esotropia may occur with amblyopia

10. True/False: A positive angle kappa (a reflex that falls nasally) of up to 5° can be physiologic and may hide a small angle esotropia *or* cause a pseudoexotropia.

11. True/False: Amblyopia precedes suppression.

12. True/False: Typically, adults have more long-standing complaints of diplopia than small children.

13. True/False: In amblyopia treatment, if you patch too much there is a high risk of permanent occlusional amblyopia.

14. True/False: The 10Δ test for amblyopia can be done by holding the prism either base-up or base-down.

15. True/False: Amblyopia should be treated before eye muscle surgery.

Answers

1. a
2. c
3. b
4. b
5. d
6. c
7. b
8. a
9. a
10. True
11. False
12. True
13. False
14. True
15. True

References

1. Strabismus. American Association for Pediatric Ophthalmology and Strabismus website. www.aapos.org/terms/conditions/100. Updated March 28, 2014. Accessed May 26, 2016.

2. Lampert R, ed. *Binocular Vision and Ocular Motility*. 6th ed. St. Louis, MO: Mosby Inc; 2006.

3. Anatomy of the human eye: extraocular muscles. Mission for Vision website. www.images.missionforvisionusa.org/anatomy/2006/03/extraocular-muscles.html. Updated March 3, 2006. Accessed May 26, 2016.

4. Costello F. Neuro-ophthalmologic manifestations of multiple sclerosis. Medscape website. emedicine.medscape.com/article/1214270-overview. Updated January 22, 2015. Accessed May 26, 2016.

5. Rogers GM, Longmuir SQ. Refractive accommodative esotropia. University of Iowa website, EyeRounds. http://webeye.ophth.uiowa.edu/eyeforum/cases/129-Accommodative-Esotropia.htm. Posted January 26, 2011. Accessed May 26, 2016.

6. Kaufman PL, ed. *Adler's Physiology of Eye: Clinical Application*. 10th ed. St Louis, MO: Mosby, 2003.

7. Duane syndrome. American Association for Pediatric Ophthalmology and Strabismus website. www.aapos.org/terms/conditions/46. Updated November 2015. Accessed May 26, 2016.

8. Wright KW, ed. *Pediatric Ophthalmology and Strabismus*. 2nd ed. New York, NY: Springer-Verlag; 2003.

9. Sixth nerve palsy. American Association for Pediatric Ophthalmology and Strabismus website. www.aapos.org/terms/conditions/98. Revised August 2014. Accessed May 26, 2016.

10. Brown syndrome. American Association for Pediatric Ophthalmology and Strabismus website. www.aapos.org/terms/conditions/29. Updated March 2015. Accessed May 26, 2016.

11. Thyroid eye disorders. American Association for Pediatric Ophthalmology and Strabismus website. www.aapos.org/terms/conditions/105. Updated November 2011. Accessed May 26, 2016.

12. Thyroid eye. American Society of Ophthalmic Plastic and Reconstructive Surgery website. www.asoprs.org/i4a/pages/index.cfm?pageid=3677. Accessed May 26, 2016.

13. Myasthenia gravis. American Association for Pediatric Ophthalmology and Strabismus website. www.aapos.org/terms/conditions/71. Updated July 2014. Accessed May 26, 2016.

14. Rowe FJ. *Clinical Orthoptics*. 3rd ed. West Sussex, UK: Wiley-Blackwell; 2012.

15. American Academy of Ophthalmology. Amblyopia preferred practice pattern. www.aao.org/preferred-practice-pattern/amblyopia-ppp--september-2012. Accessed June 19, 2017.

16. Nystagmus. American Association for Pediatric Ophthalmology and Strabismus website. www.aapos.org/terms/conditions/80. Updated April 2016. Accessed May 26, 2016.

17. Gumpert E, ed. *Management of Strabismus and Amblyopia: A Practical Guide*. 2nd ed. New York, NY: Thieme Medical Publishers; 2001.

18. Stein HA, Stein RM, Freeman MI, eds. *The Ophthalmic Assistant: A Text for Allied and Associated Ophthalmic Personnel*. 8th ed. Philadelphia, PA: Elsevier Inc; 2006.

19. Bhola R. Binocular vision. University of Iowa Eye Rounds.org website. webeye.ophth.uiowa.edu/eyeforum/tutorials/bhola-binocularvision.htm. Posted January 23, 2006. Reviewed January 6, 2013. Accessed May 26, 2016.

20. Root T. Lecture 7, pediatric ophthalmology [video]. Root Eye Network Inc, OphthoBook website. www.ophthobook.com/videos/pediatric-ophthalmology-video. Accessed May 26, 2016.

21. Vision therapy. American Association for Pediatric Ophthalmology and Strabismus website. www.aapos.org/terms/conditions/108. Accessed May 26, 2016.

22. Adult strabismus. American Association for Pediatric Ophthalmology and Strabismus website. www.aapos.org/terms/conditions/11. Updated March 2013. Accessed May 26, 2016.

BIBLIOGRAPHY

Cassin B. *Fundamentals for Ophthalmic Technical Personnel.* Philadelphia, PA: Elsevier Inc; 1995.

The figures in this chapter were contributed by the following, who are associated with this book as authors:
Al Lens: Figures 10-20, 10-22
Colleen Schreiber: Figures 10-1 through 10-19, 10-21, 10-23 through 10-39

11

RETINOSCOPY AND REFRACTOMETRY

Aaron V. Shukla, PhD, COMT

BASIC SCIENCES

A review of ocular anatomy (Chapter 2), ocular physiology (Chapter 3), and optics (Chapter 4) may be helpful prior to reading this chapter.

The role of the human eye is to converge light rays entering it so that a sharp image is produced on the fovea. In this sense the eye behaves like a plus lens. The image on the fovea is upside down, and the right side is flipped to the left. This image is transmitted to the occipital lobe of the brain by the optic nerve and visual pathway, where it is processed, turned upright, and "reflipped." A defect anywhere in this system will result in compromised vision.

CLINICAL KNOWLEDGE

Refractive Errors

A *refractive error* results when light rays from an object are not *refracted* (bent) properly by the eye and the image is not focused on the fovea, producing blurry vision. The possibilities are myopia, hyperopia, and astigmatism, all discussed in Chapter 4 (Physiologic Optics section).

It is important to note that when a person 40 years of age or older wears his/her full correction for distance vision, blurring might be produced when performing near tasks, such as looking at a computer screen or a book. This condition, called *presbyopia*, is technically not considered a refractive error but results from aging changes in the physiology of the crystalline lens and a progressive decrease in accommodative response.

Correcting Refractive Errors

The goal in correcting refractive errors is to cause images to be focused on the fovea. The role of an ophthalmic or optometric technician is to determine if a refractive error is present and, if present, to measure it by introducing corrective lenses.

Some methods of measuring a refractive error do not require a response from the patient (*objective*), whereas in other methods the patient must respond (*subjective*). The two methods described in this chapter are *retinoscopy* (which is objective) and *refractometry* (also called *refinement*, and which is subjective).

The correction of refractive errors can be looked at from several perspectives. The most common is to consider that we are using lenses to move the focal point of an image onto the retina (Figure 11-1). The purpose of

Ledford JK, Lens A, eds.
Principles and Practice in Ophthalmic Assisting:
A Comprehensive Textbook (pp 179-211).
© 2018 Taylor & Francis Group.

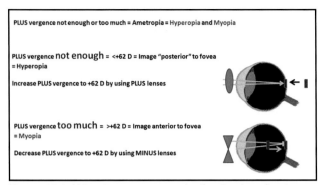

Figure 11-1. Using lenses to move the focal point of an image onto the retina in the case of refractive errors.

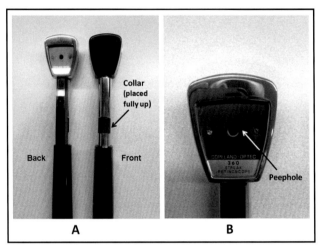

Figure 11-3. Copeland retinoscope (Stereo Optical Co), collar in the up position.

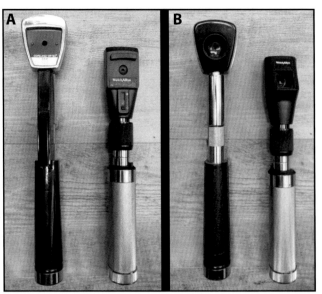

Figure 11-2. The two basic types of retinoscopes: (left) Copeland (Stereo Optical Co) and (right) Welch Allyn, (A) back and (B) front.

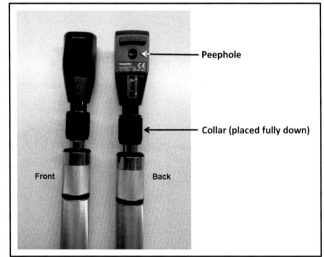

Figure 11-4. Welch Allyn retinoscope, collar in the down position.

retinoscopy and refractometry is to measure the refractive state of an eye and to place lenses in front of it so that the image falls on the fovea.

Clinical Skills

Retinoscopy

Retinoscopy is an objective method to measure (or *neutralize*) refractive errors without requiring a response from the patient. Therefore, this method is well suited for patients who are unable to respond, such as infants, toddlers, adults with speech problems, and those speaking a different language. But it is also useful for almost any patient whose refractive error is unknown.

This text describes *streak retinoscopy*, in which a slit-shaped beam of light (sometimes called the *intercept*) emerges from the instrument, causing an orange-red streak (sometimes called the *reflex*) to be observed in the patient's pupil. (The alternative is a spot retinoscope, which has mostly fallen out of use as the streak variety is much easier to interpret.)

The first streak retinoscope was developed by Jack Copeland in the 1920s and was followed by the Welch Allyn model (Figure 11-2). Both types have a peephole through which the examiner looks at the streak as reflected from the patient's eye. Both are similar in their usage and parts, and twisting the *collar* (or *sleeve*) rotates the streak 180 degrees (°). This is a key feature of the streak retinoscope.

The most important difference between the two is the position of the collar when neutralizing refractive errors. In the Copeland, the collar is placed all the way *up* (Figure 11-3), whereas in the Welch Allyn it is placed all the way *down* (Figure 11-4). In these positions the light source and condensing lens together produce *divergent* light rays (*minus* vergence) and a diffuse and unfocused intercept. This position of the collar is termed *plano*, or *plane mirror effect*, and is required for proper neutralization of refractive errors.

Moving the collar in the opposite direction (ie, *down* in the Copeland, and *up* in the Welch Allyn) emits *convergent* light rays (*plus* vergence) and a sharper intercept. This is termed *concave mirror effect*, and is used for certain advanced techniques.

The Copeland is turned on by pulling a knob at the bottom of the instrument, whereas the Welch Allyn is turned on by rotating a black ring, which also allows the examiner to vary the brightness of the light, if needed.

Set-Up and Principles

The patient is situated behind the phoropter (see Refractometry, later in this chapter). Alternately, a trial frame may be used, in which case the lenses in the following steps will have to be manipulated by hand. Both apertures in the phoropter are left open. The fixation dot is placed on the eye chart. (If a fixation dot is not available, then a similar-sized optotype may be isolated, such as a 20/60 optotype.) The patient should be directed to look at the optotype and not at the retinoscope light.

The fellow eye is blurred (called *fogging*) by adding +1.50 sphere (sph) power in the plus direction (or by inserting the "R" lens located on the auxiliary dial). Fogging helps control the accommodative response so that excess minus sphere power will not be erroneously measured trying to counteract it (quaintly known as "eating minus"). Fogging is not necessary for aphakes, pseudophakes, and patients about 72 years or older since these patients do not have an accommodative response.

The examiner sits in front of the patient, an arm's length away and slightly to the temporal side so the patient can see the chart. In this position, the dials on the phoropter are easily manipulated. The examiner holds the retinoscope in front of his/her own right eye to measure (neutralize) the patient's refractive error in the right eye, and in front of the left eye to neutralize the patient's left eye. It is a good practice for the examiner to keep both eyes open.

At this point the examiner looks through the peephole and observes the *intercept* (on the patient's eye/face) and *streak* (in the patient's pupil). The streak will be clearer in a dilated adult patient or an undilated child. The characteristics of the streak are what tell you what lenses to place in front of the eye to neutralize the refractive error.

While retinoscoping a noncyclopleged phakic eye, the patient should be encouraged *not* to look at the retinoscope but rather at the fixation dot or optotype. If the gaze wanders to the retinoscope, the pupil will constrict and accommodation may be triggered, resulting in a more myopic result. On the other hand, while retinoscoping a cyclopleged eye the patient may be encouraged to look at the instrument.

SIDEBAR 11-1
BEGINNING RETINOSCOPY HINTS

▶ When first beginning to learn retinoscopy, it is best to use a "schematic eye," which is a model (looks nothing like an eye!) that can be adjusted to simulate different refractive errors.

▶ Practice on young patients (not children!) with known refractive errors. This gives you the opportunity to learn what the reflexes look like. Or practice on young patients and dial in -3.00 sph; this will probably give you "with" motion in all meridians. Observe the reflexes.

▶ Anything that can cloud the media (corneal edema, cataracts, etc) will make it more difficult to evaluate the reflex.

▶ If the reflex looks the same in every direction, the refractive error is spherical or close to it.

▶ If you're not sure what the reflex is doing, it is probably "against" motion. Dial in +3.00 sph and see if you can get "against" motion that you can easily identify.

▶ Once you begin dialing lenses into the phoropter, your endpoint (neutral reflex) is where there is no with or against movement in the pupil at all; rather, the light fills the pupil and winks on and off as you sweep across it.

Observing the Streak and Intercept

Once the patient and instrument are properly set up, the examiner positions the retinoscope peephole in front of his/her own right eye (Sidebar 11-1). A diffuse beam is shined into the patient's right eye. Looking through the peephole of the retinoscope, the examiner sweeps the beam back and forth across the eye just enough to see any definite movement of the streak in the patient's pupil. The sweeping motion of the intercept is made *perpendicularly* (at 90°) to the streak itself (Figure 11-5). For example, in order to evaluate the 90° (vertical) meridian, one should orient the beam along the 180° (horizontal) meridian.

Ideally, the intercept and streak will be sharp and clear. But this is not always the case, and challenges may appear for various reasons. Problem reflexes are seen in irregular astigmatism (central pupil shows one type of movement, whereas the peripheral pupil shows the opposite reflex; in this case, try to use the central reflex) and corneal distortion (where the reflex looks like scissors opening and closing [*scissors reflex*]; not much can be done in this case.)

What you are looking for is the movement of the streak in the patient's pupil. The following evaluations should be made about the streak:

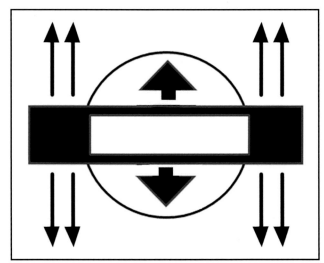

Figure 11-5. The streak is swept perpendicular to the streak and intercept.

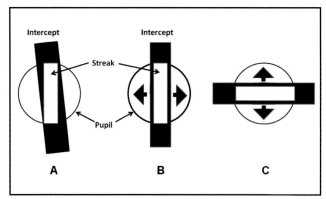

Figure 11-6. Relationship between the streak and the intercept. (A) Break phenomenon in which the streak and intercept are not aligned parallel to each other; (B) and (C) sweep direction is perpendicular to the streak.

1. Does the streak move in the *same* direction as the intercept (*with* movement)? This indicates inadequate plus vergence or hyperopia.

2. Does the streak move in the *opposite* direction as the intercept (*against* movement)? This indicates excessive plus vergence or myopia.

3. Does the entire pupil fill with light without showing any movement (*neutral* reflex)? This indicates appropriate plus vergence or emmetropia.

Additional evaluations should be made about the streak:

1. A faster, brighter, and wider streak indicates closer to neutral.

2. A slower, duller, and narrower streak indicates farther from neutral.

Begin by evaluating the streak at the 90, 45, 180, and 135 meridians. Remember to sweep perpendicularly to the streak, no matter what its axis. If the streak looks the same (in terms of movement, speed, width, and brightness) in every direction, the refractive error is spherical or close to it.

However, you may discover that the streak and the intercept are not aligned perfectly at any of these axes. If the intercept is not parallel to the streak, a *break* phenomenon will be seen, in which a break in continuity appears between the intercept and the streak (Figure 11-6). In this case, turn the streak by rotating the collar so that the intercept is aligned with the streak. This situation means that astigmatism is present, and you have just located one of the meridians. In astigmatism there are always two meridians, 90° away from each other. Once the first meridian is found, the intercept is then rotated 90° to observe the streak in the second meridian. If you have correctly determined the axis of the first meridian, then the intercept and streak in this second meridian should be parallel as well. You're looking for the two streaks and making an evaluation as to their characteristics (movement, brightness, width, and speed).

Streak and Axis Orientation

When the examiner is observing the streak along a particular orientation, the meridian being investigated is actually *perpendicular* (at 90°) to the streak and intercept. For example, when the streak and intercept are at axis 180 and the sweeping motion is vertical, the axis actually being neutralized is the 90° axis. Simply put, the *direction of the sweeping motion* indicates where the axis on the phoropter should be set. If this is not understood, the neutralizations will be off by 90°.

Neutralizing the Reflexes

At its most basic, the rule is to neutralize *against* motion by dialing in minus and neutralize *with* motion by dialing in plus. The power is changed until all meridians are neutral; that is, the streak no longer has any motion and blinks on and off as the intercept is swept across the pupil. In cases of hyperopia or myopia (ie, where there is no astigmatism), spherical lenses should be introduced until neutrality is observed. No other lenses will be needed.

But if you have discovered that astigmatism exists, the task is to neutralize the two principal meridians. The question is which meridian to neutralize first? Based on the principles of clinical optics, there are a number of ways to determine this.

First neutralize the streak representing the *sphere* portion of the refractive error with spherical lenses, and then neutralize the streak representing the plus or minus *cylinder* portion of the refractive error with cylindrical lenses. However, before cylindrical lenses are introduced, the cylinder axis on the phoropter must be set parallel to the intercept and streak (ie, 90° from the direction you are *sweeping*).

TABLE 11-1

NEUTRALIZING RETINOSCOPE MERIDIANS USING PLUS CYLINDER TECHNIQUES (WITHOUT CONVERTING ALL MERIDIANS TO *WITH* MOVEMENT)

Streak Characteristics*	Refractive Error Indicated	Neutralization Using Spherical Lenses
All meridians show similar *with* movement	Hyperopia	Neutralize with +sph lenses. All meridians will be neutralized with the same plus power.
All meridians show similar *against* movement	Myopia	Neutralize with -sph lenses. All meridians will be neutralized with the same minus power.
One meridian *neutral*; 90° away shows *with* movement	Simple hyperopic astigmatism	Make cylinder axis parallel with meridian, and neutralize *with* movement with +cyl lenses.
One meridian *neutral*; 90° away shows *against* movement	Simple myopic astigmatism	Neutralize *against* movement with -sph lenses. Other meridian will now show *with* movement. Make cylinder axis parallel with streak, and neutralize *with* movement with +cyl lenses.
Both meridians show different *with* movement	Compound hyperopic astigmatism	Neutralize *faster with* movement with +sph lenses. Other meridian will still show *with* movement. Make cylinder axis parallel with streak, and neutralize *with* movement with +cyl lenses.
Both meridians show different *against* movement	Compound myopic astigmatism	Neutralize *slower against* movement with -sph lenses. Other meridian will now show *with* movement. Make cylinder axis parallel with streak, and neutralize *with* movement with +cyl lenses.
One meridian shows *with* movement, whereas 90° away shows *against* movement	Mixed astigmatism	Neutralize *against* movement with -sph lenses. Other meridian will still show *with* movement. Make cylinder axis parallel with streak, and neutralize *with* movement with +cyl lenses.
		Note: When neutralizing a meridian representing the plus cylinder, *with* movement must be seen in order to use +cyl lenses. If *against* movement is seen, then neutralize with -sph lenses, and return to the meridian that was neutralized earlier. It will now show *with* movement indicating the plus cylinder axis. Make cylinder axis parallel with streak, and neutralize *with* movement with +cyl lenses.

*Assume working distance lens is in place (see text). Examine one meridian first and then the other, 90° away.
cyl=cylinder, sph=sphere.

The basic principles are summarized below for plus and minus cylinder methods (Tables 11-1 through 11-3). Note that these tables give instructions for "without converting all meridians to *with* movement" as well as "converting all meridians to *with* movement." This second option is provided because many examiners find it easier to see and interpret *with* movement.

Correcting for Working Distance

Because the instrument is used at arm's length, light rays emerging from the retinoscope are divergent and therefore have minus vergence when they enter the patient's eye. The light has to be corrected to plano in order to mimic infinity (Figure 11-7). This is accomplished by using a spherical *working distance* lens, usually +1.50 sph for an examiner with average-length arms. A +1.25 sph working distance lens may be necessary for a longer arm, whereas a +1.75 sph working distance lens may be necessary for a shorter arm.

The correction of a working distance lens can be made by:

1. The "R" lens on the auxiliary dial of the phoropter is a +1.50 sph lens, and may be inserted by turning the knob. At the conclusion of neutralization, it is removed and no further adjustment of the sphere is needed.

TABLE 11-2
NEUTRALIZING RETINOSCOPE MERIDIANS USING PLUS CYLINDER TECHNIQUES (BY CONVERTING ALL MERIDIANS TO *WITH* MOVEMENT)

Streak Characteristics*	Refractive Error Indicated	Neutralization Using Spherical Lenses
All meridians show similar *with* movement	Hyperopia	Neutralize with +sph lenses. All meridians will be neutralized with the same plus power.
All meridians show similar *against* movement	Myopia	Neutralize with -sph lenses. All meridians will be neutralized with the same minus power.
Add enough minus sph power to convert both meridians to *with* movement		
Both meridians show different *with* movement	Induced compound hyperopic astigmatism	Neutralize *faster with* movement with +sph lenses. Other meridian will still show *with* movement. Make cylinder axis parallel with streak, and neutralize *with* movement with +cyl lenses.
*Assume working distance lens is in place (see text). Examine one meridian first and then the other, 90° away. cyl=cylinder, sph=sphere.		

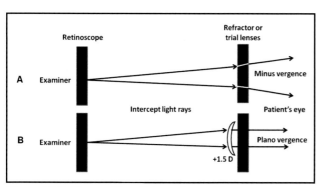

Figure 11-7. The working distance is used for convenience as well as to correct the retinoscope's vergence to plano. (A) Light rays entering the eye have minus vergence, and (B) using a working distance lens (+1.5 shown) converts the rays to plano.

2. The refractive error is neutralized without using the phoropter's retinoscopy lens *or* the sphere power may be set to +1.50 prior to beginning. However, at the conclusion of neutralization, +1.50 sph is removed by rotating the weak sphere dial in the minus direction for 6 clicks.

If you forget to remove the working distance, the patient will end up having excessive plus power equivalent to +1.50 sph, and vision will be blurry. So when the final acuity isn't what you expected, check and be sure you've removed the working lens!

Concluding Retinoscopy

After both principle meridians have been neutralized, the examiner should conclude retinoscopy with the following steps:

1. Recheck the streak in all meridians (axes). At this stage only neutral reflexes should be seen. If this is not the case, neutralizations should be rechecked.

2. Account for your working distance as mentioned above.

3. Check the patient's visual acuity. Refine using refractometry.

Using the Optical Cross to Calculate Retinoscopy Results

Using objective retinoscopy with loose trial lenses and an optical cross is a useful way for rapid measurement of hyperopia, myopia, and astigmatism in children (and other persons who cannot cooperate for subjective refractometry; Sidebar 11-2). Each streak is neutralized individually and, in cases of astigmatism, an optical cross drawn with proper axis orientations. The optical cross is then used to derive powers for spherocylindrical corrective lens.

Documenting Results

Results of retinoscopy may be noted in plus or minus cylinder form. Other notations might include whether the reading was *dry* (undilated) or *wet* (dilated). Comments about the quality and appearance of the reflex, as well as any opacities noted, should also be recorded.

TABLE 11-3
NEUTRALIZING RETINOSCOPE MERIDIANS USING MINUS CYLINDER TECHNIQUES

Streak Characteristics*	Refractive Error Indicated	Neutralization Using Spherical Lenses
All meridians show similar *with* movement	Hyperopia	Neutralize with +sph lenses. All meridians will be neutralized with the same plus power.
All meridians show similar *against* movement	Myopia	Neutralize with -sph lenses. All meridians will be neutralized with the same minus power.
One meridian *neutral*; 90° away shows *with* movement	Simple hyperopic astigmatism	Neutralize *with* movement with +sph lenses; other meridian will now show *against* movement. Make cylinder axis parallel with streak, and neutralize *against* movement with -cyl lenses.
One meridian *neutral*; 90° away shows *against* movement	Simple myopic astigmatism	Make cylinder axis parallel with streak, and neutralize *against* movement with -cyl lenses.
Both meridians show different *with* movement	Compound hyperopic astigmatism	Neutralize *slower with* movement with +sph lenses. Other meridian will now show *against* movement. Make cylinder axis parallel with streak, and neutralize *against* movement with -cyl lenses.
Both meridians show different *against* movement	Compound myopic astigmatism	Neutralize *faster against* movement with -sph lenses. Other meridian will now show faster *against* movement. Make cylinder axis parallel with streak, and neutralize *against* movement with -cyl lenses.
One meridian shows *with* movement, whereas 90° away shows *against* movement	Mixed astigmatism	Neutralize *with* movement with +sph lenses. Other meridian will now show *slower against* movement. Make cylinder axis parallel with streak, and neutralize *against* movement with -cyl lenses.
		Note: When neutralizing a meridian representing the minus cylinder, *against* movement must be seen in order to use -cyl lenses. If *with* movement is seen, then neutralize with +sph lenses, and return to the meridian that was neutralized earlier. It will now show *against* movement indicating the minus cylinder axis. Make cylinder axis parallel with streak, and neutralize *against* movement with -cyl lenses.
*Assume working distance lens is in place (see text). Examine one meridian first and then the other, 90° away. cyl=cylinder, sph=sphere.		

Troubleshooting and Errors in Retinoscopy

There are a number of phenomena that can challenge even the most experienced retinoscopist. Some of the most common problems for troubleshooting are shown in Table 11-4, along with remedies.

Errors in procedure during retinoscopy may give flawed results. Table 11-5 shows the most common, what happens when you make them, and how to correct the situation.

Advanced Concepts and Techniques

Far Point Concept

Retinoscopy is based on the principle of the *far point*, which is defined as the farthest point that is in focus in an uncorrected eye. This gives rise to three possibilities. In an emmetropic eye the far point is located at infinity. In a myopic eye the far point is located between the eye and infinity. In a hyperopic eye it is located beyond infinity and (theoretically) behind the eye.

SIDEBAR 11-2
USING THE OPTICAL CROSS

▶ Keep in mind that the streak orientation and the optical axis are oriented at 90° to each other.

▶ Hold a +1.50 sph working distance lens and examine the streaks in both eyes, keeping the retinoscope intercept parallel to the streaks. Since most children are hyperopic, the streaks most likely will show *with* motion in all meridians. Try to identify the meridians with the most and least *with* (or *against*) movement. These will be your two primary meridians.

▶ Next, choose either meridian and place an additional plus spherical lens over the +1.50 sph working distance lens. (Alternately, you can switch the +1.50 sph lens with another spherical lens with more plus power.) Examine the streak and keep increasing plus power until neutralization is achieved. Note the axis. (When a +1.50 sph working lens is not used, the power of a working lens must be subtracted from the power of the lens that yields neutralization.) Rotate the retinoscope to the other streak, and neutralize as described above; repeat for OS.

▶ In hyperopia and myopia the refractive error will be spherical, eg:

		With +1.50 sph working lens	No working lens
Hyperopia			
First streak at 90 neutralized by:		Neutralization +1.50 sph	Neutralization +3.00 sph
Second streak at 180 neutralized by:		+1.50 sph	+3.00 sph
Corrective lens power:		+1.50 sph	(+3.00) − (+1.50) = +1.50 sph
Myopia			
First streak at 90 neutralized by:		-2.50 sph	-1.00 sph
Second streak at 180 neutralized by:		-2.50 sph	-1.00 sph
Corrective lens power:		-2.50 sph	(-1.00) − (+1.50) = -2.50 sph

(continued)

With the working distance lens in place in front of an emmetropic eye, the streak will appear neutral, and the *far point* of the patient's eye will be located at the retinoscope (ie, at the examiner's eye; Figure 11-8). When the working distance lens and retinoscope are removed, the far point moves to infinity.

In a myopic eye the plus vergence (power) will be more than the +62 D required. Therefore, the far point will move closer to the patient's eye, and will be located between the examiner/retinoscope and the patient (Figure 11-9). In greater amounts of myopia the far point will move progressively closer to the patient. Therefore, an examiner may estimate the amount of myopia by simply moving forward, without adding any lenses, until neutralization is observed—the higher the myopia, the closer you must move toward the patient.

Myopia is neutralized by introducing minus lenses until a neutral reflex is observed. When the working lens is removed, the far point moves to infinity.

In a hyperopic eye the plus vergence (power) will be less than +62 D required. Therefore, the far point will move farther from the patient's eye, and will be located beyond infinity—in effect, behind the examiner's eye and retinoscope (Figure 11-10). In greater amounts of hyperopia the far point will move progressively farther from the patient and farther behind the examiner's eye. Therefore, an examiner may estimate the amount of hyperopia by simply moving back, without adding any lenses, until neutralization is observed—the higher the hyperopia the farther back you must move.

Confirming Neutralization

After a reflex has been neutralized, the far point corresponding to that reflex will be at the retinoscope/examiner. This should be confirmed by the following procedure:

1. Lean forward a few inches while sweeping the intercept and observing the reflex. If correctly neutralized, the reflex will show *with* motion in all meridians.

SIDEBAR 11-2 (CONTINUED)
USING THE OPTICAL CROSS

► If astigmatism is present, refractive errors may be derived using an optical cross. *Note that the power found using the streak is applied to the optical cross at 90° away.* For ease of illustration, the 180° and 90° meridians were used in these samples. Answers are given in both minus (-) and plus (+) cylinder. Remember, when you compose a corrective lens from an optical cross, the correct axis is the axis of the first number you use.

	With +1.50 Sph Working Distance Lens	Working Distance Lens
Compound Hyperopic Astigmatism		
▮ 1st streak at 90 neutralized by:	+2.50 Sph	+4.00 Sph (Net: [+4] - [+1.5] = +2.50)
▬ 2nd streak at 180 neutralized by:	+1.50 Sph	+3.00 Sph (Net: [+3] - [+1.5] = +1.50)
Cylinder:	1.00	1.00
Optical cross:	+2.50 ⊢ +1.50	+2.50 ⊢ +1.50
Corrective lens power:	+1.50 + 1.00 x 090 +2.50 - 1.00 x 180	+1.50 + 1.00 x 090 +2.50 - 1.00 x 180
Compound Myopic Astigmatism		
▮ 1st streak at 90 neutralized by:	-1.50 Sph	PL Sph (Net: [PL] - [+1.5] = -1.50)
▬ 2nd streak at 180 neutralized by:	-2.50 Sph	-1.00 Sph (Net: [-1] – [+1.5] = -2.50)
Cylinder:	1.00	1.00
Optical cross:	-1.50 ⊢ -2.50	-1.50 ⊢ -2.50
Corrective lens power:	-2.50 + 1.00 x 090 -1.50 - 1.00 x 180	-2.50 + 1.00 x 090 -1.50 - 1.00 x 180
Mixed Astigmatism		
▮ 1st streak at 90 neutralized by:	+1.50 Sph	+3 (Net: [3] - [+1.5] = +1.50)
▬ 2nd streak at 180 neutralized by:	-2.50 Sph	-1.00 Sph (Net: [-1] – [+1.5] = -2.50)
Cylinder:	4.00	4.00
Optical cross:	+1.50 ⊢ -2.50	+1.50 ⊢ -2.50
Corrective lens power:	- 2.50 + 4.00 x 090 + 1.50 - 4.00 x 180	- 2.50 + 4.00 x 090 + 1.50 - 4.00 x 180

Problem	Cause(s)	Remedy
Reflex not clear	Patient's tear film has dried	Have patient blink Instill artificial tears
	Media opacity	Try dilating the pupils
	Dirty lenses in phoropter	Clean lenses Have instrument serviced
	Examiner's tear film has dried	Blink Instill artificial tears
Reflex not visible	Dense media opacity	Try dilating pupils
Dark spots in reflex	Media opacities	
	Dirty lenses	Clean lenses Have instrument serviced
Curved or V-shaped streak	Broken bulb filament	Replace bulb
Reflex keeps changing	Patient is accommodating	Instruct patient to look at target
	Patient's tear film is fluctuating	Instruct patient to blink Instill artificial tears
"Scissors" reflex	Irregular astigmatism causing central and peripheral parts of streak to have different movements	Neutralize the movement of the central part of the streak
Aberrant peripheral distortion	Premium intraocular lens	
	Previous refractive surgery	
Decreased visual acuity	Failure to remove working distance lens, measurement has too much plus	Remove plus power for working distance
	Patient was accommodating during measurement, resulting in too much minus	Instruct patient to look at distance fixation target
	Axes reversed	Repeat retinoscopy

TABLE 11-4. TROUBLESHOOTING RETINOSCOPY

2. Lean backward a few inches while sweeping the intercept and observing the reflex. If correctly neutralized, the reflex will show *against* motion in all meridians.

While this procedure appears to be a simple process, it is actually an advanced skill, and will save time during refractometry.

REFRACTOMETRY

Refractometry (also termed *refinement* since it refines the measurements obtained from lensometry or retinoscopy) is one of the most important skills required in optometry and ophthalmology, and may be performed by both technicians and licensed practitioners. It is a subjective method of measuring refractive errors because it requires responses from the patient, and is well suited for patients who can comprehend verbal questions and respond appropriately.

In contrast, the term *refraction* is used when clinical judgment is exercised by a licensed practitioner in order to prescribe a spectacle or contact lens prescription. Refraction utilizes the results from refractometry and may modify them, as needed. Only a person licensed to practice may perform "a refraction"; thus, it may not be done by techs. However, as a practical matter in an eye clinic, the term *refraction* is used synonymously with *refractometry*.

Instrumentation

A *refractor* is an instrument that houses numerous rotating lenses, as well as devices used for many ophthalmic measurements, such as refractive errors, reading add powers, eye deviations, and fusion. The trade-marked name *Phoroptor* (Reichert Technologies) is often used as well, in addition to the generic term *phoropter* (note the lowercase *p* and ending in *-er* instead of *-or*), which will be used here.

	TABLE 11-5	
	ERRORS IN RETINOSCOPY	
Error	**Result of Error**	**Correction**
Fellow eye occluded	Patient pupil constricts; excess minus power measured	Open aperture of fellow eye
Retinoscope too far from examiner's eye	Reflex not clearly visible	Hold instrument against eyebrow
Examiner too close for +1.50	A shift toward more plus	Shorter working distance requires +1.75
Examiner too far for +1.50	A shift toward more minus	Longer working distance requires +1.25
Intercept too faint	Reflex not properly visible	Change retinoscope battery
Collar not positioned properly	Intercept and reflex will be sharper requiring more minus	Move collar fully up (Copeland) or down (Welch Allyn)
Intercept and sphere reflex not parallel	Reflex neutralized by inappropriate plus or minus sphere power	Ensure intercept and reflex are parallel
Intercept and cylinder reflex not parallel	Reflex neutralized by off-axis cylinder power	
Each neutralization not confirmed	Incorrect sphere and cylinder powers might be measured	Move forward and backward to confirm neutralization (see text)
Patient pupil constricts	Patient looks at retinoscope light	Encourage patient to look at fixation dot
With or *against* movement seen after neutralization	Improper neutralization	Reneutralize sphere power while observing streak 90° to the cylinder axis
		Reneutralize cylinder power while observing streak parallel to the cylinder axis

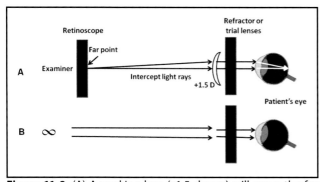

Figure 11-8. (A) A working lens (+1.5 shown) will move the far point of the patient's eye to the instrument/examiner and (B) to infinity when removed.

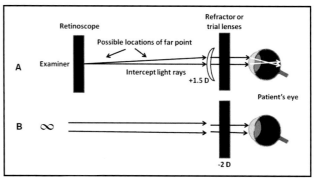

Figure 11-9. (A) The far point of a myopic eye is closer to the patient's eye, between the examiner and the patient with the working distance lens (+1.5 D) in place. (B) With the neutralization in place (shown as -2 D here), and a +1.5 D lens and retinoscope removed, the far point moves to infinity.

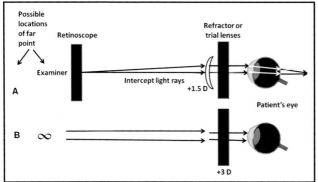

Figure 11-10. (A) The far point of a hyperopic eye is beyond the instrument and the examiner with the working distance lens (+1.5 D) in place. (B) With the neutralization in place (shown as +3 D here), and the +1.5 D lens and retinoscope removed, the far point moves to infinity.

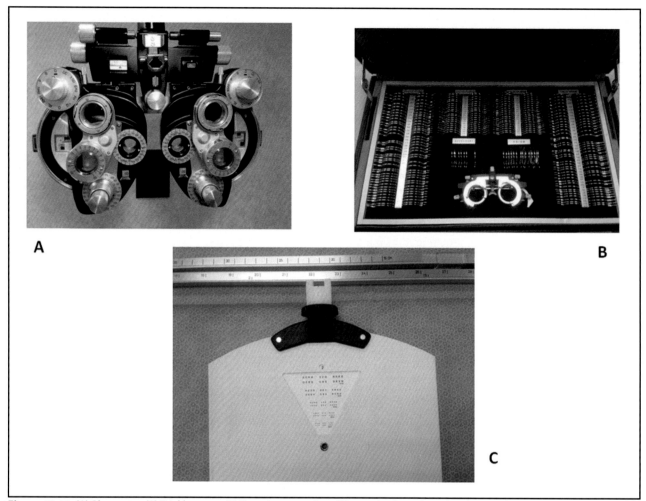

Figure 11-11. (A) Phoropter. (B) Trial lens set. (C) Rotating near chart (Nearpoint Rotochart, Reichert Technologies).

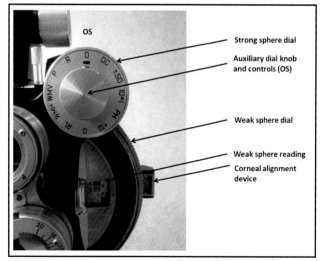

Figure 11-12. Auxiliary dials are on both sides of the phoropter.

A phoropter (or trial frame and lens set, covered later), a *Prince rule* (also called a *phoropter rod*) with a rotating near point chart, and a distance eye chart are required for this test (Figure 11-11). Examiners should be thoroughly familiar with the manuals for these instruments.

(Note: The phoropter has many parts; various features are depicted and labeled in appropriate places in this text.)

Auxiliary dials are present on the right (OD) and left (OS) sides of the phoropter to set various controls (Figure 11-12). The dials consist of two coaxial knobs located on the outer-top part of the instrument. The thin outer ring clicks in plus and minus sphere lenses in 3 diopter (D) increments, and is therefore termed the *strong sphere* dial. The inner knob introduces 12 settings useful for various tests (Table 11-6). For smaller amounts of sphere, the *weak sphere* dial enters spherical lenses in 0.25 D increments. One 0.25 D increment is often called a *click*, referring to the sound the wheel makes when the lenses move into place. Thus "four clicks" would be four 0.25 D increments, or 1.00 D.

For the purpose of measuring refractive errors, phoropters are of two principal types. *Plus* cylinder phoropters utilize plus cylinder lenses, which are marked in black. *Minus* cylinder phoropters utilize minus cylinder lenses, which are marked in red. These colored cylinder numbers are visible in a window on the face of the phoropter (Figure 11-13). (For a refresher on types of lenses, see Chapter 4.)

	TABLE 11-6		
	SETTINGS AVAILABLE ON THE AUXILIARY DIALS OF A PHOROPTER		
Notation on Auxiliary Dial	**Explanation**	**Eye**	
<u>O</u>	Open aperture	OD	OS
O	Open aperture	OD	OS
OC	Occluded aperture	OD	OS
PH	Pin hole in aperture	OD	OS
R	Retinoscopy lens (+1.50 D)	OD	OS
RL	Red lens	OD	OS
GL	Green lens		Some OS
+0.12	+1/8 D (0.125 D) lens	OD	OS
RMRV	Red Maddox rod vertical	OD	
RMRH	Red Maddox rod horizontal	OD	
WMRV	White Maddox rod vertical		OS
WMRH	White Maddox rod horizontal		OS
6ΔU	6Δ base-up	OD	
10ΔI	10Δ base-in		OS
±0.50	0.50 D cross cylinder lens with minus axis at 90°	OD	OS
P	Polarizing lens (OD axis 135° and OS axis 45°)	OD	OS

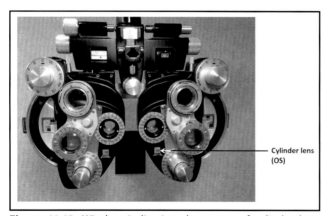

Figure 11-13. Window indicating the power of cylinder lens in the phoropter (if plus cylinder, the numbers will be black; if minus cylinder, they will be red).

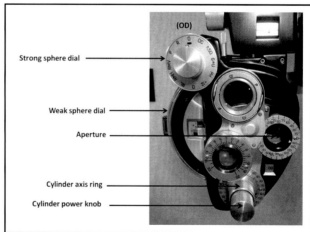

Figure 11-14. Parts of the phoropter that control the lenses.

Set-Up and Principles

Results from retinoscopy, autorefraction, or spectacle powers should be entered into the instrument as a starting point. If applicable, the *cylinder axis* and *power* should also be entered (Figure 11-14).

In cases of patients who do not wear (or did not bring) spectacles and have no previous record, or need a new spectacle prescription after eye surgery, the examiner must first perform retinoscopy (covered earlier in this chapter) or obtain a reading from an autorefractor. In a case where such instruments are not available, the

refractive error may be measured using only the phoropter (Sidebar 11-3).

For refractometry, the patient sits behind the instrument against the forehead rest, and looks through both apertures, which are set to open ("<u>O</u>" or "O" on the auxiliary dial; Figures 11-15 and 11-16). The pupillary distance (or *PD*, the distance between the optic axis of the two eyes; see Chapter 19 for more) should be adjusted so the patient's nose is not pinched and the eyes are centered in the apertures. The instrument should be leveled so that the level bubble is in the center of its window (Figure 11-17).

SIDEBAR 11-3

REFRACTOMETRY FROM SCRATCH

▶ Use clues from the patient history. Does he/she report trouble seeing up close (hyperopia)? Far off (myopia)? Both (high refractive error and/or astigmatism)?

▶ Use clues from observation and visual acuity testing. Does the patient hold the near card extremely close (myopia)? Does the patient hold the near card at arm's length (hyperopia or presbyopia)? Is there a head tilt (astigmatism)?

▶ Take the patient's age into account. If about or over 40 years, presbyopia will likely be an issue, at least once the distance refractive error is corrected.

▶ Has the patient had cataract surgery? He/she will certainly need a reading add.

▶ Check pinhole vision. Now you know what the potential final acuity is. Your measurement should improve the patient's vision at least to this point.

▶ Start by offering plus sphere. If that helps, continue adding plus sphere until the vision blurs and then go back to the previous setting.

▶ If minus sphere helps, be careful not to overminus. Make the patient "earn" more minus by reading progressively smaller and smaller letters for every change until smaller letters cannot be read even if the patient says the letters are more clear with more minus.

▶ If you are not to 20/20 yet, the patient may have astigmatism. (See text, Optional Step, in plus or minus cylinder, for a method to find cylinder axis.)

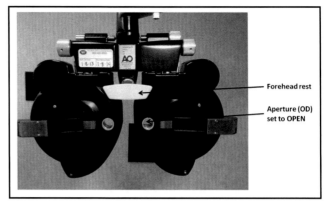

Figure 11-15. Phoropter back.

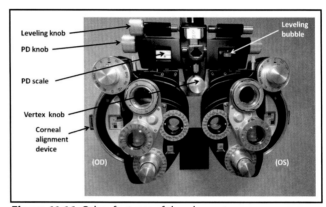

Figure 11-16. Other features of the phoropter.

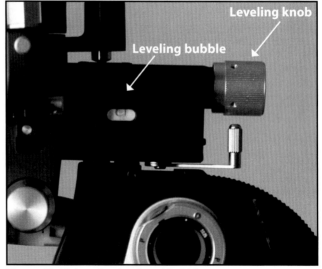

Figure 11-17. Leveling knob and bubble.

The importance of *vertex distance* (distance between the cornea and spectacle or trial lens) is discussed in Chapter 19. In most cases, the standard phoropter vertex distance of 13.75 mm should be used during refractometry. To verify the standard vertex, observe the patient's corneal profile in the alignment device (see Figure 11-12); the front of the cornea should align with the longest line in the device.

If the patient's eyelashes are brushing against the lenses, move the forehead rest back. This increases the vertex distance. Using the alignment device, observe which short line is now aligned with the corneal profile. (Each short line represents a change of 2 mm.)

In any refractive error greater than 4 D, the vertex distance should be specifically noted in the patient's record. At these higher powers, the effective power of the lens is changed if the lens is moved toward or away from the eye.

Usually the right eye is measured first, so the left eye is occluded using the "OC" setting on the auxiliary dial. The eye chart may then be presented. This author recommends using an entire screen of optotypes (Sidebar 11-4). When finished measuring the right eye, it is occluded and the left aperture is opened.

Patient Education and Involvement

Refractometry is team work involving the examiner and the patient, so the procedure should be properly explained. The patient will be asked to compare the letters through two different lenses. In some cases one choice will be obviously clearer, in other cases they may appear to be about the same. Remind the patient that your lens adjustments will be based on his/her responses.

Rushing through the measurement is one of the main reasons for failure. To get reliable results, only proceed as fast as the patient is able to cooperate.

Basic Technique

Plus and minus cylinder refractometry is performed in six steps with a possible extra step. Steps 1 through 5 (which includes an optional step) are monocular tests (one eye tested at a time), whereas Step 6 is a binocular test (both eyes open). Each step has a coordinated table of numbered hints which are referred to in the text.

▶ Step 1—Determine initial sphere power

• Optional step—Locating the cylinder axis

▶ Step 2—Refine cylinder axis

▶ Step 3—Refine cylinder power

▶ Step 4—Refine sphere power

▶ Step 5—Duochrome (red/green) test

▶ Step 6—Binocular balancing (fogging)

Plus Cylinder Refractometry

Step 1—Determine Initial Sphere Power (Table 11-7A)

The goal of this step is to determine the greatest plus sphere power (or the least minus sphere power) that provides the best vision.

▶ Determine the anchor line (the smallest line of letters that the patient has correctly identified so far), and direct the patient to look at it and not wander to larger lines.

SIDEBAR 11-4
REFRACTOMETRY AND THE DISTANCE CHART

Prior to publication, there was a lot of discussion about whether distance refractometry should be done with the patient looking at the full eye chart (this author's preference) or a single line. Each method has advantages and disadvantages.

Using the full eye chart saves the tech from having to switch lines as the test progresses. In the whole chart approach, the patient is directed to look at a particular line (the "anchor line") on the chart, then progressively smaller lines as the measurement improves vision. The tech must make sure that the patient is focusing on the desired line, and not wandering to the larger optotypes. This is the method used in this chapter.

Using a single line doesn't work if the chart is left on the same line for the entire measurement. In this technique, the chart must be changed to progressively smaller lines as the patient's vision increases, especially if working in a minus direction. The advantage lies in having more control over what size optotypes the patient is looking at.

Note: Single optotypes are not usually used, and in children can actually give erroneous results.

▶ Turn the weak sphere power in the plus direction by 0.50 D (Tip #1).

▶ Continue to add plus sphere power until the patient reports blurring; then go back to the previous setting.

▶ If additions of sphere power in the plus direction result in blurring, offer 0.25 D in the minus direction. If visual acuity improves (and patient does not report that the letters are smaller and darker), then additional 0.25 D steps in the minus direction may be given (Tip #2).

• Note: This author prefers to use 0.25 D steps during this phase of the measurement. The advantage of doing this is that minus power, given in the smallest increments, helps minimize chances of overminusing.

TABLE 11-7A
TIPS FOR DETERMINING SPHERE POWER

Tip #1	Change sphere powers by 0.25 D to 0.5 D if the visual acuity is 20/60 to 20/50 or better. This change will not be enough for the patients with vision impairment or low vision. Those patients will require choices differing by approximately 0.75 D to 1 D.
Tip #2	A good rule is that minus has to be earned. Therefore, a lesser plus power, or a greater minus, must result in improved visual acuity before it is assigned. Do not accept "…smaller and darker…" as a valid answer for assigning a power in the minus direction. With more minus power than necessary, a patient will use accommodation, which may cause problems at near, such as difficulty reading, or accommodative esotropia.

TABLE 11-7B
TIPS FOR LOCATING THE PLUS CYLINDER AXIS

Tip #3	If the current spectacle prescription for distance is spherical, it is good practice to check if cylinder correction is required.
Tip #4	This is the only time that the cylinder power (P) part of the JCC is used prior to the cylinder axis (knurled rings) part.
Tip #5	Many practitioners leave this at ".00," but +0.25 will have to be introduced for refining the cylinder axis, and is optically more precise.
Tip #6	Since +0.25 D has been dialed in, the total cylinder power at axis 180 will be +0.50 D when the white dot (Lens #1) is in place and plano (0.0) when the red dot is in place (Lens #2). Thus, you are basically inquiring if the patient prefers plus cylinder correction at axis 180 or not.
Tip #7	The axis dial is marked in 5° increments.

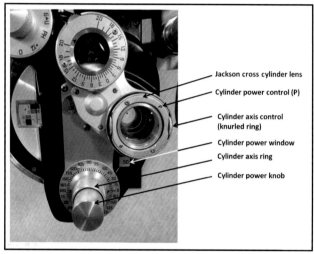

Jackson cross cylinder lens

Cylinder power control (P)

Cylinder axis control (knurled ring)

Cylinder power window

Cylinder axis ring

Cylinder power knob

Figure 11-18. The Jackson cross cylinder and related controls, plus cylinder phoropter (note black numbers in cylinder power window).

▶ The initial sphere power is determined when the greatest plus, or least minus, power that gives best acuity is reached.

▶ If the current spectacle prescription, retinoscopy reading, or autorefraction has cylinder correction, go to Step 2. If it is only spherical go to the Optional Step, locating the plus cylinder axis, next.

Optional Step—Locate the Plus Cylinder Axis (Table 11-7B)

If the patient's refractive error is unknown prior to refractometry or if the current refractive error is spherical and the vision cannot be further improved after Step 1, the patient might have uncorrected astigmatism. The goal of this step is to determine the approximate location of the plus cylinder axis by using the Jackson cross cylinder (JCC), checking for plus cylinder power at four axes: 180, 135, 90, and 45 (Tip #3 and Figure 11-18). Once this

is done, plus cylinder axis should be refined using Step 2 described below.

▶ Direct the patient to look at the anchor line. Swing the JCC into place and rotate it so that one of the dots is aligned with the axis. In this position the JCC will click into place (see Figure 11-18 and Tip #4).

▶ Rotate the outer (axis) ring on the cylinder knob so the arrows point to 180.

▶ Rotate the inner (power) cylinder knob to insert +0.25 D (Tip #5).

▶ Use the knurled ring to rapidly flip the JCC to first present the white dot at axis 180 (Lens #1) and then the red dot at axis 180 (Lens #2). Inquire if either of the two choices is clearer (Tip #6).

▶ If the patient needs plus cylinder correction at or near one of the choices of axis, then the white dot will be preferred at that location. Make a note of the axis where the patient preferred plus cylinder, but check all four positions.

▶ Repeat the process by turning the arrows to axes 135, 90, and 45 (Tip #7).

▶ If the patient chooses the red dot at all 4 axes, then no plus cylinder correction is required. Proceed directly to Step 4.

▶ When done, rotate the outer (axis) ring on the cylinder knob to the axis determined by the test. Rotate the inner ring on the JCC so that the two knurled rings are aligned with this axis and go to Step 2.

Step 2—Refine Plus Cylinder Axis (Table 11-7C)

The goal of this step is to refine the plus cylinder axis by following the white dots on the JCC. The correct plus cylinder axis is indicated either when the smallest line visible appears equally clear with the two lens choices, or the patient repeatedly goes back and forth between the two choices. The axis *must* be refined *prior* to measuring the cylinder power.

TABLE 11-7C
TIPS FOR REFINING PLUS CYLINDER AXIS

Tip #8	Inform the patient that the lens in this step checks for astigmatism and might cause blurring, but it will be removed at the end of this step.
Tip #9	Inform the patient of the goal, ie, you are looking for "sameness, not sharpness."
Tip #10	When the patient requests to repeat the choice again, it indicates that you are at or close to the correct axis. At this time offer the third choice, "Lens #1, or #2, or are they the same?"
Tip #11	It is good practice to keep changing the lens choice names, eg, #1 and #2, #3 and #4, #5 and #6, etc. It is also acceptable to use A and B as designations, alternating with the numbers. This ensures that the patient is fully engaged.

► Present a full screen of optotypes, have the patient focus on the smallest line legible. Verify this anchor line every time the axis is changed (Tips #8 and #9).

► The examiner and patient should always know which line is being viewed. This is very important, and it separates a functional process from a superior one. It will also help reduce the number of glasses rechecks.

► It is good practice to not isolate a line (see Sidebar 11-4), and definitely not a single optotype. If the patient is amblyopic, single optotypes might give erroneous results (see Chapter 8). However, if a patient is confused by numerous lines, it might be necessary to isolate a line.

► Swing the JCC into place and rotate it so that the two knurled rings are aligned with the axis. In this position the JCC will click into place. The dots will straddle the axis.

► Once the anchor line has been identified, direct the patient to look at it and not wander to larger lines. This is Lens #1.

► Use the knurled ring, rapidly flip the JCC (Lens #2) and inquire which of the two choices is sharper, or if they are the same. (Making a rapid flip will prevent an intermediate image, which might cause confusion.) If they are equally clear, the axis is correct.

► If one choice is clearer, use the outer knob on the cylinder control to rotate the axis dial by 10° (2 marks, each being 5°) in the direction of the white dot. (Make sure you remember where the white dot was on the lens of the patient's choice. Otherwise you might accidentally rotate the axis in the wrong direction.) Present the two choices again (Tip #10).

► Keep changing the axis in the direction of the white dot by 10°. When the patient's choice reverses to the other direction, change by half as much, ie, 5°, then 2.5° (Tip #11). Once the two choices appear the same, the correct plus cylinder axis has been achieved.

Go to Step 3.

Step 3—Refine Plus Cylinder Power (Table 11-7D)

The goal of this step is to measure the plus cylinder power using the JCC. The correct amount of plus cylinder is indicated either when the smallest line visible appears equally clear with the two lens choices, or the patient repeatedly goes back and forth between the two choices.

► At this stage in the process, the plus cylinder power will be at least +0.25 D as determined from an autorefractor reading, neutralization by retinoscopy or lensometry, or from the Optional Step described previously.

► Rotate the JCC so that the "P" (power) is aligned with the axis. In this position the P on the JCC will click into place (Tips #12 through #14).

► Use the knurled ring to flip the JCC so that the white dots are aligned with the P.

► Once the anchor line has been identified, direct the patient to look at it and not wander to larger lines. This is Lens #1. Rapidly change the lens by flipping the JCC so that the red dots are parallel to the axis (Lens #2).

► Ask if the vision is improved by more plus cylinder (white dots on P) or less plus cylinder (red dots on P) compared to the cylinder power initially entered (Tip #15).

► If the patient prefers more plus cylinder, turn the cylinder power knob to add +0.25 D. If the patient prefers less plus cylinder, rotate the cylinder power knob to remove +0.25 D (Tip #16).

► Continue to offer the white and red dots as choices until the patient goes back and forth between the two or they both look about the same. If the patient goes back and forth, then decrease the cylinder by 0.25 D (Tip #17).

► Once the correct plus cylinder power has been refined, rotate the JCC away from the aperture and proceed to Step 4.

	TABLE 11-7D
	TIPS FOR REFINING PLUS CYLINDER POWER
Tip #12	Inform the patient that the lens in this step checks for astigmatism and might cause blurring, but it will be removed at the end of this step.
Tip #13	Give as much cylinder power as the patient accepts. (A licensed practitioner can decide how much to actually prescribe.)
Tip #14	Typically, practitioners do not assign a great amount of cylinder power to a patient who is not used to astigmatic correction. Instead, cylinder power is incrementally increased over a period of time to allow the visual cortex to process the steadily sharpening images.
Tip #15	In Lens #1, the white dots will be parallel to the cylinder axis. Therefore, the total cylinder power in front of the patient's eye will increase by +0.25 D. In Lens #2, the red dots will be parallel to the cylinder axis. Therefore, the total cylinder power in front of the patient's eye will decrease by -0.25 D. For example, if +0.75 D was entered originally, then the total cylinder will be +1 D when the white dots are parallel to axis (+0.75 +0.25), whereas the total cylinder will be +0.5 D when the red dots are parallel to the axis (+0.75 -0.25).
Tip #16	For every two clicks of plus cylinder *added*, the sphere must be changed by -0.25 D in order to preserve the spherical equivalent. For every two clicks of plus cylinder *removed*, the sphere must be changed by +0.25 D in order to preserve the spherical equivalent.
Tip #17	It is good practice to keep changing the lens choice names, eg, #1 and #2, #3 and #4, #5 and #6, etc. It is also acceptable to use A and B as designations, alternating with the numbers. This ensures that the patient is fully engaged.

	TABLE 11-7E
	TIP FOR REFINING SPHERE POWER
Tip #18	A good rule is that minus has to be earned. Therefore, a lesser plus power, or a greater minus, must result in improved visual acuity before it is assigned. Do not accept "…smaller and darker…" as a valid answer for assigning a power in the minus direction. Assigning more minus than necessary will use accommodation, which may cause problems at near, such as difficulty reading, or accommodative esotropia.

Step 4—Refine Sphere Power (Table 11-7E)

The goal of this step is to determine the greatest plus sphere power (or the least minus sphere power) that provides the best vision.

► First, change the weak sphere power in the plus direction by 0.25 D. If visual acuity improves, offer an additional 0.25 D in the plus direction.

► If all additions of sphere power in the plus direction result in blurring, offer 0.25 D in the minus direction. If visual acuity improves (and the patient does not report that the letters are "smaller and darker"), then offer an additional 0.25 D in the minus direction (Tip #18).

► The refined sphere power is determined when the greatest plus, or least minus, power is measured.

Step 5—Duochrome (Red/Green) Test (Table 11-7F)

The goal of this step is to ensure that the measurement does not have excess plus or minus sphere power.

► Occlude one eye. Isolate optotypes twice as large as the best-corrected visual acuity (BCVA); for example, if BCVA is 20/20 then isolate the 20/40 line.

► Move the red/green filter into place on the eye chart.

► Ask the patient if the optotypes in the red and green sides appear equally sharp. If so, the sphere power refined in Step 4 is correct (Tips #19 and #20).

► If the sphere power has excess plus, the letters in the red side will be sharper. Minus sphere power is added to make both sides the same sharpness (Tip #21).

► If the sphere power has excess minus, the letters in the green side will be sharper. Plus sphere power is added to make both sides the same sharpness (Tip #22).

TABLE 11-7F
TIPS FOR THE DUOCHROME (RED/GREEN) TEST

Tip #19	The duochrome test may be performed on patients with a red/green color deficiency. In this case the patient should be instructed to use "right" and "left" side instead of red and green, respectively.
Tip #20	Optotypes in the green side form images in the vitreous, whereas those in the red side form images "behind" the fovea. If the refined sphere power is correct, both sets of optotypes will be equidistant from the fovea, and will appear equally sharp.
Tip #21	With excess plus sphere power, optotypes in the red will be closer to the fovea, thus making them sharper.
Tip #22	With excess minus sphere power, optotypes in the green will be closer to the fovea, thus making them sharper.

TABLE 11-7G
TIPS FOR BINOCULAR BALANCING (FOGGING)

Tip #23	Binocular balancing (fogging) is not necessary in children and young adults, in older presbyopes, in pseudophakes, aphakes, or if only one eye is functioning.
Tip #24	Binocular balancing (fogging) is ideally suited for hyperopes (especially presbyopic), pre-presbyopes, and first-time presbyopes.
Tip #25	Adding excess plus power moves the OD and OS images into the vitreous. If both eyes accommodate equally, both images will appear equally blurred.
Tip #26	If the OD accommodates more, its image will appear less blurry, and +0.25 D is added to relax accommodation.
Tip #27	If the OS accommodates more, its image will appear less blurry, and +0.25 D is added to relax accommodation.

Step 6—Binocular Balancing (Fogging; Table 11-7G)

The goal of this step is to ensure that both eyes accommodate equally (Tips #23 and #24).

▶ Open both apertures. Isolate optotypes twice as large as the BCVA.

▶ Add +1 D sph, OU. This will cause blurring (fogging) and relaxation of accommodation in both eyes (Tip #25).

▶ Turn the right 6Δ BU auxiliary lens (labeled 6ΔU) into the aperture OD. This will cause diplopia. (The lower image is OD and the upper image is OS.)
  • Alternate method: Since the diplopia caused by the 6ΔU lens can be uncomfortable, some examiners simply use an occluder to cover one eye at a time for the patient to compare.

▶ Ask the patient if the two blurry images appear equally blurred. If so, the refractometry result is properly balanced and you can remove the +1 D sph.

▶ If one of the images appears less blurry, add 0.25 D in the plus direction to that eye. This is an attempt to blur both eyes equally.

• If the lower image is less blurry, add +0.25 D sph to the right eye. If the upper image is less blurry, add +0.25 D sph to the left eye (Tips #26 and #27).

When done, remove the +1 D sph from both sides.

Minus Cylinder Refractometry

Step 1—Determine Initial Sphere Power (Table 11-8A)

The goal of this step is to determine the greatest plus sphere power (or the least minus sphere power) that provides the best vision.

▶ Determine the anchor line, and direct the patient to look at it and not wander to larger lines.

▶ Turn the weak sphere power in the plus direction by 0.50 D (Tip #28).

▶ Continue to add sphere power until the patient reports blurring; then go back to the previous setting.

▶ If additions of sphere power in the plus direction result in blurring, offer 0.25 D in the minus direction. If visual acuity improves (and the patient does not report that the letters are smaller and darker), then additional 0.25 D steps in the minus direction may be given (Tip #29).

TABLE 11-8A
TIPS FOR DETERMINING SPHERE POWER

Tip #28	Change sphere powers by 0.25 D to 0.5 D if the visual acuity is 20/60 to 20/50 or better. This change will not be enough for the patients with vision impairment or low vision. Those patients will require choices differing by approximately 0.75 D to 1 D.
Tip #29	A good rule is that minus has to be earned. Therefore, a lesser plus power, or a greater minus, must result in improved visual acuity before it is assigned. Do not accept "…smaller and darker…" as a valid answer for assigning a power in the minus direction. With more minus power than necessary, a patient will use accommodation, which may cause problems at near, such as difficulty reading, or accommodative esotropia.

TABLE 11-8B
TIPS FOR LOCATING THE MINUS CYLINDER AXIS

Tip #30	If the current spectacle prescription for distance is spherical, it is good practice to check if cylinder correction is required.
Tip #31	This is the only time that the cylinder power (P) part of the JCC is used prior to the cylinder axis (knurled rings) part.
Tip #32	Many practitioners leave this at ".00," but -0.25 will have to be introduced for refining the cylinder axis, and is optically more precise.
Tip #33	Since -0.25 D has been dialed in, the total cylinder power at axis 180 will be -0.50 D when the red dot (Lens #1) is in place and plano (0.0) when the white dot is in place (Lens #2). Thus, you are basically inquiring if the patient prefers minus cylinder correction at axis 180, or not.
Tip #34	Note that the axis dial is marked in 5° increments.

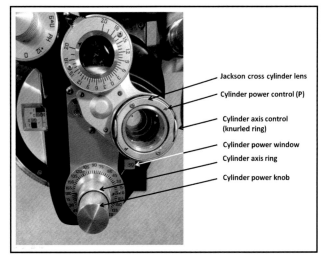

Figure 11-19. The Jackson cross cylinder and related controls, minus cylinder phoropter (note red numbers in cylinder power window).

- Note: This author prefers to use 0.25 D steps during this phase of the measurement. The advantage of doing this is that minus power, given in the smallest increments, helps minimize chances of overminusing.

▶ The initial sphere power is determined when the greatest plus, or least minus, power that gives best acuity is reached.

▶ If the current spectacle prescription, retinoscopy reading, or autorefraction has cylinder correction, go to Step 2. If it is only spherical, go to the Optional Step, locating the minus cylinder axis, next.

Optional Step—Locate the Minus Cylinder Axis (Table 11-8B)

If the patient's refractive error is unknown prior to refractometry or if the current refractive error is spherical and the vision cannot be further improved after Step 1, the patient might have uncorrected astigmatism. The goal of this step is to determine the approximate location of the minus cylinder axis by using the JCC, checking for minus cylinder power at four axes: 180, 135, 90, and 45 (Tip #30 and Figure 11-19). Once this is done, minus cylinder axis should be refined using Step 2 as described.

▶ Direct the patient to look at the anchor line. Swing the JCC into place and rotate it so that one of the dots is aligned with the axis. In this position the JCC will click into place (see Figure 11-19 and Tip #31).

▶ Rotate the outer (axis) ring on the cylinder knob so the arrows point to 180.

	TABLE 11-8C
	TIPS FOR REFINING MINUS CYLINDER AXIS
Tip #35	Inform the patient that the lens in this step checks for astigmatism and might cause blurring, but it will be removed at the end of this step.
Tip #36	Inform the patient of the goal, ie, you are looking for "sameness, not sharpness."
Tip #37	When the patient requests to repeat the choice again, it indicates that you are at or close to the correct axis. At this time offer the third choice, "Lens #1, or #2, or are they the same?"
Tip #38	It is good practice to keep changing the lens choice names, eg, #1 and #2, #3 and #4, #5 and #6, etc. It is also acceptable to use A and B as designations, alternating with the numbers. This ensures that the patient is fully engaged.

▶ Rotate the inner (power) cylinder knob to insert -0.25 D (Tip #32).

▶ Use the knurled ring to rapidly flip the JCC to first present the red dot at axis 180 (Lens #1) and then the white dot at axis 180 (Lens #2). Inquire if either of the two choices is clearer (Tip #33).

▶ If the patient needs minus cylinder correction at or near one of the choices of axis, then the red dot will be preferred at that location. Make a note of the axis where the patient preferred minus cylinder, but check all four positions.

▶ Repeat the process by turning the arrows to axes 135, 90, and 45 (Tip #34).

▶ If the patient chooses the white dot at all four axes, then no minus cylinder correction is needed. Proceed directly to Step 4.

▶ When done, rotate the outer (axis) ring on the cylinder knob to the axis determined by the test. Rotate the inner ring on the JCC so that the two knurled rings are aligned with this axis and go to Step 2.

Step 2—Refine Minus Cylinder Axis (Table 11-8C)

The goal of this step is to refine the minus cylinder axis by following the red dots on the JCC. The correct minus cylinder axis is indicated either when the smallest line visible appears equally clear with the two lens choices, or the patient repeatedly goes back and forth between the two choices. The axis *must* be refined *prior to* measuring the cylinder power.

▶ Present a full screen of optotypes, and have the patient focus on the smallest line legible. Verify this anchor line every time the axis is changed (Tips #35 and #36).

▶ The examiner and patient should always know which line is being viewed. This is very important, and it separates a functional process from a superior one. It will also help reduce the number of glasses rechecks.

▶ It is good practice to not isolate a line (see Sidebar 11-4), and definitely not a single optotype. If the patient is amblyopic, single optotypes might give erroneous results (see Chapter 8). However, if a patient is confused by numerous lines, it might be necessary to isolate a line.

▶ Swing the JCC into place and rotate it so that the two knurled rings are aligned with the axis. In this position the JCC will click into place. The dots will straddle the axis.

▶ Once the anchor line has been identified, direct the patient to look at it and not wander to larger lines. This is Lens #1.

▶ Use the knurled ring, rapidly flip the JCC (Lens #2) and inquire which of the two choices is sharper, or if they are the same. (Making a rapid flip will prevent an intermediate image, which might cause confusion.) If they are equally clear, the axis is correct.

▶ If one choice is clearer, use the outer knob on the cylinder control to rotate the axis dial by 10° (2 marks, each being 5°) in the direction of the red dot. (Make sure you remember where the red dot was on the lens of the patient's choice. Otherwise you might accidentally rotate the axis in the wrong direction.) Present the two choices again (Tip #37).

▶ Keep changing the axis in the direction of the red dot by 10°. When the patient's choice reverses to the other direction, change by half as much, ie, 5°, then 2.5° (Tip #38). Once the two choices appear the same, the correct minus cylinder axis has been refined.

Go to Step 3.

TABLE 11-8D
TIPS FOR REFINING MINUS CYLINDER POWER

Tip #39	Inform the patient that the lens in this step checks for astigmatism and might cause blurring, but it will be removed at the end of this step.
Tip #40	Give as much cylinder power as the patient accepts. (A licensed practitioner can decide how much to actually prescribe.)
Tip #41	Typically, practitioners do not assign a great amount of cylinder power to a patient who is not used to astigmatic correction. Instead, cylinder power is incrementally increased over a period of time to allow the visual cortex to process the steadily sharpening images.
Tip #42	In Lens #1, the red dots will be parallel to the cylinder axis. Therefore, the total cylinder power in front of the patient's eye will increase by -0.25 D. In Lens #2, the white dots will be parallel to the cylinder axis. Therefore, the total cylinder power in front of the patient's eye will decrease by +0.25 D. For example, if -0.75 D was entered originally, then the total cylinder will be -1 D when the red dots are parallel to axis (-0.75 -0.25), whereas the total cylinder will be -0.5 D when the white dots are parallel to the axis (-0.75 +0.25).
Tip #43	For every two clicks of minus cylinder *added*, the sphere must be changed by +0.25 D in order to preserve the spherical equivalent. For every two clicks of minus cylinder *removed*, the sphere must be changed by -0.25 D in order to preserve the spherical equivalent.
Tip #44	It is good practice to keep changing the lens choice names, eg, #1 and #2, #3 and #4, #5 and #6, etc. It is also acceptable to use A and B as designations, alternating with the numbers. This ensures that the patient is fully engaged.

Step 3—Refine Minus Cylinder Power (Table 11-8D)

The goal of this step to measure the minus cylinder power using the JCC. The correct amount of minus cylinder is indicated either when the smallest line visible appears equally clear with the two lens choices, or the patient repeatedly goes back and forth between the two choices.

▶ At this stage in the process, the minus cylinder power will be at least -0.25 D as determined from an autorefractor reading, neutralization by retinoscopy or lensometry, or from the Optional Step described previously.

▶ Rotate the JCC so that the "P" (power) is aligned with the axis. In this position the P on the JCC will click into place (Tips #39 through #41).

▶ Use the knurled ring to flip the JCC so that the red dots are aligned with the P.

▶ Once the anchor line has been identified, direct the patient to look at it and not wander to larger lines. This is Lens #1. Rapidly change the lens by flipping the JCC so that the white dots are parallel to the axis (Lens #2).

▶ Ask if the vision is improved by more minus cylinder (red dots on P) or less minus cylinder (white dots on P) compared to the cylinder power initially entered (Tip #42).

▶ If the patient prefers more minus cylinder, turn the cylinder power knob to add -0.25 D. If the patient prefers less minus cylinder, rotate the cylinder power knob to remove -0.25 D (Tip #43).

▶ Continue to offer the red and white dots as choices until the patient goes back and forth between the two or they both look about the same. If the patient goes back and forth, then decrease the cylinder by 0.25 D (Tip #44).

▶ Once the correct minus cylinder power has been refined, rotate the JCC away from the aperture and proceed to Step 4.

Step 4—Refine Sphere Power (Refer to Table 11-7E)

The goal of this step is to determine the greatest plus sphere power (or the least minus sphere power) that provides the best vision.

▶ First, change the weak sphere power in the plus direction by 0.25 D. If visual acuity improves, offer an additional 0.25 D in the plus direction (Tip #18).

▶ If all additions of sphere power in the plus direction result in blurring, offer 0.25 D in the minus direction. If visual acuity improves (and the patient does not report that the letters are "smaller and darker"), then offer an additional 0.25 D in the minus direction.

▶ The refined sphere power is determined when the greatest plus, or least minus, power is measured.

Step 5—Duochrome (Red/Green) Test (Refer to Table 11-7F)

The goal of this step is to ensure that the measurement does not have excess plus or minus power.

▸ Occlude one eye. Isolate optotypes twice as large as the BCVA (eg, if BCVA is 20/20 then isolate the 20/40 line).

▸ Move the red/green filter into place on the eye chart.

▸ Ask the patient if the optotypes in the red and green sides appear equally sharp. If so, the sphere power refined in Step 4 is correct (Tips #19 and #20).

▸ If the sphere power has excess plus, the letters in the red side will be sharper. Minus sphere power is added to make both sides the same sharpness (Tip #21).

▸ If the sphere power has excess minus, the letters in the green side will be sharper. Plus sphere power is added to make both sides the same sharpness (Tip #22).

Step 6—Binocular Balancing (Fogging; Refer to Table 11-7G)

The goal of this step is to ensure that both eyes accommodate equally (Tips #23 and #24).

▸ Open both apertures. Isolate optotypes twice as large as the BCVA.

▸ Add +1 D sph, OU. This will cause blurring (fogging) and relaxation of accommodation in both eyes (Tip #25).

▸ Turn the right 6Δ BU auxiliary lens (labeled 6ΔU) into the aperture OD. This will cause diplopia. (The lower image is OD and the upper image is OS.)

  • Alternate method: Since the diplopia caused by the 6ΔU lens can be uncomfortable, some examiners simply use an occluder to cover one eye at a time for the patient to compare.

▸ Ask the patient if the two blurry images appear equally blurred. If so, the refractometry result is properly balanced and you can remove the +1 D sph.

▸ If one of the images appears less blurry, add 0.25 D in the plus direction to that eye. This is an attempt to blur both eyes equally.

  • If the lower image is less blurry, add +0.25 D sph to the right eye. If the upper image is less blurry, add +0.25 D sph to the left eye (Tips #26 and #27).

▸ When done, remove the +1 D sph from both sides.

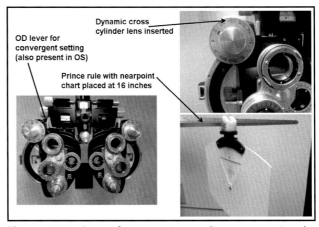

Figure 11-20. Set-up for measuring reading power using the ±dynamic cross cylinder lens method.

Measuring Reading Add Power

In presbyopic patients the reading add power must be carefully measured, especially if the distance measurement has changed and/or the patient is a hyperope or has trouble reading fine print.

A number of methods exist for measuring the add power. All involve first converging the PD levers on the phoropter, positioning the Prince rule, and placing the rotating chart at 16 inches.

±0.5 D Dynamic Cross Cylinder Lens Method

The dynamic cross cylinder (DCC) lens is this author's recommended method for measuring reading add power (Figure 11-20). The DCC is a ±0.50 D cross cylinder lens with the minus axis set at 90°. It is located on the auxiliary dial, marked "±0.5." This method is ideally suited for first-time presbyopes, medium- or high-hyperopes, patients having problems with near tasks, and glasses rechecks.

The procedure is performed as follows:

▸ The phoropter is set for near by pushing the levers toward the nose (this converges the right and left sides).

▸ Patient's distance correction is retained or entered in the phoropter and the fellow eye is occluded. (Ideally the test is done one eye at a time; binocular measurements might result in an inadequate add power, since binocular accommodative amplitudes are generally greater.)

▸ Increase the sphere power in an amount equal to the add of the patient's last spectacles.

  • Alternately, add power may be entered based on the patient's age and further refined with the DCC:

    ▪ Age 42 to 49 years: +1.0 D to +1.25 D

    ▪ Age 50 to 54 years: +1.5 D to +1.75 D

    ▪ Age 55 to 59 years: +2.0 D to +2.25 D

    ▪ Age 60 years and older: +2.5 D to +3.0 D

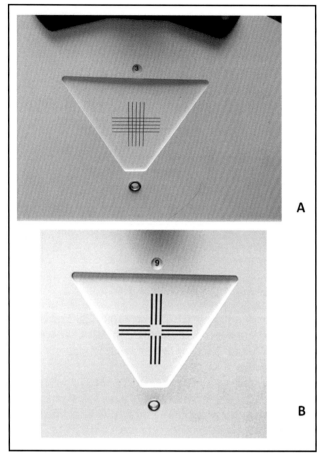

Figure 11-21. "Tic-tac-toe" or cross-hatch pattern of the rotating near chart (Nearpoint Rotochart, Reichert Technologies) for use in the ±dynamic cross cylinder method of measuring reading power.

- Insert the ±0.5 D lens and move the Prince rule into place.

- Place the near chart at 16 inches and turn it to the thin tic-tac-toe with *vertical* and *horizontal* lines (for patients with better visual acuity; Figure 11-21A), or thick tic-tac-toe with *vertical* and *horizontal* lines (for patients with decreased visual acuity; Figure 11-21B).

- If the two sets of lines appear *equally black* or *clear*, the add power is accurate.

- If the *horizontal* lines appear blacker or clearer, the current add power is not sufficient and plus sphere is added until both sets of lines are *equally black* or *clear.*

- If the *vertical* lines appear blacker and clearer, the current add power is excessive and minus sphere lenses are added until both sets of lines are *equally black* or *clear.*

- If a patient does not currently have an add but needs one, the grid will appear blurry. Plus sphere is added till both sets of lines are *equally black* or

clear. Remember that the add power is the difference between the sphere power of the distance MR and the sphere power present at the end of the DCC test.

- Repeat for the other eye.

Focal Point Method

This method is suited for patients who cannot respond adequately for the DCC method, patients who want computer glasses, and patients with other needs at near distances other than 16 inches.

- Measure the distance (in centimeters) at which the patient needs to focus. Divide 100 by the distance measured.

- Round off to the *closest, lower quarter diopter.* This will be the reading add power.

- Double-check the result in trial frames at the desired focal distance.

For example, suppose your patient needs to focus at 44 cm. Divide 100 by 44: 100/44 = 2.27. Round off to 2.25. The reading add would be +2.25 D.

Trial Frame and Trial Lenses Method

This method is suited for patients who might not be able to respond adequately to other methods.

- Take the best distance correction (preferably from today's measurement) and increase the sphere power in an amount equal to the add of the patient's current glasses. Put the result in a trial frame.

- Have the patient hold a near card at 14 inches. (Note: The visual angle of this card is based on 5 minutes of arc, which occurs at 14 inches. At other distances the near visual acuity notation will not be applicable.) Add plus power in +0.25 D increments until the vision is clear.

- Add the current add power and the additional plus power. This will be the new reading add power.

For example, suppose the patient's current reading add is +2.00; insert +2.00 into the trial frame (already loaded with the best distance correction) as the reading add. Offer +0.25 sph increments until the patient sees clearly; let's say that's +0.50 sph. Combine the add power to the additional plus power: +2.00 + 0.50 = +2.50, the new add power.

Verifying Proper Range for Add Power

The power of the reading add can be calculated mathematically as well. Have the patient hold the reading material at his/her preferred distance. Measure this and convert to metric (eg, 10 inches = 25 cm). Divide 100 by the metric value (100/25 cm = 4 D; thus, the reading add in the example is +4.0 D). In this way, add power may be measured for any preferred reading distance.

It is good practice to verify that the reading add power thus calculated is appropriate for the patient's needs. Place the latest refractometry result in a trial frame with the calculated add. Have the patient move the material slightly closer and farther until it blurs. The sharpest-appearing optotypes should be located in the middle of this range. Further adjustments may be made, if necessary, to move the range closer to (with more plus) or farther from (by reducing plus) the patient. This range of focus will be limited by the power of the add itself; that is, a weaker add will have more range of focus than a stronger add.

Adds for Other Near Tasks

Patients will frequently benefit from single vision or multifocal spectacles for computer or bench work, which is usually farther away than the standard reading distance. Other patients may need a lens or add for close work, such as knitting, carving, and jewelry crafting, where the patient will most likely hold items much closer than the typical reading distance. Bifocals can be made where the segment is for reading and the top for mid-range tasks. In these situations, the power needed must be recalculated. There are several ways to do this (Tables 11-9 and 11-10).

A final method involves simply measuring the work distances required and then set the near chart to that distance at the phoropter (Sidebar 11-5). The power needed is then obtained by adding +0.25 D at a time until the chart is clear.

Other Techniques in Refractometry

Refractometry With Trial Frames

Trial frames and loose lenses may also be used for plus and minus cylinder refractometry. The principle is the same as described for the phoropter, but the lenses are manipulated by hand.

Loose lenses corresponding to results from lensometry, retinoscopy, or autorefraction are placed in the trial frame, with the highest power lens (typically sphere) in the back clamp of the frame. If applicable, a plus or minus cylinder lens is place in the front and rotated to the proper axis. The trial frame is then placed on the patient, making sure that the temples fit snuggly. The PD, lens heights, and frame tilt are adjusted using the appropriate screws on the frame. The fellow eye is occluded.

The patient is directed to look at the eye chart. Two loose lenses are chosen, one a +0.50 sph and the other a +0.25 sph. The +0.50 sph is presented first and the +0.25 sph next, and the patient is asked to choose the clearest. If the patient prefers one of these, then proceed in the plus direction to find the greatest plus power that provides best vision. If the patient prefers to go in the minus direction, offer -0.25 sph increments, making sure the

visual acuity improves before assigning that power. As with a phoropter, the goal is to determine the greatest plus sphere (or least minus) that provides best vision.

Once the initial sphere power is determined, change the lens in the back of the frame appropriately. (It's easier to refine astigmatism without anything in front of the cylinder lens.)

A hand-held JCC is then used to refine the cylinder axis and measure the cylinder power. Such cross cylinders are available in ±0.25 D increments up to 1 D, and are marked with white and red (plus cylinder) or black and red (minus cylinder) dots. Use ±0.25 D if visual acuity is 20/40 or better, ±0.50 D for visual acuity 20/50 to 20/100, and ±0.75 D and ±1 D for visual acuities 20/200 or worse. If visual acuity improves enough during refinement, you can switch to a JCC of lesser power.

To refine the cylinder axis, the JCC is held so the *handle* is in line with the cylinder axis in the frame and then flipped to offer the two choices. The challenge is to maintain the orientation of the hand-held JCC while flipping it. The cylinder lens in the frame is rotated in 10° increments in the appropriate direction, following the white/black and red dots as when using the phoropter. Be sure to reorient the hand-held JCC to the new axis each time it is moved. The cylinder axis is correct when the two choices appear similar.

The JCC is now adjusted so the handle is at 45° to the new cylinder axis. This means that the *dots* are now aligned with the newly determined axis of the cylinder trial lens. In this position the JCC is flipped (maintaining alignment and keeping it steady), and the patient is again asked to determine which is clearer. Cylinder power is adjusted as with a phoropter.

Maintain the spherical equivalent by adjusting the sphere power by 0.25 D in the opposite direction for every 0.5 D increase in cylinder power. The proper cylinder power is determined when the two choices appear similar.

The sphere power is refined next by offering +0.25 sph. The goal is to determine the greatest plus sphere (or least minus) that provides best vision. If the +0.25 sph addition blurs the vision, try -0.25 sph. If the patient says this is an improvement, made sure he/she can actually see more clearly, and doesn't simply mean that the letters are smaller and darker.

Plus and minus cylinder refractometry may also be done with clips (eg, Halberg clips [Keeler]) attached to the patient's current glasses. Two and three shelf clips are available for this purpose.

The patient wears his/her current glasses to which the clips have been attached. The actual process of refractometry proceeds as described previously using trial lenses and hand-held JCC. When finished, the entire assembly of glasses, clips, and additional lenses are placed on a lensometer to measure the new powers and axis. Ensure that any cylinder lens, if used, is not accidently rotated during lensometry.

Step	Goal	Process	Comments
		TABLE 11-9	
		MEASURING ADD POWER FOR COMPUTER WORK	
Measure the patient's customary working distances for the computer	Determine the proper power for single vision and bifocal spectacle lenses for computer work	**Single Vision for Computer Work** The patient should sit in front of a computer screen and adjust position for the usual working distance. Using a tape measure, obtain the distance, in centimeters, from the patient's forehead to the computer screen (eg, 60 cm). Divide 100 by the distance measured. (eg, $\frac{100}{60} = \frac{10}{6} = 1.66$) Round off to the closest lower quarter (eg, +1.50 D) and algebraically add to sphere power for distance. The cylinder power and axis remain unchanged. Place trial lenses in a trial frame and seat patient in front of the same computer. Adjust as needed.	Be sure to inquire whether the patient uses a desktop or laptop.
		Bifocal for Computer Work The reading add power should be determined, as summarized above (eg, +2.75 D). The single vision power for computer work should be determined, as summarized above (eg, +1.50 D). Round off to the closest lower quarter and algebraically add to sphere power for distance. The cylinder power and axis remain unchanged. To determine the reading add power for computer work, algebraically subtract the single vision power for computer work (+1.50) from the reading add power (+2.75): (+2.75) − (+1.50) = +2.75 − 1.50 = +1.25	The total power of the top portion (+1.50) of the computer glasses and their bifocal segment (+1.25) must equal the bifocal power for reading (+2.75). Computer bifocals typically should be D-segment, and not progressive additional lenses, since clarity is not required for the short distance between the computer screen and reading. Instead of traditional D-segment, a wider D-segment will give more "reading space." If even more space is required, an executive (Franklin) bifocal may be considered.

Notes on Hyperopia

In hyperopia we know that the image has to be moved forward (using plus power) to reach the fovea. This may be achieved by accommodation of the crystalline lens and/or by using plus corrective lenses. When measuring hyperopic refractive errors, extra care must be taken to give as much plus sphere power as possible (called *pushing plus*) with lenses so that little accommodation is used for distance. Doing so in adults reserves accommodation for near tasks. In children, pushing plus helps reduce any esotropia that may be due to excessive accommodation when performing near tasks such as reading.

Accommodation introduces fluctuation into the refractive mix, and because of this there are three levels of hyperopia.

For the sake of illustration, let's take accommodation out of the picture for a moment. If this situation existed, a person with a +6.00 refractive error would require a +6.00 D lens in order to see well. This would be *absolute hyperopia*; the eye *absolutely must* have this power supplied via corrective lenses in order to have the clearest possible vision.

TABLE 11-10
MEASURING SINGLE VISION SPECTACLE POWER FOR OTHER CLOSE WORK

Step	Goal	Process	Comments
Measure the patient's customary working distances for other close work	Determine the proper power for single vision spectacle lenses for other close work	Measure the distance in centimeters from the forehead to wherever the patient holds the item for close work (eg, 23.5 cm). Divide 100 by the distance measured. (eg, $\frac{100}{23.5} = 4.2$) Round off to the closest lower quarter (eg, +4.0 D) and algebraically add to sphere power for distance. The cylinder power and axis remain unchanged.	Bifocals are not required due to the shortened working distance.

SIDEBAR 11-5
MEASURING PATIENT'S PREFERRED READING/WORKING DISTANCE

► Patient is seated comfortably in the exam chair.

► Hand patient the near reading card. Say, "If you were sitting at home in your favorite chair, show me where you would like to hold your reading material."

► If the patient moves the card around, looking for where the print is clearest, say, "Not where it's clearest right now, but where you'd like to hold it if it was clear no matter where you held it."

► You might explain that holding a book at 12 inches is one prescription; 18 inches is another, and 22 inches yet another. You are trying to focus the patient at a distance that is most comfortable for general reading.

► Use a tape measure to measure the distance from the patient's eye (NOT glasses!) to the card. This is the distance where you will put the reading chart on the Prince rule when you measure the add power.

► If the patient also needs to focus at unique distances other than for reading, measure these as well. Have the patient sit at your desk and measure the distance to the computer screen, or show you how close he/she holds jewelry when crafting. Other examples: podium, music stand, work bench, shelves, car engine, dashboard, pool table.

► Position the reading chart on the Prince rule at each working distance and measure the least amount of plus required for sharpest focus.

► If the patient is not getting a multifocal, once you obtain the add needed for the specified distance, slide the chart forward and back a few inches to emphasize that "these glasses won't work very well for anything except [whatever the task]."

Once the best vision is first achieved (the absolute hyperopia) additional plus power is introduced until the patient reports blurring. It is the *maximum* amount of plus that the *noncyclopleged* eye can accept. This amount of hyperopia is termed *manifest* or *facultative*. Lens prescriptions may or may not include the manifest power depending on the needs of the patient.

The crystalline lens, however, typically makes constant adjustments. If an eye is hyperopic and cannot focus at a distance, the lens will accommodate in an attempt to clear the blurred image. The amount of plus power provided in this way is termed *latent hyperopia*, because it is "hidden" and not directly measurable. If you did refractometry on this patient, the accommodating eye might seem to be plano.

SIDEBAR 11-6
EXAMPLE: TYPES OF HYPEROPIA

	Visual Acuity	Sphere Power Used	Hyperopia
Patient VAsc	20/40		
Patient first sees	20/25+2	Phoropter reads +1.00	Absolute = +1.00 D
Patient last sees clearly	20/25+2	+0.50 (phoropter reads +1.50)	Manifest = +0.5 D
Cycloplegic refractometry	20/25	+1.00 (phoropter reads +2.50)	Latent = +1.00 D
This patient might be given +1.00 or +1.50 for distance, but would usually not be given +2.50.			

Using eye drops to induce cycloplegia temporarily paralyzes accommodation, and latent hyperopia can then be calculated by deducting the absolute and manifest values from the cycloplegic sphere power.

Latent accommodation is typically not corrected in a glasses prescription. Since accommodation returns after cycloplegia wears off, prescribing this amount of plus power will induce myopic blurring. (Note: Some practitioners will prescribe a portion of the latent correction to "ease" a patient into lenses that will help relax accommodation at distance.)

Latent hyperopia can only "cover" for hyperopia as far as the patient's ability to accommodate. And remember, accommodation decreases with age. That means that a young patient will have more latent hyperopia than an older person. But in either case, the *absolute* hyperopia is the *least* amount of plus required to improve the vision. It is always included in a spectacle prescription.

For an example, see Sidebar 11-6.

Errors in Refractometry

The quality of results obtained from refractometry is greatly influenced by the process utilized, and when that process is not diligently followed, the results can be troublesome. Common errors in refractometry are summarized in Table 11-11.

Glasses Check

In a clinic encounter scheduled as a "glasses check," patients might complain of one or more of the following symptoms: blurry vision, eye strain, distortion, eye pain, "pulling" sensation, double vision, dizziness, or nausea. The cause(s) may be identified by checking the spectacle prescription (lensometry), retinoscopy, refractometry, and the optical fit. Steps in evaluating glasses problems are summarized in Table 11-12.

ACKNOWLEDGMENTS

The author would like to thank the following: Dinesh K. Goyal, MD, and David A. Philiph, COMT.

TABLE 11-11
COMMON ERRORS IN REFRACTOMETRY

Error	Effect on Result	Remedy/Notes
Patient forehead not on forehead rest, or forehead rest not properly set	Vertex distance not correct, which can alter sphere power 4 D and greater	Manipulate headrest knob to position patient properly
Phoropter not leveled	Cylinder axis will be inaccurate	Level instrument
Fellow eye not occluded	Better eye will reduce the actual refractive error	Occlude fellow eye
Proper instructions not given about procedure	Patient does not know what the goals are, and might not give the best answers	Process is teamwork; give proper instructions, especially for cylinder axis refinement. Remember the goal of each step.
Lens choices always named "#1" or "#2" and not varied	Patient potentially only chooses "#1" or "#2" all the time regardless of image	Alter choices, such as #1/#2, #3/#4, #5/#6,…A/B, etc
Patient continually chooses only odd-numbered or even-numbered lenses	Time wasted as you "spin the dials" trying to follow patient responses; patient confusion, inaccurate measurement, compromised final acuity	Check the patient's responses by flipping the cross cylinder so that you aren't really changing anything, monitor response after doing this; reeducate the patient
Lenses changed too fast	Patient not able to keep up; questionable responses	Proceed at a speed comfortable for the patient
Sphere not initially changed in the plus direction	Excess minus power possible	Change sphere in the plus direction first
Cylinder power measured before cylinder axis refined	Cylinder power incorrect, determined off-axis; compromised final acuity	Always refine the axis location before measuring cylinder power
Cylinder-axis dial arrows not followed properly by the red or white dots	Incorrect cylinder axis determined, and, therefore, incorrect cylinder power	Before starting, establish which dot follows which arrow
Sphere not changed by 0.25 D in the opposite direction for every two clicks of cylinder power change	Spherical equivalent not maintained	Plus cylinder: Give -0.25 D for every +0.50 D added to cylinder power Minus cylinder: Give +0.25 D for every -0.50 D added to cylinder power
Full cylinder power not measured	Blurry monocular vision due to insufficient cylinder power	Measure full cylinder power acceptable to patient (this amount may be changed in the refraction by a licensed practitioner)
Cylinder power changed using the power knob after the JCC has been removed	Erroneous cylinder power measured, since changing the power using the knob cannot mimic the efficiency of the JCC	No changes should be made to cylinder power after JCC is removed (however, in cases of impaired or low vision changing the power using the knob may be necessary)
Add power not measured with dynamic cross cylinder lens	Focal plane set to incorrect reading distance	Measure monocular powers using the dynamic cross cylinder
Refined sphere has excess minus power	Patient accommodating to offset increase in minus power	Minus power is given only if visual acuity improves ("minus must be earned")

(continued)

	TABLE 11-11 (CONTINUED)	
	COMMON ERRORS IN REFRACTOMETRY	
Error	**Effect on Result**	**Remedy/Notes**
Duochrome (red/green) not tested	Excess plus or minus sphere power possible	Duochrome is required if visual acuity is 20/50 or better; not required if visual acuity is 20/60 or worse (the difference in red and green images will not be distinguished)
Binocular balancing not tested	Eyes are not accommodating equally	Balancing is not required in children, aphakes, pseudophakes, or older presbyopes Hyperopes and first-time presbyopes should be balanced
Measurement(s) for near tasks not calculated properly	Focal planes set to incorrect distances for patient's needs	Powers of single vision and bifocal computer glasses, and glasses for other close work, should be added algebraically to the appropriate portion of the distance glasses with bifocal reading add

	TABLE 11-12		
	STEPS IN A GLASSES CHECK		
Step	**Goal**	**Process**	**Comments**
Lensometry	Verify if powers of spectacle lenses are similar to the prescription given	Neutralize distance powers of single vision, bifocal, and trifocal lenses in plus or minus cylinder form Mark progressive addition lenses (PAL) and neutralize the distance powers at the horseshoe For highest accuracy, this author recommends measuring the front vertex power of the reading add by turning the glasses around and placing them on the lensometer with the temples facing the examiner Compare with the prescription given	If powers are similar (within tolerance), then the lenses were ground correctly
Retinoscopy	Use retinoscopy to verify if the powers of spectacle lenses are appropriate	Have the patient wear the problem glasses Using an appropriate working distance lens and a standard streak retinoscope, evaluate the reflexes (see Retinoscopy)	A neutral reflex, or slight *with* or *against* motion, indicates that the powers of spectacle lenses are appropriate. On the other hand, a strong streak motion indicates residual hyperopic, myopic, or astigmatic refractive error.

(continued)

	TABLE 11-12 (CONTINUED)		
	STEPS IN A GLASSES CHECK		
Step	**Goal**	**Process**	**Comments**
Refractometry	Neutralize refractive error of patient	Measure refractive error using standard plus or minus cylinders	A change of 0.25 D of power indicates that the powers of spectacle lenses are appropriate A change of 0.5 D or more indicates that the powers of spectacle lenses are not appropriate Cylinder axis standards are different, depending on the amount of cylinder power. In general, the greater the greater the cylinder, the less the tolerance of axis variation. It will be best to consult an optical shop or lab for prevailing standards. Improper cylinder axis results in shadows and tilting (left or right) of images
Optical fit	Verify presence of induced prism (IP) by checking the optical center (OC) for decentration of spectacle lenses	Mark the OC of single vision, bifocal, and trifocal spectacle lenses on a lensometer Mark PAL spectacle lenses, showing the fitting cross and prism location (PAL templates are available from the lens manufacturers) Measure the pupillary distance (PD) Measure the patient's PD If there is a difference between the frame and patient PD, calculate the amount and direction of IP (Tips A through C) Alternatively, the patient should wear the marked glasses and gaze at a distant target. The examiner observes if the OC is in the center of the pupils. If not, the pupil center is marked and the OC displacement measured in order to calculate the amount and direction of IP (Tips A through C).	Tip A: Improper OC decentration can cause eye strain and pain, pulling sensation, diplopia, dizziness, and nausea Tip B: Prentice's rule is used to calculate the amount of IP: IP = (sphere power in diopters) x (OC decentration in cm) Tip C: Net prism is calculated by adding prism oriented in opposite directions, and subtracting prism oriented in the same direction (see Chapter 4, Prentice's Rule)
			(continued)

Step	Goal	Process	Comments
Optical fit	Verify if the glasses have the proper tilt	Inspect glasses profile from the right and left sides to ensure that the temple segments are not at 90° to the eye wire profile (Tips D and E)	Tip D: For proper pantoscopic tilt the eye wire must be tilted toward the cheeks at an angle of 4° to 15° Tip E: Proper pantoscopic tilt ensures that the distance and near vertex are similar when looking through the top or the reading add. With proper pantoscopic tilt the reading gaze also goes through the bifocal OC.
	In case of a reading add, verify if the glasses have the proper segment height	Have the patient wear the problem glasses In properly made bifocal spectacle lenses, the top of the D-segment should be level with the top of the lower eyelid (Tip F) In properly made trifocal spectacle lenses, the top of the intermediate segment should be level with the inferior pupil margin (Tip F) In properly made PALs, the fitting cross should be level with the pupil center (Tip F)	Tip F: If the segment height is not at the proper level, the full power of the reading add will not be used, and the patient will experience problems when reading
	Verify slab-off prism (see Chapter 20, Prism)	"SLAB-OFF" should be marked on the glasses prescription if there is a reading add and the distance sphere powers have anisometropia of 2.5 D or greater (Tip G)	Tip G: In "SLAB-OFF," prism is added to the reading segment and the excess material is cut (slabbed) off, thus decreasing image jump when the gaze moves from the distance part to the reading part

Table 11-12 (continued). Steps in a Glasses Check

CHAPTER QUIZ

1. The sum of all refraction in a normal human eye is similar to a:
   a. minus lens
   b. plus lens
   c. plano lens
   d. mirror

2. Total power, in diopters, of a normal adult eye (when viewing an object more than 20 feet away) is:
   a. +62
   b. +19
   c. -62
   d. +43

3. An example of the total power, in diopters, of an adult myopic eye is:
   a. +43
   b. +60
   c. +62
   d. +67

4. An objective method to measure refractive errors is:
   a. refractometry
   b. refraction
   c. trial lenses
   d. retinoscopy

5. The power, in diopters, of a working distance lens commonly used for retinoscopy is:

    a. +1.50
    b. +3.00
    c. -5.00
    d. -3.00

6. With the +1.50 D sph in place during retinoscopy, a streak oriented at 100° indicates the refractive error at axis (meridian):

    a. 100
    b. 90
    c. 10
    d. 180

7. With the +1.50 D sph in place during retinoscopy, *with* movement of one streak and *against* movement of the other streak indicates:

    a. mixed astigmatism
    b. simple astigmatism
    c. compound astigmatism
    d. presbyopia

8. Proper neutralization of a retinoscopy streak may be confirmed by:

    a. removing six clicks of plus power
    b. moving sideways
    c. adding six clicks of minus power
    d. moving forward and backward

9. Standard vertex distance of a phoropter is:

    a. 13.75 m
    b. 1.375 cm
    c. 13.75 feet
    d. 1.375 mm

10. During refractometry, vertex distance should be adjusted and noted if the:

    a. sphere power is 4 D or greater
    b. cylinder power is 3 D or greater
    c. pupillary distance is not adjustable
    d. add power is 3 D or greater

11. The power of a reading add segment may be measured most precisely using a phoropter, Prince rule, rotating near point chart, and a:

    a. Jackson cross cylinder lens
    b. cylinder power knob
    c. dynamic cross cylinder lens
    d. cylinder adjustment knob

Answers

1. b
2. a
3. d
4. d
5. a
6. c
7. a
8. d
9. b
10. a
11. c

BIBLIOGRAPHY

Cassin B, Hamed LM. *Fundamentals for Ophthalmic Technical Personnel*. Philadelphia, PA: Saunders; 1995.

Corboy JM. *The Retinoscopy Book: An Introductory Manual for Eye Care Professionals*. 5th ed. Thorofare, NJ: SLACK Incorporated; 2003.

Guyton DL. *Retinoscopy and Subjective Refraction* [DVD]. San Francisco, CA: American Academy of Ophthalmology; 1986. Reviewed for currency 2007.

Shukla AV. *Clinical Optics Primer for Ophthalmic Medical Personnel: A Guide to Laws, Formulae, Calculations, and Clinical Applications*. Thorofare, NJ: SLACK Incorporated; 2009.

Thall EH, Miller KM, Rosenthal P, et al. *Optics, Refraction, and Contact Lenses: Basic and Clinical Science Course, Section 3*. San Francisco, CA: American Academy of Ophthalmology; 2000.

The figures in this chapter were contributed by the author, Aaron V. Shukla.

12

SLIT LAMP MICROSCOPY

Sergina M. Flaherty, COMT, OSC

The wonderful world of ophthalmology expands when ophthalmic medical technicians can successfully operate the slit lamp biomicroscope. This chapter will provide an in-depth description of the slit lamp, its parts, and how to use it effectively. There are many makes and models of slit lamps in use today. However, all are based on a similar design. The two basic styles of slit lamps will be described in this chapter.

Every day, patients are evaluated with the use of the slit lamp biomicroscope, with diagnoses being made and conditions treated in offices everywhere. The slit lamp provides a three-dimensional view and concise reflection of the tissues.

The slit lamp consists of two oculars that, together, allow the observer to see stereoscopically, in fine detail, the structures of the eye as well as the exact location of foreign bodies, scars, tumors, etc. Under high magnification, even tiny changes can be observed in the cornea or lens of the eye by projecting the light beam in various directions.

To become proficient in using the slit lamp, you must use it every day. In addition, when you become proficient, you'll want to use it on every patient you see. It takes only a few minutes and can answer many questions that may come up during your initial assessment. For example, suppose you are performing refractometry on a patient and are unable to reach 20/20. You could stop and take a look at the patient with the slit lamp and discover severely dry corneas with dry spots centrally. Well, that sure can explain a decrease in best-corrected vision! As well as save you from spinning your wheels at the phoropter (pun intended).

Keep in mind that a technician's job is to gather information so the eye doctor can properly diagnose and treat eye disease. As a tech, we can *detect*, but not *diagnose*. If a patient asks, "What do you see?" or "What is wrong with my eye?" you must tell them the eye care provider will also do an exam and will convey what is going on at that time ("We'll know more after Dr. Kirby looks at you"). It is a fact that technicians become very knowledgeable as we gain experience using the slit lamp and other equipment. We can detect disease. However, we can never diagnose. Leave that discussion to the doctor.

BASIC SCIENCES

Ocular anatomy is covered in Chapter 2. Please refer to that chapter as well as chapters regarding ocular disorders, trauma, etc, to learn more about what you might observe during the slit lamp examination.

Ledford JK, Lens A, eds.
Principles and Practice in Ophthalmic Assisting:
A Comprehensive Textbook (pp 213-232).
© 2018 Taylor & Francis Group.

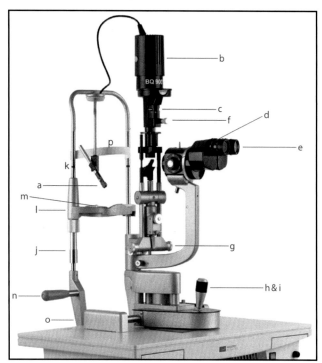

Figure 12-1. Haag-Streit slit lamp. a=external fixation light, b=lamp housing, c=filter control knob, d=magnification knob, e=oculars, f=slit beam height adjustment knob, g=slit beam width adjustment knob, h=joystick, i=joystick adjustment (up and down), j=headrest bar, k=canthus mark, l=chinrest adjustment knob, m=chinrest, n=patient grip, o=headrest base, p=headrest band. (Reprinted with permission from Haag-Streit USA.)

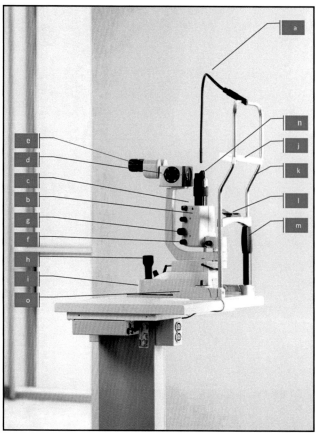

Figure 12-2. Zeiss slit lamp. a=external fixation device, b=housing lamp, c=filters, d=magnification knob, e=binoculars, f=slit beam length adjustment, g=slit beam width adjustment, h=joystick (focusing, up and down), i=base-in/out/side to side, j=patient headrest, k=ocular canthus mark, l=patient chinrest, m=chinrest knob, n=front surface mirror, o=rail covers. (Reprinted with permission from Carl Zeiss Meditec.)

CLINICAL KNOWLEDGE

Parts of the Slit Lamp (Figures 12-1 and 12-2)

External Fixation Device

Most of the time, you will ask the patient to look at your ear with the eye you are not examining. This helps the patient keep the eyes still, making it easier to perform the evaluation. (Sometimes, when the patient has difficulty seeing your ear, you may show him/her an index finger of your hand and move it until the eye you are examining is in the desired position.)

The external fixation device is used when evaluating the eye in a position other than straight ahead. It is typically attached to the slit lamp headrest, off to one side ("A" on both photos). The device is placed in front of the eye not being examined, and the patient told to look and follow the light. The examiner then moves the light until the eye being evaluated has moved into the proper position.

Lamp Housing

The lamp housing is most commonly located on the top of the illumination arm. It contains the light system of the unit. Make sure the unit is turned off for a while before trying to remove the bulb, as it gets very hot.

Filters

Filters are used to enhance the visibility of pathology. There are three filters on most slit lamps.

The *red-free* (green) filter makes red lesions and blood vessels appear black (Figures 12-3A and B). Additionally, when using a 78 or 90 diopter (D) auxiliary lens, blood on the retina will look black, and subtle changes like small hemorrhages in the retina or ill-defined exudates will be more noticeable. This filter is also used for better visualization of a Fleischer ring (a dark "ring" of metallic deposits in the peripheral corneal epithelium), as well as conjunctival inflammation associated with episcleritis (which appear as yellow spots).

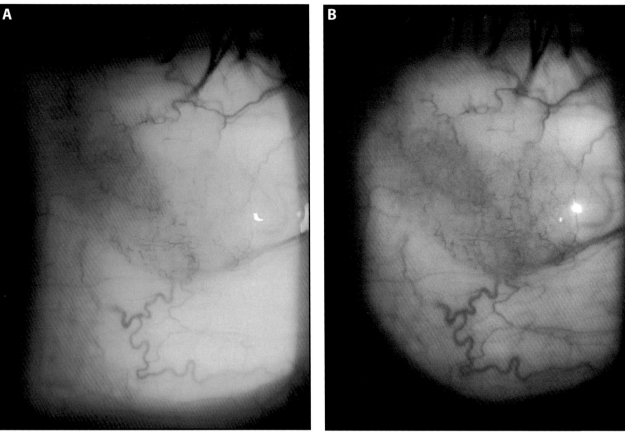

Figure 12-3. (A) Conjunctival growth, red-free. (B) Conjunctival growth without filter.

The *cobalt blue* filter is used along with fluorescein sodium drops to view disruptions in the corneal epithelium (Figure 12-4), to look for corneal or limbal wound leaks (called a *Seidel test*, where clear aqueous trickles into the dye at the site of the leak), and to perform Goldmann tonometry (see Chapter 13).

The neutral density filter present on some instruments is used to evaluate the eye under diffuse illumination by decreasing the intensity of all wavelengths of light. All structures are then equally illuminated, regardless of color.

Magnification Knob/Lever

Changing magnification varies from model to model. The basic Haag-Streit (and similar models) has a lever that swings horizontally to change from 1X to 1.6X (Figure 12-5). The Zeiss and Haag-Streit in Figures 12-1 and 12-2 have a dial to change magnification from 5X to 32X. You should start your examination on low magnification and then increase magnification as needed to view fine detail. You'll quickly note that the higher the magnification, the more that even the tiniest movement by the patient can "swish" your view around drastically.

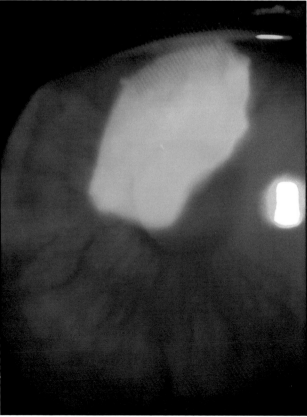

Figure 12-4. Large corneal abrasion with fluorescein staining.

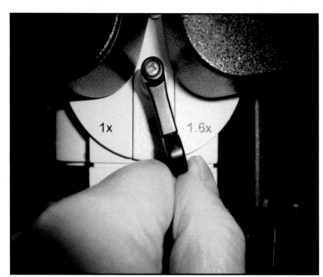

Figure 12-5. Magnification level control on a basic Haag-Streit slit lamp.

Eyepieces (Binoculars)

The eyepieces can be individually focused to the user's prescription by using a focusing rod to adjust the eyepieces (see Focusing the Oculars, later in this chapter). The eyepieces can also be exchanged for a higher/lower power, if desired.

Slit Beam

Length Adjustment

Adjustment of the length of the slit beam is controlled by turning the knob just below the lamp housing ("F" on both slit lamps), and is usually kept at its maximum length. However, when looking for cell and flare inside the anterior chamber, the length is adjusted down to a pinpoint. Another time we would change the length is when using the slit as a measuring device.

Orientation

Primarily, the slit beam is oriented vertically. However, it can be adjusted to any degree. For example, you can confirm the axis orientation of a toric intraocular lens (IOL) or contact lens by manipulating the axis orientation of the slit beam to that of the axis markings on the lens.

Width Adjustment

Adjustment of the width of the slit beam is controlled by turning the knurled knob on either side of the slit lamp illumination arm ("G" on both slit lamps). This illumination arm/column can be moved side to side to any degree desired. Generally, place your left hand on the left knurled knob when examining the right eye of the patient and your right hand on the right side when examining the patient's left eye. You will find that you'll keep your hand on this knob during most of the exam, narrowing and widening frequently as you evaluate the ocular structures.

Base: Forward, Back, and Side to Side

The base of the slit lamp ("I" on both models) slides forward, back, and side to side on a glide pad on the instrument's stage. This can be done easily with the heel of the hand while grasping the joystick.

All slit lamps have a locking screw or lever on the base that should always be tightened when the slit lamp is not in use. If it is not locked and the table is moved, the whole system can tip over and even fall off the platform.

Joystick: Focusing and Vertical Alignment

The joystick ("H" on both slit lamps) is usually manipulated with one hand and held in the vertical position when making gross movements of the slit lamp base toward the eye. Once gross focusing is accomplished, fine adjustments can be made by moving the joystick forward, backward, left, right, and diagonally while viewing ocular detail. The vertical position of the instrument is controlled by rotating the joystick itself clockwise or counterclockwise. Once the slit beam is aligned with the object of interest, this hand can be used to spread the eyelids apart, or adjust the size, width, and orientation of the slit beam.

It is preferable to keep the joystick on a central and vertical orientation at the beginning of the exam. This technique reserves plenty of play in the joystick to lower the beam by turning the joystick counterclockwise or raise it by turning clockwise. For example, if you are trying to lower the slit lamp and the joystick won't turn anymore, you have reached the endpoint. You'll need to raise your patient via the chinrest, then turn the joystick to raise the slit lamp and realign the slit beam on the eye. This problem can mostly be avoided if you make sure that the patient's outer canthus is aligned with the black mark on the sides of the headrest before you start the examination.

Headrest Assembly

The headrest ("J" on the Zeiss slit lamp and "P" on the Haag-Streit) helps to keep the patient in position. Ask the patient to place his/her head firmly against the headrest and chin firmly on the chinrest ("L" on the Zeiss and "M" on Haag-Streit) with teeth together. Keeping the mouth closed and teeth together helps prevent movement of the head during the exam, and can stop the talkative patient when the examination is underway. The patient's forehead and chin should be placed so that the head is at a vertical 90-degree (°) angle.

The canthus mark ("K" on both models) is a groove or line on the side of the headrest bar that aids in aligning the patient. While placing the patient's chin onto the chinrest, check the position of the outer canthus (corner of the eye). Adjust the chinrest up or down so that the outer canthus of the patient is in line with the groove. Misalignment will limit the range of view through the instrument.

The chinrest knob ("M" on the Zeiss and "Q" on the Haag-Streit) is located just under and to each side of the headrest. (Other models may have a "button" on the chinrest itself.) Adjusting this knob lowers or raises the patient's head.

Patient Handgrips

The handgrips (the Zeiss has hand grips only as an accessory; "N" on the Haag-Streit) are located on either side of the head and chinrest. They are intended for the patient to hold onto while being examined and help keep both the instrument and the patient in position. However, the examiner can also use these grips to maneuver the slit lamp table. Some patients will try to hold onto the table of the slit lamp, and their arms then prevent full movement of the slit lamp. If they hold onto the lower bars of the headrest assembly, the base might pinch their fingers when you move it forward. Therefore, you need to ask them to hold the handgrips. (For a child, you might call them "motorcycle handles.") If there are no handgrips, the patient can hold on to each side of the stage itself. But be careful, as the patient will often try and pull the slit lamp closer when holding onto the stage, causing you to have to move closer. This can cause difficulty, as the patient's feet are on the foot rest of the exam chair and his/her knees can block you from the eyepieces.

Rail Covers

Rail covers ("O" on both slit lamps) are used to prevent dust and dirt from damaging the rollers that allow the slit lamp base to move, and to prevent the slit lamp from rolling off the rails. The rollers should be kept covered in order to maintain smooth movement of the slit lamp base. They also prevent fingers, clothing, and other objects from coming into contact with the rollers.

Front Surface Mirror

The slit lamp employs a front surface mirror ("E" on the Zeiss and "R" on Haag-Streit). A front surface mirror provides a more pure and concise reflection of light. (A back surface mirror is not used on the slit lamp as it causes a ghosting effect.)

Auxiliary Items Used With the Slit Lamp

Tonometer

The Goldmann tonometer is mounted on the slit lamp and used to measure the eye's intraocular pressure (see Chapter 13, Tonometry). Always rotate the tonometer out of the way after use; if the microscope should quickly slide forward toward a patient and the tonometer is down, there is a potential that the tonometer unit could strike the patient in the face/eye.

Goniolens

The slit lamp is a great instrument that allows us to visualize the cornea, iris, lens, and anterior vitreous face. However, it has its limitations. One limitation is that it is impossible to view the angle, where the iris meets the cornea, because the peripheral curvature of the cornea prevents viewing. An auxiliary instrument called the *goniolens* is a three- or four-mirrored lens that is applied directly onto the cornea. The mirrors facilitate viewing of the angle structures. This lens is used primarily on patients with narrow angle glaucoma and in ocular trauma. Many ophthalmic technicians do not get to perform gonioscopy, as it is primarily a diagnostic tool performed by the practitioner. However, in order to perform anterior chamber angle photography, some technicians and photographers must master the use of the lens. Observing a person with experience performing gonioscopy and then having that person watch you will help you become proficient.

A drop of anesthetic is first instilled onto the eye. A methylcellulose-based solution (eg, Goniosol [Novartis]) is applied to the concave surface of the goniolens as a "cushion" and optical interface (Figure 12-6). Then the lens can be placed onto the cornea (Figure 12-7). Be careful to not push on the eye, as this will cause narrowing of the anterior chamber angle, making it difficult to view and photograph the angle structures.

Position the slit beam onto the mirror at 9 o'clock, and you will be viewing the angle at 3 o'clock (Figure 12-8). The 12 o'clock position on the mirror will show the angle at 6 o'clock, and so on. Figure 12-9 shows a traumatic angle iris root tear as imaged in the goniolens at 1 o'clock. (The tear itself is actually at 7 o'clock.)

There are several types of goniolenses. The Posner goniolens (Figure 12-10) has the advantage of not needing Goniosol; the lens is applied directly to the anesthetized cornea.

Hruby Lens and 90 Diopter Lens

The Hruby lens is a minus-powered lens (approximately -55 D) that neutralizes the +60 D of a "normal" emmetropic eye and magnifies by about x1. (The slit lamp provides the magnifying power.) It provides a three-dimensional, upright view of the retinal structures with a field of approximately 30°.

This lens is attached to the slit lamp at the level of the chinrest and is placed in the plate that covers the pivot hole (Figure 12-11). Once lined up with the eye, the Hruby lens can be adjusted by moving the hand lever attached to the lens.

Today, many practitioners use a hand-held 78 D or 90 D lens that provides an inverted and laterally reversed view of the retina. The lens is held in front of the cornea between the thumb and forefinger (using the right hand for viewing the left eye and left hand to view the right eye).

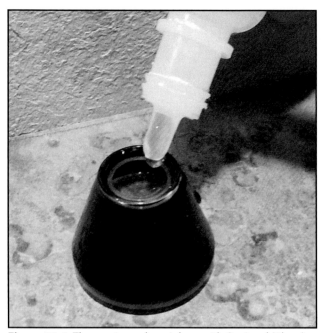

Figure 12-6. Three-mirrored goniolens with Goniosol (Alcon).

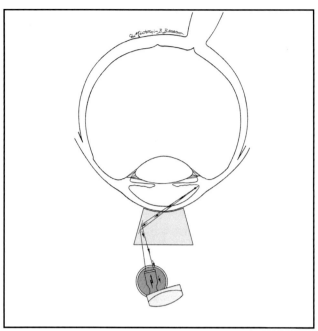

Figure 12-7. Three-mirrored lens on the eye. (Reprinted with permission from Csaba L. Martonyi, CRA, FOPS.)

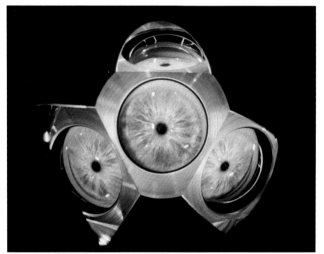

Figure 12-8. View through a three-mirrored goniolens. (Reprinted with permission from Csaba L. Martonyi, CRA, FOPS.)

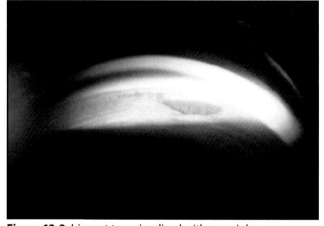

Figure 12-9. Iris root tear visualized with a goniolens.

The slit beam is aligned with the microscope (between the two oculars). The slit is narrowed to about 2 mm wide and at the height of the pupil (Figures 12-12 and 12-13). Small movements of the joystick will be needed to focus on the area of interest.

Extra Eyepieces

Generally, 10X magnification eyepieces are used. However, some slit lamps come with additional eyepieces, such as a set of 16X auxiliary eyepieces that can be used to increase magnification. Simply pull each eyepiece toward you (they will slip right out of the oculars) and replace with the 16X eyepieces. The disadvantage of using these higher powered eyepieces is the limited field of view.

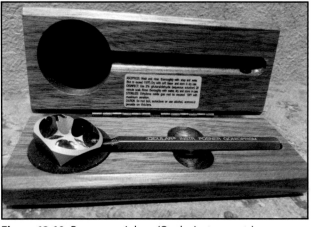

Figure 12-10. Posner goniolens (Ocular Instruments).

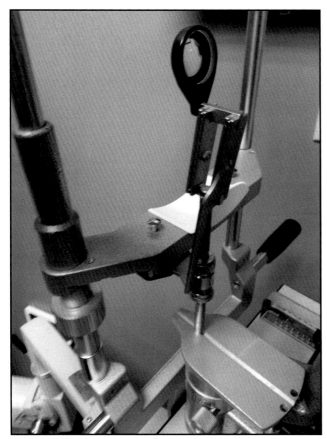

Figure 12-11. Hruby lens in place on the Haag-Streit slit lamp.

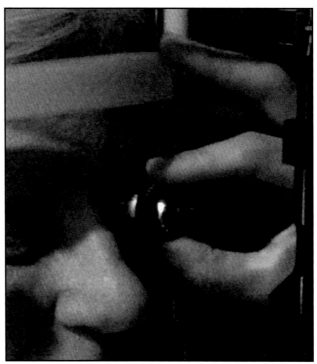

Figure 12-12. 90 D lens in use.

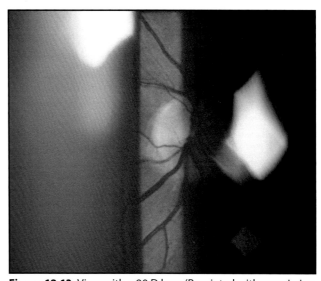

Figure 12-13. View with a 90 D lens. (Reprinted with permission from Csaba L. Martonyi, CRA, FOPS.)

CLINICAL SKILLS

Maintenance and Troubleshooting

It is very important to keep the slit lamp in good working order, and continued preventive maintenance will bring many years of use. At the end of every day, you should cover the slit lamp with a dust cover. Check with your equipment supplier and/or the owner's manual for suggested routine cleaning. A yearly cleaning by a professional is recommended.

When caring for the front surface mirror, do not touch it with a dry tissue as the silver coating can be scratched and rubbed off over time. The proper way to clean this mirror is with compressed air, a camel hair brush, or a moist lens wipe.

If the light won't come on, first try jiggling the housing unit cap. Most of the time, the problem is solved just by reestablishing the connection. Alternately, you might check all other plugs and power cords supplying the instrument and/or table.

If jiggling doesn't work, turn off the slit lamp and check the connection of the bulb. The contacts on the bulb can become corroded over time. Clean the contact gently by rubbing a pencil eraser on the connector. (You are "erasing" the corrosion and thereby improving

conductivity.) If you must replace the bulb, be sure that the old bulb is not hot. Do not touch the glass on the new bulb with your fingers because oil can cause a shadow to form and cause a premature burn-out. Handle the new bulb with a tissue. Replacement bulbs can be expensive, costing anywhere from $25 to $40 each. There are also fuses in some units that can blow. Have plenty fuses and bulbs available for replacement.

Lock the microscope stage following every use. If left unlocked, the microscope can slam forward when the

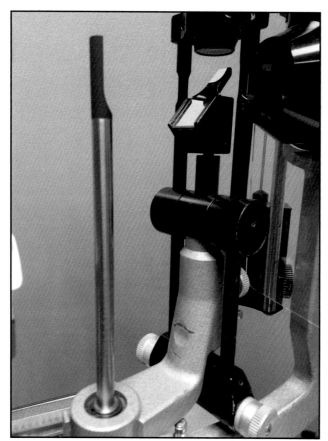

Figure 12-14. Focusing rod in pivot hole of a Haag-Streit slit lamp.

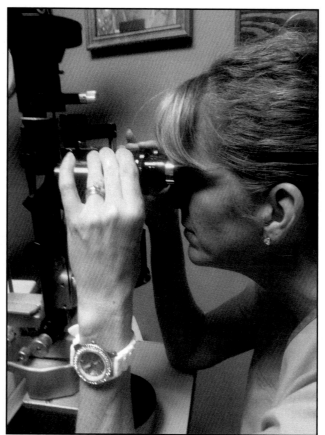

Figure 12-15. Adjusting the binocular pupillary distance.

unit is moved. This might cause the instrument to strike the patient, damage the optics of the unit, or even cause the microscope to jump off the rails. Best practice is to pull the microscope back and to your left, then lock it firmly in place before moving it away from the patient.

Focusing the Oculars

Many of the instruments we use in ophthalmology have eyepieces that are adjustable. However, many slit lamp eyepieces do not have measuring or grid lines imprinted inside on the lenses (known as *reticles* ["crosshairs"]) within the oculars to use as a focusing target. Therefore, a focusing rod comes with the slit lamp and is used to focus each ocular individually. This should be performed prior to using the instrument. (The ideal situation, of course, is to have a slit lamp that only you use. Otherwise, what usually happens is that someone sets the eyepieces and they are pretty much never changed after that!)

Remove the pivot plate and place the rod into the pivot hole with the flat side up and toward the slit lamp (Figure 12-14). Adjust the slit beam to 1 to 2 mm wide. First turn the focus ring on the eyepiece all the way

counterclockwise, then look through the ocular and turn the eyepiece clockwise in a slow, continuous movement until the slit on the rod is in sharp focus. Repeat for the other ocular. Make a note of where you stopped turning and set the oculars at this same setting each time you use the slit lamp.

The pupillary distance (PD) is adjusted by pushing both eyepieces together and then slowly separating them with both hands (Figure 12-15), adjusting until both eyes see the same image on the focusing test rod through the eyepieces. This produces a stereo view.

Methods of Illumination

The slit lamp makes it easy to visualize the ocular structures. There is no other organ in the human body that we can examine so completely. The beauty of the slit lamp is that we can adjust the brightness, size (width and length), angle, and placement of the slit beam in order to enhance our view. There are 10 separate methods of illumination described here. However, it will become apparent to the user that many of these methods will be used together during the evaluation.

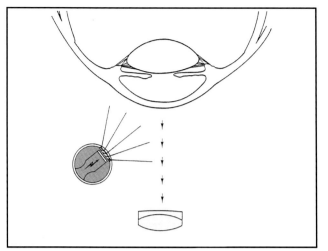

Figure 12-16. Diffuse illumination. (Adapted with permission from Csaba L. Martonyi, CRA, FOPS.)

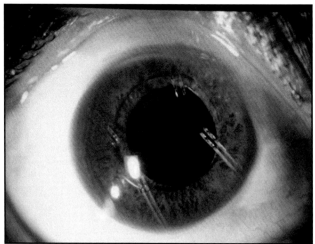

Figure 12-17. Anterior chamber intraocular lens in diffuse illumination.

Diffuse Illumination

In *diffuse illumination* the light is not projected as a slit, but is spread across the eye, which is viewed with the beam fully opened (Figure 12-16). Using a diffusing filter evens out the overall illumination. (Some slit lamps have a separate filter that is placed in front of the light source. Diffusers on other microscopes are employed just by moving a lever that flips a frosted glass over the light.)

Diffuse illumination is for viewing the general condition of the eye. The binoculars are positioned straight ahead as you evaluate the lids, lashes, conjunctiva, iris, pupil, and lens (Figure 12-17).

Direct Focal Illumination

Direct focal illumination uses a very narrow beam (the beam can be adjusted by turning the width adjustment knob; the length is adjusted by turning the knob near the lamp housing). This provides a cross-section that is especially useful in viewing the cornea and facilitates detection of foreign bodies, scars, and edema (swelling due to fluid retention). Not only is the direct view useful, but the characteristics of the beam provide information as well. Any area of corneal swelling will be evident by a thickening of the beam in that area. Conversely, if there is an area of corneal thinning, the beam will appear thinner. If the beam appears broken or not visible, that area of the cornea is perforated.

When the beam is directed at any lesion that is elevated (lid lesion, corneal cyst, iris cyst, etc), the beam will "bow out." To detect iris neovascularization (abnormal, new blood vessels), the beam must be moved from right to left and back again, otherwise this pathology could be missed completely. Figures 12-18 and 12-19 demonstrate the setting and an example of direct focal illumination.

Tangential Illumination

In *tangential illumination*, the light source is directed at the object of interest from an extreme angle, far left or far right (Figure 12-20). This causes any elevated object (such as an iris cyst; Figure 12-21) to cast a shadow, revealing its three-dimensionality.

Direct Retroillumination

Direct retroillumination, as the term implies, uses light reflected from a source behind the object you want to view (Figure 12-22). The microscope is focused on the item of interest itself. This technique is especially useful for looking at corneal pathology, such as neovascularization, "ghost vessels" (a neovascularized vessel that no longer contains blood), or epithelial ingrowth (Figure 12-23).

These three principle forms of illumination, direct focal illumination (described above), direct retroillumination off the iris, and indirect illumination off the iris, can be seen in Figure 12-24. These images show these techniques as used to photograph glass goblets and how they compare to what we see on the cornea.

Indirect Retroillumination

With *indirect retroillumination*, the beam itself is directed to the side of the object of interest, while the microscope is actually focused on the object. This uses light reflected off of a source behind the object as a backlight and may bring out subtle changes in the cornea and lens.

To use this method to view the cornea, the beam is reflected either off the iris (if peripheral) as demonstrated in Fuchs' corneal dystrophy (Figure 12-25) or can be through the pupil or off the retina (if central).

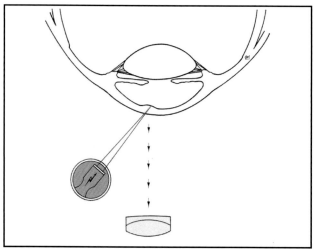

Figure 12-18. Direct focal illumination. (Reprinted with permission from Csaba L. Martonyi, CRA, FOPS.)

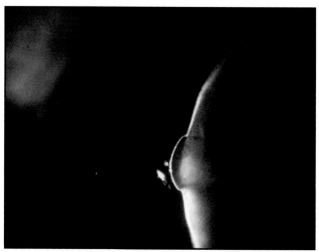

Figure 12-19. Direct focal illumination of a corneal cyst.

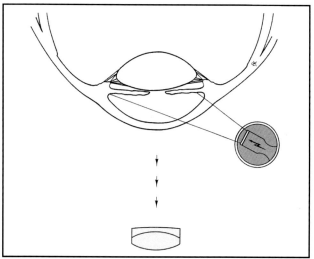

Figure 12-20. Tangential Illumination. (Reprinted with permission from Csaba L. Martonyi, CRA, FOPS.)

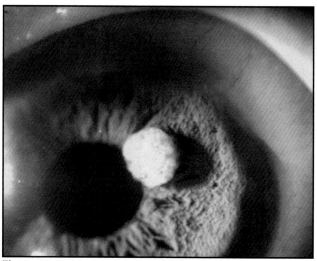

Figure 12-21. Iris cyst in tangential illumination.

We can see changes in the lens of the eye or in the capsule behind an intraocular lens implant by using direct retroillumination as well. By shining the slit beam at the edge of the pupil, the reflection off the choroid and retinal pigment epithelium (Figures 12-26A and B) or optic nerve head (Figures 12-27A and B) act as "mirrors" to light up the lens (perhaps revealing cataracts) or a multifocal intraocular lens (Figure 12-28) or the posterior capsule membrane to detect posterior capsular opacification.

Sclerotic Scatter

Sclerotic scatter is mainly used to view the cornea. The light source is positioned in such a way that it is scattered across the cornea and is reflected by any pathology. The slit beam, set at about 1 mm wide and at about half the height of the cornea, is directed onto the limbus. The

illumination arm is decentered by unlocking the knob and turning the arm to the side (Figure 12-29). Corneal macular dystrophy is seen best by sclerotic scatter (Figure 12-30). (Be courteous to the next user, and return the arm to its normal position when you're finished!)

Proximal Illumination

In *proximal illumination*, the slit beam is directed just adjacent to the entity you want to view, and your focus is set on the pathology. Set the slit beam at a 60° angle, with medium beam width and height to bring corneal or lens pathology into better view (Figure 12-31). For example, in Figure 12-32, a lenticular foreign body cannot be seen well with direct focal illumination. Using proximal illumination will allow for the best visualization of the same lenticular foreign body in Figure 12-33.

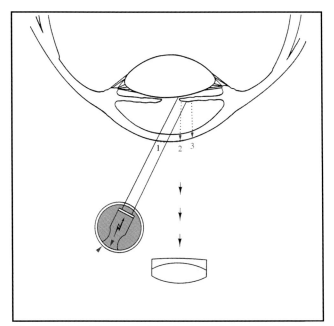

Figure 12-22. Direct retroillumination of the iris. (Reprinted with permission from Csaba L. Martonyi, CRA, FOPS.)

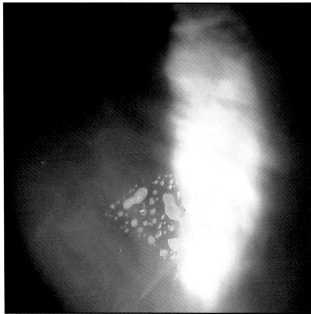

Figure 12-23. Direct retroillumination from the iris showing epithelial in-growth of the cornea after LASIK.

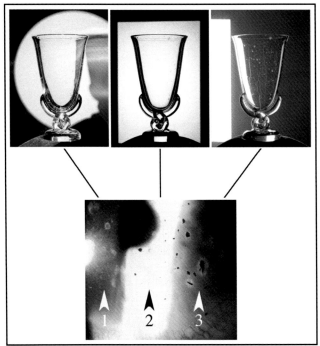

Figure 12-24. Three principle forms of illumination: (1) direct focal, (2) indirect, (3) indirect retroillumination. (Reprinted with permission from Csaba L. Martonyi, CRA, FOPS.)

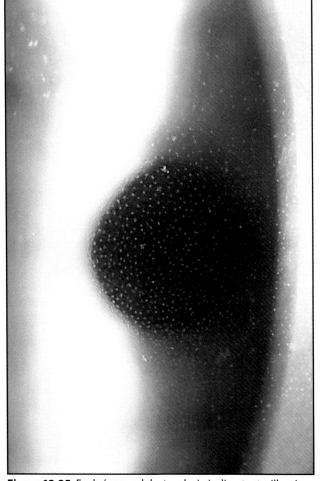

Figure 12-25. Fuchs' corneal dystrophy in indirect retroillumination.

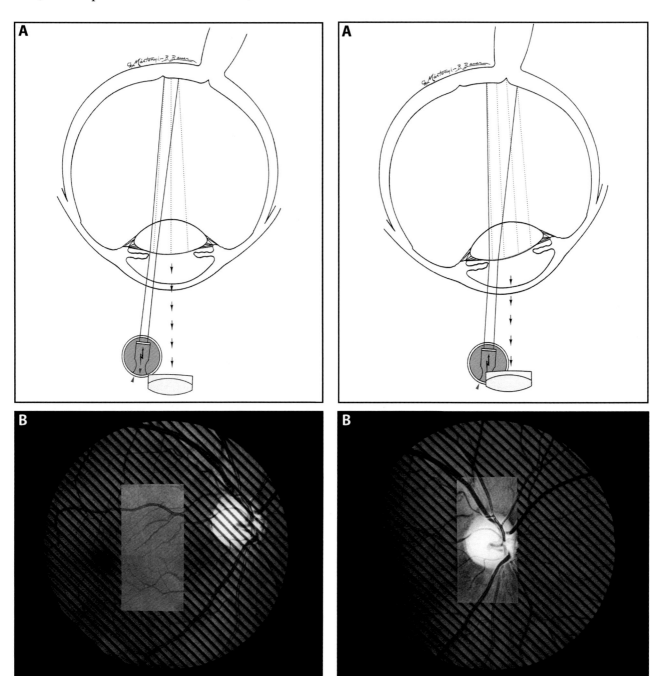

Figure 12-26. (A) Direct retroillumination using the retina. (B) Retroillumination of the retina. (Reprinted with permission from Csaba L. Martonyi, CRA, FOPS.)

Figure 12-27. (A) Retroillumination of the optic nerve. (B) Direct retroillumination using the optic nerve. (Reprinted with permission from Csaba L. Martonyi, CRA, FOPS.)

Pinpoint Illumination

Pinpoint illumination is best used to evaluate the anterior chamber. The "pinpoint" is made possible by reducing the width and height of the beam to the minimum settings and increasing brightness by turning the rheostat to the highest setting. The beam is directed through the cornea at a 45° angle (Figure 12-34). It may help to focus in and out, in the "empty" space between the back of the cornea and the front of the lens and pupil.

Normally the aqueous is optically clear, but if inflammation is present, there will be white blood cells floating in the anterior chamber. These appear as tiny dots, like dust floating in a beam of sunlight. Abnormal amounts of protein in the aqueous (known as *flare*) look like smoke and make the slit beam look hazy. (An eye at 1 day after cataract surgery might be a good practice eye for you to learn how to see cell and flare.) You may actually be able to see cells and flare moving in the anterior chamber as the aqueous circulates (Figure 12-35).

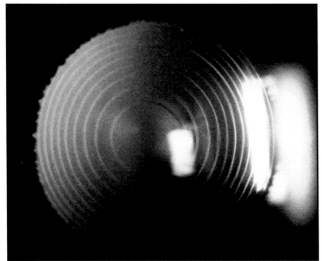

Figure 12-28. Direct retroillumination of multifocal intraocular lens.

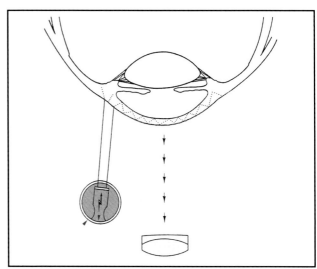

Figure 12-29. Position of the slit beam for sclerotic scatter. (Reprinted with permission from Csaba L. Martonyi, CRA, FOPS.)

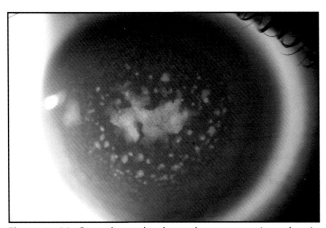

Figure 12-30. Corneal macular dystrophy as seen using sclerotic scatter. (Reprinted with permission from Dina Alismail, MSc, COMT.)

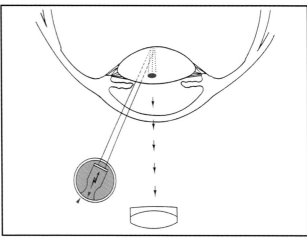

Figure 12-31. Position of the slit beam for proximal Illumination. (Reprinted with permission from Csaba L. Martonyi, CRA, FOPS.)

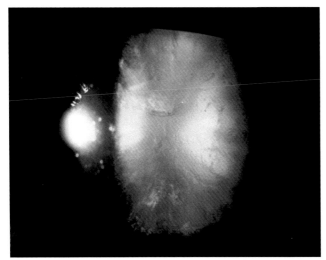

Figure 12-32. Slit beam directed on lens with foreign body. A foreign body on the lens is not very visible using direct focal illumination. (Reprinted with permission from Csaba L. Martonyi, CRA, FOPS.)

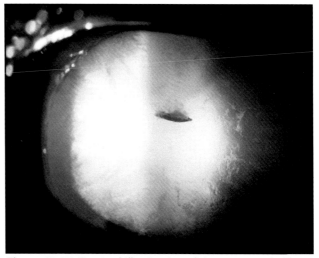

Figure 12-33. Proximal illumination of the same eye in Figure 12-32 brings the foreign body into sharp relief. (Reprinted with permission from Csaba L. Martonyi, CRA, FOPS.)

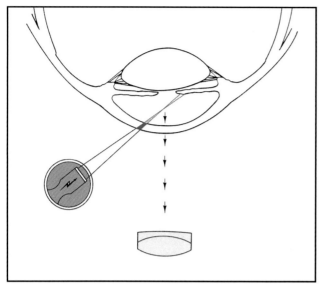

Figure 12-34. Tangential pencil of light through chamber creating a pinpoint to visualize cell and flare. (Reprinted with permission from Csaba L. Martonyi, CRA, FOPS.)

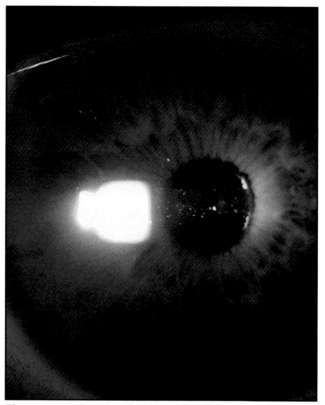

Figure 12-35. Anterior chamber cell and flare in pinpoint illumination.

Material in the aqueous is visible because of *Tyndall's phenomenon* (named after John Tyndall, British physicist, 1820-1893). This occurs when a light beam is broken up and made visible by particles suspended in the light. Imagine that you are in a dark room where someone is smoking. Someone turns on a flashlight. Now you can see the cigarette smoke moving in the beam of the flashlight.

Specular Reflection

Specular reflection occurs when light is reflected at the same angle as the observer. (An example would be the setting sun's reflection in the ocean.) In this slit lamp technique, the light source is aimed at the eye from an angle, and the oculars are swung in the opposite direction by the same number of degrees (Figure 12-36). This is a good method for observing the endothelial layer (the single-celled innermost layer) of the cornea (Figure 12-37).

Transillumination of the Iris

The integrity of the iris can best be evaluated by *transillumination*, which uses light reflected from the fundus to illuminate the iris from behind. The beam is reduced to approximately 4 X 4 mm and shone into the center of the pupil while focusing on the iris (Figure 12-38). The normal, intact iris is opaque. Openings in the iris (eg, an iris iridectomy or iridotomy) or areas where the tissue is thin or pulled away will glow orange-red with the reflected light. A patient with pigment dispersion syndrome can have transillumination defects 360°.

Performing the Slit Lamp Examination

The slit lamp is a large microscope with an illumination system. It may look difficult, but with practice it is easy to use.

The patient's chair can be moved up and down, as can the chinrest of the slit lamp, to allow your patient to be comfortable and provide optimal focusing of the instrument. Remember to adjust the chinrest so that the outer canthus of the patient's eye is in line with the mark on the headrest, as this will allow for maximum movement of the light.

Some patients want to hold onto something while you are examining them. You can ask them to hold onto the handgrips on either side of the instrument. This will keep them from grabbing the table or the rail covers, either of which can prevent smooth operation of the microscope.

Adjust your stool at a height that is comfortable for you. With your feet flat on the floor, position yourself at eye level with the binoculars of the microscope. This will help save your neck and back over the years. Then adjust the slit lamp table to your mid-torso level and look through the oculars while you are sitting straight. Next, adjust the eyepiece to your pupillary distance so that you will be able to see in three dimensions. On all slit lamps, the oculars move laterally for this purpose.

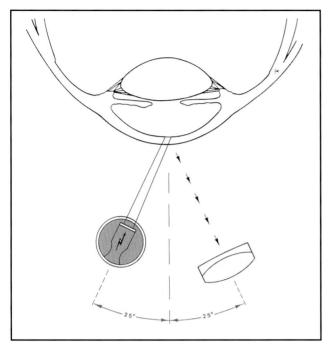

Figure 12-36. Position of the slit beam for specular reflection. (Reprinted with permission from Csaba L. Martonyi, CRA, FOPS.)

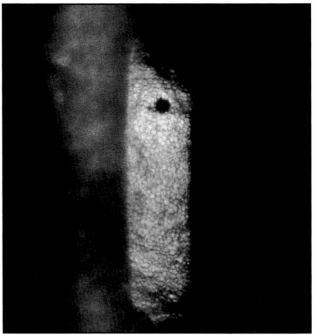

Figure 12-37. Endothelial cells with small focal alteration as viewed using specular reflection. (Reprinted with permission from Csaba L. Martonyi, CRA, FOPS.)

Focusing

Once the patient is in position, you can use one hand to slide the stage all the way forward (toward the patient) and to the far left, holding the joystick pointing straight up at 90° (Figure 12-39). There are several advantages to doing this. First, when you turn on the lamp beam, it will not be glaring right into the patient's face. Second, keeping the joystick vertical will leave you plenty of maneuverability when focusing. Finally, in this forward-most position, the only way you can focus is to pull the instrument *back* (toward yourself). This means you can avoid large "searching" motions with the microscope, making it easier for you to find the eye (and making you look more professional). With the instrument on and looking at the patient from the side (not through the oculars), just slide the stage a little to the right until the beam reaches the outer canthus. Then you can look into the oculars and fine-tune the focus. (The iris is a good place to start.)

Once grossly focused at low magnification, move the joystick forward or back slightly to adjust viewing the fine details. After mastering focusing on the iris, try a blood vessel on the conjunctiva. Keep the slit beam narrow, and increase the magnification to the highest setting, while you look at the center of the vessel and watch for the red blood cells moving through it.

Examination of the eye and adnexa should follow a step-by-step approach. Start with the lids and lashes, then palpebral conjunctiva (inside the eyelid), the bulbar conjunctiva (on the eyeball) and sclera, cornea, anterior chamber, iris, pupil edge, lens, and anterior vitreous.

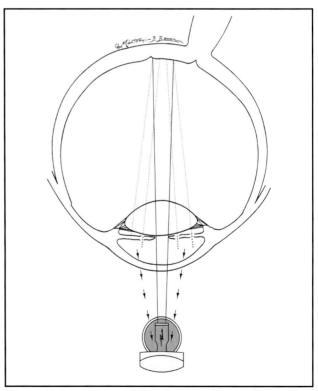

Figure 12-38. Position of the slit beam for transillumination of the iris. (Reprinted with permission from Csaba L. Martonyi, CRA, FOPS.)

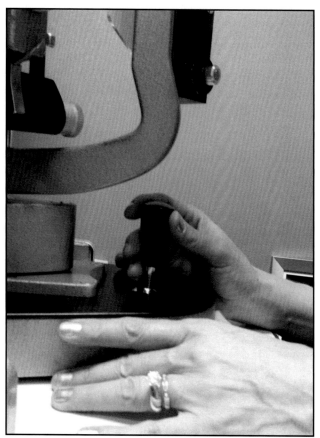

Figure 12-39. Joystick vertical 90 and base horizontal 180.

External

Note: The findings mentioned in this section are all explained elsewhere in the text. Check the Index to find more information.

With one hand on the stage and joystick, you can use the other to manipulate the light source. Start with the beam halfway open and scan the eyelids and lashes. Look for scales, lid lesions, blocked meibomian glands, and abnormal or missing lashes. The lower eyelid can be easily pulled down with a finger so the palpebral conjunctiva can be visualized. The upper eyelid must be everted if you want to see the palpebral conjunctiva. Ask the patient to look down and place the end of a wooden cotton-tipped applicator on the eyelid. Grasp the eyelashes and push down on the applicator while simultaneously flipping the lid up. Look for foreign bodies, papillae, etc.

There are several kinds of dyes that are used to evaluate the external eye through the slit lamp (Sidebar 12-1). These will be referred to at appropriate points in the text.

SIDEBAR 12-1

TOPICAL STAINS USED WITH THE SLIT LAMP

Topical *sodium fluorescein* (NaFl) will cause areas where epithelium is disturbed to stain yellow/green. It is available as a drop and a strip. Set the slit lamp beam to medium width, maximum illumination, low to medium magnification, and dial in the cobalt blue light. This causes the fluorescein to glow. NaFl has many uses:

► Fluorescein/tear break-up time (FBUT/TBUT, see Chapter 9)

► Corneal integrity (eg, abrasions, tear film, and dry eye disease)

► Foreign body assessment

► Seidel sign/test—A break in the cornea with aqueous humor leaking from the anterior chamber will look like a green waterfall on the surface of the cornea as the aqueous streams through the fluorescein

► Contact lens fitting (typically rigid gas permeable lenses, see Chapter 21)

► Goldmann applanation tonometry (GAT, see Chapter 13)

► Lacrimal drainage assessment (see Chapter 26)

Rose bengal dye will cause areas of damaged, degenerating, and dead cells on the cornea and conjunctiva to stain red. Set the slit lamp beam to medium width, high illumination, low to medium magnification, and use white light when evaluating for dry eye. It is available as both a liquid and strip.

Lissamine green is a synthetically produced organic molecule. Membrane-damaged or devitalized cells will stain green. Set the slit lamp beam to medium width, low illumination, and low to medium magnification. This dye is used to evaluate the conjunctiva in dry eye as well as in contact lens evaluation.

Conjunctiva

Evaluate the conjunctiva on the surface of the eyeball by direct illumination, looking for cysts, pinguecula, pterygia, subconjunctival hemorrhage, and abnormal growths. Move the slit beam side to side, observing the tissue from various angles.

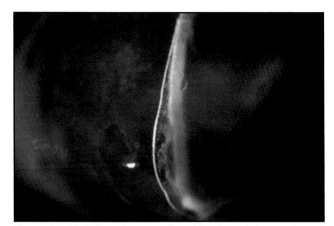

Figure 12-40. Bullous keratopathy with edema is better viewed with a narrow slit using indirect illumination. (Reprinted with permission from Dina Alismail, MSc, COMT.)

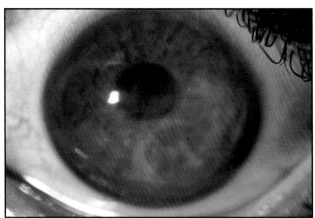

Figure 12-41. Descemet's detachment is not very obvious using diffuse illumination. (Reprinted with permission from Dina Alismail, MSc, COMT.)

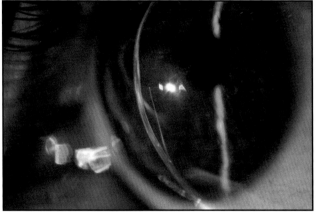

Figure 12-42. Direct focal illumination of Descemet's detachment reveals more detail. (Reprinted with permission from Dina Alismail, MSc, COMT.)

Cornea

The cornea is normally clear. When looking at the cornea with diffuse illumination, some pathology can be missed. It is important to use the slit beam to see fine detail of the corneal layers. When viewing the cornea, adjust the slit beam as narrow as possible and direct it at about a 45° angle. This setting is good for indirect illumination and will provide a view of the cornea in cross–section, making it possible to see scars, foreign bodies, or retained fluid (Figure 12-40). Direct focal illumination also brings out details not seen well in diffuse illumination (Figures 12-41 and 12-42). Abnormal blood vessels (neovascularization) can be seen with the beam set to the side of the pathology, thereby employing the indirect retroillumination technique (Figure 12-43).

The epithelium is the outermost layer of the cornea and acts as a barrier to infection. If you suspect that the epithelium is disrupted, as in a corneal abrasion, instill *sodium fluorescein dye* (see Sidebar 12-1) and use the cobalt blue filter on the slit lamp with increased illumination (Figure 12-44). If the epithelium is intact, the surface

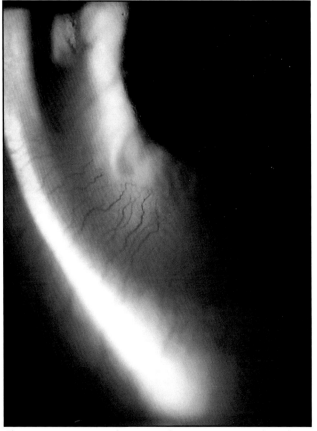

Figure 12-43. Corneal neovascularization seen with indirect retroillumination.

will look smooth and will glow bluish-green. If there is a break in the epithelium, the dye will fill in the abrasion and the area will appear brighter.

When the epithelium is degenerating, a dye called *rose bengal* is used (see Sidebar 12-1). In order to see the fine punctate staining of the surface of the cornea, use diffuse illumination with white light. The defects will then appear pink. Rose bengal is helpful in diagnosing keratoconjunctivitis sicca, better known as dry eye.

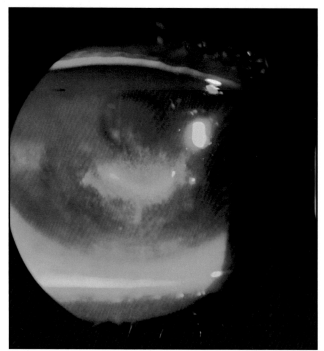

Figure 12-44. Corneal abrasion with fluorescein.

Iris

Generally, when looking at the iris, we are looking at its integrity. Use diffuse illumination for an overall view. Then narrow the slit beam to look for abnormal growths, cysts, and blood vessels. You might observe neovascularization at the pupil edge in a long-standing diabetic patient. By shining the slit beam straight through the pupil, the light will reflect off the retina and reveal any transillumination defects within the iris (areas where the light shines brighter or through, indicating missing or thinning tissue).

Anterior Chamber

The anterior chamber (AC), the space between the iris and the back of the cornea, is filled with a clear fluid called aqueous humor. If inflammation is present, blood cells and inflammatory cells may be circulating through the AC. It is a good habit to look at the aqueous humor with a very bright, pinpoint light. Try to focus somewhere between the back of the cornea and front of the iris, using the pupil as a dark background. This is best done before the eye is dilated because simply dilating the eyes can induce cells and flare in some patients.

Another common finding in the anterior chamber after trauma or injury is a hyphema (see Chapter 27). A hyphema is usually caused by injury to the root of the iris where one or more blood vessels break and bleed into the anterior chamber. Generally, the blood will accumulate at 6 o'clock in the chamber due to gravity. By adjusting the length of the slit lamp beam, it is possible to measure the height of the accumulated blood by noting the millimeter

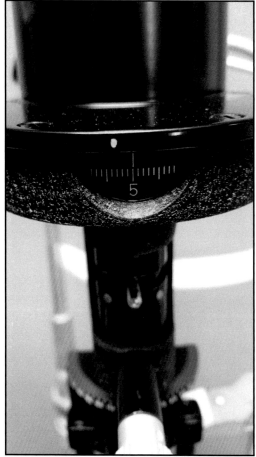

Figure 12-45. Millimeter adjustment knob and display.

reading just below the housing unit on top of the slit lamp (Figure 12-45).

A hypopyon is white- or cream-colored pus (white blood cells) that accumulates in the anterior chamber. This can occur in response to a severe infection, and can be viewed with the slit lamp in the same manner as an hyphema.

Sometimes vitreous can appear in the anterior chamber. Vitreous is most commonly seen in the anterior chamber of aphakic eyes (ie, the natural lens has been removed). Occasionally, there will be small pieces of pigment on the vitreous as well.

Estimation of Anterior Chamber Depth: The Van Herick Technique

One of the true ocular emergencies in ophthalmology is an angle closure glaucoma attack. This occurs when the angle of the eye (where aqueous drains out) becomes obstructed. Because the aqueous cannot escape, pressure builds up quickly in the eye. Typically, this patient would have severe pain (perhaps to the point of nausea and vomiting), extremely high intraocular pressure, a mid-dilated pupil, a cloudy cornea (with resultant blurred vision), and a very shallow anterior chamber with narrow or closed angles. Dilating an eye with narrow angles can actually cause such a glaucoma attack.

Sidebar 12-2
Grading Angles (Van Herick Method)

► Grade 4: Ratio of cornea to dark interval is 1:1—Open angle—The dark space between the back of the cornea and the iris is the same as (or greater than) the corneal thickness. The angle would be greater than 45°.

► Grade 3: Ratio of cornea to dark interval is 1:1/2—Open angle—The dark space between the back of the cornea and the iris is half the size of the corneal thickness. The angle is about 30°.

► Grade 2: Ratio of cornea to dark interval is 1:1/4—Narrow angle—The dark space between the back of the cornea and the iris is one-fourth of the corneal thickness. The angle would be about 20° and is at risk of possible angle closure if the pupil is dilated.

► Grade 1: Ratio of cornea to dark interval is less than 1:1/4—Dangerously narrow angle—The dark space between the back of the cornea and the iris is less than one-fourth the width of the corneal thickness. The angle would be at or near 10° and angle closure is probable; the pupil should not be dilated.

► Grade 0: Closed angle where the back of the cornea touches the iris—There is no space between the light of the slit beam on the cornea and the light falling on the iris. The back surface of the cornea is touching the iris. Check intraocular pressure and notify the practitioner, as this situation is the set-up for angle closure glaucoma (see Chapter 29).

Checking the depth of the anterior chamber is a very important task delegated to eye care techs. *An open angle must be confirmed before dilating the pupils. If a narrow angle is suspected, do not dilate!* Instead, ask the practitioner to evaluate the angles him-/herself and advise you about dilation. Carefully document this discussion in the patient's chart.

The *Van Herick technique* is designed to assess the depth of the anterior chamber with the slit beam. Set the magnification at high, position the slit beam at 60°, and place a narrow slit as close to the limbus as possible and perpendicular to the surface of cornea. Compare the thickness of the cornea (as seen by optical section) with the optically empty, dark section (sometimes referred to as the *interval*) between the front surface of the iris and the back of surface of the cornea. See Sidebar 12-2 and drawings for how to grade angles.

Posterior Chamber and Lens

Observe the lens looking for opacities and position of the lens. A normal lens in a young patient is clear; the transparency changes gradually through one's lifetime. You will most likely view the lens through a small pupil, as you generally see the patient before the doctor and before full dilation of the pupil takes effect. That being said, changes can still be observed in the central lens, such as color (clear, yellow, brown), opacities, and mother-of-pearl cataracts (see Chapter 28).

When focusing the beam farther behind the lens, you may see vitreous floaters as well as many small white particles floating in the vitreous (*asteroid hyalosis*). It is also possible, but not common, to see vitreous hemorrhages. Red blood cells in the anterior vitreous can be an indication of a retinal detachment. Both a hemorrhage and red blood cells would have to be fairly anterior in the vitreous to be seen using the slit lamp alone. However, with auxiliary hand-held lenses (as detailed earlier in this chapter) it is possible to see more deeply into the vitreous, as well as the retina.

The slit lamp examination usually ends here for technicians. In some practices, the techs may document what they observe and the physician will agree or disagree with the findings in written charts. In electronic medical records, the physician will change the findings if needed, before signing off on them.

ACKNOWLEDGMENTS

The author would like to thank the following: Csaba L. Martonyi, CRA, FOPS; Dina Alismail, MSc, COMT; and Robert Flammond, Haag-Streit Marketing Coordinator.

CHAPTER QUIZ

1. The slit lamp consists of two _____ that used together allow the observer to see stereoscopically.

2. When technicians use a slit lamp their job is to _____ disease.
   a. diagnose
   b. detect
   c. prescribe
   d. subscribe

3. The slit lamp provides a _____ view of the ocular structures.
   a. clear
   b. bright
   c. two-dimensional
   d. three-dimensional

4. When is the external fixation device used?

5. Why is asking your patient to "keep your teeth together" important when performing a slit lamp exam?

6. The canthus mark on the side of the headrest bar aids in _____ the patient.

7. Direct focal illumination uses a _____ beam.
   a. wide
   b. bright
   c. narrow
   d. dim

8. A light source directed at the object of interest from an extreme angle (far left or far right) is called _____ illumination.
   a. retro
   b. direct
   c. indirect
   d. tangential

9. Which is the best method of illumination to visualize opacities in posterior capsule of the lens?
   a. direct
   b. indirect retro
   c. tangential
   d. direct retro

10. Which method of illumination is best when visualizing the cornea?
    a. tangential
    b. sclerotic scatter
    c. proximal
    d. direct retro

11. Name the dye that is used for the Seidel test.
    a. fluorescein
    b. rose bengal
    c. tyrian purple
    d. indocyanine green

12. Which is a true emergency in ophthalmology that can often be predicted (and avoided) by performing the Van Herick estimation technique?
    a. open angle glaucoma
    b. diabetes
    c. narrow angle glaucoma
    d. age-related macular degeneration

Answers

1. Oculars
2. b
3. d
4. When we want to evaluate the opposite eye in a position other than straight ahead.
5. Helps prevent movement of the head during the exam, and can stop the talkative patient when the examination is underway.
6. Aligning
7. c
8. d
9. d
10. b
11. a
12. c

Unless otherwise noted, the figures in this chapter were contributed by the author, Sergina M. Flaherty.

13

Tonometry

Gayle Roberts, COMT, BHS

Basic Sciences

Tonometry is derived from the Greek root "tonos," meaning pressure, combined with "metria," meaning the process of measuring. It is defined as the measurement of pressure or tension. For our purposes, it is the process of measuring the pressure inside the eye, or the intraocular pressure (IOP). Instruments called *tonometers* are the devices used to quantify this measurement. They utilize either the principle of *indentation* (indent using a fixed weight) or *applanation* (flattening a specified area).

Using any of the techniques in this chapter is key in the early detection of glaucoma. Monitoring the IOPs at regular intervals, along with observing optic nerves and verifying the integrity of the patient's visual fields, contribute to successful management of the disease. Although a cure for glaucoma remains elusive, greater knowledge of the biomechanics of the eye will continually offer improved methods of detecting, monitoring and treating this vision-threatening disorder.

Anatomy

The eye contains a closed system in which fluid, called the *aqueous humor*, is produced by the ciliary body. As discussed in Chapters 2 and 3 (Ocular Anatomy and

Ocular Physiology, respectively), the aqueous flows from the ciliary body through the pupil into the anterior chamber, drains from the eye through the trabecular meshwork into Schlemm's canal, and joins the systemic bloodstream by means of the episcleral veins (Figure 13-1). This continual creation, movement, and exit of fluid contribute to the healthy homeostasis of the eye by providing nutrients to the cornea and lens. It also creates an internal pressure necessary to maintain the shape of the globe and keep it from collapsing. However, as Chapter 29 (Glaucoma) explains, sometimes the system falls out of balance, leading to optic nerve damage and a diagnosis of glaucoma.

According to the World Health Organization, glaucoma is the second leading cause of blindness in the world.[1] Early detection is key for successful treatment. Tonometry is one of a number of tests that contributes to an accurate diagnosis.

Clinical Knowledge

Historical Origins

Physicians have not always associated vision loss with elevated eye pressure. The connection became more apparent in the early 19th century. There were a lot of trial-and-error attempts to create a device that could

Ledford JK, Lens A, eds.
Principles and Practice in Ophthalmic Assisting:
A Comprehensive Textbook (pp 233-251).
© 2018 Taylor & Francis Group.

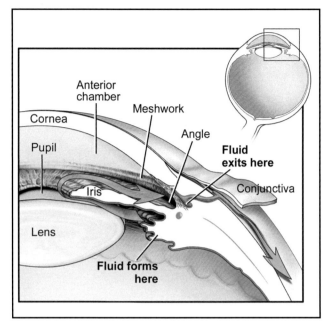

Figure 13-1. Formation and drainage of aqueous humor. (Reprinted from the National Eye Institute, National Institutes of Health [NEI/NIH].)

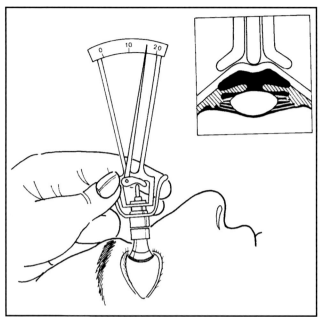

Figure 13-2. Depiction of indentation. (Image from the webpage http://www.lea-test.fi/en/eyes/images/pict13b.gif, courtesy of Lea Hyvärinen, MD, PhD, FAAP.)

more accurately assess patients' pressures. Albrecht von Graefe was one of the first to propose such an instrument in 1865.[2]

The discovery of cocaine to anesthetize the eye in 1884 allowed for the development of a corneal impression tonometer. In the early 1900s, the Schiötz mechanical tonometer was introduced. As its use proliferated, greater understanding was gained about IOP and its effect on the eye. This simple, easy to use, and fairly accurate device became the "gold standard" for measuring IOPs until the 1950s when the Goldmann applanation tonometer came into use. This became the preferred method of testing and has remained so for the past 50+ years.

Physics of Tonometry

So how does tonometry actually work? Imagine that your eye is like a water balloon. The fluid creates enough internal pressure to maintain the shape of the balloon. Otherwise, the external atmospheric pressure would act upon it, causing it to collapse. If you press your thumb into the side of the balloon, it will be met with the hydrostatic resistance of this closed system. A tonometer basically works in the same way, by either indenting (Figure 13-2) or applanating (Figure 13-3) the corneal surface. The measured resistance is a function of the IOP.

The resistance force is measured in mm Hg (millimeters of mercury), defined as a unit of pressure that can support a column of mercury 1 mm high.

Average or "normal" IOP generally falls between 10 to 22 mm Hg. (Note: sources vary on these numbers.)

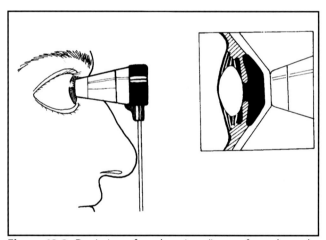

Figure 13-3. Depiction of applanation. (Image from the webpage http://www.lea-test.fi/en/eyes/images/pict13.gif, courtesy of Lea Hyvärinen, MD, PhD, FAAP.)

When IOP exceeds 22 mm Hg, but additional diagnostic testing does not detect glaucomatous changes, the condition is generally referred to as *ocular hypertension*.

Factors Affecting Intraocular Pressure
Ocular Structures

New information is continually coming to light about how the structures of the eye affect IOP.

The eye has a relatively constant volume, and a structure that is fairly resistant to changing shape. When an indentation device is applied to the corneal surface, some of the aqueous fluid is displaced; only a tiny (insignificant) amount of it manages to exit the eye. Thus, there is pressure placed on the rest of the globe. Normally, the sclera "gives" just a little under this pressure. However if the sclera is abnormally "tough," it resists and causes a falsely elevated IOP reading. This is referred to as *scleral rigidity*. Conversely, an abnormally elastic sclera (as sometimes seen in the young, high myopes, or those with exophthalmos) "gives" too much, causing a falsely low reading. Scleral rigidity is mainly of concern in Schiötz tonometry (covered later) and is not much of a factor in other, more commonly used applanation methods. (It does, however, seem to be a favorite topic on certification exams!)

It was inadvertently discovered during the Ocular Hypertension Study that *central corneal thickness* (CCT) plays an important role in the accuracy of IOP measurements and in the risk of developing glaucoma.[3]

The average CCT is about 0.55 mm or 555 μm. A thinner cornea (<555 μm) will elicit artificially low IOP measurements due to less resistance by the cornea. In contrast, a thicker cornea (>555 μm) will yield falsely high readings. This is due to more resistance by the thicker corneal tissue. Corneal thickness is particularly a concern for patients who have undergone LASIK or photorefractive keratectomy. Their corneas have been thinned to decrease a refractive error, thus artificially lowering their IOP readings. The Ocular Response Analyzer (ORA; Reichert Ophthalmic Instruments) and Dynamic Contour Tonometry (Pascal DCT; Ziemer Ophthalmic Systems AG) methods of screening IOP purport to factor in these changes in corneal thickness.[4]

In light of this breakthrough, corneal pachymetry has gained favor as part of an initial evaluation. The test employs a hand-held device that is gently touched against the central cornea after topical anesthetic is applied. In addition, CCT can easily be acquired during optical coherence tomography (OCT) or Scheimpflug imaging.

Researchers also think the recent discovery of a possible new corneal layer, called the *pre-Descemet's layer* or *Dua's layer*, could have a potential link to glaucoma.[5]

Extraocular Influences

Around-the-clock IOP testing revealed that body position influences the IOP. Pressures are lowest in a sitting position, but increase overnight when the body lies in a recumbent position. Over a 24-hour period, IOP normally fluctuates 2 to 6 mm Hg (known as the *diurnal curve*). However, the fluctuations found in glaucoma patients can be greater than 10 mm Hg.

Recent literature suggests a relationship between IOP and systemic blood pressure.[6] This is referred to as the *ocular profusion pressure* (OPP). It is theorized that when systemic blood pressure drops low, it decreases the OPP. The lower perfusion pressure leads to less oxygen and blood reaching the optic nerve, causing damage consistent with that caused by open angle glaucoma.[6] More

remains to be learned about this relationship and how to manage treatment, as it is difficult to increase OPP without inducing systemic hypertension.

New genetic discoveries will also contribute to earlier diagnosis and treatments.

CLINICAL SKILLS

Palpation

A very basic way to quickly assess the IOP is by tactile or digital palpation. In settings where tonometers (or skill in using them) are not available, this method may be used to determine how firm an eye feels, especially when angle closure glaucoma is suspected. Eyes with elevated pressure will feel more rigid and resistant to gentle palpation.

Advantages of this method include that no special equipment is needed, it can be performed in any location, and anesthetic drops are not required. It is also a simple, nonthreatening means to gauge IOP in young children. However, many noninvasive instruments have evolved for clinical use. They are more precise in estimating the IOP than palpation.

Technique

▶ Ask the patient to gently close the eyes—not to squeeze them shut

▶ Explain to the patient you are going to touch the eyes, as if giving them a gentle massage

▶ With the index and middle finger, tenderly press on the central globe through the eyelid

Indentation

The indentation method of tonometry measures the distortion of the cornea when acted upon by an external force. The amount of indention is converted to an equivalent IOP reading by using a chart.

The *Schiötz tonometer* (Figure 13-4) made its debut in the early 1900s. It is historically remembered as the premier indentation method of tonometry, which is why it earns mention in this text. Although the International Joint Commission on Allied Health Personnel in Ophthalmology (IJCAHPO) no longer holds allied ophthalmic personnel (AOP) responsible for demonstrating skill at using the Schiötz, you should still be familiar with the principles involved for potential exam questions.

The Schiötz is a cylindrical-shaped device with a concave bottom plate designed to rest on the anesthetized cornea. A plunger runs through the center of the cylinder and is attached to the scale indicator needle at the top. A small weight, typically 5.5 or 7 grams, is added to the central plunger. (These weights are supplied with the instrument; more on their use momentarily.)

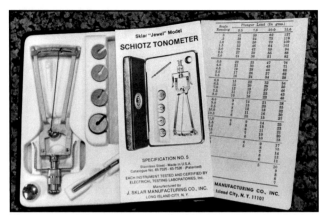

Figure 13-4. Schiötz tonometer (J. Sklar Manufacturing Co).

The weight causes the plunger to indent a small area of the cornea. The scale measures the indentation, each unit representing 0.05 mm. A conversion chart provided by the instrument's manufacturer translates the scale reading to mm Hg. When using the standard 5.5-gram weight, a scale reading between 3 to 6 mm is considered normal. If the measurement is 2 mm or less, repeat the measurement by using heavier weight. (Additional weight discs are included with the instrument and when added along with the 5.5-gram weight total 7.5, 10, and 15 grams.) If the measurement is still 3 mm or less, despite use of heavier weights, there is a higher suspicion of glaucoma.

The deformability of the cornea is a function of the IOP. The greater the indentation, the higher the reading on the scale. This indicates a softer eye and lower IOP. In contrast, with a firmer eye there will be less displacement, a lower scale reading, and thus a higher IOP.

The Schiötz tonometer has quite a few advantages. It is an inexpensive and easy to use. Probably its greatest benefit is that it is small and does not require a power source, making it very portable. Testing can be performed anywhere, including a surgical environment. Because the Schiötz comes into direct contact with the eye, it is important to sanitize or sterilize it following each use.

However, the negative effect of scleral rigidity on the accuracy of the measurements (discussed earlier in the chapter), along with the development of newer technologies, have contributed to its decline in popularity.

Checking Calibration (Adapted from Schiötz Tonometer User's Manual— J. Sklar Manufacturing Co)

▶ Prepare tonometer by checking the calibration prior to every use. Assemble the tonometer with the plunger in place and a 5.5-gram weight affixed.

▶ Inside the instrument case is a test block. Hold the tonometer by the handles and lower it until the footplate rests upon the test block. The plunger will drop,

and the needle on the scale should register a reading of zero.

▶ If the calibration is off, the device must be returned to the manufacturer to be recalibrated.

▶ Wipe the footplate with an alcohol swab and allow to air dry while the patient is prepared.

Technique (Adapted from Schiötz Tonometer User's Manual—J. Sklar Manufacturing Co)

▶ Instill topical anesthetic.

▶ Have the patient recline.

▶ If the patient needs assistance in keeping the eye open, gently spread the eyelids wider, resting your fingers on the bony orbit. (Care must be taken not to apply pressure to the globe.)

▶ At the same time, ask the patient to open the mouth and breathe slowly.

▶ With the patient holding fixation on the ceiling, hold the instrument by the handles and slowly lower the footplate perpendicularly onto the eye. The needle may pulsate.

▶ Record the measurement and use the chart to convert the reading to mm Hg. If there were pulsations, the reading is midway between the extremes.

Disinfection

Because the Schiötz comes into direct contact with the eye, it is important to practice good infection control.

▶ Following each use, disassemble the instrument.

▶ Clean the cylinder barrel with a pipe cleaner soaked in alcohol and wipe dry with a fresh pipe cleaner.

▶ The footplate and plunger tip may be cleaned with an alcohol swab.

▶ Allow to air dry before reassembling, carefully handling the parts with a clean tissue to avoid contaminating the instrument with your fingers.

▶ Alternately, the instrument can be sterilized by autoclave or other methods.

▶ Once back together, check the calibration to make certain it has not been altered during the cleaning process.

Applanation

Applanation tonometry measures the force required to flatten a standard area of the cornea. This method displaces much less aqueous in comparison to indentation.

Inventor Hans Goldmann discovered that a tonometer tip measuring 3.06 mm diameter would flatten an area of 7.35 mm², and this seemed to best balance the opposing forces inside the eye. This tip would then produce a force of 0.1 gram, which corresponded to an IOP of 1 mm Hg.

Many applanation devices have been used over the years. These can be broken down into *contact* tonometers and *noncontact* tonometers (NCT). The text will discuss the trends which are current at the time of publication.

Technicians should document tonometry readings in the patient's chart and always indicate the method used and the time the measurement was taken.

Contact Applanation Tonometry

Goldmann

Goldmann applanation tonometry (GAT) has been the gold standard in checking IOP for the past 50+ years (Figure 13-5). The tonometer tip consists of a funnel-shaped double prism with a flat applanating surface, which has a diameter of about 6 mm; the diameter of the cornea that is flattened when the correct amount of pressure is applied is 3.06 mm. The tip creates a visible ring-image when it contacts the tear film, and the bi-prism splits this into two semicircular mires when applied to the corneal surface. The prism fits into the instrument's feeler arm, which measures the pressure by leveraged weight. The arm is mounted on a housing unit containing a revolving force adjustment knob with a measuring drum. The housing unit is attached to a retractable arm on a slit lamp and can easily be moved into position.

Since slit lamps are customary pieces of equipment in the ophthalmology office, and the Goldmann is a readily available accessory on most slit lamps, it remains a very economical choice for tonometry.

On the down side, Goldmann tonometry does require training and practice. Central corneal thickness is now known to influence the validity of readings. Taking multiple IOP readings can also produce a "massage effect" that lowers the pressure. In addition, this device lacks portability. Despite these flaws, Goldmann still remains the standard.

IJCAHPO requires all three levels of ophthalmic personnel testing candidates to be familiar with the Goldmann tonometer. All will need to demonstrate knowledge of how to clean, disinfect, and check calibration of the device on their written certification exam. In addition, COT and COMT candidates will be responsible for showing competency in performing Goldmann tonometry in a practical assessment.

Checking Calibration

► The manufacturer provides a calibration weight bar with the tonometer (Figure 13-6).

► Insert the calibration weight into the receptacle on the side of the housing unit.

► Finger lock the rod into the weight at the zero position, or center hash mark.

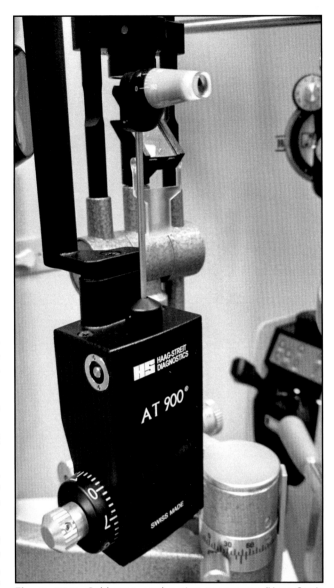

Figure 13-5. Goldmann applanation tonometer (Haag-Streit USA).

► Set the force adjustment knob indicator slightly above zero mm Hg.

► Slowly move the force adjustment knob toward "zero," watching the prism as the knob is being turned.

► The prism should shift slightly as the knob reaches the zero mm Hg setting.

► If you set the indicator at just below zero and apply more force, the prism should also slightly move as the knob reaches the zero position.

► Repeat the process by adjusting the weight to the 20 mm Hg and 60 mm Hg settings on the calibration rod. Set the force adjustment knob indicator to just above and just below the selected reading. As the prism reaches the reading, a shift in position should be detected.

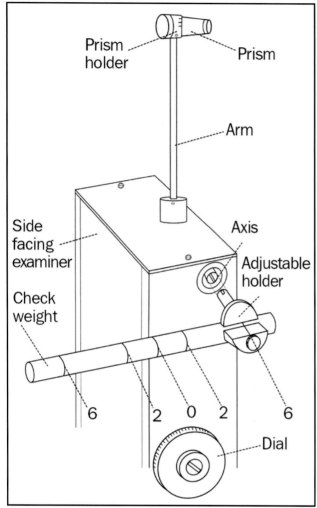

Figure 13-6. Goldmann calibration bar (Haag-Streit USA). (Reprinted with permission from Ismael Cordero, all rights reserved.)

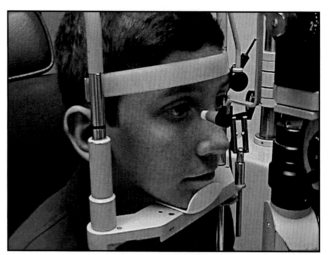

Figure 13-7. Patient position for Goldmann tonometry.

▶ If the calibration is off, the device needs to be returned to the manufacturer for recalibration.

Technique

▶ If the patient wears contact lenses, remove the lenses before commencing.

▶ Instill a combined anesthetic drop with fluorescein dye into the patient's eyes. (An anesthetic such as proparacaine, along with a moistened fluorescein strip, may be used instead.) If the combination drop is used, instill just a small amount to avoid flooding the eye with too much liquid.

▶ Seat the patient comfortably at the slit lamp with the chin down, teeth together, and forehead firmly placed against the headrest. Do a slit lamp examination to make certain the patient's corneal surface is healthy. Tonometry should be avoided if there is a suspected corneal defect; have the doctor examine the patient before proceeding with applanation and document that the defect was present prior to GAT.

▶ Swing the tonometer into position (Figure 13-7).

▶ The prism should be rotated to the 180-degree (°) position, unless there is 3 diopters or more of astigmatism. If the patient has more than 3 diopters of astigmatism, rotate the prism so the patient's refractive axis (IN MINUS CYLINDER) is at the red line on the prism holder. This is done to offset the steeper curve of such an eye.

▶ Set the magnification to the lowest power. Switch the cobalt blue filter on and open the light aperture to the brightest setting.

▶ Adjust the position of the light source so it illuminates the prism tip at a wide angle between 45° and 60°.

▶ Viewing slightly from one side, hold the joystick back so it will have more "play" and slowly bring the stage of the slit lamp forward, bringing the tonometer tip close to the patient's eye, but without touching.

▶ Once in position, look through the oculars of the slit lamp.

▶ Ask the patient focus on your ear (ie, if applanating the right eye, patient focuses on your right ear with his/her left eye and vice versa).

▶ Ask the patient to blink, continue to breathe, and hold fixation.

▶ With the joystick, gently move the prism forward. As the prism makes contact with the central cornea, the two semicircles, one above and one below the median, will glow yellowish-green. The image of the mires will appear in the left eyepiece.

▶ Adjust the position of the slit lamp as needed by slightly coming off of the eye (to avoid abrading the cornea) and reapplanating. Repeat until the semicircles are centered and equal in size.

▶ Turn the force adjustment knob on the housing unit to move the semicircles. When properly aligned, the half-circle mires will appear equal in size both above and below the prism's midline, with the inner edges of the mires just touching each other (Figure 13-8).

• If edges are too far apart, more force should be applied until they touch

• If semicircles are overlapping, less force is needed

• Sometimes the mires will pulsate (slide back and forth) with the patient's heartbeat and/or respirations

▶ Once the proper position is reached, back off of the eye and read the number on the force adjustment knob. Each mark represents 1 gram; the reading is multiplied by 10 to convert it to IOP in mm Hg.

▶ If the mires were pulsating, the correct reading is the mid-way point between the pulsations. Documentation in these cases should note that there were pulsations, and if they were excessive and/or irregular.

Disinfection and Maintenance

There has been much debate over the best method to disinfect nondisposable Goldmann tonometer prisms. Haag-Streit does not recommend using isopropyl alcohol to clean their prisms. Studies have shown that although alcohol is an effective disinfectant, it causes damage to the tips over time.[7]

Per Haag-Streit, the prism tip must first be *cleaned* with a pH neutral cleanser and rinsed with cold, running water for 30 to 60 seconds. Then to *disinfect* the tip, soak in either hydrogen peroxide 0.3% or sodium hypochlorite 10% (household bleach) for 10 minutes. Rinse for 10 to 15 minutes using cold drinking water and pat dry with a clean, soft, lint-free tissue. Store the prism in a clean, dry container so it is ready for the next use. This cleaning guide is available on the Haag-Streit website.[8]

Be meticulously thorough to rinse any disinfectant from tonometers prior to use. Failure to remove these solutions may result in a chemical burn to the patient's eye.

When the prism is not in use, make certain the swing arm that holds the prism is carefully returned to its resting position. The tonometer arm should be placed in this position at the end of the work day, prior to covering with the dust cover. Care must be exercised not to bump the arm.

Periodically inspect Goldmann prisms for cracks or chips. Replace damaged prisms to avoid abrading a patient's cornea. Pathogens can also collect in cracks. The prisms are now marked by the company with an expiration date.

Finally, establish office protocols so all staff follow the same cleaning rituals.

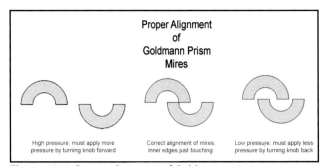

Figure 13-8. Proper alignment of Goldmann mires.

Helpful Hints

Patients often feel that the IOP check is the absolute worst part of having an eye exam. The anesthetic drops can be uncomfortable. Others feel claustrophobic and anxious at the slit lamp. And there are those who cannot suppress their fear of the tonometer tip touching their eye.

In order to make it a more pleasant experience for all involved, take a moment to describe the procedure to the patient. Explain that you will instill an anesthetic drop, which will sting initially but then numb the eyes within a few seconds so he/she can tolerate the test. Have him/her close the eyes and gently pat them dry until the stinging subsides. Also, let him/her know the eyes may feel funny, maybe heavy or sticky. This is normal. The anesthetic effect usually lasts for about 10 minutes. However, it can persist slightly, so advise the patient not to rub the eyes too firmly, even after leaving the office.

Raise or lower the slit lamp to accommodate for the patient's height. It may be easier to stand when performing tonometry on very tall patients. This is especially true if the slit lamp must be brought up beyond the height limit an exam stool can be raised in order to perform the test while seated. This technique is also helpful when attempting to obtain IOPs on shorter, heavier patients. In this instance, ask the patient to stand, and adjust the slit lamp accordingly. The patient will be more comfortable since the instrument is not crunching the knees or compressing the chest, as it might if sitting in the exam chair.

Perkins

The Perkins hand-held applanation tonometer (Haag-Streit USA) is a battery-operated, portable device that employs a counterweight, allowing it to be used on patients in an upright or recumbent position (Figure 13-9). The applanating tip uses the same double prism as a Goldmann tonometer, producing the same semicircle mires. Force is applied and the reading obtained by turning a spring-loaded scale wheel.

The principles behind how the portable Perkins works are essentially the same as those for the Goldmann tonometer. The readings are comparable to those taken with the Goldmann, within 1 mm Hg mean difference.[9] As with the Goldmann, central corneal thickness plays a role in accuracy.

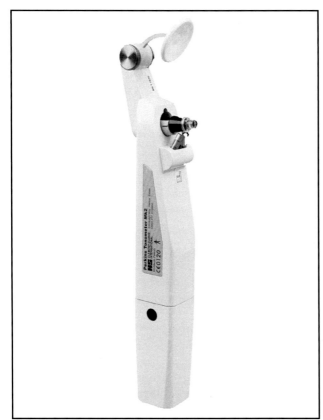

Figure 13-9. Perkins hand-held tonometer (Haag-Streit USA). (Reprinted with permission from Haag-Streit USA, all rights reserved.)

Check Calibration (Adapted from Perkins MK2 Hand-Held Instruction Manual—Haag-Streit USA)

The Perkins comes calibrated from the manufacturer; however, it is recommended that calibration be verified at regular intervals.

▸ Remove battery from housing and insert the prism in holder.

▸ Check the zero position.

• Adjust scale knob to read below zero by one full scale line; the prism should tip back.

• Adjust scale knob to read one full scale line above zero; the prism should tip forward.

▸ Check the 2-gram position.

• Lay the instrument on flat surface with tonometer prism facing up and the setting block (included with the instrument) under the body of the headrest area.

• Adjust scale knob to read below the 2 mark and place the 2-gram weight on prism; the tonometer should move fully to down position.

• Remove weight and adjust the scale knob to read just above the 2 mark.

• Place the 2-gram weight on prism; the tonometer should support the weight at this position.

▸ The 5-gram position is checked in the same manner as the 2-gram position, except using the 5-gram weight.

If calibration falls outside these limits, the instrument should be returned to the manufacturer to be recalibrated.

Technique (Adapted from Perkins MK2 Hand-Held Instruction Manual—Haag-Streit USA):

▸ Explain the procedure to the patient.

▸ Administer a drop of anesthetic combined with fluorescein dye, such as Fluress, or use an anesthetic drop along with a dab from a fluorescein strip.

▸ Ask the patient to focus on a distant target.

▸ Insert a disinfected tonometer prism, or disposable prism into holder, with the prism set at 180° position. If patient has more than 3 diopters of astigmatism, rotate the prism so the patient's refractive axis (IN MINUS CYLINDER) is at the red line on the prism holder.

▸ Rest your thumb on the scale wheel; the illumination light will turn on when the wheel is moved.

▸ Gently place the headrest against the patient's forehead at a slightly oblique angle (to avoid hitting the nose).

▸ While looking through the eyepiece, slowly apply the applanation tip to the corneal surface. If positioned correctly, two semicircles should appear.

▸ Adjust the thumb wheel to apply appropriate force until the inner edges of the semicircles coincide.

▸ Remove the device from the eye and document the reading. Large divisions on the scale equal grams; smaller divisions equal 0.2 grams. Multiply the result by 10 to convert to mm Hg.

Applying the device to the cornea with too little or too much pressure can influence the end results. This is evidenced when the device is pushed too close to the eye and the semicircles appear too large without any reduction in size when less force is applied with the scale wheel. Conversely, if the semicircles are too small and do not move when the scale wheel is turned to a higher value, then the tip is not close enough to properly applanate the surface.

Cleaning and Disinfecting

Surfaces that contact patient skin can be wiped with alcohol. The tonometer tips should be handled in the same manner as with Goldmann tonometry; see that section.

Pneumotonometer

Many companies manufacture pneumotonometers, which are a kind of hybrid applanation tonometer, utilizing principles of both applanation as well as indentation. A regulated flow of air runs from an internal pump through a tube to a probe (which contains a pneumatic sensor) attached at its end (Figure 13-10). The probe's sensor detects both the force of the air flowing through it and the force of resistance as it slightly indents the cornea. The balance of these two forces represents the IOP measurement.

Since the air flow tube is quite long, it can reach patients in most positions. The readings are quite accurate, but can be affected by central corneal thickness. Studies have shown that the pneumotonometer works well on patients with irregular corneal surfaces.[10] Readings can even be obtained through a bandage contact lens.

Check Calibration (Adapted from Reichert Model 30 Pneumotonometer User's Guide—Reichert Technologies)

▶ The Reichert Model 30 comes with a calibration verifier. Fill the calibration verifier tube with filtered water to 15 mm Hg indicator mark.

▶ Press the "Manual IOP" icon on the main screen.

▶ Touch the probe to the membrane of the calibration verifier. A low tone will signal when data are acquired. The measurement should read 15 mm Hg. The probe itself does not need to be calibrated.

Technique (Adapted from Reichert Model 30 Pneumotonometer User's Guide—Reichert Technologies)

▶ Turn on the device. Make sure there is good air flow with no kinks in the air hose (most pneumotonometers will sound an alarm if air flow is impeded).

▶ Inspect the tip; make certain there is a silicone covering in place.

▶ Administer a drop of anesthetic in the patient's eyes.

▶ Have the patient focus on an appropriate target based on the testing position:
  • If upright, look across the room
  • If reclining, focus on the ceiling

▶ Gently place the tonometer tip against the patient's central cornea. A "beep" will signal when a measurement has been obtained.

Cleaning and Disinfecting

Care must be taken to prevent spread of infection between patients. Many companies offer one-use disposable latex covers for the pneumotonometer tip.

To manually *clean* a reusable tip, proceed as recommended by the manufacturer's guidelines. Reichert Technologies, for example, recommends:

▶ Remove the silicone membrane from the tip; soak in separate baths containing 50 to 100 mL of 70% isopropyl alcohol for 5 minutes.

▶ Debris may be dislodged by either swirling the pieces in the alcohol solution or by soaking them in an ultrasonic cleaner, followed by rinsing with sterile water.

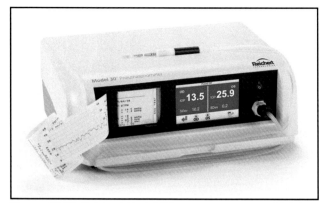

Figure 13-10. Reichert Model 30 pneumotonometer (Reichert Technologies). (Courtesy of Reichert Technologies, all rights reserved.)

To *disinfect* the tip and membrane assembly, Reichert suggests:

▶ Soak the tip and membrane in separate containers of 150 to 200 mL fresh 3% hydrogen peroxide for two rounds of 15 minutes each.

▶ Follow by rinsing with sterile water and allow the pieces to air dry at least 25 to 30 minutes before next use.

Icare

Another hand-held device is the Icare tonometer (Figure 13-11). It utilizes the principle of "rebound technology." Magnetized coils momentarily propel a tiny, disposable probe into the cornea, which then quickly bounces back, or rebounds, once it makes contact. The firmer the eye (or higher the IOP), the faster the probe rebounds.

The process happens so fast it is barely perceptible to the patient, so a topical anesthetic is not necessary. The probe is disposable and may be used for both eyes before discarding. It is recommended that six measurements be taken to eliminate user error as well as any artifact from the patient's heartbeat. Corneal curvature/shape does not affect measurements since the area of probe contact is so small. However, there are conflicting study findings as to the accuracy of the readings relative to increased central corneal thickness.[11] It is very useful as a screening tool for uncooperative patients or children. It has also been put forward as a home-monitoring device where the patient is trained to use the instrument on him-/herself.

Technique (Adapted from Icare Tonometer User's and Maintenance Manual—Icare)

▶ No calibration is needed.

▶ Anesthetic is not required.

▶ Insert a fresh probe tip into the base.

▶ Caution: Do not point the tonometer down until it has been activated, otherwise the tip may fall out.

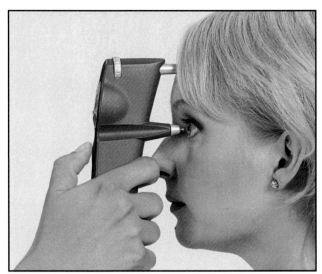

Figure 13-11. Icare tonometer (Icare USA). (Reprinted with permission from Icare, all rights reserved.)

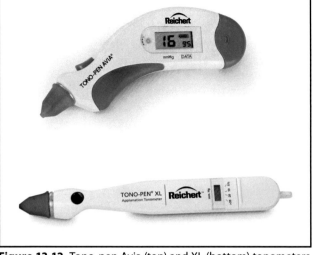

Figure 13-12. Tono-pen Avia (top) and XL (bottom) tonometers (Reichert Technologies). (Courtesy of Reichert Technologies, all rights reserved.)

▶ Activate the probe by hitting the measurement button once. "00" will appear on the display screen. Once activated the probe tip will be held in place.

▶ Adjust the forehead support so the device is aligned properly. The probe tip should be a "probe tip's" distance away from and perpendicular to the cornea.

▶ Ask the patient to look straight ahead. Press the measurement button. The tip should momentarily touch the central cornea.

▶ Six measurements are made consecutively. A quick "beep" will sound after each successful measurement.

▶ Once six measurements are obtained, the IOP reading will be displayed following a "P." If there is an error taking a reading, the device will "beep" twice and "error" will appear on the display screen.

Disinfection

Since disposable probes are used, there is no maintenance of the probes.

With use, dust particulates may collect in the base and affect movement of the probe, eliciting an error. The probe base can easily be taken out by unscrewing the catch and cleaned by injecting isopropyl alcohol with a syringe. Blow compressed air into the cavity until fully dry and reinsert the base back into the tonometer. The manufacturer recommends replacing the probe base on an annual basis.

The surface of the Icare can be wiped with a soft cloth moistened with a nonabrasive cleaner or a mixture of 70% alcohol in water. Make certain to dry the cleaned areas thoroughly with a soft cloth.

Tono-Pen

Many different versions of the Tono-pen (Reichert Ophthalmic Instruments) exist (Figure 13-12). They translate the mechanical deformation of the applanated cornea into an electrical signal, which is read by a transducer and extrapolated into a measure of the IOP. Depending on the device, up to 10 readings are taken and statistically compared. The mean IOP, as well as the standard deviation, are calculated. Some instruments require daily calibration prior to use, while others do not.

The Tono-pen is portable and easy to use on patients in any position. It requires minimal training and can be applied in a multitude of settings. The instrument tip covers (or tonocovers, dubbed Ocu-film by the manufacturer) provide protection against spread of disease. However, many studies conclude that the Tono-pen should only be used as a screening device (ie, not the only pressure method used when following patients with glaucoma) due to inconsistencies in its results.[12] It is sensitive to any corneal irregularities and not very accurate when testing in the very high or very low ranges.

Checking Calibration (Adapted from Tono-Pen XL User's Guide—Reichert Technologies)

▶ If required by device, perform daily prior to use, with a tip cover in place.

▶ Point the tip down toward the floor. Press the Operator's button twice very quickly.

▶ The Tono-pen will "beep." "Cal" should appear on display screen.

▶ Wait until the second "beep" sound and "Up" appears on display screen. Immediately invert the tip up toward the ceiling.

- If properly calibrated, "Good" will appear on display screen, followed by another "beep."

- If "Bad" appears on display screen, repeat steps for calibration.

- After "Good" is displayed, press the Operator's button once. The display screen will show "8888," then "----," then "====," followed by another "beep" tone, indicating that the instrument is ready for use.

Technique (Adapted from Tono-Pen XL User's Guide—Reichert Technologies)

- Explain the procedure to the patient.

- Administer anesthetic drops to the patient's eyes. Instruct the patient to focus on distant target, relax, and breathe normally.

- Ensure that a fresh tip cover is in place. Confirm that the patient does not have a latex allergy, as tip covers contain latex.

- While watching from the side of the patient, steady your hand on the patient's cheek and direct the tip perpendicularly to within 1/2 inch of the center of the patient's cornea. To begin measuring, press the Operator's button only once.

- "8888" will momentarily appear on display screen as a self-test. If "CAL" appears followed by "----," instrument requires calibration.

- If "====" appears followed by a "beep," begin measuring. Briefly touch then remove the tonometer tip from the corneal surface, without indenting the cornea. A "chirp" will sound when a valid IOP reading is obtained.

- After a given number of valid measurements are acquired, a final "beep" will sound. The average of the pressure readings will appear on the display screen.

- If more than 15 seconds pass without a valid measurement, the instrument will revert to pre-use status; press the Operator's button again (once) to reactivate.

- To check the opposite eye, press the Operator's button just once to reactivate device.

Maintenance

- When finished, remove the used tonocover and discard. Replace with a fresh cover before storing the instrument in its case.

- The instrument is now prepared for the next use.

The Tono-pen XL user manual recommends blowing optical quality compressed gas into the sensor end for 3 seconds to remove dust. The frequency of doing this depends on how much you use the instrument. Be aware that some commercial grade compressed dusters can leave a residue, which can be harmful to the instrument's lenses and sensors. For this reason, it is recommended to find an air duster that is filtered to eliminate any residue. One such brand is Ultrajet70 (Chemtronics). Allow the tonometer tip to return to room temperature after dusting, and calibrate the device prior to using.

Dynamic Contour Tonometry

The Dynamic Contour Tonometer (Pascal DCT; Ziemer Ophthalmic Systems AG) is designed to eliminate the errors inherent in measuring IOP caused by corneal rigidity or thickness. A microprocessor analyzes the force measurements and the ocular pulse amplitudes (OPA), which are the differences in IOP levels that occur during the systolic and diastolic heartbeats. The measurements (100 readings per second) are evaluated for quality and extrapolated into an IOP value. The DCT is attached to a retractable arm on a slit lamp, and testing is performed in much the same manner as Goldmann tonometry (Figure 13-13).

The DCT holds great promise as a technology of choice in measuring IOP. It accurately captures direct readings regardless of corneal contour. The device can be integrated for use on most slit lamps. However, obtaining measurements using DCT takes longer due to increased contact time as well as the need to repeat testing if the device detects any misalignment. It takes from 0.5 to 7.0 minutes to capture bilateral pressures with DCT in comparison to 0.5 to 3.0 minutes with GAT.[13] Another deterrent for the DCT is its price. This new technology is economically inhibiting for most general practices.

Technique (Adapted from Pascal User's Manual—Ziemer Ophthalmic Systems)

- The unit is self-calibrating.

- Place a single-use, sterile sensor cap firmly on the tonometer tip so there are no air bubbles.

- Anesthetize the cornea.

- With the patient at the slit lamp, ask him/her to look straight ahead. Advance the stage of the slit lamp holding back on joystick so the DCT comes close but does not yet make contact with the cornea. Make slight adjustments to best center on the cornea.

- Turn the unit on and slowly advance by moving the joystick until the tip makes contact with the cornea. Keep advancing until the lever arm is fully upright. (An alarm will sound if you advance too far.)

- Center the contact area in the middle of the back circle by using fine adjustments with the joystick. When properly placed, the IOP melody will sound.

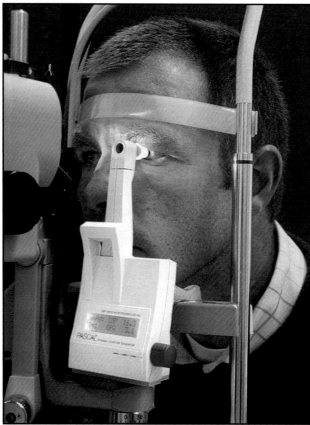

Figure 13-13. Pascal Dynamic Contour Tonometer (Ziemer Ophthalmic Systems). (Reprinted with permission from Ziemer Ophthalmic Systems, all rights reserved.)

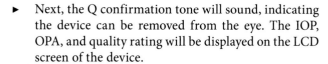

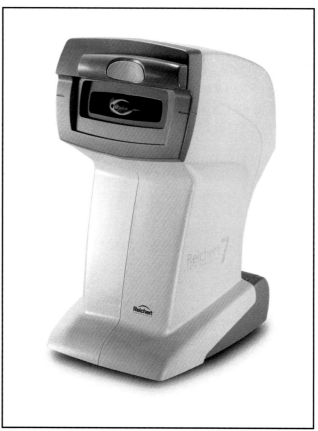

Figure 13-14. Air puff tonometer (Reichert Technologies). (Courtesy of Reichert Technologies, all rights reserved.)

▶ Next, the Q confirmation tone will sound, indicating the device can be removed from the eye. The IOP, OPA, and quality rating will be displayed on the LCD screen of the device.

Maintenance

The Pascal DCT virtually eliminates cross contamination between patients because it uses disposable covers. The device's body may occasionally be cleaned using a soft antibacterial wipe. The instrument will require periodic replacement of its 3-volt battery pack.

Noncontact Applanation Tonometry

Air Puff Tonometer

A widely used noncontact device is the "air puff." Usually an automated instrument, there are both table top and portable versions produced by multiple manufacturers (Figure 13-14). It employs infrared and photoelectric sensors to calculate the time it takes for a standardized pulse of air to flatten the cornea a specific amount. It takes a shorter amount of time to flatten a soft eye in comparison to a firmer one.

The air puff is a great screening device for health care settings in which contact tonometry may not be recommended or available. Its automated format allows for ease of use by personnel of various skill levels.

It is theorized that a fine aerosol is produced as the air puff disperses the tear film, possibly spreading viruses by an airborne route.[14] Studies regarding accuracy have found that air puff tonometers tend to read IOPs 2.7 to 3 mm Hg higher compared to GAT.[15] This may be due to a lack of the "ocular massage effect" seen with GAT. Multiple air puff readings can be performed without lowering the IOP. It is recommended to confirm suspicious measurements with GAT.

Technique (Adapted from Reichert 7 Air Puff Tonometer User's Guide—Reichert Technologies)

The air puff is factory calibrated. Since it does not come into contact with the cornea, the potential risk of a contact abrasion is eliminated, and there is no need for topical anesthesia.

▶ Seat the patient at instrument and explain the procedure. (Some instruments offer an optional "Demo" mode to demonstrate the air pulse to the patient.)

▶ Ask the patient to lean forward until his/her forehead is firmly against the headrest. (Some instruments will not operate unless "triggers" in the headrest are depressed.)

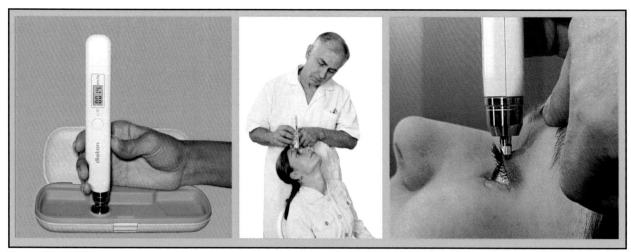

Figure 13-15. Diaton tonometer (BiCom, Inc). (Reprinted with permission from Diaton, BiCom, Inc, all rights reserved.)

▶ Press the "Measure" button or the icon on the display screen; a momentary pulse of air rebounds off of the patient's cornea.

▶ Repeat for the other eye. The measurements for both eyes will be displayed on the screen.

▶ Press the "Print" icon to print results. Otherwise, record the measurements in the patient's record, including the instrument used and the time of the test.

Disinfection

Air puff tonometers do not require special disinfection following testing other than using an alcohol swab or antibacterial cloth to wipe any surfaces that actually come into contact with the patient. Compressed air may be used to remove dust that collects near the air housing unit. Using a pipe cleaner followed by several "Demo" mode air pulses will remove debris from the air port itself.

Diaton

Another noncontact instrument is the Diaton (BiCom, Inc). This hand-held, pen-like device takes IOP measurements transpalpebrally, or through the eyelid (Figure 13-15). Even though it touches the eyelid, it is considered noncontact because it does not directly touch the cornea. The Diaton works on the "ballistic principle" of tonometry, which is similar to indentation. The elasticity of the eye is measured when a free-falling center rod with a standard weight contacts the eyelid.

The Diaton can be used on eyes with compromised corneas. Anesthetic is not required, so it is well tolerated by children. It can be performed with the patient sitting or lying down. There is minimal risk of disease transmission, and the components can be disassembled for cleaning with a cloth moistened with ethyl alcohol.

A study comparing the Diaton with GAT, however, indicated a discrepancy between the measured outcomes.[16] Accurate readings require precise placement

of the tip on the correct eyelid location. Being slightly misaligned will result in erroneous readings.

Calibration (Diaton Operational Manual—BiCom, Inc)

▶ The device should be calibrated once per day using the test plate in its storage case.

▶ With the tip facing down, see whether the free-falling center rod is present in the tip area. If so, quickly face the tip up so the rod catches inside of the tonometer and is not seen in the tip area.

▶ Return to tip down position, holding the device in proper vertical position.

▶ Press the "on" button and rest the device on the test plate. An indicator signal will sound when the reading is taken. ±2 mm of 20 mm should appear on LCD screen, meaning proper calibration.

Technique (Adapted from Diaton Operational Manual—BiCom, Inc)

▶ Prepare the tonometer prior to each measurement by "catching" the rod inside of the device.

▶ Four zeroes, "0000," will be displayed on the LCD screen when the "operation" button is pressed.

▶ An interrupted signal will sound any time the device is not held in the proper vertical testing position (measurements can only be taken in the correct vertical position).

▶ The patient can sit or recline with both eyes open, and fix on an object at a 45° angle.

▶ The upper eyelid margin should fall just above the superior corneal limbus (tester can hold the eyelid in the proper position).

▶ Stabilize the hand by resting it on the patient's forehead; lower the device onto the ciliary edge of the eyelid margin, just behind (and not touching) the

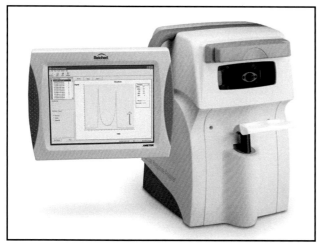

Figure 13-16. Ocular Response Analyzer (Reichert Technologies). (Courtesy of Reichert Technologies, all rights reserved.)

lashes. Take care not to apply any pressure to the globe.

▶ A short signal will sound as the rod falls, hitting the eyelid.

▶ Repeat tipping the tonometer up to catch the rod and repeat measurements until two long signals play, indicating the device has enough information to provide average.

▶ Press the "operation" button to see results.
  • An "A" with a number constantly displayed is an accurate reading
  • An "A" with a number that is pulsing is an approximate reading
  • An "A" with two zeroes means errors occurred in measuring

Cleaning and Disinfecting

Although the Diaton does not come into direct contact with the eye, the rod mechanism should be cleaned between patients.

▶ Disassemble the rod mechanism by holding it with the tip down, removing the cap, and then removing the tip with gentle force.

▶ With the screwdriver provided, loosen the brush and remove it as well as the rod.

▶ Wipe all parts with a cloth moistened with ethyl alcohol and place on a clean towel to dry.

▶ Reassemble the device and check to make sure it is functioning properly by following the directions as if preparing to take a measurement.

Ocular Response Analyzer 8

Corneal hysteresis (CH) is the ability of the cornea to absorb and dissipate energy. Studies suggest that CH may be a better indicator of the biomechanical properties of the cornea than CCT. These properties include the curvature, elasticity, and surface tension of the tissue. Cumulatively they influence the cornea's deformability, or how altering the corneal shape influences the results of the applanation process. The Ocular Response Analyzer 8 (ORA; Reichert Ophthalmic Instruments; Figure 13-16) factors in the variables of CH into its calculations.

The ORA uses force-displacement to determine the IOP. It emits a noncontact pulse of air, which pushes the cornea in past the usual depth achieved by applanation, until it becomes slightly concave. Once the air pulse ends, the cornea rebounds to its original convex shape, all in a matter of 20 ms. An electro-optical detection system captures both of these readings. The difference between these readings is the CH. These numbers are averaged and converted to a Goldmann equivalent value for the IOP.

Technique (Adapted from Ocular Response Analyzer User's Guide—Reichert Technologies)

▶ The ORA is factory calibrated.

▶ Enter/retrieve the patient's data from the Patient Selection window.

▶ Click the "Measure" icon.

▶ Loosen collars or ties, remove contact lenses. Explain there will be a gentle puff of air. (The device has a demonstration mode so you can direct a sample pulse of air against the patient's hand.)

▶ Seat the patient comfortably. The patient should lean forward with the forehead firmly against the headrest. The patient's nose and chin should almost touch the instrument. Slide the headrest fully to the right or left to properly align the eyes. The patient's eye should be level with the canthus marking on the side of the device. When properly aligned, the patient will focus on a green LED light in the center of the air tube.

▶ Instruct the patient to blink several times and then hold fixation.

▶ Click the "Measure Response" button. The results will appear in the Right or Left Eye "Data Window."

▶ Be cognizant of the "Waveform Score" (WS); the higher the WS number, the more accurate the measurement.

- ▶ Displayed information:
  - IOPcc: Corneal-compensated IOP
  - IOPg: Goldmann correlated IOP value
  - CRF: Corneal resistance factor
  - CH: Corneal hysteresis

Maintenance

Any areas that contact the patient's face may be wiped clean with an alcohol swab. The air tube may become clogged with dust, causing poor transmission of the air pulse as well as the green fixation light. A pipe cleaner can be inserted into the air hose to remove debris, followed by a few air pulses in the machine's Demo mode.

Sources of Error

There are a number of things that can influence the accuracy of tonometry measurements. Most are easily remedied if recognized. Technicians should be familiar with their impact on IOPs and try to avoid them. Table 13-1 addresses additional situations that may affect IOP readings. (Most of these apply to Goldmann tonometry, but some are pertinent to any method.)

Potential Risks

Any method of tonometry should be avoided in all cases of full-thickness corneal ulcer or orbital trauma, especially where rupture of the globe may have occurred. Whenever in doubt about checking the pressure, always ask your physician first.

Care must also be exercised when taking IOP on an infected eye, as this may facilitate the spread of the infection to the opposite eye or even to other patients.

Another potential risk is causing a corneal abrasion. Although tonometer tips are rounded, occasionally too much pressure may be applied by a novice assistant. Or a nervous patient may move excessively or squeeze his/her eyes during testing. More commonly, the patient rubs the eyes too zealously and scratches the corneal surface while drying the anesthetic drops. Take a minute to stress the importance of keeping the eyes closed while gently dabbing the corners.

Occasionally patients will react to the anesthetic drops, eyes immediately turning red, with a burning sensation and swollen lids. Previous reactions to topical anesthetics such as tetracaine or proparacaine should be documented in the patient's chart. Adverse side effects of any preservatives should also be noted, as these may be present in various eye drops.

Vasovagal Reaction

The vasovagal nerve has multiple branches, and occasionally stimulation in one area will cause a reaction in another. For example, inserting a contact lens might trigger nausea and fainting. Techs need to recognize if the patient is displaying signs of such an episode. The patient usually becomes very quiet and may suddenly feel unwell, with nausea and/or a wave of warmth. The patient may look pale or gray, and may also be sweating and clammy. AOP must remain calm and initiate first aid intervention.

First, immediately STOP trying to take the pressure. Calmly ask the patient if he/she is all right. Move any equipment out of the way. Either have the patient lower his/her head or recline the exam chair backward to bring the head at or below the level of the heart. Call for assistance, but do NOT leave the patient unattended. Remind the patient to take slow, cleansing breaths. If available, apply a cool compress to the forehead.

The patient's eyes may roll back, and he/she may lose consciousness. To prevent injury, try to assist him/her to a safe resting position until the episode passes. Vasovagal reactions usually last for less than a minute, with a full recovery. Be careful of a second reaction when the patient stands up. The blood pressure and pulse should be within a normal range before allowing the patient to leave. Finally, document this reaction in the chart for future reference.

Cleaning/Special Care of Instruments

Tonometers, for the most part, require very little maintenance. Information regarding care of specific instruments has been included in the section about each tonometer. Some general notations are pertinent.

The external casing may be wiped free of debris with a damp cloth, alcohol swab, or disinfectant wipe. A can of residue-free compressed air may be used to remove dust from lenses or sensors. Over time, batteries and fuses in some instruments may need to be replaced. To avoid injury, always turn off electrical devices and unplug them prior to replacing fuses. Many of the devices use disposable covers, tips, or prisms, which are thrown away after use. Keep a back-up supply of all these items. An instrument should be covered when not in use.

Using disposable tonometer tips or protective covers when possible is highly recommended. Tonosafe disposable prisms (Haag-Streit USA) were found to be equally accurate in measuring IOP when compared with conventional Goldmann prisms.[17] Otherwise, care must be taken to practice appropriate infection control and properly disinfect surfaces that come into contact with patients. Some cleaning products, though, may be too strong and cause damage to certain materials. The Food and Drug Administration requires equipment manufacturers to include approved cleaning/disinfection protocols in their user's guides. Consulting the owner's manual should provide detailed recommendations of proper methods to clean instruments. Unaccepted practices can potentially void a warranty or even ruin a very expensive piece of equipment.

	TABLE 13-1	
FACTORS THAT MAY AFFECT INTRAOCULAR PRESSURE		
Factor	**Effect**	**Remedy**
Amount of fluorescein dye in eye (Goldmann/Perkins)	To much: Mires will be thick, making it difficult to determine an accurate endpoint	Remove excess dye with tissue from lower fornix of patient's eye; wipe tonometer tip dry of surplus dye
	Too little: Mires will be thin, making an accurate endpoint difficult to achieve	Ask patient to blink several times to disperse dye; instill more dye
Mires not in center of cornea (Goldmann/Perkins)	If the Goldmann prism is not aligned properly (displaced up, down, nasal, or temporally), an accurate endpoint cannot be achieved	Back tonometer tip off of corneal surface and realign so tip will rest centrally on cornea
	Sometimes the mires will pulse in rhythm with the patient's heartbeat, contributing to fleeting, misaligned mires	Ask patient to take a few deep, cleansing breaths and confirm his/her chin and forehead are firmly resting in device
	Patients may back away from the device, affecting good contact with the tonometer tip	Confirm patient is resting his/her chin and forehead properly in device
Eyelid touches tonometer tip	Direct contact from the eyelids can thicken the mires	Ask patient to widely open his/her eyes
Patient squeezing eyes/pressure on globe from technician's fingers (artificially raising IOP)	Patients often reflexively squeeze their eyes shut during tonometry, anticipating pain	Try to reassure patient and encourage him/her to open widely on his/her own
	Technicians may inadvertently apply pressure to the globe when helping to hold the patient's eyelids open	Assist the patient to open his/her eyes wider by gently spreading the upper and lower eyelids apart using your index and middle fingers Make certain to rest your fingers on the bony orbit, not on the eyeball itself, to avoid raising the IOP
Patient holding breath/patient wearing tight tie or shirt collar (artificially raising IOP)	Patient reflexively performs Valsalva maneuver or holds breath as a nervous defense mechanism to avoid anticipated pain	Remind patient to take slow, cleansing breaths
	Tight shirt collar or tie inhibits blood flow to brain	Reassure patient and ask him/her to loosen the collar
High corneal astigmatism (Goldmann/Perkins)	Corneal astigmatism greater than 3 diopters creates an elliptical pattern of flattening instead of the usual circular shape	Align the tonoprism with the red line on the tonometer to correspond with the axis of the patient's astigmatism (in minus cylinder)

Reichert recommends the chin and forehead rests of their devices be wiped clean with a cloth and a mild detergent solution (1 cc of liquid dish soap to 1 L of clean, filtered water) between patients. If these areas need to be sanitized, a mixture of 1 part bleach to 10 parts water may be used. Other manufacturers suggest using an alcohol swab. Alcohol, however, can be too harsh if head positioning sensors are present on the instrument. An alternative is to use a medical-grade antibacterial wipe. The owner's manual, sales representative, or the Centers for Disease Control and Prevention's guidelines are the best resources to find the appropriate cleaning method for your particular instrument.

PATIENT SERVICES

An elevated pressure during a routine exam may be a red flag for glaucoma. AOP will be called upon to perform the testing necessary to confirm a diagnosis. Tonometry, along with other investigative tools such as OCT, formal visual fields, and corneal pachymetry, each contribute a piece of the puzzle to help determine if glaucoma is present.

Congenital or infantile onset glaucoma is a fairly rare diagnosis. It usually is not necessary to traumatize a child under age 12 by the addition of yet another eye drop to check the IOP during a routine assessment. Forcing the issue may risk losing his/her cooperation in completing the rest of the exam. Use judgment based upon the individual maturity level of the child as well as risk factors, such as family history or a previous diagnosis. A more thorough exam under anesthesia may be necessary for children who are uncooperative yet at high risk.

Physicians may recommend patients return for pressure checks at different times of the day as IOP tends to fluctuate. In certain situations, tests that study the IOP over time, called diurnal or 24-hour IOP studies, may be suggested. The purpose is to detect patterns of IOP fluctuation during the course of a day and night. The patterns can help in selecting an eye drop that may be more effective in lowering the pressure during high peaks. Such a study also gathers information about a patient's potential risk as well as a target range for maintenance of IOPs.

Usually Goldmann tonometers, as well as noncontact devices, are used for diurnal studies when the patient is upright and a Tono-pen when the patient is recumbent.[18] Consistency in performing this test requires using the same device at the same time of day each time in order to determine trends in IOP fluctuations.

Continuous IOP monitoring is being done in research settings and eliminates errors inherent in corneal contact methods. One method uses a pressure sensor either attached to an intraocular lens or directly injected into the vitreous. The transmitted frequency of the sensor is remotely monitored with an external receiver. A less invasive method currently utilized in research uses a silicone contact lens called Triggerfish (Sensimed). It transmits wireless data from an embedded microprocessor and antenna in the contact lens. It collects 144 measurements over a 24-hour period and has contributed to changes in treatment strategy. The data collected is accurate and reproducible, but the electrical signal does not directly correspond to a measurement in mm Hg.

ACKNOWLEDGMENTS

The author would like to thank the following: Barbara Cassin, MEd, CO, COMT (deceased); Diana Shamis, MEd, CO, COMT; Ella Rosamont-Morgan, COMT (deceased); and Dave Taylor, Senior Manager, Medical Marketing at Reichert, Inc.

CHAPTER QUIZ

1. The unit of measurement for intraocular pressure is:
   a. millimeters of tension
   b. millimeters of resistance
   c. millimeters of pressure
   d. millimeters of mercury

2. Accuracy of tonometry results are affected by:
   a. vitreous floaters
   b. level of AOP certification
   c. corneal thickness
   d. ciliary body contraction

3. The applanation method of tonometry flattens a small area of the central cornea measuring:
   a. 3.06 mm
   b. 5.0 mm
   c. 10 mm
   d. 6.0 mm

4. All are advantages of Schiötz tonometry except:
   a. scleral rigidity
   b. portable
   c. low cost
   d. no power source needed

5. Applanation tonometry is based on which law of physics?
   a. Murphy's law
   b. Imbert-Flick law
   c. Ohm's law
   d. Boyle's law

6. If the Goldmann tonometer is found to be out of calibration:
   a. call a repairperson to come calibrate it
   b. calibrate the unit by manipulating the weighted calibration bar
   c. continue to use the unit until a new calibration obtained
   d. return the unit to manufacturer for repair

7. All are factors that can alter intraocular pressure readings except:
   a. patient holding his/her breath
   b. patient opens the eyes too wide
   c. patient's collar is too tight
   d. examiner presses on the globe

8. All may use an alcohol prep for disinfecting the tonometer except:
   a. Schiötz
   b. Icare
   c. Goldmann prism
   d. Diaton

9. All are examples of hand-held tonometers except:
   a. Dynamic Contour/Pascal
   b. Tono-pen
   c. Schiötz
   d. Icare

10. The lines on the Goldmann tonometer calibration bar correspond to which numbers on the tension drum?

    a. 0, 10, 50
    b. 0, 20, 60
    c. 0, 20, 50
    d. 0, 10, 60

Answers

1. d, Millimeters of mercury, the same unit used in weather barometers, which measure barometric pressure.

2. c, Corneal thickness. It has been discovered that the thickness of the cornea can influence the accuracy of tonometry measurements.

3. a, 3.06 mm is the area found by Hans Goldmann which best cancelled out opposing forces during Goldmann applanation tonometry.

4. a, Scleral rigidity, or the displacement of aqueous due to indentation, can affect the accuracy of Schiötz tonometry.

5. b, The Imbert-Flick law, which states that the pressure within a sphere is equal to the force required to flatten its surface divided by the area of flattening.

6. d, Return the unit to the manufacturer for repair. Only the manufacturer is able to properly correct calibration.

7. b, Patient opens eye too wide. All of the other scenarios can artificially elevate the intraocular pressure.

8. c, Goldmann prisms can be damaged by alcohol.

9. a, The Dynamic Contour/Pascal device is mounted on a slit lamp.

10. b, The Goldmann calibration weight bar is intended to test at the 0, 20, and 60 mm Hg markings on the tension drum.

6. Karmel M. The "new" pressure for glaucoma specialists: ocular perfusion arrives. *EyeNet Magazine.* 2001; January:29-30. www.aao.org/eyenet/article/new-pressure-glaucoma-specialists-ocular-perfusion?jan-2011. Accessed July 3, 2016.

7. Friedman C, Petersen KH. *Infection Control in Ambulatory Care.* Burlington, MA: Jones & Bartlett Learning; 2004:110.

8. How to disinfect? Haag-Streit website. www.haag-streit.com/fileadmin/Haag-Streit_USA/Diagnostics/tonometry/download/disinfect.pdf. Accessed July 3, 2016.

9. Wozniak K, Köller AU, Spörl E, et al. Intraocular pressure measurement during the day and night for glaucoma patients and normal controls using Goldmann and Perkins applanation tonometry. *Ophthalmologe.* 2006;(103):1027-1031.

10. Ramakrishnan R, Krishnadas SR, Robin AL, Khurana M. *Diagnosis and Management of Glaucoma.* New Delhi, India: Jaypee Brothers Medical Publishers; 2013:121.

11. Marini M, Da Pozzo S, Accardo A, Canziani T. Comparing applanation tonometry and rebound tonometry in glaucomatous and ocular hypertensive eyes. *Eur J Ophthalmol.* 2010;21(3)258-263.

12. Stephenson M. Can you trust your IOP readings? Review of Ophthalmology website. http://www.reviewofophthalmology.com/issue/june-2011. June 13, 2011. Accessed July 3, 2016.

13. Anderson MF, Aqius-Fernandez A, Kaye SB. Comparison of the utility of Pascal dynamic contour tonometry with Goldmann applanation tonometry in routine clinical practice. National Center for Biotechnology Information. US National Library of Medicine website. www.ncbi.nlm.nih.gov/pubmed/22407393. June-July 2013. Accessed July 3, 2016.

14. Farhood QK. Comparative evaluation of intraocular pressure with an air-puff tonometer versus a Goldmann applanation tonometer. *Clin Ophthalmol.* 2013;7:23-27. www.ncbi.nlm.nih.gov/pmc/articles/PMC3534293/. Accessed July 2, 2016.

15. Blum K. Taking IOP measure beyond Goldmann. *Ophthalmology Management.* 2013;17:42-44. www.ophthalmologymanagement.com/articleviewer.aspx?articleID=107871. Accessed July 3, 2016.

16. Doherty MD, Carrim CI, O'Neill DP. Diaton tonometry: an assessment of validity and preference against Goldmann tonometry. National Center for Biotechnology Information. US National Library of Medicine website. www.ncbi.nlm.nih.gov/pubmed/21718408. May-June 2012. Accessed July 3, 2016.

17. Thomas V, Daly MK, Cakiner-Egilmez T, Baker E. Reliability of Tonosafe disposable tonometer prisms: clinical implications from the Veterans Affairs Boston Healthcare System quality assurance study. *J Eye.* 2011;25:651-656.

18. Mansouri K, Weinreb R. Continuous 24-hour intraocular pressure monitoring for glaucoma—time for a paradigm change. National Center for Biotechnology Information. US National Library of Medicine website. www.ncbi.nlm.nih.gov/pubmed/22457163. March 28, 2012. Accessed July 3, 2016.

REFERENCES

1. Kingman S. Glaucoma is second leading cause of blindness globally. World Health Organization website. www.who.int/bulletin/volumes/82/11/feature1104/en/. Accessed January 18, 2016.

2. Stamper RL. A history of intraocular pressure and its measurement. *Optom Vis Sci.* 2010;88(1):E16-E28. doi:10.1097/OPX.0b013e318205a4e7.

3. The importance of corneal thickness. Glaucoma.org website. www.glaucoma.org/glaucoma/the-importance-of-corneal-thickness.php. Last reviewed April 03, 2011. Accessed July 3, 2016.

4. Kniestedt C, Punjabi O, Lin S, Stamper RL. Tonometry through the ages. *Survey of Ophthalmology.* 2008;53(6);585. www.ncbi.nlm.nih.gov/pubmed/19026320. Accessed July 3, 2016.

5. New eye layer has possible link to glaucoma. Medical News Today website. www.medicalnewstoday.com/releases/272640.php. February 17, 2014. Accessed July 3, 2016.

BIBLIOGRAPHY

Akram A, Yaqub A, Jamal A, Fiaz D. Pitfalls in intraocular pressure measurement by Goldmann-type applanation tonometers. *Pak J Ophthalmol.* 2009;25(4). www.pjo.com.pk/25/4/Index-9.pdf. Accessed July 3, 2016.

Childhood glaucoma: facts, answers, tips and resources for children with glaucoma and their families. Glaucoma.org website. www.glaucoma.org/uploads/grf_childhood_glaucoma.pdf. Accessed July 3, 2016.

Eisenberg D. Reconsidering the gold standard of tonometry. Glaucoma Today website. http://bmctoday.net/glaucomatoday/2011/03/article.asp?f=reconsidering-the-gold-standard-of-tonometry. March 2011. Accessed July 3, 2016.

Farhood QK. Comparative evaluation of intraocular pressure with an air-puff tonometer versus a Goldmann applanation tonometer [abstract taken from National Center for Biotechnology Information. US National Library of Medicine website. http://www.ncbi.nlm.nih.gov/pmc/articles/PMC3534293/. Accessed July 3, 2016.] *Clin Ophthalmol.* 2013;7:23-27.

Frenkel REP, Frenkel MPC, Haji SA. Continuous monitoring of intraocular pressure. In: Schacknow PN, Samples JR, eds. *The Glaucoma Book.* New York, NY: Springer; 2010:59.

Glaucoma facts and statistics. Glaucoma.org website. www.glaucoma.org/gleams/high-eye-pressure-and-glaucoma.php. Last reviewed May 3, 2016. Accessed July 3, 2016.

Guideline for disinfection and sterilization in healthcare facilities, 2008. CDC website. www.cdc.gov/hicpac/Disinfection_Sterilization/3_1deLaparoArthro.html. Updated December 29, 2009. Accessed July 3, 2016.

Karmel M. New tonometry: the search for true IOP. EyeNet Magazine. American Academy of Ophthalmology website. www.aao.org/eyenet/article/new-tonometry-search-true-iop. May 2005. Accessed July 3, 2016.

Kirstein EM, Elsheikh A, Gunvant P. Tonometry—past, present and future. In: Gunvant P, ed. Glaucoma—Current Clinical and Research Aspects. InTech website. http://cdn.intechweb.org/pdfs/22969.pdf. Accessed July 3, 2016.

Malihi M, Sit AJ. Effect of head and body position on intraocular pressure. National Center for Biotechnology Information. US National Library of Medicine website. www.ncbi.nlm.nih.gov/pubmed/22341914. May 2012. Accessed July 3, 2016.

Mottet B, Aptel F, Romanet JP, Hubanova R, Pépin JL, Chiquet C. 24-Hour intraocular pressure rhythm in young healthy subjects evaluated with continuous monitoring using a contact lens sensor. JAMA Network website. http://archopht.jamanetwork.com/article.aspx?articleid=1761562. December 2013. Accessed July 3, 2016.

Stevens S. How to measure intraocular pressure: Schiötz tonometry. *Community Eye Health Journal.* 2008;21(66):34. www.ncbi.nlm.nih.gov/pmc/articles/PMC2467471/. Accessed July 3, 2016.

The importance of corneal thickness. Glaucoma.org website. www.glaucoma.org/glaucoma/the-importance-of-corneal-thickness.php. Last reviewed April 03, 2011. Accessed July 3, 2016.

Unless otherwise noted, the figures in this chapter were contributed by the following, who are associated with this book as authors:

Jan Ledford: Figure 13-7

Gayle Roberts: Figures 13-4, 13-5, 13-8

14

VISUAL FIELDS

Gayle Roberts, COMT, BHS

BASIC SCIENCES

Definitions

Perimetry (*visual field testing*) is the diagnostic technique used to establish and quantify the parameters of a patient's central and peripheral vision. The central field provides images for fine detail, color, and the ability to read. The peripheral field supplies information regarding spatial relations and helps us navigate through our environment. Certain drugs and medical conditions can impact the visual field, making perimetry a valuable tool in discovering and evaluating such problems. The science of the visual field has a language all its own (Table 14-1).

Anatomy of the Visual Pathway

Ocular anatomy is covered in Chapter 2. Please reference that material as needed.

The perception of sight begins when light that is reflected off an object stimulates nerve impulses in the retina. These impulses then travel posteriorly along the *visual pathway* (Figure 14-1). This pathway runs from the eye to the visual cortex of the brain in the occipital lobe, where the input is interpreted. There are four regions in the pathway. The first is the ganglion cells and the nerve

fiber layer (NFL). The optic nerve (ON) comprises the second. The third region encompasses the optic chiasm. The final area contains the optic tracts, lateral geniculate bodies, optic radiations, and the visual cortex. Each region will be described further in a moment.

To initiate the process of "seeing," an image must first pass through the refractive surfaces of the eye and focus on the *photoreceptor cells* (rods and cones) of the retina. This triggers an electrical impulse that stimulates the afferent sensory visual pathway, that part of the nervous system that carries sensory information toward the brain.

Each cone in the macula is paired with one *bipolar cell*, which then connects with one *ganglion cell*. This one-to-one coupling accounts for the high visual sensitivity of this area.

In contrast, in the peripheral retina many rods and cones (what few there are) synapse with each bipolar cell. Then, multiple bipolar cells synapse with each ganglion cell, diluting the photoreceptor input to the optic nerve, making it less sensitive. The lack of photoreceptors at the optic nerve explains why there is a physiologic blind spot, or nonseeing area, in the visual field.

The macular ganglion cell axons (nerve cell extensions) make up the *retinal nerve fiber layer* (Figure 14-2). These fibers form distinct areas of the retina (Figure 14-3). In the center is the *papillomacular bundle*, which

Ledford JK, Lens A, eds.
Principles and Practice in Ophthalmic Assisting:
A Comprehensive Textbook (pp 253-274).
© 2018 Taylor & Francis Group.

TABLE 14-1	
GLOSSARY OF VISUAL FIELD TERMS	
Absolute defect	Area where no target is seen no matter how bright or large
Afferent	Sensory nerve input carried to the brain
Amsler grid	Visual field test that evaluates the central 10° of field
Apostilb	Old European unit of light intensity
Arcuate	Arch-shaped visual field defect commonly seen in glaucoma affecting the retinal nerve fiber layer
Blindspot	Area of nonvision within the visual field
Cecocentral	A blind spot that extends from the optic disc to the macula, same as papillomacular
Confrontational	Visual field test in which the patient fixates on the examiner's eye while detecting the number of fingers in the periphery
Congruous	Visual field defects that are very much the same in each eye
Contralateral	Refers to the opposite side
Hemianopsia	Area of nonseeing in one half of the visual field
Heteronymous	Defect located on opposite sides of the patient's visual field
Homonymous	Defect located on the same half of the patient's visual field
Incongruous	Visual field defects that are different in each eye
Ipsilateral	Refers to the same side
Isopter	The line connecting points of the same light intensity seen on a visual field
Junctional	Chiasmal defect affecting the optic nerve of one eye and the inferior nasal fibers of the other
Kinetic	Refers to a moving target
Lumen	Unit of measurement indicating the amount of emitted light
Meridian	Straight, imaginary lines running through the macula like the spokes of a bicycle wheel
Metamorphopsia	Distorted vision (especially as seen on an Amsler grid)
Nasal step	Damage to the temporal retinal nerve fiber layer, which represents the horizontal median in one quadrant of the visual field
Papillomacular	Refers to retinal nerve fibers extending from the macula to the optic nerve (same as cecocentral)
Paracentral	Nonseeing area lying within 20° of fixation (does not involve central 5° of field)
Perimetrist	Person trained to perform visual fields
Perimetry	The process of quantifying a patient's central and peripheral visual field
Quadrantanopisa	Visual field defect affecting one-fourth of the field in one or both eyes
Relative defect	Area of reduced sensitivity in visual field that does not appreciate small, dim targets but can detect brighter, larger ones
Scotoma	An area of nonseeing
Static	Refers to a nonmoving target
Threshold	Smallest, dimmest target light the patient can detect at any one point
Visual cortex	Area in the occipital lobe that processes visual input

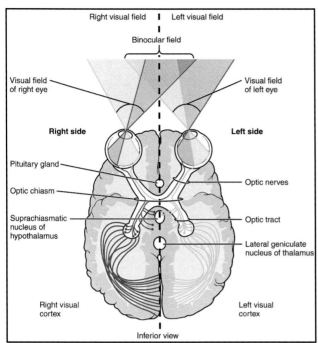

Figure 14-1. Visual pathway. (Reprinted with permission from *Anatomy and Physiology*. Download for free at http://cnx.org/contents/FPtK1zmh@6.27:KcreJ7oj@5/Central-Processing.)

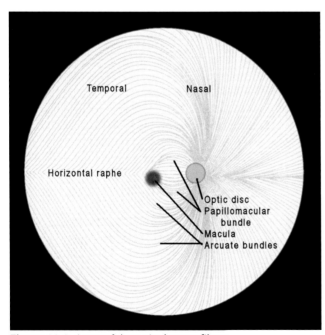

Figure 14-3. Areas of the retinal nerve fibers.

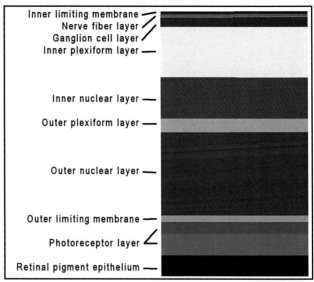

Figure 14-2. The retinal photoreceptor layer.

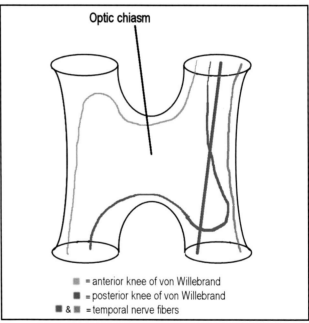

Figure 14-4. Depiction of the chiasm showing von Willebrand's knee.

includes the macula and extends to the optic nerve head. The second area of interest is temporal to the macula. It is composed of superior and inferior nerve fibers that meet at but do not cross the *horizontal raphe* (known as *respecting* the horizontal). The final area is nasal to the optic nerve. These nerve fibers fan out peripherally from the disc as *arcuate bundles*.

The *nerve fiber bundles*, composed of both nasal and temporal nerve fibers, come together at the optic disc, creating the *optic nerve*. Each optic nerve travels posteriorly through the *optic foramen* (opening) in the skull to a "crossroads" called the *optic chiasm*, located above the pituitary gland. It is at this location where most of the nasal fibers cross to the opposite side. Some of inferior nasal fibers, however, backtrack slightly anteriorly, creating what is known as *von Willebrand's knee* (Figure 14-4). The knee is comprised of the nasal and temporal nerve fibers of one eye along with the somewhat misdirected inferior nasal fibers of the opposite eye.

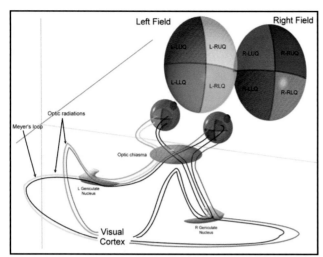

Figure 14-5. Visual pathway showing four quadrants of the visual field. (Reprinted with permission from Ratznium, Wikipedia, http://commons.wikimedia.org/wiki/File:ERP_-_optic_cabling.jpg.)

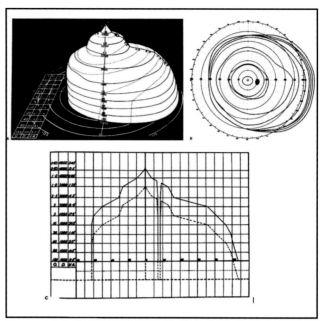

Figure 14-6. Traquair's "island of vision." (Reprinted with permission from Scott GI. *Traquair's Clinical Perimetry*. 7th ed. London, England: Henry Kimpton; 1957.)

Beyond the chiasm, the ipsilateral (same side) temporal fibers along with the contralateral (opposite side) nasal fibers continue posteriorly as the *optic tract* (one on each side). Near the midbrain, the pupillary fibers (which have been traveling with the visual fibers) leave the pathway and enter the brainstem. The visual fibers continue on to pass the neurologic impulse to the next neuron in the pathway, at the *lateral body*. The axons now form the *optic radiations*. As the name suggests, the optic radiations spread out. The inferior retinal fibers pass through the temporal lobe in an area known as *Meyer's loop*. The superior retinal fibers travel a more direct route through the parietal lobe, posteriorly until they end at the *calcarine fissure* in the occipital lobe in the part of the *visual* (or *striate*) *cortex* known as *Brodmann's area #17*.

Peripheral vision can be represented as a topographical map of the visual space perceived by the patient. Each point of the retinal nerve fiber layer can be paired with a point on a plotted visual field. The map can be divided into four quadrants: superior nasal, inferior nasal, superior temporal, and inferior temporal (Figure 14-5). Because the eye is round, each quadrant in the eye receives stimulus from opposite space. The superior nasal retina appreciates images from inferior temporal space, inferior nasal retina from superior temporal space, superior temporal retina from inferior nasal space, and inferior temporal retina from superior nasal space. Despite our brains compensating for this phenomenon, the orientation of where these points originate is key in understanding how a visual field test may be used as a diagnostic tool.

CLINICAL KNOWLEDGE
The Visual Field as an "Island of Vision"

Harry Moss Traquair first coined the analogy of "an island or hill of vision in a sea of darkness" to describe peripheral vision (Figure 14-6).[1] The perimeter of the island, or its shoreline, is the extent to which objects can be visualized. Objects beyond the shore cannot be seen. The high point of the island corresponds to the macula, or area of highest sensitivity for central fixation. As the island's terrain slopes away from the summit, it gently falls off, equating to lesser degrees of visual awareness. If the shoreline wears away, the island becomes smaller; this corresponds to a constriction of the peripheral vision. Parts of the island may erode along its equator or central axis/pole, leaving only portions intact, as if slices of a pie have been removed. "Sinkholes," or *scotomas*, may also exist, creating pits with decreased visual perception. The occasional "bottomless pit," or *absolute defect*, might also be found, an area where there is no visual perception at all.

The topography of the island extends from the central point 60 degrees (°) superiorly, 60° nasally, 75° inferiorly, and 100° temporally (Figure 14-7). Falling 15° temporal to fixation is a void measuring about 5° wide and 10° high. This is the *physiologic blind spot*. It denotes the landmark where the nerve fiber layer forms the optic nerve head. Since it lacks photoreceptor cells, vision is not detected within its limits.

Correlation of Visual Field Defects to the Visual Pathway

Lesions along the visual pathway can produce characteristic defects in the visual field based on which of the four regions they occur in (Figure 14-8). "Plotting a visual field" (*perimetry*) is like putting the pieces of a puzzle together to help identify the location and origin of such lesions. The more anterior (closer to the retina) a lesion is along the visual pathway, the less *congruous* (similar) the visual field defect in one eye will be to the other. The further posterior (closer to the visual cortex) the lesion, the more congruous the fields will appear.

Region I consists of the retina. Visual field defects found here are caused by conditions affecting the photoreceptor cells and are nonspecific. The defects often correspond to retinal damage that is visible during fundus examination, such as retinal detachment, choroidal tumors, or macular degeneration. If the macular area is involved, a central scotoma, or lack of perception of the stimulus in the central field, may occur (Figure 14-9). A slightly peripheral, ring-shaped scotoma is characteristic of the degenerative disease retinitis pigmentosa (Figure 14-10).

Region II involves the retinal nerve fiber layer and the optic nerve as it traverses back to the optic chiasm. Defects in Region II are commonly attributed to optic nerve diseases, including glaucoma (see Chapter 29, Glaucoma).

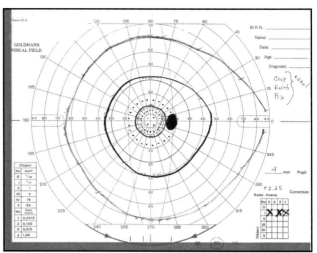

Figure 14-7. Normal parameters of the visual field as mapped on a Goldmann perimeter. The black oval just right of center is the physiologic blind spot.

Damage to the papillomacular bundle area of the RNFL may produce scotomas affecting central fixation (Figure 14-11). Also referred to as *centrocecal/cecocentral* scotomas, they generate field loss extending from the macula to the blind spot.

Arcuate scotomas occur when the arching superior and inferior temporal nerve fibers surrounding the papillomacular bundle are damaged (Figure 14-12A). These fibers do not cross the midline, thus respecting

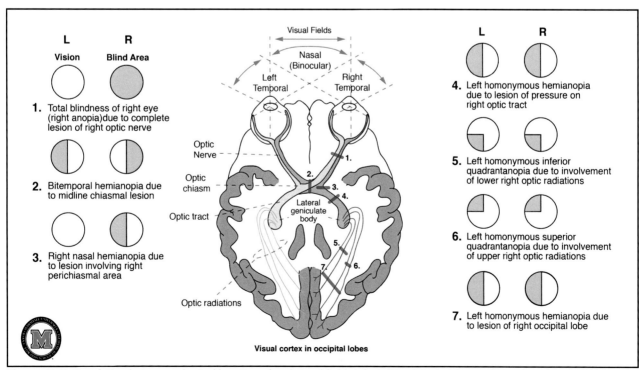

Figure 14-8. Correlation between physical location of and visual field defect. (Reprinted with permission from Marshall University Joan C. Edwards School of Medicine.)

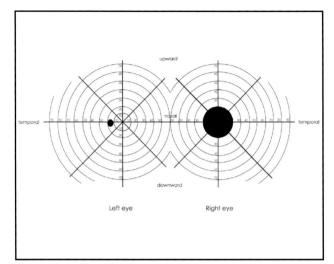

Figure 14-9. Central scotoma right eye.

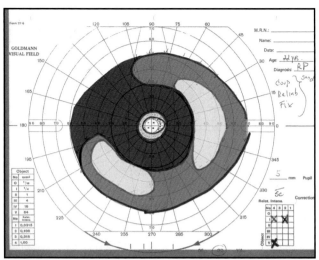

Figure 14-10. Ring scotoma caused by retinitis pigmentosa.

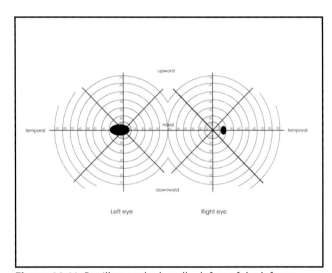

Figure 14-11. Papillomacular bundle defect of the left eye.

the horizontal meridian. They may arch off the blind spot, creating a paracentral scotoma known as *Bjerrum's scotoma* (see Figure 14-12A). Or damage may occur more peripherally, creating a *nasal step* (Figure 14-12B), where superior and inferior nerve fibers from the disc meet nasal to the optic nerve.

The final area of Region II involves the nasal radial nerve fibers. Damage here creates a *wedge-shaped defect* that fans out from the blind spot into the temporal field. Such defects are extremely uncommon.

The optic chiasm makes up Region III. This is the first location along the visual pathway where lesions produce defects in the visual fields of both eyes, since this is the intersection where temporal nerve fibers pair with contralateral nasal fibers.

The characteristic defect of Region III is a bitemporal *hemianopsia* (*hemi-* hemisphere, half of visual field; *-anopsia*, without sight; Figure 14-13). Any mass, compression, or dislocation of the chiasm places pressure on

the nasal nerve fibers, blocking transmission of sensory input. The resulting visual field produces a *heteronymous* (opposite) hemianopsia, or bitemporal defect. (It is considered "opposite" because this produces a defect on the left side in the left eye and on the right side in the right eye.) The pituitary gland sits just below the chiasm where the nasal nerve fibers cross, so a pituitary tumor can cause this type of finding.

Another defect found in this area is a *junctional* defect (Figure 14-14). It affects the area just anterior to the chiasm, where some of the nasal fibers travel slightly anterior in the opposite optic nerve before heading posteriorly with the temporal fibers. Lesions located here produce an optic nerve defect (typical of a Region II) in one eye and a temporal defect in the opposite eye (due to the backtracked, contralateral nasal nerve fibers also being affected).

Region IV, the final area of the visual pathway, includes the optic tracts, lateral geniculate bodies, optic radiations, and the visual cortex of the occipital lobe. Lesions in this region involve the temporal nerve fibers from one eye along with the nasal nerve fibers of the opposite eye. Visual field defects in Region IV tend to respect the vertical meridian. Damage in this region may be caused by brain tumors, strokes, aneurysms, trauma, and other neurologic disorders.

The nerve fibers comprising the optic tracts and lateral geniculate bodies do not have exactly paired retinal points, so the visual field defects originating from these areas are not perfectly congruous. Inferior lesions, affecting the temporal lobe, will produce a wedge-shaped defect in the superior quadrant of the field. This is commonly referred to as *pie in the sky* (Figure 14-15). Superior lesions, impinging on the parietal lobe, create a wedge-shaped deficiency in the inferior quadrant of the field. This finding is called *pie on the floor* (Figure 14-16).

Nerve fibers in the parietal and occipital lobes *do* have corresponding retinal points, producing homonymous

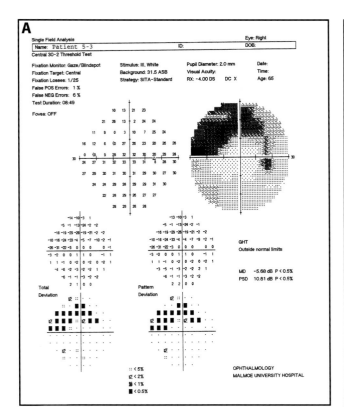
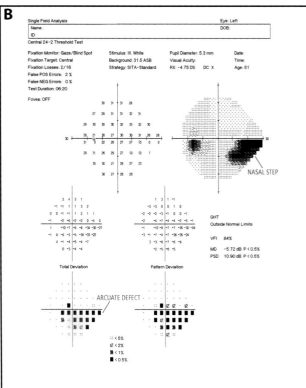

Figure 14-12. Region II field defects as plotted with the Humphrey automated perimeter. (A) Bjerrum's scotoma. (B) Nasal step. (Reprinted with permission from Heijl A, Patella VM, Bengtsson B. *Effective Perimetry*. 4th ed. Dublin, CA: Carl Zeiss Meditec, Inc; 2012.)

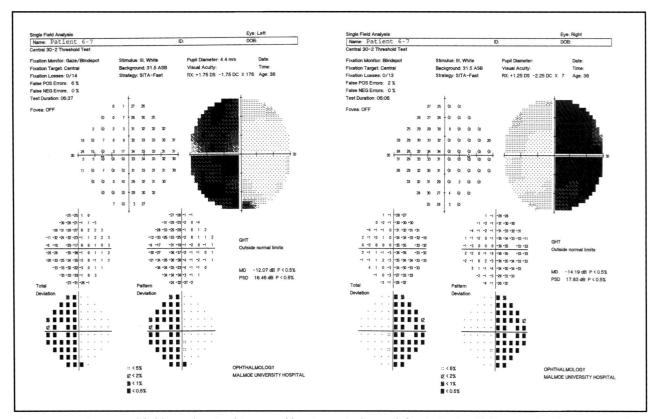

Figure 14-13. Automated field test showing bitemporal hemianopsia due to defect in Region III. (Reprinted with permission from Heijl A, Patella VM, Bengtsson B. *Effective Perimetry*. 4th ed. Dublin, CA: Carl Zeiss Meditec, Inc; 2012.)

Figure 14-14. Region III junctional defect.

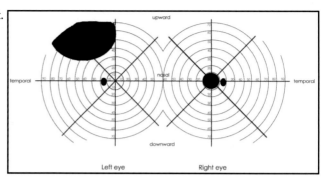

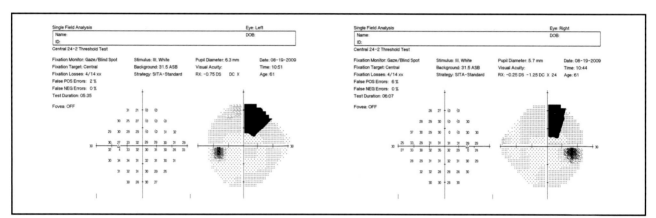

Figure 14-15. Automated field showing pie in the sky field loss. (Adapted from Heijl A, Patella VM, Bengtsson B. *Effective Perimetry*. 4th ed. Dublin, CA: Carl Zeiss Meditec, Inc; 2012.)

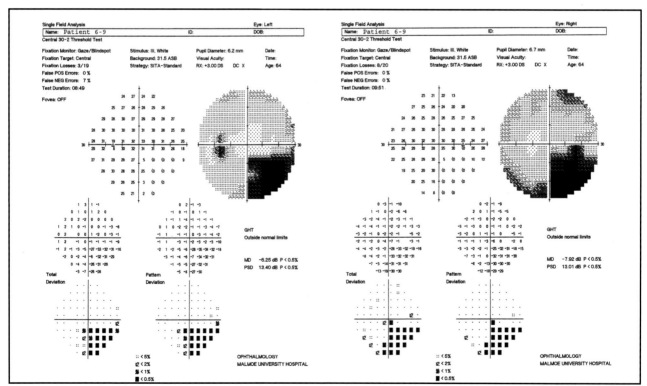

Figure 14-16. Automated field showing pie on the floor field loss. (Reprinted with permission from Heijl A, Patella VM, Bengtsson B. *Effective Perimetry*. 4th ed. Dublin, CA: Carl Zeiss Meditec, Inc; 2012.)

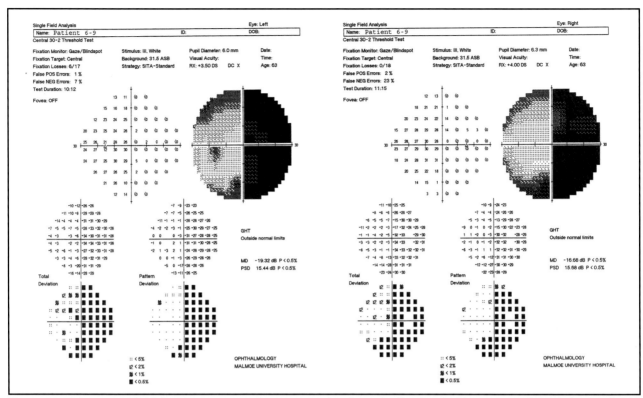

Figure 14-17. Automated field showing congruous homonymous hemianopsia. (Reprinted with permission from Heijl A, Patella VM, Bengtsson B. *Effective Perimetry*. 4th ed. Dublin, CA: Carl Zeiss Meditec, Inc; 2012.)

hemianopic defects that are considered *congruous*, or identical (Figure 14-17). The peripheral retinal nerve fibers terminate in the anterior visual cortex, while much of the posterior portion of the visual cortex contains macular nerve fibers.

Despite the central field comprising only 30° (less than one-half of the entire field), two-thirds of the entire visual cortex interprets incoming stimuli from these macular impulses. Region IV defects often involve some of the central field, close to fixation, in each eye. Although a portion of the field may be missing, the visual acuity is not reduced because half of the macular region is spared.

CLINICAL SKILLS

Before performing any method of visual field screening, it is important to determine the patient's refractive error and best-corrected visual acuity. This will give the patient the optimum vision to carry out the test, reduce artifacts from uncorrected refractive errors, and help the examiner gauge the degree of any visual deficits that may affect the patient's performance.

A quick and simple method of screening for a visual field defect during an eye exam is to perform a *confrontation field* evaluation (see Chapter 9). To test the central 10° of the field, an Amsler grid test may be done (also Chapter 9). Performing either one of these prior to formal

perimetry gives the examiner an idea of any defects that might exist, and gives the patient an understanding of fixation during the test.

To quantify the peripheral field, one of two perimetry testing strategies, kinetic or static, may be done. A combination of both methods is used in modern visual field testing. Each requires that the patient maintains fixation straight ahead on a central fixation spot and respond when a target is first perceived in the peripheral vision. The size, color, and/or intensity of the target can usually be changed.

With *kinetic* testing, a target is steadily moved from a nonseeing area into a seeing area in the patient's visual field. The point at which the stimulus is first perceived is marked. (The arc perimeter used kinetic testing, see Sidebar 14-1.) By repeating this process at regular intervals, a map of the perimeter of vision (for that particular stimulus only) can be extrapolated. Imagine horizontally slicing the island of vision at different altitudes. Each slice represents a different isopter, or line, of equal sensitivity. Dimmer, smaller lights correspond to a slice of the island at a higher altitude. Brighter, larger lights represent slices taken from a lower altitude. (The higher you go, the closer you are to the macula, which can discern tinier and dimmer lights.)

In the *static* method, the patient is presented with stationary stimuli of variable intensity in assorted locations within the field. This gives a "yes or no" response to the question, "Is the stimulus seen *here*?" The altitudinal

SIDEBAR 14-1
THE ARC PERIMETER

Probably long stashed away in the archives of retired ophthalmic equipment, the arc perimeter first appeared in the late 1860s.[2] It was a simple curved piece of metal, so that the curve maintained an equal distance from the patient's eye. The center of the curve corresponded to fixation, and etchings on the arc, denoted in 10° increments, moved out from center. The device could be rotated so that each quadrant of the patient's visual field could be measured. Testing was accomplished by occluding one of the patient's eyes at a time and slowly moving targets, of various sizes, mounted on a wand along the arc from a point outside of the patient's field of view in toward center until the patient was first able to appreciate seeing it. The results could be mapped on graph paper.

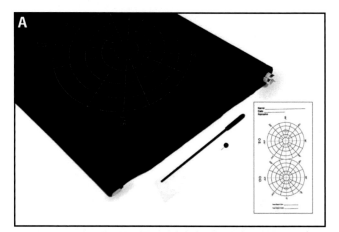

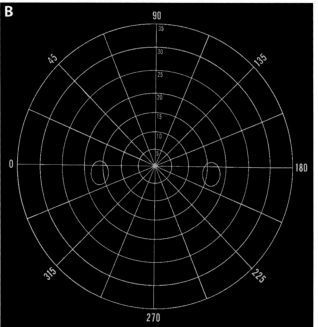

Figure 14-18. Tangent screen. (A) Tangent screen, wand, target, and recording chart (Good-Lite Company). (B) Screen as displayed for use. (Reprinted with permission from Veatch Ophthalmic Instruments/Gulden Ophthalmics, Inc.)

contour of the island is mapped by measuring the distance from a fixed point above the island to a point along the island's surface.

The diagnosis and evaluation of glaucoma is probably the main use of perimetry. Nerve damage from glaucoma usually follows a fairly standard progression, producing predictable changes on the visual field. In 1971, Mansour Armaly and Stephen Drance developed a visual field screening protocol that especially concentrates on the areas of typical glaucoma damage.[3] The *Armaly-Drance* method includes kinetic mapping of the outer isopters with extra meridians (5° and 10°) on either side of the nasal field in order to catch nasal steps. The blind spot is also mapped kinetically, looking for enlargement and/or Bjerrum's scotoma. Finally, the central 15° area is checked for scotomas in great detail, using a static (nonmoving) target presented at every meridian.

Tangent Screen

The tangent screen is a time-honored testing method that consists of a piece of black felt on which an X-Y axis is sewn using barely visible black thread (Figures 14-18A and B). Also stitched on the screen are lines radiating out in 10° increments from the central fixation, as well as concentric circles and blind spot markers. Target disks of various sizes are inserted into a long-handled black wand. The disks are white or colored on one side and black on the other. It is important to record what size and color target is used for the test.

The patient sits facing the screen usually at a distance of one meter. One eye is occluded at a time. By moving the wand, the examiner brings the target in from an outermost nonseeing area slowly toward the center at a steady rate. The patient indicates when the target is first noticed by saying "Now" or some other prearranged signal (eg, tapping a coin on the armrest of the chair). At the point where the target is seen, the examiner inserts a black-topped pin into the screen itself. Once each meridian is tested in this way, the position of each pin is marked on a preprinted paper chart and the dots are connected to form an isopter.

The physiologic blind spot is also plotted. The typical location of the right and left blind spots is marked on the tangent screen by black stitching. The blind spot of the right eye will be on the right side of the screen, and the left on the opposite side. The target is held in the center of the stitched oval with the white side down (away from the patient). The wand is then twisted so the white side is presented. If you are in the blind spot area, the patient

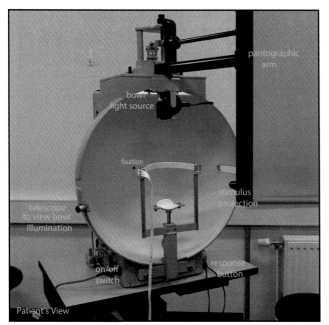

Figure 14-19. Goldmann perimeter, patient's view. (Reprinted with permission from RobertB3009, Wikimedia, https://commons.wikimedia.org/wiki/File:PatientviewGoldmannperimeter.jpg.)

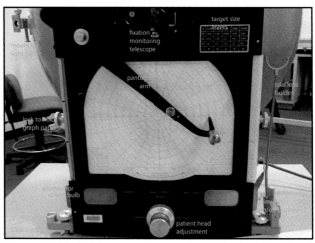

Figure 14-20. Goldmann perimeter, clinician's view. (Reprinted with permission from RobertB3009, Wikimedia, https://commons.wikimedia.org/wiki/File:ClinicianviewGoldmannperimeter.jpg.)

not require great skill. It is, however, difficult for the examiner to simultaneously monitor the patient's fixation while performing the test, and there is no way to calibrate the background lighting.

Goldmann Visual Fields

In 1945, Hans Goldmann developed an apparatus that used the kinetic technique to accurately map a patient's peripheral field.[3] Static technique is also utilized with this instrument for spot-checking specific areas. The device is a half sphere, similar in appearance to a satellite dish (Figure 14-19). From the patient side, the interior of the bowl is white, 30 cm in depth, and has a central fixation target. At the edge of the bowl is a moveable chin and forehead rest so the patient can be aligned with the fixation target. At the top of the bowl is the light source that controls the illumination inside the testing area.

On the examiner's side of the machine (Figure 14-20) is a telescope used to monitor the patient's fixation. At the top right are several levers for adjusting the target light. Marked levers move grey filters into place, which logarithmically change the size and luminance of the light stimulus. The Roman numerals represent the size of the stimulus in mm², while the Arabic numbers and letters signify the intensity or brightness of the light in apostilbs. (The *apostilb* as a way of speaking about light intensity has largely fallen out of modern use, but we seem to be stuck with it in perimetry.) The "e" intensity setting is continually used during kinetic testing. The "o" size setting is not routinely used. During testing, first the Arabic number, then the Roman numeral, are increased to plot the field (Table 14-2).

Characteristic to this instrument is a pantographic arm that is controlled by the tester. This apparatus extends from a handle (marking device) at the back of the

will not see the target. The wand is then moved slowly toward the edge of the oval until the patient reports seeing it. This spot is marked with a pin in the same way as the outer isopter. The target is again returned to the center of the blind spot, flipped over, and moved along another meridian until the patient responds. In this way the outline of the patient's blind spot can be mapped out and also transferred to the paper chart.

It is also possible to perform static spot-checking using a tangent screen by simply placing the target in different testing locations and flipping it over from the black side to the white. The patient responds that the target is seen or not seen. If it is not seen, then the parameters of this possible scotoma are plotted in the same way as the physiologic blind spot, as detailed above.

The patient may actually be tested at either 1 or 2 meters, or both. Testing both is especially useful for cases where there may be malingering or hysteria. Field defects detected with the tangent screen should expand when the testing distance is doubled. If the defects do *not* enlarge with increased distance, then malingering or hysteria is strongly suspected. Another phenomenon sometimes seen in such cases is a *spiraling* field, where the outer isopter seems to get smaller and smaller as the test goes on, collapsing in on itself even in areas where the target was previously seen.

Use of the tangent screen has both pros and cons. On the positive side, it is portable, easy to use, and more affordable than other, more sophisticated methods of visual field testing. It is fairly easy to perform and does

TABLE 14-2					
LIGHT STIMULUS SETTING FOR GOLDMANN VISUAL FIELDS					
Intensity in apostilbs	a 0.40	b 0.50	c 0.63	d 0.80	e 1.00	
Intensity in apostilbs	1 0.0315	2 0.10	3 0.315	4 1.00		
Aperture size in mm²	0 1/16	I 1/4	II 1	III 4	IV 16	V 64

machine (where the perimetrist can move it along the test graph paper), to the swing arm in front. It controls the placement of the light stimulus presented to the patient.

The test paper slides over an illuminated plate facing the tester. It is held in place by tightening knobs at the midline on both sides of the screen.

At the bottom of the instrument are knobs that allow the operator to adjust the horizontal and vertical placement of the chinrest. These assist in maintaining the proper alignment of the patient's eye with the central fixation spot, which may change as the patient takes the test. On the lower right side as the operator faces the machine is the light stimulus button. This allows the perimetrist to control whether the light stimulus is continually on or off. The button can be rotated so the light stays continually on when the button is in the up position, which is helpful when calibrating the instrument. Or, it can be rotated to the off position so the target light is only on when the button is depressed during testing.

Performing a Goldmann visual field actively connects the perimetrist with the patient. The tech must simultaneously monitor the patient's fixation through the telescope, present the stimulus in a methodical manner, and accurately document the patient's responses. The tech must play a dynamic role as detective solving a mystery by plotting out the location of any defect(s). Because of this relationship, having a solid knowledge of the visual pathway and potential defects is key in capturing a true and reproducible outcome.

Calibration of the Goldmann Perimeter

The Goldmann perimeter should be calibrated daily. Dim the room lights to the level that will be used during testing. First the stimulus, then the background illumination is calibrated.

Load a piece of Goldmann graph paper into the sleeve on the examiner's side of the instrument, aligning the placement arrows and tightening the clamp to hold it properly in place. Position the pantographic arm to 70°. There is a pin in the arm and a hole in the instrument so the arm can be pressed inward to lock it into place. Select the target setting size V4e (the largest, brightest setting). Turn the target stimulus button so the light is continually on with the button in the up position. The instrument's

light meter attaches to the holder just above the port on the left. Lift up the flag covering the port so that the full stimulus light hits the light meter. The meter should read 1430 lumens, or 1000 apostilbs. Adjustments to the illumination knob, located on the lower, left-hand side of the machine, may be needed to attain this.

If unable to adjust the illumination to 1000 apostilbs, check the light bulb. It has a special design with two sides, to provide illumination for both the background and stimulus. The glass on each side of the bulb darkens independently. This extends the life of the bulb when rotated 180° each week. If one side of the bulb does not achieve the required illumination during calibration, the other side may. When neither side reaches 1000 apostilbs, it is time to replace the bulb.

Once the target is calibrated to 1000 apostilbs, proceed to calibrate the bowl's background illumination. This should be performed with the patient sitting at the machine. (The patient's clothing reflects in the bowl and can influence the illumination.) Change the target size to the V1e setting (largest, but dim setting). Lower the flag to close the portal near the light meter so that light emanating from the arm entirely fills the space. View the flag through the small telescope mounted on the side opposite the light meter. The flag will reflect the V1e target light at 31.5 apostilbs. This is the target bowl illumination. Try to match this illumination in the sphere by adjusting the moveable sleeve covering the bulb housing unit (located at the top center of the bowl) up or down. (This is a subjective observation on your part; the meter is not used.)

It is also important to level the perimeter. There is a bubble level on the lower left side of the clinician's side of the instrument. Adjustments can be made to the leveling knobs attaching the device to the table (on the "feet") to ensure that the bowl is not tilted and will not induce an artifact (eg, normal landmarks may not plot in their correct positions).

Trial Lens Selection

Prior to testing, the working trial lens must be calculated. The power of this lens is based on the accommodative need of a patient of a specific age in order to clearly view a target 30 cm away (the distance from the patient's

TABLE 14-3 DETERMINING POWER OF TRIAL LENS	
Age	**Power**
35 to 40 years	+1.0 D
40 to 50 years	+1.5 D
50 to 55 years	+2.0 D
55 to 60 years	+2.5 D
60+ years	+3.0 D

eye to the fixation point inside the bowl) in the central 30° of field. The lens is not needed for testing the field beyond the central 30°.

The trial lens power is calculated differently than for a bifocal or reading add, since the visual field testing distance is not the same as the average reading distance. A table to determine the appropriate power for the working lens was developed based on the findings of Dr. Frans Donders, whose work demonstrated the relationship between diminishing accommodative ability with age progression.[4] The working lens power is determined by adding the spherical portion of the patient's distance refractive error to the age-appropriate add shown on the table (Table 14-3). If the patient has 1.0 diopter (D) or less of astigmatism, algebraically add half of the cylinder to the sphere of the patient's refractive error (to determine the *spherical equivalent*). If the patient has greater than 1.0 D of astigmatism, a cylinder lens is added to the spherical portion of the patient's refractive error to fully correct the astigmatism. Examples are shown in Sidebar 14-2.

The trial lens holder fits at the base of the chinrest. The device can be moved to rest comfortably in front of the test eye. It can hold both spherical as well as astigmatic lenses, with markings to align the axis. The spherical lens is usually placed closest to the patient's eye with the cylinder in the slot further away (Figure 14-21). This helps reduce any induced power shifts and prevents the cylinder lens from moving off axis. The trial lenses used must be *open aperture* (ie, have only a thin wire rim). The lenses in a typical trial lens set for refracting have a broad edge, which can create an artifact much like a ring scotoma. The thick edge can obscure the patient's vision at the 30° mark, especially if the lens sits slightly away from the patient's eye.

Performing a Goldmann Visual Field Test

To perform a Goldmann visual field, the room lights should be dim and the machine must be turned on. (The on/off toggle switch is located along the left side of the machine as the tester faces the back of the device.) A

SIDEBAR 14-2
DETERMINING TRIAL LENS POWER

Example 1: 54-year-old patient with refractive error
 OD: -0.50 + 1.00 x 180
 OS: -1.00 + 0.50 x 170
 Per the trial lens calculation table, a 54-year-old requires a trial lens of +2.00 D added to the spherical equivalent of the distance refractive error (since there is 1.0 D or less of astigmatism).
 OD: Spherical equivalent is plano, add +2.00 D = +2.00 D trial lens
 OS: Spherical equivalent is -0.75 sph, add +2.00 D = +1.25 D trial lens

Example 2: 60-year-old patient with refractive error:
 OD: +1.00 +2.75 x 175
 OS: +1.50 +1.25 x 010
 Per the trial lens calculation table, a 60-year-old requires a trial lens of +2.50 D added to the spherical part of the above distance refractive error. Because there is greater than 1 D of astigmatism, a cylinder lens is also used.
 OD: +3.50 +2.75 x 175
 OS: +4.00 +1.25 x 010

piece of Goldmann graph paper is loaded into the sleeve, aligned with the placement arrows, and clamped to hold it properly in place.

Seat the patient in front of the bowl side of the machine. Instruct the patient to keep looking straight ahead at all times at the central fixation circle. Advise the patient to press the response button whenever a small white light is seen.

Place a patch over the patient's left eye and seat him/her as comfortably as possible at the machine. The red markers on the chinrest should match the level of the patient's eye. Warn the patient not to sit back suddenly, as there is a risk of being hit by the swing arm as you move it during the test.

The fundamentals of performing a Goldmann visual field are fairly simple. With the working lens in place, the tester must first determine the smallest, dimmest light that the patient is able to perceive. (Experienced perimetrists may have different techniques for finding this—one is not necessarily more correct than another.) Using the stimulus settings at the top right on the testing side of the instrument, place the stimulus to the I4e setting. This is a small but very bright light. With the left hand controlling the pantographic handle and the right hand simultaneously resting on the light stimulus knob on the right lower side, move the handle so that it falls within the central 10°. Press down on the light stimulus knob to display the light

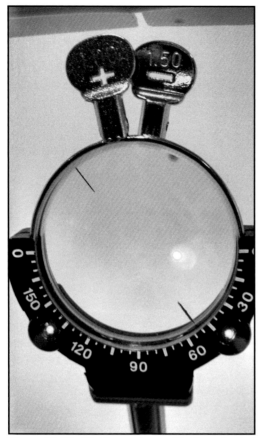

Figure 14-21. Trial lens set-up, with the spherical lens closest to the eye.

and ask if the patient notices it in the center of the bowl. If yes, repeat this step, but decrease the illumination to the I3e and then the I2e stimuli if he/she continues to detect the light. The smallest, dimmest light that the patient can appreciate is the stimulus you will use to begin the actual testing.

Begin plotting the central field by steadily moving the pantographic handle on either side of the radial markings on the graph from nonseeing to seeing areas. When the patient responds, place a mark on the graph at the location using a colored pencil. (There is a place on the chart to document what color is being used for which stimulus setting.) Once 360° have been checked using one stimulus, connect the marks. This line of connected dots is called an *isopter*.

Every light stimulus produces a different isopter and represents an area of equal retinal sensitivity to light in the visual field. Each isopter should be color-coded when recorded on the graph according to the size and intensity of the target used. (A color-coding system should be standardized to your clinic, to promote consistency in documentation.) The test proceeds in this fashion, first increasing target illumination and then size, until the parameters of the patient's peripheral field are determined.

The physiologic blind spot falls approximately 15° temporal to fixation. It is plotted from nonseeing to seeing by placing the stimulus handle in the anticipated center of the blind spot and moving the stimulus light outward along several meridians (looks like spokes on a wheel) until the parameters are determined by the patient's responses.

Static testing is employed in the central 30° of field to search for blind spots, or scotomas, centrally and along the superior or inferior arcades (the arching superior and inferior retinal nerve fibers, which do not cross the median). If any are found, they are plotted similarly to the physiologic blind spot. Once the central 30° have been successfully plotted, remove the working lens to test the peripheral field.

Usually a minimum of two isopters are plotted: the I2e and I4e. Additional isopters may be done to further evaluate the depth of a defect.

When a scotoma is discovered, it must be quantified. This is done by placing the stimulus in the center of the scotoma, turning it on, and slowly moving outward to plot the extent of the defect. This is repeated several times, rather in the shape of an asterisk, to find the border and shape of the defect. As the stimulus is made brighter and larger, the *depth* of the scotoma is determined. It may be a *relative defect*, in which case with each successive isopter the defect will become smaller. For example, a shallow defect might "respond" to a larger, bright target but not to a small, dimmer one. This would be comparable to a ditch in the island of vision. Or, if the defect persists through the course of the test, it is considered an *absolute* defect. In this case the patient does not respond to any light (not even the largest and brightest) inside the scotoma *on that particular perimeter*. This is analogous to a "bottomless pit" in the island of vision, such as the natural blind spot where the optic nerve enters the eye.

Special attention should be paid to the nasal meridian to detect a nasal step if the patient has (or is suspected of having) glaucoma. The same diligence should be given the vertical meridian with possible neurologic pathology.

When performing Goldmann perimetry, try to move the stimulus at a constant speed that is not too slow or too fast (about 2° to 4° per second). It is key to continue steadily moving the stimulus without stopping or slowing down in anticipation of the patient's response.

To avoid patient fatigue, remember that the smaller, dimmer lights won't be seen until they get closer to the center of the field. Bringing such small lights in from the far, outermost parameters tires both patient and examiner. It also increases the patient's temptation to peek. These dim targets can be started closer to the center. If the patient responds when you first turn on the light, turn it back off and move a little farther away from the middle.

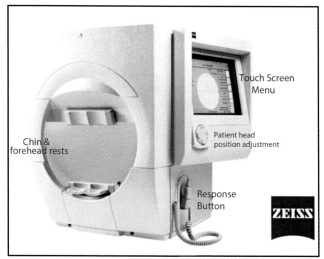

Figure 14-22. Humphrey Field Analyzer. (Reprinted with permission from Heijl A, Patella VM, Bengtsson B. *Effective Perimetry.* 4th ed. Dublin, CA: Carl Zeiss Meditec, Inc; 2012.)

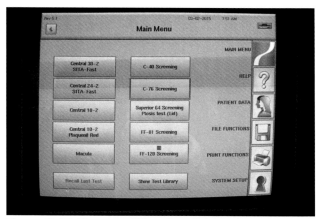

Figure 14-23. Directory of Humphrey Field Analyzer tests.

Cleaning/Maintenance of the Goldmann Perimeter

Patient contact surfaces (ie, chin and forehead rests, response button) should be wiped between patients with an alcohol swab or disposable antibacterial cloth. The graph paper sleeve may be cleaned using a soft cloth and lens cleaner. The pantographic swing arm joints may require a small drop of lubricating oil after years of use to keep them moving smoothly. Cover the instrument nightly with the manufacturer's dust cover to prevent accumulation of debris in the bowl. Maintain an inventory of testing graph paper, pencils, and colored markers. Back-up bulbs for the perimeter bowl and graph screen should be on hand as well.

The perimeter bowl itself can be cleaned by blowing canned, condensed air in the bowl to remove dust particles. Avoid touching the surface of the bowl with bare fingers.

Automated Visual Fields

Unfortunately, many techs were not formally trained to perform Goldmann perimetry, resulting in variable outcomes. To help standardize testing strategies and generate reproducible results, automated perimetry was developed. Hundreds of normal visual field exams were collected to formulate algorithms to develop computerized programs for comparison. The early devices were physically quite large, often occupying an entire room. They were also costly and the testing laborious, taking as long as 30 minutes or more per eye. As technology advanced, the instruments were streamlined, as were the testing strategies. Several devices evolved over the years to address the need for standardization, such as the Octopus (Haag-Streit USA) and Humphrey Field Analyzer (Carl Zeiss Meditec).

The *Humphrey Field Analyzer* (HFA; Figure 14-22) has become the gold standard computerized threshold static perimeter. Consult the user's manual for full information, as only basics are covered here.

The Swedish Interactive Thresholding Algorithm (SITA) standard is the most frequently used strategy. This program employs statistical averages to quickly evaluate a patient's visual field. Usually a size III white target light, of varying illumination, is briefly presented in a range of locations in the central 24° of the patient's visual field. (Most glaucomatous and neurologic pathology appear within the central 24°, as it represents 66% of the retinal ganglion cells and 83% of the visual cortex function.[5])The threshold, or the stimulus intensity seen 50% of the time, is determined at each test location.

Testing Strategies

The Humphrey is very versatile, offering many different test strategies, including both static and kinetic (Figure 14-23). It can perform 120° full field screenings as well as superior-field-only evaluations (to document lid anomalies such as dermatochalasis or ptosis). The 24-2 SITA test is the most commonly used test for glaucoma and neurologic disorders. Larger fixation and target sizes may be used for those who are visually impaired. What's more, specific tests for central foveal sensitivity are available. These utilize a red light stimulus to assess the central 10° of field for subtle changes caused by medications that can be toxic to the macula. It is helpful for allied ophthalmic personnel (AOP) to familiarize themselves with these alternate tests.

Calibration of the Humphrey Field Analyzer

The HFA eliminates any skew that may occur during the calibration process by performing an internal series of automated system checks when it is first powered on. The background illumination is verified by an internal light meter and standardized to measure 31.5 apostilbs. The stimulus projection and brightness are also automatically confirmed.

The device uses separate bulbs for background and target illumination. The stimulus projection bulb can be replaced by following the guidelines set forth in the operation manual. The background illumination bulb must be replaced by an authorized Carl Zeiss Meditec field service engineer. A pop-up message will appear if either of the bulbs needs to be replaced. The life of the bulbs can be extended by powering the machine on and leaving it on for the course of a clinic day. Repeatedly turning the machine on and off reduces this life expectancy.

Performing the Test

To carry out a Humphrey visual field, it must first be powered on. It will automatically run through calibration tests before the menu screen illuminates. It is important that the room lighting during this warm-up period be the same as the illumination will be during the test.

The test selections on the initial screen can be set up at time of the instrument's instillation, depending on the needs of the practice. Since booting up takes several minutes, the AOP should take this time to verify which test will be performed. Once the machine is ready, this test can be chosen by touching the appropriate icon on the screen. By convention, the right eye is usually tested first. However, if the left eye is the visually stronger of the two, it will be tested first.

Prompts appear on the screen to guide the AOP through entering the patient's identification data, such as name, date of birth, and medical record number if this is a new patient. (It is important to establish a protocol for entering patient names, as the instrument will only identify exact matches for repeat testing.) If the patient has had previous testing, "recall previous patient data" may be selected to bring forward this information. The final piece of data entered is the patient's refractive error to determine the trial lens. The Humphrey calculates the appropriate "add" based on Donder's table and will indicate which lens to use. These steps may be done with or without the patient sitting before the machine. The next prompt will be to begin testing.

At this point, instruct the patient how to perform the test (Sidebar 14-3). The test is done one eye at a time, and a patch is placed over the nontesting eye. The patient is asked to always look straight ahead into the center of the sphere at the black hole with the yellowish light inside. (On the other side of this hole is a camera and you will be monitoring fixation to make certain there is no peeking.) In different areas of the bowl, a small white light will appear. Sometimes it will be very bright and obvious. Other times, it will be quite dim and more difficult to perceive. Give the response button to the patient with directions to press the button any time the light is noticed. Remind the patient to not look around the bowl for the light, but to remain looking straight ahead. Confirm the patient understands before proceeding.

Once the patient knows what is expected, it is time to comfortably seat him/her at the instrument. The patient will need to rest the chin on the left side of the chinrest in order to test the right eye, and the right side of the chinrest when testing the left eye. Place the forehead against the headrest. Explain that contact with the machine must be maintained at all times as there are sensors in both of these pressure points.

The table that the machine sits on can be raised or lowered, as can the chinrest, to make certain the patient is not straining the neck or back and is properly aligned. As the patient is adjusted to a comfortable posture, the eye being tested should be visible on the fixation screen and remain centered throughout the test. Subtle adjustments may be made during the test to maintain this positioning (Figure 14-24).

The trial lens is moved close to the testing eye, but not so close that the eyelashes come into contact with it. Press the Start button on the screen. There will be a prompt indicating that the machine is initializing the patient's fixation, which takes about 3 seconds. Once this is complete, a Begin Testing button will appear and testing can commence. Keep monitoring the patient's gaze by closely watching the eye on the fixation screen. Fine tune the patient's position if need be to keep the eye centered.

On average, a 24-2 standard test takes about 4 to 8 minutes per eye. Once the test is finished, a prompt to save the test will appear. *Be certain to save the examination, otherwise it will be not be archived in the machine's memory.* At this point, move the patch to the opposite eye and allow the left eye to adjust to the lighting. In the meantime, print the results from the right eye. Now the Test Other Eye button may be selected and steps repeated to test the left eye.

Printout

The Humphrey Single Field Analysis printout provides much information. The false positive and false negative percentages let the physician know how reliable the test results are. A *false positive* occurs when a patient gets "trigger happy" by falling into a rhythm of pressing the response button even when a stimulus has not been presented. A *false negative* happens when a previously seen test location is not detected by the patient when retested with a brighter light stimulus. This is considered to be a sign that the patient is "falling asleep."

The gaze tracker feature indicates how steady the patient's fixation was. As the test progresses, a light stimulus is periodically presented in the blind spot to check whether the patient is maintaining fixation on the central point. If the patient responds to a stimulus here it is recorded as a *fixation loss*. This tally of fixation losses also contributes to the overall reliability of the test.

SIDEBAR 14-3
HOW TO PERFORM A HUMPHREY VISUAL FIELD

▶ Seat patient at machine.

▶ "This is a test to measure your peripheral vision. It takes about 4 to 8 minutes to complete.

▶ In a moment, you will sit with your chin on the chinrest.

▶ During the test, you will focus straight ahead at the larger black circle with the yellow light in it.

  • On the other side of this circle is a camera, and I will be watching to make certain you are not peeking during the test.

▶ As you are looking straight ahead, a little white light will come on in different areas. Some of these lights will be very bright and obvious, while others will be dim and you may not feel as confident you see them. There may even be times when you do not see any lights at all. This is perfectly normal, as you not supposed to be able to see them all.

  • The machine tries to find the dimmest light you are able to see at every point it checks. Sometimes it goes dim beyond what you are able to perceive and will gradually become brighter until you see it again.

  • Any time you see one of these lights, even if you think you are guessing, press the button to let the machine know you see it (demonstrate pressing the button as you hand the patient the response button).

▶ Remember to blink as you normally would.

  • Your eye may dry if you do not blink, making it harder to see the little light.

  • Do not be afraid of missing the light if you blink, as the machine is programmed to double check if you do miss a target.

▶ This test is done one eye at a time. We will place a patch over the left eye and test the right eye first. [Pirate jokes are allowed as you cover left eye.]

▶ Do you have any questions? If not, please sit forward with your chin down and your forehead in contact with the machine.

  • Are you fairly comfortable?

  • I am moving a lens into place which will help you see the little lights.

  • You may feel slight adjustments to your head position during the test. This is to help keep your eye centered."

▶ Begin test.

  • "Please keep looking straight ahead at the yellow light in the black circle.

    ▪ Please hold still for a few seconds as the machine calibrates to begin testing the right eye.

  • We will start the test now. Remember to keep looking at the yellow light in the black circle. Remember to blink. And, remember to resist the urge to look for the little white lights.

  • Here we go..."

▶ Periodically encourage the patient. When maybe a dozen points remain to be plotted, let the patient know that the test will be over in a minute or so.

▶ Once the right eye is completed, immediately save the test and shift the patch over to the opposite eye. This allows the left eye to adjust to the bowl illumination. (You can use this moment to print the results for the right eye.)

▶ Repeat test on the left eye.

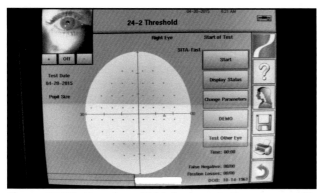

Figure 14-24. Humphrey Field Analyzer testing screen with patient properly aligned.

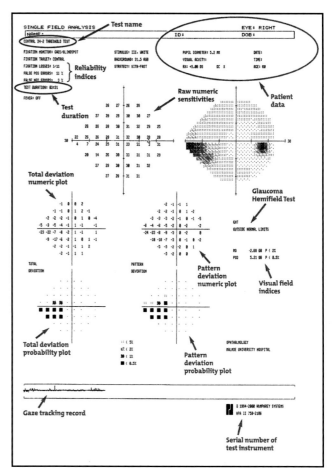

Figure 14-25. STATPAC single field analysis explanation. (Reprinted with permission from Heijl A, Patella VM, Bengtsson B. *Effective Perimetry.* 4th ed. Dublin, CA: Carl Zeiss Meditec, Inc; 2012.)

The gray scale of the printout offers a pictorial representation of areas where the patient could see the stimulus. The numeric sensitivities shows the decibel value of each stimulus detected by the patient; higher numbers indicate appreciation of dimmer stimuli. The mean deviation depicts how much the overall field departs from the model. The pattern standard deviation shows more specific defects in the field that vary from the norm (Figure 14-25).

Aside from the single field analysis, the HFA offers other printout options. The overview printout allows an analysis of field tests over a period of time. This can demonstrate progressive field loss from one year to the next. This feature can be used for the 30-2, 24-2, and 10-2 tests.

Another helpful printout shows the glaucoma change probability. This focuses on changes in the sensitivities of individual test points of repeat field tests based on the patient's test-retest variability. It uses an algorithm to mathematically calculate field progression. The program uses the first two tests from the patient's history of exams to establish the best baseline for comparison. A true worsening is demonstrated by considerable and reproducible deterioration relative to the baseline studies.

Less commonly used printouts include defect depth and change analysis. Also known as the three-in-one, the defect depth is a basic illustration of how profound a defect is. A change analysis can depict progression with all disease modalities. This printout includes mean and pattern standard deviation plots over time, as well as the mean deviation regression. (The mean deviation regression is a linear analysis showing variation in the mean deviation slope over time.)

Cleaning/Maintenance for the Humphrey Field Analyzer

It is recommended to perform weekly back-up of the hard drive to retain test results. System back-up on the HFA has evolved over the years from older models, using floppy disks or cassette tapes, to current machines utilizing USB storage devices. The back-up prompts can be accessed from the File Functions screen by pressing

Back-Up/Restore. Next, choose Hard Drive as the Source. Connect a USB device to the USB port on the HFA. Select the corresponding USB device as the Destination. Hit the Proceed prompt to begin backing up the hard drive. Once the back-up has finished, press the OK button to return to the main testing menu. The USB device should be removed and stored in a safe place.

The external panels and table may be wiped with a cloth and an ammonia-free glass cleaner. Patient contact surfaces (ie, chin and forehead rest as well as the response button) should be wiped between each patient with an alcohol swab or disposable antibacterial cloth. The touch screen monitor should be dusted using a soft cloth and ammonia-free glass cleaner when the device is powered off. Cover the instrument nightly with the manufacturer's dust cover to prevent debris from collecting in the perimeter's bowl.

The bowl may be dusted with a clean, dry cotton cloth. Use gentle downward strokes to push any dust particles to the bottom of the sphere near the base of the lens holder. When the machine is operating, avoid placing items on top of the device that may cover the fan motor's vents, causing the instrument to overheat. The instrument should be operated in a cool, dust-free room with a temperature than does not exceed 40°C (104°F).[6]

Replacements for fuses, bulbs, and the patient response button may be purchased from the manufacturer. Carl Zeiss Meditec recommends plugging the device into a 450-volt or high-surge protector to avoid electronic damage should a brown-out occur.[6] The appearance of a red line on the printed test results acts as a warning that the thermal paper is beginning to run low. A pop-up warning will indicate when the paper is out and needs replacing. Keep a back-up supply of thermal paper in inventory to replace as needed. The back-up USB storage device and the floppy disc drive are highly sensitive to electromagnetic energy. They should be kept at least 5 feet away from anything producing a magnetic field.

Helpful Hints for Performing Any Visual Field Test

Patients often feel anxious when performing visual fields. They worry that this is a "pass-or-fail" examination, and if they do not provide the correct response, they may be diagnosed with a vision-threatening disease. Thoroughly explaining the procedure can help alleviate some of their apprehension. It empowers them to understand what is expected and usually results in greater cooperation and test reliability.

Inform the patient of the approximate duration of the test. During the test, encourage the patient now and again. Tell the patient when the halfway point has been reached, and when the test is almost finished. This helps immensely in keeping the patient's momentum going. Never leave a patient alone when performing an automated test.

Remind the patient to continually maintain central fixation and use the peripheral vision to detect when the stimulus light appears. The urge to glance about should be resisted, as this lessens the validity of the test. Let the patient know you are constantly monitoring fixation and will observe when he or she peeks. Encourage the patient to blink normally. Staring in anticipation of the light may cause the eye to dry and blur the vision, making it more difficult to perceive the light.

Factors That May Affect Outcome

Poor fixation during any type of visual field testing reduces the validity of the exam. When the patient glances about, seeking out the stimulus, peripheral vision is not being used, but rather central vision. This makes the purpose of the test moot.

Fixation losses are checked when performing automated perimetry such as the Humphrey by periodically presenting a stimulus in the physiologic blind spot area. If the patient continually responds, it may indicate a slight variation in the location of the patient's blind spot. This

can often be remedied by rechecking fixation and replotting the blind spot.

Be sure to confirm that an eye is properly occluded. Failure to place a patch over one eye will lead to fixation losses as well as the inability to successfully plot a blind spot. Even the most experienced perimetrist forgets to apply a patch now and then. Laugh it off and tell the patient, "Now that you understand the concept, let's try that one eye at a time!"

Failing to use the proper trial lens can impact the outcome of a field test. Without the proper lens power, the patient may be less sensitive to lower light intensities, or thresholds, potentially indicating a false deficit in the results.

Not placing the trial lens close enough to the patient's brow may produce an artifact in the test results (Figure 14-26). This can appear as an overall constriction in the field. Using a thick-rimmed trial lens can also obscure the patient's view, creating a *ring scotoma* with a sudden drop-off in sensitivity from adjacent test points. On the contrary, placing the lens too close will cause it to rub against the patient's eyelashes and may become a source of distraction or smear the lens.

Improper head placement can also lead to artifacts. A patient may lean to one side, back the forehead away from the machine, or open the mouth, causing the head to rise up. The technician must be cognizant of the patient's body position. This can be observed when monitoring the patient on the fixation observation window. Automated tests have pressure sensors in the head- and chinrests. If the patient strays away, an alarm may sound or a pop-up warning may appear on the test screen. Gently remind the patient to return to the appropriate testing position. Sometimes it may be necessary to gently hold the patient's head in place during the test.

Drooping upper eyelids can cause an artifactual field loss in the upper half of the visual field. Unless the field test is being performed in order to document lid position (explained shortly), it is necessary to move the lid out of the way in order to expand testing into this part of the field. Often simply asking the patient to open wide will suffice. If the patient is unable to open the eye sufficiently, then the upper lid may have to be taped up.

Diagnostic Uses of Visual Field Testing

Perimetry is often ordered along with other tests when narrowing down a differential diagnosis, and may involve collaborative interpretation not only by the eye care practitioner, but also physicians from other disciplines.

Due to the characteristic appearance of certain visual field defects, plotting visual fields can contribute to pinpointing the exact location of a deficit along the visual pathway. Damage due to tumors, aneurysms, strokes, and trauma can all be demonstrated. Outcome of testing may

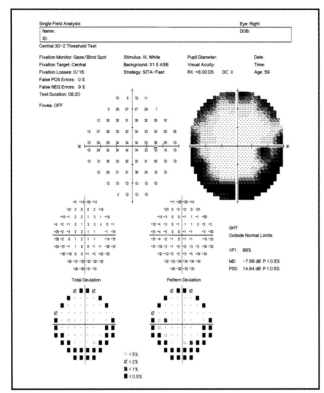

Figure 14-26. Artifact from trial lens. (Reprinted with permission from Heijl A, Patella VM, Bengtsson B. *Effective Perimetry*. 4th ed. Dublin, CA: Carl Zeiss Meditec, Inc; 2012.)

prompt referral to a neurologist for further evaluation. If any treatment is needed, field testing before treatment, as well as after, can serve to document changes. Perimetry can also be used to monitor progression in defects over time.

As mentioned earlier, the tangent screen may be employed to quickly evaluate a patient's peripheral vision. Remember, if a true defect is discovered, it will double in size when the test is performed at twice the distance (known as the *distance phenomenon*). This is a helpful diagnostic tool with patients who may be malingering, or feigning a loss of vision for an ulterior motive such as avoiding military service or trying to gain financial compensation. Malingering patients will claim to be incapacitated by their visual loss, yet they often ambulate normally. They might exhibit nontypical visual field defects, but the ruse may be exposed when these defects fail to double in size when tested at both 1 and 2 meters.

Retinal pathology can be visualized by the ophthalmologist during funduscopic examination, but the extent of how these problems affect the patient's vision can be mapped through visual field examination. For example, distortion present on Amsler grid testing may alert the physician to early changes due to macular degeneration. Or, visual fields may be requested to plot any islands of vision still present in patients with retinitis pigmentosa. This degenerative disease can affect the rods in the peripheral retina, causing tunnel vision. As the disease progresses, the cones may become involved leading to

blindness. This information is valuable to occupational therapists and low vision specialists in formulating visual aid therapies for patients.

Hydroxychloroquine (Plaquenil) is a medication which was first used to treat malaria. Although it is not fully understood how, hydroxychloroquine also has the ability to relieve the pain and inflammation found in many autoimmune disorders, such as rheumatoid arthritis, systemic lupus, and multiple sclerosis.[7] It is usually well tolerated, but in rare instances may cause subtle visual changes, which can be detected by Amsler grid and central 10° Humphrey field testing (using a red stimulus). Field testing using these strategies is often part of the recommended follow-up care of patients who take this medication.

Visual fields are part of a repertoire of tests used to diagnose glaucoma (covered in detail in Chapter 29). Glaucoma is a group of conditions that cause damage to the optic nerve. This damage can be observed on funduscopic exam as characteristic cupping of the optic nerve head. A corresponding visual field may show enlargement of the blind spot and possible defects along the superior or inferior arcades. Or damage to the retinal nerve fibers that arch around the macula and do not cross the horizontal meridian may produce a Bjerrum's scotoma and/or a nasal step. Subtle changes detected by the Humphrey analyzer may determine early management of the disease. A Humphrey visual field also allows for comparative studies over time to detect any progression of disease. Such changes may elicit modifications in treatment such as which pharmaceuticals are being used or if more invasive action should be taken.

Visual fields may also be used to help qualify a patient for insurance coverage for *blepharoplasty* (plastic surgery to repair drooping eyelids). Many patients develop *dermatochalasis*, or excess folds of upper eyelid skin, due to the aging process. Herniated orbital fat may also add weight to this tissue, causing it to create a "hood" that can obscure the patient's vision. Either a Goldmann or Humphrey visual field machine can be used to perform what is called a *ptosis field*. This test quantifies whether drooping eyelids restrict the patient's peripheral field. The test focuses on the nasal, temporal, and especially superior fields using a bright light stimulus, such as an I4e. It is performed with the patient's upper eyelid in its natural, drooped state and then repeated with the upper eyelid taped, to simulate how the vision would improve if this tissue was surgically removed. A visual field test demonstrating an expansion of the patient's field may determine that eyelid surgery is medically indicated, in which case the patient's insurance may contribute to paying for the operation (instead of being considered a cosmetic procedure that the patient would be financially responsible for). There are no guarantees, though, that insurance companies will pay for this expense.

Patients with limitations in their peripheral vision may not meet the conditions to pass a driver's license examination. In the United States, each state has different requirements, which can vary for personal and commercial licenses.[8] Canada requires private drivers to possess at least 120° of field along the horizontal meridian and at least 15° above and below fixation binocularly.[9] These standards, too, may vary from province to province.

ACKNOWLEDGMENTS

The author would like to thank the following: Barbara Cassin, MEd, CO, COMT (deceased); Diana Shamis, MEd, CO, COMT; Ella Rosamont-Morgan, COMT (deceased); and Dave Taylor, Senior Manager, Medical Marketing at Reichert, Inc.

CHAPTER QUIZ

1. The line connecting detected points of equal sensitivity to a single target is called a(n):

    a. scotoma
    b. depression
    c. isopter
    d. slope

2. The physiologic blind spot can be found in the _____ field.

    a. temporal
    b. central
    c. nasal
    d. inferior

3. True/False: Computerized visual field testing is the standardized method used to detect visual field defects.

4. The method of visual field testing where the brightness of the target is gradually increased until first detected by the patient is called:

    a. tangent screen
    b. threshold perimetry
    c. Goldmann perimetry
    d. arc perimetry

5. The best visual field test to detect a central retinal defect is:

    a. Amsler grid
    b. tangent screen
    c. confrontation
    d. Goldmann

6. Label the visual pathway using the following choices: optic tract, optic nerve, lateral geniculate body, visual cortex, optic chiasm, optic radiations.

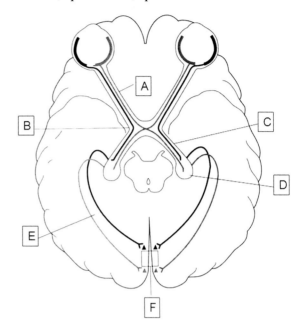

7. True/False: The target in kinetic stimulus perimetry is more difficult for the patient to perceive than that of static stimulus perimetry.

8. A defect in the superior nasal retinal nerve fibers will affect the:

    a. superior temporal field
    b. superior nasal field
    c. inferior temporal field
    d. inferior nasal field

9. Factors that contribute to errors in the outcome of visual field testing include all of the following *except*:

    a. uncorrected refractive errors
    b. technician capability
    c. patient limitations
    d. temperature of testing room

10. The visual field in both eyes will be affected if the defect occurs in all of the following *except*:

    a. optic chiasm
    b. optic nerve
    c. occipital cortex
    d. optic radiations

Answers

1. c
2. a
3. True
4. b
5. a
6. a. optic nerve, b. optic chiasm, c. optic tract, d. lateral geniculate body, e. optic radiations, f. visual cortex
7. False
8. c
9. d
10. b

REFERENCES

1. Trobe J, Glaser J. *The Visual Fields Manual*. Gainesville, FL: Triad Publishing Company; 1983:59.

2. Measurement of the visual field limits: the perimeter. Imaging and Perimetry Society website. www.perimetry.org/PerimetryHistory/3-perimeter.htm. Accessed September 18, 2016.

3. The age of standardization: Hans Goldmann 1945. Imaging and Perimetry Society website. http://www.perimetry.org/index.php/the-age-of-standardization-hans-goldmann-1945. Accessed July 9, 2017.

4. Wade N, Piccolino M, Simmons A. Frans Cornelis Donders 1818-1889. Portraits of European neuroscientists. http://neuroportraits.eu/portrait/frans-cornelis-donders. Accessed September 18, 2016.

5. Yaqub M. Visual fields interpretation in glaucoma: a focus on static automated perimetry. *Comm Eye Health*. 2012;25(79 & 80):01-08. www.ncbi.nlm.nih.gov/pmc/articles/PMC3678209/. Published June 4, 2013. Accessed September 18, 2016.

6. Artes PH. Manual for the Humphrey field analyzer II series. Dublin, CA: Carl Zeiss Meditec; 2012. www.scribd.com/doc/112839436/Humphrey-Field-Analyzer-Manual-5-1-for-Series-II-instruments. Accessed September 18, 2016.

7. Hydroxychloroquine (Plaquenil). American College of Rheumatology website. www.rheumatology.org/Practice/Clinical/Patients/Medications/Hydroxychloroquine_%28Plaquenil%29/. Accessed September 18, 2016.

8. State vision screening and standards for license to drive. Prevent Blindness website. http://lowvision.preventblindness.org/daily-living-2/state-vision-screening-and-standards-for-license-to-drive. Accessed September 18, 2016.

9. Vision standards for driving in Canada. Canadian Ophthalmological Society website. www.cos-sco.ca/advocacy-news/position-policy-statements/vision-standards-for-driving-in-canada/. Accessed September 18, 2016.

BIBLIOGRAPHY

Barton J, Sexton B. Examination of the visual field. In: Albert DM, Miller JW, Azar DT, Blodi BA, eds. *Albert & Jakobiec's Principles & Practice of Ophthalmology*. 3rd ed. Philadelphia, PA: Saunders; 2008.

Carroll JN, Johnson CA. Visual field testing: from one medical student to another. EyeRounds.Org website. www.eyerounds.org/tutorials/VF-testing/index.htm. Accessed July 4, 2016.

Choplin NT, Edwards RP. *Visual Fields*. Thorofare, NJ: SLACK Incorporated; 1998.

Garber N. Tangent screen perimetry. *J Ophthalmic Nurs Technol*. 1994;14(2):69-76.

Garber N. *Visual Field Examination*. Thorofare, NJ: SLACK Incorporated; 1988.

Goldmann Perimeter 940 Manual. www.scribd.com/doc/97438343/20159193-Goldmann-Perimeter-940-Manual#scribd. Accessed July 4, 2016.

Grzybowski A. Harry Moss Traquair (1875–1954), Scottish ophthalmologist and perimetrist. *Acta Ophthalmol*. 2009;87:455-459. http://onlinelibrary.wiley.com. doi:10.1111/j.1755-3768.2008.01286.x/pdf. Accessed July 4, 2016.

Herrin MP. *Instrumentation for Eyecare Paraprofessionals*. Thorofare, NJ: SLACK Incorporated; 1999.

Incesu AI. Tests for malingering in ophthalmology. *Int J Ophthalmol*. 2013;6(5):708-717. www.ncbi.nlm.nih.gov/pmc/articles/PMC3808926/. Published October 18, 2013. Accessed July 4, 2016.

JCAHPO criteria for certification and recertification. JCAHPO website. http://documents.jcahpo.org/documents/Certification/Criteria_For_Certification.pdf. Accessed July 4, 2016.

Johnson CA, Ketner JL. Optimal rates of movement for kinetic perimetry. *Arch Ophthalmol*. 1987;105(1):73-75.

Ophthalmic Medical Assisting: An Independent Study Course. 3rd ed. San Francisco, CA: American Academy of Ophthalmology; 2002.

Ramulu P, Griffiths D, Salim S. Standard automated perimetry. American Academy of Ophthalmology website. http://eyewiki.aao.org/Standard_Automated_Perimetry. Accessed July 4, 2016.

Trobe J, Glaser J. *The Visual Fields Manual*. Gainesville, FL: Triad Publishing Company; 1983.

Unless otherwise noted, the figures in this chapter were contributed by the following, who are associated with this book as authors:
Al Lens: Figures 14-2, 14-3
Gayle Roberts: Figures 14-4, 14-7, 14-9 through 14-11, 14-14, 14-21, 14-23, 14-24

15

OPHTHALMIC PHOTOGRAPHY

Sarah M. Armstrong, CRA, OCT-C, FOPS

Ophthalmic photography is used to document, determine and confirm diagnoses, and guide the treatment plan for ophthalmic diseases. It is important to have a basic understanding of ocular anatomy and physiology prior to performing photography. Review these topics in Chapters 2 and 3. In addition, most of the disorders mentioned in this chapter can be found in the Index if more information is required.

FUNDUS PHOTOGRAPHY

Basic Sciences

There are many different vendors that manufacture fundus cameras. There are two categories of camera design: traditional and the scanning laser ophthalmoscope (SLO, covered in Chapter 16). The difference between the two is the light source. The traditional camera design uses a flash system where the image is captured with a flash of white light, just like traditional indoor photography. As the name suggests, the light source for SLO cameras are designed on a laser system. Be aware of which type of system you are using as they can create different types of artifacts.

Parts of a Camera

Similar to different makes and models of cars, each fundus camera will be designed slightly different from the next, but the basic parts are largely the same (Figure 15-1):

- ▶ Chinrest: The patient places his/her chin here for stabilization.
- ▶ Eyepiece (if equipped): The photographer looks through the eyepiece to view the patient's retina. It is important to set the eyepiece for your vision, as this will vary between photographers. To set the eyepiece, spin it completely counterclockwise. Then look through the eyepiece as if looking down a long road (at infinity). While turning the eyepiece slowly clockwise, stop when you notice the crosshairs in the reticle (grid inside the eyepiece) come into focus. To ensure the correct setting, note your location and repeat this step a couple of times. Once you are getting the same location repeatedly, the eyepiece has been set for your vision. Note: This is only found on traditional camera systems. More modern cameras have only a monitor.
- ▶ Illumination: Controls the intensity of the light that is used to view the retina.
- ▶ Exposure: Controls the intensity of the light that is used to capture (photograph) the retina.

Ledford JK, Lens A, eds.
*Principles and Practice in Ophthalmic Assisting:
A Comprehensive Textbook* (pp 275-296).
© 2018 Taylor & Francis Group.

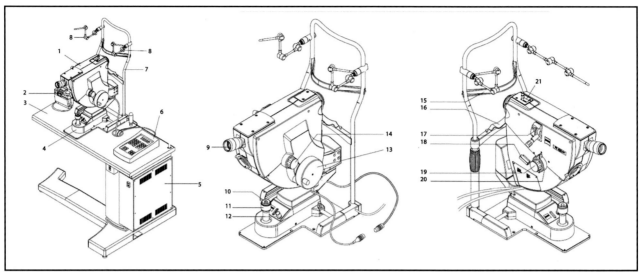

Figure 15-1. Parts of a Zeiss fundus camera. 1=camera, 2=camera back, 3=instrument table, 4=instrument base, 5=power supply, 6=control panel with exposure and some filter controls, 7=headrest, 8=external fixation lights, 9=eyepiece, 10=release button, 11=joystick, 12=illumination, 13=hand wheel for tilt, 14=focus, 15=forehead rest, 16=chinrest, 17=astigmatism correction, 18=slider for filter, 19=focus, 20=viewing angle, 21=internal fixation device. (Reprinted with permission from Carl Zeiss Meditec.)

► Camera back: Contains the digital sensor that records the image.

► Focus: Knob used to get the retina in focus.

► Joystick: Controls the up, down, left, right, in, and out motions of the camera and is used to obtain the proper alignment.

► Viewing angle: Controls magnification.

► Filters: Used to modify the wavelength of light that is recorded on the digital sensor.

► Astigmatism correction: Used to enhance the sharpness and to correct visually elongated vessels in a patient with astigmatism or when imaging in the periphery. (Note: This feature is only found on traditional systems and is usually an "extra" not included on the base model.)

► Fixation devices: All fundus cameras will have both internal and external fixation devices. These are used to give the patient a place to fixate so the photographer can capture the image at the proper place in the eye.

Mydriatic vs Nonmydriatic Systems

An important distinction between fundus cameras is if they are mydriatic (pupil dilation required) or non-mydriatic (dilation not required). While dilation is not required for a nonmydriatic camera, imaging will still be easier on a dilated eye and is recommended if more than two or three images per eye are needed. Capturing stereo images (covered later) can be a challenge, and often is not possible through an undilated pupil on a nonmyd-riatic system. To help the pupil dilate naturally, turn off the room lights and ask the patient to close his/her eyes

between images. Because a larger pupil is often necessary to allow space to maneuver around media opacities (eg, cataracts), dilation is ideal for these patients. If performing a fluorescein angiogram on a nonmydriatic system, dilation is still required as well.

While each system is unique, the majority of non-mydriatic systems do not allow movement of the camera from side to side (swing) or up and down (tilt). When a camera is capable of swinging, it will have a pivot point near the front of the camera allowing the back side of the camera to swing right and left. This allows the photographer to adjust the view in the nasal to temporal directions. When a camera can be tilted, it will pivot near the center of the camera allowing the back side of the camera to tip up and down. This allows the photographer to adjust the view in the superior to inferior directions. Both of these features can be helpful when imaging in the far periphery or when the patient has a difficult time with fixation.

Another difference between the systems is that most nonmydriatic systems do not have an eyepiece. Focus is usually more automated and confirmed on the computer monitor rather than through the eyepiece. This makes nonmydriatic systems easier to use for beginners as focus is one of the most difficult parts of using a mydriatic system. In general, nonmydriatic cameras are more soft-ware-driven rather than user-driven. Controls for illumination, exposure, viewing angle, filters, and fixation tend to be done with a mouse rather than a knob/button on the side of the camera. Photographers with experience using a mydriatic system may feel like they want more control over the automated features of a nonmydriatic camera. However, beginners and technicians performing fundus photography less frequently tend to be able to use an automated system more easily.

TABLE 15-1
DISORDERS COMMONLY DOCUMENTED WITH FUNDUS PHOTOGRAPHY

Diagnosis	Technique	Field of View
Macular degeneration	Standard	50° and 35°
Glaucoma	Stereo	35° and 20°
Diabetic retinopathy	Wide field/montage	Wide field/montage
Nevus in posterior pole	Standard	50°
Nevus in periphery	Wide field/montage	Wide field/montage
Occlusions	Wide field/montage	Wide field/montage

Clinical Knowledge

Fundus photographs are generally taken for documentation. Since the images are the same as what the physician sees during the clinical exam, fundus photography is usually requested so the physician can compare today's image to what the patient's eye looks like at the next appointment. To document pathology properly, it is important to first understand the normal retina; please review Chapters 2 and 3 for this.

When ordering fundus photographs, the physician needs to indicate the area(s) of interest so the photographer can capture the proper images. Table 15-1 shows disorders commonly documented with fundus photography. It is the photographer's responsibility to understand what the physician is requesting. It is ideal to keep an ophthalmology textbook with images nearby to look up new or rare diagnoses. If you are unable to find the pathology, ask the physician to review the images while the patient is still in front of the camera so another photo can quickly be taken, if necessary.

A standard set of terms are used to describe the location of retinal pathology. Understanding these terms is critical to properly locating and documenting abnormalities. The terms are based on imaginary quadrants within the eye: superior=up, inferior=down, nasal or medial=toward the nose, temporal or lateral=toward the temple. Each of these quadrants can be visualized in two ways:

1. Change the patient's fixation
2. Change the swing/tilt of the camera (if available)

When imaging into the far periphery, it is helpful to use both the patient's fixation and swing/tilt to image the pathology properly (Sidebar 15-1). While this may sound confusing, after enough repetition, it will become second nature.

Decades ago, a study on diabetic eye disease called the Early Treatment Diabetic Retinopathy Study (ETDRS) used these descriptive terms to define "seven standard

---

SIDEBAR 15-1
SWINGS AND TILTS

To photograph in the superior quadrant, the patient should look up. To get farther into the superior periphery, tilt the camera so the back goes down and the lens goes up. To photograph in the inferior quadrant, the patient should look down. To get farther into the inferior periphery, tilt the camera so the back goes up and the lens goes down. When imaging in the inferior, it is almost always necessary to retract the eyelids to get a better view.

To image the nasal quadrant of the right eye, the patient should look to his/her left. To get further into the nasal periphery, the patient should look further to his/her left and the camera should swing so the back moves to the photographer's left and the lens is pointing more to the photographer's right. To image the temporal peripheral on the right eye, the patient should look to his/her right. To get further into the temporal periphery, swing the camera so the back goes toward the photographer's right and the lens is pointing more to the photographer's left. Left/right moves will be reversed when imaging the left eye.

---

fields" that would be imaged for the study (see Figure 30-1). At the time, the standard magnification was 30 degrees (°). As cameras have evolved to have variable magnification, most fields are now captured at the widest field of view available (45° to 60°). As the optic nerve and macula are the two parts of retinal anatomy most often imaged, a view called the *posterior pole* is used to document both of these in one image (Figure 15-2).

When preparing the camera to take pictures, there are several settings that should be modified based on the imaging plan (Sidebar 15-2).

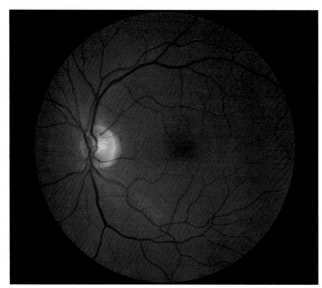

Figure 15-2. Posterior pole.

Clinical Skills
(Step-by-Step Fundus Photography)
Plan

Prior to bringing the patient into the room, review the patient record to know the diagnosis, location of pathology, and his/her visual acuity. When the pathology is not located in the posterior pole, it is helpful if the physician draws a quick image describing where the pathology is located. With this information, plan the imaging sequence.

Since the macula and the optic nerve are the most important parts of the fundus, the posterior pole should always be captured in both eyes. Plan to take additional images to document all of the pathology requested by the physician. When the pathology covers a large area of the retina, many physicians request images to be merged together into one large image (*montage*). When capturing images for a montage, overlap the images by about 10% to 20% so the software can use the vessel structure to match up the images and stitch them together.

Prepare

Prepare the camera by entering patient demographics, setting the eyepiece, and selecting the proper settings for the imaging plan (proper camera back, viewing angle, exposure, and viewing light; see Sidebar 15-2). Prepare the patient by informing him/her about the photographs, confirming that the eyes are dilated, and adjusting the height of the chair and/or the table to make sure that the chin/forehead rest can be reached comfortably. An uncomfortable patient will be less cooperative, which will make the imaging session take longer than necessary.

Perform

Start by establishing patient fixation with the external fixation device. If the patient is unable to follow it, use the internal fixation device. Once the patient is fixating, move the fixation device so his/her eye is directed to the proper field of view according to the imaging plan.

Next move the base of the camera forward to the "sweet spot" for proper working distance. (Working distance is the distance between the optics and the patient's eye.) You've found the sweet spot when the image is illuminated evenly across frame. Another way to confirm that that you've found the sweet spot is to move the joystick to the right or left and view the crescent of light that will appear just as you move off the right place. Then move back until the crescent just disappears.

Next, establish focus. When looking through the eyepiece, make sure the crosshairs of the reticle are in focus at the same time as the retina. (Try to relax your own vision as if you are looking into the distance, in order to prevent accommodation.) Be sure to focus on the area of interest. If focusing on the macula, the goal is to get the smallest vessels in focus. If the optic nerve is the point of interest, the goal is to focus on the rim. Adjust the settings to avoid any artifacts and quickly capture the image by engaging the shutter release button. Review the image on the computer monitor to ensure that you obtained the proper field with even saturation, exposure,

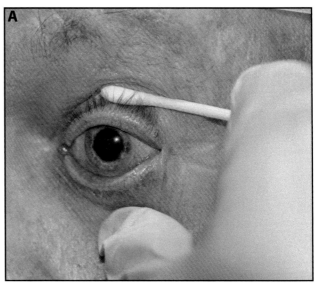

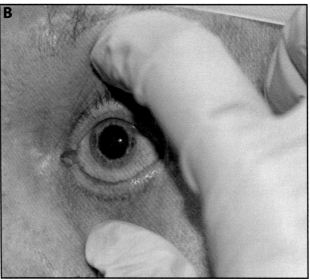

Figure 15-3. Lid holding techniques. (A) Cotton-tipped applicator and finger. (B) Fingers only. (Reprinted with permission from Houston P. Sharpe III, COT, OCT-C.)

and focus, and that the photo is free of artifacts (Sidebar 15-3). Continue capturing images according to the imaging plan. Be sure to delete any duplicates or images with artifacts prior to sending to the physician.

Patient Management

A successful photographer will be able to work with patients, even the most difficult ones, to capture the images requested by the physician.

A common challenge during fundus photography is establishing fixation for a patient with poor vision. When reviewing the patient's record, remember which eye has better vision and be especially aware of an eye with vision worse than 20/400, as the patient will likely have a hard time using fixation devices. It is best to start with the external fixation device and, if the patient is unable to follow it, change to the internal fixation device. The internal fixation device is more difficult to use because it needs to be flipped out of the way just prior to capturing the image. This can cause the patient to follow the movement and lose the initial fixation placement.

If the patient is following the internal fixation light as it flips, or if he/she can't see it at all, simply tell the patient which way to look. When verbally instructing a patient, start with straight ahead. Use the swing of the camera to document the fields on the central axis. Next, ask the patient to look up and swing the camera to document the superior fields. Lastly, ask the patient to look down and swing the camera to document the inferior fields. If your camera is a model that does not swing, simply tell the patient where to look. Alternately, you might post small

glow-in-the-dark stickers in the room and on the table to act as fixation points for specific protocol photos.

It can be difficult to get images when long lashes or droopy lids get in the way. A colleague may assist or you can manage lids/lashes yourself with either a cotton-tipped applicator or your finger. (Some photographers prefer to use a cotton-tipped applicator as they can usually spin it to get a better grip on the upper lid than they can with a finger.) If the cotton-tipped applicator isn't working, try using your pointer finger on the upper lid and thumb on the lower lid (Figures 15-3A and B). Patients may offer to hold their own lids. Sometimes this is successful, but often they will pull so hard on their upper lid that the lower lid will then get in the way (or vice versa). Any patient will be more cooperative if given

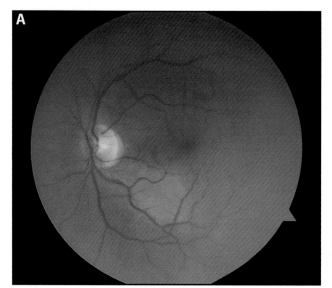

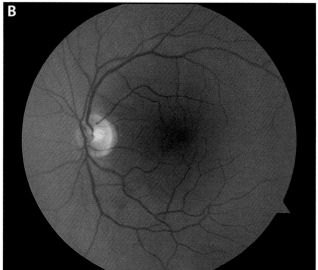

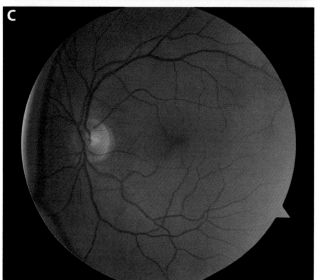

Figure 15-4. (A) Working distance too close, yellow borders. (B) Working distance not close enough, blue borders. (C) Crescent at proper working distance (although right and left must be adjusted to eliminate crescent).

enough opportunities to blink and even close the eyes for a few seconds throughout the imaging session.

Working with patients with decreased auditory ability can challenge even the most experienced photographer. When working with a patient who has some difficulty hearing, find out which ear he/she hears better with and instruct the patient loudly with short commands toward that ear. It may also help to deepen your voice. You may feel like you are barking orders, but this will help you both get through it with the least amount of frustration for everyone. You might establish signals for "blink/don't blink," for example, tapping on the patient's hand to communicate that it's time to blink and on the shoulder to communicate it's time to keep the eyes open wide.

Common Artifacts

Understanding how artifacts originate is the first step to correcting the mistake. Figures A, B, and C in Figure 15-4 demonstrate several common artifacts.

If the camera is not at the proper working distance, the image will be unevenly saturated. When the camera is too close, the borders of the image are yellow, and when the camera is too far away, the borders of the image are blue. A trick to knowing if the camera is at the proper working distance is if a crescent is visible when the camera is moved slightly to the right or left. If the camera is out of position, the crescents may show up in the image as an artifact.

It is a challenge to photograph the retina when there is a media opacity. The most common media opacity is a cataract. Corneal opacities, blood in the vitreous, and asteroid hyalosis are other examples. Rotate the joystick up and down, or left and right, to try to get a better view

of the retina. After photographing the retina as best as you can, take another photo focusing on the opacity itself. This image communicates to the physician why the image of the retina may be of poor quality.

One of the main challenges in fundus photography is imaging through a small pupil. If the patient's eye has pathology preventing the pupil from dilating very well, move the position of the camera until you have the clearest view, increase the exposure a few intervals, and capture the image. If the image is underexposed, move the camera to the side to include the crescent in the image. The crescent will block some of the image, but it will also provide extra light. Then move the camera in the opposite direction and capture another image. (The crescent will now be on the other side.) With two partial images from a patient with a small pupil, the posterior pole can be documented (Figures 15-5A through C).

The ultimate small pupil challenge is to capture images using a traditional mydriatic camera system on an

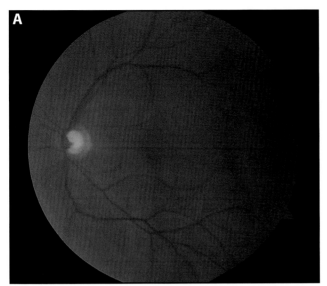

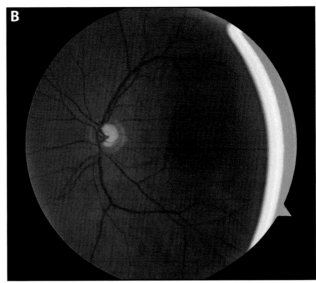

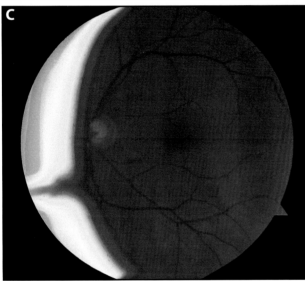

Figure 15-5. Imaging through a small pupil. (A) With a straight-ahead approach, there is a shadow cast by the pupil's edge. (B) and (C) combine to give the full picture by moving the pupil's shadow from one side to the other.

faster with the flash system of a traditional set-up, motion artifacts are not a concern.)

Camera Maintenance

Proper maintenance of the camera is a part of a photographer's job. Standard instrument care should be followed (eg, cover when not in use, clean the lens, and archive images).

When the lens gets dirty from tears or nose prints, cleaning is necessary to eliminate potential debris artifacts. As each camera may have different materials coating the lens, reference the user manual to get the best instructions for cleaning the lens. The Ophthalmic Photographers' Society (opsweb.org) has an online collection of user manuals for many ophthalmic instruments from a variety of manufacturers, although one must be a member in order to access them.

When working with a traditional fundus camera, you may notice that over time it becomes necessary to use a higher exposure to capture images. This is an indication that the flash bulb is approaching the end of its life. Remove the panel for the light bulb and examine it without touching. If the bulb is burned or whitened, it should be replaced. A supply of extra bulbs and fuses should be kept on hand.

In order to keep a copy of the fundus photographs safe and ensure there is enough space on the capture station hard drive to allow for new photographs, set up the fundus camera software to archive. Each system will archive differently, so review the user manual and work with your information technology support team to identify the best method for archiving in your clinic.

eye that will not dilate. An undilated pupil will also continue to constrict with the bright light of the flash. As it may only be possible to capture one image, start with the most critical field of view. In addition to the above suggestions, turn off the room lights, position the camera, and ask the patient to close both eyes to allow them to dilate as much as possible. Then instruct the patient to open the eyes and quickly capture the picture.

Debris on the surface of the camera lens may appear in images, especially when imaging in the periphery. Occasionally a digital camera may get debris internally, which must be removed by the manufacturer. (White artifacts on images are from debris on the surface of the lens; black artifacts are from internal debris.)

Imaging with an SLO system can create artifacts that occur when the patient moves the eye while the image is being captured. To correct this, ask the patient to look only at the fixation device. (Because the image is captured

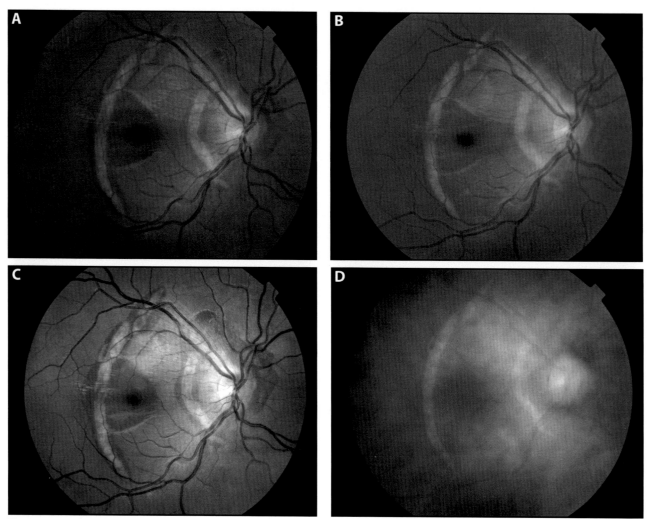

Figure 15-6. Choroidal rupture as seen with (A) color, (B) blue filter, (C) green filter, and (D) red filter. (Reprinted with permission from Timothy J. Bennett, CRA, OCT-C, FOPS.)

Special Techniques

Monochromatic Imaging

Color is the standard for fundus photographs. Color photography uses three wavelengths of light (red, green, and blue). When using monochromatic imaging, only one wavelength is used at a time by placing a filter in the path of the light. There are times when it is clinically beneficial to use filters that highlight certain portions of the retina. Because light scatters more at shorter wavelengths than at longer wavelengths, the blue filter (shortest wavelength) will highlight the nerve fiber layer, the green filter (medium wavelength) will highlight the retina, and the red filter (longest wavelength) will highlight the choroid. Using these filters can document pathology in a manner that can sometimes show the physician more information than a color photograph (Figures 15-6A through D).

Stereo Imaging

When we look at photographs, they are generally viewed in two dimensions. However, there is a special technique for capturing and viewing photographs in three dimensions. This is generally done to document pathology with large topographical changes. Instead of calling this three-dimensional like you would for a movie, in ophthalmology this is called *stereo imaging*. Stereo imaging is most commonly used for glaucoma patients. The optic nerve naturally has elevated contours, and these can increase based on the degree of cupping a glaucoma patient has. Other conditions that are better viewed with stereo imaging include papilledema (optic nerve swelling), retinal detachment, and macular edema.

The general technique of stereo imaging is to quickly capture two images with a slight lateral shift in camera position. When capturing stereo images, start by getting in position for a normal fundus photograph. Then move the joystick to one side past the crescent, and then to the other, observing the view. Usually one side will provide a slightly darker, yet clearer image and the other side will be mostly dark. Once the side with

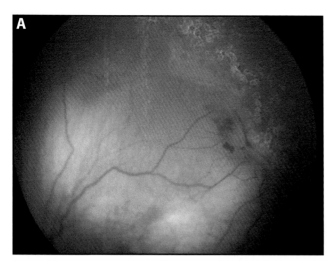

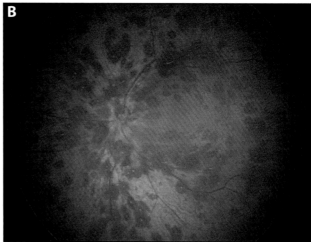

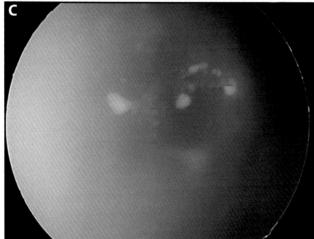

Figure 15-7. Images taken using a hand-held camera. (A) Retinopathy of prematurity. (B) Trauma (shaken baby syndrome). (C) Infectious disease (fungal endophthalmitis).

Wide Angle Imaging

Pathology can often cover a large area of the retina. The most common need for wide angle imaging is in diabetes. Other conditions that photograph well using wide angle imaging include uveitis, retinitis pigmentosa, blood vessel occlusions, and central serous retinopathy. Capturing images to cover these larger areas of pathology can be performed either with a system that has a larger viewing angle or by taking multiple images to merge together for a montage (see Table 15-1).

Hand-Held Imaging

There are a few systems designed specifically for imaging the fundus with a hand-held device. These can be helpful in the operating room on sedated patients, babies in the neonatal intensive care unit, or patients who are unable to leave the hospital. Recently, specialty lenses were developed to modify smart phones to capture images of the fundus as well. Conditions that might be documented with hand-held systems include retinopathy of prematurity, injuries and trauma, and infectious diseases (Figures 15-7A through C).

Patient Services

Ergonomics

A patient will be most cooperative when comfortable. Once the patient is sitting on the chair, adjust the height of the table so he/she can place the chin on the chinrest. It is helpful to have the table slightly lower so gravity will help keep the forehead pressed against the forehead rest. Most devices will have a mark on the vertical bar of the headrest to indicate where the patient's canthus should be aligned. This is necessary so there is enough room to

the clearer view has been identified, line up accordingly. (So if the clearer view is on the left, the first image is taken just past the crescent on the left. Move the joystick to the right a few millimeters to find the center of the pupil and take the second image. If the clearer view is on the right, take the first picture in the center of the pupil and then move the joystick a few millimeters to the right past the crescent to take the second picture.) It is important to take them in this sequence so the three-dimensional affect shows in the proper direction. (If you get it backward, then the pathology will be viewed backward; ie, an elevated area will instead appear sunken.) After capturing these images, review them with a stereo viewer to make sure that the three-dimensional view is obvious. Also keep in mind that capturing stereo images on a small pupil is nearly impossible. During image capture, encourage the patient to remain still; the patient's fixation must remain stable during sequential stereo imaging. If the patient's fixation changes between capturing the first and second images, the stereo images will not fuse appropriately.

move the joystick up and down and still be able to photograph the patient's eye.

When working with a child who is not tall enough to sit at the camera properly, be creative to get him/her in position. For a younger child, ask him/her to sit on a parent's lap. An older child may be able to stand on the floor or on a small step stool to be at the appropriate height.

Obese and/or large-chested patients can be a challenge to position at the fundus camera. Raise the height of the chair and scoot it away from the camera a few inches to allow them space to lean forward. Ask the patient's guest or a colleague to stand behind the chair to support it from slipping.

Patients who are unable to get out of a wheelchair will often be sitting too low to reach the chinrest. You can either raise them by putting reams of paper or a telephone book beneath them. Some chairs and power scooters have a feature that raises the entire unit.

Blinking

While capturing images, it is necessary to give the patient some time to blink and even close the eyes. If a patient says his/her eyes feel like they are burning, they have been open too long. This can lead to dryness, which can blur the entire image. It can also result in watering, which can spatter on the camera lens and cause artifacts in the images. It is ideal to have the patient blink between every picture and close the eyes any time you are reviewing images or changing a setting. Asking a patient to blink just before an image is taken will also help prevent blink artifacts.

FUNDUS AUTOFLUORESCENCE

Basic Sciences

Fundus autofluorescence (FAF) imaging requires no injections of dye. Instead, it captures the fluorescence that some structures of the eye have naturally (such as optic nerve drusen), as well as certain chemicals that are byproducts of some disease processes. Most notably, FAF records the presence of *lipofuscin*, a pigment that occurs as part of the metabolic processes in the retinal pigment epithelium (RPE). Ideally, the cells in the RPE resorb this material. But as we age, the lipofuscin (also appropriately called *age pigment*) tends to build up and remain as tiny granules that are toxic to the tissue. A build-up can also occur if the retina is under oxidative stress, where there is an imbalance between free radicals and the antioxidants that detoxify them.

Because it can image the fluorescent lipofuscin, FAF reveals the health of the retina at a cellular level. This information is used by the physician to help diagnose diseases, determine treatment plans, and sometimes to help predict disease progression. It is important to have a basic understanding of retinal anatomy (see Chapter 2) prior to performing FAF.

FAF imaging uses the same equipment as fundus photography with the addition of an excitation filter (488 to 580 nm depending on the system) and a barrier filter (500 to 715 nm depending on the system). The excitation filter transmits blue-green light at the peak excitation range of fluorescein. The barrier filter blocks all visible wavelengths except for the color of fluorescein. Most base-model fundus cameras do not include the filters necessary to produce FAF images. As not all systems use the same wavelength, when following a patient with FAF over time, it is important to use the same system at each visit for the most accurate comparison. As the light is brighter for FAF than for color fundus photography, dilation is required to perform this study even on a nonmydriatic system. (Still, the blue light for FAF is rather low intensity; high intensity blue light can be very uncomfortable for the patient, as well as potentially harmful to the retina.) When using the Spectralis HRA (Heidelberg Engineering), the best FAF images are created when multiple still images (frames) are averaged together using Heidelberg's software to form an image with more contrast.

Clinical Knowledge
Normal Findings

When performing any test, it is important to recognize what a normal result looks like. When autofluorescence filters are used to capture images in a healthy eye, the optic nerve and blood vessels appear black and the posterior pole displays a range of grays with a gradual decrease to the darkest shade of gray at the heavily pigmented fovea.

Pathology

In an unhealthy eye, increased autofluorescence will appear a brighter gray and even white at its highest intensity. This is thought to indicate cells that will soon die. Decreased autofluorescence due to degenerated RPE will appear a darker gray, and areas where there is absence or death of RPE will appear black. While the initial set of images are helpful, the best use of FAF is to track disease progression by capturing images over time. Common conditions captured with an FAF include age-related macular degeneration, optic disc drusen, Plaquenil (hydroxychloroquine) toxicity, central serous chorioretinopathy, intraocular tumors, and genetic diseases.

Clinical Skills

FAF can vary a good bit depending on the specific device that is used. The skills for FAF are the same basic skills for fundus photography. Each system will be slightly different in how the exciter and barrier filters are

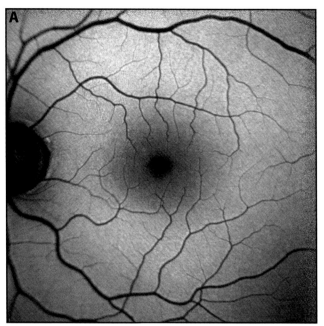 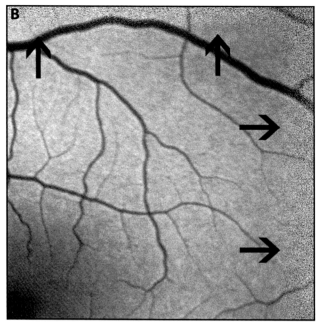

Figure 15-8. (A) Fundus autofluorescence imaging with scanning laser ophthalmoscope showing edge artifact. (B) Same image cropped to highlight edge artifact (arrows).

engaged. It is also necessary to increase the intensity of the exposure when capturing FAF images.

When taking autofluorescent images on an SLO device that uses image averaging, patient movement can create artifacts on the edge of the image (Figures 15-8A and B). To prevent artifacts, encourage the patient to fixate while the image is averaging. To track disease progression, some vendors include measurement tools in the software. Refer to the user manual for step-by-step instructions for this feature.

If using FAF for research purposes, be mindful that retinal bleaching can alter the measurement of the density of the pixels that create the image. Retinal bleaching occurs when the retina is exposed to the FAF light for a period of time prior to capturing the image. This is done in order to establish a standard for measuring pixel density for research and serial imaging of a patient. When performing quantitative analysis, it is important to be consistent with retinal bleaching.[1,2] Otherwise, the intensity of pixel density can vary. Discuss the expectations and safety of retinal bleaching with the physician prior to beginning a study, because extended exposure to blue light can cause retinal damage. Without a healthy RPE, bleaching can become permanent, meaning that the normal visual pigments stop being renewed.

Patient Services

This test can be uncomfortable for patients because the light intensity needs to be very high. To lessen patient discomfort, capture images as accurately and quickly as possible.

If using the Spectralis HRA, this author recommends the following steps: When performing optical coherence tomography (OCT) and FAF, perform the OCT first in both eyes. To begin the FAF, use the infrared wavelength to find the appropriate position. Next, ask the patient to close his/her eye and then engage the FAF light. Ask the patient to open the eyes, and quickly focus the image (it is usually approximately 1 diopter off from the infrared image). Next, ask the patient to close the eyes for a few seconds, then open for capturing the image. While the image is averaging, capture the image around 10 frames, then 25 frames and, if the patient is cooperative, at 50 frames. You will notice a point where the image quality doesn't appear to be improving. There is no need to continue averaging beyond at that point.

FLUORESCEIN ANGIOGRAPHY

Basic Sciences

Fluorescein angiography (FA) is an invasive diagnostic test that uses an intravenous injection of fluorescein sodium (NaFl) to reveal the flow of blood in retinal vasculature. It is important to have a basic understanding of retinal anatomy and physiology prior to performing an FA. Please review these topics in Chapters 2 and 3.

Fundamentals

There is a misconception that NaFl is a "vegetable dye." It is actually a mineral-based synthetic dye. The FA technique uses a blue exciter filter (490 nm) and a green

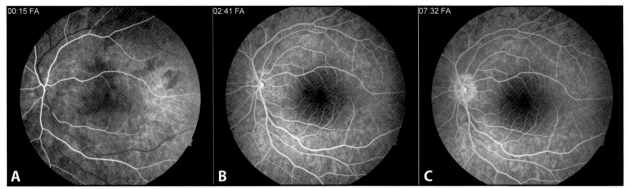

Figure 15-9. (A) Early phase FA, normal. (B) Mid-phase FA, normal. (C) Late phase FA, normal.

barrier filter (525 nm) to best view the NaFl in the eye. Several systems have a special feature that allows not only fluorescein images to be captured but also video. This can be especially helpful for vascular disorders where the timing of the dye entering the retinal blood vessels is critical.

On traditional fundus cameras, the exciter and barrier filters can degrade overtime, becoming less effective. This causes an artificial glow called *pseudofluorescence*. It is standard to take a picture at the moment the dye is being injected. This *control frame* is taken to start the timer and allow the physician to see what the eye looks like without any dye in it, but it can also indicate breakdown of the filters. The control frame should be completely black. If it is a diffuse gray, the filters may be degrading and a call should be made to the vendor. Be sure not to confuse this with autofluorescence (covered in the previous section).

Clinical Knowledge

When performing any test, it is important to recognize what a normal result looks like.

FA images are captured to document the flow of blood in retinal vasculature. It is critical to know the potential diagnosis prior to beginning the FA, as this may change the imaging plan. Without this information, the most important images for the diagnosis may be missed. Common disorders captured with an FA include age-related macular degeneration, diabetic retinopathy, and vascular occlusions.

Fluorescein Sodium

Injectable NaFl is available in 10% and 25% concentrations. The 10% concentration requires that a larger volume of dye (5 mL) to be injected than the 25% concentration (2 mL). Read the product information insert for dosage amounts for adults and children, and follow your physician's instructions.

It is the responsibility of the person injecting the dye, as well as the physician requesting the test, to be aware of the side effects, adverse reactions, and complications of NaFl. These will be discussed momentarily under Patient Services. Even though the FA study will go smoothly the majority of the time, be prepared to handle any problems. Discuss and plan with your physicians and coworkers how your clinic plans to manage severe adverse reactions so everyone can handle it calmly and professionally, if one ever occurs.

Descriptive Interpretation

The phases of the angiogram describe the location of the dye in the vessels and the timing of the FA. After the dye is injected, the *early phase* of the FA occurs (also called the *transit phase*; Figure 15-9A). The early phase is broken down into four sections: choroidal flush, arterial phase, arteriovenous phase, and venous phase.

The choroidal vessel network is separate from the retinal vessels, and because the choroid is posterior to the retina, the *choroidal flush* appears as diffuse or patchy shades of gray in the background. Next, the dye flows from the central retinal artery that enters the eye through the optic nerve and quickly reaches the smaller branches of arteries and into the capillaries. The *arterial phase* occurs when the dye is only in the arteries. From the capillaries, the dye transfers into surrounding tissue and then through the veins. When dye enters the veins, it initially flows along the edges of the vein. This is called *laminar flow*. The *arteriovenous phase* occurs when the arteries still contain dye and the veins are in laminar flow. Once the middle of the veins fill and are brighter than the arteries, the *venous phase* has been reached. In a normal eye, the four parts of the transit phase take place in approximately 40 to 45 seconds after the dye is injected.

The *mid-phase* starts 2 minutes after the NaFl injection (Figure 15-9B). The dye will have an even intensity between the arteries and veins during this phase. This is an ideal time to photograph the periphery. This phase is also referred to as the *recirculation phase* as the dye is recirculating through the entire body before returning to the eye.

The *late phase* (also called the *lates*) generally begins at 5 minutes (Figure 15-9C). As the dye continues to

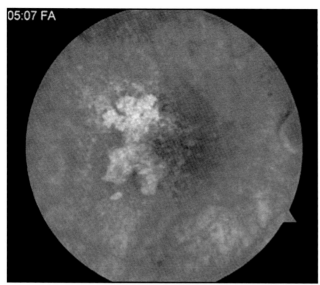

Figure 15-10. FA window defect. (Reprinted with permission from Rona Lyn Esquejo-Leon, CRA.)

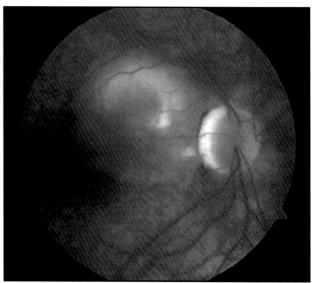

Figure 15-11. FA pooling.

diffuse into the surrounding tissue, the contrast of the vessels next to the retinal tissue is reduced and will be noticeable in the images. Each physician has a preference how long to document into the late phase, and it is often specific to the patient's diagnosis. Choroidal serous retinopathy is one example of a diagnosis that benefits from going out to 10 minutes as the view of the pathology continues to change over time.

Abnormal Angiogram

To be consistent when interpreting FAs, terminology was created to describe the abnormal angiogram.

Hyperfluorescence is the general term for "more than expected" fluorescence. *Autofluorescence* and *pseudofluorescence* are forms of hyperfluorescence that can be seen without NaFl, and have been previously described.

A *transmission defect* occurs at an area where the retina is thin or missing pigment, causing hyperfluorescence when the choroidal vessels fill during the early phase. This defect has a clearly defined shape. The shape and size of hyperfluorescence don't change, but rather it becomes dimmer during the lates. This is also appropriately described as a *window defect* (Figure 15-10). It most commonly occurs in macular degeneration with geographic atrophy.

Leakage occurs when the retinal vessels fail to function properly or when new, abnormal, weak vessels grow into the retina. Areas of leakage will appear bright during the early phase and continue to become brighter throughout the angiogram. The area of dye will also expand as it is absorbed into surrounding tissue. Leakage most commonly occurs in macular degeneration with choroidal neovascularization, as well as in diabetes with macular edema or proliferative retinopathy.

Pooling occurs after leakage when there is a collection of dye during the late phase in one well-defined location, as in central serous retinopathy (Figure 15-11). *Staining* occurs when tissues absorb the dye over time. During the FA, a stain will start out dim and become brighter in the late phase. Like a transmission defect, a stain has a specific shape that doesn't change (in shape or size) except in intensity. In a normal eye, the optic nerve stains during the late phase. In an abnormal angiogram, staining commonly occurs with drusen.

Hypofluorescence is the general term for "less than expected fluorescence." A *filling defect* occurs when the dye is unable to continue its path to fill in a vein or an artery. This happens with vascular occlusions and ischemic diseases. It is most critical to capture the early phase photos when documenting a filling defect. *Blocking defects* occur when there is something obscuring the view and the dye can't be seen (Figure 15-12). They most commonly occur when there is blood just above the retina blocking the view of retinal vasculature or subretinal blood blocking the view of the choroidal vessels.

Clinical Skills

Prior to performing FAs, it is necessary to be comfortable and confident performing fundus photography. Review the previously described step-by-step instructions.

Plan

During the planning stage, the FA supplies need to be prepared. These supplies should include NaFl dye, syringe, filter needle, saline, butterfly needles (25, 23, and 21 gauge), gauze/cotton ball, medical tape/adhesive bandage, tourniquet, elbow rest, and alcohol prep pads. Make sure that the emergency kit is accessible. In addition,

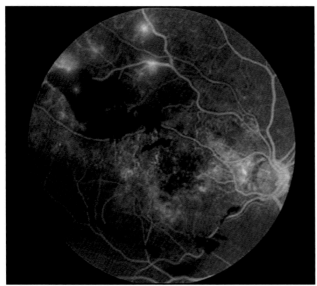

Figure 15-12. FA blocking defect. (Reprinted with permission from Rona Lyn Esquejo-Leon, CRA.)

because only one eye can be photographed during the fast-paced transit phase, a decision must be made as to which eye will be imaged in this manner.

Prepare

When reviewing the test with the patient, ask about any allergies, pregnancy status, and relevant systemic diseases. Explain the test to the patient, answer any questions, and obtain consent.

Perform

Prior to the injection of the dye, it is standard to begin with color fundus photography. The specific steps discussed previously in the chapter are recommended for color photography with a traditional fundus camera. After capturing the color images, continue with the steps in Table 15-2 to perform the FA.

Quality Concerns

Because the FA is a time-sensitive test, it is imperative that the proper images are captured the first time. If images aren't taken during a critical portion of the test, the physician may not have all of the information required to properly diagnose or treat the patient. When learning how to perform FAs, it can be best to begin by photographing the mid and late phases *after* an experienced photographer has captured the early phases. This is a great introduction to viewing through the exciter filter, as the dimmer view can be a challenge for new photographers. The first solo FA should be on a diagnosis where the early phases are not as critical to the physician for treatment decisions, such as central macular edema.

Low-contrast images may be caused by cataracts and media opacities. They can also be caused by topical NaFl on the corneal surface. If topical NaFl has been used to

check the corneal surface prior to performing an FA, it should be washed out prior to beginning the FA.

Role of the Angiographer

The role of the angiographer in regard to the injection of the dye is a somewhat controversial topic. Some states have specific legislation that only nurses and physicians may inject the dye. However, the majority of states are silent on the matter leaving the decision up to your employer and (hopefully) you. Be sure to know the guidelines in your state. Regardless of who injects the dye, the photographer is always the patient's advocate. Some patients may be too sickly to perform the test, and it is the responsibility of the photographer to discuss this with the physician.

Patient Services

This section will review the most common and important side effects, adverse reactions, and complications of NaFl. Consult the product insert in the NaFl package for additional information. When obtaining consent from a patient, he/she must be advised of possible reactions. If you aren't comfortable with answering patient questions, involve the physician in the discussion.

Side effects from NaFl occur within minutes of injecting the dye. Patients with a light complexion will notice their skin will have a slight yellow tone for a few hours after. The patient's urine will be a bright yellow-orange for a day or two. While these side effects are not harmful, patients can drink more fluids to flush the dye out of their bodies more quickly. The appearance of side effects does not generally warrant the physician's attention, but he/she should be made aware of any adverse reactions or complications.

Adverse reactions are negative responses from the dye that are classified as mild, moderate, severe, and death. As NaFl has limited uses, it is likely that only a patient who has previously had an FA will know if he/she is allergic to it or not. The Fluorescein Angiography Complication Survey reported the frequency of moderate reactions 1 out of 63 FAs, severe reactions 1 out of 1900, and death 1 out of 222,000 FAs.[3]

The most common of all reactions is the mild effect of nausea and vomiting. Consistently, this starts 30 to 90 seconds after the injection and only lasts for 1 or 2 minutes. Most patients are able to continue the test after the feeling passes. To help a patient through nausea, ask him/her to take deep breaths. Sometimes having the patient inhale the smell from an alcohol prep pad will help. While the primary concern is always the patient, if the patient begins to feel nauseous, cover the camera lens and turn him/her in the direction of a trash can.

Another common mild reaction in patients who have a fear of needles is dizziness and lightheadedness. If the patient seems anxious about the needle or mentions a fear

TABLE 15-2
STEPS IN PERFORMING A FLUORESCEIN ANGIOGRAM

Capture Monochromatic Images
1. Engage the green filter
2. Increase the flash intensity
3. Take monochromatic images of the nontransit eye
4. Take monochromatic images of the transit eye

Perform Fluorescein Angiography
5. Engage exciter and barrier filters
6. Increase the flash power
7. Set the FA timer
8. Position patient for procedure including chin/forehead firmly in place
9. Injector finds vein
10. Align camera on transit eye
11. Cue injector to begin
12. As the dye first enters the vein, take the control photograph
13. When the injector announces the dye is all in (5 to 10 seconds), take the second photograph
14. Early transit images captured every 2 to 3 seconds of posterior pole until about 30 seconds
15. Capture posterior pole photo of the nontransit eye
16. Check in with the patient to make sure he/she is doing OK; respond to any adverse reactions
17. If pathology requires, continue capturing images in the periphery
18. Capture mid-phase photographs of posterior pole of both eyes 2 to 4 minutes after the injection
19. Capture late-phase photographs of posterior pole of both eyes 5 to 6 minutes after the injection

of needles, distract him/her with conversation during the stick, or draw attention to the fixation light instead of the needle.

The second most common of all reactions is the moderate reaction of urticaria (hives). Patients with a lot of discomfort or any itchiness near their mouth/throat should be treated with an antihistamine. Patients with a history of hives can be premedicated with an antihistamine prior to performing the test.

Severe reactions include difficulty breathing or talking, loss of consciousness, seizures, cardiac arrest, and anaphylaxis. A physician should be called into the exam room if any severe reaction occurs, and a system should be in place to reach emergency medical services, as it is possible for any of these severe reactions to end in death. Thankfully, these reactions are rare, but everyone involved in performing FAs should be prepared to help if one occurs. CPR training is recommended for the staff, and emergency medical supplies should be located close to any room where FAs are performed.

Complications occur when there is a problem finding a vein strong enough to support an injection of NaFl. When a failed injection results in excess blood or dye infiltrating the tissue surrounding the injection site, the tissue may bruise and become painful. As NaFl has a salt component, the patient will feel sharp pain similar to when salt touches an open wound. Ice packs can provide some relief, but it generally passes in about 5 minutes. Care should be taken to ensure that the injection is being performed in a vein (dark red blood) and not an artery

(bright red blood). Arterial injections send the dye down the arm to the fingers and can be extremely painful.

INDOCYANINE GREEN ANGIOGRAPHY

Basic Sciences

Indocyanine green angiogram (ICGA) is an invasive diagnostic test that uses an intravenous injection of indocyanine green dye to reveal the flow of blood in the choroidal and retinal vasculature. It is important to have a basic understanding of retinal anatomy and physiology prior to performing ICGAs. Please review these topics in Chapters 2 and 3.

Fundamentals of Indocyanine Green Angiography

Indocyanine green is a synthetic, dark green powder that is mixed with sterile water to create an injectable dye. Because ICG dye has a higher molecular weight than NaFl, this dye binds to the blood more tightly than NaFl, allowing for a clear view of choroidal vasculature with infrared light (805 nm absorption, 835 emission). By comparison, NaFl has a lower molecular weight, causing the dye to diffuse more in the retinal tissue and blocking the view of the choroidal vasculature.

Because ICGAs provide different information than FAs, they are often performed in conjunction with FAs. It is possible to mix the dyes to perform both tests simultaneously or to use a device called a stopcock that allows multiple syringes to be attached to the tubing for the butterfly needle. (That way the tests can be performed sequentially.)

ICGAs can be performed on traditional fundus cameras with the proper filters and digital sensor. Some ICGA cameras can capture video as well. This can be especially helpful for diagnoses of vascular problems where the change in flow happens so quickly it can be missed during traditional ICGAs.

Clinical Knowledge

Pathology

ICG images document the flow of dye in both choroidal and retinal vasculature. As the imaging plan can change based on the diagnosis, it is important to know the diagnosis prior to beginning. Without this information, the most important images for the diagnosis may be missed. Common diagnoses captured with ICG include age-related macular degeneration, central serous retinopathy, retinal angiomatous proliferation (RAP; seen in wet macular degeneration where abnormal blood vessels form in the choroid), and polypoidal choroidal vasculopathy (PCV; a disorder characterized by choroidal hemorrhaging).

Side Effects, Adverse Reactions, and Complications

It is the responsibility of the photographer, physician, or nurse who may inject the dye, as well as the physician requesting the test, to be aware of the side effects, adverse reactions, and complications of ICG dye. This section will review the most common and important. Consult the product insert for additional information. When obtaining consent from the patient, be sure to advise him/her of possible reactions. If you aren't comfortable with patient questions, involve the physician in the discussion.

ICG dosage for adults is 40 mg in 2 mL of aqueous solvent.[4] In comparison to NaFl, ICG is much better tolerated by the patient. One study reported the frequency of mild reactions to ICG at 0.15%, moderate reactions 0.2%, severe reactions 0.05%, and zero deaths.[5]

The only side effect of ICG dye is green staining of the stool. The mild reactions are nausea, vomiting, and lightheadedness. A moderate reaction to ICG dye is hives. Fainting may occur in patients who are especially anxious. Severe adverse reactions from ICG dye are incredibly rare, but the precautions outlined in the FA section above apply to ICG dye as well. ICG complications occur when there is a problem finding a vein strong enough to support an injection of dye; however, failed ICG injections (where dye infuses into the tissue) are not painful to the patient.

There is a misconception that patients with an allergy to iodine (commonly found in shellfish) will also be allergic to ICG dye. The heart of this confusion is between the words *iodide* and *iodine*. There is a small amount of a sodium iodide ion in ICG dye; this does *not* cause a reaction in patients with an iodine allergy.[6]

Descriptive Interpretation

In 1973 when Drs. Flower and Hochheimer first published on ICG, they described the phases of the test.[7]

Even though ICGA focuses on choroidal vasculature, the phases of ICGA are described based on the location of dye in the retinal vasculature (consistent with FAs). After the dye is injected, the early phase of the ICGA occurs (the *transit phase*; Figure 15-13A). The early phase is broken down into four sections: choroidal flush, arterial phase, arteriovenous phase, and venous phase.

The *choroidal flush* will appear with more detail during an ICGA than during an FA because of the higher molecular weight of ICG dye and the use of infrared light. This allows a clearer view of the choroidal vasculature. The dye will fill the small to medium-sized choroidal vessels first and shortly after fill the larger choroidal vessels. This happens simultaneously with the rest of the transit phase. It is normal to find areas of delayed choroidal filling, referred to as a *watershed area*.

As the choroidal flush is occurring in the choroidal vasculature, the dye flows from the central retinal artery that enters the eye through the optic nerve and quickly reaches the smaller branches of arteries and into the capillaries. The *arterial phase* occurs when the dye is only in the arteries. From the capillaries, the dye transfers into surrounding tissue and then through the veins. In comparison, ICG dye is not as apparent in the retinal capillaries as FA dye. When dye enters the veins, it initially flows along the outer edges of the vein. This is called *laminar flow*. The arteriovenous phase occurs when the arteries still contain dye and the veins are in laminar flow. Once the middle of the veins are filled and brighter than the arteries, the *venous phase* has been reached. In a normal eye, the four divisions of the transit phase take place during the 40 to 45 seconds after the dye is injected.

The *mid-phase* starts 2 minutes after the injection (Figure 15-13B). The dye will have an even intensity between the arteries and veins during this phase. This is an ideal time to photograph the periphery. This phase is also referred to as the *recirculation phase*, as the dye is recirculating through the entire body before returning to the eye. The retinal vessel fluorescence will be very dim, and the choroidal vessels will have a more homogenous appearance.

The *late phase* (also called the *lates*) generally begins around 10 minutes (Figure 15-13C). Due to the dye no longer being present, the retinal structures will no longer be visible and the optic nerve will appear dark. The dye will begin to leave the choroidal vasculature as well, and the

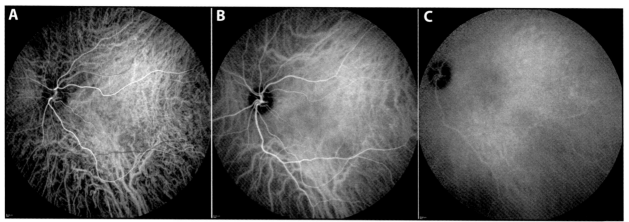

Figure 15-13. (A) Early/transit phase ICG, normal. (B) Mid-phase ICG, normal. (C) Late phase ICG, normal. (Reprinted with permission from Glen Jenkins, COA, CRA.)

larger choroidal vessels will appear dark in comparison to the smaller surrounding ones. (Some refer to the ICG late phase as the *inversion phase* due to this reversing of fluorescence.) Each physician has a preference for how long to document into the late phase, and it is often specific to the patient's diagnosis. Some physicians will request imaging as late as 20 to 30 minutes to be able to follow the inversion process to the end.

Clinical Skills

The step-by-step instructions for performing FAs can also be used for ICGAs with a few changes. Make sure that the proper infrared filters are engaged, use the correct dye, and focus on the choroid instead of the retina. Be sure to reduce exposure during the early phase to capture detail in the choroid. Since the inversion phase happens during minutes 10 to 20, communicate with the physician about how far out he/she would like the lates to be captured.

Performing an ICGA simultaneously with an FA, either by mixing the dyes or using a stopcock, adds another layer of complexity to capturing high quality FA/ICGAs. Be sure to adjust exposure and focus throughout the procedure (Table 15-3).

EXTERNAL PHOTOGRAPHY

Basic Sciences

A basic understanding of the anatomy and physiology of the brow, eyelid, and eye muscles is helpful when performing external photography. Please review these topics in Chapters 2 and 3.

There are many different manufacturers of digital cameras that can be used for external photography. While a point-and-shoot camera (or camera phone) with a built-in flash can be used to capture acceptable external images, the lack of controls for focus and illumination make them inferior to a digital single lens reflex (SLR) camera with a macro lens and ring flash.

Clinical Knowledge

External images are captured to document pathology to allow the physician to compare the images on future visits. Before and after surgery images can be especially helpful with patient education. External photos are also used to prove medical necessity to insurance companies for surgeries that can also be performed for cosmetic reasons. Some clinics take a headshot to include in every medical record for patient identification.

The two subspecialties in ophthalmology that routinely use external photography are plastics and neuro-ophthalmology. Plastic surgeons will most often request external images of ptosis (droopy lids), dermatochalasis (excess eyelid skin), or larger lesions on the lid, brow, nose, or face. Neuro-ophthalmologists will request images on patients with nerve palsies, muscle disorders, and thyroid eye disease.

Clinical Skills

Plan and prepare for the patient prior to performing external photography. While planning, mentally step through the image sequence. Should the magnification setting be wide enough to cover the entire face in the frame or narrow enough to just capture one eye at a time? Which direction should the patient's face (straight head, oblique, side) and head (straight, chin tilted down, or chin tilted up) be positioned? Should the patient's eyes be opened or closed? Is there enough three-dimensional information to justify taking stereo images as well?

It is important to have a consistent, blank background for external photography to provide distraction-free images and for documenting before/after shots. The

TABLE 15-3
STEPS FOR SIMULTANEOUS FLUORESCEIN AND INDOCYANINE GREEN ANGIOGRAPHY

Injector's Set-Up for ICGA and FA With Stopcock
1. Reconstitute the ICG dye and pull up into a syringe
2. Pull up FA dye into a syringe
3. Attach both syringes of dye and a syringe of saline to a four-way stopcock
4. Push the saline through all parts of the stopcock
5. Attach the butterfly needle to the stopcock and push the saline through it

Perform ICGA Earlies
6. Engage exciter and barrier filters for ICG
7. Increase the flash power
8. Set the ICG timer
9. Position patient for procedure including chin/forehead firmly in place
10. Injector finds vein
11. Align camera on the transit eye while focused on the choroid
12. Cue injector to begin
13. As the ICG dye first enters the body, take the control photograph
14. When the injector announces the dye is all in (5 to 10 seconds), take the second photograph
15. Early transit images captured every 2 to 3 seconds of posterior pole until about 30 seconds
16. Capture posterior pole photo of the nontransit eye
17. Check in with the patient to make sure he/she is doing OK; respond to any adverse reactions

Perform FA Earlies and Alternate Between FA and ICGA
18. Repeat Steps 6 through 17 (omitting Step 10), but with the FA filters, timer, and dye, and focus on the retina
19. After the FA earlies, switch back to ICG settings/focus for the ICG mids
20. After the ICG mids, switch back to the FA settings for the FA mids
21. After the FA mids, switch back for ICG lates round 1
22. After ICG lates, switch back to FA lates
23. After FA lates, switch back to ICG lates round 2

ideal set-up is one with a blue or white photographic backdrop made of a material designed to absorb the flash. Blue is often used in medical settings as it provides a nice contrast to the color of skin.

Before capturing images of the patient, take a photo of the patient's demographic sheet from the chart. Then perform photography following the imaging plan or protocol. Always start with lower magnification images first and increase magnification throughout the image series. Establish patient fixation with verbal commands. As most people naturally have a subtle head tilt, instruct the patient to straighten out his/her head. When using a macro lens, focus is determined by your working distance while rotating the ring that changes magnification. For each image, establish the magnification first and then slowly move forward and backward to find the proper focus prior to snapping the photo. To properly expose the image, adjust the aperture, shutter speed, ISO, and flash settings until the desired exposure has been found (Sidebar 15-4). Be sure to have the room lights on when capturing external images. Review images for quality and recapture until satisfied.

For diagnoses that are imaged frequently, discuss a standard imaging protocol with the physician. In order for the physician to compare images over time, a standard protocol is ideal. One standard protocol in neuro-ophthalmology is the nine directions of gaze. (See Figure 10-9 for an example.)

There are several challenges to capturing external photographs. A patient with ptosis or dermatochalasis will often tilt his/her chin up and even tighten the forehead muscles to lift the eyebrows in order to see. If necessary, show the patient in a mirror what this looks like and encourage him/her to keep the brows, lids, and chin down. Another challenge is that some patients may blink in the middle of every picture. Use the "blink trick" to capture blink-free images: Get everything set up, then ask the patient to close his/her eyes and open just before taking the picture. After a few tries, a blink-free image can usually be achieved.

are also part of a photo slit lamp set up. A reticle (grid, ruler, or other target) is inside the eyepiece as a tool for focusing the image (Sidebar 15-5).

Clinical Knowledge

When performing any test, it is important to recognize what a normal result looks like. Please review anterior segment anatomy (eyelids, conjunctiva, cornea, pupil, and lens) in Chapter 2. Understanding normal anterior segment anatomy is important in order to document what the physician requests.

Of the many subspecialties in ophthalmology, three routinely request slit lamp images. Plastic surgeons will most often request slit lamp images of lid lesions. Cornea ophthalmologists often document dry eye, corneal ulcers, cataracts, and postoperative complications. Glaucoma specialists may request images of malfunctioning blebs and occasionally narrow angles.

Clinical Skills

Similar to previous imaging modalities described in this chapter, plan and prepare for the patient prior to photography. When planning the image series, use a standard sequence to prevent missing any images. Such a protocol may need to be established with the physician for diagnoses that he/she requests most often. It's ideal to begin with lower magnification and diffuse lighting to capture the overall subject prior to using high magnification and special techniques to highlight the area of interest.

SLIT LAMP PHOTOGRAPHY

Basic Sciences

Slit lamp photography is a noninvasive method of documenting anterior segment pathology. It is considered by many to be the most challenging imaging modality because it is the only instrument that all physicians know how to use, and they expect the pictures to look the same as the view through the microscope.

There are multiple manufacturers of slit lamps; some of the systems are capable of capturing video in addition to images. As image quality has improved with mobile devices, there are also options to adapt these to a slit lamp.

The parts of the clinical slit lamp have been reviewed in Chapter 12. In addition to the basic slit lamp, a few parts are added specifically for imaging. A *beam splitter* is added to direct the image to both the eyepiece and to the camera. To allow for better spread of light, a *diffusing filter* is placed in front of the slit beam. There is also a *fill flash* feature that is designed to fill in the background of the image with diffuse light. The camera back and often a computer with software to save and organize the images

TABLE 15-4
SLIT LAMP PHOTOGRAPHY LIGHTING TECHNIQUES[8]

Technique	Area of Interest	Flash Intensity	Background Intensity	Background Angle	Slit Beam Width	Filter Position	Position of Slit
Diffuse	Conjunctiva	Low	50%	30° to 45°	Fully open	Diffusing	30°
	Lids	Low	50%	30° to 45°	Fully open	Diffusing	30°
	Cornea	High	50%	30° to 45°	Fully open	Diffusing	30°
Direct: Narrow slit	Conjunctiva	High	25%	30° to 45°	0.1 mm	N/A	45°
	Cornea	High	0% to 10%	45°	0.1 mm	N/A	45° to 60°
	Lens	High	25%	45°	0.1 mm	N/A	45°
	Vitreous	High	0% to 10%	45°	0.1 to 1 mm	N/A	45°
Direct: Wide slit tangential	Cornea	High	0% to 25%	45°	Fully open	N/A	60° to 80°
	Iris	High	0% to 10%	45°	Fully open	N/A	80°
	Lens	High	10%	45° to 60°	2 to 6 mm	N/A	45° to 60°
Indirect	Conjunctiva	High	10%	30° to 45°	2 to 4 mm	N/A	Decentered
	Iris	High	0% to 10%	N/A	1 to 2 mm	N/A	Decentered
Retro: From iris	Cornea	High	0%	N/A	1 to 2 mm	N/A	Decentered
Retro: From fundus	Lens	High	0%	N/A	2 mm	N/A	Decentered

Reprinted with permission by Haag-Streit International.

To perform slit lamp imaging, start by establishing the patient's fixation. If the slit lamp doesn't have a fixation device, ask the patient to look at your ear. Then if you want the patient to look to the side, either use your finger as a fixation device or give verbal instructions. Working distance (the space between the optics and the patient's eye) determines the focus. Move the base of the slit lamp forward in order to focus on the area of interest. Adjust the lighting according to protocol and capture the image using the shutter release.

Review images for quality to make sure the patient is looking in the proper place, the image is in focus, the exposure is set properly, and that the lighting technique has highlighted the pathology in the proper manner. Make changes to the settings and recapture the image if necessary. Exposure can be changed in several ways on a slit lamp: intensity of the fill light, intensity of the slit light, and aperture of the slit beam. While both the width and height of the slit beam are primarily used to shape the beam for the desired lighting technique, the shape of the slit also contributes to the exposure. As there are a variety of lighting techniques for slit lamp imaging, it's important to master each of them and know when it is best to apply them (Table 15-4).[8] (See also Chapter 12.)

In this chapter we will refer to only four basic types of illumination: diffuse, direct, indirect, and retro. In diffuse illumination the slit lamp beam is covered by the diffusing filter, and the fill flash is used to create even illumination over the subject. This is best used for low magnification overview images. Direct illumination uses a centered slit beam, and the focus is on the same plane as the slit beam light. This lighting technique is most commonly used to identify pathology. Indirect illumination is created by decentering the slit beam, but the focus is on a different plane from the slit beam light. This is often used to detect subtle changes in the cornea. Retroillumination is a type of indirect illumination where the light is reflected off of the fundus or iris to illuminate pathology from behind. This is most often used to view the lens or subtle changes in the cornea. Please refer to Chapter 12 for slit lamp photos of various ocular findings using different illumination techniques.

As pathology of the anterior segment can sometimes have a lot of dimension to it, capturing images in stereo can be helpful. Using diffuse light, capture the first image with the joystick to the left and the second image with the joystick moved to the right. No other changes should be made to the settings of the camera or the patient's fixation. View the images with stereo viewers to confirm a good three-dimensional view.

Topical stains can highlight subtle pathology to give the physician a better idea of the extent of damage. Apply the dye to the conjunctiva. To capture the best images with stains, take the pictures immediately after the patient blinks a couple of times to spread the dye over the eye. Corneal pathology stained with NaFl will appear yellow-green when imaged using a blue filter. The images are more saturated when the fill light is turned off, if you

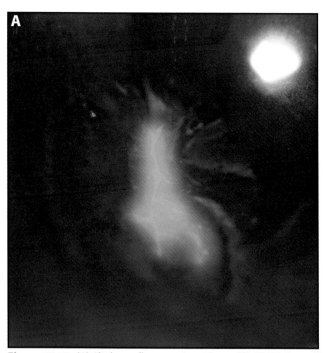 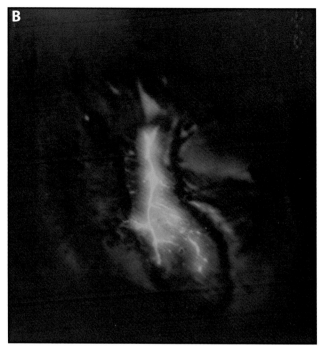

Figure 15-14. (A) Slit lamp fluorescein without fill. (B) Slit lamp fluorescein with fill.

are imaging pathology stained with NaFl (Figures 15-14A and B). Corneal and conjunctival pathology appears pink in color when stained with rose bengal and green when stained with lissamine green, both under diffuse white light.

ACKNOWLEDGMENTS

The author would like to thank the following: Debra Cantrell, COA; Rona Lyn Esquejo-Leon, CRA; Houston P. Sharpe III, COA, OCT-C; Timothy J. Bennett, CRA, OCT-C, FOPS; James Gilman, CRA, FOPS; Glen Jenkins, CRA, COA; and Michael P Kelly, FOPS.

CHAPTER QUIZ

1. True/False: Illumination controls the intensity of light that is used to capture the retina.

2. True/False: Dilation is not required for a mydriatic fundus camera.

3. When trying to set the reticle for fundus photography, it is best to look:
   a. into the distance
   b. at the magnification knob
   c. at the joystick
   d. at the computer

4. To establish patient fixation, it is best to start with:
   a. verbal commands
   b. the internal fixation device
   c. the external fixation device
   d. your ear

5. During fundus photography, if the image is unevenly saturated, you need to change the:
   a. focus
   b. working distance
   c. exposure
   d. illumination

6. If your fundus photographs have soft white circular artifacts on them, you need to clean the:
   a. internal lenses
   b. camera chip
   c. eyepiece
   d. lens

7. In monochromatic imaging, green light will highlight the:
   a. nerve fiber layer
   b. retina
   c. choroid
   d. sclera

8. It is best to capture digital stereo images in this sequence:
   a. left to right
   b. right to left
   c. front to back
   d. back to front

9. Using fundus autofluorescence imaging, the optic nerve and vessels of a normal patient appear:
   a. white
   b. black
   c. gray
   d. red

10. Fluorescein sodium is a:
    a. synthetic dye
    b. vegetable dye
    c. green dye
    d. shellfish dye

11. Which of the following is a type of hyperfluorescence?
    a. leakage
    b. pooling
    c. staining
    d. all of the above

12. Indocyanine green angiography is performed to view the:
    a. choroid
    b. optic nerve
    c. sclera
    d. iris

Answers

1. False, Exposure controls the intensity of light that is used to capture the retina.
2. False, Dilation is required for a mydriatic fundus camera.
3. a
4. c
5. b
6. d
7. b
8. a
9. b
10. a
11. d
12. a

REFERENCES

1. Morgan JIW, Pugh, EN. Scanning laser ophthalmoscope measurement of local fundus reflectance and autofluorescence changes arising from rhodopsin bleaching and regeneration. *Invest Ophthalmol Vis Sci*. 2013;54:2048-2059.

2. Yamamoto K, Zhou J, Hunter JJ, Williams DR, Sparrow JR. Toward an understanding of bisretinoid autofluorescence bleaching and recovery. *Invest Ophthalmol Vis Sci*. 2012;53:3536-3544.

3. Yannuzzi LA, Rohrer KT, Tindel LJ, et al. Fluorescein angiography complication survey. *Ophthalmology*. 1986;93(5):611-617.

4. IC-Green [package insert]. Lake Forest, IL: AKORN; 2012.

5. Hope-Ross M, Yannuzzi LA. Adverse reactions due to indocyanine green. *Ophthalmology*. 1994;101(3):529-533.

6. Morris P, Larsen C. Is indocyanine green choroidal angiography safe for diabetic patients taking metformin? *J Ophthalmic Photography*. 1998;20(2):43-44.

7. Flower RW, Hochheimer BF. A clinical technique and apparatus for simultaneous angiography of the separate retinal and choroidal circulations. *Invest Ophthalmol*. 1973;12(4):248-261.

8. Haag-Streit International. *Slit Lamp Imaging Guide: BX900 Photo Slit Lamp*. http://pdf.medicalexpo.com/pdf/haag-streit-diagnostics/imaging-guide-bx900/70767-91393.html. Bern, Switzerland: Haag-Streit International; 2005. Accessed July 4, 2016.

Unless otherwise noted, the figures in this chapter were contributed by the author, Sarah M. Armstrong.

16

DIAGNOSTIC IMAGING

Al Lens, COMT

Ophthalmic medical personnel are the primary users of diagnostic imaging equipment in ophthalmology. Advances in technology have really enhanced this aspect of ophthalmology. These tests are a vital part of patient care, and have been embraced by the eye care community.

LASER INTERFERENCE BIOMETRY

Basic Sciences

Laser interference biometry (LIB) has almost replaced the ultrasound A-scan to measure the axial length of the eye (from anterior cornea to retina). Because LIB is an optical form of biometry, some of the flaws of ultrasound are eliminated. For example, the speed of ultrasound varies in different media. This can be a problem if the patient has had previous intraocular surgery that changed the eye's natural structures, such as surgery to remove a cataract (with or without an intraocular lens [IOL]) or a procedure to replace the vitreous with silicone oil. LIB has proven to be more accurate in these situations. However, ultrasound is still useful in cases where the optical media (cornea/lens) have dense opacities, because the LIB has difficulties measuring in these cases. (Roughly 10% of eyes cannot be measured with LIB because the optical media is not sufficiently transparent.)

Another advantage of LIB is the increased likelihood of measuring the axial length to the macula rather than some other part of the eye. Using LIB, the patient views a fixation light with the eye that is being measured, so the measurement follows the line of sight. With ultrasound, it is quite possible to be off axis, causing an inaccurate measurement (especially in myopic eyes with a staphyloma [a bulge due to the tissues being stretched as well as to degeneration]) and a coinciding "refractive surprise" after surgery.

Built into the LIB is a method to measure corneal curvature, so separate keratometry is not necessary. Other measurements typically done using these instruments include white-to-white (corneal diameter) and anterior chamber depth. Some also measure corneal thickness, lens thickness, and pupil diameter.

There are various models of LIB available, including IOLMaster (Carl Ziess Meditec), Lenstar (Haag-Streit USA; Figure 16-1), Aladdin (Topcon Medical Systems, Inc), and AL-Scan (Nidek). The IOLMaster was first on the scene and enjoyed a monopoly for many years. Now, the competition is fierce, and this list may be incomplete as we go to press.

Ledford JK, Lens A, eds.
Principles and Practice in Ophthalmic Assisting:
A Comprehensive Textbook (pp 297-306).
© 2018 Taylor & Francis Group.

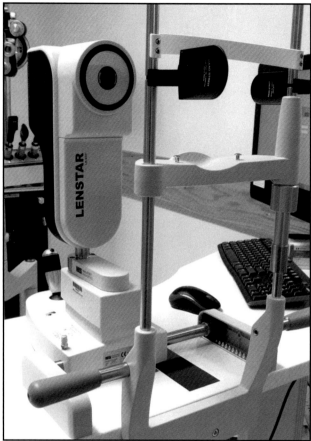

Figure 16-1. Lenstar laser interference biometer (Haag-Streit USA). (Reprinted with permission from Kim McQuaid, COMT.)

Clinical Knowledge

While modifications to the eye can affect LIB measurements as mentioned, it is not on the same magnitude as for ultrasound. For a pseudophakic eye, it is not necessary to know what type of material the IOL is made of when using LIB; just measure in the pseudophakic mode.

The LIB measures to the retinal pigment epithelium, which is a bit deeper than ultrasound (which uses the inner limiting membrane for its measurement). Most LIBs will make an adjustment for this difference so that the measurements are on par with ultrasound and can maintain the accuracy of IOL formulas. Practices switching from ultrasound to LIB should reassess their IOL constants (used in the formulas for IOL power selection), especially if a contact ultrasound probe was used (because the axial length may measure longer with the LIB).

IOL formulas are installed on the LIB unit, so IOL powers can be calculated without using a separate computer. However, if the preferred formula is not available on the LIB, then the data will need to be transferred to a separate computer. Some computer programs, however, can import the data directly from the LIB if they are connected.

Clinical Skills

All measurements are done without contacting the eye. For an eye that has a high refractive error and cannot see the fixation target, it may be better to measure through the patient's spectacles. Do not measure through a contact lens, because this will add the thickness of the contact lens to the axial length measurement.

The patient's sole task in the measurements is to look at the fixation target (which may change during the procedure). Central vision may be deficient if the patient has macular pathology, and the patient may struggle to fixate. Ultrasound biometry is more reliable in these cases.

CORNEAL TOPOGRAPHY

Basic Sciences

The average cornea has about 43 diopters of focusing power at its center. The cornea is aspheric, where the central curvature is the steepest and gradually gets flatter toward the edge of the cornea. Thus there is less focusing power in the periphery. The keratometer measures the corneal curvature, but only gives information at two points just off center. (See Chapter 21 for keratometry.) This is adequate if the cornea has no irregularities. However, for cases that are outside the norm or for a detailed study, a corneal topographer is the instrument of choice. As the name implies, it gives a topographical map of the cornea, providing a lot more information than keratometry.

The principle for *corneal topography* (also known as *photokeratoscopy* and *videokeratoscopy*) began as a simple Placido disk. The cornea reflects the concentric rings of the disk, and the examiner looks at the reflected rings to see if they are closer or farther apart in any area. When the space between the rings is narrowed, the curvature is steeper. Unfortunately, the examiner had to be fairly observant to notice subtle changes in the space between rings. So, corneoscopy was invented. This instrument combines an illuminated Placido disk and a Polaroid camera (PLR IP Holdings, LLC). This allows the examiner to view the Placido reflection in more detail (possibly with the help of a magnifying glass) and provides a photo for the patient's record. Still, most examiners could not detect mild abnormalities.

The next step was a computer that could analyze the photograph and assign numerical values to the rings, representing the radius of curvature in 72 points (along eight radial lines). However, the examiner was required to plot the edge of the rings and significant errors could occur.

Finally, computers took over the whole process (except basic alignment functions). Along with this evolution came the appearance of color topographical maps and the ability to diagnose conditions like keratoconus,

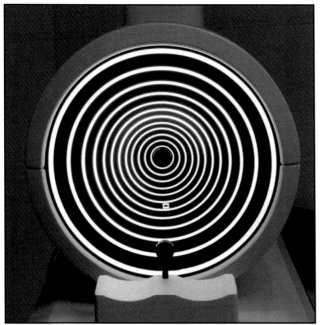

Figure 16-2. Placido disk-based topographer. (Reprinted with permission from Kim McQuaid, COMT.)

pellucid marginal degeneration (a type of corneal degeneration), and post-surgery ectasia (a bulging forward of a cornea that was thinned by surgeries like photorefractive keratectomy and LASIK). Such mapping is also excellent for contact lens fitters and refractive surgeons. Early models were based on the Placido disk; some current models still use this design (Figure 16-2). The more advanced systems use either a scanning slit or Scheimpflug imaging (a complex imaging system that creates a sharp image across the eye despite the curvature of the cornea); these allow mapping the posterior corneal curvature and determining corneal thickness.

Clinical Knowledge

Placido-based systems are useful tools to have in practices that do not offer refractive surgery. Because these instruments require a reflection of the disk to do their calculations, the cornea must be clear of any pathology or condition that inhibits its reflective characteristics. Thus, a dry eye can be problematic. Some Placido-based corneal topographers perform curvature calculations beginning with the innermost ring and then each subsequent ring; if a portion of one ring is missing, the adjacent rings cannot be calculated. Other than being lower priced than other systems, Placido topography units also have the advantage of capturing images very quickly.

Elevation-based systems use either a scanning slit or a rotating Scheimpflug camera (Figure 16-3). Both types take a couple of seconds to acquire the images and provide information about the anterior and posterior curvatures of the cornea, as well as corneal thickness across the

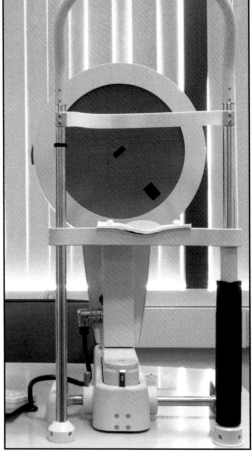

Figure 16-3. Elevation-based corneal topographer. (Reprinted with permission from Kim McQuaid, COMT.)

entire cornea. Technically, these should be called corneal *tomographers* rather than topographers since they gather cross-section images of the cornea. Unless combined with a Placido disk (like the Galilei [Ziemer Group]), these methods are not influenced by the tear film and provide more accurate results in dry eyes.

Clinical Skills

Obtaining measurements varies quite a bit between instruments, although the basic task is to align the instrument and obtain clear focus. Instruments with a larger Placido disk will require a larger palpebral fissure (ie, patients need to open their eyes wide). If the patient cannot elevate the upper lid adequately, then the examiner may use a finger to do so. (Do not allow the patient to do this.) Care must be taken to not exert any pressure on the eyeball as this will distort the shape of the cornea. It may be necessary to turn the patient's nose away from the disk in order to prevent the nose from blocking the reflection.

Once the measurement has been obtained, the results need to be displayed as a printout or digital file. Most physicians will have a preferred display for the majority of

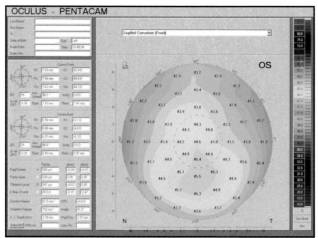

Figure 16-4. Corneal topography sagittal map (Oculus Inc, USA).

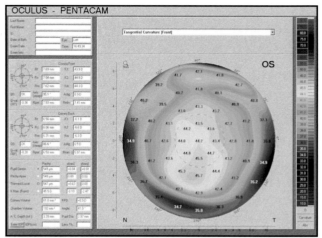

Figure 16-5. Corneal topography tangential map (Oculus Inc, USA).

cases. There are two display scales: absolute and relative. Absolute (or standardized) scales apply the same colors to the same range of curvature for every eye: green on the map represents a normal curvature (compared to the average cornea), hotter colors are for steeper than normal curvatures, and colder colors for flatter.

If using the relative (normalized) scale, the examiner will be able to adjust the amount of curvature change required to alter the map's colors. A 0.25 diopter step between color changes will show lots of detail as long as there is not a huge range from the flattest to steepest parts of the cornea. It may be necessary to use larger steps (0.50 or 1.0 diopters, or more) when there is a diverse range of curvatures.

Some units are equipped with software that has specialized data related to keratoconus. This is beneficial to use whenever there is steepening of the cornea below the visual axis (referred to as *inferior steepening*).

Another change that can be made to the display is switching between tangential and sagittal algorithms. Sagittal (axial) maps (Figure 16-4) are based on changes compared to a perfect sphere. They are not as sensitive to abnormalities as the tangential maps. The tangential algorithm (Figure 16-5) calculates the curvature of the cornea on a more localized level, making it more sensitive to irregularities, but can make it less reproducible on repeated measurements.

Patient Services

Dry eye or any other corneal surface irregularity can pose a problem with Placido disk systems. It is best to instill balanced salt solution (BSS) or a saline solution prior to testing rather than artificial tears because BSS does not have the viscosity (thickness) of artificial tears and is less likely to alter the outcome of topography. If

BSS or saline is not available, use an artificial tear with low viscosity.

Patients will often express an interest in the print-outs from corneal topography. Discussing these reports on a purely technical level is permissible, but care must be taken to not discuss any possible diagnosis. You may describe what the colors mean (eg, hotter colors representing a steeper curvature), but you should refrain from comparing the patient's result to what is considered normal. Diagnoses and comparisons are the physician's purview.

OPTICAL COHERENCE TOMOGRAPHY
Basic Sciences

Optical coherence tomography (OCT) uses near-infrared light to create high-resolution cross-section imaging of the retina. Anterior segment OCT uses a higher wavelength of light that allows analysis of the sclera, conjunctiva, cornea, anterior chamber, iris, and angle structures. Because the instrument uses light for its imaging, media opacities (eg, dense cataract or vitreous hemorrhage) can interfere with the image quality.

OCT can be performed in either time domain or spectral domain. Most new OCT models are spectral domain (Figure 16-6), which uses a spectrometer and collects signals from all depths of the tissue simultaneously. This shortens the image capture time and thereby decreases artifacts due to patient movement. It also collects more information than the time-domain models.

For anterior segment OCT, there are benefits to the time-domain modality, mainly that it can penetrate more deeply (up to 6 mm compared to about 2 mm for spectral domain). This is effective for assessing the iris and structures behind it. However, the trade-off for the deeper penetration is that there is less resolution.

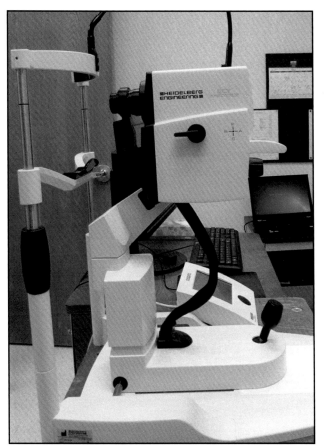

Figure 16-6. Spectral domain optical coherence tomographer (Heidelberg Engineering). (Reprinted with permission from Kim McQuaid, COMT.)

OCT is most commonly done to assess the macula for various pathologies such as a macular hole or pucker, macular degeneration, central serous retinopathy, macular edema, or vitreomacular traction. It can also be used to assess optic nerve disorders like glaucoma.

Anterior segment OCT is not as commonly performed as posterior segment OCT. It may be needed to evaluate the position or status of the haptics (flexible stabilizing "arms") of an IOL, look for ruptured zonules, examine corneal pathology (especially after LASIK or corneal transplant surgery), analyze tumors or cysts, and assess the anterior chamber's angle structure.

Clinical Knowledge

Normal Findings

A normal OCT has a characteristic appearance (Figure 16-7). The vitreous is not reflective, so it is represented as a large dark space. The fovea is easily identified as a depression. The retinal epithelium and nerve fiber layers are highly reflective and display as a hotter color (usually red). The layers between the nerve fiber layer and

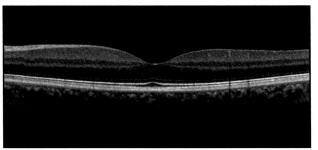

Figure 16-7. Normal OCT scan of the macular area.

retinal epithelium are not very reflective and are not easily identified in the OCT scan. There is a dark space just in front of the retinal pigment epithelium that represents the photoreceptor layer.

Common Abnormalities

Macular pathology is sometimes easily visible, but not always. The OCT is used to follow the presence and progression of retinal disease and aid in the diagnosis of more subtle macular pathology.

Macular edema shows decreased reflectivity in the macular area and thickening of the retina (Figure 16-8).

A *macular hole* will be seen as a dark space in the area of the rupture (Figure 16-9). There is also some thickening in the area around the macular hole.

An *epiretinal membrane* shows a highly reflective, thin membrane in front of the retina. The OCT can reveal the membrane's thickness and the location where it adheres to the retina (Figure 16-10).

In the case of *vitreomacular traction*, the vitreous that is pulling away from the retina will show a thin line of vitreous in front of the retina that is not present in front of the macula (Figure 16-11).

The retinal pigment epithelium is highly reflective, so when it detaches from Bruch's membrane (*pigment epithelium detachment*), the red/orange line on the OCT will separate/bulge away from the underlying retina, leaving a dark space beneath it (Figure 16-12). Of course, the overlying tissue will bulge forward, too.

There are three primary types of *retinal detachment*: exudative, tractional, and rhegmatogenous, with the last being the most common. An OCT is not required in order to diagnose the retinal detachment, but it is useful to determine if the macula is "on" or "off" (ie, whether the retinal detachment has involved the macula or not; Figure 16-13) as that impacts the urgency of treatment.

The OCT can be used to monitor the progression of glaucoma. It has somewhat limited capabilities in discriminating early stages of glaucoma, but can detect more advanced glaucoma. The retinal nerve fiber layer thickness is measured with the OCT; a sign of glaucoma is a thinning of the retinal nerve fiber layer. Glaucoma is covered in detail in Chapter 29.

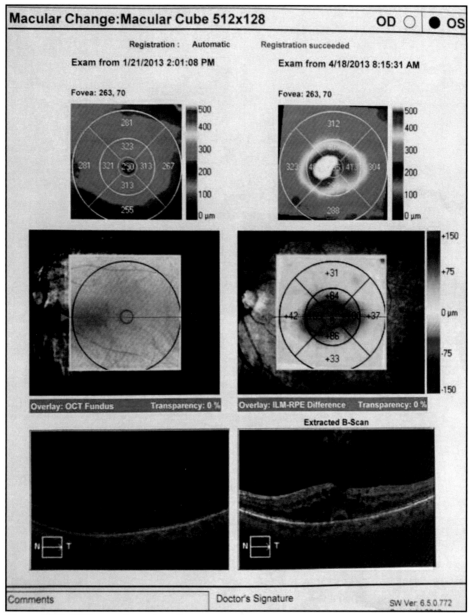

Figure 16-8. OCT scan of macular edema.

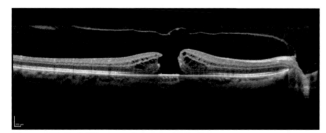

Figure 16-9. OCT scan of a macular hole.

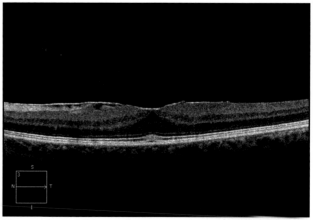

Figure 16-10. OCT scan of an epiretinal membrane.

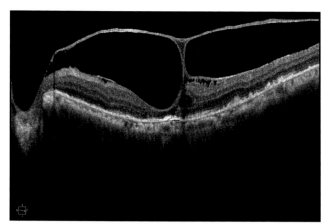

Figure 16-11. OCT scan of vitreomacular traction. (Reprinted with permission from Amy Désirée Goldstein, CRA, OCT-C.)

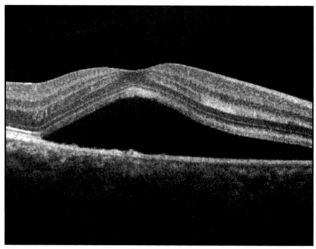

Figure 16-12. OCT scan of pigment epithelium detachment.

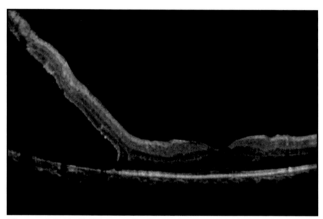

Figure 16-13. OCT scan of a "macula on" retinal detachment.

Clinical Skills

After turning on the OCT's computer, the scanning software may launch automatically, or you might need to select the appropriate icon to initialize the instrument. Enter the patient's information into the program.

Position the patient comfortably on the chinrest with forehead against the headrest. Adjust the height of the chinrest so the lateral canthus is aligned with the canthus marker on the support, and raise or lower the table height as needed for the patient's comfort.

Direct the patient to look at the fixation target. Use the joystick to align the camera, centering on the area of interest (usually the macula or optic disc). Then use the fine-tuning adjustment (micromanipulator) knobs to refine the centering. Use the focus knob(s) to adjust for the patient's refractive error. Choose the acquisition pattern desired, and use the control to activate the scan.

CONFOCAL SCANNING LASER OPHTHALMOSCOPY

Basic Sciences

Two primary features of glaucoma are thinning of the retinal nerve fiber layer and an enlarged and/or notched optic disc cup. In some cases, early thinning of the retinal nerve fiber layer precedes visual field defects. The Heidelberg Retina Tomograph (HRT; Heidelberg Engineering; Figure 16-14) is a confocal scanning laser ophthalmoscope (SLO) mainly used to analyze the retinal nerve fiber layer (RNFL) and cupping of the optic disc. It can be used to help confirm the diagnosis of glaucoma as well as aid in following the progression of the disease.

The HRT can also be equipped with a retina module for imaging the macula. Using this module, it is possible to detect subtle swelling (edema) in the macula. In the absence of an OCT, this is a useful tool to have for assessing the macula.

Clinical Knowledge

The confocal scanning laser ophthalmoscope uses laser light (670 nm) to scan the retina. To increase the sharpness of the image, the reflected light is directed through a pinhole placed at the focal point of the lens. Unless the pupil is very small, dilation is not required. The series of two-dimensional images collected during the scan are then transformed into a three-dimensional image by the unit's software.

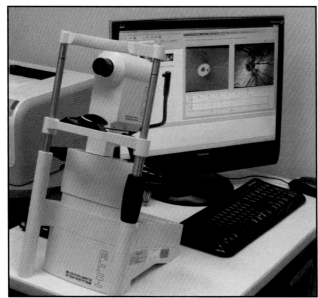

Figure 16-14. The Heidelberg Retina Tomograph (Heidelberg Engineering).

Using the glaucoma module, the software can analyze the results and compare them to a database of the normal population. This comparison is reflected in the printout. The optic nerve head is divided into six sectors, each displayed with a green check mark, a yellow exclamation point, or a red X, denoting if that sector is within normal limits, borderline, or outside normal limits, respectively.

With the retina module, the software can assess edema (even if it is not visible using conventional methods), retinal thickness, and retinal reflectance.

Clinical Skills

Conducting the Scan

Enter (or recall) patient data, select desired acquisition. Affix the appropriate cylinder lens over the aperture, if needed to correct astigmatism. Align the patient with the scanner's lens about 10 mm from eye, patient looking straight ahead.

A small pupil or opaque media will likely require dilation. Dry eye often causes decreased vision and reduces the quality of images. Artificial tears may be useful prior to the scan.

For the glaucoma module, the patient is asked to look at the red box, then inward (toward the nose) to find the green light.

Adjust the focus, and press the acquisition button. The instrument automatically continues to collect images until three useful images are captured.

Image Analysis

Using the computer mouse, mark out the edge of the optic disc (also referred to as *drawing the contour line*). It is recommended to plot six to eight points on the edge of the optic disc, selecting the same number of points on each side. Print the physician's desired reports.

When at least two images are captured from separate visits, the software can be used to compare changes between visits. When three or more images are available for an eye, a progression analysis can be performed.

SPECULAR MICROSCOPY

Basic Sciences

Corneal anatomy is covered in Chapter 2. The layer of the cornea assessed with the specular microscope is the endothelium. This layer is responsible for drawing moisture out of the cornea to help maintain its clarity. Unfortunately, these cells are not capable of reproducing. As endothelial cells die through aging or trauma, the remaining cells enlarge to compensate for the lost cells. The human cornea has 3000 to 4000 cells/mm² at birth. When the cell population falls below 500/mm², there is a high risk of corneal swelling that impairs vision and can cause pain.

Ideally, endothelial cells are hexagonal in shape and uniform in size. *Polymegathism* (Figure 16-15) exists when the cells have variable sizes. Because there is a natural loss of cells over time, there is a certain amount of polymegathism that is expected, more so later in life. This usually occurs in conjunction with *pleomorphism* (Figure 16-16), which is a variation in shape as the cells morph to fill empty spaces.

Clinical Knowledge

While the endothelium is visible with the slit lamp microscope, there is not adequate detail to properly analyze the cells. *Specular microscopy* is performed to assess the population, size, and shape of the endothelial cells. It also provides a record for the patient's file so changes can be noted over time.

Specular microscopes utilize specular reflection to illuminate the mirror-like surface of the endothelium. (This is in contrast to diffuse reflection, which is the reflection of light from a rough surface such as clothing.) The space between the cells appears as a dark line, making it possible to view the shape and size of each cell using the high magnification of the microscope.

Specular microscopes come in contact and noncontact varieties. Some are automatic, requiring very basic skills by the operator. Others are manually operated. Some specular microscopes have larger fields of view than others.

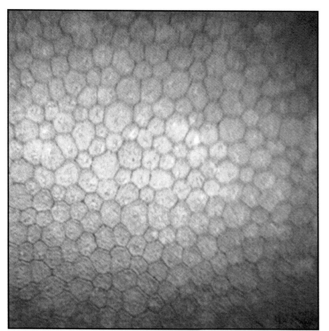

Figure 16-15. Specular microscope photo showing polymegathism, where cells are of varying sizes but retain their hexagonal shape.

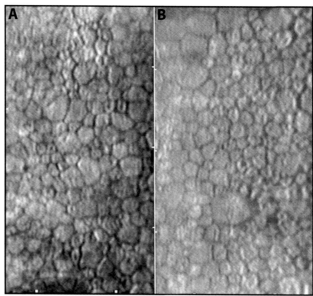

Figure 16-16. Specular microscope photo showing (A) polymegathism with variable cell sizes and (B) pleomorphism, where cells vary in shape in order to fill empty spaces.

Indications for a scan include any endothelial abnormality, thicker than average corneas, preoperatively for intraocular or refractive surgery, postoperative management, and extended contact lens wear.

Clinical Skills

Conducting the Scan

Instill anesthetic eye drop if using the contact method. Position the patient in the chinrest with the forehead against the headrest. Instruct the patient to hold still and look at the fixation target.

Focus and capture images in the center, mid-periphery, and periphery. Analyze the image for size, shape, and number of cells.

There are situations where there may be difficulties in obtaining a scan. It may be poor fixation, a thickened cornea, or corneal opacities that prevent a clear view. The presence of guttata (nodular-shaped collagen secretions) causes dark areas absent of visible cells. In the case of pathology, it may be possible to get a better view by moving to a different area of the cornea.

Image Analysis

There are several methods of counting the cells: the frame method (also called fixed or variable), center-to-center method, corner method, and comparison method (Figure 16-17).

Counting cells with the *frame method* involves selecting a frame size on the computer then counting the cells within the frame. Cells that touch the edge of the frame are counted on two adjacent edges and ignored on the other two. Accuracy increases with the size of the frame.

The *center-to-center method* is the most common technique. The examiner selects the center of each cell within a certain area. The number of cells counted is chosen by the examiner (minimum 150 is recommended), but all adjacent cells must be marked. Accuracy improves with the number of cells chosen. The software will determine the cells per square millimeter after the cells are marked.

The *corner method* determines the cell area by selecting the corners of each cell. The analysis software then determines the size and dimension of the cells. The *comparison method* compares the cell pattern to a known honeycomb pattern for various cell densities.

The most common reason for inaccurate results is related to improper analysis of the captured image. The examiner may miss some cells, or perhaps count some cells more than once. If the device has automated analysis, the examiner needs to recognize when the software has traced the cell borders inaccurately. Another source of error is a poor quality image, making it difficult to correctly identify cells.

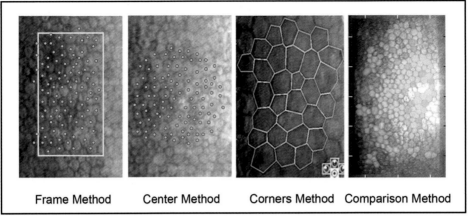

Figure 16-17. Cell-counting methods using specular microscopy.

CHAPTER QUIZ

1. Laser interference biometry is used to measure:

    a. axial length
    b. retinal nerve fiber layer
    c. macular pathology
    d. all of the above

2. Which of the following is *true* regarding the "absolute scale" in corneal topography?

    a. it reveals irregularities in the cornea that are not otherwise detectable
    b. it is required for all display outputs
    c. it utilizes the tangential algorithm
    d. it matches the same colors to the same range of curvature for every eye

3. Optical coherence tomography is most commonly used for:

    a. corneal topography
    b. axial length measurement
    c. macular pathology
    d. crystalline lens opacity quantification

4. What is the density of endothelial cells of the average cornea at birth?

    a. 500 to 1000 mm²
    b. 1000 to 2000 mm²
    c. 2000 to 3000 mm²
    d. 3000 to 4000 mm²

5. What causes dark areas in specular microscopy?

    a. improper technique
    b. guttata
    c. pleomorphism
    d. polymegathism

6. The primary use of the Heidelberg Retina Tomograph is:

    a. retinal topography
    b. optic disc/retinal nerve fiber layer analysis
    c. assessing severity of retinal detachment
    d. retinal blood flow analysis

Answers

1. a
2. d
3. c
4. d
5. b
6. b

Unless otherwise noted, the figures in this chapter were contributed by the following, who are associated with this book as authors:
Sergina M. Flaherty: Figures 16-8, 16-12
Al Lens: Figures 16-4, 16-5, 16-14 through 16-17
Adeline Stone: Figures 16-7, 16-9, 16-10, 16-13

17

OPHTHALMIC ULTRASOUND

Monique Rinke, COMT
Laura Barry, BSc, COMT

Ophthalmic ultrasound has been around since approximately 1956.[1] Prior to that, the development of ultrasound can be traced back to the Currie brothers in the late 1880s,[2] and more fine-tuning of the art of diagnostic medical ultrasound was done in the 1940s and 1950s.[3]

The practice of using ultrasound in ophthalmology as a diagnostic tool is called *echography* or *ultrasonography*. These terms can be used interchangeably. Ophthalmic ultrasound is an important diagnostic tool. The various types of ophthalmic ultrasounds are invaluable for imaging through opaque media, quantifying lesions, and measuring ocular structures and dimensions. This chapter will discuss the basic physics of ophthalmic ultrasound, as well as various instruments and examination techniques. A-scan biometry, B-scan, ultrasound biomicroscopy (UBM), standardized A-scan, and pachymetry will be included. (Optical biometry, a method of measuring axial length using light instead of sound, is discussed in Chapter 16.)

BASIC SCIENCES

Physical Principles of Ultrasound

Ultrasound has many applications in both everyday life and the medical field. For example, some denture cleaners, jewelry cleaners, and instrument sterilizers use ultrasound. These devices, used on inanimate objects, tend to have low frequencies and high powers. Ultrasound used in medicine can be therapeutic and diagnostic. Physiotherapy, for example, uses a therapeutic frequency to treat soft tissue injuries. In this case, the frequency is low but the intensity is high to produce the acoustic wave, which in turn creates heat. The amount of energy or power can be adjusted as needed. Diagnostic ultrasound, on the other hand, uses a higher frequency with low power that cannot be adjusted, and does not create heat.

Ophthalmology uses diagnostic ultrasound. The frequency of ophthalmic ultrasound is high and the wavelength is short, allowing for greater visualization of ocular structures without damaging any tissue. In order to have a basic understanding of how ultrasound works and why images and results look the way they do, there are some principles and physics that need to be discussed.

Sound and Frequency

Sound is formed by waves that bounce off of a surface. As these vibrations form, the oscillating waves hit the ear, and sound is perceived. The normal human ear is able to perceive sound with a frequency of less than 20 KHz. (One hertz is 1 oscillation/second [o/s]; 20 KHz is 20,000 o/s.) Ultrasound uses frequencies much higher

Ledford JK, Lens A, eds.
Principles and Practice in Ophthalmic Assisting:
A Comprehensive Textbook (pp 307-334).
© 2018 Taylor & Francis Group.

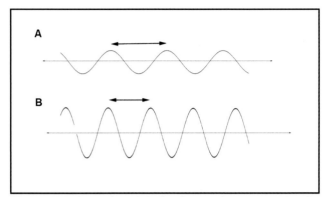

Figure 17-1. A wavelength is the distance between peaks of a waveform. (A) A long wavelength and (B) a short wavelength.

TABLE 17-1	
VELOCITIES AND DENSITIES	
Structure	**Velocity (m/s)**
Lens	1641
Aqueous/vitreous	1532
Average (aphakic)	1550

than 20 KHz. Abdominal ultrasound is in the range of 1 to 5 MHz (megahertz, or one million hertz). Ophthalmic ultrasound ranges from 8 to 20 MHz for A-scan biometry, B-scan, and standardized A-scan, and up to 100 MHz for high-frequency ultrasound, which images the anterior segment. (This is commonly referred to as *ultrasound biomicroscopy* [UBM] and usually uses 35 to 50 MHz.)

Wavelengths

Different ultrasound frequencies produce different wavelengths. A *wavelength* is defined as the distance between any two similar points on two consecutive cycles of a sound wave (Figure 17-1). Higher frequencies have shorter wavelengths and, in turn, increased absorption and resolution (both discussed momentarily). A shorter wavelength will gather more information as it moves forward, because the wave passes through more of the structure. Therefore, the visualization of small ocular and orbital anatomy is possible. Due to the increased absorption, the penetration into the tissue is low, which is good in the case of ocular structures since they are located close to the surface of the body. In other areas of medicine, ultrasound is used to image larger structures in the abdomen, pelvis, chest, and throat. These instruments use lower frequencies, have longer wavelengths, and therefore the sound waves penetrate deeper since they are not absorbed as well.

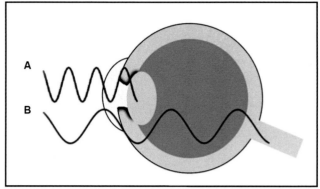

Figure 17-2. (A) A high frequency probe (35 to 40 Mhz) creates a shorter waveform that does not penetrate as deeply into the tissue. (B) A lower frequency probe (10 mHz) has a longer wavelength, and therefore penetrates more deeply.

Resolution

Resolution is the quality or sensitivity of the image based on the structure's size and distance from the wave source. It is the smallest distance between two interfaces that can be displayed, and is dependent on the type of transducer that is used. A *transducer* is the part of an ultrasound probe that sends and receives sound waves. The higher the frequency of the transducer, the shorter the wavelength emitted, the better the resolution achieved, and the less the penetration of the sound wave through the tissue (Figure 17-2).

Attenuation and Absorption

As sound moves through structures, some of the energy is *attenuated* (lost). Attenuation can depend on the medium the sound passes through, the frequency of sound, and absorption and/or reflectivity. A high amount of absorption creates heat in the exposed tissues. During ophthalmic diagnostic ultrasound, the amount of energy absorbed is extremely low, and therefore does not harm the ocular structures. In addition, the velocity of sound through a tissue or structure also plays a role in the amount of absorption. Higher velocities and greater tissue thickness result in greater absorption of the sound waves.

Velocity

Velocity is the speed at which sound travels through media. (This would be tissue when discussing ultrasound.) As the sound waves pass through the interface (junction) of two tissues, the velocity changes based on the density of the medium (Table 17-1). For example, water (which is very compressible) causes sound to travel relatively slower than less compressible materials such as bone, through which sound travels very quickly. The product of density and velocity of a tissue is known as *acoustic impedance*. As a sound wave travels through the eye, each interface it encounters will produce an echo.

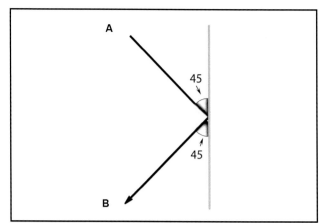

Figure 17-3. The angle of incidence (A) is equal to the angle of reflection (B).

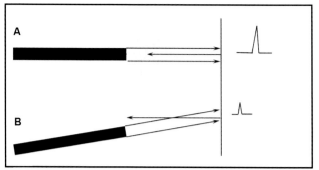

Figure 17-4. (A) High echo from sound beam that is perpendicular to the surface. (B) Lower echo from sound beam oblique to the surface.

The strength of the echo will depend on the difference in the acoustic impedance between the two interfaces. A strong echo is produced if the difference between tissues is high, because more energy is returned or reflected back to the probe.

Reflectivity

Reflectivity is defined as the strength of the echo produced when a sound wave passes through various interfaces. In addition to acoustic impedance, there are a number of other factors that affect the strength or reflectivity of the echo or image. The amount of reflectivity affects how much sound is attenuated.

The direction or angle at which the sound beam is directed through a tissue will affect the strength of the echo. Remembering that the angle of incidence equals the angle of reflection (Figure 17-3). The more perpendicular the incident sound wave is to the interface, the higher the strength of the echo will be because most of the energy is reflected back to the probe (Figure 17-4). The opposite is true if the incident sound beam is oblique to an interface. More energy is being reflected away at the oblique angle, producing a weaker echo.

The size, shape, and smoothness of an interface influence the strength of the echo. For example, very small particles or a bumpy surface will scatter most of the incident sound beam. What is reflected back is very weak, producing a weak echo. This is what happens when sound waves are directed through a vitreous hemorrhage. If the interface is smooth and flat, like the retina, then most of the sound is reflected, producing a stronger echo (see Figure 17-4).

Gain

Gain is the adjustment of the amplification of the echoes (in decibels [db]) displayed on the screen. Simply put, it is like adjusting the volume on a stereo. Sound is present as long as the stereo is on and therefore volume can

be adjusted. Changing the gain is changing the intensity or sensitivity of the image that has already been produced. If the gain is high, there is lots of information on the screen (ie, lots of volume from the stereo). If the gain is turned down, weaker echoes lose definition. Gain is frequently adjusted when performing A-scan biometry and B-scan ultrasound to better visualize the image. Decreasing the gain will improve resolution but decrease sensitivity. The only time gain is not adjusted and is set at a standardized number is when performing standardized A-scan. Standardized A-scan is used to evaluate tissue (pathology).

Ultrasound in Ophthalmology

Ocular ultrasound is a quick, cost-effective, painless technique used to visualize the eye and orbit. Since ultrasound reflects off tissue, it is widely used to examine structures not easily seen because they are obscured by other structures or pathology. Ultrasound can also be used for accurate measurements of length or thickness of structures, for inspecting the anatomy in the eye and orbit, and to assess tissue characteristics and pathology.

There are a multitude of instruments available to perform ophthalmic ultrasound. The manner in which the images are processed and displayed is unique to each of them. There are two common types of displays used, the A-scan and B-scan.

A-scan is *amplitude* modulated and produces a one-dimensional, linear image. As the single beam passes through the ocular tissues, a single echo is produced for each interface. A-scan biometry is used for axial length measurement, with a focused beam of 10 to 12 mHz. B-scan is a *brightness* modulated image represented by a series of dots, or multiple A-scans. It is a two-dimensional image produced by a focused, oscillating transducer in the range of 10 MHz, or at a higher frequency in the range of 35 to 100 MHz. The difference in A and B probes is demonstrated in Figure 17-5. A- and B-scans will be discussed at length in the following sections. Finally, standardized A-scan has a special probe that uses an unfocused or parallel beam to assess, differentiate, and measure tissue.

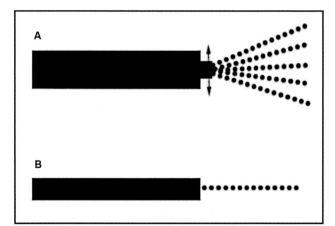

Figure 17-5. (A) B-scan transducer oscillates back and forth producing multiple A-scans over a surface. (B) Biometry (A-scan) probe measures to one point on a surface.

All instruments that use ultrasound for examination require a transducer in the form of a probe, a system to receive the information, a processor, and a screen to display the information.

The probe is required to emit a pulse of energy, pause (for microseconds), and then receive echoes back. This is called a *pulse-echo system*. In order for this to occur, a *piezoelectric element* must be present. This element is generally in the form of a small, thin piece of quartz or a thin ceramic plate. When electricity is applied to it, the element bends or vibrates and the reverse is true: Vibrations cause electrical energy to be produced. The initial vibration sends sound waves through the medium. Then as the transducer pauses, it can receive the reflected waves back, which cause the element to vibrate and create electrical energy. This electrical signal is sent to the receiver, where it is processed, amplified, and then displayed on a screen as an image. All of this occurs very quickly and is very complex.

There are two other important points about the probe. Resolution is not only dependent on the frequency of the transducer, but also on the size of the structures as well as spatial resolution. *Spatial resolution* describes how far apart structures must be in order to show up as separate entities. Ophthalmic ultrasound uses a probe with short pulses and high frequency (more cycles per second); therefore, more points on the interface will be imaged. This improves axial resolution (the ability to display two separate structures along the axis of the directed sound beam). Second, the transducer produces either a focused beam or parallel beam. A focused beam requires a lens placed close to the transducer to help focus the beam. The focal length of this lens will vary with instruments. The image will be most clear in the focal zone (defined as the *depth of field* [DOF]). For regular 10 MHz B-scan the focal length will usually be about the distance from the cornea to the retina. The DOF will be a certain distance in front and behind the retina. For a 50-MHz probe the focal length will be more anterior, like the iris margin, and the DOF will be a distance in front

and behind that. A focused beam produces better lateral resolution, which is the ability to display structures that are side by side, or perpendicular to the sound wave. A parallel beam, like that of the standardized A-scan probe, shows structures that are side by side as one image, yielding poor lateral resolution.

In more recent years, three-dimensional high-frequency B-scan instruments are becoming more widely used. These instruments commonly image the anterior segment and are in the range of 20 to 100 MHz. This is called *ultrasound biomicroscopy* (UBM). The most common frequencies are in the range of 35 to 50 MHz. There is also a posterior segment high-frequency probe that uses a 20-MHz frequency. The 20-MHz posterior segment probe provides somewhat better visualization and resolution of smaller pathology like retinal tears and macular pathology.

Color Doppler imaging (CDI) has been an important development in ultrasonography for detecting blood flow. Movement of the blood in relation to the transducer reveals the direction of blood flow. This blood flow pattern is displayed as color, usually red and blue, which signifies either flow toward or away from the transducer. This color image can be superimposed with the B-scan image, which aids in localization.

While fluorescein angiography is excellent at imaging and assessing retinal vascular disorders, conventional B-scan ultrasonography is useful for evaluating membranes as well as intraocular and orbital tumors. In some of these cases, further information can be provided using CDI. Small blood vessels, vascular tumors, and other vascular structures can be easily assessed with CDI. For example, in central retinal artery occlusion, CDI can show calcification of the blood vessel walls. It can provide information on the blood flow of the posterior ciliary artery in patients with primary open angle glaucoma. CDI may also be helpful in preoperative assessment of large vessels in orbital lesions. CDI is not commonly available in most ophthalmology clinics. Therefor,e it is not discussed further in this chapter.

CLINICAL KNOWLEDGE

A-Scan Biometry

The eye is an optical system; the power of the cornea, the power of the lens, as well as the axial length, contribute to the overall refractive state of the eye. A-scan biometry is used to measure the axial length of the eye. (The *axial length* is the length of the eye, from the cornea to the macula, ideally measured through the visual axis.) Axial length is part of the data used to select the power of intraocular lens (IOL) that is implanted during cataract surgery (see Chapter 28) or in other procedures where the natural lens of the eye is removed and an IOL put in its place. See Sidebar 17-1.

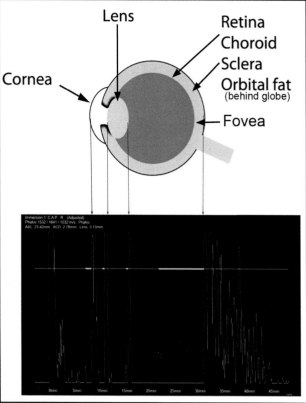

Figure 17-6. Probe aimed toward the eye, demonstrating sound traveling through the eye. The spikes (echoes) represent the interfaces of the eye.

The relatively simple geometry of the eye allowed ophthalmic biometry to be one of the first ultrasounds used on the body. By the mid-1970s, A-scan biometry became an essential component of cataract surgery, and two techniques evolved: immersion and contact.

Patient expectations after cataract surgery are often high, and accurate axial length measurements are required. More recently, biometry is also used to calculate for clear lens extraction surgery. This type of refractive surgery involves replacing a patient's natural noncataractous lens with an IOL to correct the patient's refractive state.

There are two types of axial biometry performed today. The first is biometry using ultrasound waves, and the second is biometry using light waves and laser interference biometry (eg, IOLMaster, discussed in Chapter 16).

Ultrasonic pachymetry, the measurement of the thickness of the cornea, uses the same principles of A-scan biometry. Stand-alone and hand-held pachymeters are available. There are other pachymeters that do not use ultrasound, such as OCT and topographers.

Principles of A-Scan Biometry

As discussed previously, A-scan biometry is a one-dimensional sound wave that represents only one point in space. When a biometry probe is placed on the eye, the ultrasound beam travels through the ocular structures. This process produces the one-dimensional amplitude-related image on the display that shows upward deflections from the baseline of the scan. These upward

deflections, or spikes, are known as *interfaces*, and represent the change of the ultrasound wave from one tissue to a tissue of a different density.

To acquire an accurate and reproducible axial length measurement, the ultrasound beam must be perpendicular to the ocular structures and travel through the visual axis. Perpendicularity is verified when the on-screen spikes are all the same height, are 100% reflective, and have a 90-degree angle with the baseline.

The distance between the on-screen spikes represents the distance between the structures in the eye. A-scan biometry determines the axial length by measuring the anterior chamber depth, the thickness of the lens, and the length of the posterior chamber. Depending on the status of the eye (phakic, pseudophakic, or aphakic), the number of interfaces will differ. Each interface requires the placement of a measuring *caliper* or *gate*. The gates are used to quantify the distances between interfaces, and these distances are then calculated using the proper velocities of each media type. This is expressed in the equation distance = velocity x time (D= V x T).

The cornea, anterior chamber, lens, vitreous, and retina/choroid/sclera/orbital fat complex are all interfaces seen on an A-scan (Figure 17-6). Although the retina, choroid, sclera, and orbital fat each produce an individual spike, the axial length is measured only to the internal

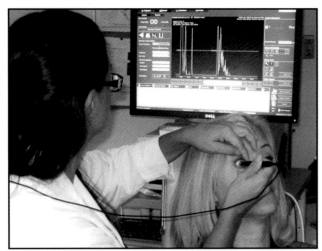

Figure 17-7. The probe is aligned with the visual axis, and comes into light contact with the cornea. The examiner sits so the patient and the screen are easily visible at all times.

surface of the retina, and therefore, the choroid, sclera, and orbital fat spikes do not require a gate. Having said this, to ensure that the scan is representative of the visual axis, the pattern of the choroid, sclera, and orbital fat must still be evaluated for proper alignment.

The optimal gain setting is the lowest setting that allows for 100% reflectivity of spikes, a double-peaked cornea spike, and visual separation between the retina and choroid spikes. On occasion, the sound vibrations will be absorbed more than usual by a structure, such as a dense cataract. In this case, the gain will need to be set higher to achieve 100% reflective spikes beyond the cataract (because a higher gain will penetrate more deeply).

A-Scan Biometry vs Optical Biometry

There are multiple published papers on the increasing accuracy and popularity of optical biometry over immersion and contact biometry. The internal fixation light and that the axial length is measured directly to the photoreceptors layer of the retina help achieve accurate axial length measurements. Point-and-shoot technology that is not operator-dependent, and the fact that it requires no anesthetic drop, makes optical biometry a popular choice. The advantage on the surgery side is that all calculations can be performed on the machine, and the data can be transferred to a computer-assisted surgery unit to assist with toric IOL placement.

There is still room for ultrasound biometry, however. While upward of 95% of eyes can be measured using optical biometry, traditional A-scan biometry is still relied upon for patients who cannot fixate, have dense cataracts, or cannot sit at the machine.[4]

CLINICAL SKILLS

Equipment

There are a few pieces of equipment, as well as some supplies, that you will need to perform either immersion or contact biometry. The first is a probe. The biometry probe has a frequency of 10 to 12 MHz and emits a one-dimensional *focused beam*. There are two types of probes that can be used in A-scan biometry: a standardized A probe or a biometry probe. The standardized A-scan probe uses a *parallel beam*. Either probe will produce an acceptable reading. If performing contact A-scans, some examiners prefer the concave end of the biometry probe, as well as the fixation target located on the end of this probe. These types of probes are specific to their particular instrument.

A stable chair is essential for performing any type of biometry because even the tiniest of movements can prevent a perfect scan. The need for a fluid-filled shell placed on the eye for immersion biometry makes a reclining chair most practical. Contact and optical biometry are often performed while the patient is sitting upright.

The supplies needed depend on the type of biometry being performed. Immersion and contact biometry both involve touching the surface of the eye, and therefore require a local anesthetic drop. In contact biometry the probe itself touches the eye. Immersion biometry requires a "shell" to be placed on the sclera to create a fluid-filled medium, although the probe itself does not contact the eye.

Biometry Procedures

Immersion and contact biometry can be successfully performed on most eyes, and are portable to places such as the operating room. Any measuring or testing that requires a clear cornea (eg, keratometry, topography) should be performed prior to the A-scan. Immersion and contact biometry can measure any length of eye and will measure to increments of 0.01 mm.

Contact Biometry

Contact biometry is performed by placing a probe directly on the cornea and aiming the beam through the visual axis (Figure 17-7). This method requires no fluid medium other than the tear film. The examiner must take precautions not to compress the cornea. Corneal compression will cause erroneously short readings, commonly up to 0.3 mm. Therefore, contact A-scan should only be used as a last resort. Gels should never be applied to the probe when performing contact biometry, as this can cause a fluid bridge, resulting in an erroneously long reading. Contact biometry can be performed with a handheld probe while the patient is upright or supine, or at a

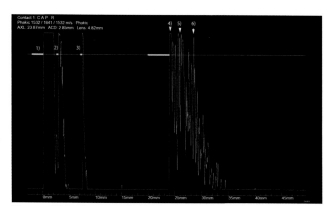

Figure 17-8. Contact phakic A-scan. 1=probe/cornea, 2=anterior lens capsule, 3=posterior lens capsule, 4=retina/choroid, 5=sclera, 6=orbital fat pattern.

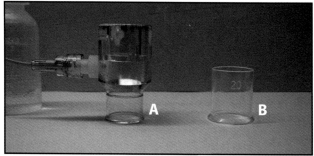

Figure 17-9. Immersion shells. (A) Praeger shell. (B) Hansen shell.

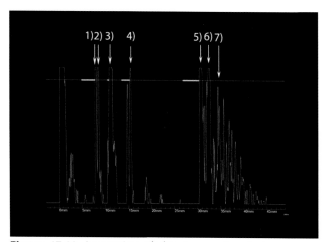

Figure 17-10. Immersion phakic A-scan. 1=anterior cornea, 2=posterior cornea, 3=anterior lens capsule, 4=posterior lens capsule, 5=retina/choroid, 6=sclera, 7=orbital fat pattern. The echoes preceding the anterior lens are from the immersion fluid.

slit lamp using a probe that is suspended like a Goldmann tonometer tip.

The contact scan of a phakic eye will have four interfaces. The probe and cornea will represent the first spike. Ideally the gain should be set so there is a separation of the spike, although the separation will not continue to the baseline. The second and third spikes represent the transition from the aqueous to the anterior capsule and the transition from posterior lens capsule to the vitreous. The final group of spikes represent the retina, choroid, sclera, and orbital fat complex. In a good quality scan, all spikes should have 100% reflectivity and meet the baseline at a 90-degree angle (Figure 17-8). Depending on the opacification of the lens, it may be difficult to maximize the posterior lens capsule echo, and the gain may need to be increased to maximize the spike. Scan appearance in situations other than phakic will be discussed momentarily.

To perform contact biometry, place an anesthetic drop in each eye. (It is common practice to measure both eyes to ensure the measurement is correct, because most of the time the eyes are relatively similar.) To perform contact biometry, have the patient fixate in the distance. (Some clinics tape an X or dot on the wall for this purpose.) Assess where the patient is looking, and imagine you are aiming the sound beam directly through the patient's line of sight. An alternate way to assess the direction of the visual axis is to have the patient look at a penlight and aim the beam toward the reflection in the pupil. The patient may be positioned sitting up or supine.

Just before coming into contact with the cornea, activate the probe by pressing the foot pedal. Once the probe comes into contact with the cornea, the spikes will display on the screen. Some trial and error will occur to achieve perpendicularity of the spikes. If the scan does not initially meet the criteria, remove the probe from the cornea to make adjustments. To freeze and save the scan, press the foot pedal again. To prevent injury, ensure that the probe does not come into contact with the cornea for more than 15 seconds, and that the probe is not moved while on the cornea. Encourage the patient to blink between readings to ensure the cornea does not dry out.

Immersion Biometry

During immersion biometry, the probe does not come into direct contact with the eye, and therefore requires a fluid medium for the sound waves to travel through. This fluid medium is formed by placing a plastic shell on the sclera between the eyelids and filling it with a balanced salt solution or artificial tears. (Never use tap water as it can contain microbes that could cause an eye infection.)

There are several types of immersion shells (Figure 17-9). The Prager shell (ES) is specific to the type of probe, and is designed to hold the probe while allowing the examiner to deliver the fluid via a tube. The Hansen shell (Hansen Ophthalmic Development Laboratory) comes in many sizes and is filled by pouring the fluid into the top of the shell.

The immersion scan of a phakic eye also has four interfaces (Figure 17-10). The first spike represents the cornea because the probe is not in direct contact. The remaining spikes are the same as contact biometry: the interfaces between the aqueous and anterior capsule, the posterior lens to the vitreous, and the vitreous to the retina/choroid/sclera/orbital fat complex (Sidebar 17-2).

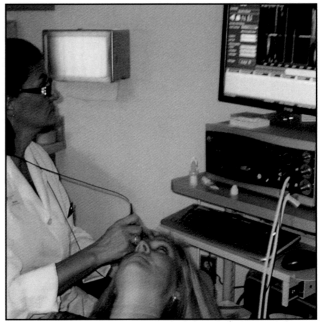

Figure 17-11. Immersion biometry is performed while the patient is supine. A shell is inserted between the lids.

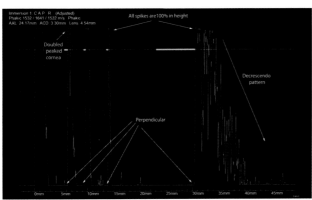

Figure 17-12. Reliable scan. All spikes perpendicular from baseline with 100% reflectivity. Reliable scans also have double-peaked cornea spikes and a decrescendo posterior to the retina spike.

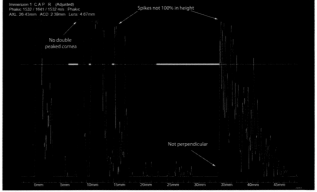

Figure 17-13. Poor scan. Spikes are not perpendicular from baseline and are not 100% reflective. The cornea spike will be poor or absent, and there is an absence of a uniform decrescendo pattern.

Immersion biometry is performed while the patient is in the supine position. An anesthetic drop is placed on the eye, and a shell is inserted between the upper and lower eyelids. Balanced salt solution is then used to fill the shell, and the probe is held or suspended perpendicularly in the fluid to get the reading (Figure 17-11). Like contact biometry, perpendicularity is important to achieve a reliable scan. Immersion biometry can be more difficult to learn, but will produce more reliable (and less variable) readings (Figures 17-12 and 17-13).

Biometry Results

The Phakic Eye

The scan of a phakic eye will have four distinct spikes, representing the cornea (immersion) or cornea/ probe (contact), the anterior lens capsule, the posterior lens capsule, and the retina/choroid/orbital fat complex. The ultrasound beam travels at different velocities through these media; therefore, it is imperative that the setting on the ultrasound machine is set on "phakic." The phakic setting will measure the distances from the cornea to the anterior capsule using a velocity of 1532 m/s (the speed of sound in aqueous or vitreous), the distance from the anterior capsule to the posterior capsule will be measured at 1641 m/s (the speed of sound through the lens), and the distance from the posterior capsule to the retina/ choroid/sclera/orbital fat complex will be measured using 1532 m/s. Each of the four spikes will be marked with a gate that the examiner places on the ascending portion of the spike. These gates are used to measure the different sections of the eye (see Figure 17-10).

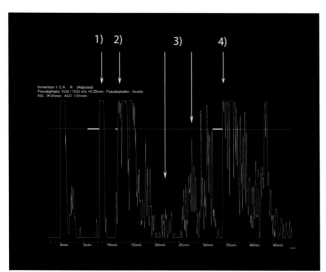

Figure 17-14. Pseudophakic scan. 1=anterior/posterior cornea, 2=anterior surface of intraocular lens, 3=reverberations/artifacts from intraocular lens, 4=retina/scleral/orbital fat pattern.

The Pseudophakic Eye

There are a few situations when a biometry measurement is taken on a pseudophakic eye. Pseudophakic patients may need biometry performed if cataract surgery on the fellow eye is planned, or if the patient has a dislocated IOL. A postoperative refractive "surprise" may require an A-scan to determine if the correct IOL was inserted. By remeasuring the corneal power and axial length, the correct (ie, optimal) power of IOL can be calculated and compared to the original power of lens that was implanted.

The lens spike is the only part of the pseudophakic scan that differs from the phakic scan. A highly reflective spike from the anterior portion of the IOL will be present, followed by multiple small spikes or reverberations (Figure 17-14). This pattern will vary depending on the type of IOL material (polymethyl methacrylate, acrylic, etc).

There are three gates in the pseudophakia setting; this is because there is no posterior capsule spike. The first gate is placed in front of the corneal spike, the second in front of the anterior lens spike, and the third in front of the retina/choroid/sclera/orbital fat complex. The velocity settings for the anterior chamber and vitreous are the same as the phakic eye, at 1532 m/s. The lens velocity is set for the material of the patient's IOL.

Alternately, the scan can be measured on phakic mode with a correction factor added to the scan to account for the IOL material. The optical biometer can also be set to a variety of lens velocity settings.

The Aphakic Eye

The scan of an aphakic eye also has a unique appearance. Since there is no IOL or natural lens, there are fewer interfaces. Biometry will show a corneal as well as

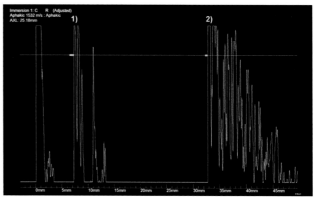

Figure 17-15. There are only two gates on an aphakic scan: 1=the cornea, 2=the retina.

a retina/choroid/orbital fat complex spike (Figure 17-15). Frequently, there is a third spike in the area where the lens would be; this may represent the aqueous/vitreous interface, lens capsule, or iris. The velocity used for the aphakic eye is the average tissue velocity of 1532 m/s. There are two gates for the aphakic scan; they are placed in front of the cornea and in front of the retina/choroid/sclera/orbital fat complex.

Silicone Oil

In some types of retinal detachment repair, the vitreous is removed and replaced with silicone oil. Silicone oil has a low velocity; sound therefore takes longer to travel through the eye. This results in the false appearance of a very long eye (Figure 17-16). Low viscosity silicone oil has a velocity of 980 m/s and high viscosity silicone is 1040 m/s. Extra calculations may need to be performed if there are multiple variables (such as pseudophakia and silicone oil in the same eye) since biometers have a limited number of settings. The optical biometer (eg, IOLMaster) is more accurate than either contact or immersion methods when measuring an eye with silicone oil.[5]

Completing the Exam/ Putting It All Together

Patient History

A few questions should always be posed to the patient before beginning the examination.

First, it is important to know if the patient has had previous ocular surgery or eye conditions. If he/she has had retina surgery, there could be oil or gas in the eye, which would require a different velocity setting. If the eye has a scleral buckle, it may measure longer than the other due to compression (and therefore elongation) of the globe. A diabetic eye may have swelling at the posterior pole, which can cause a shorter reading. Conversely, if the patient has a history of myopia, one or both eyes may be longer than average. A staphyloma (an outpouching

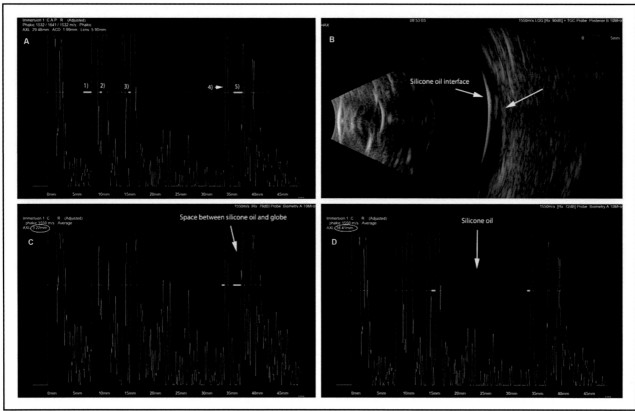

Figure 17-16. Silicone oil. (A) 1=cornea, 2=anterior lens capsule, 3=posterior lens capsule, 4=interface of silicone bubble, 5=retina/sclera/orbit fat pattern. The axial length is measured as 29.34 mm, which is a falsely long reading due to the silicone oil. The gain is set high (72 dB) to achieve a retina spike through the silicone oil. (B) On B-scan the interface of the silicone oil is visible. (C, D) Because the scan is measuring the vitreous cavity at 1532 m/s and not the velocity of silicone (980 m/s), the examiner must manually set the calipers to measure the portion of the vitreous cavity that represents the space between the silicone oil and the globe (the bubble = 3.22 mm) and the silicone oil (18.41 mm) to calculate the actual length of the eye. Note when using the two-caliper setting to measure, the velocity is automatically set to 1550 m/s. The true length of the eye is lens (5.90 mm) + anterior chamber depth (1.99 mm) + bubble (3.22 mm) + silicone oil calculated at the velocity of silicone oil, and not the velocity of vitreous (18.41 * 980/1550 = 11.64 mm). The true axial length is 22.75 mm.

or slope to the macula) may also be found in a myopic eye, and this may make it more difficult to aim the beam perpendicularly.

Second, it is important to know if the cornea has been altered in shape, by either refractive surgery or contact lenses. If the patient has had refractive surgery, the keratometer may under- or overestimate the corneal power, and a different IOL formula may be required.[6] If the patient wears contact lenses, they should not be worn 2 weeks prior to keratometry readings for hard contacts and 1 week prior for soft contacts (or according to your office policy). Contact lenses temporally change the curvature of the cornea and can lead to erroneous readings if the lenses are not removed for the recommended amount of time prior to measurement.

Lastly, for contact and immersion biometry, it is important to ask the patient if he/she has any allergies, because a topical anesthetic is used.

Positioning

Giving a quick layperson's explanation of why the test is required, what you are measuring, and what the patient will experience will help put the patient at ease. A cooperative patient will help achieve quick and reliable results.

To set up, move the ultrasound unit just behind the patient. Position your chair so that you are facing the screen for easy viewing. You want to be able to see both the screen and the patient. If using manual mode, make sure the foot pedal is within reach for freezing scans. If your right hand is dominant, seat yourself on the patient's right side. Sit on the patient's left side if you are left-handed.

Using a stable hand position will allow you to get repeatable results more quickly, and make the patient more comfortable throughout the procedure. For contact biometry, rest the nondominant hand on the patient's forehead and use your thumb to hold the upper lid. Hold the probe between the thumb and index finger in the

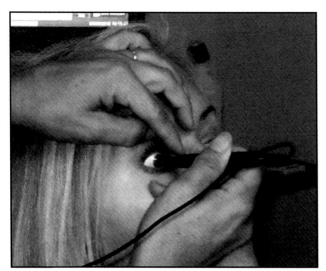

Figure 17-17. Contact hand position.

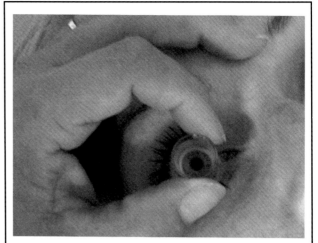

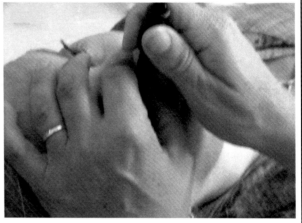

Figure 17-18. Immersion hand positions.

dominant hand, and rest the heel of the hand on the lower cheek (Figure 17-17).

While performing immersion biometry, rest the heel of the nondominant hand firmly on the patient's forehead. Using the thumb of your nondominant hand, lift the patient's upper eyelid and have him/her look down. Gently insert the edge of the shell underneath the upper eyelid. Then instruct the patient to look straight, and use your dominant thumb to pull down the lower eyelid and insert the other edge of the shell. With the nondominant thumb and index finger encircling the shell, apply slight pressure—just enough to avoid any leakage from beneath the shell. Rest the heel of the dominant hand on the patient's cheek, and hold the probe in the thumb and index finger of that hand (Figure 17-18). Keeping your hands steady will allow you to make micro-adjustments to achieve perpendicularity.

Patient Fixation

Having the patient fixate correctly makes it much easier to acquire an accurate contact or immersion A-scan. For contact biometry, have the patient fixate in the distance and look down a few degrees off axis. If you are having difficulty acquiring a scan, assess the patient's fixation and adjust the probe accordingly.

Always instruct the patient to keep both eyes open during the measurement. Once one eye closes, the other eye wants to close as well. Closing also evokes Bell's phenomenon, where the eyes roll upward, making it a challenge to scan through the pupil. Closing the eyes during immersion biometry also makes it uncomfortable for the patient, because the shell is being squeezed between the lids.

Auto and Manual Acquisition Settings

Most contact and immersion biometry machines have two acquisition settings: automatic and manual. The automatic setting will save any scan that meets the criteria of the type of eye (phakic, aphakic, etc) for which it is set. The automated setting can be frustrating to the examiner because the machine may freeze a scan that is displaying the proper spikes, but may be missing other crucial characteristics such as perpendicularity. Most biometrists prefer the manual setting because they can freeze the scan the moment it looks optimal.

Gating

Each echo must be marked with a gate to ensure accurate axial length. Most ultrasound machines require the gate to be placed on the ascending portion of the echoes, but on some machines, the gates are placed on the top of the echoes. These gates must be placed properly in order for the correct velocities to be used.

Quality Checks and Reproducibility

As a rule, both eyes should always be measured for comparison to each other. A series of 5 to 10 consistent readings should be collected per eye. Keep a mental note of the range of measurements during the scanning process. For acceptable immersion and contact biometry

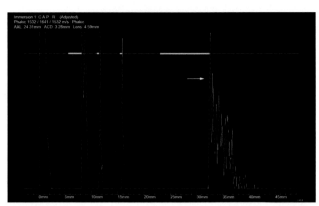

Figure 17-19. The arrow represents the optic nerve. Notice the absence of the typical decrescendo pattern behind the optic nerve spike.

readings, the intereye (comparing the two eyes) measurements should be within 0.3 mm of each other, and acceptable intraeye measurements (repeated measurements on the same eye) must be within 0.2 mm.

For ultrasound biometry where the intereye readings vary by more than 0.3 mm, check for proper probe placement and alignment. If scans still appear to be consistent but a greater than 0.3 mm difference between eyes is present, you must determine the cause (Sidebar 17-3). A B-scan screening of the macula or an OCT may also be needed to ensure there is no pathology causing the intereye difference. A larger difference in axial length between eyes may exist in anisometropia, where there is a refractive difference (of 2 diopters or more) between the two eyes. As a general rule, 0.3 mm of axial length is equivalent to 1 diopter of power.

Landmarking

Landmarking is a vital technique to check that the scan is properly aligned to the macula. First, achieve a scan where the sound is going through the cornea and anterior and posterior part of the lens. Once the anterior spikes are established, aim the sound beam nasally to find the optic nerve spike. The area of the optic nerve is demonstrated when one single spike is displayed in the area of the retina complex. The optic nerve does not have any orbital fat behind it, and will appear as a single spike (Figure 17-19).

Once the optic nerve has been located, aim the beam temporally toward the macula until the descending pattern of the retina, choroid, sclera, and orbital fat complex is visible; this is the area of the macula.

Conversion of Measurements

A-scan biometry may require manual calculations in some instances, such as a patient who has had previous refractive surgery or who has silicone oil in the eye. When converting a measured distance from one velocity to another, simple cross-multiplication is needed (Sidebar 17-4).

Erroneous Readings

Inaccurate readings may result from multiple sources. Contact A-scan biometry is notorious for resulting in shortening the axial length due to corneal compression. A fluid bridge, due to tears between the cornea and the probe, may contribute to a falsely longer axial length. If the proper velocities are not set or calipers are not in the correct position, the axial length may be artificially long or short. If an eye filled with silicone oil is scanned on the 1532 m/s setting for the vitreous instead of 980 m/s for the oil, the length will be erroneously long.

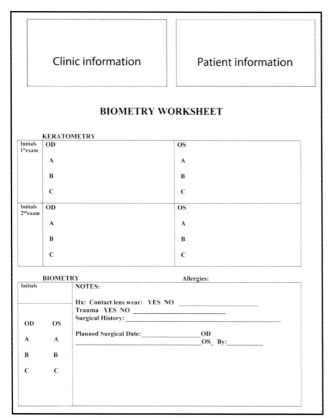

BIOMETRY WORKSHEET

Figure 17-20. A biometry worksheet should include patient demographics, keratometry, previous eye surgeries and laser treatments, allergies, surgery date, and contact lens use, as well as examiner notes.

Documentation

As with any testing, scanning, and observations we make in the eye clinic, documentation must be accurate and complete. It may be helpful to develop a form (Figure 17-20) to record the answers to the patient history questions, as well as the K values. The sheet can also be used to grade the confidence and difficulty of the scan.

Standardized B-Scan Examination and Techniques

When a designated protocol or universal technique is implemented, this is called *standardized echography*. Standardized echography requires an understanding of intraocular anatomy and physiology, and the ability to quickly process the information on the display. The B-scan will provide a topographic picture of intraocular and orbital pathology. The examiner must be able to think in a three-dimensional way while observing the flat, two-dimensional screen. In order to achieve a proper exam, specific techniques have been developed. Echography is reliable and repeatable as experience is achieved. The echographer can provide valuable information to the

ophthalmologist, who can interpret the findings in order to develop a reliable diagnosis.

B-scan ultrasonography is used to assess the eye where the media is cloudy or opaque, or through clear media in cases where tissues require further assessment or measurement. The sound waves are able to pass through the opaque media, such as a dense cataract, corneal scar, or vitreous hemorrhage, to give an ultrasonic view of the posterior segment. It is useful for evaluation of intraocular lesions, intraocular foreign bodies, and retinal detachments, as well as other ocular conditions. The list of indications is long (Sidebar 17-5).

The brightness modulated B-scan probe uses a focused oscillating transducer in the range of 10 MHz. The image produced is two-dimensional and represented by a series of dots of varying brightness (Figure 17-21). The transducer of the probe is covered by a thin membrane. This makes it possible for the probe to be placed directly on the lids or globe using a coupling medium, such as methylcellulose or tear gel. One section of the eye is examined at any single point relative to the placement of the probe on the eye. This section can be anywhere from 45 to 60 degrees, depending on the probe design. A marker on the probe is used for orientation and indicates the direction of the oscillating transducer inside the probe (ie, the transducer moves in a line toward and away from the marker). This movement produces a fan-like scanning beam.

Patient and Examiner Positioning and Probe Orientation

Most often the patient is reclining. Sometimes, due to restrictions, limitations, or a specific need, the patient may be in an upright position. It is important for the echographer to be comfortable as well. This usually means the examiner is seated so that the screen and patient are easily viewed at the same time. The dominant hand is used to hold the probe, like a pen, with the pinky finger supported on the patient's cheek. The other hand rests on the patient's forehead helping to open the lids and also supporting the probe (Figure 17-22). This technique helps to stabilize the probe and keep it from sliding around while the examiner watches the screen. A foot pedal is used to start the scan. When ready, the image is saved, again using the foot pedal. Most instruments have a mechanism to save and label the images (labeling is discussed shortly).

The patient is given anesthetic drops. A coupling medium is required to increase contact and provides better sound propagation. Ultrasound does not travel well in air and poor contact gives way to poor image quality and artifacts. After liberally applying methylcellulose, tear gel, or other coupling medium to the probe face, the probe is placed either on the eyelids or directly on the globe. Examination through the lids does not allow the examiner to observe the patient's fixation, however, and the lids

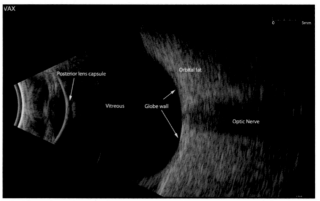

Figure 17-21. Normal B-scan.

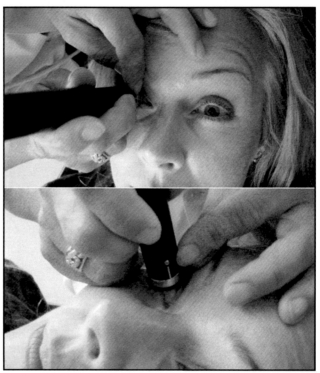

Figure 17-22. B-scan examination hand position. The probe marker is clearly visible in the bottom photo.

also attenuate some of the sound waves. This technique is used for children or patients with recent surgery or trauma. Placing the probe directly on the cornea or sclera is most common and allows for better and more accurate examination. This is especially true when assessing the vitreous cavity for mild vitreous hemorrhage. Special care must be taken to avoid abrasions when the probe is placed directly on the cornea.

Over time, experts in the field of echography have developed examination techniques and labeling methods that are universally used. Correct labeling aids in documentation, diagnosis, and follow-up. A systematic screening approach is used to examine the entire eye/orbit.

It is important to understand and remember that the *left* side of the display screen represents the contact of the B-scan probe to the eye. The top part of the display on the screen corresponds to the orientation of the marker on the probe. The bottom part of the display corresponds to the side of the probe opposite the marker. The center of the right side of the display corresponds to where the center of the sound beam is directed (Figure 17-23).

It is important to constantly be aware of where the marker is oriented during the examination because it indicates the area of the eye/orbit being scanned, as well

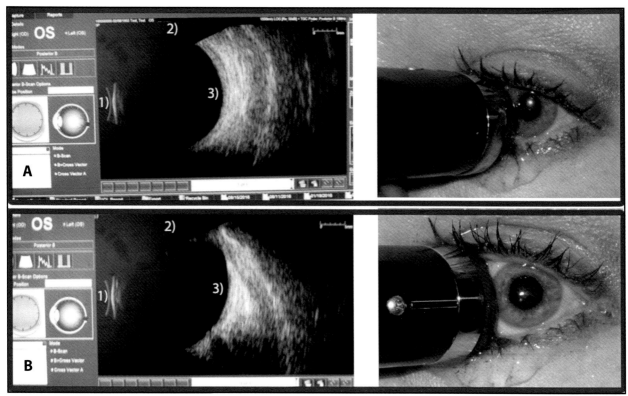

Figure 17-23. Orientation of B-scan image. 1=The probe face on the eye corresponds to the left side of the screen. 2=The marker corresponds to the top of the screen. 3=The right side of the screen is the area of the globe imaged. (A) The marker is oriented vertically for a transverse scan. (B) The marker is oriented nasally for a longitudinal scan. Point 1 is the same in both scans. However, points 2 and 3 are 90° from each other.

as how the image is labeled. Imagining the eye as a clock face will help with orientation and labeling. For example, nasal in the right eye is 3 o'clock, and nasal in the left eye is 9 o'clock (Figure 17-24).

Most often the B-scan exam is done transocularly, meaning across the globe. The probe is placed on the eye in a position opposite the area of the globe to be examined. For example, to examine the nasal retina, the probe is placed temporally.

A para-ocular B-scan exam is sometimes done when examining the anatomy and pathology of the orbit. In this technique the probe is placed directly over the area to be examined (eg, when looking at the lacrimal gland). Other orbital assessments such as muscles and optic nerve use the transocular approach. When assessing the orbit it is important to image and compare both eyes.

There are three basic orientations of the B-scan probe. These are axial, transverse, and longitudinal (radial). Axial scans are really a type of transverse scan and are generally oriented vertically and horizontally, but can also be oblique. The marker is always oriented upward or toward the nose for axial and transverse scans. (Never point the marker down for these positions.) For longitudinal (radial) scans, the marker always points toward the cornea. The only time the probe is placed directly on the cornea is for an axial scan.

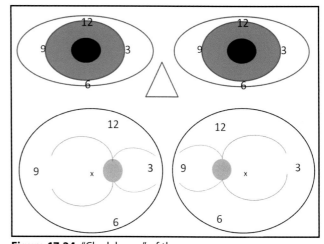

Figure 17-24. "Clock hours" of the eye.

Axial Scans

Axial scans (AX) go through the visual axis. The probe face is placed on the cornea with the patient looking straight ahead; the sound beam is directed to the posterior pole, through the pupil and lens. Most commonly the marker is either pointing up (vertical scan—labeled as VAX) or toward the nose (horizontal scan—HAX). It can also be oriented in an oblique fashion (ie, toward 10, 11, 1, or 2 o'clock, but the marker will never be pointed

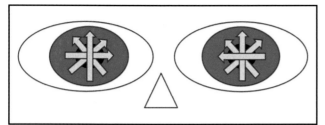

Figure 17-25. Marker orientation of axial scans.

downward toward 4, 5, 6, 7, or 8 o'clock; Figure 17-25). The documented reference would be the clock hour the marker points to, followed by "AX" for axial.

The image produced in all cases will have the optic nerve shadow centered in the middle of the image on the right side of the display (Figure 17-26). Scanning through the optic nerve produces a tubular-looking (V-shape pattern) defect referred to as the *optic nerve shadow* or *defect*. This is not really a defect but rather an acoustic void: an absence of echoes. This is because the optic nerve is basically homogenous and absorbs much of the sound, plus the sound beam is oblique to the edge of the optic nerve. This appearance of the optic nerve on the image aids in positioning and reference.

If the patient is phakic, the lens echo will appear in the center of the left-hand side of the display. If the patient is pseudophakic, artifacts from the artificial lens are produced. These artifacts are known as *reverberation echoes* (Figure 17-27). In a horizontal axial scan (probe on the cornea, marker toward the nose) the sound is sweeping from the nasal retina, through the optic nerve to the temporal retina. The image will show the nasal retina on the top half of the right side of the screen, the optic nerve in the center, and the temporal retina on the bottom half. This image is labeled HAX. With the marker toward the nose, all HAX scans will show the macula just below the optic nerve shadow. A vertical axial scan (VAX) images from 12 o'clock through the optic nerve to 6 o'clock (superior retina to inferior retina).

Axial scans are helpful in orientation of pathology in relation to the posterior pole. When an IOL is present and artifacts are produced, the image quality can be poor. Axial scans should not be used to assess optic nerve pathology, such as drusen and fluid. Longitudinal and transverse scans are best for this.

Transverse Scan

The *transverse scan* can be oriented vertically, horizontally, or obliquely as well. In simple terms, approximately 4 to 6 "clock hours" are being examined at any one time (remember the beam produced is moving like a fan as it scans).

The probe is placed on the sclera opposite to the area being examined. For example, to obtain a vertical transverse exam of the nasal quadrant or retina of the right

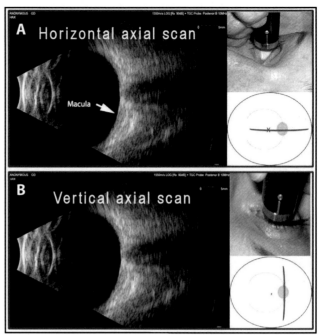

Figure 17-26. (A) In this horizontal axial scan, the marker is oriented toward the nose. The scan goes horizontally through the optic nerve, and the macula is slightly below the optic nerve shadow. (B) In this vertical axial scan, the marker is oriented up. The scan goes vertically through the optic nerve. The scanned area above the optic nerve represents the superior retina, and the area below represents the inferior retina.

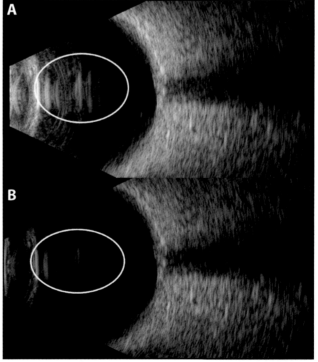

Figure 17-27. Reverberation artifacts with (A) high and (B) low gain from the intraocular lens (circle) in a pseudophakic patient.

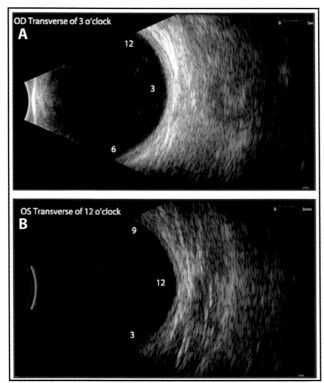

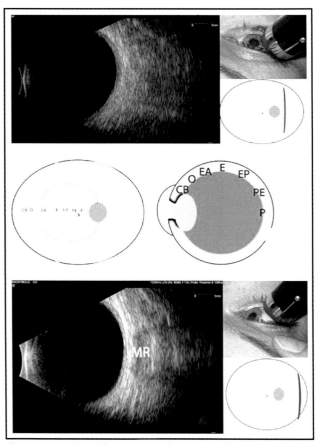

Figure 17-28. The transverse scan is a cross-sectional scan that includes 4 to 6 clock hours. (A) Scanning the globe of the right eye produces an image from 12 o'clock to approximately 6 o'clock, with 3 o'clock in the center. (B) The superior retina scan produces an image from 9 o'clock to 3 o'clock with 12 o'clock in the center.

Figure 17-29. In addition to the clock hour, the transverse scan label must also include the position scanned. P represents posterior retina, PE is slightly more anterior than P, EP is just posterior to the equator, E represents the equator, EA is anterior to the equator, O is the ora seratta, and CB is very anterior close to the ciliary body. For a transverse scan of the nasal retina of the right eye, 3 o'clock is in the center, 12 o'clock is at the top, and 6 o'clock is at the bottom. A cross-section of the medial rectus muscle (MR) can be seen. In a more posterior scan (P), the medial rectus is not easily visible. Scanning more anteriorly (E), the cross-section of the muscle becomes more visible and is closer to the eye wall.

eye, the probe face is placed on the temporal sclera near the limbus (9 o'clock) and the marker is oriented up. The scanning will occur from 12 o'clock to 6 o'clock, with 3 o'clock in the center. With the marker up, 12 o'clock is represented on the top of the image on the display and 6 o'clock is at the bottom (Figure 17-28). This will provide a lateral aspect of pathology.

Examination must include the entire eye. So, while the probe is still at the 9 o'clock limbus, for example (which is scanning more posteriorly), the patient looks away from the probe, in this case left, and the examiner then tilts (sweeps) the probe laterally into the fornix, which moves the direction of the sound beam more anteriorly. The center of the image is still 3 o'clock.

For the transverse exam, the labeling is achieved by the clock hour at the center of the display and by the posterior-anterior orientation of the image (Figure 17-29). For the above example, if evaluating the nasal quadrant and the probe is directed posteriorly, just anterior to the optic nerve, the label would be 3P (3 o'clock is in the center, and P for posterior). If the sound beam is directed more anteriorly (say, near the equator), the label would be 3E (equator). In some clinics the position is preceded by the letter T to indicate "transverse" (eg, T3E).

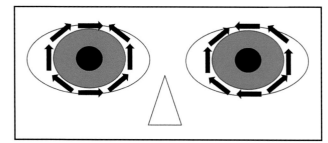

Figure 17-30. Transverse marker orientation.

Transverse scans can be taken of any clock hour. The method is the same. If the exam is horizontal, the marker is toward the nose. If it is oblique, the marker is pointed upward (never down) as much as possible (Figure 17-30).

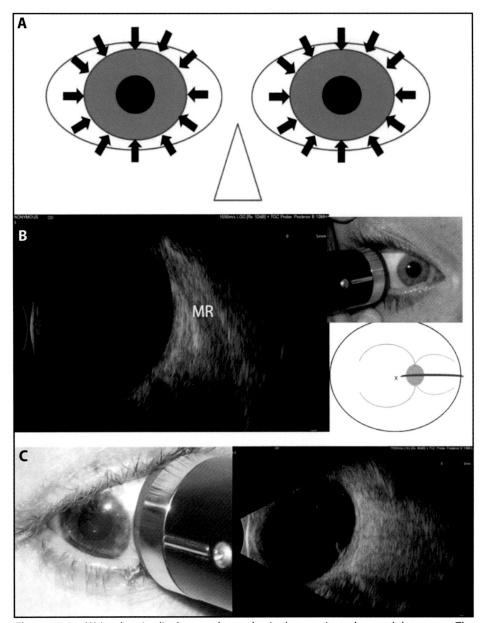

Figure 17-31. (A) In a longitudinal exam, the marker is always oriented toward the cornea. The optic nerve pattern will be seen in the bottom of the image, and long sections of recti muscles will be imaged at 12, 3, 6, and 9. (B) Longitudinal scan of the nasal globe of the right eye shows the long section of the medial rectus (MR) muscle. (C) Longitudinal scan of the macula of the right eye (L9) images the macula well and can show pathology.

Longitudinal Scan

Longitudinal scans are scans of one "clock hour" or one meridian, from the optic nerve anteriorly. Longitudinal scans are achieved by placing the probe face on the sclera near the limbus with the marker always directed toward the cornea as the patient looks in the opposite direction. These exams give the radial (or posterior-to anterior) aspect of pathology. Think of this scan like looking at one hour on a clock, following the little hand from the center as it points to a particular clock hour. When labeling these views, the clock hour that is being examined is proceeded by the letter "L" to signify longitudinal. For example, if the nasal retina of the right eye is being examined longitudinally, the probe is placed temporally on the sclera, near the limbus, with the marker toward the cornea. The label is L3. The optic nerve shadow will be in the bottom of the image (Figure 17-31), and will sometimes disappear if the probe is tilted more posteriorly or the patient looks further away. This will achieve a more anterior longitudinal (radial) view. Longitudinal scans are a great way to assess the optic nerve and look for retinal tears in the presence of vitreous hemorrhage.

Screening Technique

When screening a patient's eye, generally all the techniques are used so that no pathology is missed. It is a good idea to have a protocol or a systematic approach so the exam is done the same way every time. If pathology is found, more attention should be given to that area. Usually the axial views are done first, then transverse scans of the four quadrants (horizontal and vertical), and finally longitudinal scans are done. Not all clock hours need to been examined longitudinally. Typically the macula is examined, then superiorly, inferiorly, and nasally. In this way all quadrants will be thoroughly scanned. In most cases a screening exam is fairly quick.

When scanning it is important to try to remain perpendicular to the area being examined. When assessing a membrane, for example, perpendicularity will produce the strongest echo. Or when assessing a lesion for shape and thickness, being perpendicular will provide the most accurate reading. Scanning a lesion obliquely can produce a falsely thick reading when measuring with on-screen calipers.

The exam should be dynamic. Sometimes the probe is moving to obtain a more posterior or anterior exam. Other times the patient is asked to move the eyes or head to see if there is any movement of pathology. For example, this technique is helpful when trying to differentiate between a posterior vitreous detachment (PVD) and a retinal detachment (RD). The PVD will have more movement than the RD.

Another feature of the dynamic exam means that the gain is constantly being changed. For example, high gain is needed to appreciate a vitreous hemorrhage. Lower gain is used to improve resolution, and also better outlines pathology.

Using these techniques allows the examiner to define the topography of the pathology being studied. Shape, size, contour, and position can be determined.

It is essential to label scans correctly, as outlined above. This is important for documentation and follow-up examination. Also, if a different examiner or the ophthalmologist looks at the images, proper labeling makes it clear how the image corresponds to the eye.

Finally, the echographer needs to describe what was seen. This includes documenting the status of the lens, the appearance of the vitreous cavity and posterior pole, and the contour of the globe, as well as if any elevations, tears, membranes, or detachments were imaged. It takes practice to master the probe positioning and labeling and to understand the image produced by thinking three-dimensionally. See Figures 17-32 through 17-35 for a few examples of various pathologies as imaged with B-scan.

Sometimes artifacts are apparent on the image (Figures 17-36 and 17-37). Artifacts can be caused by something simple, such as poor contact and pseudophakia, or by something more difficult to interpret, such as reverberation echoes from a foreign body, air, or gas.

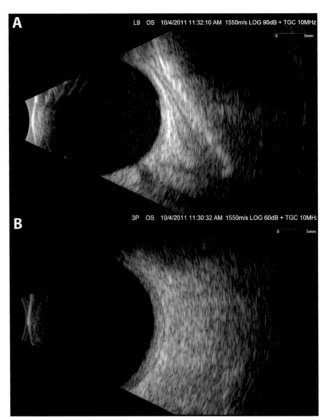

Figure 17-32. B-scan of vitreous hemorrhage. (A) Fine dot-like opacities are noted in the vitreous cavity with high gain. These opacities are mobile and often demonstrate convectional movement in new hemorrhages or hemorrhage after vitrectomy. (B) The opacities appear to disappear with lower gain as blood has low reflectivity.

Shadowing can occur as well, which could be due to an entity that is highly reflective, such as calcified sclera or an osteoma (a bone-like tumor). Silicone oil used in retinal detachment surgery causes the sound to travel slowly, and therefore the image is abnormally elongated.

Standardized A-Scan

In conjunction with performing diagnostic B-scan and using standardized techniques, standardized A-scan can be used to aid in the assessment of tissues and diagnosis of lesions (Figures 17-38 and 17-39). This technique is less commonly used as it requires a very experienced echographer. The A-scan probe used for this is different than the A-scan biometry probe. To perform standardized A-scan, an 8-MHz, unfocused, parallel beam is required. A predetermined gain setting is needed for standardized A-scan. This is achieved by using a tissue model. The standardized A-scan probe is placed on the model, and the gain is adjusted to produce a specific echo pattern. This gain setting is in decibels (db) and is referred to as *tissue sensitivity*.

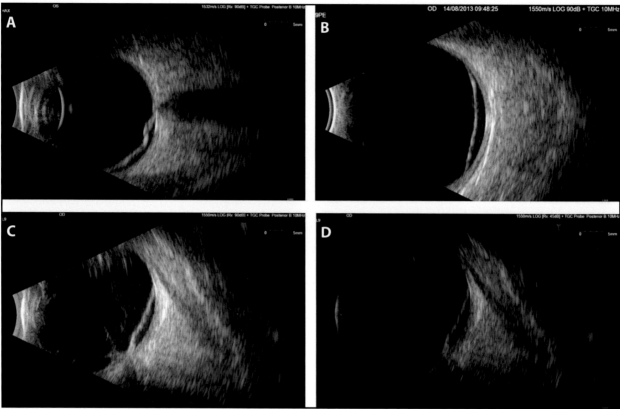

Figure 17-33. (A) Retinal detachments are highly reflective, nonmobile membranes. HAX view of a macula off retinal detachment. (B) Transverse view of a retinal detachment. (C) Longitudinal view of a tractional retinal detachment, in a patient with proliferative diabetic retinopathy, on high gain. (D) The retinal detachment persists on low gain.

Figure 17-34. (A) Longitudinal and (B) transverse scan of a choroidal nevus. Elevations can be measured with on-screen calipers.

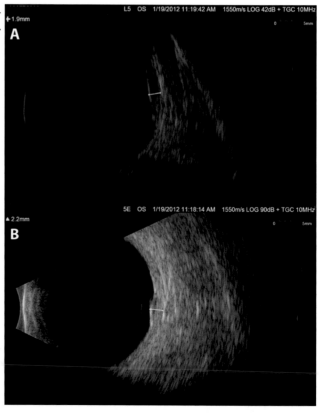

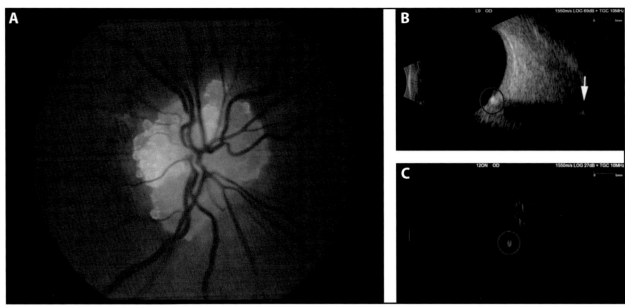

Figure 17-35. (A) Optic nerve head drusen appear as highly reflective, discrete, round, nonmobile opacities in the optic nerve head and (B) produce a reduplication echo in the orbit (arrow). (C) Drusen persist on low gain.

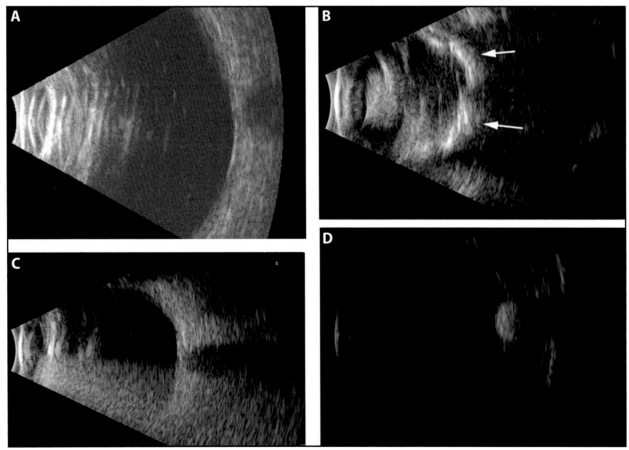

Figure 17-36. Artifacts. (A) Elongated image produced from scanning through silicone oil. (B) Calcification of the eye wall producing attenuation of sound, likely in a phthisical eye. (C) Intraocular gas used in retinal detachment surgery causes reverberation artifacts causing blurring on the ultrasound image. (D) An indentation artifact is imaged on a patient with a previous scleral buckle procedure for retinal detachment surgery.

Figure 17-37. An intraocular foreign body is noted on an ultrasound exam. The foreign body is highly reflective and produces a subtle reverberation echo (arrow).

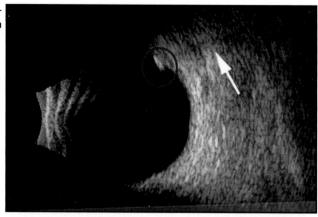

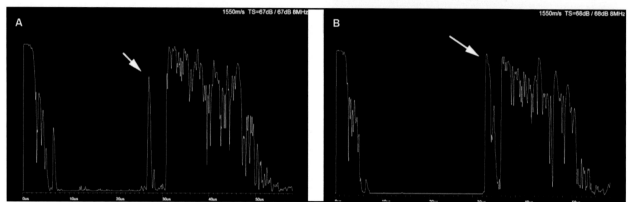

Figure 17-38. Standardized A-scan of posterior vitreous vs retinal detachment. Membranes (arrows) can be assessed with standardized A-scan when gain is set at tissue sensitivity. (A) Posterior vitreous detachments have lower reflectivity but can exhibit slightly more reflective membranes when hemorrhage is present. (B) Retinal detachments produce 100% reflective spikes.

The probe placement is generally opposite the area being examined (transocular), and the probe beam is directed perpendicular to the area/pathology being examined.

When the standardized A-scan probe is used with correct tissue sensitivity (gain), certain characteristics of a structure, tissue, or lesion can be identified because of the image pattern. For example, the echographer can assess the reflectivity of a membrane (eg, retina vs PVD) or evaluate the internal structure of a choroidal nevus vs a choroidal melanoma (high vs low internal reflectivity, respectively). Tissue movement and vascularity can also be assessed. This is quantitative echography, so measurements of the thickness of lesions can also be made. (For this, the gain is sometimes decreased.)

Standardized A-scan is helpful for measuring muscle thickness in cases of thyroid orbitopathy and myositis (inflammation of a muscle). Other uses include differentiating a wide range of intraocular tumors and orbital tumors, quantitative assessments of membranes, and evaluation of the optic nerve (such as drusen and edema/fluid).

A valuable test in the hands of a skilled sonographer is the *30-degree test*. This test was developed by Carl Ossoinig. It is used to evaluate whether or not there is increased cerebrospinal fluid around the optic nerve. The goal is to measure the *perineural sheaths* (connective tissue around the nerve) anteriorly and posteriorly using the standardized A-scan probe, while the patient is in primary gaze. The patient is then asked to look about 30 degrees toward the probe, and the measurements are taken again. The test is positive if the measurement decreases (by at least 10%) when the patient looks laterally. The idea is that when the eye moves to the side, the optic nerve stretches a bit and redistributes the fluid.

Anterior Segment Examination: Ultrasound Biomicroscopy

One area where B-scan ultrasonography was somewhat lacking was the assessment of anterior segment anatomy and pathology. Using a stand-off or immersion B-scan, some details of the anterior segment could be appreciated, but the image lacked good resolution and detail. A very high frequency ultrasound (35 to 100 MHz) was developed to address this area. These frequencies allow imaging of the anterior segment at a near-microscopic level (Figure 17-40).

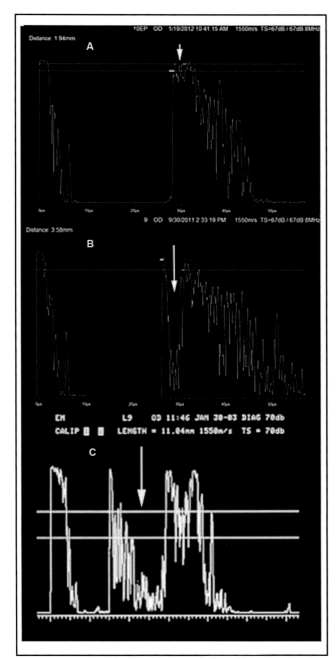

Figure 17-39. Standardized A-scan of choroidal nevus vs choroidal melanoma. Internal reflectivity (arrows) can be assessed with standardized A-scan with gain set at tissue sensitivity. (A) A choroidal nevus demonstrates a high internal reflectivity, and (B and C) a melanoma commonly demonstrates a low internal reflectivity with decrescendo pattern.

The term given to this type of imaging is *ultrasound biomicroscopy* (UBM). Small structures such as zonules, the scleral spur, ciliary processes, and cells in the anterior chamber are easily imaged with this technique. Tumors and lesions of the anterior segment are effortlessly imaged and followed. Structural abnormalities causing some forms of glaucoma can be identified, such as those in pupillary block and plateau iris syndrome. The

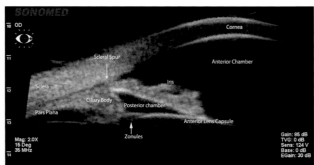

Figure 17-40. Anterior segment anatomy seen with UBM. A longitudinal image at 3 o'clock gives excellent detail of the cornea, scleral spur, iris, posterior chamber, ciliary body, anterior lens capsule, zonules, anterior chamber, sclera, and pars plana. The angle is open.

anterior chamber depth can be measured, and angles can be evaluated in narrow angle glaucoma suspects. Previous laser peripheral iridotomies can be checked for patency. Zonules can be imaged and assessed in conditions such as Marfan syndrome or in patients with previous blunt ocular trauma.

The main pitfall with UBM is the lack of penetration due to the high frequency. For example, 35- and 50-MHz probes would have a penetration depth of approximately 12 to 15 mm with a focal point of about 10 to 11 mm. In contrast, the 10-MHz B-scan probe has a penetration of 45 to 50 mm. The axial resolution of the 35 MHz is around 0.02 mm, and the 50-MHz probe has a resolution of 0.015 mm (meaning the UBM can differentiate microscopic anatomy/pathology). The 10-MHz B-scan probe has an axial resolution of about 0.10 to 0.20 mm (ie, an object/entity needs to be about 100 to 200 mm before it can be differentiated as separate). With such a shallow focal point of UBM, the depth of field where the sound is focused is narrow with high frequency.

Due to the high frequency, the transducer does not have a membrane covering it, as this would cause distortion. Therefore, the exam requires the patient to be supine, and an immersion technique is used. Commonly a scleral shell is used. The shell is placed on the anesthetized sclera, between the upper and lower lid. The shell is filled with fluid, such as sterile balanced salt solution. The probe is then immersed into the fluid (Figure 17-41). Care is taken to avoid contact with the cornea, as the uncovered transducer is moving. Good hand positioning is very important. Place the nondominant hand on the patient's forehead to hold the shell in place with the thumb and either the pointer finger or the middle finger. The other (dominant) hand holds the probe and should be braced by placing the pinky finger on the patient's cheek or nose and using the forefinger of the hand on the forehead to stabilize the probe (Figure 17-42).

Alternately, some manufacturers make disposable probe attachments with thin membranes that don't cause

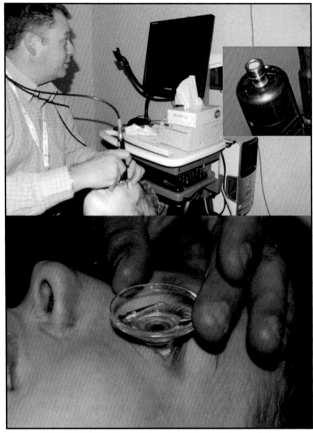

Figure 17-41. UBM set-up. The patient is supine, and the examiner sits comfortably so the patient and the screen are both visible, and the foot pedal is within reach.

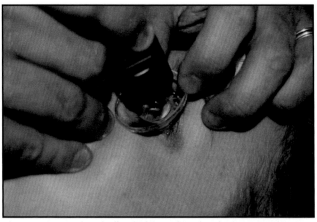

Figure 17-42. The shell is held in place by the examiner's nondominant hand, while the probe is in the dominant hand. The probe is immersed in the fluid, but does not come into contact with the eye.

distortion. An attachment called a ClearScan (ESI, Inc) is an acoustically invisible cover that is filled with saline and fits over the probe. The sac is then place directly on the eye. This method can make the UBM more pleasant for some patients, and can be used with the patient in a seated position.

Similar to the 10-MHz B-scan probe, axial, transverse, and longitudinal scans can be performed with the UBM probe. The main difference in scanning technique between a traditional 10-MHz B-scan probe and a UBM probe is that the UBM probe is placed directly over the area to be imaged. Axial scans are centered over the cornea and labeled either HAX or VAX, or (if oblique axial scans) then the clock hour of the scan followed by AX (eg, 2AX; Figure 17-43). Some settings also allow for a wide view and show a cross-section from one angle to the opposite angle and include the posterior capsule (Figure 17-44). Longitudinal or radial scans are of a single clock hour. The anatomic angle is best viewed with this technique (Figure 17-45). Transverse scans show a cross section of the area scanned (eg, the iris or the ciliary processes; Figure 17-46).

There are two other types of B-scan probes. One is a 20-MHz anterior segment probe, and the other is a 20-MHz posterior segment probe.

The 20-MHz anterior segment probe is an open probe system similar to the UBM, but with a lower frequency and less resolution. The application is similar to the UBM. The probe must be covered with a latex tonocover. (Immersion in fluid using a shell can be used, but this limits how far posterior the probe can be placed.) The technique is the same as the UBM with the probe placed directly over the pathology to be imaged. UBM is still the preferred choice in most anterior segment examinations, but the 20-MHz B-scan probe for anterior segment has a good application with patients who can't lie down, or sometimes with children who may cooperate better with contact imaging vs immersion. It also works very well to image pathology, such as anterior lesions that are too posterior for UBM, but too anterior for 10-MHz B-scan (Figure 17-47).

The 20-MHz posterior segment probe provides a higher resolution image than the standard 10-MHz B-scan probe. The images are similar, but a bit more detail is provided with the 20-MHz B-scan as the images of the retina and optic nerve look slightly larger and are in better focus (ie, higher resolution). The technique is the same as with the traditional 10-MHz probe. Some users consider the 20-MHz posterior segment B-scan probe as superior when imaging posterior pole and orbital pathology.[7] It may be worthwhile to use the 10 MHz as a screening exam for its superior sensitivity in imaging the vitreous cavity.[7]

Cleaning, Disinfection, and Maintenance

Infection prevention and control have become hot topics. The standards for disinfection have increased drastically in recent years. Items that touch the eye are considered semi-critical items. (Semi-critical items are those that come into contact with a mucous membrane [such as the conjunctiva/eye] and must be high-level disinfected [HLD] at a minimum.)

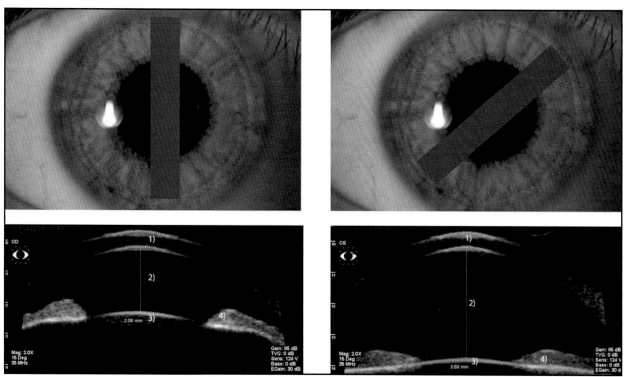

Figure 17-43. Axial UBM. Using the immersion technique, the probe is held in the fluid above the center of the cornea. HAX, VAX, and oblique scans will look the same. In the VAX image (left set), the probe scans from 12 o'clock to 6 o'clock. Oblique scanning (right set) occurs from 2 o'clock to 7 o'clock. The (1) cornea, (2) anterior chamber, (3) anterior lens capsule, and (4) iris are well-imaged in this view. Anterior chamber depths can be measured very accurately.

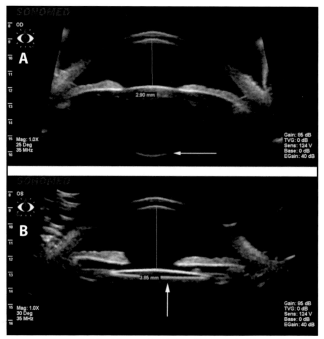

Figure 17-44. Axial wide-angle UBMs. (A) In a phakic patient the posterior capsule is well imaged. (B) In a pseudophakic patient the intraocular lens is seen and its position assessed. Both anterior chambers appear well formed and deep.

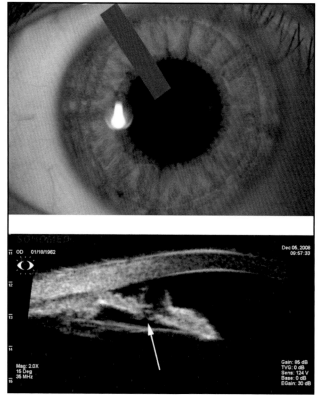

Figure 17-45. In this longitudinal image of 11 o'clock on angle view, a disruption in the iris (arrow) is imaged consistent with a previous peripheral iridotomy.

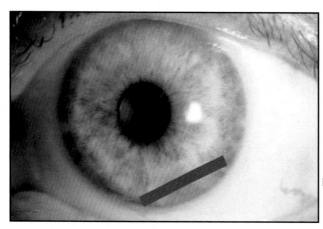

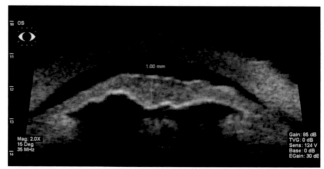

Figure 17-46. Cross-section of an iris lesion using transverse UBM.

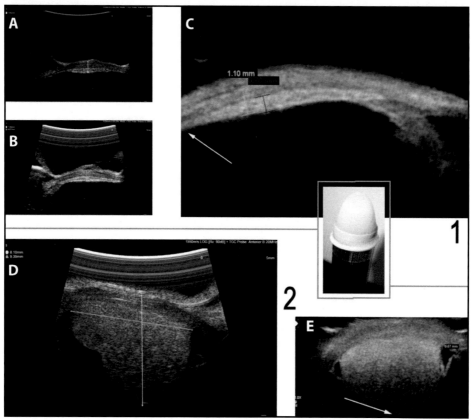

Figure 17-47. 20-MHz B-scan image vs UBM of anterior lesions. (1) The 20-MHz probe (inset). A small anterior lesion is imaged (A) transversely and (B) longitudinally with 20 MHz. All borders of the lesion are easily and well imaged. A longitudinal UBM (C) images the lesion, but does not show the most posterior edge (arrow). (2) (D) All borders of a large lesion including the apex are imaged with 20 MHz, allowing the height to be measured. (E) The apex cannot be imaged with UBM due to the limitation of wavelength penetration (high frequency).

There are generally five steps involved in the reprocessing of a medical device. The first step is a mechanical clean, using friction and a mild low-foaming cleaner at the point of contact to remove debris. Dried residual debris on a probe or shell can become very difficult to remove. The next step is disinfection, which involves soaking in a high-level disinfectant such as glutaraldehyde. (Note: Many hospitals prohibit the use of certain high-level disinfectants. Moreover, these high-level disinfectants must be used in a fume hood or room that meet adequate air exchanges. Proper personal protective equipment must also be worn to ensure the handler is safe.) The third step is a sterile rinse. Rinsing is a crucial step in HLD to ensure that all chemical residues are removed. If a rinse is not feasible, a series of three 1-minute sterile water soaks may be used. The fourth step is drying the probe/

shell, which should be done with a clean, lint-free cloth. The final step is inspection. It is important to ensure that the probe/shell has not been damaged and that it has been thoroughly disinfected.

Due to the delicate nature of the probes, sterilization is never recommended. Consult the manufacturer for cleaning and disinfectant instructions. Manufacturers often do not have instructions for HLD. In this case, one would have to decide whether or not to comply with HLD guidelines and risk damaging the probe (which will probably not be covered by the manufacturer, since their recommendations were not followed). HLD should always be done away from patient care areas.

When removing the probe from the unit, care must be taken because the connections are very delicate. Never drop the probe or place the probe on its face. This can damage the transducer, the piezoelectric plate, and/or the membrane. Always inspect the probe prior to use, making sure the membrane of the B-scan is not punctured. (Oil in the probe can leak out.)

It is always recommended to perform routine back-up of data to ensure no exams are lost. It is also important to stay current on software upgrades. Work with your sales representative or clinical application specialist to keep the equipment current and in working order.

CHAPTER QUIZ

1. Explain the advantages of immersion biometry over contact biometry.

2. Will an eye containing silicone oil measure as artificially long or short?

3. Explain the different between biometry and standardized A technique.

4. How many gates are required in the following situations?
   a. immersion technique on a phakic eye
   b. immersion technique on an aphakic eye
   c. contact technique on a pseudophakic eye

5. Name several factors that affect image quality.

6. What does the "B" in B-scan stand for?

7. If the optic nerve is centered in the image produced by a B-scan, what scanning technique is being used?
   a. transverse
   b. axial
   c. longitudinal
   d. immersion

8. True/False: A radial (longitudinal) scan is a sector image of approximately 6 clock hours.

9. When should the gain be adjusted when doing a B-scan?

10. Small, fine, dot-like opacities in the vitreous cavity could be an example of what?
    a. retinal detachment
    b. tumor
    c. vitreous hemorrhage
    d. vitreous detachment

11. A thin, highly reflective, nonmobile membrane that attaches into the optic nerve could be an example of what tissue?

Answers

1. Advantages of immersion biometry over contact biometry: not touching the cornea and no corneal compression.

2. An eye containing silicone oil will erroneously measure longer because the oil has a low velocity and sound takes longer to travel through the eye.

3. Biometry is used to measure the length of a tissue by measuring the distance between interfaces and velocities. Standardized A-scan techniques allow the examiner to determine the sensitivity or reflectivity of a tissue.

4. a. four gates, b. two gates, c. three gates

5. Multiple variables affect the quality of an image: transducer frequency (a high frequency gives a better resolution but has less penetration), penetration, gain (high gain gives more information but less resolution), resolution (which depends on frequency and gain), probe contact (poor contact produces artifacts), proper fluid medium (for immersion techniques), the tissue being examined, and the interfaces involved.

6. The B in B-scan stands for "brightness" modulated. The B-scan is made of many tiny dots and is a two-dimensional image (in most cases, unless you are using three-dimensional ultrasound).

7. b

8. False, A radial scan is an image of one clock hour or one meridian at one time. It is a scan from the optic nerve anteriorly in a single meridian. The optic nerve shadow is usually at the bottom.

9. During B-scan, the gain is constantly being adjusted. It is best to use high gain to image the vitreous cavity (ie, for hemorrhage) and for doing the screening exam. The gain should be decreased when assessing pathology and measuring with calipers. For biometry, the gain is set where the spikes (interfaces) are best.

10. c

11. Clinical correlation would be required, but based on the sonogram, this could be an example of a retinal detachment.

REFERENCES

1. Byrne SF, Green RL. *Ultrasound of the Eye and Orbit.* 2nd ed. Philadelphia, PA: Jaypee Brothers Medical Publishers Ltd; 2010.

2. Fisher Y. Essential lectures in ophthalmic ultrasound [video]. Vimeo website. http://vimeo.com/album/2640067/video/78740879. Accessed April 8, 2016.

3. Bellis M. The history of ultrasound in medicine. About.com website. http://inventors.about.com/library/inventors/blultrasound.htm. Updated June 29, 2015. Accessed April 8, 2016.

4. Emerson JH, Thompkin K. *IOLMaster: a practical operational guide* [user's guide]. Dublin, CA: Carl Zeiss Meditech; 2009.

5. Kunavisarut P, Poopattanakul P, Intarated C, Pathanapitoon K. Accuracy and reliability of IOLMaster and A-scan immersion biometry in silicone oil-filled eyes. *Eye.* 2012;26:1344-1348. doi:10.1038/eye.2012.163.

6. Tang M, Li Y, Avila M, Huang D. Measuring total corneal power before and after laser in situ keratomileusis with high-speed optical coherence tomography. *J Cataract Refract Surg.* 2006;32(11):1843-1850.

7. Hewick SA, Fairhead AC, Culy JC, Atta HR. A comparison of 10 MHz and 20 MHz ultrasound probes in imaging the eye and orbit. *Br J Ophthalmology.* 2004;88(4):551-555.

BIBLIOGRAPHY

Astbury N, Ramamurthy B. How to avoid mistakes in biometry. *Community Eye Health Journal.* 2006;19(60):70-71.

Byrne SF. *A-Scan Eye Length Measurements: A Handbook for IOL Calculations.* Mars Hill, NC: Grove Park Publishers; 1995.

Canadian Standard Association. Medical device reprocessing. Z314.0-13-2013.www.freestd.us/soft4/2090775.htm. Accessed April 8, 2016.

Cassin B. *Ophthalmic Technical Personnel.* Philadelphia, PA: Saunders; 1995.

Cook D, Kreutzer TC, Armin W, Haritoglos C. Variability of standardzed echographic ultrasound using 10 MHz and high resolution 20 MHz B-scan in measuring melanoma. *Clin Ophthalmol.* 2011;5:477-482.

Holladay JT. Ultrasound and optical biometry. *Cataract and Refractive Surgery Today Europe.* 2009;November/December:18-19.

Kendall CJ. *Ophthalmic Echography.* Thorofare, NJ: SLACK Incorporated; 1990.

Lizzi FL, Coleman DJ. History of ophthalmic ultrasound. *Journal of Ultrasound in Medicine.* 2004;23(10):1255-1266.

Pavlin CJ, Foster FS. *Ultrasound Biomicroscopy of the Eye.* New York, NY: Springler-Verlag; 1995.

Prager TC. Fixed immersion shell improves axial measurement. *Rev Ophthalmol.* 2005;5(1).

Shammas HJ. *Intraocular Lens Power Calculations.* Thorofare, NJ: SLACK Incorporated; 2004.

Shammas HJ. A comparison of immersion and contact techniques for axial length measurement. *American Intra-Ocular Implant Society Journal.* 1984;10(4):444-447.

Velázquez-Estades LJ, Wagner A, Kellaway J, Hardten D, Prager T. Microbial contamination of immersion. *J Ophthalmol.* 2005;112(5):13-18.

The figures in this chapter were contributed by the authors, Monique Rinke and Laura Barry.

18

ELECTROPHYSICAL TESTING

Jacob P. McGinnis, BA, COT

BASIC SCIENCES

Over the past few years, dramatic increases in computer technology have resulted in an evolution in electrophysical testing. What once may have required sending a patient to a neurological practice or a research university can now be done in-office, saving clinical staff and patients valuable time, and promoting a more accurate and earlier diagnosis of pathologic conditions that affect eyesight.

We often do not think of the interconnectivity of our brains and eyes. We forget about the distance and structures through which a light signal must travel, first from being perceived by our photoreceptor cells, then along the optic nerves, the optic chiasm, the optic tract, into the occipital lobe, and back out the optic radiations. Thus, the stimulus finally reaches the visual cortex, where all the information is decoded and put into a neat little image for us to recognize as a cat or other object.

Prior to reading this chapter, it may be helpful to review ocular anatomy (Chapter 2) and physiology (Chapter 3).

CLINICAL KNOWLEDGE AND SKILLS

Each light flash, each object we perceive, is converted into an electrical signal and interpreted by our brains. Occasionally it is difficult to determine the specific cause of vision loss in a patient. Because of the electrical charges involved, some visual problems can be evaluated by means of electrophysical tests (Sidebar 18-1).

Nerve tissue is the primary structure of our nervous system, which controls and regulates the body's functions. The brain's electrical charge is maintained by a specialized cell type called a *neuron*, which generates and conducts nerve impulses.

Neurons generally have two functions: 1) they respond to stimuli, and 2) they transmit electrical impulses within the body. Neurons constantly exchange ions from inside to outside their cell membrane, which changes the membrane's electrical charge. Ions of similar charge repel each other, and when neurons push away numerous ions, those ions push along other ions, and so on, forming a wave. This is known as *volume conduction*. Cumulatively, when these ion waves reach the scalp and any electrode attached to that scalp, they can affect the electrons on the metal of the electrodes. This change is easily detectable by a gauge called a *voltmeter*, and the recording of this measurement over time is known as an *electroencephalogram* (EEG).

Ledford JK, Lens A, eds.
Principles and Practice in Ophthalmic Assisting:
A Comprehensive Textbook (pp 335-343).
© 2018 Taylor & Francis Group.

SIDEBAR 18-1

USES/INDICATIONS OF ELECTROPHYSICAL TESTS IN OPHTHALMOLOGY

▶ Visual evoked potential (VEP): Optic nerve atrophy, ischemic optic neuropathy, papilledema, optic disc drusen, color vision deficiencies, visual field defects, subjective visual disturbances, pituitary tumor, lesions pressing on the optic nerve, idiopathic vision loss, retinal pigment epithelium dystrophies, ocular injuries involving the optic nerve and visual pathways, retrobulbar neuritis

▶ Electroretinography (ERG): Cone dystrophy, retinitis pigmentosa, color vision deficiencies, macular dystrophies, sickle cell retinopathy, carotid artery occlusion, vitreoretinopathy, siderosis, central and branch artery and vein occlusions, certain medication toxicities, certain vitamin deficiencies

▶ Electro-oculography (EOG): Retinal pigment epithelium disorders, evaluation of eye movements, implications in ocularly controlled mechanisms for the physically disabled, age-related macular degeneration and other types of macular dystrophy, Stargardt's disease, choroideremia

▶ Dark adaptometry: Retinal degeneration, night blindness, cone dysfunction, macular degeneration, Stargardt's disease, retinitis pigmentosa

▶ Electronystagmography (ENG): Oculomotor nerve function, nystagmus, vertigo, Meniere's disease, Usher syndrome

An EEG is a noninvasive testing modality that measures electrical signals given off by the brain. An EEG can be done on most any patient. (Certain medical conditions may be contraindicated, and it is important to take that into consideration. Often this is related to underlying neurological disorders like epilepsy.) As the eyes work in conjunction with the brain to encode visual stimuli into meaningful images, the electrical signals given off by this interpretation are measurable with specialized subgroups of EEGs. In ophthalmology, EEGs are particularly useful on young children who frequently are unable to describe the exact nature of their vision problems.

Having an EEG does require that sensors be placed on the scalp, often in conjunction with a conductive paste, which can occasionally be bothersome to patients. But the process is generally brief and has no long-lasting effects.

The Visual Evoked Potential

"Vision" is not solely a product of the eyes. The electrical signals produced by the eyes are transferred via the optic nerve to the occipital region of the brain, and there they are converted into images that we interpret. There are a variety of diseases that can affect the visual pathway, and there is no reliable noninvasive method to visually inspect damage beyond the retina and disc. However, there are tests available to clinicians to determine if there is ongoing damage to the optic nerve tract or the occipital region of the brain.

Visual evoked potentials (VEPs) are electrophysiologic responses to a set stimulus, measuring the electrophysiological activity being transmitted in the visual cortex. The test evaluates a small portion of the total electrical output of the brain as measured by an EEG. VEP results demonstrate the efficiency of a patient's visual pathway from the anterior segment to the retina, optic nerve, optic chiasm, lateral geniculate nucleus, and visual cortex. It is also sometimes referred to as the *visual evoked response* (VER) or *visual evoked cortical potential* (VECP).

Due to the nature of the eye, any problem that may cause a loss of or depression in electrical activity may require this mode of testing. For example, a patient who presents with glaucoma or glaucoma-like symptoms may benefit from having this test, as it will show whether or not there is depressed electrical function from the eye to the brain. Alternately, a patient with dry eyes could also benefit from this test, as it may indicate a loss of electrical signal due to a loss of focal power at the cornea.

Visual Evoked Potential Stimuli

Various levels of light are used in conduction of a VEP test. One of the earliest methods utilized a diffuse flashing light. This method is rarely used in current testing methodology due to its widely variable results. It is, however, useful in testing infants and individuals with poor acuity.

The International Society for Clinical Electrophysiology of Vision (ISCEV) states that the preferred method for investigation of the visual pathway is a pattern reversal stimulus. Typically presented in a checkerboard pattern (Figure 18-1), the image's segments reverse from white to black and black to white, maintaining a constant light output. Occasionally a different image may be used, such as a circle of white and black stripes (Figure 18-2) that reverse pattern. Regardless whether the target is a checkerboard or stripes, the images are equal in measure and provide more consistent results than the diffuse flashing light method.

The images are typically presented via a computer monitor placed in front of the patient, who is wearing electrodes connected to a voltmeter. Defer to the manufacturer's instructions and training on the type of stimuli to be used.

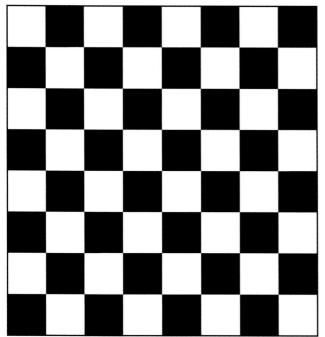

Figure 18-1. VEP checkerboard stimulus.

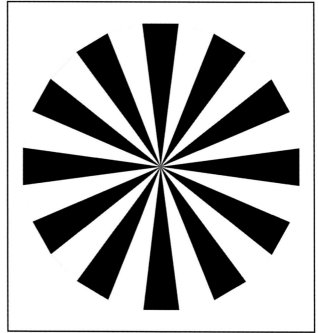

Figure 18-2. Alternate VEP stimulus.

Visual Evoked Potential Waveforms

VEP results are displayed as a waveform. Waveforms are visual representations of the variation in a current over time; specifically we are concerned with bidirectional waveforms. Bidirectional waveforms, also known as alternating waveforms, vacillate from a positive direction to a negative direction crossing over a zero axis point. Bidirectional waveforms can accurately indicate the difference in amplitude.

A typical pattern-reversal VEP waveform consists of a *N75-P100-N140* complex. In patients with no pathology the first negative peak (N) should occur at the 75 ms mark, or 75 ms after the beginning of the waveform. The first positive peak (P) should occur around the 100 ms mark, and the second major negative peak should occur near the 140 ms mark. A patient's waveform will change dependent on testing conditions and the patient's pathology.

Amplitude

The waveform *amplitude* is the amount of electrical energy that is reaching the visual cortex. Amplitude is calculated as the difference between the first negative peak (N) and the first positive peak (P). Thus amplitude = P – N.

Amplitude is often indicative of the status of the patient's eyes; generally an increase in amplitude correlates to better health. (Normal amplitude using the formula above of P – N should be around 25 ms.) This can be helpful in determining the stage of a patient's condition. Generally speaking, if a patient has difficulty in seeing the stimulus, there would be a lower electrical response and lower amplitude results.

Latency

Latency is the measure of time that it takes the electrical signal to travel from the retina to the visual cortex. It is marked by the first positive peak on the waveform. The overall health of the eyes will affect the amount of time that it takes for that signal to reach the visual cortex; a longer latency is an extremely reliable indicator of significant pathology. A normal value for the first positive peak is 100 ms; therefore, an increase in damage due to pathology would extend that time. So anything over 100 ms should be considered abnormal or delayed.

Electrode Placement

The placement of the electrodes is extremely important to provide a stable, artifact-free VEP response (Sidebar 18-2). The number of electrodes is dependent on the manufacturer's design, and it is useful to consult their instructions. The strongest impulses are generated along the *calcarine fissure* in the brain (the "line" that divides the occipital lobe into left and right halves). Thus, it is important to ensure that an electrode is located close to the *inion*, the projection from the occipital bone at the base of the skull, which is near this fissure (Figure 18-3). The electrode is to be placed 2.5 cm above the inion. (It is useful to locate the inion with a finger and then measure one finger-width above it.)

Other electrodes are often required, and their placement is dependent on the manufacturer's instructions. Frequently a *reference electrode* is placed in the center of the forehead, where if a line were traced from it backward, the skull would be perfectly divided in two. This particular electrode is used to provide a stable,

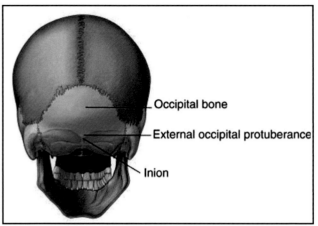

Figure 18-3. Back of the skull showing location of inion for proper placement of VEP electrode.

reproducible electrical current to which the other electrodes can be compared.

Performing the Test

- Refer to the manufacturer's guidelines for specifics in testing.
- Educate the patient about the test. Explain the purpose of the test, what he/she may experience, how to respond if need be, and the average length of the test. Make the patient aware that the test's quality is adversely affected by movement, inattention, and fatigue.
- Ensure that the screen or testing mechanism is the appropriate distance from the patient (no closer than 70 cm).
- The patient should be properly refracted and corrected for the testing distance.
- Minimize any possible distractions to the patient. Limit the room to one patient (unless the patient is a child). Reduce any noises and nonessential movement.
- Unless otherwise specified, do not instill any drops prior to testing, as any alteration of the patient's eyes can skew test results. For example, if you're testing to determine if there is a latency being caused due to the dry eye, giving the patient a drop to moisten the eyes would alter your end results.
- Apply electrodes as per manufacturer's instructions.

- Ensure that the testing room is dimmed during the evaluation.
- Some VEP devices allow for variation in testing size and testing patterns. It may be useful to utilize these options based on a particular patient's needs. For example, a patient with low vision might require larger fixation targets.
- Any visual field defects should be noted in the patient record. Such defects may need to be accounted for in evaluation of the test results. For example, a patient who has suffered a stroke may automatically have delayed latency.
- Run the test according to the manufacturer's directions.

Results

With modern computer technology, most test results are averaged automatically. They filter out other electrical signals that are created by the brain during testing. There is a generalized normal result (Figure 18-4); anything that differs from this is considered abnormal.

Electroretinography

The electroretinogram (ERG) analyzes electrophysiologic responses to a set stimulus. It evaluates the activity generated by neural and non-neural cells in the retina. ERG measurements are obtained by a variety of electrodes that interpret the electrical activity of the retina as evidenced at the surface of the cornea. ERGs are important in diagnosing pathological issues within the retina. Common reasons for testing a patient with an ERG are diseases that affect the retinal tissue, such as macular degeneration, diabetic retinopathy, and retinitis pigmentosa.

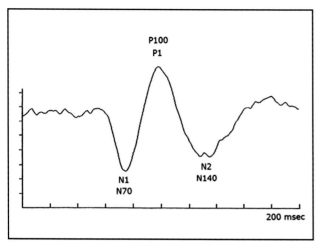

Figure 18-4. A normal result for VEP testing.

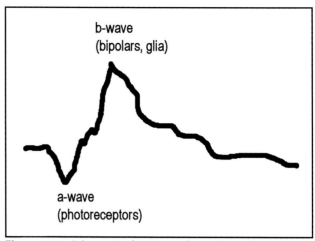

Figure 18-5. Schematic of ERG waveform. (Note: The c-wave is not usually seen, especially in conjunction with a b-wave.)

Electroretinogram Stimuli

The *flash/full field* is the most frequently used ERG test. It evaluates the photoreceptor cells within the retina (the rods and cones) as well as other cells that process light. Cones, primarily located in the macula, provide information correlated to detailed vision. Rods provide information in low-light scenarios. There are more rod cells than cone cells.

During the test a brief, flashing light is used (often < 4 ms) to illuminate the entire retina. The test often requires the patient to be dark adapted prior to beginning.

A *pattern reversal* stimulus is used to test the macula. The pattern reverses at a set interval, but maintains the same level of luminance.

Electroretinogram Waveforms

The test measures three types of electrical waves given off by the retina: a-waves, b-waves, and c-waves. The a-wave is represented in the waveform by a negative dip, where the b-wave is the positive peak. The c-wave is a slower positive wave (Figure 18-5). Each wave results when chemical byproducts are formed in the eye during light reception and processing.

As with the VEP waveform, there is an initial negative peak, followed by a positive peak, and another negative peak (which is actually a slower positive wave that, therefore, registers in a negative direction). The amplitude of the b-wave is measured from the valley of the a-wave to the peak of b-wave. This is often used to indicate overall health of the retinal tissue.

Types of Recording Electrodes

The type of electrode used when performing an ERG differs based on the manufacturer's design. The electrodes fall into three categories, dependent on the surface of the eye that they contact. It is important that you become knowledgeable about the type of electrode that you use to ensure that appropriate contact and positioning are maintained, giving reliable test results.

Corneal electrodes come in contact with the cornea and provide the most stable test results, but also cause the most discomfort. They require a lid speculum to ensure that the electrode is not blinked out, anesthetic drops to ensure that discomfort is kept to a minimum, and wetting solution to ensure the eye doesn't dry and distort the test results. There are several types (Figure 18-6).

Bulbar conjunctival electrodes come in contact with the conjunctiva and provide reliable test results, however, can cause a high amount of testing defects due to an increased desire to blink. There is better patient comfort because no lid speculum is needed, but it does require an anesthetic and wetting solution.

Skin electrodes come in contact with the skin of the lower eyelid. Due to lower amplitude readings, testing is less reliable, and a longer testing duration is needed to ensure a reliable signal average. However, this type of electrode has excellent patient comfort as no contact is made with the eye.

Performing the Test

► Refer to the manufacturer's guidelines for specifics in testing.

► Educate the patient about the test, explain its purpose, what he/she may experience, how to respond if need be, and the average length of the test. Make the patient aware that the test's quality is adversely affected by movement, inattention, and fatigue.

► Ensure that the screen or testing mechanism is the appropriate distance from the patient (a patient should be not be closer than 70 cm).

► The patient should be properly refracted and corrected for the testing distance.

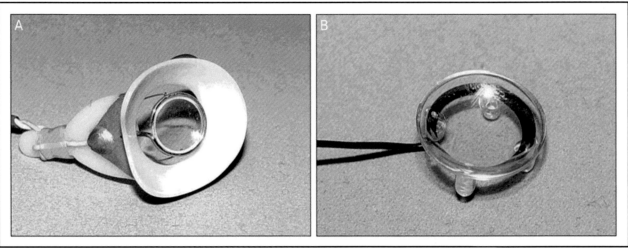

Figure 18-6. (A) Burian-Allen contact lens electrode. (B) ERG-Jet disposable lens with a gold-plated ring.

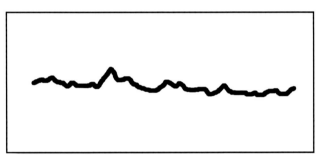

Figure 18-7. Schematic of ERG waveform in retinitis pigmentosa showing overall retinal degradation. The ERG is almost extinguished due to photoreceptor dysfunction, resulting in a fairly flat graph.

► Minimize any possible distractions to the patient. Limit the room to one patient (unless the patient is a child). Reduce any noises and nonessential movement.

► Follow proper protocol per the physician or manufacturer to determine whether or not a patient's eyes should be dilated.

► Apply electrodes as per manufacturer's instructions.

► Ensure that the testing room is darkened prior to the evaluation. Appropriate dark adaptation should take no less than 20 minutes, although some testing specifications may vary based on design.

► Any visual field defects should be noted in the test results to ensure that all modifying factors are taken into account before evaluation of the test results.

► Run the test according to the manufacturer's directions.

Results

Most test results are averaged automatically, and other electrical signals created by the brain during testing are filtered out. The results give an idea of the overall health of the retina and can be used to detect and monitor the progression of retinal disorders, such as retinitis pigmentosa (Figure 18-7 and Table 18-1).

Electro-Oculography

The electro-oculogram (EOG) is an electrophysical test designed to evaluate the function of the outer retina and retinal pigment epithelium (RPE). Changes in the electrical potential of the RPE are measured and recorded over several periods of dark and light adaptation.

The corneo-fundal potential is the difference in the electrical charge from the front to the back of the eye. It is mainly influenced by the electrical charge that occurs due to the ion permeability of the RPE. The EOG determines the standing potential of this membrane in the dark, and then again the maximum potential in the light. This difference is referred to as the *Arden ratio*, or the difference from the maximum potential in the light and the standing potential in the dark.

This test is particularly useful in testing abnormalities of the retina, particularly those affecting the macula and the choroid. Specifically, the EOG is used to evaluate any toxic reaction caused by chloroquine as well as diagnosing and following Best disease. (Best disease is one of several types of genetic juvenile macular degeneration.)

Electro-Oculogram Stimuli

The electrical potential of the front of the eye, which is positively charged, differs from that located at the back of the eye. Two electrodes placed on either side of the eye can measure the change from the front to the back.

An EOG should be performed using a full-field dome or Ganzfield Stimulator. There should be a comfortable head- and chinrest for the patient, as well as two fixation lights located 15 degrees to the left and right of center. The fixation lights will be bright during the light adaptation process and dim to barely visible in the dark.

TABLE 18-1

ELECTRORETINOGRAM RESULTS IN SEVERAL OCULAR DISORDERS

Ocular Disorder/Entity	Electroretinogram Form
Cone dystrophy	Significantly depressed photopic response
Cancer-associated retinopathy	Reduced amplitudes of a- and b-waves
Retinitis pigmentosa	A- and b-wave amplitudes are minimal
Congenital red/green color deficiency	Normal
Best vitelliform macular dystrophy	Normal
Adapted from Ramkumar HL, Epley KD, Karth PA, Kumar UR, Shah VA. Electroretinogram. American Academy of Ophthalmology's EyeWiki website. http://eyewiki.aao.org/Electroretinogram. Accessed August 8, 2017.	

Electro-Oculogram Waveforms

The height of the eye's adaptation in light is represented by a rise called the *light peak*, which is reached in about 10 minutes. The height of the eye's adaptation in the dark is indicated by a dip called the *dark trough*, which takes about 8 to 12 minutes. (Adaptation varies naturally according to age.) These are compared to each other as the Arden ratio, mentioned previously.

Electrodes

The test uses small skin electrodes, such as those used during standard VEP tests. They are placed by the side of the nose nearest the eye and the outer canthi.

Performing the Test

▶ Explain the procedure fully. Head position should be maintained throughout the test; specifically, moving the eyes does not require any movement of the head. It is also important to let patients know not to anticipate the movement of the fixation lights. It is suggested you practice with the patient.

▶ The dark adaptation test should take place in total darkness; the fixation lights should be only be bright enough to adequately produce fixation.

▶ Darkness should be maintained based on the manufacturer's specifications.

▶ During the light adaptation portion of the test, the dome should be evenly lit and appear white. The room the test is being performed in may be lit as well, so long as the luminance is not equal to or greater than that of the dome.

▶ Patients, particularly those with poor ocular motility, central vision impairment, or diplopia, may have difficulty fixating on the lights. Modifications can be made for these patients. It is helpful for patients with diplopia to focus between the fixation lights.

▶ Due to the length of the test, patient fatigue is likely to occur. Common causes of test error include the

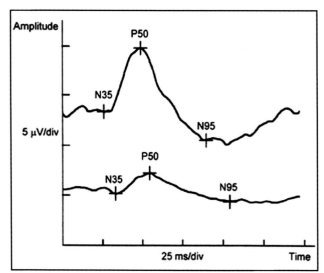

Figure 18-8. Normal EOG test (with slight variances).

patient tilting the head away from the dome and erratic eye movement. Remind the patient of the importance of staying alert.

Results

Most test results are averaged automatically and the instrument filters out other electrical signals that are created by the brain during testing (Figure 18-8). A normal Arden ratio is 2:1 when comparing the light peak to the dark trough. A ratio of less than 1.8:1 if the patient is under 60 years old, and less than 1.7:1 if the patient is over 60, is considered abnormal.[1]

Dark Adaptometry

Dark adaptometry is a test that is often performed to determine how well someone's vision functions at night. When exposed to light, the photochemicals in the retina are activated. However, exposure to bright light causes these pigments to bleach out. Thus, when subsequently exposed to a dark environment, it then takes the eye a

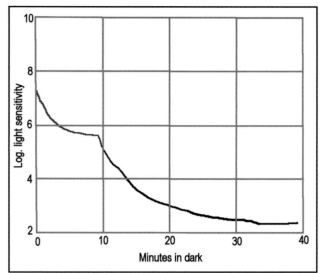

Figure 18-9. Typical dark adaptation curve. The red line indicates the time when cones are most sensitive. The black line represents when the rods are most sensitive.

while to reproduce the spent pigment. Dark adaptometry measures the eye's ability to recover from this bleaching phenomenon. It is useful to determine the extent of some hereditary or genetic retinal diseases that may interfere with an individual's ability to see in dimly lit areas.

An instrument called an adaptometer is used. The test is monocular so one eye is occluded, and the patient places his/her chin and forehead into the instrument's headrest. The patient is left in full darkness for 2 minutes, then exposed to a bright light for about 4 minutes. Then he/she is again exposed to darkness. The examiner begins to reintroduce lighting at varying levels with a control on the instrument, and the patient indicates whether or not the light is seen. The patient's responses are mapped out as a curve on a graph and compared to a normal dark adaptometry result to determine if there is any retinal damage (Figure 18-9). The results can be tracked over time.

Electronystagmography

Electronystagmography (ENG) is a diagnostic procedure used to measure involuntary muscle movements of the eye. It also determines how well the vestibular nerve (CN VIII, which runs from the brain to the ears) and the oculomotor nerve (CN III, which runs from the brain to the eyes) are working within the brain. In primary care settings, the ENG is used to evaluate dizziness and balance issues.

The test is performed by attaching four electrodes around the eyes (on each side, as well as above and below) and a reference electrode placed in the center of the forehead. The electrodes are attached to a computer to monitor the electrical output.

There are several versions of the test. To evaluate nystagmus (involuntary, repeated movements of the eyes) the patient is asked to look directly at a fixation light, which may be positioned straight ahead or to the left or right. The test results can indicate the magnitude of the movements as well as if the movement increases or decreases in any position of gaze.

The test can also be performed to test voluntary eye movements. A set of three objects are affixed or projected onto the wall, one object in center and two on either side. The patient is then directed to shift his/her gaze from one object to the other while the instrument tracks the movements. In the optokinetic version of the test, the patient is told to keep his/her head still while tracking a quickly-moving light.

CHAPTER QUIZ

1. Testing modalities such as VEP, ERG, and EOG measure what type of signal produced by the body?
   a. motor
   b. electrical
   c. auditory
   d. visual

2. Neurons exchange what from their outer membrane to inner membrane to change their electrical charge?
   a. electrons
   b. protons
   c. neutrinos
   d. ions

3. With VEP testing, an increase in amplitude usually signifies:
   a. better health of the visual system
   b. a problem with the ocular media
   c. progressive glaucoma damage
   d. VEP does not use amplitude as an indicator

4. What type of sensor provides the most stable test results for the ERG?
   a. skin electrode
   b. corneal contact electrode
   c. conjunctival electrode
   d. reference electrode

5. Which test requires a patient to experience light adaptation and dark adaptation?
   a. VEP
   b. ERG
   c. EOG
   d. EEG

6. Which test can be used to evaluate both voluntary and involuntary eye movements?

    a. VEP
    b. ERG
    c. EOG
    d. ENG

7. The EOG is an electrophysical test designed to evaluate:

    a. the integrity of the nerve fibers in the chiasm
    b. the amplitude of corneal sensation
    c. the function of the outer retina and retinal pigment epithelium
    d. the function of the visual cortex

8. A patient with retinitis pigmentosa might be tested by performing an:

    a. EOG
    b. ERG
    c. ENG
    d. none of the above

Answers

1. b
2. d
3. a
4. b
5. c
6. d
7. c
8. b

REFERENCE

1. Creel DJ. The electroretinogram and electro-oculogram: clinical applications by Donnell J. Creel. The Organization of the Retina and Visual System website. http://webvision.med.utah.edu/book/electrophysiology/the-electroretinogram-clinical-applications/. Accessed November 11, 2016.

BIBLIOGRAPHY

Arden GB, Barrada A, Kelsy JH. New clinical test of retinal function based on the standing potential of the eye. *Br J Ophthalmol.* 1962;46:449-467. www.ncbi.nlm.nih.gov/pubmed/18170802. Accessed November 11, 2016.

Cobb WA, Morton HB. A new component of the human electroretinogram. *J Physiol.* 1954;123:36-37.

Introduction to dark adaptometry psychology essay. UKEssays website. www.ukessays.com/essays/psychology/introduction-to-dark-adaptometry-psychology-essay.php?cref=1. Published March 23, 2015. Accessed November 11, 2016.

Kerber KA, Baloh RW. Neuro-otology: diagnosis and management of neuro-otological disorders. In: Daroff RB, Fenichel GM, Jankovic J, Mazziotta JC, eds. *Bradley's Neurology in Clinical Practice.* 6th ed. Philadelphia, PA: Saunders Elsevier; 2012:chap 37.

Lawwill T, Burian HM. A modification of the Burian-Allen contact-lens electrode for human electroretinography. *Am J Ophthalmol.* 1966;61:1506-1509. www.ncbi.nlm.nih.gov/pubmed/5938319. Accessed November 11, 2016.

Marmor MF, Brigell MG, McCulloch DL, Westall CA, Bach M. ISCEV standard for clinical electro-oculography (2010 update). *Doc Ophthalmol.* 2011;122(1):1-7. doi:10.1007/s10633-011-9259-0.

McCulloch DL, Marmor MF, Brigell MG, et al. ISCEV standard for full-field clinical electroretinography (2015 update). *Doc Ophthalmol.* 2015;130:1-12. doi: 10.1007/s10633-014-9473-7.

Perlman I. The electroretinogram: the ERG by Ido Perlman. The Organization of the Retina and Visual System website. http://webvision.med.utah.edu/book/electrophysiology/the-electroretinogram-erg/. Accessed November 11, 2016.

Sutter EE. Noninvasive testing methods: multifocal electrophysiology. In: Dartt DA, ed. *Encyclopedia of the Eye.* Vol 3. Oxford, England: Academic Press; 2010:142-160.

Underwood C. Electronystamography. Healthline website. www.healthline.com/health/electronystagmography#Overview1. Accessed November 11, 2016.

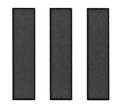

OPTICAL SKILLS

19

OPTICAL PROCEDURES

Sumáya "Sumi" Rodríguez, COT, OSC, ABO-AC, FNAO, USN (Ret)

Patients will often present with prescription glasses or some kind of visual aid meant to provide them with 20/20 vision. Knowing the prescription a patient is wearing is valuable to the doctor during examination, and is therefore an essential requirement of the patent's preliminary assessment. But even though eyewear production has greatly advanced over the years, 20/20 is not always the case. Patients will frequently have concerns or complaints about their eyewear and they will often voice that complaint to the doctor's office where they got the prescription. Therefore, it falls to optometric and ophthalmic paraprofessionals to have the skills to measure, evaluate, and verify eyewear prescriptions. Failing to recognize a faulty pair of glasses can put both the doctor's and the practice's reputation at risk.

BASIC KNOWLEDGE

Lens Power

What exactly gives a lens its "power"? To answer that question, we must first observe the nature of light as we know it and how it interacts with the human eye. For the purposes of basic optics, we consider that light travels in straight, parallel lines from an energy source at infinity. When rays of light travel from infinity, they do not have any appreciable vergence (ie, spreading apart or merging together). They will continue to travel in straight lines until interrupted or blocked by a medium such as water, a mirror, an eye, or an ophthalmic lens.

If the rays of light come in contact with a lens that is plano (flat, with no curves) the lens will allow the parallel rays of light to pass right through, undisrupted. If the lens has a "bend" or curve on the front or back surface, then the rays of light will also "bend" or *refract*. Thus, when parallel light rays from infinity come in contact with a lens with curves, the lens makes the light rays bend. So it can be said that the bent surfaces of a lens have exerted "power" or force on the rays of light. This is where a lens gets its power, from the precise shape or curvature of its front and back surfaces that cause light to bend. How much the light is bent equals the value of the lens power, measured in diopters (D).

For more details on these topics, see Chapter 4.

Optical Center of a Lens

The optical center of a lens is very important. This is the one point of every ophthalmic lens where light is *not* bent or refracted. When obtaining the measurements for prescribed spectacles or when crafting a pair of spectacles, it is very important to ensure that the optical center

Ledford JK, Lens A, eds.
Principles and Practice in Ophthalmic Assisting:
A Comprehensive Textbook (pp 347-362).
© 2018 Taylor & Francis Group.

of each lens is set directly in front of the patient's visual axis when the patient is looking straight ahead at a distant target. If the optical centers of the patient's lenses are not in line with the patient's visual axis, the patient may experience headaches or eye strain and discomfort due to the prismatic effect created. (See Chapter 4 for more on this topic, the section entitled Induced Prism.) For example, if the distance between the patient's pupils (the patient's *pupillary distance* or *PD*, discussed in more detail later) is 62 mm while looking straight ahead, then the optical centers of the right and left lenses must be set 62 mm apart as well. It is important to note that the *optical center* of a lens might not be positioned in the *geometric center* of the frame's eyewire.

When a patient is reading, the eyes converge (ie, both move inward) and the distance between the pupils decreases. Therefore, the "reading PD" will always be less than the PD measured while the patient is looking straight ahead. For most people, the near PD is about 3 mm less than the distance PD, but can be as little as 2 mm for narrow and up to 4 mm for wide PDs.

CLINICAL SKILLS
The Format of a Spectacle Prescription

Written glasses prescriptions (Rx) will usually consist of up to 10 digits per lens representing spherical power, cylinder power, and cylinder axis.

Examples:

+16.00 -1.00 x 090

-6.00 +7.00 x 180

The first number denotes the sphere power of a lens in diopters. The second number indicates the amount of cylindrical power in the lens (to correct astigmatism), also in diopters. The third number is the axis of the lens (tells where the cylinder is positioned). The axis value is limited to 001 to 180 degrees. (A perfectly horizontal axis is always designated 180, never 000.)

The degree symbol (°) should be avoided when writing a prescription as it can be easily mistaken for the number zero (0) and cause miscommunication between the ophthalmic practice and optical laboratory. It is also a good idea to cross the number 7 (7) so it is not confused with the number 2.

Transposition

An ophthalmic lens prescription can be written in plus cylinder or minus cylinder form. This conversion is referred to as *transposing* a lens prescription, where the transposition does not change the value of a prescription (or the power of the lens), but simply changes the lens's numerical presentation. To transpose a spherocylindrical lens prescription from plus to minus form or vice versa, use the following process:

1. Add the sphere and cylindrical powers algebraically. (An answer of zero [+0.00] is noted by the word plano, meaning flat, or no power.) If you need a refresher on basic algebra, see Appendix A.

2. Change the sign of the cylinder (without doing anything else to the number value).

3. Change the axis by 90°. If the result exceeds 180°, then subtract 90° from the axis value instead. (Another way to say this is that if the axis is 0 to 90, and then add 90. If the axis is 91 to 180, then subtract 90.)

Some examples are given in Chapter 4.

Manual Lensometry

Manual lensometry is an important task for eye care personnel. Reading the prescription of corrective lenses (also known as *neutralizing* the lenses) is a primary source of baseline optical data unique to each patient. In order for this information to be as precise as possible, the skills used to gather this data must be dependable. Even with today's increasing technological advances, such analytical data should not be left solely to automated machinery that can be susceptible to miscalibration, making manual lensometry highly valuable to every optometric, ophthalmic, and optical practice.

Parts of the Manual Lensometer

It would be impractical to try and describe every type of available lensometer (also called a lensmeter). Each lensometer comes with a user's guide and operations manual. Nevertheless, most lensometers have the same basic parts (Figure 19-1).

▶ Eyepiece and reticle: The *reticle* (also spelled *reticule*) is the set of black lines, circles, and numbers visible inside the eyepiece. This is superimposed over the lens when viewed through the eyepiece, and is used to help center the lens being read, as well as identifying prism. There are two knobs on the eyepiece. The focusing knob is for adjusting the reticle focus (explained below). The reticle turning knob is for rotating the reticle in the eyepiece. This feature is used when superimposing the black reticle lines over the lines of light (*mires*) seen in the lensometer. Once the black reticle lines and the mires are properly superimposed, the details of a lens can be obtained, including the optical center and the amount of prism found in the lens.

▶ Stage: Every manual lensometer has a *stage* (or *spectacle table*). When reading spectacles it is important to keep the spectacles flat and level against the stage; that is, the bottom part of both lenses/frames must rest against the stage. This is to ensure proper

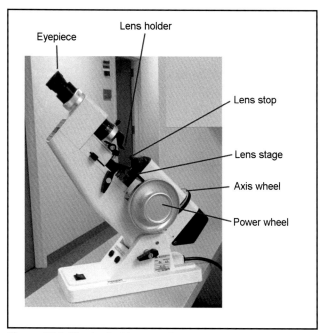

Figure 19-1. The typical lensometer.

Eyepiece
Lens holder
Lens stop
Lens stage
Axis wheel
Power wheel

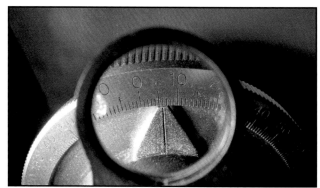

Figure 19-2. Close-up of the axis wheel, here reading axis 006.

measurement of cylinder axis and to compare the height of the optical center in each lens. If the stage "rocks" or has "see-saw" play in it, it cannot be used to read lenses and must be sent for repair. The lensometer stage is maneuvered up and down via a lever.

▶ Lens stop: Once the frame is flat and level on the stage, care must be given to rest the lens on the *lens stop* of the lensometer. It is important that the lens lay flat against the lens stop in order to get an accurate reading of the lens. Do not let the temples, nosepieces, or any other objects interfere with the lens's lying flat on the lens stop and flat on the stage. The lens stop actually touches the lens, so to avoid scratches you should ensure that the lens stop is clean and free of nicks. The scratching of a lens is unprofessional. A patient's spectacles are private property and should be handled with care.

▶ Lens holder gimbal: After the frame is positioned against the stage and stop, the *gimbal* is gently lowered against the lens using the lens holder handle, to hold the lens and frames in place. It actually touches the lens and can also cause scratches; therefore, it should be kept clean and free of nicks. Because the lens holder hinges on small screws, it is commonly the part of the lensometer that becomes worn and loose. Care should be given to maintain the gimbal in good functioning order. Never allow the lens holder gimbal to slam or clap onto a lens. Always keep control of the gimbal, allowing it to slide and rest on the lens.

▶ Power drum: The lens power is read either directly off the *power drum* (the large numbered wheel, usually on the right side of the instrument) or within the eyepiece. The drum is essentially a number line.

▶ Axis wheel: The *axis wheel* (Figure 19-2) adjusts the position of the axis when reading a toric lens. (If a spherical lens is being handled, the axis wheel will not need to be employed.) Its exact use is detailed below. Most lensometers have a small magnifier attached to make it easier to see the axis scale. If your lensometer has the axis scale *inside* the instrument's scope, be sure to read the scale as the user's manual directs.

The accuracy of the axis is especially crucial in lenses with high cylinder power. The higher the cylinder power (±1.50 or more), the more accurate the axis value must be to provide patient comfort and best-corrected vision. An inaccurate axis can cause the patient to experience discomfort and eye fatigue as well as less-than-optimal vision.

▶ Filter and filter lever: Most lensometers have a green *filter* that is operated by a lever. The green filter gives a more accurate measurement because it reduces color aberrations. Technicians who spend lots of time at the lensometer also like the green filter setting to reduce eye strain. The non-green filter setting is reserved for handling lenses that are tinted (dark sun wear, highly mirrored lenses, etc), in order to see the reticles and mires more clearly. The brighter filter setting may also be used in high-powered lenses (in plus or minus) or high-index lenses where light is more strongly refracted.

▶ Marking device and ink pad: All lensometers have ink pads and a corresponding *marking device* (Figure 19-3). The ink marking device is usually a set of three parallel pins that are touched to the ink pad then tapped onto a lens, creating three parallel dots across its surface. The middle dot marks the optical center and helps identify the amount of prism in lenses.

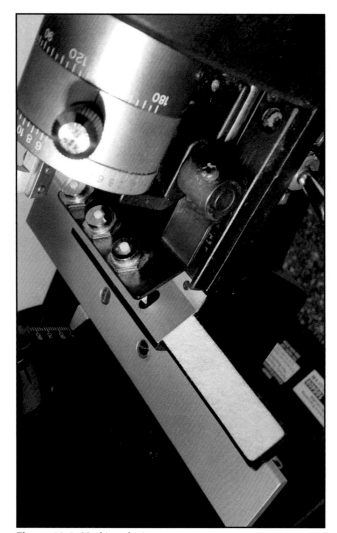

Figure 19-3. Marking device.

The inkpad may be a flat piece of felt inserted in a slot. Other ink pads are pieces of absorbent material wrapped around a small bar. A twist of the bar lifts ink from a well, ready for the marking pins to pick up. Consult your instrument's manual for further details.

▶ Marking pins: Lensometer *marking pins* are precision instruments, set into place at equal intervals, making dots across the surface of a lens at 180°. Made of either metal or industrial plastic, each pin is held in constant tension by a spring, allowing each pin to move in and out of its housing. Test the marking pins to make sure each of them slides in and out firmly, without rocking side to side.

Observe the marking pins as you tap them onto a lens (Figure 19-4). Ensure that all three pins make contact with the lens, and only at a 90° angle. If any of pins have side-to-side play, the pin(s) will splay out, creating unequal distances between the dots and therefore false measurements. Also, the misaligned pins may scratch the lens surface.

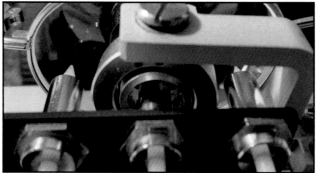

Figure 19-4. Marking the centers of a lens (as seen from above).

▶ The ink: The ink used to mark up (sometimes referred to as "dotting up") lenses is usually water based or acrylic based. Water-based ink (or India ink) creates clean, neat, and small (0.5 to 1 mm) dots that provide great accuracy when measuring to the half millimeter. The downside of using a water-based ink is that it is very easily smudged, especially if the lens has some sort of coating.

Acrylic-based inks create small and neat dots but rarely to a half-millimeter accuracy. The dots are usually approximately 1 mm, which is still desirable and accurate. The benefit of acrylic-based ink is that it dries well on most surfaces and does not smudge as easily.

The color of ink used to mark up lenses is left to the preference of the technician, depending on the lighting of the examination area and the needs of the practice. Common lensometer ink colors are red, green, yellow, and black. It is recommended that the chosen color is not easily filtered out by dim, bright, or colored lighting.

Warning: Regardless of the type of ink chosen for use in a lensometer, care must be taken to ensure that *permanent ink* is never used, as this will damage lenses permanently.

If ink is allowed to build up on the pins, this will create large, disproportioned dots that can lead to false measurements. To ensure consistent size, gently wipe ink residue from the tips of the marking pins as needed.

Ink should be added to the pad without overflowing the well or pan using an eye drop or industrial needle. If the well or pan become dry, add enough water or ink to rewet the ink. Eventually, the ink pad will have to be replaced, and the well or pan will have to be emptied and cleaned out. Having fresh supplies of ink and pad material is recommended.

▶ Prism compensating device: When the amount of prism in the lens shifts the mires out beyond the scope of the lensometer (usually more than 5 D), the *prism compensating device* (PCD) is used to bring

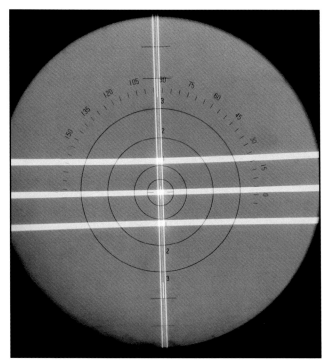

Figure 19-5. Mires of a spherical lens, showing the three narrow and three wide lines are clear together. (Green filter not in place.)

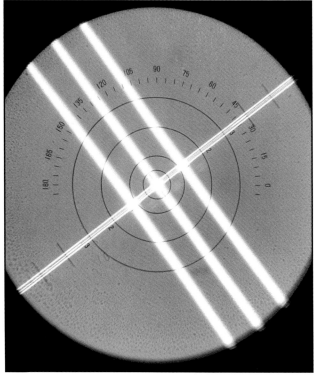

Figure 19-6. Narrow mires are clear; wide mires are blurred. This indicates that cylinder is present.

the mires back into view. Different lensometers have specific ways of operating the PCD, so be sure to refer to the user manual.

▶ Mires: With the power drum set at "0," you will see two sets of lighted lines (*mires*) inside the instrument (Figure 19-5). One set has three thin lines (for reading the sphere power), and the second set has three thick lines (for reading the cylinder power). These sets of lines are always perpendicular to each other. If the lens you are reading is spherical, both sets of mires will be sharp at the same time. If the lens is spherocylindrical (toric, for astigmatism) then only one set of mires will be sharp at a time, each at a different power setting. The mires are rotated by the use of the axis wheel, clockwise and counterclockwise.

Using the Manual Lensometer

Adjust the Eyepiece

The eyepiece must be in focus for your own vision, whether you wear corrective lenses or not. The eyepiece must be adjusted before every use by a different tech, or any time you switch back and forth from wearing your own lenses. (Note: If you are performing manual lensometry as part of a practical exam and do not adjust the eyepiece first, you will fail the test.) Try to train yourself to keep both eyes open when using the instrument.

Start by rotating the eyepiece counterclockwise until the reticle is blurred. Slowly turn the eyepiece clockwise just until the reticle appears sharp and in focus, then stop.

Do NOT turn the eyepiece back and forth trying to find this point of focus or you may induce your own accommodation. If you miss the point of focus, look away for a minute (to relax accommodation), then start over.

Place the Frames in the Instrument

Place the frame flat on the stage, temples away from you, and rest the lens flat against the lens stop. (By convention the right lens is usually handled first.) Looking through the eyepiece, find the optical center of the lens (where the reading will be most accurate) by carefully adjusting the position of the lens (taking care to lift the lens off the lens stop to avoid scratching) until the mires are centered in the middle of the reticle. (If you cannot see the mires, turn the power wheel a bit until you find at least one set.) Gently lower the gimbal onto the lens.

Neutralize the Lens

Looking in the lensometer, turn the power drum until the mires (or at least one set of them) come into clear focus. If the three thin lines and the three thick lines focus at the same power setting, then the lens is spherical.

If both sets of lines will not focus together, there is cylinder present (Figure 19-6). In this case, you must know whether you want to read the lens power (prescription) in plus or minus cylinder form (Sidebar 19-1).

Looking into the lensometer, turn the power drum until the *three thin lines* of light come to clear focus and stop. You may notice the thin lines seem "broken" or as if there are "open gates" on the lines (Figure 19-7). If so,

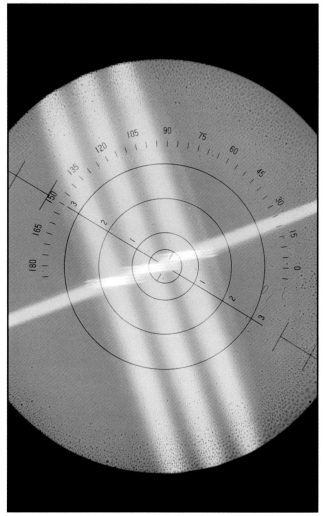

Figure 19-7. Note "broken" lines: Narrow mires are not aligned.

turn the axis wheel to "close the gates" and create straight lines. Readjust the position of the lens to center the mires in the reticle if needed, and ensure the frames are against the stage. After the thin lines are in focus, quickly check if the three thick lines would come into focus by rotating the power drum toward the plus or toward the minus.

Once the thin lines are clear and you have determined the proper position for plus or minus cylinder, refocus the thin lines (if necessary) and read the power on the power drum. This is the sphere power of the lens. Then turn the power drum until the three thick lines come into focus. The *difference between these numbers* is the cylinder power. (It is a common mistake to read the cylinder power directly off the power drum. If you need a refresher on the number line and basic algebra, see Appendix A.) The cylinder axis is read directly off the axis wheel. Sidebar 19-2 shows a sample lensometry reading.

It is also important to note that the quality of the mires may indicate the quality of the lens (Sidebar 19-3). The mires should be bright, sharp, and crisp, and at a 90° angle from each other. If they are not, this may indicate that the lens manufacturing is poor, or that the lenses are warped or otherwise marred.

Identify and Measure ADDs (If Present)

Segmented Multifocals

Multifocal lenses come in various forms. These lenses contain both distance and reading sections, and sometimes intermediate portions as well. The distance part is usually at the top of the lens, the intermediate near the center, with the reading portion at the very bottom. (Refer to Chapter 20 for more on lenses and types of lenses.) The reading portion of a lens is referred to as the reading segment or "ADD." It is important to note that the reading segment adds plus to (or reduces minus from) only the *spherical* power of a lens; the *cylinder* power remains unchanged.

If the lens has visible segments, it is easily identified as being a bifocal or trifocal (two or three sections to the lens, respectively). Once the top/distance part of the lens has been read and noted, lift the gimbal and move the lens stage to slide the lens up on the lens stop. Center the mires for the bottom-most segment if possible. (Sometimes the segment is very small, and centering the mires in the reticle is difficult.) Turn the power wheel toward yourself

SIDEBAR 19-2

LENSOMETRY EXAMPLE

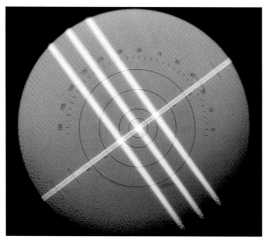

Step 1. Focus the three thin mires. Note the "closed gates" and the clear, sharp images.

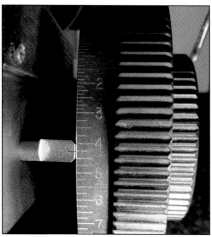

Step 2. Note the three thin lines (mires) come into focus at -4.25 D.

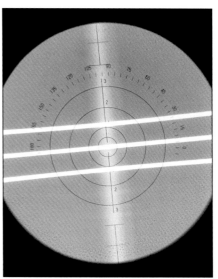

Step 3. Next focus the three thick mires, which also have "closed gates."

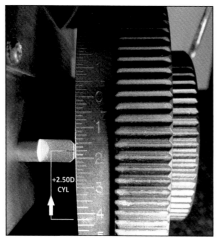

Step 4. Note the reading of the power drum where the three thick lines (mires) come into focus at -1.75 D. The algebraic difference between these two points on power drum is the lenses' cylinder (CYL) power in diopters: 2.50 D. Because you went from -4.25 to -1.75 (toward the plus direction), the cylinder is in the "plus" form, in this case: +2.50 D CYL.

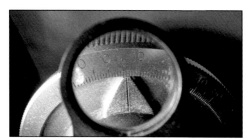

Step 5. Note the cylinder axis on the axis wheel, 006.

The prescription is -4.25 + 2.50 X 006.

SIDEBAR 19-3
LENSOMETRY AND THE WARPED/INFERIOR LENS

When a technician comes across a poorly manufactured lens, it can be very confusing, as these lenses seem to defy known laws of optical physics. The following are common in the poorly manufactured lens:

1. In a toric lens, the thin and thick mires will not center onto the black reticles at the same point of focus (the optical center is not going through the lens at 90°).

2. Thin and/or thick mires appear to come into focus but are doubled (you see up to six thin and/or thick lines), and no amount of focusing can correct for this.

3. The mires are blurry and will not exactly focus at one point on the power drum. The lens surfaces are worn, scratched, or manufactured with uneven back/front surfaces.

4. The axis wheel cannot "close the gates" at the same time. Even when the gates seem closed, the mires remain wavy, blurry, or doubled. No amount of focusing or lens repositioning can correct for this.

5. The power (sph or cyl) will not come to a precise point of power in the power drum. Each of the smallest, dash-lines on the power drum measure 0.125 D. If the sph power of a lens measures 10.875 D (neither 10.75 D nor 10.00 D) this can be a source of discomfort to a patient, especially in higher-powered Rx's.

6. The coating on the surface of the lens (back or front surface) has worn down, is damaged, peeling away, or was applied unevenly. This will cause light to be distorted (both for the patient and the lensometry mires) and thus change the intended Rx.

These are practical lens problems that can be spotted in the clinic setting at any time. Under these conditions, the patient's spectacle Rx cannot be clinically obtained. The solution in each of these conditions is to obtain new lens(es) for the patient.

SIDEBAR 19-4
IS THIS LENS A PROGRESSIVE ADDITION LENS?

There are several ways you might identify a PAL.

▶ Hold the glasses above a line of print and move them up and down. The letters will look larger toward the bottom of the lens if this is a PAL.

▶ Hold the glasses out from you and look at a straight line and move them up and down. You can often see the distortion as the lens power changes from top to bottom.

▶ Hold the glasses up to a strong light and see if you can find any etchings.

▶ Use a PAL ID instrument to see if you can find any etchings.

▶ Put the lens on the lensometer, with the upper part of the lens on the lens stop. Find the sphere power, then move the frame so the lower part of the lens is on the lens stop. If these are PALs, there should be more plus (less minus) toward the bottom of the lens vs the top.

▶ Ask the patient.

Progressive Addition Lenses

The progressive addition lens (PAL) is a subtype of multifocal lens. In its most simple terms, the power of a PAL "progresses" from the distance section at the top, then morphs gradually with more plus power (or less minus, which is the same thing) as you go down the lens until the bottom part of the lens, which contains the strongest reading power (Sidebar 19-4).

Progressive lenses may at first appear to be single vision lenses with no reading segment, and indeed, this is one of the benefits of the PAL—its cosmetic value. To know the power of the reading portion of a PAL, one need only find the etchings placed on the lens by the manufacturer. The power of the ADD is usually found toward the temporal part of the lens, but some manufacturers only etch two numbers on the lens. Thus a +2.00 ADD would be noted on the lens as 20, a +2.25 ADD as 22, and a +2.75 as 27.

The manufacturer may also etch the company's logo onto the lens near the ADD etching or opposite from it. Once the logo is visualized, you can identify the maker in a "Progressive Identifier" catalog. Knowing the manufacturer will allow you to find the appropriate layout template for marking up the lenses.

If you need to find the power of a PAL using the lensometer, the point on the lens called the "fitting cross" must be found. First, locate the manufacturer's etchings.

until the thin mires clear for the spherical power of the ADD. Note the reading; the *difference* between the two spherical values (*not the actual numeric reading on the power wheel*) is the ADD power of the reading segment. The reading ADD is usually the same for both eyes. The intermediate segment is usually half that of the reading ADD, but can be read individually if desired.

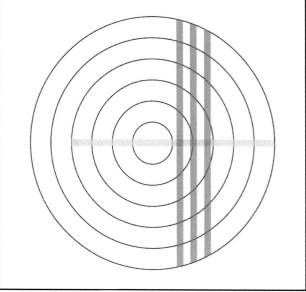

Figure 19-8. Schematic of decentration of mires where the lens has prism. In this case, the mires cross on the first circle from the center, so there is 1 D of prism. If this were the right lens, then the prism is base-in; if the left lens, then base-out.

These may be a symbol + or °. Using a *nonpermanent* ink marker, mark or "dot up" the etchings. Then find the appropriate Progressive Lens Layout Template provided by the manufacturer of the lenses. These templates are readily available from the manufactures via catalogs and online sources. Lay the spectacles onto the template and line up your etching marks. Next, carefully trace the fitting cross, the distance portion (the "setting sun" symbol), and the reading portion (in the form of a circle).

Now you are ready to put the lenses into the lensometer. Following the steps above, read the distance prescription by placing the setting sun marker over the lens stop and gently lower the gimbal. Remember to keep the spectacles flat against the lens stop and flat across the stage. This is the distance lens power or prescription. Then place the reading circle against the lens stop and verify the reading power of the ADD.

Identify Prism (If Present)

Prism is sometimes added to a prescription lens in order to deviate light rays in a particular direction. This causes the eye(s) to shift, and is used to prevent double vision. The direction of the prism is noted by the location of the prism base, and is thus designated as base-in (BI), base-out (BO), base-up (BU), or base-down (BD). (See Chapter 10 for more on prism use in strabismus.) Prism that is added to a lens does not affect the lens's power.

Prism can be incorporated into a lens either by grinding it in or by shifting the optical centers of the lenses away from the patient's pupillary distance (*decentering*). Prism caused by decentering is called *induced prism*. There are also temporary prisms (Fresnel prisms) that can be stuck onto a lens and peeled off later. Either way, light is deviated away from the visual axis. Unless prescribed, induced prism must always be identified and

corrected, as it can cause significant patient discomfort and/or double vision (Sidebar 19-5).

Prism can be identified with the manual lensometer. If the prism is ground in (vs decentered), you will notice that it is impossible to center the mires in the reticle. (Note: If the lens is toric, neither set of mires will center.) No matter how you move the lens around on the lens stop, the mires are off-set and stay in the same off-center location on the reticle. The orientation of the mires and where they fall on the reticle tells you the power of the prism (in diopters) as well as its position (BU, BD, BI, or BO, or some combination of vertical and horizontal).

The concentric circles in the reticle have numbers that tell how many diopters of prism is in the lens. Observe the spot where the two sets of mires cross and at which circle the center of the mires is located. The number on that circle denotes the power of the prism (Figure 19-8).

The location of the mires tells you the orientation of the prism base. If the center of the mires is located above the center of the reticle, then you have found BU prism. If the center of the mires is located below the center of the reticle, then you have found BD prism.

To check for induced vertical prism, first center and measure the distance portion of the right lens. Then *do not move the stage up or down as you move the left lens over onto the stage*. If the mires of the left lens are not centered in the reticle, take note of how many rings above or below they are from the reticle's center.

Horizontal induced prism (ie, base-in or -out) can be trickier to find and evaluate. In this case the lens mires *will* center, but not in the expected place. To measure the amount of induced prism, you must mark and measure the centers of the lenses and compare this measurement to the patient's pupillary distance (covered later).

One may also measure the amount of prism with the *prism compensating device* (PCD) on the lensometer's eyepiece. When the amount of prism in the lens shifts the mires center out of the scope of the lensometer, the PCD is used to bring the mires back into view. This may need to be done before the power of the lens can be read.

To use the PCD, bring any visible mires into focus. If the mires are displaced vertically, rotate the PCD's knob and bring the target of the mires to the center of the reticle. If the mires are horizontally displaced, grasp the knob of the PCD and swing the device so the knob is at 90°. Then rotate the knob to bring the targets onto the reticle. The power of the prism and the base direction is read from the two scales on the PCD collar. Once the mires are centered, read the lens prescription as usual. If you use the PCD, be courteous of the next user and turn it back to zero when you're done.

Induced horizontal or vertical prism in PALs is very difficult to find unless you mark up the lenses. Once you've marked the lenses using the appropriate template, proceed as above.

Automated Lensometry

The standard automated lensometer (see Figure 5-14) provides a considerable amount of information concerning a lens, including sphere power, cylindrical power, cylinder axis, ADD power (if present), and prism (if present).

Automated lensometers should be used in accordance with the manufacturer's operational manual. Just like the manual lensometer, the spectacles must be kept flat against the lens stop and flat across the stage. The user must indicate if the desired reading should be plus or minus cylinder by pressing a button on the instrument's panel. Most models provide a printout of the reading, if desired.

One thing an automated lensometer will not provide is information that a lens is irregular or poorly manufactured. The mires of a manual lensometer still provide the best visual evaluation regarding the quality of a given lens.

Measuring Pupillary Distance

The patient's *pupillary distance* (PD) is the measurement in millimeters from the optic axis of one pupil to that of the other, on a 180° plane, while the patient is looking at a distance of 6 meters or 20 feet (ie, optical infinity). This is the patient's distance PD. The patient's PD is also measured while looking at a near object, 12 to 20 inches away. This is the patient's reading PD. Because the eyes converge when looking at near, the reading PD is always smaller than the distance PD. In the case of prescribing

progressive lenses, mono PD's (from one pupil to midline of face) at both distance and near must be provided in order to complete the prescription.

The patient's PD is a baseline measurement used when selecting frames. An accurate PD must be obtained in order to craft a comfortable, precision set of spectacles. An inaccurate PD can cause induced prism, giving the patient double vision or eye strain.

Several methods can be used to obtain a patient's PD and are discussed below.

Pupillometer

When possible, an electronic pupillometer is utilized to obtain a patient's PD. The instrument utilizes corneal reflection created by a light that reflects off of the cornea as the patient looks at a central target.

To operate, have the patient hold the device up to the eyes like a set of binoculars. Look into the other end of the device and slide the appropriate levers on either the top or the bottom of the instrument to *Distance PD, Near PD,* or *Mono PD*. Then measure the PD by sliding the vertical black hairline over the small white light reflected on the patient's cornea so that it bisects the pupil. Measure each eye and then read the desired PD from the digital readouts on the outside of the pupillometer; record in the patient's chart.

Pupillary Distance Ruler

When no other tools are available, a PD ruler is used to measure the PD. This method is an essential skill for all optometric and ophthalmic technicians, and requires a straight 6-inch ruler (approximately 150 mm).

▶ Method 1—PD ruler: The examiner should be positioned directly in front of the patient and at the same vertical level, at a distance of no more than 16 inches. Ensure that the ruler does not bend, bow, or arc during the measurement. The ruler is held with the thumb and forefinger while resting the other three fingers gently against the patient's head. Place the ruler on the bridge of the patient's nose at a plane of 180°.

Ask the patient to look straight at your open left eye. Using your left eye and with the right eye closed, place the edge of the ruler, where it reads 000 mm, beneath the center of the pupil of the patient's right eye. Once proper alignment is achieved, close your left eye, and with your right eye, observe the patient's left eye. The patient is asked to look straight ahead at your open (now right) eye. Read the measurement just beneath the center of the patient's left pupil and record the result in millimeters.

▶ Method 2—PD ruler: For patients with dark irides, the center of the pupil is not always clearly visible. In cases like this, using a penlight may brighten the iris but it may also constrict the pupil, making it more difficult to see the ruler. Also, it may sometimes be necessary to take a PD measurement when the patient is dilated. In such a case, the technician may use the PD ruler as indicated above, but measuring from the *outside* edge of the right limbus to the *inside* edge of the left limbus. This distance is roughly the same as the distance between the pupils.

▶ Method 3—Englemann method: The Englemann method of measuring a patient's PD makes use of a straight edge (hairline) to bisect the patient's pupils. You will need two rubber bands, a set of frames with no lenses in them, and two "hairlines" (any stiff, straight-line object that is tall enough to sit against the frame). Straightened metal paperclips are exactly 1 mm thick (in diameter) and therefore make good hairlines as they will not be bent by the rubber bands, and are easily measured to the half millimeter.

A rubber band is positioned across each eyewire at a position of 180°. The vertical hairline is positioned at 90° within the rubber band so that it is held fast. The frame is then placed on the patient's face, and the hairlines are slid over until they bisect the pupils (Figure 19-9). The distance between the right and left hairlines is the patient's PD.

This method is recommended for use when a "functional PD" is necessary, such as when measuring for low vision devices, occupational scopes, or binoculars.

Since the malfunction of any of these pieces could potentially injure the patient's eyes or face, ensure that your straight-line objects are long enough to not slip off the top and bottom of the eyewire while measuring or so weak that they can crack or snap in two. Also, ensure that the rubber bands are new and sturdy.

Frame and Lens Measurements

Mark and Measure the Centers

If the optical center of a lens needs to be verified, use the inking mechanism on the lensometer. Once the lens mires are centered in the instrument, push the lever of the marking device (above the stage) onto the lens surface. "Dotting up" the lenses in this manner should produce three small dots, the middle dot representing the optical center of the lens. The three dots together, which should be on the same plane, represent the horizontal meridian of the lens. If the dots are not aligned, an error has been made in the dotting process.

Once both lenses are "dotted up," use a millimeter scale or ruler to measure from the center dot of one lens to the other. This measure is known as the *distance between the optical centers* (DBOC). It is important that the ink dots on lenses are crisp and sharp, about 1 mm in diameter. Be care to not bend or "arc" the ruler across

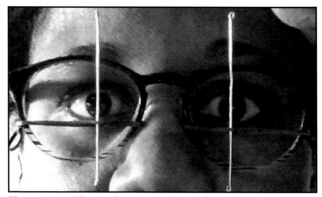

Figure 19-9. The Englemann method of measuring a patient's pupillary distance.

the lenses. If the ruler must be bent, then a set of straight calipers should be used to measure the DBOC instead. Bowing the ruler will provide a false reading.

Calculating Induced Prism

While looking through the optical center of a lens, the patient will experience no prismatic effect. However, if a patient is looking above or below, to the left or right of the optical center of the lens, he/she will experience *induced prism*. The farther away the eye looks from the optical center of a lens, the greater the prismatic effect will be. Sometimes prism is induced intentionally as prescribed by a practitioner. However, if this is not the case, induced prism can be a real problem for the patient (see Sidebar 19-5).

The formula used to calculate the amount of prism is known as *Prentice's rule* and is as follows:

P = (h)(D)

P = prism power, in prism diopters

h = the distance between the optical center of the lens and the position where the eye is looking through the lens, in *centimeters*

D = the power of the lens, in diopters

The power of the lens (in diopters) is directly associated with the amount of prism induced (Sidebar 19-6). This is to say the higher the power of the lens (in either plus or minus), the easier it is to create large amounts of induced prism with just a small shift between the optical center of the lens and the position where the eye is looking through the lens. See also Prentice's Rule in Chapter 4, Optics.

The Boxing System

The *boxing system* is the method by which frame and lens measurements are designated (Sidebar 19-7). The boxing system is also used to obtain industrial/official frame measurements. When manufacturers, designers, and research developers construct new frame and lens cut models, the boxing system is used to produce

---

You are looking 3 cm below optical axis on a
- 2.00 D lens. How much prism is induced?

$P = h\,D$

$P = (3)(2) = 6$ pd BD

You are looking 5 mm above the optical axis of a
+6.00 D lens. How much prism is induced?

$P = hD$

$P = (0.5)(6) = 3$ pd BD

You are looking 3 cm below optical axis on a
- 2.00 D lens. How much prism is induced?

$P = h\,D$

$P = (3)(2) = 6$ pd BD

You are looking 5 mm above the optical axis of a
+6.00 D lens. How much prism is induced?

$P = hD$

$P = (0.5)(6) = 3$ pd BD

The boxing system is not the same as the datum system, which is older than the boxing system. First established for the measuring of bifocal heights and placements of lens optical centers and comprised mostly of horizontal lines, the datum system soon evolved into our current boxing system. Ultimately, the boxing system is based on figuratively placing a set of frames into a "measuring box" and obtaining various dimensions in millimeters.

---

the blueprints and drawings, making this technique an industry standard.

In our fast-growing digital industry, where the measurements are becoming more and more precise down to the half and quarter millimeter, a solid understanding of lens and frame measurements is vital to the proper handling of optical wear.

The measurements given by the boxing system apply to a specific frame and also refer to the lenses that are ground specifically to fit in that frame. (The parts of a frame are covered in Chapter 20. Important for this discussion is the eyewire or rim, the open part of the frame where a lens is inserted. See also Figure 20-24.) These dimensions include:

▶ A size: The *A size* is the widest horizontal measurement across the eyewire (rim) of a frame (also referred to as the *eye size*). Regardless of the frame's shape or fashion design, the A size is the frame's longest horizontal distance from temple to nasal, measured on a 180° line. This includes the depth of the bevel cut into the lens. (The bevel on a lens is the V-shape of the edge that is "gripped" by the frame.)

A bevel cut can be as much as 2 mm, depending on frame design. The A size is important in measuring the distance between the optical centers of lenses and the distance between the geometric centers of frames (discussed momentarily).

▶ B size: The B size is the tallest vertical measurement of the eyewire. Regardless of the frame's shape or design, the B size is the tallest vertical distance from the top of the eyewire to bottom, measured at 90°. (Again include the depth of the lens bevel.) This dimension is vital in measuring segment heights during fitting, as well as determining the placement of a progressive lens fitting cross during grinding. It is also instrumental in determining vertical imbalances/unwanted vertical prism.

▶ Geometric center/point C: The *geometric center* (C, or point C) of the eyewire or the mounted lens is the point where the A size line intersects the B size line, creating a point that is the geometric center of the eyewire and lens. Point C is not to be confused with the optical center of the lens, which can only be found using the lensometer.

▶ Effective diameter: The *effective diameter* (ED) of a lens is the diameter of the smallest circle that completely encloses the cut and beveled (ground prescription) lens, where the center of the circle coincides with the point C of the lens. This generally makes the ED the longest measurement from one side of the lens to the other. The ED is used to estimate the smallest lens blank (uncut lens) to use for that particular frame. This is desirable in order to provide the patient with premium optics.

▶ Distance between the lenses: The *distance between the lenses* (DBL) of a frame is the shortest distance between the mounted lenses. This measurement is determined with precision calipers, measuring from the inside bevel of one eyewire to the inside bevel of the other eyewire, on a 180° plane. (This measurement is not to be confused with the frame bridge size [which does not include the eyewire] or the distance between lens centers.)

▶ Box number: The "size" of a set of frames is the box number stamped on the frame in question, usually on the bridge, nose pad, or a temple. All prescription frames have a box number. If a pair of frames does not have a box number, it is probable that the manufacturer did not intend for that set of frames to receive prescription lenses.

The box number is two numbers separated by a box-like symbol, for example 58☐16. The first number denotes the A size of the eyewire and the second denotes the DBL, in millimeters. The box symbol denotes that these measurements were determined by use of the standard boxing system. Added together, the two numbers provide the distance between the geometric centers of the frame.

The box number is used to determine the official frame size that is used in frame identification. Being able to identify a frame by box number is important because it is possible to have the same color, design, and style of frame available in several different frame sizes.

▶ Frame distance between centers: The distance between point C of each eyewire is the frame's *distance between centers* (DBC). This measurement is mostly used in manufacturing and lens fitting. In an ideal situation, the patient would choose a frame where the distance between the frame centers is close to his/her PD. This means that the optical center of each lens does not have to be decentered more than just a few millimeters.

▶ Lens distance between optical centers: The *distance between optical centers* (DBOC) of the lenses is distance from the optical center of one mounted lens to the other. (Don't confuse this with the frame DBC, which measures between the geometric centers.) This measurement must be the same as the patient's PD and aligned with the patient's visual axis. If it is not, then the patient is not getting the full optical value of the lenses, and vision will not be as sharp as it could be. In addition, such misalignment can cause unwanted induced prism.

Measuring Vertex Distance

Vertex distance (VD) is the distance from the surface of the cornea to the back surface of a lens as it sits in a frame, trial frame, or phoropter. Thus, the VD will vary from one frame to another and one instrument to another. The VD is important for high-powered eye wear prescriptions (≥ 3 D) because of the properties of minus and plus lenses. If a lens is moved further away or closer to the eye, the focal point of that lens shifts. This can adversely

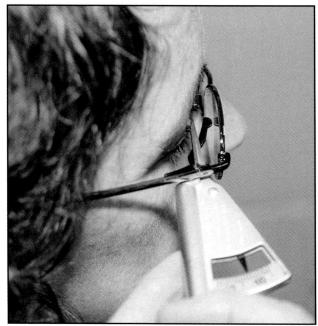

Figure 19-10. Using the distometer to measure vertex distance. (Reprinted with permission from Ray Mok, COMT, CRA.)

affect vision if the image is moved off the fovea. While the actual power of the lens is fixed and does not change, the patient's perception is that it no longer provides the intended visual result. This is because the *effective power* of the lens has been altered by shifting it.

To ensure that the correct lens power is ordered, VD needs to be measured at the time of refractometry. VD can also be measured when a patient returns with a glasses problem, to rule out any problems with the effective power of the spectacles.

The most commonly used device to measure VD is the *distometer* (also called *vertexometer*). Note that the distometer does not initially point to zero; this is because the instrument compensates for the thickness of the patient's eyelid. For patient safety, ensure that he/she keeps both eyes closed for the measurement. Do not contact the globe with the footplate.

Ensuring that the patient's eyes are closed, place the stationary footplate of the distometer on the center of the closed upper eyelid. (If the patient has redundant skin on the upper eyelid, gently pull the skin up so that you are only measuring one thickness. Make sure the lids are still closed.) Press the plunger until the moveable foot just touches the lens (Figure 19-10). The measurement in millimeters is read right off of the distometer as the VD. If recalculation of lens power is necessary, use the rotating chart that comes with the instrument or consult published charts to find the appropriate change. When finished, the footplate should be sanitized, as it is a point of patient contact.

Most phoropters have a viewing scale on each side (called the corneal alignment device) where one can view

---

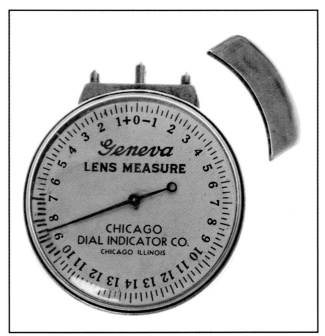

Figure 19-11. Geneva lens clock (Chicago Dial Indicator Co).

the distance from the lens to the apex of the patient's cornea. Place the patient to the phoropter, and then look into the alignment device. In order to avoid parallax error (ie, error induced by an oblique angle of the observer), align the V notches with the zero point (heavy vertical line). If the apex of the patient's cornea falls on the zero point, the VD is the standard 13.75 mm. If the cornea falls to the right of the zero point, each line in the device represents 2 mm, which would be added to the standard 13.75 mm. Phoropters vary, so check your user's manual.

Trial frames have a VD scale on each side of the frame. Use a penlight for better visibility (the scale is small), and be sure to view the patient from a perpendicular position. Reading the scale at an angle can give an erroneous result.

Measuring Spectacle Lens Base Curve With the Geneva Lens Clock

The *Geneva lens clock* or *measure* (also simply called the lens clock; Figure 19-11) can be used to measure the *base curve* of a lens, which is on the front (ie, outer) surface of modern lenses. The average base curve is usually about +6.00. If a patient receives new glasses with a different base curve than he/she is used to, this may be a source of discomfort and eye strain. The only way to know the base curve of a lens is to measure it. It is important to note that a lens clock is calibrated for either glass or plastic lenses; thus, a change in lens material can also cause patient discomfort. Refer to the clock manufacturer's guide prior to use.

The lens clock is a precision instrument that should not be exposed to extreme heat, cold, or direct sunlight.

The clock itself has a face with a single moving hand and two number scales, one in red and one in black and/or one inside the other. The clock's hand is not exactly at zero when not in use. This is the normal starting position (usually about 2 D off zero) unless otherwise indicated by the user manual. The base of the instrument has three pins; the outer pins are stationary but the center pin is spring-loaded and moves the hand. A cap is provided to protect the pins.

To verify the lens clock's calibration, place the device on a smooth, flat surface such as a mirror or glass countertop with all three points touching. (Wood and plastic surfaces may suffice but are not ideal.) With the instrument held perpendicularly on the surface, note where the clock hand is pointing. If the hand points precisely to zero (plano), then the clock is in calibration. If it stops at a place other than zero, it needs to be reset. (Instructions on how to do this may be found at http://ep.yimg.com/ty/cdn/yhst-591685299959315/HOWTOCALIBRATEALENSCLOCK.pdf.) If the center pin sticks or does not move properly, the device should be replaced.

Note: The prescription of a lens may be ground on the front or back surface, but most modern lenses are ground on the back surface. This means that the front surface is spherical, ideal for measuring the base curve. For the purpose of this discussion, it is assumed that the lens in question has the prescription on the back surface.

Surface power readings can be taken on either side of the lens, but if all you need is the lens's base curve, reading the front surface is enough. To read the base curve, the three pins of the clock are placed against the front surface of the lens, ensuring that the middle pin is on the center and the instrument is perpendicular. The lenses' base curve (or surface power) is read directly from the face of the lens clock in diopters of power as indicated by the black or *inner* number scale. (If you want to read the back surface of the lens, the above process is repeated, except the red or outer numbers on the dial are used.)

During use, the clock must be held at 90° (perpendicular) to the front lens surface. Tilting just 10° can give a reading that could be up to 2 D off. Once the instrument is properly applied to the lens, the clock hand will point to the base curve reading, indicated by the black or inside number scale. A reading cannot be taken on progressives, aspheric lenses, or on lenses with a warped surface. A multifocal segment can be read if all three pins will sit on the segment.

The lens clock can be used to discover if a lens is warped. With the lens clock against the front surface and facing you, hold it steady in one hand as the other hand rotates the lens 180°. Keep the three pins in contact with the lens during the entire rotation. Observe the lens clock hand. If it remains on the same gauge number throughout the rotation, that surface is spherical, as it should be. If the hand moves erratically as the lens is rotated, then the lens is warped.

Estimating Lens Power With the Geneva Lens Measure

The lens clock can also be used to estimate the lens's surface power, determine if the lens is toric or spherical, and to roughly locate the axis of a toric lens. The steps are as follows:

- Test calibration by zeroing out the lens clock.

- Measure the base curve of the front surface and record (F1).

- Apply the clock to the back surface of the lens and rotate, using the center pin as the fulcrum. Be careful to hold the clock perpendicular to the surface and maintain the center pin in the center of the lens. Watch the dial as you rotate the clock.
  - If the clock reading does not change as you rotate it, then the lens is spherical. Write down this number (F2). Adding F1 and F2 will give you the lens power.
  - If the hand moves as you rotate the clock, the lens is toric (ie, has cylinder).

- Note the position (axis) of the clock at both the highest and lowest measurements. Record the axis and power at each.

- The approximate prescription of the lens can be calculated by use of the optical cross (Sidebar 19-8).
  - Note: If during this operation you notice that the lens clock hand is erratic in its rise and fall (ie, high reading and low reading are not 90° away from each other), the lens may be warped or damaged.

ACKNOWLEDGMENTS

The author would like to thank the following: Catherine Horan, BA, COMT, and Teresa (Anjali) Narayan, OD.

CHAPTER QUIZ

1. Why is it important to place optical center directly in front of the patient's pupil or visual axis?

2. A spectacle prescription can be transposed to plus or minus cylinder. Transpose the following prescriptions:
   a. +2.50 -1.00 x 132
   b. -3.25 +0.75 x 056

3. Explain the difference between reticles and mires.

SIDEBAR 19-8
FINDING A LENS PRESCRIPTION USING THE GENEVA LENS CLOCK

Example 1
The clock reading on the front surface of the lens (F1) is +2.50. The clock reading on the back surface of the lens (F2) is -4.50 at axis 90 and -2.50 at axis 180, indicating that cylinder is present. Because the lens power is equal to F1 + F2, the power of each surface is put onto an optical cross and combined:

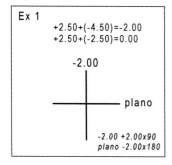

Example 2
The clock reading on the front surface of the lens (F1) is +6.00. The clock reading on the back surface of the lens (F2) is +2.25 at axis 135 and -0.75 at axis 045, indicating that cylinder is present. Because the lens power is equal to F1 + F2, the power of each surface is put onto an optical cross and combined:

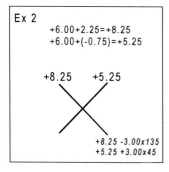

---

4. What can be done to avoid inducing one's own accommodation while adjusting the eyepiece, before beginning lensometry operations?

5. When neutralizing a lens with the lensometer, what is indicated when the three thin lines and the three thick lines of light come into focus at the same power setting?

6. During lensometry, the three thin lines come into focus at -1.50 D and the three thick lines come into focus at -4.75 D. What does this information tell us about this lens?

7. What is the standard power for an intermediate segment of a trifocal lens?

8. A progressive lens has "27" laser etched on to the front surface of the lens. What does this tell you about this lens?

9. Why is it important to keep spectacles flat against the lensometer stage at all times while neutralizing?

10. When calculating induced prism, what do each of the formula variables represent in the following equation: $P = (h)(D)$

11. What is the difference between the optical center of a lens and the geometric center of a lens?

12. Name three ways of obtaining a pupillary distance measurement.

Answers

1. If the optical centers of the patient's lenses are not in line with the patient's visual axis, the patient may experience headaches or eye strain and discomfort due to the prismatic effect created (induced prism).

2. a. +1.50 +1.00 x 042, b. -2.50 -0.75 x 146

3. The reticle is the set of black lines and circles visible inside the eyepiece. This is superimposed over the lens when viewed through the eyepiece, and is used to help center the lens being read, as well as identifying prism. Mires are any set of lines, produced by light, seen inside of a scope.

4. To focus the lensometer's eyepiece, start by rotating the eyepiece counterclockwise until the reticle is blurred. Slowly turn the eyepiece clockwise just until the reticle appears sharp and in focus, then stop. Do NOT turn the eyepiece back and forth trying to find this point of focus or you may induce your own accommodation.

5. If the lensometer lines come into focus together, this indicates that the lens is spherical and no cylinder power is present.

6. The lens is toric (corrects for astigmatism or has cylinder power). The cylinder power is 3.25 D, indicated by the difference between the two points of focus.

7. The intermediate segment of a trifocal is usually half that of the reading ADD.

8. This tells us that the reading or near portion of the lens has an ADD power of +2.75 D.

9. Keeping the spectacles flat on the lensometer stage ensures proper measurement of the cylinder axis (if present). It also ensures an accurate measurement of prism (induced or prescribed).

10. $P = (h)(D)$. P = prism power. h = the distance from the optical center of the lens to the position where the eye is looking through the lens, in centimeters. D = the power of the lens in diopters.

11. The optical center is the point on the lens where light is not deviated, diverged, or converged. This point on the lens can only be determined by the use of a lensometer. The geometric center of the lens is measured with a ruler and indicates the center of the diameter of the lens.

12. 1) PD ruler: Measuring from center of pupil to center of pupil. 2) PD ruler: Measure from the outside of the right limbus to the inside left limbus. This distance is roughly the same as the distance between the pupils. 3) Pupillometer: The technician measures each eye, one at a time, and then reads the desired PD from the digital read-outs on the outside of the instrument.

BIBLIOGRAPHY

Brooks CW, Borish IM. *System for Ophthalmic Dispensing.* 2nd ed. Waltham, MA: Butterworth-Heinemann Ltd; 1996.

Dowaliby M. *Practical Aspects of Ophthalmic Optics.* 3rd ed. Waltham, MA: Butterworth-Heinemann Ltd; 1988.

How to use a lens clock to determine the base and the power! Ophthalmic Lenses blog. ophthalmiclenses.blogspot.com/2011/08/how-to-use-lens-clock-to-determine-base.html. August 8, 2011. Accessed March 4, 2016.

Meister D. Ophthalmic lens design. Online Optical Continuing Education website. www.opticampus.com/cecourse.php?url=lens_design/. Accessed March 4, 2016.

Stoner E, Perkins P, Ferguson R. *Optical Formulas Tutorial.* 2nd ed. Philadelphia, PA: Elsevier Health Sciences; 2005.

Zelada AJ. *A Dispensing Optician Manual: An Introduction to Vision Care for the New Ophthalmic Technician.* Springfield, IL: Charles C Thomas Pub Ltd; 1987.

20

EYEWEAR
SPECTACLES AND LENSES

Anne West-Ellmers, COT, OSC, LDO, NCLEC, AAS

Sir Elton John. Tom Cruise. Sarah Palin. Malcolm X. Jacqueline Kennedy Onassis. These notable individuals became synonymous with the now-iconic frame styles that each wore and popularized.

Today's eyeglass frames are both fun and fashionable. As eye care professionals, we are challenged with balancing these first two aspects with that of a most important third: its functionality.

Patients focus on the fun colors, shapes, and other fashionable aspects of their eyewear, but we must be cognizant of the functionality of the frame choice, in addition to its good looks. How well a frame fits a given patient will determine how well he or she sees. Its position on the face affects the optics of the lenses and can make or break the refractionist's best efforts.

BASIC KNOWLEDGE

Essential to the understanding of frames and lenses is a working knowledge of refractive errors and optics. These are covered in Chapter 4.

CLINICAL KNOWLEDGE

Frames

Eyeglass frames are optical devices used to suspend prescription quality lenses in front of the eyes as a means to compensate for refractive errors and/or accommodative and convergence dysfunctions, thereby improving vision. (Prescription/optical quality lenses are precisely manufactured to eliminate inherent or otherwise unwanted distortions. This is not the case with inexpensive, mass-produced readers and sunglasses.)

Frames can also be employed to hold prisms for reducing or eliminating double vision. They position lenses with antireflective coatings and light-polarizing films to reduce or eliminate disabling glare, or colored lens filters that permit the color blind to more easily discriminate between previously indistinguishable colors. Frames are also used to secure impact-resistant safety lenses for work or sports, in addition to hearing aids and various prosthetics.

Ledford JK, Lens A, eds.
Principles and Practice in Ophthalmic Assisting:
A Comprehensive Textbook (pp 363-377).
© 2018 Taylor & Francis Group.

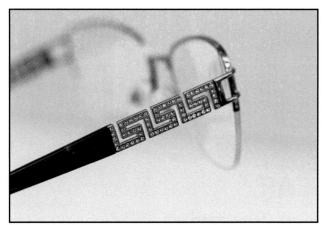

Figure 20-1. Rhinestone-studded decorative temple.

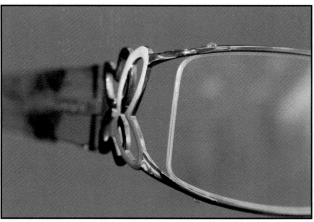

Figure 20-2. Enameled endpiece on a semi-rimless mounting.

Composition

Contemporary spectacle frames are produced or manufactured from an array of suitable materials that provide beauty, tensile strength (for durability and resilience), corrosion resistance (to oils, salts, and perspiration), and feather-light weight (for comfort). Materials are often distinguished by our patients simply as "metal" or "plastic."

For our purposes, the "plastic ones" are actually proprietary blends of epoxy resins, polymers, copolymers, carbon fibers, Kevlar (DuPont), polycarbonate, cellulose acetate (plastic mixed with plant fibers), or cellulose acetopropionate. Even wood, nylon, and rubber get in on the game. Some materials are extruded and then cut or milled into shape, while others are injection molded. The goal is to provide strength and impact resistance along with shape and color retention, and to prevent flammability.

The "metal ones" are a bit less complicated until we get to the alloys (metals mixed with other metals or even nonmetals). Alloys are created by combining chemical elements of various purities, whose resultant properties prove superior to those of its constituent components. Gold was once the predominant metal from which eyeglass frames were crafted, sometimes mixed with a base metal, other times used to plate or "cover" a base metal. With gold prices on the world market exceeding $1200 an ounce, it's no surprise that gold has now been replaced by less expensive metals.

Today's corrosion-resistant, durable, hypoallergenic metal frames are commonly produced from titanium, stainless steel, anodized aluminum, bronze, and other alloys. Frame trends today incorporate a combination of metal and plastic parts in addition to a mixture of colors and patterns within a single frame. Cut-outs, rhinestones (Figure 20-1), and enameling (Figure 20-2) add to their variety and appeal.

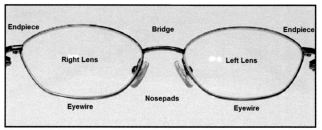

Figure 20-3. Diagram of a frame front.

In the 1980s, advocates of color theory and color "seasons" dictated appropriate frame color choices for individuals. Today, we espouse a philosophy of *patient preference*. If patients like them, they'll wear them! This holds true for both children and adults.

Frame Parts

The *frame front* (Figure 20-3) holds the prescription lenses and is composed of *eyewires* (or *rims*, Figure 20-4), which encircle or otherwise attach to the lenses. The *endpieces* (Figure 20-5) are the points of attachment of the *temples* to the frame front at its widest point, on opposite sides of the lenses. They might or might not be hinged.

The bridge of the frame is the area of attachment between the lenses that rests upon the nose. Three major types exist—saddle, keyhole, and nose pads. A *saddle* bridge follows the contours of the nose and evenly distributes the weight of the frame along the top or top and sides of the nose. It may be constructed of metal (Figure 20-6) or plastic (Figure 20-7), often with a flared section at the base of each side for increased contact and comfort. *Keyhole* bridges (Figure 20-8) apply weight only on the sides of the nose. The sensitive top of the nose is spared any contact through a little "cut-out" area reminiscent of a keyhole in a door. *Nose pads* (Figure 20-9)

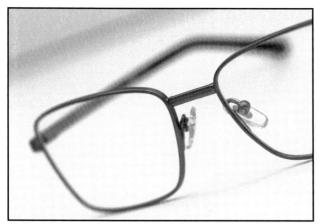

Figure 20-4. Metal eyewires or rims.

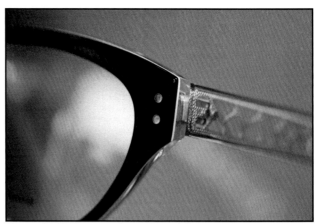

Figure 20-5. Frame and temple endpieces.

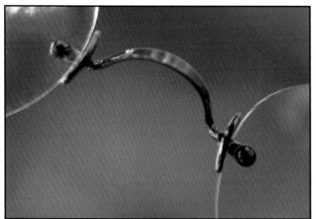

Figure 20-6. Metal saddle bridge.

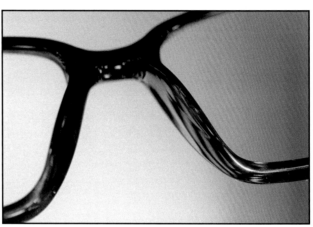

Figure 20-7. Plastic saddle bridge.

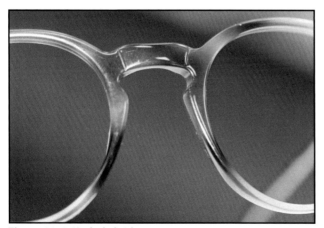

Figure 20-8. Keyhole bridge.

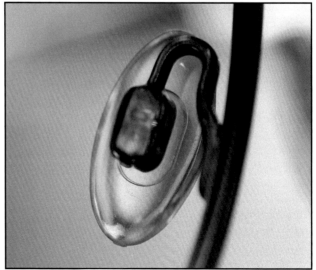

Figure 20-9. Guard arm and nose pad.

are commonly round or oval in shape; are constructed of rigid plastic or soft, slip-resistant silicone; are attached to the eyewires by means of metal *guard arms*; and support the majority of a frame's weight upon the nose at just two points of contact.

Hinges, if present, connect the frame front to the temples. They may employ *barrels*—odd-numbered, interlocking, stacked loops through which a screw passes to

hold the unit together (Figures 20-10A and B). A *spring* hinge mechanism (Figure 20-11) allows flexure of the temples, ensuring a longer-lasting fit and greater resistance to breakage—a perfect combination for active children and adults. Hingeless frames have a seamless design

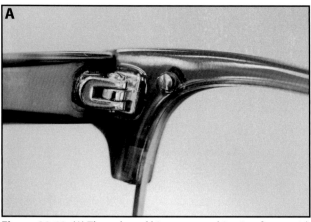
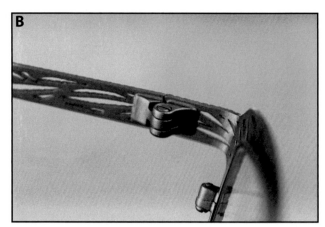

Figure 20-10. (A) Three-barrel hinge on combination frame with metal rims and plastic temples. (B) Three-barrel hinge and eyewire screw.

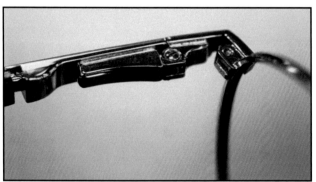

Figure 20-11. Spring hinge.

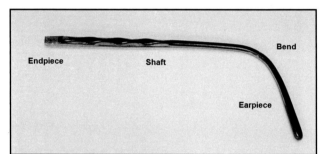

Figure 20-12. Parts of a temple.

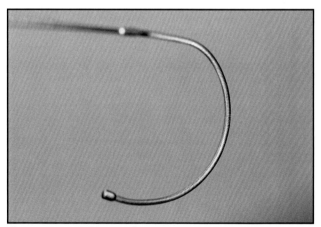

Figure 20-13. Cable temple.

with temple covers on one end and endpieces at the other. They attach directly to the lenses with pins and washers or screws and nuts.

The *temples* (Figure 20-12) are the most confused and misnamed parts of a frame. Our patients call them stems, wings, arms, earpieces, etc. The temples begin at the endpiece and extend either beyond or around the ears. There are many styles and lengths. *Cable* (Figure 20-13) and *riding-bow* temples (Figure 20-14) completely encircle the ear. The former is metal, designed for adults, and the later is plastic-coated wire, made for children. Frames designed for infants employ elastic straps that attach at the temple ends and wrap around behind the head to help prevent frame slippage and removal. *Skull* temples follow the contour of the patient's skull, stopping just short of the earlobe (Figure 20-15). *Library* temples (Figure 20-16) are fairly straight and are meant for quick removal without having to tug the frames over the ears.

Temples function to distribute the weight of the frames behind the ears rather than solely on the bridge of the nose. Friction keeps them in place and careful adjustments may be needed every few months, depending on use, to maintain the initial proper fit and positioning of the spectacle lenses.

Frame Styles

Eyeglass frames may be further differentiated by their type or style, independent of composition.

Full frames consist of a front (or *chassis*) and a pair of temples. *Rimless frames* are composed of a bridge-assembly, endpieces, and two temples. These attach to a pair of prescription lenses by means of screws (Figure 20-17), clips, or pins (Figure 20-18), after first drilling or notching the lenses to hold them.

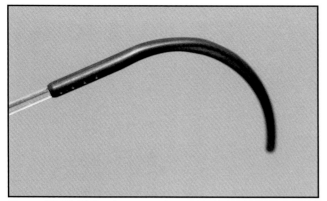

Figure 20-14. Riding-bow temple.

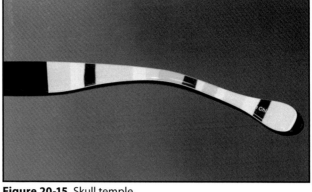

Figure 20-15. Skull temple.

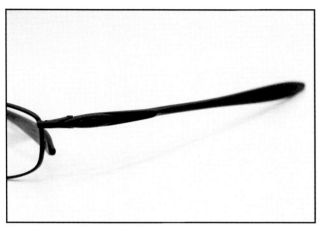

Figure 20-16. Library temple.

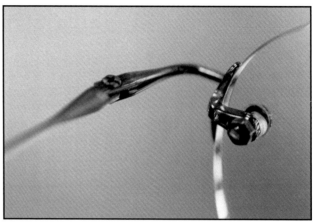

Figure 20-17. Rimless mounting with screws and nuts.

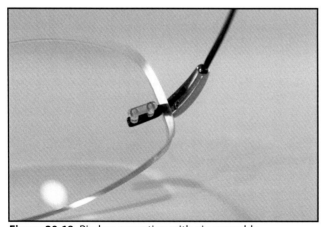

Figure 20-18. Rimless mounting with pin assembly.

The lenses of a *semi-rimless* mounting have a channel in the lens edges. A nylon cord fits into this channel and is affixed to the superior rim of the frame front/eyewire, thus suspending the lenses (Figure 20-19). A pair of endpieces and temples completes this frame type.

Half-eyes are usually readers, and have a shallow vertical dimension. These styles customarily sit farther down the nose, permitting the user to view distant objects by looking over the top rim. There is a variation of this style, where the rims are hinged at the bottom, allowing each lens to flip down out of the way. This is ideal for those who need near correction when applying makeup.

Sports styles, such as Rec-Specs (Liberty Sport, Inc), provide superior protection for athletes (Figure 20-20). They have protective cushions at the bridge and endpieces, and remain securely in place during movement by an elastic strap that wraps around the head. They are fitted with break-resistant lenses to deflect fingers, elbows, and high-velocity projectiles, such as tennis and racquet balls.

Clip-on frames attach a secondary pair of rims and lenses to an existing pair of eyeglasses by means of clips or magnets. These often incorporate sunglass tints or polarizing filters, but can be used to hold various other types of lens options.

Safety eyewear is mandated for use within industrial occupations and provides far superior impact resistance and breakage protection than that of dress eyewear or even sports styles. Specially produced, treated, and tested, impact-resistant frames and lenses reduce the risk of ocular injuries due to projectile or splash hazards. Side shields are constructed of metal or resin, and serve to deflect objects or liquids from passing behind the lenses and into the eyes (Figure 20-21).

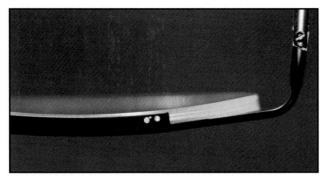

Figure 20-19. Semi-rimless mounting with nylon cord.

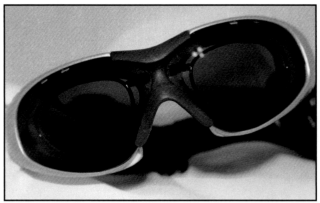

Figure 20-20. Sports goggles with prescription lenses.

Fitting Considerations

The proper sizing of a frame affects a patient's overall quality of vision in addition to overall comfort.

Frame fronts must match the width of an individual's face or they will constantly fall forward, applying pressure on the sensitive ears and sides of the head. In addition, multifocal lenses would be rendered useless as they would no longer sit at the correct height.

Temples create a problem if too short, because the weight of the glasses will not be balanced and will cause the eyewear to constantly slip down the nose and pinch the tops of the ears. Again, multifocal lenses will drop down as well. When the temples are too long, the excess length will extend beyond the ears and down onto the neck.

Human face and bridge shapes, as you might expect, vary wildly. Our goal is to aesthetically balance facial characteristics with frame styles that accentuate a person's best features.

Angular frames provide structure and definition, while round or oval frames suggest softness. Tiny frames can preclude the use of multifocal lenses. Those which are excessively large can deemphasize wide-set eyes but will make near-set eyes appear closer still. An overly large frame may also cause unwanted prism and increased lens-edge thickness.

Frame Markings

Eyeglass frames are imprinted with specific product information that includes the frame name or model number, manufacturer and country of origin, eye and bridge sizes, temple length, gold content (if any), and color.

Safety frames must include a designation of Z87 or Z87-2, in addition to the manufacturer's name or identifying mark, stamped on the temple, side shield, and frame front (Figures 20-22 and 20-23). In the absence of these identifying marks, the glasses will not meet the American National Standards Institute (ANSI) safety standards and are not safety eyewear.

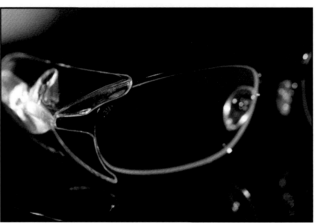

Figure 20-21. Safety frame with side shields.

Frame and Lens Dimensions

Lenses are sized to fit into frames through a system of measure referred to as the *boxing system* (Figure 20-24).

Imagine that a lens (of any shape or size) is enclosed by a square or box. The width of that box is called the "*A*" box measurement, and equals the lens width or frame eye size in millimeters. The height of the box and corresponding lens or frame size is called the "*B*" box measurement.

If you divide the box/square into four quadrants, the bisecting horizontal line is referenced as the *datum line.* The bisecting vertical line remains nameless, but is again equal to the length of the "*B*" measurement. The point of intersection between both bisecting lines is called the *geometric center* of the lens or frame opening.

When you draw a diagonal line from the geometric center of the lens shape to the eyewire edge at its longest dimension then double the length of that segment, you have measured the *effective diameter* of the lens. This value is used to determine the smallest uncut prescription lens blank that will successfully fit into the frame's eyewires without leaving gaps or causing unwanted prismatic effects through improper lens decentration.

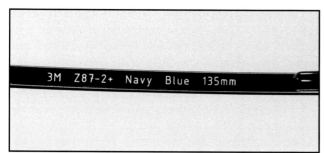

Figure 20-22. Safety temple with ANSI designation.

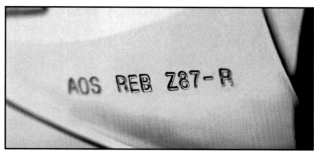

Figure 20-23. Safety shield with ANSI designation.

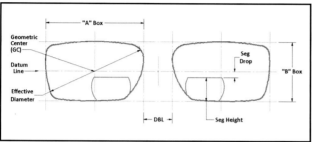

Figure 20-24. The boxing system. (Drawing by Charles M. Ellmers.)

Safety vs Dress Eyewear

Dress eyewear is manufactured to be worn in everyday situations while *safety eyewear* is intended for use in the workplace or while performing at-risk tasks. Safety frames must pass strict testing and be imprinted with Z87 or Z87-2, indicating that the frame can handle either regular or high-impact safety lenses with a central thicknesses of 3 mm or 2 mm, respectively.

Spectacle Lenses

Prescription spectacle lenses are produced in many forms and of numerous materials. Each has very specific properties and uses to improve a patient's visual acuity. They function to alter the path of light rays coming from an object and placing or redirecting an actual or virtual image upon the macula within the retina. "Actual images" are formed by light rays that emanate from a distant target and then converge upon the retina by means of an optical system of natural and/or man-made lenses. "Virtual images" are extrapolated by tracing the path of divergent light rays from their apparent origin in front of a spectacle lens. (See Chapter 4.)

LENS FORMS

Spherical lenses compensate for simple myopia, hyperopia, and presbyopia, while cylindrical lenses compensate for astigmatism in its numerous forms. *Spherocylindrical* lenses, then, are a combination of two types or forms to compensate for multiple refractive errors within the eye. (See Chapter 4 for information on refractive errors.)

Plano lenses are produced with a net power of zero. The front surface power is equal to that of the back surface. *Planoconvex* lenses have a front surface power of zero and a back surface of plus power. *Planoconcave* lenses, as you might expect, have a front surface power of zero and a back surface of minus power. If the lens is spherical, the back surface has just a single curve. For astigmatism, there are two different curves (the base curve and a second cross curve) on the posterior side of the lens.

Biconvex lenses are made with two plus-powered convex surfaces, while *biconcave* lenses are made up of two

The *optical center* (OC) of a lens is that specific point in a lens through which light will pass *without* bending or deviating. Prismatic power will be induced within a spectacle lens if the OC is not directly in front of the patient's pupil and, hence, along the optical axis. This could be done intentionally to achieve prism power as specified within the Rx, or inadvertently through carelessness during manufacture. In the later case, the patient may experience headaches, eye strain, or diplopia.

After marking the OC of each lens at the lensometer (see Chapter 19), measure across the bridge of the frame from one optical center to the other to derive the *distance between optical centers* (DBOC). This value (in millimeters) should be equal to the patient's pupillary distance (the distance between the center of each pupil).

The *seg drop* is the distance between the datum line and the top of the bifocal segment, in millimeters. The distance from the bottom of the frame or lens to the top of the bifocal line is called the *seg height*. Failure to note and duplicate these two measurements (in addition to replicating the distance of the OC from the top of the segment itself) when planning and fabricating a single replacement lens within the patient's frame will cause the OCs and the multifocals to be at differing heights, thus inducing a vertical imbalance between the images that the wearer experiences as vertical double vision.

A frame's bridge size can be referred to as the *distance between lenses* (DBL) and is equal to the distance between the right and left lens boxes. Its width is measured with a millimeter ruler held at the narrowest point between the two inside bevels of the nasal eyewires.

minus-powered concave surfaces. *Meniscus* lens forms combine a plus-powered front surface with a minus-powered back surface. The resultant overall power may be of minus or plus power. Most of today's eyewear is made using this type of lens form.

Bitoric lens designs have cylinder power ground on both the front and back surfaces of the lenses. This combination allows the creation of greater magnification in one power meridian vs another on the front surface of the lens. The back curves are then modified to compensate for the alteration in power upon the front surface.

Free-form lens design is a new method of producing patient-specific PALs with more precise steps of increasing power, wider reading zones, and specific back-of-lens curvatures designed to reduce or eliminate both oblique astigmatism and peripheral lens aberrations (inherent flaws within a PAL which were formerly unmanageable).

Index of Refraction

The physics of light, its reflection, and refraction are discussed in Chapter 4. Remember that light rays travel at different speeds when moving through air as compared to other substances, including lenses. In addition, different lens materials permit light to pass through at differing rates or speeds. The speed with which light can pass through a substance is that material's *index of refraction*. The higher the index of refraction of a particular lens material, the thinner the spectacle lens.

Thinner lenses equal happier patients because of improved cosmesis. As a result of high-index lens materials, minus-powered lenses can have thinner edges within a frame of appropriate size, and plus-powered lenses can have thinner centers vs traditional lens materials. High-index lenses are available in both glass and plastic. Because glass is heavier, it has a more limited use.

Materials

The most commonly produced glass ophthalmic lens is *crown glass*. This material possesses a low index of refraction, a high density, and very little chromatic aberration. (Chromatic aberration is one of two types of color dispersion, or the unwanted break-up of white light into its component colors, reducing clarity and producing annoying color fringes.) Crown glass is thicker and heavier than some plastic lens materials, but it has very good optics and resists scratching, pitting, and chemical splashes. As such, it is usually reserved for safety eyewear within the United States.

In other countries, there still exists a preference for using high-index glass for higher minus prescriptions, due to its ability to be made quite thin (although heavy) as compared to traditional crown and standard resin lenses. Crown and high-index glass lenses may be dinosaurs... but they're not yet extinct!

Crown glass lenses can be made with ultraviolet, light-sensitive crystals incorporated into the molten glass to make them *photochromic* and darken outdoors. These lenses are heavier than their resin counterparts, but retain the sworn allegiance of those individuals who have worn this material for more 40 years.

Pittsburgh, Pennsylvania is home to more than steel and football. During World War II, the Pittsburgh Plate Glass Corporation developed resin alternatives to glass materials used within the aerospace industry. In the late 1940s, with a surplus of their new materials on hand, PPG sought to find a peace-time use for their remaining stock. They developed Columbia resin, batch number 39, for use as a spectacle lens material.

CR-39, once the most commonly produced and used plastic spectacle lens material, is nearly half the weight of crown glass lenses. It has a higher refractive index and optics that rival that of its glass competitor. It is less scratch resistant, however, necessitating the use of anti-scratch coatings to make it more durable. This material accepts tints and antireflective coatings, and can be made into very large lens-blank sizes. CR-39 became the industry leader with few exceptions.

Lenses of increasingly higher refractive index have been developed. Many such lenses incorporate softer materials that increase their impact resistance. Polycarbonate is one such material, initially developed in the 1950s for use in the canopies of jet airplanes. It was further developed and became the first safety and sport lens on the market. It is still in use today for children's eyewear and industrial safety eyeglass lenses, as well as the lens of choice for monocular patients (to afford the greatest protection to their seeing eye).

Trivex (PPG Industries, Inc) high-index lenses became available in 2002, after first being developed as a window material for military vehicles including helicopters and fighter jets. It proved to have very good optics, breakage resistance that rivals that of polycarbonate lenses, is extremely lightweight, and can be drilled without splitting or cracking (as when used in drill-mounted frame styles).

Lens Types and Designs

Spectacle lenses are further classified as to the purpose(s) they serve.

Single vision or monofocal lenses compensate for visual deficiencies at one fixed focal length (eg, at near only, distance only, or computer only). They may be composed of spherical power alone, cylindrical power and corresponding axis orientation, or in spherocylindrical combination with prismatic power if prescribed.

Multifocal lenses employ various designs to focus at two or more focal lengths, most commonly distance (20 feet and beyond) and near.

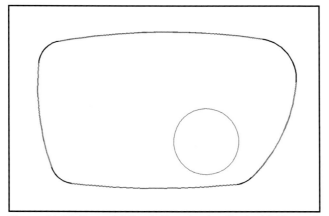

Figure 20-25. Kryptok bifocal. (Drawing by Charles M. Ellmers.)

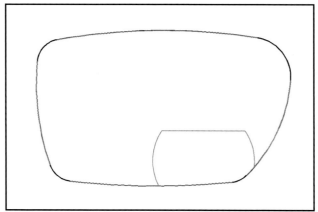

Figure 20-26. Flat top 28-mm bifocal. (Drawing by Charles M. Ellmers.)

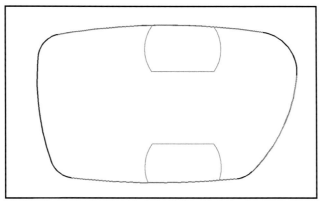

Figure 20-27. Occupational bifocal. (Drawing by Charles M. Ellmers.)

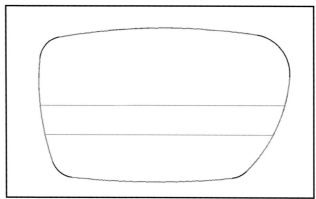

Figure 20-28. Executive trifocal. (Drawing by Charles M. Ellmers.)

Bifocals are types of multifocals that contain two separate lens powers, usually adding plus power to the lower part of the lens to give the boost necessary to see at near. Depending on the lens material used and the shape of the near portion (*segment*), they may be manufactured by fusing or gluing the bifocal to the bottom of the main lens. Another method produces *single-piece* multifocals, easily identified by a raised ledge on the front surface of the lens.

Bifocal segments can vary in shape and size. They may be fashioned as a strip or a circle (Figure 20-25), narrow or wide, curved or *flat-top* (Figure 20-26), or with a straight line that crosses the lens as with an *executive* style.

Occupational style multifocal lenses position multiple segments within the lens, usually with a near segment at both the top and bottom of the lens (Figure 20-27), thus permitting the wearer to also see close detail while working above the head (think plumbers, mechanics, and such).

Trifocal lenses incorporate a third lens power above the reading addition. It comes in the same shapes and styles as the lined bifocals, including executive style (Figure 20-28). This middle segment is focused at "midrange," usually half the power of the lower segment (known as a *50% trifocal add*). For example, if the patient needs a +2.25 add to read at 16 inches, then the middle segment is probably going to be set at +1.12.

Progressive addition lenses (PALs), or no-line lenses, are produced with varying curvatures of increasing plus power on the front surface of the lens. It is, in fact, a trifocal lens with additional powers in between. This type of lens allows the wearer to enjoy the next best thing to natural vision at multiple ranges from distance through near, by adjusting the position of the head and eyes to view objects through the power corridor that runs from below the patient's optical axis to the inner corner of the lenses. The corridor length and width of a PAL can now be specified to suit the reading and working needs of the wearer. For example, a patient who reads a lot will probably do better with a wider reading area at the bottom of the lens.

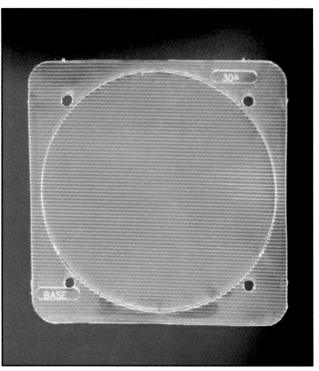

Figure 20-29. Fresnel press-on prism (The Fresnel Prism and Lens Co).

Prism

Prismatic power within a lens may be intentional and prescribed, or unintentional and problematic. A prismatic effect occurs when the eyes look through any point of a lens other than the optical centers. (See Chapter 4.)

Ocular muscles normally work in teams, or more specifically in yoked pairs, to rotate and direct our eyes and gaze, providing binocular vision, fusion, and thus stereopsis (see Chapter 10). If one lens of a pair is inadvertently displaced, then the eyes may not be able to yoke, or work together because prism is induced (Sidebar 20-1; see also Chapter 19 and Sidebar 19-6). If the displacement is horizontal, one eye will converge or diverge while the other eye moves too much, too little, or in the opposite direction. This unfortunate patient then sees side-by-side double images, at least part of the time. The lenses should be remade at the laboratory to eliminate the horizontal disparity.

When a multifocal lens wearer requires a distance prescription of moderately to greatly unequal powers between the eyes (known as *anisometropia*), the patient may experience a vertical imbalance and see up-and-down double images. In such a case, a technique called *slab-off grinding* can be applied to the lenses to eliminate the vertical diplopia by intentionally adding a base-up prism to the lower half of just one lens. (A base-down prism is used for a *reverse* slab-off grind.)

Another method of compensating for diplopia is a *Fresnel prism* (Figure 20-29). This type of prism is a thin, lightweight, flexible sheet of horizontally stacked prisms that, when viewed from the side, resemble the tooth pattern of a saw blade. It's commonly called a *press-on prism* because the sheet can be cut to match the size and shape of a spectacle lenses, and then be applied to either the front or back surface.

There are several advantages in using Fresnel prisms compared to conventionally prepared prisms in that they are lightweight and comfortable to wear, are inexpensive, can be easily cut and applied at the clinic providing instant trial feedback to the prescriber (especially handy prior to having an optician fabricate new replacement lenses), come in a variety of prism powers, and may be removed and reused if the condition warrants.

Safety Lenses

Since 1971, the Food and Drug Administration (FDA) has required that all spectacle lenses, clear or tinted, be impact resistant and of minimum thickness to provide safety to the wearing public.

Additionally, ANSI set forth manufacturing, thickness, quality, and impact-resistance standards for eyewear (ANSI Z80.1). These standards were adopted by the Occupational Safety and Health Administration (OSHA), the federal agency responsible for regulating and administering safety policies and practices within workplaces, schools, and other institutions.

ANSI Z80.1 standards are federally required of all safety eyewear. After passing quality assurance testing, lenses must be marked at their outside corner or top edge with an identifying logo, or logo and plus sign, to signify compliance with the standards (Figure 20-30). The plus sign designates certification as a high-impact–resistant lens.

The impact resistance of a spectacle lens is regulated and measurable. Lenses may be tested individually or within batches, in preshaped or unshaped form (as designated by their future use), and as appropriate to their respective materials (per ANSI regulations). Testing is done by dropping steel balls of increasing weight and diameter one at a time from a height of 50 inches onto the front surface of the lens. Appropriately, this is called a *dropped-ball test*. If the lens breaks, it is not approved and cannot be used.

Unlike resin lens materials, glass spectacle lenses must be specially treated (by the application of heat or chemicals) to properly harden them in order to produce increased impact and breakage resistance that can withstand drop-ball testing.

Lens Tints and Coatings

The eyes need to be protected from the cumulative harmful effects of ultraviolet radiation and nuisance glare. Long-term exposure to ultraviolet light hastens the formation of cataracts, development of macular degeneration, aging of the skin, and the incidence of melanoma.

Clear ophthalmic lenses inhibit ultraviolet light either by the inherent physical properties of the lens material or by the application of topical coatings deposited on the surface. Sunglasses must block light wavelengths of the visible spectrum (which produce debilitating glare) and also those of the invisible or ultraviolet light spectrum (namely UVA, UVB, and UVC). Glare is commonly reduced or eliminated through the use of filters, tints, or coatings.

In most discussions of lenses, we primarily consider their transmissive properties with respect to the visible light spectrum. Light hits the surface of the lens, is refracted, it travels on, end of story. But *absorptive* lenses, which are most often tinted, allow for the selective transmission of energy waves of both the visible and invisible spectra…absorbing certain frequencies of light, reflecting others, and transmitting the rest. Ultimately, as the total amount of light they absorb increases, the actual amount of light transmission through them decreases.

Lens thickness, density, and refractive index are also factors that affect light transmission, given that as tinted glass lenses increase in thickness, they naturally transmit less light. (The same holds true for resin lenses, but to a lesser extent.) High-index materials decrease light transmission due to reflections on both the front and back lens surfaces. Also, lens tints and mirror coatings further impede light transmission, compounding the effect.

Now, imagine this scenario. An elderly patient with a sight-limiting ocular disease, wearing a high-plus or high-minus spectacle Rx with tinted, high-index lenses and a pair of mydriatic sunshields, leaves your office with

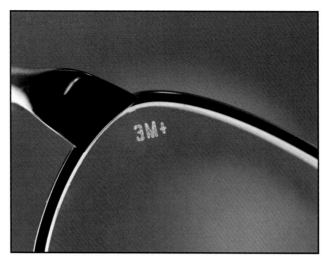

Figure 20-30. Safety lens with ANSI designation.

dilated pupils and gets behind the wheel of his car (which, by the way, also has a tinted windshield). This is a recipe for disaster! With so many compounding factors limiting a patient's vision, it is beneficial to suggest that your patients have a driver to safely take them home after their appointments.

However, not all absorptive lenses cause problems. Some solve them! As was discussed earlier, ultraviolet filters absorb or "filter" short, high-energy wavelengths of the visible spectrum (ultraviolet radiation) up to 400 nanometers, protecting the eyes from long-term exposure and, potentially, the formation of macular degeneration and cataracts. Some practitioners, usually in low vision clinics and optometry colleges, support the use of infrared-absorbing lenses for their patients. These adaptive lenses are available with multiple transmission characteristics (and in over 50 colors).

Gray polarized and plum-colored lenses are recommended to decrease overall light transmission and reduce glare. Yellow tints improve contrast and block blue light, which is especially helpful for patients with early cataract development or those who drive at dusk, dawn, or in the rain. The color orange seems to help glaucoma patients who have experienced ganglion nerve fiber losses, green for retinitis pigmentosa sufferers, and amber or brown for individuals with macular degeneration. The goal is to help regain some of the functional vision lost to disease processes. These deficits may occur in the forms of debilitating glare, night blindness, decreased contrast sensitivity, loss of peripheral vision, increased requirements for additional illumination, and even the inability to benefit from increases in magnification within the spectacle prescription.

When sandwiched between two tinted surfaces, *polarizing light filters* act like a sieve for light. They block rays traveling along a horizontal plane (where light reflections produce glare and distortion), but allow them to

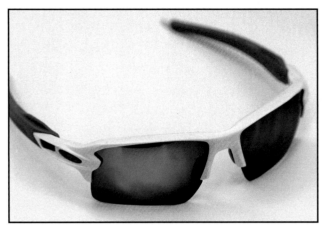

Figure 20-31. Mirrored sunglasses.

pass along a vertical plane. This provides clearer images and eliminates the glare reflected off surfaces such as water, sand, snow, and pavement.

Photochromic or *Transitions* (Transitions Optical, Inc) lenses darken with direct exposure to ultraviolet light, and are prescribed as either comfort lenses or sunglasses. They provide a reduction of visible light and an increase in comfort, but afford no protection from glare unless teamed with a back surface antireflective coating and a light-polarizing filter. In addition, since the windshields of vehicles incorporate ultraviolet filtering, some lenses do not turn dark in the car. I recommend that your patients discuss current lens options with the optician.

Antireflective coatings reduce glare and the associated eyestrain caused by artificial light sources, such as fluorescent and incandescent bulbs, car headlights, and computer screens. They are most often combined with scratch-resistant coatings to improve the durability of the lenses. They are also cosmetically appealing because they eliminate surface reflections and give an "invisible" appearance to the lens surface, thus permitting the ability to better see the wearer's eyes.

Mirrored-surface coatings (Figure 20-31) can be applied to one or both surfaces of a tinted lens to provide a fashion look or to control the extreme glare that skiers or water enthusiasts must contend with. Law enforcement and military personnel sometimes use mirrored lenses for the "intimidation factor" that comes from the inability to see the wearer's eyes.

PATIENT SERVICES

Position of Multifocal Segments

Although this chapter doesn't aim to teach you how to fit and dispense eyewear, it's beneficial to know a little about bifocal/trifocal segment placement in order to better troubleshoot patient complaints during the patient history or before performing refractometry.

The average lined bifocal segment is usually positioned at the margin of the patient's lower lid, and that of a lined trifocal at the bottom of the patient's pupil. However, a one-size-fits-all approach is not appropriate for every patient.

If a patient complains about the location of the segment(s), observe the patient's head carriage and posture. If the body and chin are carried noticeably erect and high, then an otherwise normally placed bifocal will be too high for the patient's use. Similar situations are faced by extremely tall persons who must constantly look down at shorter people or desks and such. You could suggest a slightly lower bifocal segment height to the prescriber.

The opposite would be true in the case of low chin position or stooped shoulders. The bifocal will be too low as the patient looks through the very top of his/her frames. Wheelchair-bound patients could benefit from a higher bifocal placement as much of their work and world is above eye level.

If you work with a pediatric patient base, you may see a notation of "split pupil" on a child's eyeglass prescription. This directs the optician to raise the height of the bifocal segment within the chosen frame to a level that bisects the center of the pupil. This helps a child with a convergence insufficiency to more easily use the bifocal as prescribed without simply looking above it while reading. In most instances the doctor will recommend a wide, flat-topped segment to more nearly fill the bottom of the child's frame, allowing for the eyes to scan in any direction with complete comfort and proper vision. If you are unsure whether the line is positioned properly, use a transilluminator or penlight to check the height against the corneal light reflex.

Vertex Distance

Vertex distance (VD) is a notation in millimeters of the distance from the front of the cornea (as measured over a closed eyelid) to the *ocular* or *back surface* of a lens.

Spectacle frames position the lenses closer to a patient's eyes than most trial frames or phoropters, so VD should be measured with a *distometer* (a hand-held measuring tool designed for the purpose, see Chapter 19), and noted on the patient's prescription. This is important whenever the manifest refraction reaches 5 diopters (some sources say 3 diopters) or more in strength. The dispensing optician then measures the VD of the sample eyewear selected by your mutual patient, and compensates for the difference in VD when fabricating the new glasses.

If the measurement is neglected or forgotten, your patient will notice a change in the *effective power* of the lenses and not see as well with his/her new eyeglasses as he/she did when the refraction was performed. In other words, the lens will not have the same effect on incoming light, will not refract light onto the retina, and thus vision will not be optimal (Sidebar 20-2). The unfortunate consequences of this are chair time lost to spectacle rechecks, costly remakes of the lenses, and unhappy patients.

Frame Tilt

When patients complain that they have difficulty seeing out of their eyewear, and especially mention issues with their multifocal lenses, observe the patient in profile for horizontal and vertical misalignments of frame position.

If the frame sits closer to the patient's forehead than to the cheeks, then the frame has too much *retroscopic angle* or *tilt*. This error in fitting causes a misalignment of the multifocal, forcing the patient to use the mid-range (or intermediate) lens power for distance viewing by lifting it higher than normal; induces the effect of an oblique astigmatism since the patient now views objects off-axis (no longer along the true optical axis of their lens); and alters the effective power of the prescription by decreasing the VD.

Conversely, if the bottom of the frame presses into the cheeks while the top sits quite far from the forehead, then too much *pantoscopic* tilt exists. This deviation forces the patient to view above the optical axis; can also induce an oblique astigmatism; drops the reading area so low that it's impossible to locate the bifocal area without tipping the head back and lifting the chin; and changes the effective power of the prescription, this time by increasing the VD.

A third misalignment is excessive *wrap* or *face form*, which induces a prismatic effect that might be mild in low-power prescriptions but becomes significantly greater in higher-power ones. In every case, make a note of your observations and share them with your physician.

Care and Cleaning

Adjustments and repairs of spectacles are more complex than they appear and, as such, should be left to the professional competencies of duly licensed, trained, and experienced optician. A well-intentioned attempt to "help" by an otherwise well-meaning technician or assistant can easily backfire, causing ill-will toward the practice and unnecessary expense to your patient or employer in the form of replacement costs.

Limit your service to the patient by properly cleaning his/her lenses. Remember that modern eyewear is expensive and lenses scratch easily. It's common for patients to spend hundreds of dollars on their custom eyewear.

After first rinsing the lenses under warm, running water to remove particulate matter, apply liquid dish soap and gently rub with your fingers. Rinse the cleaned glasses again, shake the excess water from them, and (here's the key thing) carefully BLOT the lenses once or

---

> ### SIDEBAR 20-2
> ### EFFECTIVE POWER
>
> It might help you visualize the concept of effective power if you think about how we correct vision after cataract surgery. There are three options: glasses, contact lenses, and intraocular lens (IOL) implants.
>
> If you correct with glasses, the standard would be about +12.00 D. If you move onto the cornea with a contact, the power needed is around +14.00 D. If you go closer yet to the retina and use an IOL, the necessary power would be around +22.00 D. Each of these lenses, at its particular distance from the retina, has the same effective power because each one focuses an image at the same place—on the retina.
>
> However, if you prescribed a contact lens the same power as that needed for glasses (+12.00 D), the contact would not be strong enough. By moving the +12 D lens closer to the retina, you have changed its effective power.
>
> In the same way, if you took the +22 D power of the IOL and put it into spectacles (moving the lens away from the retina), you have changed the effective power of the +22 D lens.
>
> Bottom line: By moving a strong lens closer to or away from the retina, the effective power of that lens is changed.

---

twice with a clean towel (cloth or paper). Never, ever, rub the lenses!

Today, some ophthalmologists have incorporated an optical dispensary within their practice. Your ability to work alongside the optician will definitely increase your skill in serving your patients, and will also increase your value to your physician(s). If you are interested in furthering your knowledge of eyewear dispensing, you may serve a formal apprenticeship under the guidance of a licensed or certified optician. (Regulations vary by state.) There are instructional materials, tutorials, and classes available online, through junior colleges, and from your state or national professional organizations, licensing bodies, or certifying boards.

Remember: If you do your best for the patients, you serve not only their needs, but also those of your employer and community at large.

ACKNOWLEDGMENTS

The author would like to thank the following: Anna L. Katz-Schloss, OD (Low Vision Specialist, Cleveland Sight Center, Cleveland, Ohio); and Deborah M. Kogler, LDO (President/Owner, Magnifiers and More, Mentor, Ohio).

CHAPTER QUIZ

1. True/False: Department store sunglasses and pre-made reading glasses are made to the same exacting standards that prescription eyewear must meet.

2. True/False: Modern spectacle frames are produced from one of two materials: metal or plastic.

3. Name three metal alloys commonly used in the manufacture of eyeglass frames.

4. Name two methods by which the frame front can hold prescription lenses.

5. The weight of a frame is distributed behind the ears by means of the ____ .

6. Nose pads are attached to the frame front by means of:
   a. guard arms
   b. sergeant at arms
   c. hinges
   d. pad extenders
   e. a and d

7. Cable, riding bow, skull, and library are types of ____ .

8. Name the part of a safety frame that serves to deflect objects or liquids from passing behind the lenses and into the eyes.

9. Frame markings include the designations of frame name, model number, manufacturer, and country of origin in addition to:
   a. thickness
   b. color
   c. eye and bridge sizes
   d. temple length
   e. b and c
   f. b, c, and d

10. What conditions must be met in order for safety eyewear to meet ANSI standards?

11. The term *boxing* refers to:
   a. prize-fighting
   b. a public holiday within the United Kingdom
   c. a form-fit adjustment of a frame
   d. a system of measure used when sizing lenses to fit a frame
   e. none of the above

12. The optical center of a lens is that specific point in a lens through which light will pass without ____ or ____.

13. Name four important differences between glass and resin spectacle lens materials.

14. True/False: Photochromic lenses are only available in crown glass.

15. Name two high-index lens materials that were first developed and used within the field of aviation and by the US military.

16. True/False: A trifocal has a middle segment or area that is focused at "mid-range," and is usually three-quarters of the strength of the add power within the bifocal.

17. A prismatic effect occurs when the eyes look through any point of a lens other than the ____ ____ .

18. Name the type of prism that is available as thin, light-weight, flexible sheets.

19. Long-term exposure to ultraviolet light hastens the formation and/or development of which of these conditions?
   a. cataracts
   b. retinitis pigmentosa
   c. macular degeneration
   d. melanomas
   e. all of the above
   f. all except b

20. The notation of "split pupil" on a spectacle lens prescriptions is a directive by the physician to:
   a. perform surgery
   b. check pupil functions
   c. observe the corneal light reflex
   d. bisect the pupil with a lined bifocal segment
   e. none of the above

21. A notation in millimeters of the distance from the front of a cornea (as measured over a closed eyelid) to the back surface of a lens is called:
   a. effective power
   b. vertex power
   c. vertex distance
   d. viewing distance

Answers

1. False, Prescription/optical quality lenses are produced so as to eliminate inherent or otherwise unwanted distortions. This is not the case with inexpensive, mass-produced readers and sunglasses.

2. False, In addition to resins and metals, frames can be fashioned from wood, nylon, rubber, carbon fibers, and mixtures of resins with other plant fibers in the form of cellulose.

3. Possible answers: Titanium, stainless steel, anodized aluminum, bronze, and other alloys.

4. Possible answers: Eyewires (or rims), nylon cords, screws and nuts, clips, or pins.

5. Temples

6. a

7. Temples

8. Side shields

9. f

10. Safety eyewear must include a designation of Z87 or Z87-2 in addition to the manufacturer's name or identifying mark stamped on each lens, temple, and frame front. This indicates that the eyewear meets ANSI safety standards. The lenses may be produced of either hardened crown glass or polycarbonate, with a minimum thickness of 3 mm or 2 mm, respectively, and survive inspection through dropped-ball testing.

11. d

12. Possible answers: Bending, deviating, or refracting.

13. Possible answers: Crown glass possesses a low-index of refraction, a high density, and very little chromatic aberration. It has good optics and resists scratching, chemical splashes, and pitting. It naturally inhibits ultraviolet wavelengths, and can be tinted or coated. Drawbacks include increased weight and easier breakability than polycarbonate resin lenses, even when safety hardened. Resin lenses have higher indices of refraction, are more shatter resistant and lighter in weight than their glass counterparts, easily accept tints and coatings, possess excellent optics, and can be produced in larger sizes than glass to fit a larger variety of frame choices. Drawbacks include ease of scratching, need to incorporate ultraviolet filter, and increased chromatic aberrations as compared to crown glass.

14. False, Photochromic lenses are available in both glass and resin.

15. Polycarbonate and Trivex

16. False, The intermediate area or zone is usually one-half or 50% of the strength of the bifocal add-power.

17. Optical center

18. Fresnel or press-on prism

19. e

20. d, "Split pupil" refers to the bisection of a child's pupil by the bifocal segment of his/her eyeglasses. This forces the patient to read using his/her bifocal, rather than the distance portion of the lens.

21. c

BIBLIOGRAPHY

ANSI standards Z80.1-2010 prescription ophthalmic lens tolerance recommendations. Ophthalmic Lenses Blog [Internet]. http://ophthalmiclenses.blogspot.com/2011/07/ansi-standards-z801-2010-prescription.html. Posted July 5, 2011. Accessed July 4, 2016.

Brooks CW, Borish IM. *System for Ophthalmic Dispensing.* 3rd ed. St. Louis, MO: Butterworth-Heinemann; 2007.

Ditchfield C. *The Story Behind Plastic.* Chicago, IL: Heinemann Library; 2012.

NoIR Medical Technologies and Noir Laser Co. NoIR website. www.noir-medical.com/index.html. Accessed September 6, 2017.

Rhode SJ, Ginsberg SP. *Ophthalmic Technology: A Guide for the Eye Care Assistant.* New York, NY: Raven Press Books, Ltd; 1987.

Stein HA, Stein RM, Freeman MI. *The Ophthalmic Assistant: A Text for Allied and Associated Ophthalmic Personnel.* 9th ed. Philadelphia, PA: Saunders; 2013.

Unless otherwise noted, the figures in this chapter were contributed by the author, Anne West-Ellmers.

21

CONTACT LENSES

Wendy M. Ford, BS, COMT, FCLSA, NCLEM

Contact lenses can be a successful mode of vision correction for many patients, providing an alternative to wearing glasses—for sports, activities, hobbies, or cosmesis. Contact lenses can also provide visual and prosthetic rehabilitation, and can be used in the management of some ocular surface diseases. With improved manufacturing techniques, designs, and materials, many patients who formerly were not considered good contact lens candidates can successfully wear them today. This chapter is an introduction and overview to contact lens fitting.

BASIC SCIENCES

Anatomy and Physiology

Contact lens fitting requires the knowledge of ocular anatomy, physiology, and pathology (especially that of the anterior segment). These topics are covered in Chapters 2, 3, and 26, respectively. Since the contact lens involves the anterior surface structures, an in-depth knowledge of the lids, lashes, precorneal tear film, bulbar and palpebral conjunctiva, cornea, and sclera are important. Understanding normal vs abnormal will aid the contact lens fitter in patient selection, lens choice, fitting assessment, and management of contact lens-related complications.

Contact Lens Optics

Contact lenses are refracting lenses that sit directly on the eye. The optics of the lens is affected by the tear layer of the eye, the refractive vertex distance, corneal and lenticular astigmatism, and the interaction of the eyelids.

Transposition and Spherical Equivalent

Contact lenses are manufactured, fit, and prescribed in minus cylinder form. By convention, plus-cylinder prescriptions must be transposed prior to contact lens fitting. Please see the section on transposition in Chapter 4.

For prescriptions with less than a diopter of cylinder, the spherical equivalent power is used in soft contact lens fittings. Please see the section on spherical equivalent in Chapter 4.

Vertex Distance

The refractive power of the contact lens must be adjusted to accommodate the shorter focal distance of the contact lens to the retina. Unlike spectacles with an average distance of 12 mm from the surface of the eye, the vertex distance (VD; see Chapter 19) of a contact lens is 0 (zero). Therefore, additional plus (converging) power is needed in the contact lens to focus light rays onto the retina. This is termed *vertex distance compensation*.

Ledford JK, Lens A, eds.
Principles and Practice in Ophthalmic Assisting:
A Comprehensive Textbook (pp 379-415).
© 2018 Taylor & Francis Group.

TABLE 21-1 VERTEX DISTANCE CONVERSION CHART						
Rx* ±	CL +	CL −	Rx* ±	CL +	CL −
4.00	4.25	3.75	11.25	13.00	9.75
4.25	4.50	4.00	11.50	13.50	10.00
4.50	4.75	4.25	11.75	13.75	10.25
4.75	5.00	4.50	12.00	14.00	10.50
5.00	5.25	4.75	12.25	14.25	10.75
5.25	5.50	5.00	12.50	14.75	10.75
5.50	5.75	5.25	12.75	15.00	11.00
5.75	6.00	5.50	13.00	15.50	11.25
6.00	6.50	5.50	13.25	15.75	11.50
6.25	6.75	5.75	13.50	16.25	11.50
6.50	7.00	6.00	13.75	16.75	11.75
6.75	7.25	6.25	14.00	17.00	12.00
7.00	7.50	6.50	14.25	17.25	12.25
7.25	8.00	6.75	14.50	17.75	12.50
7.50	8.25	7.00	14.75	18.00	12.50
7.75	8.50	7.00	15.00	18.50	12.75
8.00	8.75	7.25	15.25	18.75	12.75
8.25	9.00	7.50	15.50	19.00	13.00
8.50	9.50	7.75	15.75	19.50	13.25
8.75	9.75	8.00	16.00	19.75	13.25
9.00	10.00	8.25	16.25	20.00	13.50
9.25	10.50	8.25	16.50	20.50	13.75
9.50	10.75	8.50	17.00	21.50	14.00
9.75	11.00	8.75	17.50	22.50	14.50
10.00	11.50	9.00	18.00	23.00	14.75
10.25	11.75	9.00	18.50	24.00	15.00
10.50	12.25	9.25	19.00	25.00	15.25
10.75	12.50	9.50	19.50	26.50	15.50
11.00	12.75	9.75	20.00	27.00	16.00

To use the chart: 1) Locate the amount of the spherical spectacle (refractive) power on the left (*at an average spectacle vertex distance of 12 mm). 2) Determine the adjusted contact lens power for either a minus or plus lens to the right.

Compensating for the change in VD with a contact lens is only necessary with prescriptions greater than ±4.00 D. The simplest method is to use a vertex conversion chart (Table 21-1).

Diopter/Radius Conversion

Contact lens curvature, or *base curve* (BC), is the *fitting curve* of a contact lens. It is the part of the lens that fits against the cornea. This is usually expressed as millimeters of radius of curvature. It can also be expressed in its keratometric diopter equivalent (D). These two measurements are interchangeable and inversely proportional. To convert from the dioptric equivalent to radius of curvature, either a table (Table 21-2) or formula (Sidebar 21-1) can be used.

Lacrimal Lens

The *lacrimal lens* is the tear film between a rigid contact lens and the cornea. While the refractive effect of the tear film is negligible in soft contacts (because the lens rests or "drapes" across the cornea), it plays an important role in rigid lens fittings. The lacrimal lens can fill in and neutralize corneal astigmatism and irregularities. It is, in effect, another refractive lens on the eye. It can take the shape of a plus or minus lens, depending on the base curve of the rigid lens.

The power of the lacrimal lens is determined by the base curve of the contact lens and the *K-readings*. (The K-readings are a measurement of the curvature of the cornea's front surface, as measured with a keratometer.) The flattest keratometric value is often termed "flat-K" or just "K." Because the lacrimal lens neutralizes most corneal astigmatism less than 3 D, only the relationship

TABLE 21-2
DIOPTER RADIUS CONVERSION CHART

Diopter	mm	Diopter	mm	Diopter	mm	Diopter	mm
36.00	9.375	41.25	8.181	46.62	7.239	51.87	6.506
36.12	9.343	41.37	8.158	46.75	7.219	52.00	6.490
36.25	9.310	41.50	8.132	46.87	7.200	52.12	6.475
36.37	9.279	41.62	8.109	47.00	7.180	52.25	6.459
36.50	9.246	41.75	8.083	47.12	7.162	52.37	6.444
36.62	9.216	42.00	8.035	47.25	7.142	52.50	6.428
36.75	9.183	42.12	8.012	47.37	7.124	52.62	6.413
36.87	9.153	42.25	7.988	47.50	7.105	52.75	6.398
37.00	9.121	42.37	7.965	47.62	7.087	52.87	6.383
37.12	9.092	42.50	7.941	47.75	7.068	53.00	6.367
37.25	9.060	42.62	7.918	47.87	7.050	53.12	6.353
37.37	9.031	42.75	7.894	48.00	7.031	53.25	6.338
37.50	9.000	42.87	7.872	48.12	7.013	53.37	6.323
37.62	8.971	43.00	7.848	48.25	6.994	53.50	6.303
37.75	8.940	43.12	7.826	48.37	6.977	53.62	6.294
37.87	8.912	43.25	7.803	48.50	6.958	53.75	6.279
38.00	8.881	43.37	7.784	48.62	6.941	53.87	6.265
38.12	8.853	43.50	7.758	48.75	6.923	54.00	6.250
38.25	8.823	43.62	7.737	48.87	6.906	54.12	6.236
38.37	8.795	43.75	7.714	49.00	6.887	54.25	6.221
38.50	8.766	43.87	7.693	49.12	6.870	54.37	6.207
38.62	8.738	44.00	7.670	49.25	6.852	54.50	6.192
38.75	8.708	44.12	7.649	49.37	6.836	54.62	6.179
38.87	8.682	44.25	7.627	49.50	6.818	54.75	6.164
39.00	8.653	44.37	7.606	49.62	6.801	54.87	6.150
39.12	8.627	44.50	7.584	49.75	6.783	55.00	6.136
39.25	8.598	44.62	7.563	49.87	6.767	55.12	6.123
39.37	8.572	44.75	7.541	50.00	6.750	55.25	6.101
39.50	8.544	44.87	7.521	50.12	6.733	55.37	6.095
39.62	8.518	45.00	7.500	50.25	6.716	55.50	6.081
39.75	8.490	45.12	7.480	50.37	6.700	55.62	6.068
39.87	8.465	45.25	7.458	50.50	6.683	55.75	6.054
40.00	8.437	45.37	7.438	50.62	6.667	55.87	6.041
40.12	8.412	45.50	7.417	50.75	6.650	56.00	6.027
40.25	8.385	45.62	7.398	50.87	6.634	56.50	5.973
40.37	8.360	45.75	7.377	51.00	6.617	57.00	5.921
40.50	8.333	45.87	7.357	51.12	6.602	57.50	5.869
40.62	8.308	46.00	7.336	51.25	6.585	58.00	5.819
40.75	8.282	46.12	7.317	51.37	6.569	58.50	5.769
40.87	8.257	46.25	7.300	51.50	6.553	59.00	5.720
41.00	8.231	46.37	7.280	51.62	6.538	59.50	5.672
41.12	8.207	46.50	7.258	51.75	5.621	60.00	5.625

between the flat-K and the base curve of the contact lens need be considered. For base curves fit *flatter than K*, the lacrimal lens takes on a shape of a minus lens. For base curves fit *steeper than K*, the lacrimal lens takes on the shape of a plus lens (Figure 21-1). A simplified formula for determining lacrimal lens power is shown in Sidebar 21-2.

The lacrimal lens plays a role any time the base curve of the rigid lens is adjusted. When a base curve is flattened, a minus lacrimal lens is induced. To compensate for this optical power change, additional plus power must be added to the contact lens prescription. The acronym *FAP* (flatter add plus) is used. For each dioptric amount the contact is flattened, plus power in the same dioptric amount is added to the contact lens prescription (Sidebar 21-3).

SIDEBAR 21-1
DIOPTER TO RADIUS CONVERSION FORMULA

D = dioptric value (D)
r = radius value (mm)
D = 337.5/r or r = 337.5/D

Example 1. A lens with a base curve of 7.50 mm has a corneal dioptric value of:
D = 337.5/7.5
D = 45.00 D

Example 2. A lens with a base curve of 44.00 D has a radius of curvature value of:
r = 337.5/44.00
r = 7.67 mm

SIDEBAR 21-2
DETERMINING LACRIMAL LENS POWER

base curve (D) – flat-keratometry reading (D) = lacrimal lens power (D)

Example. Rigid gas-permeable lens BC = 7.50 mm (45.00 D)
K = 45.50 D/46.50 D
Lacrimal lens = 45.00 D – 45.50 D = -0.50 D
The lacrimal lens is concave, inducing a minus power of -0.50 D.

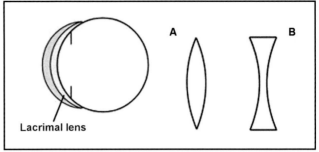

Figure 21-1. Lacrimal lens. (A) Fit steeper than K, the lacrimal lens is convex (plus). (B) Fit flatter than K, the lacrimal lens is concave (minus).

SIDEBAR 21-3
FLATTER ADD PLUS (FAP)

Example. Initial lens parameters: BC 7.89 DIAM 9.4 POWER -3.75
If the base curve of this lens needs to be flattened by 0.50 D (0.9 mm, using the diopter/radius conversion), the power would also need to be adjusted by +0.50. The new lens parameters would be:
BC 7.98 DIAM 9.4 POWER -3.25

SIDEBAR 21-4
STEEPER ADD MINUS (SAM)

Example. Initial lens parameters: BC 7.89 DIAM 9.4 POWER -3.75
If the base curve of this lens needs to be steepened by 0.50 D (0.9 mm, using the diopter/radius conversion), the power would also need to be adjusted by -0.50. The new lens parameters would be:
BC 7.80 DIAM 9.4 POWER -4.25

Whenever a base curve is steepened, a plus lacrimal lens is induced. To compensate, additional minus power must be added to the contact lens prescription. The acronym *SAM* (steeper add minus) is used. For each dioptric amount the lens is steepened, minus power in the same dioptric amount is added to the contact lens prescription (Sidebar 21-4).

Residual Astigmatism

Astigmatism can be either regular (with meridians 90 degrees [°] apart) or irregular (meridians that are not 90° apart or perpendicular).

Regular astigmatism can be corneal, lenticular (on the natural lens of the eye), or both. Any astigmatism that is left over after a contact lens is fit to the eye is termed *residual astigmatism*. Residual astigmatism is measured by a spherocylindrical overrefraction of the contact lens. (Note: A spherical overrefraction is done with loose trial lenses or at the refractor while the patient is wearing the contacts, and involves changing sphere lenses *only*, in an attempt to improve vision. A spherocylindrical overrefraction also employs cylinder [axis and power, as usual] to obtain best-corrected vision.)

Residual astigmatism in a soft lens can be lenticular and/or corneal, as there is no lacrimal lens to correct corneal astigmatism. In either case, residual astigmatism greater than 1.00 D must be addressed in the soft contact lens design by changing from spherical to toric (has incorporated cylinder to correct the astigmatism) or by changing the lens design altogether. However, residual astigmatism with a rigid lens is going to be lenticular unless there is a high degree of corneal astigmatism (>2.5 D). For residual astigmatism less than 1 D, the spherical equivalent of the overrefraction can be added to the sphere power of the lens if the patient finds the correction satisfactory.

Evaluating the keratometry and refractive values of each eye can help determine if residual astigmatism will be present. (Keratometry is covered later in this chapter.) This may help streamline the fitting process by going directly to a toric lens or different lens design (Sidebar 21-5).

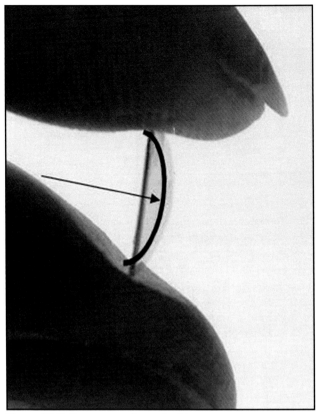

Figure 21-2. Base curve of a contact lens.

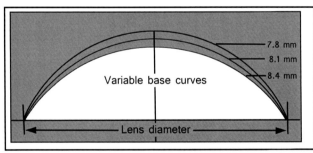

Figure 21-3. Base curve changes also affect the lens vault.

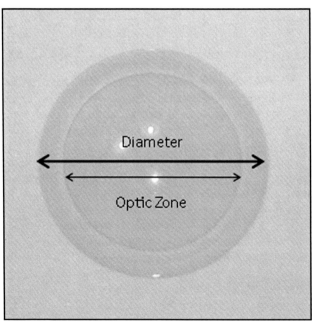

Figure 21-4. Diameter and optic zone diameter of a rigid gas-permeable lens.

CLINICAL KNOWLEDGE

Physical Characteristics of Contact Lenses

Base curve (BC) is the radius of curvature of the central posterior surface of the contact lens (Figure 21-2). It is also known as the *central posterior curve* (CPC). Steepening the base curve of a lens increases the *lens vault* or *lens curvature depth*. Conversely, flattening the base curve decreases the lens vault (Figure 21-3). Either of these values may need to be adjusted during fitting.

Diameter (D) is the overall width of the contact lens from edge to edge (Figure 21-4) in millimeters (mm). Diameter selection is based on the overall horizontal visible iris diameter (HVID) of the patient's cornea and varies according to contact lens type and design. Increasing

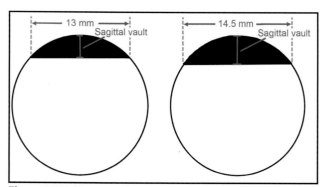

Figure 21-5. Diameter changes.

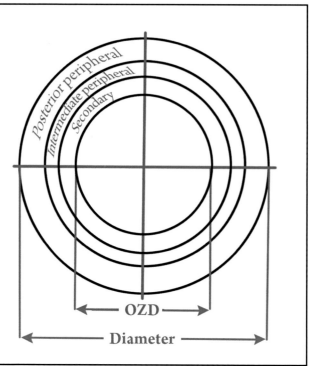

Figure 21-6. Peripheral curve system of a rigid gas-permeable lens.

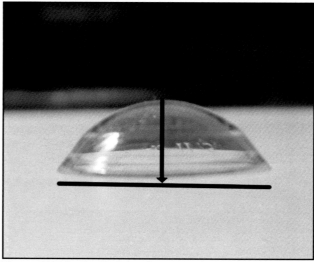

Figure 21-7. Sagittal height of a contact lens.

lens diameter will increase the lens vault, thus steepening the lens, and vice versa (Figure 21-5).

Power refers to the prescription of the lens in diopters (D). Power can be spherical or spherocylindrical, and can include presbyopic corrections as well. Contact lens prescriptions are written in minus cylinder form.

The *optic zone* (OZ) is the diameter (in millimeters) across which the base curve extends over the posterior surface of a contact lens. It is the "power zone" of the lens, where the prescription of the lens is located (see Figure 21-4). Increasing the optic zone diameter increases the lens vault and steepens the lens. Decreasing the optic zone diameter decreases the lens vault and flattens the lens. Additional surface power, as with some anterior toric and aspheric lens designs, can be added to the front surface optical zone of the lens as well.

Peripheral curves pertain primarily to rigid lenses since peripheral curves of a soft contact are not customizable. Peripheral curves are defined as any curve that is applied outside of the optical zone of the posterior lens surface. Just as the base curve is the fitting curve of the lens, the peripheral curves are the "landing curves" of the lens. The peripheral curves control the tear flow under the lens and contribute to lens comfort. Peripheral curves can vary in number and width. The primary peripheral curves are the secondary curve, intermediate curve, and posterior curve (Figure 21-6). The *secondary curve* is applied just outside of the base curve of the lens and is flatter than the base curve. The *intermediate peripheral curve* is between the secondary and posterior curve. It is flatter than the secondary curve. The final curve is the *posterior peripheral curve.* It is the outermost, flattest curve of the lens. All of the curve junctures are blended for smoothness and comfort.

Dk refers to the oxygen permeability of a lens material. *D* is the diffusivity or the ease with which oxygen moves through the material, and *k* is the solubility of the material, or how much oxygen is inherently contained in the material. Dk values can range from 0 (no oxygen permeability) to over 150 (hyper-Dk materials). Dk/t refers to the oxygen permeability of a lens at a specific thickness (t), as increased lens thickness can hinder the ability of oxygen to diffuse through the material. Lens material, water content, and lens thickness, as well as proteins and deposits on the lens surface, can all affect the oxygen permeability of a contact lens.

Sagittal depth or *height* is the distance between the central base curve of the lens to a flat surface (Figure 21-7). It is also referred to as the *vault* of the lens. A lens with a higher vault will have a steeper curve; a lens with a lower vault will have a flatter curve. The vault of the contact lens should approximate the vault of the cornea. Larger diameter corneas may require larger and/or steeper contact lenses.

Lens thickness will vary as to the lens material and the power of the lens. This is important to remember regarding the Dk value of various lens powers, as permeability decreases with increased lens thickness.

A minus lens will be thinner in the center and thicker on the edge. A plus lens will be thicker in the center and thinner at the edge. A high minus rigid lens can be designed with a *hyperflange*, or plus lens carrier, added to the peripheral curve to make the thick edge of the concave lens more thin. Alternately, a *myoflange*, or minus lens carrier, can be added to the peripheral curve of a high plus rigid lens to thicken the peripheral edge. This may be needed to aid in upper lid attachment of the lens, better alignment, and overall lens centration of a rigid lens.

Center thickness is also important in rigid lens fittings. As the center thickness of the lens decreases, the lens is more prone to flexure. Flexure can be induced from the blink action of the eyelids and the amount of corneal astigmatism present, and can cause fluctuating visual acuity and blurred vision.

Wetting angle describes how the tear film spreads across the surface of a contact lens. A low wetting angle will allow the tears and eyelid to glide across the lens surface, thus increasing the wettability of the lens. A high wetting angle will cause a lens to not wet well. A surface that is dry will continue to attract other hydrophobic materials, such as lipids and mucins, creating a cycle of poor wetting and dryness.

Contact Lens Advocacy

In July 2004, the *Contact Lens Rule*, formally known as the Fairness to Contact Lens Consumers Act (FCLCA), was established to ensure fair and safe contact lens practices among providers and sellers for the benefit of the patient (Sidebar 21-6). It was designed and is enforced by the Federal Trade Commission (FTC). The rule provides consumers with certain rights regarding their contact lens prescription as well as protects the public from illegal contact lens sales. It allows patients to obtain a copy of their written contact lens prescription from the eye care provider and to purchase the lenses at the place of their choice. The prescription must then be verified by the seller prior to contact lens dispensing.

Reference Materials

There is a variety of resources available for additional information and guidelines. Publications such as *Tyler's Quarterly* and websites such as TheRightContact.com offer a full listing of soft and rigid lens materials and manufacturers. Educational societies and websites such as Contact Lens Society of America (CLSA), Scleral Lens Education Society, and Gas Permeable Lens Institute (GPLI) offer online education. Government websites, such as the Food and Drug Administration (FDA) and

---

> ### SIDEBAR 21-6
> ### FAIRNESS TO CONTACT LENS CONSUMERS ACT PROVISIONS
>
> ▶ Prescribers are required to give the patient a copy of his/her contact lens prescription at the end of the contact lens fitting.
>
> ▶ Patients are not required to purchase contact lenses from the prescriber.
>
> ▶ Contact lenses can only be purchased with a valid prescription presented either by a person, email, or fax.
>
> ▶ Sellers must verify a contact lens prescription before selling the lenses if no prescription is presented at time of ordering. Verification by the prescriber can occur by phone or fax. The seller cannot alter a prescription or fill a prescription that has been denied by the prescriber.
>
> ▶ The prescriber has 8 business hours to confirm or deny the contact lens prescription before it is filled by the seller.
>
> ▶ The prescriber can set the expiration date of the contact lens prescription based on the medical needs of the patient and applicable state contact lens laws. Typical expiration is 1 year from the date the prescription was written.
>
> ▶ The seller must maintain records for 3 years.

Centers for Disease Control and Prevention (CDC) have specific guidelines and information regarding safe contact lens wear. Contact lens manufacturers' websites offer a wealth of information on their lenses, designs, and fitting guidelines.

Soft Contact Lenses

A soft contact lens (SCL) is a soft, flexible, plastic lens that molds to the shape of the eye, providing comfort and vision correction without glasses. SCLs can correct for myopia, hyperopia, astigmatism, presbyopia, aphakia, and irregular astigmatism.

Materials

Soft lenses are fabricated from two basic material types: hydrogel and silicone hydrogel.

Hydrogel (or *2-hydroxyethyl methacrylate* [HEMA]) lenses are the original soft lens material, made from plastic polymers that bind with water to form a *hydrophilic* (water-loving) lens (Table 21-3). The characteristics of these different plastic polymers can vary as to water content, oxygen permeability, material stiffness, wettability, and deposit resistance.

TABLE 21-3	
HYDROGEL LENS PROS AND CONS	
Pros	**Cons**
▸ All the benefits of a soft contact lens (see Table 21-6) ▸ Better initial lens comfort than a high modulus silicone hydrogel lens	▸ Limited maximum oxygen permeability (Dk), which limits extended wear applications ▸ Prone to protein deposits ▸ Flimsy with increased water content, difficult for patient to handle ▸ Risk of microbial keratitis

TABLE 21-4	
SILICONE HYDROGEL LENS PROS AND CONS	
Pros	**Cons**
▸ All the benefits of a soft contact lens (see Table 21-6) ▸ Increased oxygen permeability (Dk) ▸ Decreased water content ▸ Increased lens stiffness/modulus (better handling) ▸ Less limbal redness, corneal edema, and neovascularization than with hydrogel lenses[1] ▸ Less prone to protein deposits ▸ Less prone to drying	▸ Same risk of microbial keratitis as with hydrogel lenses[1,2] ▸ Increased risk of contact lens-induced giant papillary conjunctivitis with increased lens modulus[2] ▸ Increased risk of noninfectious corneal infiltrates than with hydrogel lenses[1] ▸ More prone to mucin balls

In general, as the water content of a hydrogel lens is increased, so is the Dk. However, as more water is introduced into the lens matrix, the lens becomes more fragile and prone to surface deposits. The oxygen permeability of a hydrogel lens is limited by the water content of the lens.

Silicone hydrogel soft lenses are a newer lens material made from silicone hydrogel polymer combinations that provide a low water content lens with increased oxygen permeability (Table 21-4). Silicone is naturally oxygen permeable and can have relatively high Dk values, yet still maintain its stability and deposit resistance. However, silicone alone is hydrophobic (water-fearing). To overcome the wettability issues, silicone materials are combined with hydrogel materials.

The FDA has sorted soft lenses into various classifications to help describe lens material interactions with proteins (deposit resistance) and to minimize solution incompatibilities with certain materials.

The FDA divides contact lens materials by the water content of the material and the surface ionic charge. As water content increases, the lens becomes more fragile and more prone to deposits, yet more oxygen permeable. The ionic charge refers to the surface charge of the lens material. When the surface is referred to as ionic, it has a negative surface charge that can attract positively charged proteins and deposits, and can have biocompatibility problems with some cleaning/disinfecting solutions. A

surface that is nonionic does not react nor does it readily attract proteins.

Manufacturing

Each soft lens manufacturer has its own proprietary design and production technique for its lenses, although all soft lenses are produced by spin-casting, cast- or injection-molding, lathe-cutting, or a combination of these techniques.

Spin-casting is the original soft lens manufacturing method. With spin casting, the liquid plastic is spun in a mold at high speeds, creating the desired power and shape of the lens. It is highly reproducible, easily mass produced, and delivers a comfortable lens. However, the design is limited by the power parameter range and the lack of a precise fitting alignment to the cornea. All spin-cast lenses are aspheric (ie, no cylinder to compensate for astigmatism).

With *cast-* or *injection-molding*, the liquid lens material is precision-injected into computer-designed molds under pressure, then solidified with ultraviolet radiation, removed, and finished. Each lens parameter must have its own specific mold, thus creating high-quality, reproducible lenses. Cast molding is efficient, cost effective, and the most common method of soft lens manufacturing.

The final soft lens manufacturing technique is *lathe-cutting*. A dry disk button is mounted on a spinning shaft and cut to precision using a computer-controlled lathe. The lens edges are then polished, and the lens undergoes hydration and finishing. Complex lens designs and higher levels of precision can be achieved, allowing more parameter choices and high-quality custom soft lenses.

Rigid Contact Lenses

A rigid contact lens is a hard, plastic lens that provides a stable refractive surface over the cornea. Between the rigid lens material and the cornea, a *lacrimal tear lens* is created, providing an additional optical surface for correcting myopia, hyperopia, astigmatism, presbyopia, and irregular astigmatism.

Materials

Polymethylmethacrylate (PMMA, also called acrylic) was the original plastic lens polymer for rigid corneal lenses. However, the Dk of the material is less than 1, making it unable to "breathe." The lens had to have a small diameter and be able to pump tears beneath the lens in order to supply oxygen to the cornea. *Cellulose acetate butyrate* (CAB) was the first-generation gas-permeable rigid lens material. It provided oxygen permeability, and the lenses could be made in larger diameters. However, it is not as durable as PMMA, and although it provides some oxygen permeability, it is minimal. *Silicone acrylate* (S/A) was the second generation of gas-permeable rigid lens materials. These lenses were a mix of silicone and PMMA, which provided a stable lens with increased Dk values. They were the first successful gas-permeable lens, but there were still some drawbacks. These included poor lens wetting, deposit formation, susceptibility to scratches, and increased flexure and warpage.

Fluoro-silicone acrylate (F-S/A) is the modern-day rigid gas-permeable lens material, a combination of silicone acrylate polymers and fluorine. With the addition of fluorine, less silicone can be used, increasing the overall lens stability, oxygen permeability, and lens surface wettability. F-S/A lenses have variable Dk values from low (Dk >20) to hyper-Dk (>100). Hyper-Dk materials are used in extended wear, orthokeratology (explained later), and scleral lens designs.

F-S/A lenses can also be combined with hydroxyethyl methacrylate (HEMA) to create a modified gas-permeable lens material that optimizes surface wettability, such as Hydro-2 material (by Innovision). This material, along with ONSI-56 (by Lagado), a silicone hydrogel rigid material, is particularly beneficial for patients with dry eyes.

Manufacturing

Rigid gas-permeable contact lenses (RGPCL, or RGP) are custom designed and produced using advanced *computer-controlled lathe technology*. Each lens is custom cut and finished by polishing the surfaces and smoothing the edges. The lens can be plasma treated to improve overall surface wettability and comfort. Plasma treatment involves the application of low-temperature oxygen plasma to the surface of the lens, changing the surface ionization, and thus decreasing the wetting angle and super cleaning the lens surface.

Specialty Contact Lenses

A specialty contact lens is any lens that is uniquely customized for an individual patient (ie, "made to order"). A custom lens is indicated for those individuals whose ocular measurements fall outside of the standard inventoried contact lens parameters. It also includes medically necessary contact lenses, such as those used to treat irregular corneal conditions that are not correctable with spectacles.

Custom latheable soft lenses can fabricate virtually any custom parameter the fitter may require. Base curve, power (sphere and spherocylindrical corrections), diameter, lens thickness, optic zone, lens stabilization (prism ballasting), and multifocal optics can all be customized to the patient's special needs. These lenses are especially useful for adult and pediatric aphakia.

Scleral rigid lenses are designed to vault an irregular corneal surface and rest on the sclera beyond the limbus, creating a protected environment for the corneal surface. This makes them especially useful for patients with irregular corneas and ocular surface diseases. Scleral lenses tend to be very comfortable due to the large diameters, which can vary from 14 to 20 mm. They can also be used with normal corneas in cases of corneal RGP lens intolerance where vision is not satisfactorily corrected with soft lenses.

Hybrid lenses are the combination of an RGP lens surrounded by a soft lens "skirt." These large-diameter lenses provide the sharp optics and lacrimal tear lens correction of a rigid lens, but the comfort of a soft lens in the periphery. Hybrid lenses can be used for ametropia as well as irregular corneas.

Soft lenses for keratoconus are thicker than traditional soft lenses, eliminating the "draping" nature of a regular soft lens. (Draping is a disadvantage in keratoconus because the lens conforms to the irregular shape of the cornea, thus providing no optical correction.) Lens thickness ranges from 0.3 to 0.6 mm. This allows the soft lens to create a new optical surface much like a rigid lens, correcting mild to moderate amounts of corneal irregularity.

Orthokeratology is corneal reshaping with RGPCLs for the purpose of refractive vision correction. The flat-fitting lenses are worn only while sleeping, changing the corneal shape, and thus correcting mild to moderate amounts of myopia. If the night-time schedule is discontinued, the cornea will eventually return to pretreatment status.

Reverse geometry lenses are primarily made from RGP materials, but are available in a few soft lens configurations as well. This design is used in cases where the corneal surface has been altered and the central cornea is now flatter than the peripheral cornea, as seen after refractive surgery. Contacts with reverse geometry optics have a flatter central base curve with a steeper mid-peripheral curve and a flatter peripheral curve.

Piggyback lenses are a combination fitting of an SCL and then a separate corneal RGP lens over that. This technique is used in cases of irregular astigmatism where the patient cannot tolerate the discomfort of a rigid lens. The soft lens acts as a foundation lens for comfort, and the rigid lens provides the crisp optics and lacrimal lens for correcting irregular corneal conditions such as keratoconus.

A *bandage lens* is a therapeutic plano soft lens that is applied to the cornea as a dressing or protective measure following injury, trauma, or corneal procedures. Bandage lenses are worn as extended wear, and only certain lenses are approved for this use. (A listing can be found in *Tyler's Quarterly*.)

Prosthetic lenses can be made of both soft and rigid lens materials. These fit over a disfigured eye to mask pupil abnormalities and corneal opacities, and is painted or tinted to look like a "normal" eye. Prosthetic lenses also provide a psychological benefit to the patient. In some cases, such as severe photophobia and irregular pupils, there can be visual benefits as well. Soft prosthetic lenses have options that include transparent or opaque backgrounds, clear or black pupils, and hand-painted iris color-matching. Additional prosthetic contacts include theatrical lenses, sports-tinted lenses, and color-vision enhancing lenses.

CLINICAL SKILLS

Instrumentation

Slit Lamp Biomicroscope

The slit lamp biomicroscope is the primary diagnostic tool for evaluating contact lenses. A careful slit lamp examination is also necessary to rule out preexisting ocular problems that could interfere with contact lens success. The techniques most commonly used with contact lens evaluations are diffuse, direct focal (including parallelepiped and optic section) and sclerotic scatter. These are covered in detail in Chapter 12, but a few features that pertain to contact lens fitting are appropriate here.

Diffuse illumination provides a general view of the contact lens on the eye. By sweeping the light across the surface, any gross abnormalities can be noted. Lens movement, centration, and sodium fluorescein (NaFl) dye patterns can be observed.

The *parallelepiped* or *broad beam* illumination uses a narrower beam to view specific detail of the contact lens fit and the lens's relationship to the eye.

The *optic section* illumination provides a block of light with a cross-sectional view for visualizing the contact lens thickness, the tear film thickness under the contact lens, and the corneal thickness. This is important in proper evaluation of the lens to cornea relationship, including vault, in the more advanced contact lens designs.

Lastly, *sclerotic scatter* illumination can be used for viewing contact lens irregularities, as well as possible corneal edema related to contact lens wear.

Various filters are used in conjunction with vital stains to evaluate contact lenses with the slit lamp. Commonly used filters are the cobalt blue filter and the Wratten #12 yellow filter (Figure 21-8).

The three stains used for ocular evaluation include NaFl, rose bengal, and lissamine green. During the pre-fit exam, rose bengal and lissamine green are used for evaluation of conjunctival staining, while NaFl is best used to evaluate corneal staining. However, only NaFl is used when evaluating contact lenses on the eye.

NaFl is an orange-yellow dye that fluoresces green under the cobalt blue light. It highlights the tear film under the contact lens, allowing visualization of fitting patterns (covered later). It also will cause hyperfluorescence (or staining) of the ocular surfaces where tissue is compromised or disrupted.

NaFl is best applied using a single-use, sterile impregnated paper strip. The strip can be wet with sterile saline or irrigating solution then tapped to remove excess fluid. The wet strip is touched to the superior bulbar conjunctiva or to the inferior palpebral conjunctiva. It can also be applied directly to the surface of an RGPCL using a gentle, light touch.

A combination liquid anesthetic and NaFl should be avoided in patients wearing contact lenses. The dye can penetrate the lens matrix of an SCL and stain the lens. (If this occurs, repeatedly rinse and soak the lens in saline solution to flush the lens.) A high molecular weight NaFl dye (ie, fluorexon) is recommended for use with soft and hybrid contact lenses. This is available as a strip or single-use liquid ampule.

After the dye is applied, the eye can be evaluated using a white light, the blue cobalt light, and/or the Wratten #12 filter. The white light can be used with an optic section technique as described above to measure the vault of a rigid scleral lens. The white light can also be used to view toric lens markings, lens orientation markings, surface defects, and deposits. The blue cobalt light along with a diffuse or parallelepiped beam can be used to evaluate the fit and fluorescein patterns of a rigid or a specialty SCL, and to look for surface staining related to contact lens complications (covered later). By adding the Wratten #12 filter over the slit lamp objective along with the blue cobalt filter, an enhanced or highlighted fit pattern can be visualized.

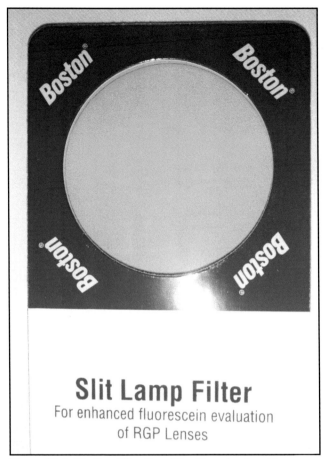

Figure 21-8. Wratten #12 yellow filter (Bausch + Lomb).

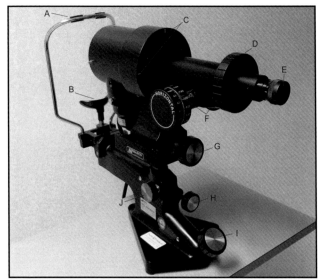

Figure 21-9. Parts of the keratometer (Marco). A=forehead rest, B=chinrest, C=axis marking, D=axis rotation knob, E=eyepiece, F=measuring drums, G=focus knob, H=chinrest height adjustment knob, I=instrument height adjustment knob, J=lock knob.

The Burton Lamp

The Burton lamp is an ultraviolet fluorescent lamp for use with NaFl. It is a hand-held unit consisting of a magnifying lens and dual ultraviolet lamps. The magnifier is large enough to allow simultaneous viewing of both eyes. When evaluating rigid lens patterns with the lamp, it is important to view the patient at eye level.

Keratometer

Keratometry is the measurement of the base curve of the corneal surface as well as the curvature of the two principal (flat/steep) meridians. These readings (called *K-readings*) quantify the amount of corneal astigmatism present. This information is needed for contact lens fitting as well as for intraocular lens implant selection prior to cataract surgery (see Chapter 28).

The manual keratometer (Figure 21-9) can also be used to evaluate corneal irregularity (irregular astigmatism) and the quality of the tear film. In addition, one can evaluate proper fit of an SCL through this instrument. An automated keratometer will only give a curvature reading and no information on the quality of the corneal surface.

However, keratometry only measures approximately 3 mm of the central cornea cap, and while this is useful

information, it is not representative of the entire corneal surface and provides no information on the peripheral cornea (necessary for more advanced contact lens fittings). In such a case corneal topography is necessary (discussed momentarily).

Taking K-Readings

▶ Apply a thin artificial tear to the patient's eye and let it "settle" while you are preparing the instrument. (More helpful hints are in Sidebar 21-7.)

▶ Set the eyepiece for your eye by focusing the crosshairs. Position the white occluder in front of the instrument and turn the focusing knob counterclockwise as far as it will go. Look into the instrument and slowly turn the knob clockwise until the crosshairs just come into sharp focus, then *stop*. Do not fine tune by moving the dial back and forth.

▶ Ask the patient to bring the chin into the chinrest and the forehead against the band. It is important that he/she keep the back teeth together and breathe slowly through the nose to minimize movement. Align the lateral canthus to the canthus mark on the instrument. When looking at the patient from the side, the "donut" light of the keratometer should be centered on the cornea.

▶ Occlude the fellow eye with the occluder. Ask the patient to look straight ahead at the fixation light (if your instrument has one) or at the image of his/her own eye inside the instrument.

▶ Keep the crosshair aligned in the bottom right circle (Figure 21-10A). This ensures the optical axis of the instrument is aligned to the visual axis of the patient.

SIDEBAR 21-7
DO IT BETTER: KERATOMETRY

- ▶ If the patient has trouble finding proper fixation, you can shine a penlight into the ocular. Ask the patient to maintain this position even after the penlight is turned off.

- ▶ If you are having trouble "finding" the eye, shine a penlight into the ocular and look at the patient's eye from the side. Adjust the instrument so that the reflection you see is centered on the patient's cornea.

- ▶ Encourage the patient to blink frequently during the measurement.

- ▶ Dimming the lights can help you see the mires better.

- ▶ Double check your endpoint by having the patient blink while refocusing your mires.

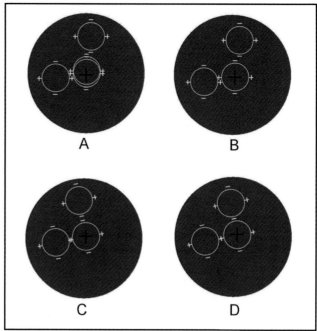

Figure 21-10. Mire alignment. (A) Doubling of mires indicates unfocused mires. (B) Focus adjusted, but "plus signs" on side of mires not aligned indicating misaligned axis. (C) Axis aligned, but plus and minus signs do not overlap indicating incorrect curvature measurement. (D) Horizontal and vertical measurements adjusted for correct measurement; plus and minus signs are superimposed.

Use the focusing knob to keep the circles in focus (Figure 21-10B). Lock the instrument once alignment is achieved.

- ▶ Use the vertical and horizontal adjustment knobs to pull the plus/minus signs apart.

- ▶ Align the axis by turning the barrel until the ends ("posts") of the plus signs of the bottom two circles are aligned (Figure 21-10C).

- ▶ Once axis alignment is achieved, move the vertical and horizontal knobs until the plus/minus signs are aligned and merged (Figure 21-10D). A good endpoint is when the plus/minus signs are aligned, the crosshairs are in the bottom right circle, and the mires are single and crisp.

- ▶ Record the results. Results are written by taking the horizontal drum reading with the corresponding horizontal axis reading and the vertical drum reading with the corresponding vertical axis reading. Then, any distortion of the mires can be graded on a scale of 1 to 4, and recorded (eg, H 42.00 x 180/V 44.00 x 090 [2+ distortion]). Some prefer to record the results in terms of flat and steep K-readings with flat-K being the lower K-reading and steep-K being the higher K-reading. In that case, the above example would be 42.00/44.00 x 090.

When the mires are distorted without a contact lens on the eye, it could represent a dry eye or an irregular cornea. Applying a thin artificial tear can enhance the tear film and smooth out the mires if the tear film is irregular. If the cornea is irregular, the mires will remain distorted (Figure 21-11).

When the mires are distorted with an SCL on the eye, it could represent an improper fit. If the mires blur after the patient blinks, the lens could be too loose and thus moving too much. If the mires are clearer after the patient blinks, the lens could be too steep. An acceptable fit is when the mires remain unchanged through a patient blink.

Sometimes the actual corneal readings extend beyond the range of the instrument (36 D to 51 D). The range of the keratometer can be extended using a trial lens and then the actual drum value corrected by using a conversion chart (Table 21-5). If the cornea is less than 36 D, tape a -1.00 D sphere trial lens over the keratometer aperture to extend the range by 6 D. If the cornea is steeper than 52 D, tape a +1.25 D sphere trial lens over the keratometer aperture to extend the range another 9 D.

Corneal Topography

Corneal topography has become a very useful tool in fitting contact lenses. Topography has advantages over keratometry in that it plots the curvature into the periphery. It also provides information on the shape of the cornea, the location and elevation of irregularities, as well as simulated keratometry readings of the central cornea (Figure 21-12). Corneal topography is the primary diagnostic tool for detecting and mapping the extent of

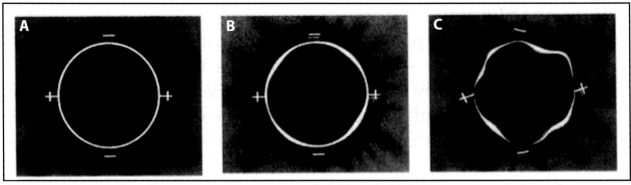

Figure 21-11. (A) Normal crisp keratometry mires. (B) Mires are a little blurry/doubled. (C) Mires are grossly distorted.

TABLE 21-5			
EXTENDED KERATOMETRY RANGE CONVERSION CHART			
Extended Keratometer Range With +1.25 D Lens		**Extended Keratometer Range With -1.00 D Lens**	
Actual Drum Reading (Diopters)	*Extended Value (Diopters)*	*Actual Drum Reading (Diopters)*	*Extended Value (Diopters)*
45.00	52.46	36.00	30.87
45.25	52.76	36.25	31.09
45.50	53.05	36.50	31.30
45.75	53.34	36.75	31.51
46.00	53.63	37.00	31.73
46.25	53.92	37.25	31.95
46.50	54.21	37.50	32.16
46.75	54.51	37.75	32.37
47.00	54.80	38.00	32.59
47.25	55.09	38.25	32.80
47.50	55.38	38.50	33.02
47.75	55.67	38.75	33.23
48.00	55.96	39.00	33.45
48.25	56.25	39.25	33.66
48.50	56.55	39.50	33.88
48.75	56.84	39.75	34.09
49.00	57.13	40.00	34.30
49.25	57.42	40.25	34.52
49.50	57.71	40.50	34.73
49.75	58.00	40.75	34.95
50.00	58.30	41.00	35.16
50.25	58.59	41.25	35.38
50.50	58.88	41.50	35.59
50.75	59.17	41.75	35.81
51.00	59.46	42.00	36.02

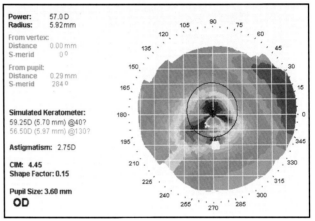

Figure 21-12. Corneal topography of a steep cornea, typically seen in a keratoconus or post-LASIK ectasia patient.

keratoconus. The size, shape, elevations, and location of the cone can be visualized on topographical displays.

Topography can be used to design and simulate RGPCLs on the eye. Many instruments offer contact lens fitting programs. Simulated fluorescein patterns of different lens designs and parameters can help reduce trial and fitting time of rigid lenses. The various displays can aid in lens selection, troubleshoot complications (such as corneal warpage), and provide information beyond the limits of keratometry. Some contact lens manufacturers also design lenses from topographical maps.

When viewing the display, cool colors (blue, green) represent flat areas on the cornea, while warmer colors (red, orange) represent steeper areas. The *axial map* view displays an axial representation with the central radius on the central axis. The map is a generalized or average dioptric value of the cornea. The *tangential map* displays a true dioptric representation of the cornea with every data point detailed. An *elevation map* displays the relative height or elevation of the cornea as referenced from a best-fit sphere, and can be compared to the fluorescein pattern of a rigid lens. The *refractive map* displays the refractive power of the cornea at any given point and is useful for determining the optical quality of the cornea.

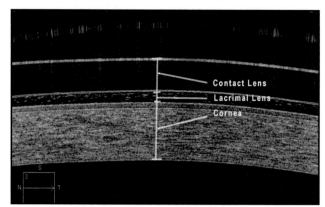

Figure 21-13. OCT image of a scleral rigid gas-permeable lens on the eye.

Performing the Scan

Topography units vary—Familiarize yourself with your instrument and the various printouts available.

To minimize artifacts, apply a thin artificial tear to the patient's eye and align the patient carefully. Have the patient blink frequently until you are ready to capture the image.

Missing data points and incomplete rings could be the result of a dry eye or droopy eyelid. Instruct the patient to blink and open the eyes wide.

The more irregular the cornea, the more missing data points there will be; take multiple images if necessary.

Optical Coherence Tomography

Optical coherence tomography (OCT) is principally used to evaluate the eye's interior (see Chapter 16), but is also one of the newest diagnostic tools used in contact lens evaluations. Anterior segment OCT can capture *sagittal height* values of the cornea, which takes into consideration, among other things, overall corneal diameter and the central corneal radius. These data are important because certain contact lens designs are based on corneal vault vs base curvature measurements.

The OCT is also useful for evaluating the lens-to-cornea relationship of rigid and scleral lenses, as well as visualizing the conjunctival landing zone of a scleral contact lens. A cross-sectional OCT image of the cornea can show the contact lens on the eye. The exact vault of the lens, the fluid reservoir beneath the lens, and the landing of the lens can all be imaged with the OCT (Figure 21-13). While it is not essential to utilize OCT with these specialty lens designs, it can provide more precise measuring and troubleshooting capabilities (Sidebar 21-8).

Radiuscope

The *radiuscope* (Figure 21-14; also known as a *radius gauge* or *microspherometer)* is used to measure the base curve of a rigid contact lens, including spherical and toric lens designs, and can determine if a rigid lens is warped.

SIDEBAR 21-8
DO IT BETTER: PERFORMING AN OCT ON A CONTACT LENS PATIENT

▶ The patient can be scanned with the contact lens in situ (on the eye).

▶ Anterior segment OCT can vary, so familiarize yourself with your machine and the various scan settings.

▶ If your machine is not a full anterior segment OCT, then utilize the anterior segment functions of the machine to obtain a limited view of the area being measured (ie, choose an Anterior Segment Cube or an Anterior Segment HD 5-Line Raster to visualize the cornea).

▶ Take multiple images or use the machine to view the corneal vault and landing zone of the contact lens on the eye.

▶ Use the measuring tool within the program to measure sagittal depth, much like you would measure corneal thickness in optical pachymetry.

Procedure

▶ Make sure the lens is clean and dry.

▶ Select the large aperture (for a wider field of view) and align the objective (microscope lens). Make sure the light is focused in the middle of the lens mount.

▶ Remove the lens mount. Add drop of saline solution to the lens mount and float the lens on it, concave side up. (Avoid excess fluid or any fluid on the concave side of the lens. A tissue can be used to siphon excess fluid from the mount.)

▶ Replace the lens mount and align the light source on the middle of the lens.

▶ Use the course focusing knob to focus the internal "star." The objective should be at its lowest position and the star centered.

▶ Calibrate the internal scale to your eye by adjusting the ocular focus knob until the scale is sharp and clear.

▶ Zero out the scale by turning the hairline position knob until the scale is set on zero. This must be done on every lens. If you are unable to zero it out, set the scale on the nearest whole number. You will adjust by this amount when recording your final reading.

▶ Use the course focusing knob to raise the objective. You will pass through the light filament image until the second star comes into focus.

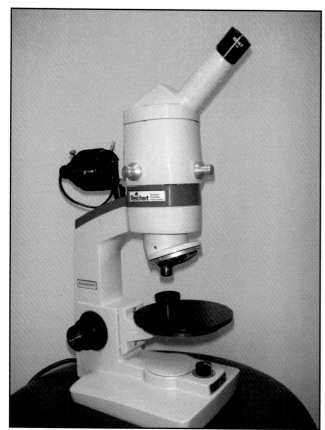

Figure 21-14. Radiuscope (Reichert Technologies).

► Measure the base curvature here by using the fine adjustment knob to sharpen the star. All of the spokes should focus clearly if the lens is spherical and not warped.

► Read the base curvature on the scale. If the lens would not calibrate at zero, remember to subtract your starting point from the reading.

Some radiuscopes use a clock dial on top of the instrument instead of an internal number scale. While the technique is similar, please refer to the manual for specifics about your instrument.

When there is toricity or the lens is warped, the spokes of the star will not come into focus in the same plane. If the lens is toric, the spokes should come into focus 90° apart. Measure the base curvature of each meridian. If the lens is warped, the spokes will focus at various axes with no clear, obvious base curve reading.

Lensometer

The *lensometer* is used to measure the optical power of a contact lens. Basic lensometry is covered in Chapter 19. Contact lenses are read similarly to spectacles. Spherical, toric, and warped lenses can be identified.

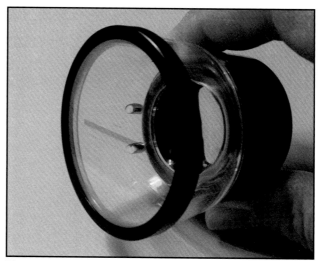

Figure 21-15. Reticle magnifier.

How to Read a Rigid Contact Lens
► Focus the reticle eyepiece to your eye.

► Make sure the lens is clean and dry.

► Use a smaller aperture if available (<6 mm; some lensometers come with removable apertures—one for spectacles and smaller one for contact lenses). You can use a contact lens holder to position the lens, or use your thumb and index finger to gently hold the lens over the aperture. Be careful not to pinch and flex the lens.

► Most contact lenses are read and labeled with back vertex power. (If in doubt, check with the contact lens lab on their design.) Hold the lens with the convex side facing you and the concave side facing the lens stop.

► Read the power as you would with spectacles.

Reticle Magnifier

A *reticle magnifier* is used to measure the diameter of a contact lens, and can be used to inspect the lens for deposits and irregularities. It is a hand-held magnifier (7x to 10x) with a number line (reticle) on one end and an inspection magnifier on the other (Figure 21-15). Using a bright light as background, a rigid lens is placed concave side down on the ruler, aligned to zero on one edge. The diameter is read on the other edge. The optical zone diameter, segment heights of translating bifocals, and sometimes peripheral curve widths can also be measured using this technique. The reticle can then be flipped and the magnifier on the other end used to inspect the lens for deposits, chips, scratches, and edge irregularities.

Diameter Gauge (V-Gauge)

A *diameter* or *V-gauge* is used to measure the diameter of a rigid contact lens. It is a type of ruler with a progressively narrow channel in which a rigid lens is

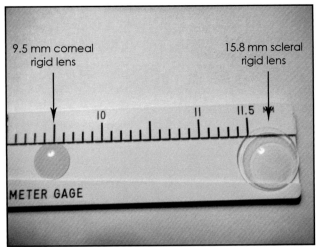

Figure 21-16. Contact lens diameter gauge. (Note that the scleral lens is too large for the gauge.)

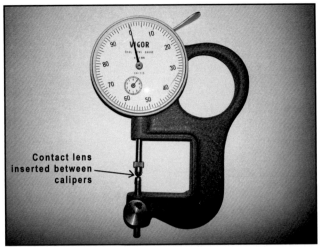

Figure 21-17. Center thickness gauge (Vigor Optical).

placed concave side down. The lens is then slid down the channel until it stops. The diameter is read off the scale at the widest portion of the lens (Figure 21-16). Take care not to force the lens in the channel or apply pressure to the lens surface.

Center Thickness Gauge

A *center thickness gauge* is used to measure the center thickness of a rigid contact lens. The lens is placed concave side up at the exact center, between the two calipers. The center thickness is read on the dial (Figure 21-17). By moving the lens to the periphery, the edge thickness can also be read.

Verifying Soft Contact Lenses

SCL verification is difficult, often inaccurate, and not very practical in an office setting. However, some parameters can be evaluated using tools and techniques readily available.

The slit lamp examination can provide information on edge and surface irregularities of a soft lens on the eye. The diameter can be checked using a reticle magnifier, and the power can be approximated using a lensometer (blot off excess solution first).

When fitting a new lens from a trial set, always double-check the base curve, diameter, power, ADD power, and any other pertinent parameters on the packaging before opening the lens. If the lens is not performing as expected, confirm that it is properly inserted on the correct eye, then check the lot number and try a lens from a different lot. If in doubt, always try another lens.

If a patient comes in wearing lenses and complaining of poor vision, or is not sure if the lenses have been switched, a simple check and swap can often confirm

which lens is which. Check the vision of each eye and perform an overrefraction, then swap lenses and check again.

A *Soft Lens Analyzer* can assess the base curvature, diameter, center thickness, and edges of soft lenses. The lens is placed in a wet cell and submerged in saline so the lens can be evaluated in a hydrated state. While this is a useful tool, it is not common in most eye care practices.

Additional Instrumentation

Modification Unit

There are certain changes that can be performed in the office on rigid lenses using a *modification unit*. These modifications include modifying and blending peripheral curves, polishing edges and surfaces, and changing lens power by ±0.50 D. The modification unit is a motor-driven spindle attached to a splash bowl with various spindle tools and polishing pads. Polishing compounds containing a mild abrasive are used for lens polishing and modification (as well as lubrication), to protect the surface wetting properties of the lens, and to reduce heat build-up during manipulation. Take caution when modifying newer, higher oxygen permeable rigid materials—they crack and break more easily than lower Dk materials. Modification of rigid lenses is best taught with a hands-on course.

Shadowgraph or Projection Magnifier

A *shadowgraph* or *projection magnifier* projects light through a rigid contact lens mounted on a stage to create a magnified image of the shadow of the lens. It resembles an enlarged reticle magnifier in which various parameters can be measured, including overall diameter, optic zone diameter, peripheral curve system, blends, and surface imperfections. The lens can also be rotated sideways to view the edges.

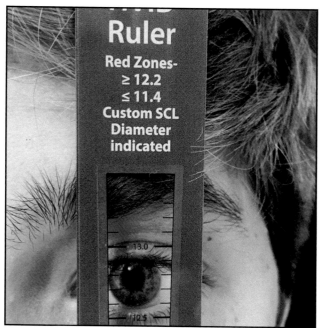

Figure 21-18. Measuring corneal diameter or horizontal visible iris diameter with a diameter gauge.

Profile Analyzer

A *profile analyzer* is a modified radiuscope used to evaluate the blending of the peripheral curve system of a rigid lens. The lens is mounted so the edge profile of the lens is visible through the microscope. The lens edge blending and any irregularities will be visible.

Pre-Fit Evaluation

A baseline of ocular measurements needs to be obtained prior to contact lens fitting. These measurements include visual acuity, a careful refraction, keratometry using the keratometer or topographer (or both), and a measurement of corneal diameter.

Corneal diameter or *horizontal visible iris diameter* (HVID) is the measurement of the cornea along a horizontal axis from limbus to limbus. This measurement is used to determine the appropriate diameter for soft and rigid contact lenses.

There are many different ways to measure HVID. While accuracy may vary, a few methods include reticles that fit into the ocular of a slit lamp biomicroscope, some autorefractors and topographers, as well as hand-held devices such as white-to-white cornea gauges, calipers, or rulers (Figure 21-18).

For contact lens fits and evaluations, a pre-fit ocular evaluation is necessary to rule out ocular complications that could preclude successful contact lens wear. For information on specific entities/disorders mentioned, kindly consult the Index.

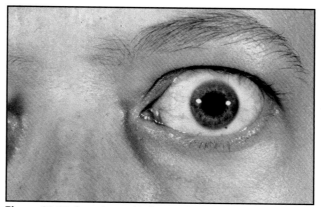

Figure 21-19. Superior and inferior scleral show.

Slit Lamp Exam

Prior to fitting contacts, a thorough slit lamp exam is necessary to evaluate the patient's eye while asking the question, "Will this patient be able to wear contact lenses safely?" The lids and lashes should be clean and free of debris or crusts, without missing lashes or abnormal growths. Blepharitis and meibomian gland dysfunction can affect the quality of the tear film which can lead to dryness, lens discomfort, and deposits. Lid hygiene, warm compresses, and artificial tear supplements may be necessary to maintain a clean environment for a contact lens.

The lid margins should be smooth and touch the globe. There should be no entropion or ectropion. Palpebral fissures (the opening between the superior and inferior lid margins) and the position of the upper and lower eyelids should be evaluated. An upper eyelid that is above the limbus (*superior scleral show*) may not hold an RGPCL in place adequately or may lead to dryness due to overexposure of the corneal surface (Figure 21-19). A lower eyelid that is below the limbus (*inferior scleral show*) can also affect contact lens fit and comfort, especially for some presbyopic contact lens designs.

An upper lid that is too loose may not hold a rigid lens in place or allow for its removal due to the lax tension. An upper lid that is too tight may eject a rigid contact lens, cause torsional rotation of a soft toric contact lens, and make it difficult to insert a contact lens (especially one with a larger diameter).

The normal blink rate is 10 to 15 blinks per minute.[3] A blink rate less than normal or incomplete blinking (where the upper and lower lid margins do not meet during the blink) can result in a poor precorneal tear film, overexposure of the ocular surface, and dry eyes. They can also affect the fit of a rigid contact lens.

The precorneal tear film provides moisture to the hydrophilic soft lens and the lacrimal lens between a rigid contact lens and the eye. A poor tear film can cause symptoms of dry eye, poor contact lens wetting, increased surface deposits, blurred vision, and lens bearing (rubbing on the corneal surface, which can lead to corneal

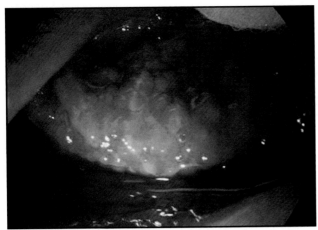

Figure 21-20. Giant papillary conjunctivitis. (http://webeye. ophth.uiowa.edu/eyeforum/atlas/pages/Giant-Papillary-Conjunctivitis.html. The author/editors and publisher acknowledge The University of Iowa and EyeRounds.org for permission to reproduce this copyrighted material.)

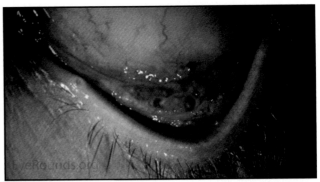

Figure 21-21. Follicles. (http://webeye.ophth.uiowa.edu/eye-forum/atlas/pages/follicular-conjunctivitis/follicular-conj-1-LRG.jpg. The author/editors and publisher acknowledge The University of Iowa and EyeRounds.org for permission to reproduce this copyrighted material.)

pathology). The tear film should be tested using one of the methods in Chapter 9.

The bulbar conjunctiva should be white and transparent with no redness, swelling, or discolorations. Growths such as pterygia and pingueculae can interfere with contact lens centering and comfort. Large growths can lead to *dellen* formation (corneal thinning due to tissue drying out). The conjunctiva should be checked for staining with rose bengal or lissamine green dye if moderate to severe dry eye symptoms are present.

The palpebral conjunctiva should be evaluated for papillae and follicles. *Papillae* are tiny, red elevations with raised vascular cores commonly seen as an allergic immune response or a response to an ocular foreign body. Prior contact lens wearers should be screened for *giant papillary conjunctivitis* (GPC; Figure 21-20), an allergic reaction of the superior palpebral conjunctiva to contact lens deposits. It produces large, sometimes scarred, cobblestone papillae on the lid surface, making contact lenses uncomfortable and unstable. *Follicles* are small, clear lymphoid elevations (Figure 21-21) common in inflammation (such as viral infections and topical medication allergies).

The cornea should be clear, smooth, and without irregularities. The light beam from the slit lamp should reflect with a sharp, shiny reflex from the corneal surface, and should be even across the surface without distortion. The layers of the cornea should be checked for neovascularization, haze, old scars, epithelial dystrophy, or other abnormalities. The cornea should also be checked for epithelial staining with NaFl dye. The cornea can be affected by ocular surface diseases, such as dry eye, blepharitis, and meibomian gland dysfunction. These disorders should be managed prior to contact lens fitting.

Contact Lens Fitting

Patient Selection

Patient selection is the most important first step in fitting any contact lens. Selecting the right lens for the patient requires investigation into a variety of factors.

Patient Expectations

Discuss the motivation behind the patient's desire for contact lenses and how he/she intends to use the lenses. Discuss replacement rates, wearing expectations (daily vs extended wear), hygiene, and expected visual outcome. For younger patients, discuss proper care and responsibility of contact lens wear with both the child and the parent. Distribute office information, such as a contact lens guide or contract, explaining proper wearing expectations, the fitting process, time involved, cost of the fitting and of the lenses, as well as lens replacement costs.

Recreational Hobbies

Discuss any hobbies or sports during which the patient intends to wear the lenses. Soft, hybrid, and scleral rigid lenses are less likely to become dislodged during contact sports. Swimming is not recommended with any lens, but if necessary, a daily disposable soft lens with immediate replacement after the activity can be an option. Remind the patient that contact lenses are not a replacement for goggles or recreational safety glasses.

Work Environment

The patient's occupation and work environment can affect contact lens usage and comfort. Long-term computer use can be accompanied by ocular drying. Environments with dust and debris may not be a good place for most contact lens wear, especially rigid corneal lenses where debris is easily trapped between the lens and cornea. Chemical fumes in the air can cause toxicity to the lens and the eye. (A daily disposable SCL might be an option in such cases.) Talking through the patient's needs and expectations will aid in the best lens selection for that

TABLE 21-6
SOFT LENS PROS AND CONS

Pros	Cons
▶ Immediate comfort and quick adaptation ▶ Can be used for intermittent/flexwear use ▶ Good for sports ▶ Daily, weekly, monthly, quarterly replacement ▶ Good for rigid lens failures (ie, comfort issues, tight lids) ▶ Easy to fit/in-office dispensing trials ▶ Good for children ▶ Standard and custom lens options	▶ Deposit build-up/durability ▶ Risk of contact lens-induced giant papillary conjunctivitis ▶ Hydrophilic nature can contribute to ocular dryness ▶ Larger, softer lens can be harder to handle for some individuals ▶ Limited applications with irregular astigmatism and ocular surface disease ▶ Inability to modify or verify parameters ▶ Poor alignment with oblique astigmatism

TABLE 21-7
RIGID LENS PROS AND CONS

Pros	Cons
▶ Excellent visual acuity/sharpness ▶ Longer lens life/replacement rate ▶ Custom fit for the individual patient ▶ Suitable as medically necessary lens for irregular cornea and severe ocular surface disease ▶ Increased comfort with newer scleral lens designs ▶ Less deposit build-up/lens material interaction ▶ Easy to handle secondary to rigid nature ▶ Ability to modify and verify lens parameters	▶ Increased initial lens awareness in new wearers ▶ Longer initial adaptation period ▶ Not recommended for intermittent wear ▶ Not recommended in dusty environments ▶ Smaller lens designs less stable in individuals with tight lids or in contact sports ▶ Poor alignment with high against-the-rule astigmatism

patient. Emphasize that contact lenses are not a replacement for safety glasses in high-risk activities.

Medical History and Medications

Many conditions and medications can change the surface tear chemistry, inducing dryness. Allergies, pregnancy, menopause, thyroid conditions, autoimmune diseases, and the patient's own physical capabilities could potentially challenge successful contact lens wear. Diabetics can be prone to infections and poor healing. Medications associated with ocular dryness include antihistamines, decongestants, some acne medications, diuretics, hormone replacement therapies, anti-anxiety/depressants, beta blockers, and chemotherapy drugs.

Ocular History and Refractive Error

A review of the patient's ocular history and examination is necessary prior to contact lens fitting. Evaluate visual acuity, HVID, refraction, keratometry, topography, and perform a slit lamp examination. For patients currently wearing contact lenses, gather information on current lens parameters, wearing schedule, replacement rate, and care regimen.

Choosing a Lens

Contact lenses come in a variety of modalities. Choose a lens that will 1) best correct the patient's refractive error, 2) provide comfort for all-day wear, and 3) best fit into the patient's lifestyle needs. Consider whether a soft or rigid lens would be the best choice, and choose the best material for the patient's needs (Tables 21-6 and 21-7).

Fitting a Soft Lens

The majority of soft lens fittings will fall within the typical stock lenses provided by SCL manufacturers. Most standard parameters will work on normal-sized corneas between 11.3 to 12.3 mm in diameter, keratometry values of 41.00 D to 47.00 D, and refractive errors from +6.00 D to -12.00 D. Any parameters outside these ranges will most likely require a custom soft lens.

Basic Guidelines for Soft Spherical Lens Fitting

▶ *Select diameter.* Lens diameter should be at least 2 mm larger than the HVID, enough to cover the corneal and limbal surfaces completely. Larger diameters offer more stability; smaller diameters lead to limbal irritation.

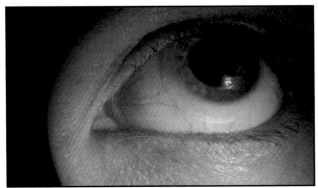

Figure 21-22. A flat soft contact lens fit, decentering in upgaze.

▶ *Select base curve.* Choose the flattest base curve available first. For a custom base curve, subtract 4 D from the flat-K value to determine a starting base curve selection. Follow the manufacturer's guidelines for lens fittings with both standard and custom lens designs.

▶ *Select power.*
  • Convert spectacle prescription to minus cylinder
  • Determine spherical equivalent
  • For prescriptions with greater than 1.00 D of cylinder power, a toric lens will most likely be needed
  • For prescriptions ±4.00 D, you will need to take vertex distance into account (see Chapter 19)
  • Place calculated lens on the eye and perform overrefractometry for best prescription

▶ *Evaluate fit.* Put the lens on the patient. The contact should be allowed to settle on the eye long enough for the lens to equilibrate and the initial reflex tearing to subside (~5 minutes). Toric lenses should be given time to rotate into position (~10 minutes). The lens should drape over the eye with a 3-point touch—the center of the lens on the cornea and opposite edges resting on the sclera. The lens should center on the eye with at least 1 mm overlap onto the conjunctiva. Lens should move 0.5 to 1.5 mm in upgaze without edge fluting. A steep lens will have minimal/no movement. A flat lens will decenter in upgaze and/or ripple at the edge (Figure 21-22). A steep lens will feel more comfortable than a flat lens.

If movement is less than 0.5 mm, gently place the finger on the lower eyelid and push the lens upward. There should be no resistance and the lens should move. If not, the lens is too tight and you should choose a lens with a flatter base curve. If there is too much movement, the lens is too loose, and you will need to choose a lens with a steeper base curve.

▶ *Evaluate vision.* Perform overrefractometry with loose spherical lenses for best vision. If spheres do not correct vision completely, spherocylindrical overrefractometry may be needed. To determine spherocylindrical starting point, autorefract or perform retinoscopy over the lens. Adjust the contact lens power or move to a toric lens as needed.

Vision should remain stable with blinking. If vision *blurs* after a blink, the lens could be too loose. Manual keratometry over a loose lens will show blurry mires after a blink. If vision *clears* after a blink then blurs again, the lens could be too steep. This happens because blinking pushes the optical zone of the contact down onto the cornea, but the lens pops back off the cornea once again right after the blink. Manual keratometry over the lens will show mires that are clear right after a blink but then blur. A well-fit lens will show no change in keratometry mires or vision before or after blinking.

▶ *Adjust fit.* For a lens that is too flat, the base curvature could be steepened or the diameter of the lens increased. This will increase the vault of the lens on the eye and tighten the fit. For a lens that is too steep, the base curvature could be flattened or the diameter of the lens decreased. This will decrease the vault of the lens on the eye and loosen the fit.

Fitting a Soft Toric Lens

A soft lens will "mask" small amounts of corneal cylinder because of the lens's rigidity and thickness, but if the patient's refractive astigmatism is greater than or equal to 0.75 D to 1.00 D, then a toric soft lens will be indicated. (Remember, the lacrimal lens power in a soft lens is zero due to the draping effect of the lens.)

Soft toric lenses are marked to show lens positioning on the eye and the amount of lens rotation (Figure 21-23). A soft toric lens needs to be stabilized on the eye to maintain proper axis orientation. They work best with against-the-rule corneal astigmatism (ie, within 30° of horizontal). Tight lids and oblique astigmatism can lead to lens instability and rotation. Stabilization methods of soft toric lenses are shown in Sidebar 21-9.

When fitting a soft toric lens, follow the basic soft lens fitting guide above, with the following differences:

▶ *Select power.*
  • Convert the patient's refraction into minus cylinder form
  • For prescriptions ±4.00 D, you must take vertex distance into account (see Chapter 19)
  • Choose the lowest cylinder power option closest to the patient's prescription

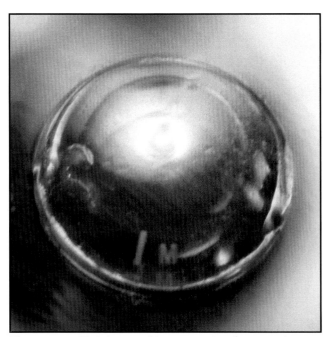

Figure 21-23. Toric lens marking on a toric soft contact lens.

- Place selected lens on the eye and perform over-refractometry with loose spherical lenses for best vision
- If spheres do not correct vision completely, spherocylindrical overrefractometry may be needed

▶ *Evaluate and adjust fit.* Allow lens to stabilize on the eye for a minimum of 10 minutes. Lens markings vary but are usually intended to be at the 6 and 12 o'clock or 9 and 3 o'clock positions on the eye. (Check for specifics with the manufacturer or in *Tyler's Quarterly* for details on lens marks.)

A well-fit lens will not rotate. If the lens is rotated, the cylindrical power of the lens will be moved off-axis and the patient's vision will be blurred. To check lens rotation, evaluate the position of the toric lens marking. Generally, for every "clock minute" the lens is skewed, there are 6° of axis rotation. Calculating rotation can be done by estimation, using an axis calculator wheel, by rotating a reticle mounted on the slit lamp, or by adjusting the slit lamp beam to the corresponding axis alignment (Sidebar 21-10). Once the degree of rotation is determined, the power of the lens can be adjusted by using the "left/add, right/subtract" (LARS) principle (Sidebar 21-11) or by consulting the manufacturer or online toric lens calculators. The LARS principle repositions the lens so that its axis is better aligned with the refractive axis. *Keep in mind that once a lens power is recalculated for lens rotation, the lens will continue to rotate in the same position as before.*

Fitting a Rigid Lens

Rigid lenses are custom made for each individual patient. Lenses can be fit *empirically* or *diagnostically*.

To fit a lens empirically, a lens is ordered based on the patient's ocular data. The lens is then placed on the patient's eye, overrefractometry performed, fit evaluated, and the lens is dispensed if satisfactory. If the fit and/or vision is not acceptable, the necessary changes are calculated, and a new lens is ordered.

To fit a lens diagnostically, a fitting set of trial lenses is used, and the optimal fit is achieved by trying the lenses on the patient. In this initial step, vision is not important; the goal is to find the lens that physically fits the best. Once the fit is satisfactory, overrefractometry is performed to obtain the patient's prescription, and the lenses are ordered with the specific parameters for that patient. The trial lenses must be cleaned and disinfected following every use and stored dry.

When fitting rigid lenses, the lacrimal lens layer between the contact lens and the eye neutralizes up to 2.5 D of corneal astigmatism. All that remains is the spherical component of the refraction. Rigid lenses fit best in "with-the-rule" astigmatism (steep axis within 30° of vertical) as all rigid lenses gravitate to the steeper corneal

---

SIDEBAR 21-10
CALCULATING SOFT TORIC LENS ROTATION

▶ Estimation—A gross estimation of rotation can be calculated by visualizing clock hours on the cornea. For every "clock minute" the lens is skewed, there is approximately 6° of axis rotation. If the lens is skewed "clockwise," that is considered "left," so additional degrees are added (see LARS principle, Sidebar 21-11). If the lens is skewed "counterclockwise," that is considered "right," so additional degrees are subtracted.

▶ Axis wheel calculator—This is a hand-held protractor that can be used at the slit lamp for measuring axis rotation.

▶ Slit lamp reticle—This is an attachment reticle that replaces one of the oculars of the slit lamp. It slides into the ocular and has a degree alignment for measuring axis rotation.

▶ Slit lamp beam alignment—Some slit lamps have a protractor with axis degree markings at the base of the illumination housing. By rotating the housing unit, the slit lamp beam can be adjusted along the protractor from a vertical to a horizontal beam. The beam can be aligned with the rotation of the soft toric lens, and the degree of misalignment calculated.

SIDEBAR 21-11
LARS PRINCIPLE (LEFT ADD, RIGHT SUBTRACT; ALSO KNOWN AS THE CLOCKWISE/COUNTERCLOCKWISE RULE)

▶ If a soft toric lens mark at 6 o'clock is rotated to the practitioner's left (or clockwise), the number of degrees of rotation is *added* to the patient's refractive axis to determine new lens axis.

Example 1
CL axis: 90°
Refractive axis: 90°
Lens rotation: 10° to the left (or clockwise)
New CL axis: 100°

▶ If a soft toric lens mark at 6 o'clock is rotated to the practitioner's right (or counterclockwise), the number of degrees of rotation is *subtracted* from the patient's refractive axis to determine new lens axis.

Example 2
CL axis: 100°
Refractive axis: 100°
Lens rotation: 5° to the right (or counterclockwise)
New CL axis: 95°

▶ For lens rotations greater than 20°, a different lens design/stabilization method will be required.

▶ For spherocylindrical overrefractions and a rotated lens, use a toric lens calculator or consult with the lens manufacturer for the new power. Many manufacturers' websites and optical apps have toric lens or cross cylinder calculation programs to compute these complex overrefractions. These apps can also be used to determine best initial lens selection using data from the patient's refractive error.

---

meridian, thus the up and down movement with a blink. High "against-the-rule" astigmatism (steep axis within 30° of horizontal) will cause the lens to rock from side to side.

Rigid lenses are generally fit using a *corneal alignment fitting philosophy*[3,4] or *lid attachment fit*. This involves fitting a larger, flatter lens that tucks under the upper eyelid. However, when the palpebral fissure is wider or the upper lid margin does not properly touch the superior cornea, an *apical clearance fit* may be necessary. This utilizes a smaller, steeper lens that fits intrapalpebrally (ie, between the lids without resting on either upper or lower).

There are many fitting nomograms available for fitting RGPCLs. A fitting nomogram is a formula or chart in which the initial lens parameters can be chosen using available patient data. Additional fitting resources include the manufacturer's guide as well as online resources.

Basic Guidelines for Fitting Rigid Spherical Lenses (Corneal Alignment)

▶ *Choose initial diagnostic lens* according to the nomogram (Table 21-8). Clean and place selected lens on the eye.

▶ *Evaluate fit.* Evaluate the *fluorescein pattern* under the lens. When the tear film is stained with NaFl, the lacrimal lens layer becomes visible under the lens.

Any areas of increased vaulting or bearing of the lens on the cornea can be seen.

Evaluate the pattern following a blink. Optimal lens alignment produces an even, smooth NaFl pattern from edge to edge. When a lens is too steep, a pooling of NaFl (where the lens vaults the cornea) will be visible. When a lens is too flat, areas of nonfluorescence or lack of NaFl (where the lens contacts the cornea) will be seen.

▶ *Flat fit.* A flat-fitting lens will rest on the central corneal cap. This will produce a dark center with a brighter NaFl pattern in the periphery. The

TABLE 21-8
CORNEAL ALIGNMENT FITTING NOMOGRAM[5]

Keratometric Corneal Cylinder	Example: 9.4 Diameter Base Curve
0.0 to 0.75 D	0.50 D flatter than flat-K
1.00 D to 1.25 D	0.25 D flatter than flat-K
1.50 D to 1.75 D	On flat-K
2.00 D to 2.25 D	0.25 D steeper than flat-K
> 2.50 D	Bitoric lens design

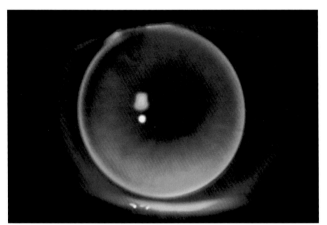

Figure 21-24. A flat/loose-fitting rigid gas-permeable lens. Notice the dark center with excessive NaFl in the periphery.

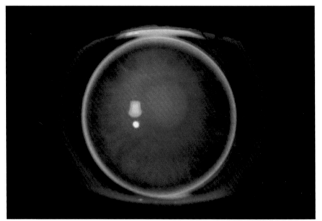

Figure 21-25. A steep/tight-fitting rigid gas-permeable lens. Note excessive NaFl in the center.

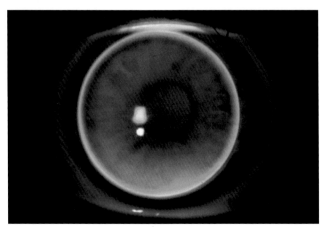

Figure 21-26. An acceptable rigid gas-permeable fit.

peripheral curve band will show an excessive amount of NaFl (Figure 21-24). A loose lens will often decenter, move excessively with a blink, and the inferior edge may lift off the cornea after blinking. There can be central corneal staining as well as peripheral conjunctival staining caused by the lens rubbing and decentering.

▶ *Steep fit.* A steep-fitting lens will result in excessive NaFl over the corneal cap. There can be mid-peripheral touch on the cornea and a thin peripheral edge band because the lens fits tight in the periphery (Figure 21-25). Steep lens fits can produce bubbles under the lens with resultant dimple veiling (indentations in the cornea caused by the bubbles). Steeper lenses will not translate (or move) well with blinking. There can be staining in the corneal mid-periphery or at 3 and 9 o'clock.

▶ *Astigmatic fit.* Spherical lenses that are fit on a moderate-high toric cornea can exhibit a dumbbell-shaped band on NaFl evaluation. With-the-rule astigmatism will produce excessive NaFl in the vertical meridian with touch at the flatter 3 and 9 o'clock positions. Against-the-rule astigmatism will produce excessive NaFl in the horizontal meridian with touch at the 12 and 6 o'clock positions.

▶ *Optimal fit.* The optimal lens will center under the upper lid and will translate with eye movements. There will be an even NaFl pattern from edge to edge with an even peripheral curve band (Figure 21-26). There should be no corneal or conjunctival staining present.

▶ *Adjust lens fit.* When adjusting the lens fit, it is important to make changes that will be significant enough to be seen on evaluation (Sidebar 21-12).

▶ *Select power.* Determine power once best diagnostic lens fit is achieved.

- Perform overrefractometry with loose spherical lenses for best vision.

- If spheres do not correct vision completely, spherocylindrical overrefractometry may be needed. If residual astigmatism is less than 1.00 D, the spherical equivalent of spherocylindrical overrefractometry can be used. If greater than 1.00 D, the patient may have residual blurred vision and a toric/bitoric lens will be necessary.

- For overrefractions greater than ±4.00 D, you will need to take vertex distance into account before adding the overrefraction amount to the lens power.

► *Determine peripheral curves.* Most manufacturers have standard curves they apply to their lenses. On average, the secondary curve is approximately 1.0 D flatter than the base curve and the peripheral curve is 1.5 D to 2.5 D flatter than the base curve. The widths of the curves are standard but can be adjusted if wider/narrower peripheral curves are desired for improved lens stability.

► Determine final lens parameters for ordering (Sidebar 21-13).

Fitting a Rigid Toric Lens

For corneal astigmatism greater than 2.50 D or for residual astigmatism, a toric rigid lens will be indicated. The stabilization methods for rigid lenses are somewhat different from soft toric lenses (Sidebar 21-14).

Fitting Designs

A *bitoric* rigid lens is the most common toric lens design for the correction of moderate to high astigmatism (>2.5 D). It applies a toric correction to both the front and back surfaces of the lens, hence correcting not only corneal but also any residual astigmatism. Bitoric lens designs can be calculated by using the *Mandell-Moore Bitoric Lens Guide*, consulting GPLI's online calculators, or fit empirically by collaborating with your lab consultant.

Front surface toric designs apply the toric correction to the front surface of the lens, leaving the back surface spherical. It is mainly used for lenticular or residual astigmatism when the corneal surface is spherical.

Back surface toric designs apply the toric correction to the back surface of the lens; the front surface is spherical. It is best used when the residual astigmatism is greater than the corneal astigmatism by approximately 40%.[5] It is not a common fitting method.

Presbyopic Lenses

Presbyopia is the loss of accommodation at near (see Chapters 3 and 4).

There are many options to provide vision at various distances. Multifocal correction is now available in low to high refractive error corrections, with multiple ADD selections and even toric multifocal lenses.

SIDEBAR 21-14
STABILIZATION METHODS FOR RIGID TORIC CONTACT LENSES

▶ Prism ballast—A prism ballast lens is a low-powered prism (usually 1.5 D base-down) added to the lens mass, increasing the weight of the lens inferiorly to prevent rotation.

▶ Truncation—The inferior segment of the lens is removed. This can be combined with other stabilization methods including prism ballast. The lens is aligned to rest on the lower eyelid, which provides rotational stability. A normally positioned lower eyelid is critical for a truncated lens to work.

▶ Corneal toricity—Corneal toricity uses the front surface corneal curvature to align with the back surface contact lens curves to maintain alignment.

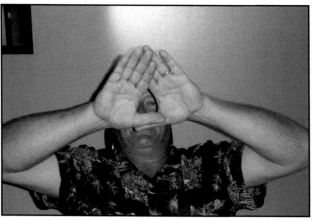

Figure 21-27. Checking for dominant eye.

SIDEBAR 21-15
DO IT BETTER: FITTING PRESBYOPIC CORRECTIONS

▶ Push plus power during refractometry.

▶ Start with lowest ADD as suggested by manufacturer's fitting guide.

▶ Allow the trials lenses to settle for a minimum of 10 minutes.

▶ Do not use the reading card. Instead give the patient typical reading material (eg, magazines, newspaper, computer, cell phone) to test the vision.

▶ Overrefract in 0.25 D steps. Even the smallest change can make a significant improvement in multifocal designs.

▶ Encourage binocular vision. With presbyopic designs, the eyes are meant to work together in tandem. Instruct the patient not to compare the vision between the eyes.

▶ Do not make too many changes at once. Allow the patient to take the lenses home to try in his/her natural environment.

The key for patient selection is motivation. Discuss the fitting process for the lenses (including the potential for extra chair time during the fitting), the lens options available, and reasonable expectations. Explain that while presbyopic lenses will be good for most visual activities, they will not be perfect for every activity. Discuss the patient's activities and visual needs.

Sometimes presbyopic contact lens correction requires that a specific lens be worn on the patient's dominant eye. To check for *eye dominance*, have the individual focus on the eye chart at distance and extend the arms to create a small "frame" between the hands. Have the patient bring the hands toward the eye while still gazing at the eye chart (Figure 21-27). The patient will naturally bring the hands to the dominant eye.

Review medical history, medications, and ocular history carefully. Older individuals may have additional medical and/or ocular complications that could affect contact lens wear. Set realistic expectations for patients with cataracts or other visual limitations.

Evaluate pupil size. The size of the pupil and the location of the visual axis can be key in obtaining optimal vision correction with multifocal lenses. Patients with smaller pupils may report blurred distance vision in center-near designs, while a large pupil can cause halos and glare with night vision activities.

Evaluate lid alignment. In some designs, such as translating bifocals, the position of the lids to the cornea is crucial to proper lens alignment. Patients with a high degree of superior or inferior scleral show may not be good candidates for certain lens types.

Presbyopic correction is available in multiple forms that can vary between soft and rigid contact lens designs. Follow the manufacturer's fitting guide for the specific lens chosen to achieve best results. Also, see the pearls in Sidebar 21-15.

Presbyopic Lens Options and Designs
Distance/Reading Glasses
The simplest option for patients needing presbyopic correction at near is to use reading glasses over their contact lenses. This option requires no change to their current lens modality and maintains binocular vision at distance and near without compromise. For those patients who do not mind depending on glasses for close work, it is a successful solution.

Monovision
Monovision allows the patient to maintain the current lens modality. The dominant eye remains corrected

for distance vision, while the nondominant eye is corrected for reading. It is a visual compromise, resulting in some loss of stereopsis. To evaluate a patient for monovision tolerance, perform the *swinging plus test*. Take a +1.50 D trial lens and hold it up to the nondominant eye. If the patient can tolerate the lens at both distance and near, he/she will most likely be a successful monovision candidate. If there is disorientation, nausea, or blurring, choose a different presbyopic correction modality.

Monovision is most successful with early presbyopes, but as presbyopia increases and the disparity in correction between the two eyes increases, later presbyopes can have problems adjusting. One solution is to provide spectacle correction over the monovision to provide binocular vision when desired for extended near or distance related tasks (eg, driving at night). While monovision was the presbyopic modality of choice in the past, it has been largely replaced by multifocal lenses.

Multifocal

Multifocal lens options (both SCL and RGP) have improved to become the standard in presbyopic lens management. The benefits of multifocal lens designs include maintaining binocular vision and the correction of intermediate vision often lost in monovision technique.

▶ Soft: The majority of multifocal SCLs are aspheric with either a center-near or center-distance configuration. The center of the lens is either a spherical distance or spherical near zone with an aspheric or progressive transition of power from the center of the lens to the periphery. The patient is unaware of these transitions as the eye naturally focuses at the appropriate distance.

▶ Rigid

- Translating: *Translating* designs, also called *alternating*, rely on the movement, or translation, of the rigid lens as the patient looks down to read. Several physiological changes happen while reading. There is miosis of the pupil, accommodation of the natural crystalline lens (which may be limited or absent in the presbyopic patient), and convergence (moving inward) of the eyes. Translating lenses can be segmented much like bifocal spectacles, and can provide sharp vision if properly fit. While viewing distance, the patient looks through the top or distance portion of the lens. For reading, the eyes converge and the lens translates upward, positioning the bottom, or reading segment, in front of the pupil. The reading segment can vary in size, design, and position. The lens must be stabilized by using prism ballasting or lens truncation in order to prevent rotation.

- Aspheric: An *aspheric* rigid lens design is a progressive lens in which there is an increase in plus power from the center of the lens to the periphery.

Because rigid lenses translate upward in downgaze, rigid multifocals tend to be more successful than their soft lens counterparts. Lens power can be placed on the back surface of an aspheric lens, on the front surface, or both if additional presbyopic correction is needed. However, using back surface aspherics can change the fitting characteristics of the lens, so follow manufacturer's suggesting fitting guidelines.

▶ Modified monovision: *Modified monovision* can be a creative solution to correcting presbyopia. There may be times when standard presbyopic fitting protocols are unsuccessful, or the patient wants better vision at a specific distance and is willing to compromise at others. Modified monovision may involve using a multifocal lens in both eyes, but providing the better distance correction in the dominant eye and the better near correction in the nondominant eye. It can also involve using a standard lens in the dominant eye for distance and a multifocal lens for reading in the nondominant eye (or vice versa), depending on the patient's visual requirements.

Identifying Complications of Contact Lens Wear

Lens Complications

The contact lens surfaces and edges need to be inspected on every visit. Some common contact lens complications include:

▶ Chips/scratches/tears: Chips can occur on the edges of both soft and rigid lenses. Small surface cracks in an SCL are often caused by pinching a dry lens from the eye or rough handling. Thin lenses and soft lenses with a high water content can tear more easily. The patient may be asymptomatic or have a foreign body sensation if the rough areas irritate the cornea. A lens with any defect should be replaced.

Usually if rigid lenses tear, they crack into multiple pieces. Rigid lenses can also develop scratches on the surface caused by mishandling or scraping the lens on the bottom of the case or other surface. Polishing the lens surface can help with minor scratches, but most of the time the lenses should be replaced. Scratches and irregularities on a rigid lens surface are opportunities for deposits to develop, may harbor bacteria, and affect surface wetting.

▶ Crazing: *Crazing* is diffuse, interconnecting surface cracks on an RGPCL that cause a haze. It can occur in the material during the manufacturing process (especially if excessive heat was used). A crazed lens should be replaced.

▶ Deposits: Both rigid and soft lenses can develop deposits. The composition of the deposits can vary

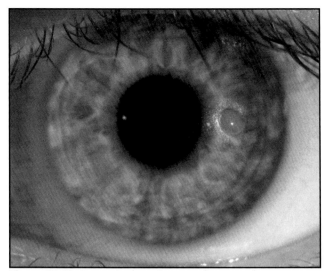

Figure 21-28. A protein deposit on a soft contact lens.

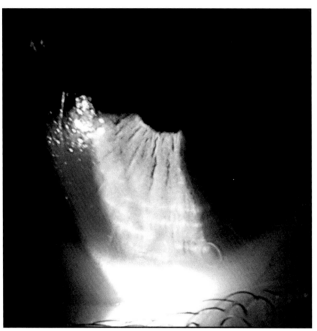

Figure 21-29. Poor surface wetting of a soft contact lens.

by the material of the lens and the tear quality of the patient. Contact lens deposits (Figure 21-28) can be made up of tear proteins, lipids, mucins, calcium, makeup, fungi, or residue from hand cleansers with additives (eg, oils, lanolin, lotions).

Patients with blepharitis and meibomian gland dysfunction tend to have more lipid deposits. Hydrogel materials, especially high water content lenses, tend to deposit more proteins, while silicone hydrogel materials tend to deposit more lipids and mucins. Hard calcium deposits can be seen on rigid lenses of advanced age.

Deposits can be addressed by managing underlying contributory ocular conditions, changing lens material, replacing the lens more often, and/or by adjusting cleaning/disinfecting methods. Adjustments in cleaning include rubbing the lens, adding a daily cleaner, and/or adding an enzymatic cleaner. For rigid lenses, adding a heavy-duty solvent such as Menicon Progent (Menicon Products), can help remove heavy deposits and proteins.

▶ Warpage: Contact lens warpage can cause distorted vision, poor fit of the lens, or both. Warping of rigid lenses can be seen under the radiuscope and lensometer, where the mires will be unfocused or multiple. Warped soft lenses do not fit as expected, often are too loose or have irregular edges. Warped lenses should be replaced.

▶ Hazing/poor wetting: Wetting problems are more common in hydrophobic rigid lenses, but can also occur in soft lenses, especially as the lens surface dynamic changes through the course of the day. Poor wetting can be a function of tear film quality, lens surface quality, and wetting angle of the lens (Figure 21-29). A clean, hydrated lens wets better. Soaking

rigid lenses in a disinfecting/wetting solution overnight will aid in lens wetting. Using approved contact lens rewetting agents can also be beneficial. In chronic cases, changing lens solutions or lens materials can be helpful.

There is a new surface treatment available for SCLs and RGPCLs. Tangible Hydra-PEG (Tangible Sciences LLC) is a high-water, hydrophilic, permanent surface coating applied to the contact, increasing wettability.[6] The purpose of the coating is to decrease lens dryness, friction, clouding, and deposits.[6] Care must be taken with handling and cleaning of the Hydra-PEG surface, so consult manufacturer's guidelines.

▶ Lens discolorations: SCLs can become discolored by certain preservatives such as sorbic acid, which can cause yellowing. Medications and solutions not approved for SCLs use can also lead to lens discoloration. Some medications, such as laxatives, urinary tract infection treatments, tetracycline, and rifampin can cause lens discoloration due to systemic excretion into the tears.[7]

Solution Reactions

Solution reactions can present with a multitude of problems from mild, such as dryness and decreased lens tolerance, to more severe reactions with diffuse punctate epithelial keratopathy (tiny erosions), redness, GPC, and contact lens-induced superior limbic keratoconjunctivitis (SLK).

Delayed hypersensitivity to solutions is common and can occur months after starting a new care system.

Further investigation into the patient's care products is essential as patients may frequently change their disinfection solutions, especially when using an "all-in-one" system. Switching the patient to a hydrogen peroxide system (for both rigid and soft lenses) or switching to a daily disposable soft lens can help eliminate solution sensitivities.

Ocular Complications

Ocular complications of contact lens wear can be induced from a poor fitting contact lens, surface deposits, an irregular contact lens surface, a reaction to solutions, poor lens care and hygiene, and contact lens overwear. The patient should be evaluated on every follow-up visit for possible lens-related complications. Any ocular complication associated with contact lens wear should be addressed and managed by the prescribing eye care provider.

Lids and Lashes

▶ Giant papillary conjunctivitis (GPC) is a surface allergic reaction of the superior palpebral conjunctiva to contact lens deposits. It is more common in soft lens wearers who form lens deposits. GPC produces large, sometimes scarred, cobblestone papillae on the lid surface, making contact lenses uncomfortable and unstable (see Figure 21-20). The papillae also can cause decentration of the lens along with decreased wearing time and increased mucous discharge. The upper lid must be everted to be evaluated.

Conjunctiva

▶ Hyperemia: An eye wearing a well-fitting contact lens should be white and quiet. Hyperemia (redness) is usually a sign of an underlying condition. Hyperemia can be present with dryness, solution irritation, lens tightness, poorly fitting lens (causing limbal irritation), *contact lens-associated red eye* (CLARE, discussed momentarily), *contact lens overwear syndrome* (OWS), and neovascularization.

▶ CLARE: See above. This problem is an inflammatory reaction that occurs after overnight SCL wear. Patients present with diffuse conjunctival hyperemia (redness in no particular pattern), photophobia, and discomfort. Peripheral subepithelial infiltrates of the cornea can also be present in some cases. The underlying causes, though varied, can include hypoxia (lack of oxygen) of the corneal tissue and toxic reaction to certain microbial contaminants (specifically gram-negative bacteria) on the surface of the lens. Lens wear should be discontinued until symptoms resolve. The patient should be educated on the risks of overnight wear, instructed in proper wear and disinfection of the lenses, and should not sleep in lenses that are not approved for extended wear.

▶ Lens indentation: Indentation of the conjunctival surface by an SCL is visible at the slit lamp with diffuse illumination using NaFl dye and the cobalt blue filter. This finding can indicate a tight-fitting lens. It can also occur with a silicone hydrogel material worn overnight. It may not be visible with the lens on the eye. Lens fit and material should be reevaluated.

▶ Limbal epithelial hypertrophy (LEH): Limbal changes are often seen due to mechanical irritation of a lens. LEH results in a furrowed appearance of the peripheral limbus, with an associated ring-like pooling of fluorescein in the furrows. It can be due to a thick soft lens material with poor alignment to the cornea and/or poor movement of a thick lens. LEH can be a precursor to corneal neovascularization. Lens fit, material, and wearing time should be reevaluated.

Cornea

▶ Mechanical rubbing of the limbus by a contact lens can lead to ocular irritation, redness, decreased epithelial cell health, and neovascularization.

▶ Lens imprinting: Corneal lens imprinting is most often seen with rigid corneal lenses, but can also be caused by the optic zone transition of a thick SCL. When the lens is removed, a circular lens imprint will still be visible on the cornea while viewing with the blue cobalt filter. Lens imprinting with rigid lenses can be caused by the lens binding to the cornea and/or a steep lens, and refitting is indicated.

▶ 3-and-9 staining: *3-and-9 staining* is a complication seen with rigid corneal contact lenses. Using diffuse illumination with NaFl and the blue filter, localized staining patterns and hyperemia at the 3 and 9 o'clock hours are visible on the conjunctiva and cornea. It is caused by mechanical irritation of the lens. As the irritation advances, a *vascularized limbal keratitis* (VLK) can develop. This additionally results in scarring and a nodular-like appearance of the corneal tissue at 3 and 9 o'clock. Causes include a rigid lens with poor peripheral corneal alignment, dry eye, incomplete blinking, and either a thick or thin lens edge. Treatment includes reevaluating the rigid lens fit, addressing any underlying dry eye conditions, and/or refitting the patient with a soft lens.

▶ Dimple veiling: *Dimple veiling* refers to circular indentations on the cornea where NaFl pools when a rigid contact lens is removed. This is not true corneal epithelial staining, but rather an imprint left by tiny trapped air bubbles caught in the lacrimal lens layer between the cornea and lens, usually due to a steep-fitting rigid lens. The bubbles can be seen with the lens in place, and the dimple veil staining when the lens is removed.

▶ Neovascularization: The cornea normally is an optically clear tissue with no blood vessels. *Corneal neovascularization* is the in-growth of blood vessels into the cornea from the peripheral limbus. Neovascularization can be found superficially at the limbus in mild cases, and deeper into the stromal tissues with more advanced cases. In the worst case scenario, contact lens use must be discontinued.

Neovascularization is an inflammatory response either to a lack of oxygen to the cornea (*hypoxia*) or as a result of limbal epithelial trauma from contact lens wear. Overwear and extended wear use of contact lenses, low-Dk lenses, high-powered lenses with thick centers and peripheral edges, and poorly fit lenses can all contribute to neovascularization. This problem should be monitored and measured as to the extent of vessel growth into the cornea.

▶ Lens abrasion/foreign body tracks: Scratches to the cornea can be induced by a rigid contact lens, a tear in a soft lens, or from a foreign body trapped between a lens and the ocular surface. A foreign body in the superior palpebral conjunctiva can also cause linear corneal tracks. These tracks appear as striate epithelial abrasions that stain with NaFl. Oftentimes the foreign body is no longer in the eye, but the lens should be removed and the corneal tissue and palpebral conjunctiva inspected. A soft lens can act as a bandage over a corneal foreign body reducing patient symptoms, and the patient may postpone needed treatment.

▶ Arcuate corneal staining: Staining of the peripheral corneal epithelium in a localized, arcuate shape (after lens removal) is termed a *superior epithelial arcuate lesion* (SEAL) if located superiorly, and *smile* staining if located inferiorly. These arcuate breaks in the epithelial surface can be caused by mechanical irritation of a contact lens, especially in dry conditions, and with incomplete blinking. It can also be seen with a poor lens-to-cornea relationship, as with a stiff soft lens material like silicone hydrogel. Refitting the patient with a different lens material, ensuring the best fit, and addressing dry eye symptoms are recommended.

▶ Hypoxia: *Hypoxia* is a sign that the cornea is not receiving enough oxygen through the lens material, either from a low-Dk lens or extended wear overnight use. (*The minimum Dk requirement for an overnight lens material is between 87 to 125 Dk/t.*[3]) Hypoxia can present with neovascularization of the cornea, corneal edema or swelling of the stromal tissues (inducing a haze or striae), or as corneal microcysts. *Microcysts* appear as tiny, round, clear cysts in the epithelium. These cysts can persist for months after a hypoxic event, often appearing worse before resolving.

▶ Infiltrates/ulcers: The presence of *infiltrates* or *ulcers* in the cornea with contact lens wear is a serious

complication that needs immediate attention. The patient often presents with severe pain, redness, tearing, and photophobia. On examination, there is an ulcerative corneal lesion with an epithelial defect and stromal haze. It is important that treatment is immediate and aggressive. If the patient is later able to return to contact lens wear, a carefully prescribed course of limited wearing time, proper lens wear and care, and close follow-up are necessary.

The severity of the condition can vary depending whether the lesions are sterile (noninfectious) or microbial (infectious). An infiltrate is the collection of white blood cells in the corneal tissue due to inflammation. Infiltrates located peripherally are usually sterile, while more centrally located infiltrates tend to be infectious. An ulcer involves the breakdown of corneal tissue causing an epithelial defect with involvement into the stroma. While ulcers can be inflammatory, they are often infectious due to bacterial, viral, or fungal microorganisms.

• Sterile corneal lesions such as a *contact lens peripheral ulcer* (CLPU) and *infiltrative keratitis* (IK) are an inflammatory, hypersensitivity response to hypoxia or contact lens solutions. A sterile lesion may also form in response to bacterial toxins (specifically gram-positive bacteria) generated from a dirty contact lens, ocular surface disease, poor hygiene, etc.[3] (In this case, the inflammatory response is to the toxins and is not an "infection" per se.) They produce subepithelial, whitish lesions that generally occur in the peripheral cornea. The epithelium is usually intact. The patient's symptoms can vary from nonsymptomatic to symptoms of redness, foreign body sensation, photophobia, and tearing. Management includes discontinuation of lens wear and proper treatment by the eye care provider. The underlying cause of the inflammation should be addressed, perhaps by changing solutions and/or reinstructing the patient in proper lens wear and care.

• Microbial (infectious) ulcers are one of the most serious complications of contact lens wear, and can be sight-threatening. Microorganisms most commonly associated with contact lens-related microbial keratitis include bacteria (eg, *Pseudomonas aeruginosa, Serratia marcescens*), parasites (eg, *Acanthamoeba*), and fungi (eg, *Fusarium*).[8] (See Chapter 23 for more on microbiology.) Causes include improper disinfection techniques, poor hygiene, contaminated contact lens cases and/or solutions, tap water or well water use, homemade saline use, swimming/bathing in lenses, and overnight contact lens wear.

PATIENT SERVICES

Dispensing Contact Lenses

When dispensing contact lenses, it is important to include thorough instruction in application and removal techniques (Sidebar 21-16); a detailed explanation of lens cleaning and disinfection, including recommended solutions for the patient's lens type; a typical wearing schedule; and a list of important guidelines are vital to successful contact lens wear. For first-time wearers, this training often sets the groundwork of a lifetime of good contact lens habits and hygiene. Provide both verbal and written instruction (Sidebar 21-17) and have the patient repeat important information and cleaning techniques back to you. Reinforcement during follow-up visits is key to long-term contact lens success.

Insertion

There are several techniques to apply a lens to the eye. The patient will often find the best technique for him/her through trial and error. Insertion is the same for both SCLs and standard RGPCLs (Sidebar 21-18).

Application and removal for specialty lenses, especially scleral rigid lenses, is vastly different. Consult the manufacturer for specific cleaning and handling of these types of lenses. A good resource on scleral lens handling, application, and removal can be found at specific manufacturers' websites: www.gpli.info and/or www.scleral-lens.org.

Two-Handed Lid Hold Technique

In this approach, the nondominant hand holds the upper eyelid by the lashes and the dominant hand pulls down the lower lid with the third or fourth finger, and with the index or middle finger, applies the contact lens to the cornea (Figure 21-30).

One-Handed Lid Hold Technique

This technique uses one hand to hold both the upper and lower eyelids. Using a one-handed technique may be easier for patients with poor coordination.
1. The thumb and index finger of the nondominant hand holds the eyelids open while the lens is applied with the dominant hand.
2. Make sure the patient is holding the lids against the upper and lower orbital bones, and not applying pressure to the globe itself.

Insertion by the Fitter

Steps for inserting a lens on a patient:
1. Have the patient sit upright and look at the eye chart (or some other fixation point) at the end of the room. It is important for him/her to keep both eyes open.
2. Stand to the side of the patient and use a two-handed approach, one hand holding the upper lid and the other holding the lens and the bottom lid.
3. Apply the lens to the cornea.
4. If you're having difficulty inserting a soft lens, try having the patient look up or down and apply the lens to the conjunctiva. The lens will usually center itself or can be slid into place.

Removal

The removal of soft and standard rigid contact lenses is not the same. The flexibility of a soft lens allows it to be pinched or rolled out of the eye. A rigid lens uses the tension of the eyelids for expression from the eye.

SIDEBAR 21-17
PATIENT GUIDELINES FOR SUCCESSFUL CONTACT LENS WEAR

► Thoroughly clean hands using soap without oils, lotions, or perfumes prior to handling the contact lenses. Avoid products with aloe, lanolin, or coconut oils, which can put a film on the lenses. Dry hands completely before handling lenses.

► A soft lens can fold and get stuck to itself during insertion. Never try to pull a soft lens apart, but rather rub it gently with sterile contact lens solution to release the lens.

► A soft lens can flip inside out. A simple test, called the *taco test*, is to place the lens on the tip of the finger or in a fold in the palm of the hand. Gently flex the lens. If the edges want to roll in (like a taco), it is correct. If the edges want to roll out and flip, the lens is inside out. It may be difficult to tell, especially with thinner lenses. A lens that is inside out will fit loosely on the eye and will oftentimes be felt. Vision may also fluctuate or blur. If in doubt, remove, rinse with appropriate solution, flip, and reinsert the lens.

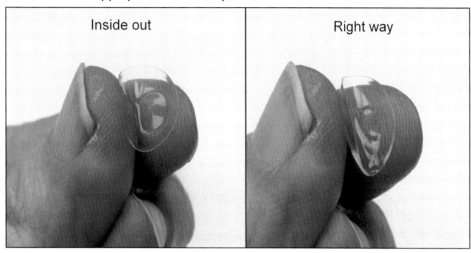

► Gently "swirl" a soft lens on the eye to remove trapped debris if a foreign body sensation is felt after insertion. If no improvement, remove the lens, rinse with appropriate solution, and reinsert. For a rigid lens, remove the lens, rinse with appropriate solution, and reapply.

► A quick way to ensure the lens is in place and on the cornea is to check vision. Cover the opposite eye, and if the vision is clear, the lens is on the eye and centered. If not, check for dislocation on the eye or on the work surface.

► Wet the eye with a lubricating drop prior to contact lens removal to avoid difficulty in removing the lens and to prevent minor surface cracks to a dry lens.

► Keep the case clean at all times. Rinse with disinfecting solution, wipe with a lint-free tissue, and allow the case to air dry when not in use between cleanings. Cases can be cleaned in boiling water or soaked in hydrogen peroxide once a week. Replacing the case frequently is also recommended.

► Do not substitute tap water, well water, distilled water, or saliva for sterile contact lens solution.

► For gas-permeable solutions, try not to store the lens dry. It will be more comfortable and wet better if soaked in solution overnight. Do not rinse with water after disinfection. If necessary, rinse with wetting solution.

► Soft lenses cannot be stored dry. If found dry in the case, rehydrate with appropriate solution for 15 minutes prior to inserting lenses. Note: Even though the lens may rehydrate, the optics may be ruined. Blurred vision is the signal that this has happened.

► Apply makeup after inserting lenses. Shield eyes from hairspray or use it prior to inserting lenses.

► Contact lenses cannot "get lost behind the eye." For a lens that has folded or decentered on the eye, apply wetting solution and gently massage the lens down for removal.

(continued)

SIDEBAR 21-17 (CONTINUED)
PATIENT GUIDELINES FOR SUCCESSFUL CONTACT LENS WEAR

► Always wear protective goggles while playing contact sports, working under machinery, or doing work where there may be flying debris. Contact lenses are not a substitute for safety glasses.

► Do not substitute disinfectant solutions to avoid toxicity and possible solution sensitivity.

► Always use fresh, sterile solutions each day. Do not top off solutions in the case. Dump out the solution from the case in the morning, rinse with appropriate solution, allow the case to air dry, and use fresh solution each day.

► Daily worn lenses must be cleaned and disinfected once a day (unless they are daily disposables, which are discarded). Extended wear lenses must be cleaned/disinfected or discarded every 7 days.

► Don't wear lenses if they have suddenly or consistently become uncomfortable, or if the lens is ripped, torn, split, or chipped.

► If you fall asleep in your lenses, don't remove them immediately upon awakening. Always lubricate with rewetting solution prior to removal.

► Do not shower, swim, or use a hot tub while wearing any contact lens.

► Using prescription ocular medications or over-the-counter artificial tear drops not approved for contact lenses (while wearing the lenses) can result in soft lens discoloration, medication toxicity, and surface filming. Apply these types of drops when the contact lenses are removed.

SIDEBAR 21-18
HINTS FOR LENS INSERTION

► Place the lens concave side up (like a bowl) on the tip of the finger with all edges up and off of the finger.

► Keep both eyes open and use the other eye for alignment.

► Keep the lens and the tip of the finger slightly moistened with solution, but not too wet, or the lens will adhere to the finger when brought close to the eye.

► For a soft lens, once it is applied to the eye, swirl the lens a little bit to settle it on the eye and to remove air bubbles and debris.

► For a soft lens, close eye and gently massage out any air bubbles.

► A soft lens can be applied to the conjunctiva and slid onto the cornea.

► A gas-permeable lens needs to be applied directly to the cornea.

► If a gas-permeable lens lands on the conjunctiva, close the lid and gently massage the lens in the direction of the cornea to center, or use the lids to manipulate the lens into place.

► For some patients, it is easier to place the lens on the right hand for the right eye and the left hand for the left eye for insertion.

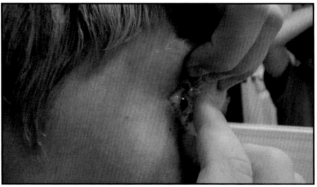
Figure 21-30. Two-handed lid hold application technique.

Soft Lens Removal
Slide and Pinch
1. Have the patient look up and, using a two- or one-handed lid hold technique as described above, take the index finger of the dominant hand and gently touch the contact lens.
2. Apply firm pressure and slide it off of the eye and into the inferior conjunctival fornix.
3. Twist the hand slightly, using the thumb and index finger, and pinch the lens out of the eye using the pads of the fingers (never the fingernails).

This should eventually be practiced without the use of a mirror so the patient can remove the lens in any situation.

J-Roll

1. Using the same technique to hold the eyelids, place the index finger of the dominant hand on the lens and apply firm pressure.

2. Slide the lens off of the eye inferiorly, making the shape of the letter J.

3. The lens should fold into the inferior fornix for removal.

Removal by Fitter

Steps for removing a lens for a patient:

1. Have the patient sit upright and look at the eye chart at the end of the room. It is important to keep both eyes open.

2. Stand to the side of the patient and use a two-handed approach with one hand holding the upper lid and the other holding the lens and the bottom lid.

3. Touch the lens and slide inferiorly off the cornea.

4. Using thumb with index or third finger, pinch the lens off the eye.

Rigid Lens Removal

Lid Pop

Rigid lenses can be dislodged by using the tension of the eyelids to pop the lens out. To remove the lenses:

1. Have the patient place the middle or index finger into the lateral canthus.

2. Open the eyes wide and apply an outward and upward pull with the finger.

3. Blink and the lens should pop out.

This method does not work well for eyelids that are overly loose or lax.

Lid Squeeze or Scissor Method

This method uses the lid margins of the upper and lower eyelids to apply pressure to the lens and dislodge it. To remove the lens:

1. Place one finger of one hand on the upper eyelid and another finger of the other hand on the lower eyelid at the position of the lid margin.

2. Open wide.

3. Gently push the lids inward and together using the lid margins to catch the edge of the lens.

4. The lens should pop out.

Contact Lens Plunger

The contact lens plunger is a device that can be used to remove a rigid lens when other methods fail. It is also the preferred method for fitter removal. To use the plunger:

1. Moisten the eye and the plunger with an approved lubricating drop.

2. Make sure the rigid lens is central on the cornea.

3. Bring the plunger parallel to the lens (Figure 21-31).

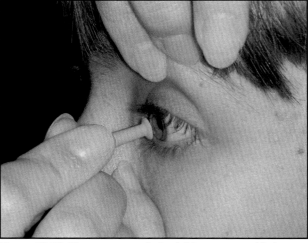

Figure 21-31. Plunger removal of a rigid gas-permeable lens.

4. Gently press the plunger into the lens.

5. The lens should adhere to the plunger and release from the eye.

6. Slide the lens off the plunger.

The plunger can also be used to remove a decentered rigid lens from the conjunctiva, as long as the lens can be visualized. *Never "fish" for a lens using the plunger.*

Wearing Schedules

Normal adaptation symptoms can include lens awareness, increased blinking and tearing, and lens handling issues. These can be more pronounced in rigid lens wearers and it may take 2 to 4 weeks to fully adapt to the lenses. New lens wearers should build up their wearing time to ease these symptoms in the first week.

Providing a chart with the number of hours of wear for each day during adaptation is a simple way to keep the patient on track. Start the patient with just a few hours a day, typically 2 to 4 hours/day for rigid lenses and 4 to 6 hours/day for soft lenses, and add a few hours every day (provided that no problems have surfaced) until he/she is wearing the lenses full time. The lenses could be worn a few hours on and a few hours off, until the full wearing time is reached. The average wearing time for most lenses is 10 to 12 hours/day.

Always ask returning patients how many hours they wear their lenses and if they sleep in them. If the lenses are used for overnight wear, determine the number of days the patient sleeps in the lenses before removing and cleaning and/or replacing the lens. Make sure the lens is approved for overnight use (appropriate Dk value) and that the patient is adhering to the recommended replacement schedule.

The American Academy of Ophthalmology (AAO) recognizes that extended wear of contact lenses can be a safe and useful modality of lens wear when properly selected and monitored by an eye care professional.[9] The

AAO recommends that practitioners instruct the patient in proper lens hygiene, including best practices of contact lens care and handling, and review the risks and possible ocular complications associated with overnight contact lens use. In accordance with the FDA, the AAO also recommends that any extended wear lens be removed weekly and cleaned or disposed of, according to the replacement schedule of the lens manufacturer, and the eyes allowed to rest overnight without lenses.

Lens Care

The purpose of contact lens care is to minimize microbial contamination, reduce deposits, and to maintain an adequately clean lens, whether it is a disposable or conventional replacement lens. Lens care includes cleaning, disinfection, protein removal, and lubrication. It is important that daily wear lenses be cleaned and disinfected every day. Lens care solutions should be used as directed and replaced as recommended or if expired. If contamination is suspected, solutions should be discarded.

Cleaning

Cleaning is the physical act of removing debris, mucus, makeup, and build-up from the surface of a contact lens. Cleaning solutions can be part of a multipurpose solution or a separate surfactant, which is then rinsed from the lens. The concentration of surfactant in a multipurpose solution may not be enough for patients with high surface deposits, however. Adding a separate cleaner may be necessary.

Cleaning involves applying a few drops of the cleaner, manually rubbing the lens with the finger (preferably in the palm of the hand) with a counterclockwise motion (which actually reduces excess force on the lens) for about 10 seconds or as recommended by the solution manufacturer. (Note: Many practitioners recommend this type of manual cleaning even if "no-rub" solutions are used.) It is recommended that cleaning be performed when the lenses are removed at the end of the day and prior to disinfection. Cleaning prepares the lens for disinfection, removing large debris and microorganisms, so the disinfecting agent can be more effective.

Once a lens is cleaned, it should be rinsed completely. For soft lenses, rinse with a saline or multipurpose solution according to the manufacturer's guidelines. *Water should never be used on a soft lens.* For rigid lenses, rinse with saline or water prior to disinfection. *Water should not be used on a rigid lens once it has been disinfected.* Rigid lens cleaners can be either abrasive or nonabrasive. Abrasive cleaners are not recommended on high-Dk rigid lenses or rigid lenses that have been plasma treated.

Disinfection

Disinfection is an antimicrobial process that reduces the levels of microorganisms on a lens to an acceptable level. It is not a sterilization process, but rather decontamination process. It is important to follow the manufacturer's guidelines on disinfection techniques and soaking duration to achieve the maximum disinfection benefit. Disinfection can be effective against a wide variety of microorganisms, including bacteria, fungus, protozoa, and amoeba.

Thermal/Ultraviolet/Ultrasonic Disinfection

Thermal disinfection achieved popularity in the early years of SCL wear, though it is not a common soft lens disinfection method today. The lenses are placed in the unit's chamber with nonpreserved saline solution and exposed to a temperature of 80° to 90° C for at least 10 minutes. Thermal disinfection is not recommended on high-water content soft lenses (> 55%).

Ultraviolet/ultrasonic cleaners can be used on soft and rigid lenses. It involves ultraviolet exposure and subsonic turbulence over a period of time to disinfect the lenses. It is used with nonpreserved solutions. It is not a common form of disinfection.

Chemical Disinfection

Chemical disinfection is the most common form of contact lens decontamination. This method works well for both soft and rigid contact lenses, although the solutions are different. A majority of soft lens solutions can be used on rigid lenses, but the reverse is not true. Chemical disinfectants can be found as stand-alone soaking solutions or as multipurpose solutions. Multipurpose solutions accomplish cleaning, rinsing, and storage/disinfection all in one product.

Disinfecting agents can vary from older generation solutions and preservatives, especially those in generic equivalents, to the new dual disinfection preserved systems found in many brand-name solutions today. In any case, the lenses must be soaked for at least the minimum time required by the manufacturer to achieve disinfection. Most chemical and multipurpose solutions are good for long-term storage from 7 to 30 days (varies by manufacturer). Due to the preservatives and disinfectants found in these chemical solutions, they may not be the best choice for patients with hypersensitive eyes or allergic symptoms.

Oxidation

Oxidation disinfection uses a microfiltered, buffered 3% hydrogen peroxide solution to disinfect both rigid and SCLs. Hydrogen peroxide systems require neutralization of the solution either by using a one-step platinum catalytic disc or a two-step, separate neutralization tablet. Incomplete neutralization can result in residual hydrogen peroxide in the case, causing a mild superficial chemical burn (with burning and irritation) when the lenses are inserted. Educate the patient to replace the catalytic disc (case) as recommended and to not use the solution directly in the eye. (There are red caps and warning labels on all solution bottles of this type.)

Hydrogen peroxide is not approved for long-term lens storage, so patients who wear their lenses on a part-time basis may not be good candidates for this type of disinfection. Hydrogen peroxide systems, however, can be a suitable choice for patients with hypersensitivity to other solutions.

Ophthalmic grade hydrogen peroxide is recommended by the CDC for in-office disinfection of trial lenses. The CDC recommends 10-minute disinfection in a 3% hydrogen peroxide solution.[10]

Protein Removal

Protein removal utilizes an enzymatic cleaner to break down surface protein deposits on both rigid and soft lens materials. It is an additional step to daily cleaner and disinfecting solutions, performed approximately once a week for lenses with increased protein deposits or for lenses that are not replaced frequently. Protein removal is often not necessary on disposable soft lenses.

Rinsing Agents

Rinsing agents are saline solutions (preserved and nonpreserved) used for irrigating the lens after use of a daily cleaner and/or after disinfection prior to application. Rinsing agents are *not* disinfectants and should not be used as such.

Preserved saline solutions are packaged in large squeeze bottles. Nonpreserved saline solution can be packaged in large aerosol containers (packaged under pressure, and with a longer expiration date), in smaller 4-ounce squeeze bottles with a short (< 7 days) expiration date, or in single-use 5-mL sterile saline ampules. Patients should be instructed to discard unused saline (especially nonpreserved, smaller dose units) as recommended to prevent microbial contamination.

Patients should be warned against the use of tap water, well water, or homemade saline solutions for rinsing soft lenses to avoid the risk of microbial contamination and serious eye infections.

Wetting Agents

Wetting agents are applied to the eye while wearing a lens for occasional dryness and irritation. Some brands are specific for a rigid or soft lens; others can be used with either. These lubricants usually contain preservatives, some of which may be dissipating (disappearing on contact with the ocular surface). They can also have added surfactants for cleaning the lens surface and reducing build-up.

SIDEBAR 21-19
EXAMPLE FOLLOW-UP SCHEDULES

▶ A typical follow-up schedule for daily wear lenses:
- Initial fitting
- 2-week follow-up
- 1-month follow-up
- Annual eye exam thereafter

▶ Extended wear lenses require closer monitoring:
- Initial fitting
- 1 day following overnight wear
- 1-week follow-up
- 1-month follow-up
- 3-month follow-up
- 6-month follow-ups thereafter

Follow-Up Care

Proper follow-up care after contact lens fitting and dispensing is necessary to monitor the eye for lens adaptation and tolerance to both the contact lenses and the solutions. It can also minimize possible contact lens-related complications and maximize the success of the fitting by addressing lens-related vision and fit issues before they become a problem.

Contact lens follow-up should be tailored to each individual patient based on his/her ocular history and needs (Sidebar 21-19). All patients wearing contact lenses should have a routine eye exam annually.

On follow-up exams and annual assessments, ask the patient about any problems, issues, or concerns with the lenses or wearing time. Determine the number of hours per day and/or number of days the lenses are being worn. For disposable lenses, determine how frequently the lenses are being replaced. For conventional lenses, determine the approximate age of the current lenses. Verify the brand of solutions being used and specific hygiene habits (eg, "Do you rub the lenses?").

Check visual acuity and perform overrefractometry if necessary. First, see if vision can be improved with spheres. If vision remains poor there may be residual astigmatism, so refractometry with sphere and cylinder may be necessary.

Using the slit lamp, evaluate the fit, movement, and cleanliness of the lens. For rigid lenses instill NaFl to stain the tear film to evaluate the fit pattern. Check the bulbar conjunctiva and the inferior and superior palpebral conjunctiva for any allergic reactions. Remove the lens and check the cornea for any punctate epithelial keratopathy associated with lens wear. Check the limbus for any signs of neovascularization.

Assess the information gathered and make necessary plans to change the lens or to continue with the current lens and care system. Always educate patients regarding proper lens wear and hygiene—remember the more they hear it, the more likely they are to follow your carefully determined guidelines. Lastly, determine the next date of return.

CHAPTER QUIZ

1. The vertex distance of a contact lens is ____ , therefore more ____ power is needed in prescriptions ≥ +/-4.00 to focus light rays onto the retina.
   a. 12 mm, plus
   b. 0 mm, plus
   c. 12 mm, minus
   d. 0 mm, minus

2. When converting diopters into radius of curvature for base curve measurements, a radius of curvature of 8.30 mm is ____ a radius of curvature of 8.90 mm.
   a. steeper than
   b. flatter than
   c. the same as
   d. smaller than

3. Sagittal depth is important in contact lens fitting because:
   a. smaller diameter corneas may require a steeper contact lens
   b. a lens with a lower vault will have a steeper curve
   c. as the corneal diameter increases, the vault decreases
   d. larger diameter corneas may require a larger/ steeper contact lens

4. Soft contact lenses are made from what two basic materials?
   a. hydrogel and silicone hydrogel
   b. hydrogel and silicone acrylate
   c. polymethylmethacryate and silicone hydrogel
   d. silicone acrylate and silicone hydrogel

5. What material are modern day rigid gas-permeable lenses made from?
   a. cellulose acetate butyrate
   b. hydroxyethyl methacrylate
   c. fluoro-silicone acrylate
   d. silicone acrylate

6. Which two instruments can be used to measure corneal surface curvature and astigmatism prior to contact lens fitting?
   a. radiuscope and keratometer
   b. radiuscope and lensometer
   c. corneal topographer and lensometer
   d. corneal topographer and keratometer

7. Which of the following basic measurements are needed before fitting contact lenses?
   a. refraction, keratometry, and tonometry
   b. refraction, keratometry, and pupil diameter
   c. refraction, keratometry, and iris diameter
   d. refraction, iris diameter, and pupil diameter

8. When fitting a soft contact lens, the lens diameter should be at *least* ____ mm larger than the horizontal visible iris diameter.
   a. 2
   b. 3
   c. 1
   d. 0

9. Using the LARS principle, when a soft toric contact lens rotates to the right (or counterclockwise), you should:
   a. add the degree of lens rotation to the lens cylinder axis
   b. add the degree of lens rotation to the refractive cylinder axis
   c. subtract the degree of lens rotation from the lens cylinder axis
   d. subtract the degree of lens rotation from the refractive cylinder axis

10. What signs will a flat-fitting rigid gas-permeable lens exhibit?
    a. central fluorescein pooling, mid-peripheral touch, and dimple veil
    b. central fluorescein absence, lens decentering, and inferior edge lift
    c. central fluorescein pooling, lens decentering, and inferior edge lift
    d. central fluorescein absence, lens decentering, and dimple veil

11. Which contact lens-induced complication can be caused by contact lens overwear and low-Dk lenses?
    a. foreign body tracks
    b. dimple veiling
    c. neovascularization
    d. 3-and-9 staining

12. Which contact lens-related complication is the most serious and requires immediate attention by an eye care provider?

    a. microbial keratitis
    b. hypoxia
    c. neovascularization
    d. CLARE

13. What is the process that reduces the level of microorganisms on a lens making it safe to wear?

    a. cleaning
    b. disinfection
    c. enzymatic cleaning
    d. lubrication

14. Using well water and/or home-made saline, or wearing contacts while showering, swimming, or using a hot tub can all increase the risk of:

    a. neovascularization
    b. sterile ulcers
    c. microbial keratitis
    d. giant papillary conjunctivitis

15. True/False: Lenses that are not replaced daily should be cleaned and disinfected daily with fresh solution in a clean case.

Answers

1. b
2. a
3. d
4. a
5. c
6. d
7. c
8. a
9. d
10. b
11. c
12. a
13. b
14. c
15. True

REFERENCES

1. Wilcox M. Microbial adhesion to silicone hydrogel lenses: a review. *Eye & Contact Lens.* 2013;39(1):61-66.

2. French K, Jones L. A decade with silicone hydrogels: part 2. *Optometry Today.* 2008;48(18):38-43.

3. Bennett ES, Henry VE. *Clinical Manual of Contact Lenses.* 4th ed. Philadelphia, PA: Lippincott Williams & Wilkins; 2014.

4. Contact Lens Society of America. *Contact Lens Manual: A Comprehensive Study and Reference Guide.* Vol 1. St Paul, MN: Contact Lens Society of America; 1999.

5. Contact Lens Society of America. *Advanced Contact Lens Manual: A Comprehensive Study and Reference Guide.* Vol 2. St Paul, MN: Contact Lens Society of America; 2003.

6. Tangible Science website. www.tangiblescience.com/copy-of-technology-1. Accessed September 3, 2017.

7. Silbert J. Medications and contact lens wear. *Contact Lens Spectrum.* May 2002. www.clspectrum.com/articleviewer.aspx?articleID=12149. Accessed July 4, 2016.

8. Weibel K, Miller W, Nichols J. Microbial keratitis and contact lens wear. *Contact Lens Spectrum.* 2013;28(6):24-40.

9. American Academy of Ophthalmology. Extended wear of contact lenses. www.aao.org/assets/c53ade92-e496-41a9-9689-4c682b-9fe8b8/635110637373130000/extended-wear-of-contact-lenses-may-2013-pdf. Published May 2013. Accessed July 4, 2016.

10. Centers for Disease Control. Recommendations for prevention of HIV transmission in health-care settings. *MMWR.* 1987;36 (suppl no. 2S). www.cdc.gov/mmwr/preview/mmwrhtml/00023587.htm. Accessed July 4, 2016.

Unless otherwise noted, the figures in this chapter were contributed by the following, who are associated with this book as authors:
Wendy M. Ford: Figures 21-1 through 21-16, 12-18, 12-19, 12-22, 12-24 through 12-31
Anna Kiss: Figure 21-17
Al Lens: Figure 21-23

IV

OPHTHALMIC MEDICAL SCIENCES

22

PHARMACOLOGY

Peter D. Anderson, Pharm D, BCPP, CMI-IV
Gyula Bokor, MD

BASIC SCIENCES

The pharmacological definition of a drug is any substance other than food that alters the physiology of the body via chemical means.[1] Drugs include medications, substances of abuse, and poisons.

The distinction between food and drugs is not always clear cut. When higher doses of vitamins are used than needed for nutrition, they are considered a drug. For example, if niacin is used in the treatment of elevated cholesterol, it is a drug rather than a food. Nutrients administered by injection are considered drugs rather than foods (eg, when vitamin B_{12} is given as an injection). This is because sterility and greater quality control procedures are needed for injections than foods.

The legal definition of a drug, such as used by the Food and Drug Administration (FDA), differs from the pharmacological definition. The FDA states that drugs are "articles intended for use in the diagnosis, cure, mitigation, treatment, or prevention of disease" and "articles (other than food) intended to affect the structure or any function of the body of man or other animals."[2]

Any drug used therapeutically has a chemical name, a generic name, and a brand name. The *chemical name* is derived from the structure of the drug's molecule. A *generic name* is a simplified chemical name of a drug.

The *brand name* is a trademark of a specific manufacturer. N-acetyl-p-aminophenol is the chemical name for an over-the-counter drug used to treat fever and minor pain. Acetaminophen is its generic name. Tylenol is brand name of acetaminophen produced by McNeil Consumer Healthcare. Acetylsalicylic acid (ASA) is the chemical name of a nonprescription medication used for pain, fever, and inflammation, and in the prevention of heart attacks. Aspirin is the generic name for ASA, and Anacin is the brand name of aspirin produced by Insight Pharmaceuticals.

The Controlled Substances Act (CSA) regulates drugs with potential for abuse. The lead agency for enforcing the CSA is the Drug Enforcement Administration (DEA). Drugs with abuse potential are classified into one of 5 schedules. Schedule I substances are drugs with a high potential for abuse and no accepted medical uses. Schedule I substances include phencyclidine and heroin. Schedule II are with drugs with a high potential for abuse, but have accepted medical uses. Morphine, oxycodone, cocaine, and amphetamines are examples of Schedule II substances. The DEA forbids refills on Schedule II substances, thus a written prescription is always required for them except in a bonafide emergency. Schedule III substances have less of a potential for abuse than Schedules I and II, and have an accepted medical use. Examples of

Ledford JK, Lens A, eds.
Principles and Practice in Ophthalmic Assisting:
A Comprehensive Textbook (pp 419-438).
© 2018 Taylor & Francis Group.

Schedule III drugs include barbiturates and acetaminophen with codeine. Schedule IV substances have less of a potential for abuse than Schedule III, and have accepted medical uses. Schedule IV substances include benzodiazepines and zolpidem (Ambien). Schedule V substances have less potential for abuse than Schedule IV, and have accepted medical uses. Cough syrups containing a small amount of codeine are an example of a Schedule V substance.

Identification of Ophthalmic Drugs

With so many eye medications on the market, a system for identifying certain classes of prescription drugs by the color of the bottle cap has evolved (Table 22-1). Over-the-counter eye drops do not necessarily adhere to this scheme. When asking a patient about his/her eye drops, knowing the color of the cap is useful, but not always accurate. Patients should be asked to bring their medications with them to every visit.

Definitions

There are several definitions related to medications that are important to understand.

An *active ingredient* is the chemical in the pharmaceutical product that is biologically active and exerts the therapeutic effect.

The other ingredients in a pharmaceutical product are considered *inactive ingredients*. The role of such ingredients include flavorings, binders, diluents (makes a mixture more liquid), preservatives, and stabilizers. Inactive ingredients, although generally considered therapeutically inert, can cause hypersensitivity or allergic reactions in susceptible individuals.

The *shelf-life* of a medication refers to the drug quality over a specified period of time. A key factor with the shelf-life is drug *stability*, which is the ability of the pharmaceutical dosage form to maintain the physical, chemical, therapeutic, and antimicrobial properties during the time of storage. Penetration of a sterile vial of an injectable product shortens the shelf-life. Thus, a common practice in hospitals is to discard vials of injectable medications 28 days after the vial is penetrated.

The *expiration* relates to the quality and safety of a medication at a specific point in time. Every pharmaceutical product manufactured in the United States is granted an expiration date by the manufacturer. The expiration date of a medication indicates the date to which the manufacturer guarantees the full potency and safety of a drug. The expiration date is only valid if the drug is stored in the original container and at an appropriate temperature. The main risk with using expired products is decreased potency. However, some products can become toxic when expired, such as tetracycline. In addition, sterile products may no longer be sterile after the expiration date.

When a drug is approved for use by the FDA, the product is granted approval for a specific indication (eg, disease state). This is referred to as a *labeled indication*. For example, modafinil (Provigil) is indicated for the treatment of narcolepsy. However, many clinicians use modafinil as a treatment for attention deficit hyperactivity disorder (ADHD). This is an *unlabeled* or *off-label indication*. The manufacturer, granted the license by the FDA, may only advertise and market the product for labeled indications. Prescribers, however, may use the product for off-label conditions.

A *prodrug* is a medication that is administered in a pharmacologically inactive form but is then converted to an active form by a normal metabolic process in the body. An example of a prodrug is levodopa, which is administered orally to treat Parkinson's disease. The levodopa is metabolized in the brain into dopamine. Dopamine, if administered in the same way, would not be able to cross the blood–brain barrier so that is why the prodrug levodopa is used.

Compounding is a technique used by pharmacists to prepare pharmaceutical preparations of products that are not commercially available. Vancomycin is an intravenous medication to treat a variety of difficult infections. It is sometimes needed to treat corneal ulcers, but is not commercially available in an ophthalmic dosage form. A properly trained pharmacist is able to compound vancomycin eye drops from the injectable version. Most community pharmacies are *not* able to do ophthalmic compounding.

Characteristics of Medications

Medications are administered by a number of routes, including oral, inhalation, injection, and topical. Orally administered medications include tablets, capsules, and liquids.

Inhalation routes include nebulizers and inhalers, which are commonly used when treating disorders involving the lungs. For example, albuterol is prescribed to expand the airways during an asthma attack. Inhalation medications have also been used for systemic effects, such as administering albuterol by nebulizer to correct elevated potassium levels.

Medications may be injected intravenously (in the veins), intra-arterially (in the arteries, a technique rarely used), intramuscularly (into the muscle), and subcutaneously (below the surface of the skin). Ophthalmic injections include intravitreal injections, subconjunctival injections, and periocular injections. Intravitreal injections involve diluted concentrations of drugs introduced into the vitreous humor, such as vancomycin to treat endophthalmitis. Subconjunctival injections are deposited underneath the conjunctiva, such as 5-fluorouracil

TABLE 22-1
CAP COLOR SCHEME FOR COMMON PRESCRIPTION EYE DROPS*

Drug Type	Cap Color	Purpose	Generic (Trade) Names
Alpha-adrenergic agonists	Purple	Glaucoma treatment	brimonidine (Alphagan) apraclonidine (Iopidine)
Anti-infectives	Tan	Infections	Antibiotics: ciprofloxacin (Ciloxan) erythromycin (Ilotycin) moxifloxacin (Vigamox) ofloxacin (Ocuflox) tobramycin (Tobrex) Antifungals: natamycin (Natacyn) Antivirals: trifluridine (Viroptic)
Beta blockers (beta-adrenergic antagonists) Nonselective	Yellow	Glaucoma treatment	carteolol (Ocupress) levobunolol (Betagan) metipranolol (OptiPranolol) timolol (Timoptic)
Beta blockers (beta-adrenergic antagonists) Selective	Light blue	Glaucoma treatment	betaxolol (Betoptic)
Carbonic anhydrase inhibitors (CAI)	Orange	Glaucoma treatment	brinzolamide (Azopt) dorzolamide (Trusopt)
CAI/adrenergic agonist combinations Alpha Beta	Light green	Glaucoma treatment	brinzolamide/brimonidine (Simbrinza) brinzolamide/timolol (Azarga [outside United States])
CAI/beta blocker combinations	Dark blue	Glaucoma treatment	brimonidine/timolol (Combigan) dorzolamide/timolol (Cosopt)
Cycloplegics/ mydriatics	Red	Pupil dilation: Diagnostic Pain control in inflammation Penalization in amblyopia treatment	cyclopentolate (Cyclogyl) phenylephrine (Neo-Synephrine) tropicamide (Mydriacyl, Tropicacyl)
Immunomodulators/ suppressants	Olive green	Allergic conjunctivitis, dry eye treatment, corneal graft rejection	tacrolimus (Protopic)
Miotics	Dark green	Glaucoma treatment, dilation reversal	dipivefrin (Propine) echothiophate (Phospholinelodide) epinephrine (Eppy/N) pilocarpine (Isopto Carpine, Pilocar)
Nonsteroidal anti-inflammatories	Gray	Inflammation	ketorolac (Acular) diclofenac (Voltaren)
Prostaglandin analogues	Turquoise/teal (patients may call it green or blue)	Glaucoma treatment	bimatoprost (Lumigan) latanoprost (Xalatan) tafluprost (Zioptan) travoprost (Travatan)
Steroidal anti-inflammatories	Pink	Inflammation	fluorometholone (FML, Flarex) loteprednol (Lotemax, Alrex) prednisolone (Pred Forte, Pred Mild)

*Note: Manufacturers of prescription medications generally go with this color scheme. Some over-the-counter medications, however, use container and cap colors indiscriminately.

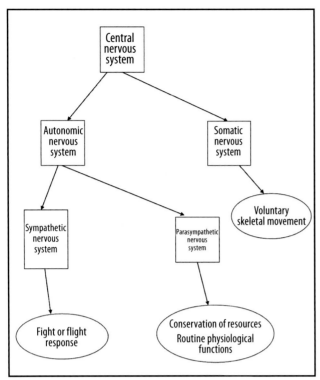

Figure 22-1. Breakdown of the central nervous system.

given to treat glaucoma. A periocular injection is injected into tissues around the eye (vs the eye itself). For example, botulinum is injected into extraocular muscle to treat strabismus.

Topical medications include nasal sprays, ear drops, ophthalmic drops, and ointments or creams applied to the skin. These may be applied for either a local effect (eg, hydrocortisone 1% to treat a rash) or systemic effect (eg, nitroglycerin paste to treat angina).

The most common topical ophthalmic medications are solutions, suspensions, and ointments. Ophthalmic *solutions* contain the drug in a dissolved form. In ophthalmic *suspensions*, the drug is in particle form suspended in the liquid, and thus must be shaken well prior to use. Ophthalmic *ointments* and *gels* are thicker and used when prolonged contact is needed, such as erythromycin for conjunctivitis. Less commonly, ophthalmic medications might be administered by ocular inserts. Innovative ophthalmic medication delivery includes using contact lenses to release a constant supply of mediations.

The pharmaceutical requirements for ophthalmic medications are much stricter than those used on the skin. Eye drops and ointments must be sterile and have narrow pH limits. Ophthalmic solutions must also be isotonic. These characteristics will be discussed next.

Preservatives are added to multiuse containers of ophthalmic medications to prevent microbial contamination. Examples of preservatives include benzalkonium chloride (BKC), chlorobutanol, phenylmercuric nitrate or acetate, methylparaben, thimerosal, and propylparaben.

Preservatives such as sodium bisulfate or ethylenediaminetetraacetic acid (EDTA) are also used to prevent oxidation of the drug, extending the shelf-life. Allergies or hypersensitivities have been reported with preservatives. A case in point is allergic contact conjunctivitis from thimerosal.

The *pH* is the concentration of hydrogen ions in a solution. (See Appendix A for more.) A pH of 7 is considered neutral. An acid is a solution with a pH below 7. A base is a solution with a pH above 7. The tears are a weak base with a pH of 7.4. Ocular preparations typically need to have a pH of between 7.0 and 7.7. In other words, most ophthalmic medications need to be a weak base-in order to be compatible with the eye. *Buffering agents* are added by the manufacturer to adjust the pH of ophthalmic solutions. Buffering agents include hydrochloric acid, sodium bicarbonate, potassium borate, potassium phosphate, and sodium citrate.

Tonicity refers to the concentration of salts in a solution, and can affect the movement of fluids into and out of tissues. Ophthalmic medications generally need to be *isotonic* (iso- means equal) with the tear film, or equivalent to 0.9% of sodium chloride. The eye can generally tolerate a sodium chloride concentration between 0.5% to 1.8%. If the tonicity of an eye medication is too far outside these boundaries, it will sting and burn. Agents such as sodium chloride, buffering salts, dextrose, glycerin, and mannitol are used to produce isotonicity.

Other inactive ingredients in ophthalmic products include viscosity enhancers, which help create the thickness of a medication. Viscosity enhancers function to prolong the contact time of the pharmaceutical solution on the external ocular surface. Water-soluble polymers (polymers are made up of long chains, sheets, or networks of molecules) are employed as viscosity agents. Cellulose (plant-based) derivatives including methylcellulose, carboxymethylcellulose, and hydroxypropyl methylcellulose are commonly used. Noncellulose (not plant-based) viscosity agents include polyvinyl alcohol, dextran, and propylene glycol.

Drugs and the Central Nervous System

The central nervous system (CNS; Figure 22-1) consists of the *somatic nervous system* and the *autonomic nervous system*. The somatic nervous system (*soma* referring to body) contracts voluntary muscle movements, predominantly skeletal muscle. The autonomic nervous system (ANS) controls "automatic" activity such as breathing, digestion, and heart rate.

There are two divisions of the autonomic nervous system: sympathetic and parasympathetic. The sympathetic nervous system is responsible for the "fight or flight" response, as when a person is danger. Activation of the sympathetic nervous system increases heart rate,

TABLE 22-2
ADRENERGIC RECEPTORS

Receptors	Location	Result of Activation	Agonists	Antagonists
α-1	Blood vessels	Vasocontriction, increased blood pressure, contraction of radial muscle in iris producing mydriasis	Phenylephrine	Prazosin
α-2	Presynaptic neurons	Decreased output of norepinephrine	Clonidine	Yohimbine
β_1	Heart	Increased heart rate and force of contraction	Dobutamine	Atenolol
β_2	Lungs, blood vessels	Bronchial dilation, vasodilation resulting in lowering of blood pressure	Albuterol	Propranolol (blocks β1 and β2)

widens the bronchial airways, and dilates the pupils. The parasympathetic nervous system is responsible for conservation of the body's resources, such as slowing of heart rate, constriction of pupil, and promotion of digestion. The parasympathetic system is a complementary system to the sympathetic system, essentially doing everything opposite of what the sympathetic system does.

In the nervous system, information is relayed by chemicals called *neurotransmitters*. These chemicals flow between the synapses (gaps) and act on receptors. The receptors are typically proteins located on a cell membrane or cell surface. Activation of a receptor initiates a chemical cascade in the cell that produces a physiological response. The primary neurotransmitter of the sympathetic nervous system is *epinephrine* (adrenaline). The primary neurotransmitter of the parasympathetic nervous system is *acetylcholine* (noradrenaline).

Most drugs work in the body by acting on receptors. A drug that activates a receptor is an *agonist*. A drug that inhibits a receptor is an *antagonist*. For example, there are beta receptors in the heart. Activation of a beta receptor increases the heart rate and force of contraction. Antagonism of the beta receptor slows the heart rate and decreases the force of contraction.

There are different types of receptors. Adrenergic receptors are involved with the sympathetic nervous system. Cholinergic receptors are predominantly linked to the parasympathetic nervous system. However, some cholinergic receptors are involved with sympathetic nervous system. For example, cholinergic receptors are needed for sweating. Cholinergic receptors are also found in the ganglia of the sympathetic nervous system. Agonists of the adrenergic receptors include epinephrine and norepinephrine. The two main types of adrenergic receptors (Table 22-2) are alpha (α) and beta (β), and each of these have several subtypes.

There are two types of cholinergic receptors (Table 22-3). *Muscarinic* receptors are located in the heart, smooth muscle, and iris. The *nicotinic* receptors are located at muscles and in the ganglia of the sympathetic nervous system.

TABLE 22-3
CHOLINERGIC RECEPTORS

Receptor	Anatomical Location	Function	Agonist	Antagonist
Muscarinic (M)	Heart, sweat glands, smooth muscle	Slowing of heart rate, narrowing of airways, and constriction of pupil; fluid functions including sweating, urination, and defecation; contraction of sphincter in iris producing miosis	Pilocarpine, muscarine	Atropine
Nicotinic neuronal (NN)	Autonomic ganglia	Release of epinephrine	Nicotine	Trimethaphan
Nicotonic muscular (NM)	Neuromuscular junction	Constriction of skeletal muscle	Nicotine	Tubocurarine

The activity of drugs in the body is the science of pharmacology. The action of drugs on the receptors and on the tissues is referred to *pharmacodynamics.* *Pharmacokinetics* is the study of the absorption, distribution, metabolism, and excretion of drugs. Thus, pharmacodynamics is what the drug does to the body, and pharmacokinetics is what the body does to the drug. The primary organ for drug metabolism is the liver. The primary organ for drug elimination is the kidney.

Drugs are modified chemically to exhibit selectivity for certain receptors in the body. This often leads to greater efficacy and fewer side effects. Selectivity for a receptor, however, does not mean exclusivity for the receptor. For example, atenolol is selective for β_1 receptors so is better tolerated in patients with asthma than propranolol, which has equal activity on β_1 and β_2 receptors. However, at higher doses atenolol does activate the β_2 receptors.

Allergic Reactions and Side Effects

A *side effect* of a medication is any effect of the medication other than the intended effect (ie, why it was administered). For example, diazepam may be administered to stop muscle spasms. The diazepam produces tiredness, which is a side effect.

While side effects often become known during drug testing, sometimes complications arise. A *complication* is when the patient has an unexpected reaction.

An *adverse drug reaction* (ADR) is a noxious reaction to a medication when administered at normal therapeutic doses and can be thought of as a severe side effect. (Effects from an excessive dose of a medication is a *poisoning*, not an adverse reaction.) For example, if one became unconscious after taking diazepam that would be an adverse reaction.

A *type A* ADR is an adverse reaction that is an exaggerated reaction from the normal pharmacology of the drug. (For example, a benzodiazepine normally makes a person sleepy. Unconsciousness from a benzodiazepine would be type A ADR.) A *type B* ADR is a reaction that is not typical from the normal pharmacology of the drug, including idiosyncratic (ie, peculiar to that individual) and allergic reactions. *Allergic reactions* are immune-mediated reactions with symptoms that vary from mild itching and rash to anaphylactic shock (anaphylaxis). Allergic reactions to medications are always considered ADRs and not side effects.

Anaphylaxis is an acute, fatal, or potentially fatal hypersensitivity (allergic) reaction. The clinical presentation of anaphylaxis includes flushing, hives, itching, angioedema (rapid swelling of skin and mucosa), airway constriction, and severe hypotension. An *anaphylactoid* reaction is a reaction resembling generalized anaphylaxis but is caused by a nonimmunologic mechanism. Common triggers of anaphylactic reactions are penicillin and peanuts. Examples of substances that produce anaphylactoid reactions include aspirin and fluorescein. Anaphylaxis requires the prior exposure of the trigger, whereas anaphylactoid reactions can occur with first exposure to the substance.

More common adverse reactions are detected in the clinical trials of medications. Less common adverse reactions may not be detected years or even decades after the drug enters the market. New ADRs or suspected ADRs can be reported directly to the manufacturer or to the FDA through the MedWatch Program (at www.fda.gov/Safety/MedWatch/). Clinicians may also report in-depth findings via case reports in peer-reviewed journals.

CLINICAL KNOWLEDGE

There are many ophthalmic medications available, both over the counter (OTC) and by prescription. It is impossible to cover them all. Appendix D, Common Ophthalmic Medications, is a table listing many ocular drugs first by brand/trademarked name and then giving the generic name and general use of the drug. Diagnostic drugs used in the clinic are not included on the list, as they are mentioned in this chapter.

Anesthetics

An *anesthetic* is a drug that causes a reversible loss of sensation. Anesthetics typically work by blocking the sensation of pain from passing along the nerves to the brain. Anesthetics are not to be confused with pain killers, which work by relieving pain without stopping sensation.

Topical Anesthetics

As the term implies, local anesthetics are applied externally to the tissue. In eye care, patients often refer to these as "numbing drops." They are used for in-office procedures that involve contacting the cornea and sometimes other ocular tissues, as well as cataract surgery. Allergic reactions to topical anesthetics are rare.

Cocaine is the only naturally occurring topical anesthetic in clinical use. All other topical anesthetics are synthetic compounds. Cocaine is not commercially available as an ophthalmic formulation, but can be compounded by a specially equipment pharmacy. Cocaine 10% is used in the diagnosis of Horner's syndrome (see Chapter 25).

Commercially available ophthalmic anesthetics include tetracaine, benoxinate, and proparacaine.

Tetracaine comes as a 0.5% solution and is used in tonometry and minor procedures involving the cornea or sclera. The primary side effects of tetracaine are stinging and burning upon instillation. A potential adverse reaction to tetracaine is corneal compromise.

Benoxinate is only commercially available with dyes such as sodium fluorescein (Fluress) or disodium fluorexon. The primary use of benoxinate products is applanation tonometry.

Proparacaine (Alcaine, AKTaine) is commercially available as a 0.5% solution. Proparacaine has less corneal penetration than tetracaine and produces less compromise to corneal structure. Proparacaine appears to cause less pain on instillation than tetracaine. It is also available in combination with fluorescein (Flucaine).

Prolonged use of these topical anesthetics will break down corneal integrity and interfere with the healing process. Patients should never be given a prescription for them, or given a bottle from the office for home use.

Local Anesthetics

More complex and invasive ophthalmic procedures require the use of injectable anesthetics, such as procaine, lidocaine, mepivacaine, bupivacaine, or etidocaine, to produce a local nerve block. Many minor office procedures (chalazion incision, lid surgery, growth excision, etc) call for a local anesthetic.

Epinephrine is often mixed with injectable anesthetics for invasive surgical procedures to prolong the duration of anesthesia, to reduce systemic effects, and to control local bleeding.

Local anesthetics are injected into tissues at the site to be numbed. This might be done externally (such as the lids) or even behind the eye (retrobulbar).

General Anesthesia

General anesthesia is when the patient receives drugs for amnesia, analgesia, muscle paralysis, and sedation. (Patients often refer to this as being "knocked out.") Drugs used to induce general anesthesia include anesthetic gases, pain killers, anti-anxiety/relaxation agents, and paralytic agents. In ophthalmology it is usually reserved for surgery on infants, children, and others who may have difficulty remaining calm and still during a procedure. It is administered via inhalation or intravenously.

Mydriatics and Cycloplegics

Mydriatics are drugs that dilate the pupil either by paralyzing the iris sphincter muscle or stimulating the iris dilator muscle.

The iris sphincter muscle (which constricts, or makes the pupil smaller) is innervated by the parasympathetic system (Sidebar 22-1). If we want to block this system in order to dilate the eye, a *parasympatholytic* agent (eg, tropicamide, or Mydriacyl) is used, which paralyzes the iris sphincter along with the ciliary muscle used for accommodation. (The suffix -*lytic* implies the destruction of something.)

The iris dilator muscle is innervated by the sympathetic system, thus one of the actions of the sympathetic system is pupil dilation. If we want to mimic the action of

---

SIDEBAR 22-1

TERMS AND COMBINING FORMS FOR SPEAKING ABOUT THE AUTONOMIC NERVOUS SYSTEM

▶ -olytic: Lysis refers to the decomposition of something

▶ -mimetic: To "mime" is to mimic or copy or to be like something else

▶ Sympathomimetic: Mimicking (having the same action as, or causing the same reaction as, or stimulating of) the sympathetic (nervous system)

▶ Sympatholytic: Causing the decomposition (break down) of the sympathetic (nervous system), thus having a parasympathetic effect

▶ Parasympathomimetic: Mimicking (having the same action as, or causing the same reaction as, or stimulating of) the parasympathetic (nervous system)

▶ Parasympatholytic: Causing the decomposition (break down) of the parasympathetic (nervous system), thus having a sympathetic effect

---

the sympathetic system, a drug called a *sympathomimetic* is used (eg, phenylephrine, or Mydfrin).

Phenylephrine is strictly a mydriatic agent, which means it will dilate the pupil but will not affect accommodation. (It can, however, still cause slightly blurred vision due to the enlarged pupil.) Dilation occurs in 20 to 30 minutes and lasts 3 to 8 hours. This drug is available in 2.5% and 10% strengths.

Only the 2.5% strength of phenylephrine should be used in infants, children, and the elderly due to possible systemic absorption and its effect on the body. The physician should be consulted before instilling phenylephrine in patients with cardiovascular or cerebrovascular disease. It is common to use 2.5% in conjunction with tropicamide to obtain maximal pupil dilation, especially in older patients or those with diabetes.

Phenylephrine also causes vasoconstriction, which is helpful in certain circumstances (such as limiting blood leakage during LASIK on corneas with abnormal peripheral blood vessels). However, if a patient is complaining of a red eye, it is helpful for the ophthalmologist to see the patient before phenylephrine is instilled so the degree of redness can be determined.

Because phenylephrine dilates by stimulating the iris dilator, its effect can be mostly reversed by using a parasympathomimetic drop (such as pilocarpine) that stimulates the iris sphincter muscle, which is stronger than the dilator muscle. Combining pilocarpine with phenylephrine can cause shallowing of the anterior chamber, increasing intraocular pressure.

Hydroxyamphetamine (Paredrine) is a sympathomimetic drug that causes pupil dilation in 15 to 60 minutes. It is most commonly used to determine if a confirmed case of Horner's syndrome is pre- or post-ganglionic, as dilation is poor in post-ganglionic cases.

Cycloplegic drugs are parasympatholytic and thus block the effects of the parasympathetic system. In addition to their mydriatic effect, cycloplegic drops also reduce or paralyze accommodation. Most clinics use tropicamide (0.5% or 1.0%) routinely for dilation. Its action is apparent in 15 to 30 minutes and lasts for 4 to 6 hours.

When a stronger cycloplegic agent is required for a cycloplegic refraction, cyclopentolate 1% (AK-Pentolate or Cyclogyl) is commonly used. It takes effect in 25 to 60 minutes. Pupil dilation can last a few days, but accommodation recovery occurs in 6 to 24 hours. When using cycloplegic drops for the purpose of cycloplegic refractions, it is important to note that inhibition of accommodation does not usually occur simultaneously with pupil dilation. The effect on accommodation can be verified by placing the manifest refraction in front of the patient and ask if the near vision is blurred.

If pupil dilation is desired for therapeutic reasons (eg, uveitis), scopolamine 0.25% (Hyoscine), homatropine 2% or 5%, or atropine 0.5%, 1%, or 2% can be used. Scopolamine has a shorter duration than atropine, but has a stronger action. It affects accommodation for about 3 days. Homatropine is only about one-tenth as potent as atropine and lasts for 1 to 3 days. Atropine has a duration of up to 2 weeks.

Cycloplegic agents should not be used in eyes with narrow- or closed-angle glaucoma.

Dyes

Dyes are important tools for diagnosis in ophthalmology. Dyes used topically on the eye are *vital stains*, which can safely be applied to living tissue.

Fluorescein

The most widely known dye is *fluorescein sodium* (NaFl). Topical application of NaFl permits the detection of corneal lesions and abnormalities including edema, abrasions, and ulcers. Fluorescein directly stains diseased corneal cells. Epithelial defects appear in vivid green fluorescence when the cobalt blue filter of the slit lamp is used (see Figure 12-4). The detection of foreign bodies in the eye is enhanced by dye. It is also a tool for evaluating the lacrimal system, including tear break-up time and lacrimal obstructions. Leakage from wounds in the anterior segment can be detected by observing a tiny, clear stream of aqueous moving through fluorescein dye at the slit lamp (*Seidel's sign*, see Chapter 12). Furthermore, NaFl is

used in applanation tonometry. (For these applications, please see appropriate chapters or check the Index.)

Greater care to avoid contamination is needed with liquid fluorescein than many other ophthalmic pharmaceuticals. NaFl drops are highly susceptible to contamination with *Pseudomonas aeruginosa*.[3] This is one reason fluorescein strips are widely used. These are filter strips impregnated with the dye, which leaches off the strip when moistened.

Fluorescein is used in evaluating the fit of rigid gas-permeable contact lenses by permitting visualization of the tear film under the lens. It can, however, damage soft contact lenses. The eye should be rinsed free of any fluorescein before soft contact lenses are inserted.

Fluorexon is an alternative dye for patients using soft contact lenses as well as hybrid design lenses. It has a larger molecule that is not as easily absorbed as regular NaFl. However, it is also prone to microbial contamination so it is made available in single-dose pipettes. Fluorexon can stain soft contact lenses if it remains on the lens for more than a few minutes, but can often be removed by repeated rinsing with saline. It should not be use in contacts with a water content greater than 60% because of potential permanent colorization.

An intravenous formulation of NaFl is used in ophthalmology for evaluating vascular abnormalities of the retina including macular lesions, central serous choroidopathy, disciform macular degeneration, and diabetic retinopathy (see Figures 30-3 through 30-5). Intravenous fluorescein is also sometimes used to assess anterior segment blood flow, such as vessel abnormalities of the iris. Investigation of aqueous flow is another clinical application of intravenous NaFl.

The most common adverse reaction with intravenous fluorescein is nausea, with vomiting occurring less frequently. Other adverse reactions include fainting, urticaria, and pain on injection. Patients need to be asked about past histories of allergies, including reactions to previous angiography procedures. Emergency kits should be readily available in the case of a more serious adverse reaction.

Rose Bengal and Lissamine Green

Rose bengal dye is widely used in ocular diagnosis. The application of rose bengal produces a vivid pink or magenta staining of damaged or dead tissue when viewed with the slit lamp. Rose bengal is used in the differential diagnosis of dry eye syndromes. Other uses include corneal abrasions and ulcers, conjunctival lesions, and detection of foreign bodies. Rose bengal may be more toxic than other dyes, causing cell death.[4] It can easily stain clothes and soft contact lenses. It may also interfere if used prior to taking a tissue sample to culture for Herpes viruses.

Lissamine green stains mucus, dead cells, and degenerated cells a green to bluish color. It is replacing rose bengal as the preferred agent for conjunctival staining because it causes less local discomfort.[5] The staining effects may be longer lasting than rose bengal, and its clinical uses are similar.

Other Dyes

Indocyanine green (ICG) is an intravenous dye used for retinal and choroidal angiography. ICG angiography employs a diode laser illumination system with an output of 805 nm and barrier filters at 500 and 810 nm. The vasculature of the choroid is more pronounced using indocyanine than fluorescein. However, severe allergic reactions have been reported.

Methylene blue stains devitalized cells, mucus, and corneal nerves. It is meant for external use only. Clinical uses of methylene blue include assessment of the lacrimal sac before dacryocystorhinostomy, by irrigating the sac with the dye. It is also used to outline glaucoma filtering blebs. The area to be treated is "painted" with the methylene blue. Next an argon laser is targeted to the selected site. Side effects can include local irritation to the degree that a topical anesthetic is required. (See Chapter 29 for details about glaucoma.)

Antiglaucoma Agents

Untreated glaucoma leads to visual impairment and blindness. Pharmacotherapy of glaucoma focuses on lowering the intraocular pressure (IOP) by reducing aqueous humor production and/or enhancing aqueous outflow. (See also Appendix D, Common Ophthalmic Medications.)

For most patients, the first-line treatment of glaucoma is *prostaglandin analogues*. Prostaglandin analogues are physiologically similar to hormones. However, hormones are secreted into the blood for distant targets, whereas prostaglandins act in the anatomical vicinity of their secretion. Prostaglandin eye drops increase the outflow of aqueous and are used once daily (typically at bedtime). Drops in this category can cause a change in eye color (especially for lighter colored eyes) and often cause eyelash growth. A more serious side effect is *prostaglandin-associated periorbitopathy* (PAP), where the orbital fat breaks down and the globe sinks back into the orbit (enophthalmos). Some patients will complain of the redness caused by these drops. Latanoprost (Xalatan), travoprost (Travatan), and bimatoprost (Lumigan) are commonly used prostaglandin analogues.

Second-line glaucoma agents are beta blockers, alpha-2 agonists, topical carbonic anhydrase inhibitors, or a combination drop with two of these three agents.

Antagonism (blocking) of the beta receptors in the ciliary body results in the lowering of IOP. *Beta blocker* drops work by decreasing production of aqueous humor (rather than increasing outflow). Five beta blockers have FDA approval in ophthalmic formulation: timolol (Timoptic), levobunolol (Betagan), betaxolol (Betoptic), metipranolol (Betanol), and carteolol (Ocupress). Beta blockers often need to be administered twice a day, but for some patients, once a day is effective. Local effects with topical beta blockers include allergic reactions, corneal anesthesia, cataract progression, and uveitis.

The major concern with beta blockers is the systemic side effects. Beta blockers can cause bradycardia (slow heart rate), hypotension, and bronchoconstriction (narrowing of airways). Beta blockers are contraindicated with a preexisting bradycardia or a greater than first-degree heart block (when impulses through the heart are slowed). Beta blockers (with the exception of betaxolol) are also contraindicated in patients with asthma. Betaxolol is selective for β_1 receptors. Since the lungs have β_2 receptors, betaxolol may be safely used in many patients with asthma. However, betaxolol is less effective at lowering IOP than other topical beta blockers.

Activation of alpha-2 (adrenergic) receptors in the ciliary body reduces the production of aqueous humor and increases drainage. Brimonidine (Alphagan) is the most commonly used *alpha-2 agonist*. (An agonist activates the receptors.) The typical dosage is three times daily when used by itself, but often just twice a day when used with other glaucoma drops. Local side effects include burning, stinging, hyperemia (redness), foreign body sensation, and a slight miotic effect. Because of the miosis, brimonidine is sometimes prescribed for postoperative laser refractive surgery patients who suffer from night vision effects (such as halos and low-contrast visual acuity). This keeps the pupil smaller, decreasing the degree of aberrations.

Aqueous humor production requires the presence of bicarbonate. Carbonate anhydrase is a key enzyme in the formation of bicarbonate in the ciliary epithelium. By inhibiting the carbonate anhydrase, the synthesis of bicarbonate is retarded, resulting in a decrease in aqueous humor production. Drugs that inhibit carbonate anhydrase are termed *carbonic anhydrase inhibitors* (CAIs).

The first CAIs were administered systemically to treat blood pressure, and are acetazolamide (Diamox) and methazolamide (Neptazane). Numerous systemic side effects can occur with acetazolamide, including numbness and tingling of the toes and fingers, a metallic taste, and gastrointestinal upset. The gastrointestinal upset can usually be minimized by taking it with food. Because bicarbonate is also key in keeping the blood plasma at the proper pH, metabolic acidosis (too much acid in the blood) can occur, typically with acetazolamide. A potential severe complication is renal calculi producing kidney stones. Contraindications for taking oral CAIs include severe renal or hepatic disease, severe chronic obstructive pulmonary disease (COPD), and a history of a major allergic reaction to sulfonamides. Methazolamide may be better tolerated in patients with COPD, and is less likely to cause renal calculi than acetazolamide.

The routine use of oral CAIs for treating glaucoma has been replaced by topical CAIs, including dorzolamide (Trusopt) and brinzolamide (Azopt). The usual dose is three times a day. Local side effects include stinging, foreign body sensation, blurring of vision, and superficial punctate keratitis (tiny erosions on the corneal surface). The topical CAIs do not achieve the same magnitude of IOP as oral CAIs. Therefore, some patients are still treated with acetazolamide or methazolamide. There is no additive therapeutic advantage when taking topical CAIs along with oral CAIs.

Sometimes a patient may benefit from a combination of a beta blocker and alpha antagonist or CAI. To make this easier for the patient, combination drops exist. Combigan consists of timolol and brimonidine, and Cosopt contains timolol and dorzolamide. The dosage of either drop is twice per day.

The *Rho-associated protein kinase* (ROCK) *inhibitors* are an emerging treatment for glaucoma. ROCK is an enzyme involved in the maintenance of the cytoskeleton of the cell. (The physiological functions of the cytoskeleton include cellular movement, migration, and adhesion.) Smooth muscle contraction is thus regulated by ROCK. In the trabecular meshwork, ROCK stimulates tissue contraction, resulting in decreased aqueous humor drainage thus increasing IOP. ROCK inhibitors cause relaxation of the trabecular meshwork, lowering ocular pressure. Another potential benefit of ROCK inhibitors is improvement of blood flow to the optic nerve (creating a neuroprotective effect) which is an area in glaucoma that current pharmacotherapy does not address. An obstacle with developing ROCK inhibitors for ocular use is creating agents that are selective for the ocular tissues (to minimize side effects). Nevertheless, these drugs are undergoing clinical trials to evaluate their safety and effectiveness in the treatment of glaucoma.

An older class of medications used to treat glaucoma is the cholinergic agonists. Topical cholinergic agonists are also called miotics because they cause miosis (pupil constriction). Pilocarpine (1%, 2%, or 4%) is a direct-acting agonist for muscarinic receptors in the iris sphincter muscle and in the ciliary body. (Remember, there are two types of cholinergic receptors: muscarinic and nicotinic.) Stimulation of the ciliary body causes the scleral spur to widen the trabecular spaces, thus increasing aqueous outflow. Pilocarpine also directly stimulates the outflow tissue even in the absence of an intact ciliary muscle. Pilocarpine needs to be administered four times a day. A gel form of pilocarpine is available that can be applied once a day at bedtime.

Blue irides respond more to pilocarpine than dark eyes. In younger patients, pilocarpine causes spasms of the ciliary body, producing unwanted accommodation (making the eye temporarily nearsighted). Use of this drop also brings an increased risk for detached retina.

Systemically, pilocarpine activates cholinergic receptors in the lungs, precipitating an asthma attack in susceptible patients. Pilocarpine can also directly stimulate cholinergic receptors in the heart, producing bradycardia.

Pilocarpine 0.125% is also used for diagnosing third-nerve palsy (see Chapter 10). The 0.125% strength can be made by a pharmacy, or in the office by combining one drop of pilocarpine 2% with 15 drops of sterile saline 0.9%.

Hyperosmotics

Hyperosmotic agents are used in the acute treatment of angle-closure glaucoma. They work by osmosis, a process by which molecules of a solvent (fluid in which a substance is dissolved) pass through a semipermeable membrane from a less concentrated solution (of solvent) to a more concentrated solution. Hyperosmotics increase the osmolarity of the blood and thus "pull" water from the eye into the blood. The loss of fluid in the eye (especially from the vitreous humor) reduces the IOP. The reduction in IOP starts in 15 minutes to 2 hours. The effects only last approximately 6 to 8 hours so they are for temporary use. Hyperosmotic agents include mannitol (Osmitrol), glycerin (Osmoglyn), and isosorbide (Ismotic). Mannitol is administered intravenously, whereas glycerin and isosorbide are given orally. (It is sickly sweet, so is served over ice to be sipped slowly.) Increased urination results from the administration of hyperosmotics. Contraindications to hyperosmotics include renal failure, severe dehydration, pulmonary edema, and congestive heart failure.

Anti-Infective Agents

Infections are caused by microorganisms including bacteria, viruses, fungi, and protozoans. Drugs used to fight infection are antimicrobials or anti-infectives. For information on microbes and their identification, see Chapter 23.

Antibacterials (Antibiotics)

Antibacterials treat bacterial infections. In clinical practice, the term antibiotic is used as a synonym for antibacterial, and here we will use these terms interchangeably.

Fortified antibiotics are made by compounding pharmacies by adding injectable antibiotics into the commercially available topical products. Their use decreased substantially with the introduction of the ophthalmic fluoroquinolones but are sometimes used to treat corneal ulcers. These preparations must be handled carefully and expiration dates (as set by the pharmacist) must be strictly adhered to.

Penicillins

Penicillin is the prototype antibiotic. The term "penicillin" refers to the antibiotics penicillin V and penicillin G. "Penicillin" also refers to the class of antibiotics containing molecular derivatives of the penicillin molecule. The penicillin class belongs to a broader class of antibacterials known as the *beta lactams*. Beta lactams work by impairing the cell wall of bacteria and work mainly against the genus *Streptococcus* and certain gram-negative bacteria.

Penicillin G is not absorbed orally and must be given by injection. Penicillin V is effective orally. Over the years, the original penicillin molecule was modified to expand the spectrum of activity or to fight resistant bacteria. Many strains of *Staphylococcus* began to synthesize penicillinase to destroy penicillin's structure, providing resistance to that drug. Methicillin, oxacillin, dicloxacillin, and nafcillin were developed to overcome the action of penicillinase. Ticarcillin, piperacillin, and mezlocillin are penicillins with activity against *Pseudomonas aeruginosa*. The main clinical side effects of penicillin are allergic reactions ranging from rash to anaphylaxis.

Cephalosporins

Cephalosporins are another class of beta lactam antibiotics. Although no cephalosporins are commercially available as ophthalmic formulations, they are used in oral and injectable forms to fight ocular infections.

There are five generations of cephalosporins. The first generation includes cefazolin (Kefzol, Ancef) and cephalexin (Keflex). The antibacterial activity of cefazolin and cephalexin is primarily against gram-positive organisms such as *Staphylococcus* and *Streptococcus*. Cefazolin eye drops, which need to be compounded by the pharmacist, are used for treating corneal ulcers.

Second-generation cephalosporins include cefaclor (Ceclor), cefuroxime (Ceftin), cefprozil (Cefzil), cefoxitin (Mefoxin), and cefotetan (Cefotan). Second-generation cephalosporins have increased activity against gram-negative bacteria including *Haemophilus influenzae*. Cefotetan has activity against bowel anaerobes (bacteria not requiring oxygen).

Third-generation cephalosporins have reduced gram-positive coverage, but more activity against enteric gram-negative bacteria. Third-generation cephalosporins include cefixime (Suprax), cefdinir (Omnicef), cefotaxime (Claforan), cefditoren (Spectracef), ceftazidime (Fortaz), and ceftriaxone (Rocephin). Ceftazidime has antipseudomonal activity. Intravenous ceftazidime, in combination with intravenous vancomycin, is used to prevent infections secondary to rupture of the globe.

The fourth-generation cephalosporin is cefepime (Maxipime). Cefepime has activity against beta lactamase-producing bacteria and *Pseudomonas*. Ceftaroline (Teflaro) is a fifth-generation cephalosporin with activity against methicillin-resistant *Staphylococcus aureus* (MRSA) and gram-positive bacteria. Cross-sensitivity allergic reactions with cephalosporins and penicillins can occur because they are both beta lactams. The cross sensitivity is approximately 1% between cephalosporins (first and second generation only) and penicillins.

Other Antibiotics

Bacitracin is a topical antibiotic with activity against *Staphylococcus* and *Streptococcus*, but virtually no gram-negative coverage. Topically, it is used to treat skin infections. Ophthalmic bacitracin is used for superficial eye infections such as blepharitis. Bacitracin inhibits the movement of mucopeptides into the cell wall. (Mucopeptides are responsible for the structure and integrity of the bacterial cell wall.) The main side effect of topical bacitracin is hypersensitivity (rare).

Aminoglycosides have activity against *Staphylococcus aureus*, but not *Streptococcus*. The main clinical use of aminoglycosides is against gram-negative organisms. Aminoglycosides work by inhibiting protein synthesis in the bacteria, and include neomycin, streptomycin, gentamicin, tobramycin, and amikacin. Neomycin is often combined with bacitracin in commercial preparations to add gram-negative coverage. A drawback of neomycin is a high rate (approximately 4%) of hypersensitive reactions.[6] Both gentamicin and tobramycin are commercially available as ophthalmic solutions. The main side effects with local aminoglycosides are local irritation and toxicity.

Tetracyclines include tetracycline, oxytetracycline, demeclocycline, doxycycline, and minocycline. Tetracyclines work by inhibiting protein synthesis. A special niche for tetracyclines is the treatment of infections caused by intracellular bacteria (ie, bacteria that penetrate into the host cells), such as *Chlamydia*. Oral tetracyclines are used as a treatment for acne. Tetracycline and doxycycline are used to treat noninfected corneal ulcers. Tetracyclines are contraindicated in patients who are pregnant or breast feeding. They are also contraindicated in children younger than 8 years because of the potential to cause permanent tooth discoloration. Numerous food interactions occur with tetracycline, and patients should discuss these interactions with their pharmacist.

Macrolides are a group of antibiotics that include erythromycin, clarithromycin (Biaxin), and azithromycin (Zithromax). Erythromycin is used against gram-positive cocci, *Mycoplasma pneumonia*, *Chlamydia trachomatis*, *Chlamydia pneumoniae*, and *Borrelia burgdorferi*. Azithromycin and clarithromycin have activity against *H. influenzae*. Topical erythromycin ointment is commonly used for treating staphylococcal infections of the eyelid. The most common side effect with oral macrolides is gastrointestinal upset, and they should be administered with food. Erythromycin and clarithromycin have numerous cytochrome drug interactions. (Cytochromes are enzymes that help detoxify matter that is absorbed by or administered in the body, including many drugs.)

Sulfonamides are a group of antibiotics that inhibit the bacterial synthesis of folic acid. By blocking folic acid synthesis, the production of DNA and protein is impaired. The most common sulfonamide is sulfamethoxazole. Allergic reactions, including Stevens-Johnson syndrome, are a concern with the sulfonamides. Photosensitivity is another side effect. Adequate hydration is needed when patients are on sulfonamides to prevent crystals forming in the urinary tract.

Trimethoprim is a nonsulfonamide drug that also inhibits folic acid synthesis. It is combined with sulfonamides in the products Bactrim, Bactrim DS, Septra, and Septra DS. The sulfonamide/trimethoprim combination is used to treat *Toxoplasma gondii* infections of the eye.

The *fluoroquinolones* are a group of antibacterial drugs that inhibit bacterial DNA synthesis. Fluoroquinolones include ciprofloxacin (Cipro), ofloxacin (Floxin), levofloxacin (Levaquin), lomefloxacin (Maxiquin), norfloxacin (Noroxin), gatifloxacin (Zymar), and moxifloxacin (Avelox). Common uses of fluoroquinolones include urinary tract infections, upper respiratory tract infections, and lower respiratory tract infections. Oral fluoroquinolones should not be administered at the same time as calcium, iron, magnesium, and antacids because they impair absorption of the antibiotic. A potentially serious complication of fluoroquinolones is rupture of the tendons; elderly patients may be more at risk for this. Routine use of fluoroquinolones is not recommended in children or pregnant women.

Topical fluoroquinolones are used in the treatment of conjunctivitis and corneal ulcers. Ciprofloxacin (Ciloxan), ofloxacin (Ocuflox), besifloxacin (Besivance), moxifloxacin (Vigamox, Moxeza), and gatifloxacin (Zymaxid) are commercially available as ophthalmic preparations.

Vancomycin is a drug that inhibits synthesis of the bacterial cell wall. The antibacterial activity of vancomycin includes staphylococci, streptococci, and *Clostridium difficile*. Vancomycin is not absorbed orally, so the only indication for oral vancomycin is treatment of pseudomembranous colitis from *C. difficile*. Vancomycin is used intravenously to treat suspected or confirmed cases of MRSA. Intravenous and intravitreal vancomycin is used for treating endophthalmitis. Vancomycin is not commercially available in ophthalmic formulations, but can be compounded by a pharmacy that has equipment for handling sterile solutions. Topical vancomycin is used for treating corneal infections. Complications of intravenous vancomycin include ototoxity (toxicity to the ear, including loss of hearing) and renal damage. A common hypersensitivity reaction from vancomycin is the "red man syndrome," which includes itching and a red rash on the face, neck, and upper torso. Red man syndrome is not a true allergy.

Antivirals

Antiviral drugs are used for treating viral infections, and have been developed to treat HIV, herpes viruses, hepatitis, and influenza. The goal of an antiviral is to treat (ie, ease the symptoms) rather than cure infection. Most antivirals work at the nucleic acid level.

Acyclovir is commercially available in capsules, topical ointment (dermal), and intravenous formulation. Acyclovir works by incorporating itself into the viral DNA. It is used to treat genital *Herpes simplex* (HSV), *Herpes zoster* (shingles), HSV encephalitis, and *Varicella zoster* (chicken pox). Acyclovir is used off label to treat ocular HSV infections and varicella zoster viral infections of the eye, including keratitis, blepharoconjunctivitis, retinal necrosis, and uveitis. The most common side effect of acyclovir is gastrointestinal intolerance, including nausea, vomiting, abdominal pain, and diarrhea. Rarer side effects include photosensitivity, dizziness, lethargy, and hallucinations.

Cytomegalovirus (CMV) is a type of Herpes virus. However, acyclovir has no significant clinical activity against CMV. *Ganciclovir* (Cytovene) was the first drug approved for treating CMV retinitis. Ganciclovir has a mechanism of action similar to acyclovir, but is more toxic.

Valganciclovir is prodrug of ganciclovir that is rapidly metabolized to ganciclovir by enzymes in the liver and intestine. It is commonly used outside of ophthalmology to reduce the risk of infection in patients with organ transplants.

Foscarnet (Foscavir) inhibits DNA synthesis. Foscarnet has activity against CMV strains that are resistant to ganciclovir. The major drawback with foscarnet is kidney dysfunction and the need for hydration. Changes in electrolytes, including potassium, calcium, magnesium, and phosphate levels, are a common reaction to foscarnet. *Cidofovir* (Vistide) is another antiviral that works against resistant CMV infections of the retina. Its mechanism of action is inhibition of viral DNA enzymes, affecting DNA replication. However, cidofovir is very toxic to the kidneys.

Topical antivirals for use in the eye center mainly around the treatment of corneal infections caused by *Herpes simplex*, *H. varicella*, and *H. zoster*. *Trifluridine* drops (Viroptic) and *vidarabine* (Vira-A) drops and ointment are commonly used for this purpose. Side effects include burning and stinging. Redness, irritation, itching, swelling, and blurred vision have also been known to occur.

Antifungals

Antifungal drugs fight fungal infections. Many antifungal drugs work by inhibiting ergosterol, a key component of the fungal cell membrane. Ergosterol does not occur in plant or animal cells, making it an attractive "target" for these drugs.

The *azoles* are a common class of antifungals that includes clotrimazole, ketoconazole (Nizoral), miconazole, itraconazole, and fluconazole. Ketoconazole's primary activity is against *Candida albicans*, with weaker activity against *Aspergillus*, but it can have potential deadly interactions. Itraconazole (Sporanox) largely replaced the use of ketoconazole in general medicine but has poor ocular penetration.

Fluconazole (Diflucan) has good ocular penetration with oral or intravenous use.[7] It has good activity against *Candida* and *Cryptococcus*, but weak activity against *Aspergillus*. Fluconazole eye drops are used to treat keratitis and endophthalmitis caused by susceptible organisms.

Amphotericin B is a drug used in general medicine to treat systemic life-threatening infections of *Aspergillus*. Amphotericin B increases the permeability of the fungal cell membrane, causing electrolyte imbalances, but it is not effective orally. A topical ophthalmic formulation of amphotericin B is not commercially available, but can be prepared by a compounding pharmacy to treat corneal fungal infections. Intravitreal injections of amphotericin B have been used to treat endophthalmitis due to fungi.

Natamycin 5% (Natacyn) is the antifungal agent commercially available in an ophthalmic preparation. Natamycin has activity against *Fuscarium*, *Aspergillus*, *Curvularia*, and *Acremonium*. Natamycin works by binding with an essential compound in the cell walls of the fungus.

Anti-Inflammatory Drugs

Drugs used to treat inflammation include corticosteroids and nonsteroidal anti-inflammatory drugs (NSAIDs). Both corticosteroids and NSAIDs work by inhibiting the activity of prostaglandins (hormone-like compounds that are produced by injured tissue, causing inflammation). Corticosteroids inhibit the production of arachidonic acid, which is necessary for prostaglandin formation. NSAIDs directly inhibit the synthesis of the prostaglandins.

Corticosteroids

Corticosteroids, most of which are derivatives of cortisol, are not to be confused with anabolic steroids (testosterone derivatives), which are used to build muscle mass. The prototype corticosteroid is hydrocortisone. Corticosteroids suppress the immune system, making them useful for treating a variety of autoimmune disorders including allergies. Other ophthalmic uses for topical corticosteroids include reduction of inflammation after surgery and in chemical burns, acne rosacea keratitis, scleritis, retinal vasculitis (inflammation of blood vessels associated with the retinal artery), compressed optic nerve, and ocular myasthenia gravis. Anterior chamber disorders typically respond well to topical corticosteroids. Deeper diseases involving the optic nerve, posterior segment, or orbit typically require either oral or intravenous therapy.

Prednisolone acetate is commercially available in 1% (Pred Forte) and 0.125% (Pred Mild). Dexamethasone is available as 0.1% ophthalmic suspension (Maxidex). Loteprednol etabonate is a derivative of prednisolone and is available in a 0.5% ophthalmic gel (Lotemax Gel) and an ophthalmic ointment (Lotemax). Altrex is a 0.2% formulation of loteprednol etabonate. Rimexolone (Vexol) is another derivative of prednisolone. It has FDA approval for treating uveitis and postoperative inflammation.

Fluorometholone (FML) is a structural derivative of progesterone rather than cortisol. It is less likely to elevate IOP than dexamethasone or prednisolone (see next paragraph). However, dexamethasone and prednisolone have greater potency than fluorometholone. Medrysone is another derivative of progesterone, and is the weakest topical steroid for ophthalmic use.[8]

Topical steroids are commonly used in ophthalmology. However, they have numerous adverse reactions, including suppression of the immune system's response to bacterial, viral, and fungal infections. Corticosteroids are also well known to cause posterior subcapsular cataracts. Prolonged corticosteroid use can raise IOP and even lead to glaucoma. The typical onset for development of elevated IOP is 2 weeks, but may take several more.

Nonsteroidal Anti-Inflammatory Drugs

NSAIDs also inhibit inflammation. Most of the NSAIDs also inhibit coagulation (blood clotting).

The most well-known NSAID is aspirin. In the past, aspirin was used to treat fever in children. However, aspirin was linked to Reye's syndrome (a potentially fatal condition involving swelling of the brain and liver) when used in children or teenagers with influenza or chicken pox. Thus, the most frequent use of aspirin today is prophylaxis of heart attacks in adults. Common uses of other NSAIDs include treatment of fever that does not respond to acetaminophen and pain (especially affecting the musculoskeletal system). Potentially serious adverse reactions to systemic NSAIDs include gastrointestinal bleeding and renal failure.

Overall, topical NSAIDs are less effective than steroids at decreasing inflammation, but NSAIDs do not increase IOP. The first ophthalmic NSAID was flurbiprofen 0.3% solution (Ocufen), which was FDA approved to maintain pupil dilation during cataract surgery. Suprofen 1% suspension and diclofenac (Voltaren) were later approved for the same purpose. Bromfenac 0.09% solution (Xibrom) received FDA approval for treating post surgical pain associated with cataract surgery. Ketorolac (Acular) 0.5% is indicated for treating allergic conjunctivitis. Acular LS is a 0.4% solution with FDA approval for treating pain following corneal refractive surgery. Acular LS has less concentration of benzalkonium chloride and edetate disodium than Acular. The lower concentrations of inactive and active ingredients are to reduce the stinging in postoperative patients.

Nepafenac 0.1% (Nevanac) is a prodrug that is converted to amfenac (also an NSAID) in the anterior chamber. The advantage of using a prodrug is that higher intraocular concentrations are achieved than with other topical NSAIDs.

Off-label indications of topical NSAIDs include treatment of pain after cataract or refractive surgery (in some drugs), treatment of inflammation associated with glaucoma, and treatment of corneal abrasions. Topical NSAIDs have minimal side effects but can cause local irritation.

Immunosuppressives

The purpose of *immunosuppressive* drugs is to decrease activity of the immune system. Cyclosporine A is an immunosuppressive agent that works by inhibiting the production and release of proteins that boost the immune system. The original use of cyclosporine was the prophylaxis of organ rejection in transplants involving the kidney, heart, and liver by blocking the immune response. Cyclosporine was also used to treat severe cases of rheumatoid arthritis.

Ophthalmic cyclosporine (Restasis) is indicated for treating decreased tear production due to keratoconjunctivitis sicca-associated ocular inflammation. Cyclosporine A is used off label to treat allergic conjunctivitis. A compounded cyclosporine A 2% has been used to treat certain types of superficial punctate keratitis.

Medications Used for Allergies

A number of drugs are used for treating the symptoms of allergies, including antihistamines, decongestants, and mast cell stabilizers.

Histamine is a compound in the body (released by mast cells) that regulates the inflammatory and immune response as well as acid activity in the stomach. It functions as a neurotransmitter, binding with specific proteins (receptors) of cells in the body. These receptors are designated as H_1 through H_4. The most relevant histamine receptors pharmacologically are the H_1 and H_2 receptors. Physiological effects of histamine include bronchial constriction, dilation of blood vessels, increased permeability of blood vessels, and sensory nerve stimulation. *Antihistamines* work by blocking histamine.

H_2 receptor antagonists are often used in combination with H_1 antagonists and epinephrine to treat severe reactions, including anaphylactoid events.

Commercially available ophthalmic antihistamines include antazoline, pheniramine, ketotifen (Zaditor), olopatadine (Pataday, Patanol), and emedastine (Emadine). Some of these are available in combination with a decongestant (see next paragraph). Side effects of topical antihistamines are generally limited to mild irritation.

Decongestants are drugs that relieve congestion (swelling, inflammation, and mucus production) by constricting of blood vessels. Common oral decongestants include pseudoephedrine and phenylephrine. Side effects of decongestants include increased blood pressure, nervousness, and insomnia. Caution is warranted when used by patients with hypertension, certain heart problems, hyperthyroidism, and diabetes mellitus.

A potential serious adverse reaction of both topical and systemic decongestants is precipitation of an acute angle-closure glaucoma attack. In this case, the decongestant has caused a degree of pupil dilation and subsequent blockage of the structure in the eye that drains aqueous. IOP can build up quickly, and can cause irreversible damage to the optic nerve. (For more on this topic, see Chapter 29). Thus topical decongestants are contraindicated in patients at risk for angle closure glaucoma.

Topically applied ophthalmic decongestants that are commercially available include phenylephrine, naphazoline, oxymetazoline, and tetrahydrozoline. There are many brand names, and some are combined with antihistamines. A common use of ophthalmic decongestants is in the treatment of allergies, including allergic conjunctivitis. Transient stinging is the most common local reaction. *Rebound redness* can occur with prolonged use. However, what is considered "chronic use" is not clear. One study found no rebound vasodilation after 10 days' use of naphazoline and tetrahydrozoline.[9] The effectiveness of tetrahydrozoline, however, was reduced after the 10-day period.[9] In addition, these drops are counterproductive in patients with dry eye, since the chemicals act to dehydrate the eye further.

As discussed above, mast cells produce histamine. *Mast cell stabilizers* act to quiet the mast cells to prevent histamine release. Those available for ocular use include cromolyn (Opticrom), lodoxamide (Alomide), nedocromil (Alocril), and pemirolast (Alamast). Mast cell stabilizers are used to treat allergic conditions of the eye affecting the conjunctiva and cornea. Side effects are generally limited to mild local irritation.

Drugs for Retinal Disease

A number of drugs are used for treating retinal diseases, including photodynamic agents, antiangiogenesis agents (prevent formation of new blood vessels), and monoclonal antibodies (immune cells that [among other things] bind only to one specific receptor).

Photodynamic therapy (PDT) uses nontoxic light-sensitive agents that become toxic once exposed to light in the presence of oxygen. The toxicity is the result of the generation of free radicals. PDT is used to kill diseased cells. A common use of PDT outside of ophthalmology is for treating cancer.

Verteporfin (Visudyne) is used in PDT for treating abnormal growth of blood vessels in age-related macular degeneration. The procedure involves administering verteporfin intravenously. A red laser light is then targeted to the affected areas of the eye. Off-label uses of verteporfin include pathologic myopia, multifocal choroiditis (inflammation of choroid, retina, and vitreous), angioid streaks, and choroidal rupture. Common side effects include burning or swelling at the site of injection, back pain, dry eyes or skin, itchiness of the eyes, and muscle pain. Protection from light, including high-intensity indoor light, is needed for 5 days. Serious adverse reactions include anaphylaxis.

Angiogenesis is the physiological process by which new blood vessels are generated from existing blood vessels. Proteins needed for angiogenesis include vascular endothelial growth factor (VEGF). Inhibition of VEGF, the prevue of *antiangiogenesic* drugs, has become an important pharmacological weapon for treating retinal disease.

Pegaptanib (Macugen) is a nucleic acid derivative that is a VEGF antagonist (anti-VEGF). It has FDA approval for treating wet age-related macular degeneration and is administered by intravitreal injection. Minor side effects include ocular pain and swelling, blurred vision, and visual disturbances. A potential complication from these injections is endophthalmitis.

Monoclonal antibodies have also been developed to seek out and inhibit VEGF. Because they bind only to one specific receptor, they can be targeted to specific cells. Ranibizumab (Lucentis) and aflibercept (Eylea) are approved for treating wet age-related macular degeneration. They are administered as an intravitreal injection usually once a month. Bevacizumab (Avastin) is a monoclonal antibody for metastatic colorectal cancer, certain types of lung cancer, and glioblastoma (aggressive tumors of the brain and spinal cord). Bevacizumab has been studied off-label as a treatment for AMD, macular edema, and diabetic retinopathy.

Dry Eye Treatment

Dry eye is actually a complex disorder. At its most simple, it results from a decreased production of tears or an increased evaporation of tears. It is often complicated, however, by underlying or resultant inflammation of the ocular tissues.

Artificial Lubricants

A variety of agents are used as artificial lubricants. The primary ingredient in artificial tears is water. Additional ingredients are added to improve viscosity, maintain isotonicity, maintain sterility, adjust pH, and promote tear stability. Polymer-based lubricants are the most frequently used product for treatment of dry eye. (Polymers are made up of chains of large molecules.) The polymers include methylcellulose, dextran, propylene glycol, polyethylene glycol, povidone, and polyvinyl alcohol. The most common polymers are cellulose-based. (Cellulose is the main component in the cell walls of plants.)

The primary difference among artificial tear solutions is the *viscosity* (how easily a liquid flows). Patients with a mild dry eye often prefer a less viscous (more watery) product whereas patients with more severe dry eye may prefer a more viscous agent. The higher viscosity agents stay on the ocular surface longer but blur the vision more. Higher viscosity agents can also trap allergens on the eye.

Frequent use of preserved artificial tears may produce toxicity to the cornea. Patients using artificial tears more than four times a day should use preservative-free. In addition, preservative-free eye drops may be better tolerated by post surgical patients. The disadvantages of preservative-free solutions are increased cost and more manual dexterity to handle the tiny, single-dose containers. Preservative-free solutions are also prone to microbial contamination, so it is important to discard any unused portion. Another option for patients who are sensitive to regular preservatives is the use of tear drops with preservatives that dissipate upon exposure to light, such as Blink Tears.

Gel formulations can be considered for patients with persisting symptoms after a trial with artificial tears. Nonmedicated tear ointment is indicated for moderate to severe dry eye. Ointments are retained in the eye longer than the liquid-based lubricants and thus are generally only used at bedtime because of blurred vision. Ointments should be avoided in patients with corneal abrasions or lacerations.

Prescription Treatments

Ophthalmic cyclosporine (Restasis) is a prescription preparation indicated for treating decreased tear production due to ocular inflammation, and is not a lubricant. Lifitegrast (Xiidra) binds to protein on the surface of white blood cells. It blocks the adhesion of T-cells (which are part of the immune response) and blocks the release of cytokines (molecules that stimulate inflammatory cells to report to the affected locality).

Sealants

Ophthalmic sealants are used to prevent fluid leaks. ReSure Sealant, consisting of polyethylene glycol, has received FDA approval for use in the prevention of post-surgical fluid leaks from incisions following cataract surgery. This polyethylene glycol product serves as an alternative to sutures. Other sealants are used off-label. Cyanoacrylate is used to seal perforated corneal ulcers. Fibrin glue is used to secure conjunctival tissue in pterygium surgery.

Botulinum

Botulinum is a toxin produced naturally by the bacterium *Clostridium botulinum* and related species. The disease botulism results from poisoning with botulinum toxin. Botulinum inhibits the release of acetylcholine from motor neurons, producing paralysis in muscles. Ophthalmic uses of botulinum include strabismus following extraocular muscle surgery, CN VI palsies, esotropia, CN III palsies, and certain types of diplopia.

Commercially available botulinum, under the brand names Botox and Oculinum, comes in a freeze-dried form and needs to be reconstituted with saline solution. The physician injects the product into the relevant muscle. Muscle paralysis lasts for several weeks because a nerve axon on the nerve terminal needs to be generated in order for the effects to wear off. The main risk of botulinum injection is the spread of the toxin beyond the targeted site of action. For example, spread of the toxin to the medial rectus produces a ptosis. Systemic absorption could cause symptoms of botulism including respiratory difficulties, trouble swallowing, and blurred vision.

OCULAR EFFECTS OF SYSTEMIC DRUGS

While the focus of this chapter is ocular pharmacology, it bears mentioning that some systemic medications affect the eyes. In certain cases, this is what we desire (as in hyperosmotics or pain relief). In other cases, however, these ocular side effects can be quite serious. Table 22-4 provides an overview of some common medications that can have a marked effect on the eye and/or vision.

ACKNOWLEDGMENTS

The authors would like to thank the following: Kathryn Pokorny, PhD; Steven M. Cohen, BA; and David Chu, MD.

TABLE 22-4
OCULAR EFFECTS OF SELECT SYSTEMIC MEDICATIONS

Medication	Class	Clinical Use	Ocular Effects
Alendronate (Fosamax)	Biphosphates	Osteoporosis	Conjunctivitis, episcleritis, scleritis, uveitis
Amiodarone (Cordarone)	Anti-arrhythmic	Atrial fibrillation	Whorl-like opacities of the cornea
Amphetamines (Dexedrine, Adderall), methylphenidate (Ritalin), pseudoephedrine (Sudafed)	Stimulants	Attention deficit hyperactivity disorder, narcolepsy, congestion (pseudoephedrine)	Precipitation of angle-closure glaucoma
Atovaquone (Mepron)	Antiprotozoal	Treatment or prophylaxis of *Pneumocystis jiroveci* pneumonia	Whorl-like opacities of the cornea
Atropine, glycopyrrolate, benztropine	Anticholinergic	Hypersalivation, treatment of side effects of antipsychotics	Dry eyes, precipitation of angle-closure glaucoma
Busulfan (Myleran)	Chemotherapy	Chronic myeloid leukemia	Cataracts
Carbamazepine (Tegretol)	Mood stabilizer/ anticonvulsant	Bipolar disorder, epilepsy	Double vision
Chloroquine (Aralen), hydroxychloroquine (Plaquenil)	Quinolines	Rheumatoid arthritis, systemic lupus erythematosus	Whorl-like opacities of the cornea
Chlorpromazine (Thorazine)	Phenothiazines	Antipsychotic	Corneal pigment changes, anterior subcapsular cataract
Digoxin (Lanoxin) and digitalis	Cardiac glycosides	Congestive heart failure, atrial fibrillation	Snowy vision, alterations in color vision
Etanercept (Enbrel)	Tumor necrosis factor blocking agent	Rheumatoid arthritis, plaque psoriasis	Ocular inflammation
Ethambutol (Myambutol)	Antitubular agent	Pulmonary tuberculosis	Optic neuritis
Indomethacin (Indocin)	NSAID	Anti-inflammatory	Whorl-like opacities of the cornea
Isotretinoin (Accutane)	Vitamin A derivative	Acne	Corneal opacities, neovascularization of the cornea, blepharoconjunctivitis
Lithium	Mood stabilizer	Bipolar disorder	Lateral gaze nystagmus
Morphine, oxycodone, hydrocodone, hydromorphone	Opiates	Painkillers	Pinpoint pupils in overdose (although mydriasis occurs if hypoxia is present)
Prednisone (Deltasone), dexamethasone (Decadron)	Corticosteroids	Anti-inflammatory	Subcapsular cataracts
Rifabutin (Mycobutin)	Antitubular agent	Prevention of disseminated *Mycobacterium avium* complex	Uveitis
Tamoxifen (Nolvadex)	Estrogen receptor antagonist	Breast cancer	Retinopathy with crystalline deposits in inner retina
Tamsulosin (Flomax)	Alpha-1 blocker	Benign prostatic hypertrophy	Intraoperative floppy iris syndrome
Topiramate (Topamax)	Anticonvulsant	Epilepsy	Acute-onset myopia

CHAPTER QUIZ

1. Preservatives and stabilizers are considered:
    a. buffers
    b. inactive ingredients
    c. anti-infectives
    d. too toxic to be used in ophthalmic medications

2. When a drug is granted Food and Drug Administration approval for a specific disorder, this is considered a(n):
    a. off-label indication
    b. labeled indication
    c. unlabeled indication
    d. illegal use

3. An advantage of an ophthalmic medication in ointment form is:
    a. prolonged contact
    b. promotes clear vision
    c. increases potency of the drug
    d. decreased viscosity

4. Which of the following is *not* a preservative?
    a. benzalkonium chloride
    b. thimerosal
    c. EDTA
    d. polyvinyl alcohol

5. Buffering agents are added to eye drops in order to:
    a. add color
    b. adjust the pH
    c. adjust the tonicity
    d. increase the shelf life

6. The eye can generally tolerate an eye medication with a sodium chloride tonicity of:
    a. 0.3 to 2.7 parts per million
    b. 20 to 40 mg
    c. 0.5% to 1.8%
    d. 3.0% to 5.9%

7. Which of the following is *not* an example of an allergic reaction?
    a. itching
    b. rash
    c. anaphylaxis
    d. drowsiness

8. Which of the following is a cycloplegic?
    a. tropicamide
    b. phenylephrine
    c. cyclopentolate
    d. cyclosporine

9. Which of the following are *not* used to treat glaucoma?
    a. prostaglandin analogues
    b. carbonic anhydrase inhibitors
    c. beta blockers
    d. mydriatics

10. Anti-infective agents include all of the following *except*:
    a. antibiotics
    b. antisteroids
    c. antivirals
    d. antifungals

11. Which of the following might be used to treat HIV?
    a. antiviral drugs
    b. antifungal drugs
    c. anti-VEGF drugs
    d. mast cell stabilizers

12. Drugs used to fight inflammation include:
    a. antihistamines and decongestants
    b. alpha and beta blockers
    c. corticosteroids and NSAIDs
    d. mydriatics and cycloplegics

13. Which of the following is *not* used for treating the symptoms of allergies?
    a. antihistamines
    b. decongestants
    c. mast cell stabilizers
    d. hyperosmotics

14. Macugen and Lucentis are used to treat:
    a. wet age-related macular degeneration
    b. fungal infections
    c. HIV in the eye
    d. cytomegalovirus

15. Which of the following might be beneficial in treating a patient with dry eye who uses artificial tears more than four times a day?
    a. steroid-enriched tear drops
    b. preservative-free tear drops
    c. lower viscosity tear drops
    d. sodium chloride drops

16. Contraindications for beta blockers include:
    a. tachycardia (fast heart rate)
    b. asthma
    c. chronic obstructive pulmonary disease
    d. high blood pressure

17. Which anticholinergic is commonly used for dilated ophthalmoscopy?

    a. atropine
    b. scopolamine
    c. tropicamide
    d. homatropine

18. When are prostaglandin inhibitors typically administered?

    a. in the morning
    b. in the afternoon
    c. around bedtime
    d. four times a day

19. Which dye is used when evaluating soft contact lenses?

    a. fluorescein
    b. rose bengal
    c. indocyanine green
    d. fluorexon

20. What antibiotic has activity against methicillin-resistant *Staphylococcus aureus*?

    a. ciprofloxacin
    b. vancomycin
    c. nafcillin
    d. cefepime

21. Complications of cortisosteroids can include:

    a. cataracts
    b. glaucoma
    c. infections
    d. all of the above

Answers

1. b, Inactive ingredients include preservatives, stabilizers, flavorings, binders, and diluents.

2. b, When the FDA approves a drug, it is for a specific use. This is the labeled indication of the drug. (Off-label and unlabeled indications are the same thing. It is not illegal for a physician to use medications off-label.)

3. a, Because an ointment is thick (with increased viscosity), it stays on the eye longer, increasing the time that the drug is in contact with the tissues. One drawback of ointments is that they cause blurred vision.

4. d, Polyvinyl alcohol is not a preservative; it is a viscosity agent.

5. b, The purpose of buffering agents is to adjust the pH of a solution.

6. c, Tonicity refers to the concentration of salts in a solution. The eye can tolerate a sodium chloride level of 0.5% to 1.8%.

7. d, Drowsiness would be a side effect, an unintended result of a drug.

8. c, Of the four listed, only cyclopentolate is a cycloplegic. Tropicamide and phenylephrine are mydriatics, and cyclosporine is an immune suppressant.

9. d, Mydriatics dilate the pupil, and are not used in treating glaucoma.

10. b, There is no drug class known as the antisteroids.

11. a, Antiviral drugs such as acyclovir are used in treating HIV infection.

12. c, Corticosteroids and NSAIDs are both anti-inflammatory drugs.

13. d, Hyperosmotics are used to draw fluid out of the eye in order to lower intraocular pressure.

14. a, Lucentis and Macugen are used in the treatment of wet age-related macular degeneration.

15. b, If a patient is using artificial tears more than four times a day, using a preservative-free tear drop is a good idea to prevent toxicity.

16. b, Blockade of the β_2 receptor in the airways can induce an asthma attack. The presence of COPD warrants precaution before giving a beta blocker, but it is not an absolute contraindication.

17. c, Atropine and scopolamine are too long acting to be used for routine ophthalmic dilated examination. Homatropine is not potent enough for an effective view of the retina. Tropicamide is short acting and potent.

18. c, Prostaglandin inhibitors for glaucoma are administered once a day, usually at bedtime.

19. d, Fluorescein can damage soft contact lenses. Fluorexon is used for soft contact lenses, but exposure time should be limited to a few minutes.

20. b, Vancomycin is the only drug on the list with meaningful activity against MRSA. Ciprofloxacin has mainly gram-negative coverage with limited gram-positive coverage. Nafcillin works against penicillinase-producing bacteria but not MRSA. Cefepime covers mainly gram-negative organisms such as *Pseudomonas*.

21. d, Cataracts, glaucoma, and infections (especially fungal infections) are all possible complications of corticosteroids.

REFERENCES

1. Benet LZ. General principles. In: Hardman JG, Limbird LE, Molinoff PB, et al, eds. *Goodman & Gilman's The Pharmacological Basis of Therapeutics.* 9th ed. New York, NY: McGraw-Hill; 1996:1-2.

2. Is it a cosmetic, a drug, or both? (or is it soap?). Food and Drug Administration website. www.fda.gov/cosmetics/guidanceregulation/lawsregulations/ucm074201.htm. Accessed May 30, 2016.

3. Claoue C. Experimental contamination of Minims of fluorescein by *Pseudomonas aeruginosa. Br J Ophthalmol.* 1986;70(7):507-509.

4. Paush JR. Dyes. In: Bartlett JD, Jaanus SD, eds. *Clinical Ocular Pharmacology.* 5th ed. St. Louis, MO: Butterworth Heinemann Elsevier; 2008:283-294.

5. McDonnell C. Lissamine green [available to subscribers only]. *Optician.* May 2010. Opticianonline.net website. www.opticianonline.net/assets/getAsset.aspx?ItemID=3921. Accessed February 15, 2016.

6. Yolton DP, Haesaert SP. Anti-infective drugs. In: Bartlett JD, Jaanus SD, eds. *Clinical Ocular Pharmacology.* 5th ed. St. Louis, MO: Butterworth Heinemann Elsevier; 2008:175-220.

7. Savani DV, Perfect JR, Cobo LM, Durack DT. Penetration of new azole compounds into the eye and efficacy in experimental Candida endophthalmitis. *Antimicrob Agents Chemother.* 1987;31:6-10.

8. Sendrowski DP, Jaanus SD, Semes LP, Stern ME. Anti-inflammatory drugs. In: Bartlett JD, Jaanus SD. *Clinical Ocular Pharmacology.* 5th ed. St. Louis, MO: Butterworth Heinemann Elsevier; 2008:139-174.

9. Abelson MB, Butrus SI, Weston JH, Rosner B. Tolerance and absence of rebound vasodilation following topical ocular decongestant usage. *Ophthalmology.* 1984;91(11):1364-1367.

The figure in this chapter was contributed by the following, who is associated with this book as an author: Jan Ledford: Figure 22-1

23

MICROBIOLOGY

Catherine Horan, BA, COMT

BASIC SCIENCES

Microbiology is the study of microorganisms: their activity, structure, metabolism, and identification. We may think of microscopic organisms primarily in terms of their ability to cause and transmit infectious disease. That's not surprising, as infectious diseases remain an important cause of morbidity (illness) and mortality (death) worldwide. However, it may be surprising to learn that only a very small percentage of microorganisms (probably between 1% and 3%) are pathogenic (disease-causing), and that a far greater proportion are actually beneficial or essential to life on Earth.[1]

The ability to study microorganisms at the molecular and genetic level has revolutionized the science of microbiology. It is now estimated that hundreds of thousands of microbial species exist. Microbial communities are found everywhere on the planet. Microbes are environmental scavengers, decomposing dead organisms and the waste products of living organisms. Microbes capable of photosynthesis produce more oxygen than plants, and are important links in the food chain of the ocean. Human, animal, and plant life require microorganisms for many essential functions. Modern biotechnology uses the unique properties of microbes for a great variety of purposes, including clearing industrial waste, food and beverage production, and the manufacturing of vaccines and medications.

An intensively studied microbial community is the one that lives in and on the human body. The human body contains trillions of microorganisms, which actually outnumber the human cells in our body by a factor of at least 3 to 1.[1] They (and their byproducts) contribute to the body's metabolism, immune system, and inflammatory response, and even help produce certain vitamins, enzymes, and neurotransmitters.[2]

Measuring Microbes: The Metric System

The microbial world is populated by exceptionally large numbers of exceptionally small organisms. The human body carries as many 100 trillion (100,000,000,000,000) microbes,[1] some so small that their size is expressed in metric units called *nanometers.* A nanometer is one *billionth* part of a meter (0.000000001 meters). Scientific notation more easily expresses such very large and very small numbers using exponents: 100,000,000,000,000 is written as 10^{14} and 0.000000001 meters becomes 10^{-9} meters.

Scientific measurements use the metric system (Table 23-1). Bacteria, fungi, and protozoa (the cellular microorganisms) are measured in micrometers (microns). Most

Ledford JK, Lens A, eds.
*Principles and Practice in Ophthalmic Assisting:
A Comprehensive Textbook* (pp 439-457).
© 2018 Taylor & Francis Group.

TABLE 23-1
SCIENTIFIC MEASUREMENTS USED IN MICROBIOLOGY

Metric Unit and Symbol		Fraction of a Meter		Decimal Notation	Scientific Notation
Decimeter	dm	One-tenth of a meter	1/10 meter	0.1 m	10^{-1}
Centimeter	cm	One-hundredth of a meter	1/100 meter	0.01 m	10^{-2}
Millimeter	mm	One-thousandth of a meter	1/1000 meter	0.001 m	10^{-3}
Micrometer or micron	μm	One-millionth of a meter	1/1,000,000 meter	0.000001 m	10^{-6}
Nanometer	nm	One-billionth of a meter	1/1,000,000,000 meter	0.000000001 m	10^{-9}
Angstrom	Å	One-ten billionth of a meter	1/10,000,000,000 meter	0.0000000001 m	10^{-10}

SIDEBAR 23-1

BINOMIAL NOMENCLATURE

The scientific names of organisms are written following specific rules of nomenclature.

▸ The first term (genus name) is always capitalized; the second term (species name) is never capitalized. Example: *Escherichia coli*.

▸ The full genus and species name are written the first time the name is used in a publication (eg, *Escherichia coli*). After this, the generic initial (capital letter) and species name may be used. Example: *E. coli*.

▸ The abbreviation "spp" (species) is used when referring to numerous species within a genus. For example, *Mycobacterium* spp. refers to a group of *Mycobacteria* species. ("sp" is the singular form. Note that the abbreviation is not italicized.)

▸ The scientific name is generally printed in italics.

---

bacteria are 0.2 to 10 microns. Most fungi and protozoa are typically 10 to 100 microns. Viruses, the smallest microbes, are measured in nanometers. Nanometers are much smaller than microns (1 micron = 1000 nanometers). Most viruses are between 20 and 300 nanometers in diameter.

Naming Microbes: Binomial Nomenclature

Note: The various types of microorganisms mentioned in this section will be covered later.

Biologists use a binomial (two-name) nomenclature system for living organisms (Sidebar 23-1). For example, in the bacterium *Staphylococcus aureus* the first term identifies the genus and the addition of the second identifies the species. Sometimes the genus is represented by a single letter, as in *S. aureus*.

A genus may include multiple species (abbreviated "spp" [not italicized]). The genus *Staphylococcus* has more than 30 species of which *S. aureus* is one. A species may also have strains or subtypes (eg, methicillin-resistant *S. aureus* [MRSA] is a strain of *S. aureus*).

Viewing Microbes: Microscopy

The unaided human eye with good vision can see objects as small as 0.1 mm, one-tenth of a millimeter. Viewing microorganisms requires a microscope (Figure 23-1). Microscopy provides magnification to increase the size of the image presented to the eye, and resolution to maximize image clarity and detail.

Light Microscopy

The most commonly used microscope in the clinical microbiology lab is the standard compound light microscope. Visible white light is transmitted through a specimen; the observer views the image against a bright background. Since most biologic specimens are nearly transparent, low contrast is a limitation of bright-field microscopy. Staining techniques improve contrast but kill the microorganism. (Stains are covered later in this chapter.)

Variations of the compound light microscope may use fluorescent light, polarized light, ultraviolet light, and other properties of light to produce the specimen image. Dark-field microscopy, for example, uses light directed obliquely onto the specimen, brightly outlining it against a dark background. This is useful for very thin microbes that are difficult to see with staining techniques, such as the causative agent for syphilis, *Treponema pallidum*.

Phase-contrast microscopy, another variation of compound light microscopy, enhances contrast and internal cellular details without the need for staining. The specimen can be viewed live allowing observation of motility, which is useful in species identification.

Microscopes using light as an illumination source have a maximum image resolution of about 200 nanometers (0.2 microns). This is suitable for viewing bacteria, fungi, and protozoa. Most viruses, however, are smaller than 200 nanometers and require a more powerful type of microscope.

Electron Microscopy

Microscopes using electrons as the illumination source can magnify up to 500,000 times and resolve images of viruses and particles as small as 0.1 nanometers. Electron microscopy requires highly specialized equipment and extensive specimen preparation.

Microbes and Infectious Disease
The Host–Microbe Relationship

The human body is host to a fairly stable population of microbes. These *resident* or *indigenous* microbes generally benefit the body and do not ordinarily cause disease. They are also referred to as *commensal organisms* or *normal flora*. The skin, upper respiratory tract, gastrointestinal tract, urinary and reproductive tracts, external ear, and external eye (lids and conjunctiva) are all colonized with a resident microbiota that is specific to the site. The types of microbes living on the surface of the skin are different from the microbes living in the gut or the nasopharynx.

The body also has a *transient* complement of microbes, whose composition varies depending on exposure to the external environment. These microbes may be eliminated by host defenses or by actions such as hand washing.

The body has sites that are sterile or nearly sterile, including the internal organs and tissues, the internal body cavities, and internal body fluids (ie, the circulating blood, lymph and cerebrospinal fluid). The interior of the eye, including the aqueous and vitreous fluids, is a sterile environment.

Transient microbes may cause infectious disease if they are able to evade or break down the host's defenses. Resident or transient microbes entering normally sterile body sites can become disease-causing agents.

Pathogens

Microbes with the potential to cause infectious disease are called *pathogens*. Pathogens may be *exogenous*

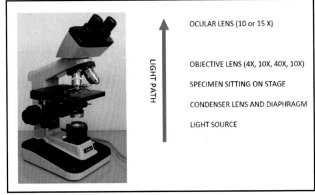

Figure 23-1. Typical microscope (Nikon Corporation) used in microbiology.

OCULAR LENS (10 or 15 X)
OBJECTIVE LENS (4X, 10X, 40X, 10X)
SPECIMEN SITTING ON STAGE
CONDENSER LENS AND DIAPHRAGM
LIGHT SOURCE
LIGHT PATH

(acquired from environmental sources, animals, or other persons) or *endogenous* (acquired from microbes already present in the body).

A *true pathogen* can cause disease in a healthy individual with a normal immune system. True pathogens can evade the host's immune system and cause infectious disease with fewer invading cells (*infectious dose*). True pathogens are called *virulent* and have factors that promote their infectious ability.

An *opportunistic pathogen* is a microorganism that is usually harmless but has caused an infectious disease because the host is weakened or immunocompromised, or because the microbes have gained entry to a normally sterile area of the body. Commensal organisms and generally nonvirulent microorganisms may become opportunistic pathogens in these circumstances.

Infectious Disease

The presence of pathogenic organisms does not necessarily result in infectious disease. The process of infectious disease requires a specific series of events.

1. Pathogens must find a portal of entry to the body. The skin is a portal when penetrated by cuts, abrasions, surgical wounds, or catheters. The corneal epithelium and the conjunctiva may become portals when penetrated by breaks in the epithelial barriers. Some pathogens are invasive and create their own entry portals via toxins that they produce.

2. Pathogens, after entry, must attach to and colonize susceptible host tissue.

3. Pathogens must overcome host defenses and multiply.

4. Pathogens must damage cells and tissues, causing symptoms of infectious disease.

Some pathogens cause direct damage by entering and disrupting the host cell. Many pathogens cause damage to host cells indirectly by secreting toxins and enzymes, by consuming nutrients needed by the host, or by causing a harmful inflammatory reaction.

Pathogens may be present in the body without causing disease. A number of factors influence the likelihood of whether the pathogen will cause infectious disease.

Pathogenic factors include:

▶ The virulence of the organism. A highly virulent organism has a higher likelihood of causing disease. Virulence factors are properties of the microorganism that facilitate adherence to the host cells and evasion of the host defenses. Capsule formation and biofilms are examples of virulence factors.

▶ The infectious dose of the organism. The *infectious dose* (ID) is the number of microorganisms required to cause an infection in the host. Pathogens with a low ID require fewer organisms to cause disease in the host.

Host factors that influence disease include:

▶ An immune-compromised state is an important risk factor in ocular infectious disease. Possible causes for a weakened immune system include old age or very young age (birth/infancy), malnutrition, any general state of debilitation, HIV/AIDS, chemotherapy, diabetes, diseases of the bone marrow, cancers, viral infections, and use of immunosuppressive medications after organ transplant.

▶ Recent surgery, organ transplants, and implants in the body are risk factors.

▶ Breaks in the first-line defense of the body are risk factors, including abnormalities in the epithelial body surfaces of the skin, mucous membranes, or cornea.

▶ Other infections in the body put a potential host at higher risk.

▶ Immunity from prior exposure to the pathogen is a *protective* factor.

Host Defenses: The Immune System

The immune system is the set of tissues, cells, molecules, and processes that protect the body from infection and disease. Immune defenses are directed against infectious agents such as microbes, toxins, and parasites; against foreign substances and foreign cells such as organ transplants; and against abnormal cells such as cancer cells and body cells infected with viruses.

The immune defense has two components: innate immunity and adaptive (or acquired) immunity. The innate response is immediate; acquired or adaptive immune response may take days to develop.

Innate immunity is a nonspecific defense system meaning that it operates against all invaders in the same way. Its components are always in place and ready to mobilize. The innate response system uses physical and chemical barriers as a first-line defense and specialized immune cells and proteins circulating in the blood and lymph as a second-line defense.

The epithelial cells of the body are a first-line physical and chemical barrier to invasion. The cornea, skin, and mucous membranes of the digestive, respiratory, urinary, and reproductive tracts are all surfaced with tightly joined epithelial cells that block entry of pathogens. In addition, epithelial cells secrete substances with antimicrobial properties. Tears, saliva, nasal secretions, and perspiration contain lysozyme, an antibacterial enzyme.

Microbes clearing the first-line defenses encounter specialized cells circulating in the blood and lymph. Some of these cells surround and destroy invaders, others recognize and kill cancer cells and infected cells, and some release chemical mediators for inflammation and allergic reactions. Innate immune cells also help prepare the body for adaptive immunity.

Acquired or *adaptive immunity* is a highly specific defense mechanism. The basis of adaptive immunity is the antigen-antibody reaction, the process protecting the body from invasion and damage. Adaptive immunity identifies a specific invader (antigen) and designs specific cells (antibodies) to eliminate the antigen at this encounter and to protect the body from future encounters with this antigen.

Antigens are invaders. Anything recognized as "nonself" or abnormal produces an antigenic response—the production of antibodies. *Antibodies* are defenders. These immune cells and blood proteins are tailor-made by the immune system to neutralize the specific invading antigen.

Once activated, the cells and components of the adaptive response generate great numbers of antibodies to seek out and destroy the antigen invader. Adaptive response to the first encounter with an antigen may take 4 to 7 days. This first encounter creates "memory" cells that remain in the body. Future exposures to the antigen activate those cells quickly, leading to a rapid antibody response.

Acquired immunity is cumulative and becomes stronger with each exposure to the antigen. In contrast, innate immunity is not cumulative and has no "memory."

Immune system disorders include *autoimmune* illness in which the immune response attacks the body's own cells and tissues. The cause may be a genetic defect or the cause may be unknown (idiopathic). Autoimmune diseases are well known to ophthalmologists and include thyroid eye disease and multiple sclerosis as well as collagen vascular disorders, such as lupus and rheumatoid arthritis.

Allergy is an abnormal immune response to a substance that is harmless to most people. Almost any substance can be an allergen (can cause an allergic response). The exposure may be through direct or airborne contact, ingestion, inhalation, or injection. The allergic response may be mild to moderate or severe and life-threatening.

Symptoms of mild allergic response include varying degrees of localized redness, rash, and itching. *Localized* is the key word. In an ophthalmology office we may see such symptoms in persons allergic to the adhesive in surgical tape or to medicated ointment applied to the lids or face. Allergy to topical ophthalmic medications applied to the eye may present as allergic conjunctivitis characterized by redness (injection), tearing, and swelling of the conjunctiva (chemosis) and the periocular tissues. Hypersensitivity reactions to ophthalmic eye drops and contact lens solutions are often a response to the preservative rather than the active compound. However, by far, the most common causes of allergic conjunctivitis are seasonal and environmental triggers such as pollens, dust mites, molds, and pet dander.

Moderate to severe allergic response is disseminated (widespread, not localized to the exposure site). Symptoms of moderate reaction may include hives, tingling of the mouth and swelling of lips, face, and eyes. Such symptoms are treated without delay as the response can rapidly increase in severity.

In allergy, the first exposure to the allergen does not provoke allergic symptoms, but it does sensitize the immune system. Once a person is sensitized, even a small exposure to the allergen can trigger a serious reaction.

Anaphylaxis is a potentially fatal, severe allergic response with multisystem involvement. Onset may be within seconds of exposure, but may also be delayed. It may present with a combination of signs and symptoms. The most common include hives (urticaria) and flushing; swelling of the lips, eyelids, and hands; shortness of breath; and wheezing due to upper airway swelling. Fluids flood out of the blood vessels causing a severe drop in blood pressure and acceleration of heart rate. Collapse of the cardiovascular and respiratory system can occur. Untreated anaphylaxis can lead to death quickly.

The most common causes of anaphylaxis are food allergies and insect bites. In a medical setting, latex and medications are other potential anaphylaxis triggers. In the ophthalmic medical setting, the possibility of anaphylactic reaction to intravenous fluorescein angiography is a special concern. An emergency protocol must be in place to minimize risk and manage complications. An office crash cart should include epinephrine (adrenaline), which counteracts the reaction.

Persons with a history of asthma, allergy, previous anaphylactic reaction, or with family history of severe hypersensitivity reaction in the parents may be at increased risk for anaphylaxis.

Host Defenses: The Inflammatory Response

Inflammation is the body's response to cellular injury, including physical injury or cell damage from microbial invasion and microbial toxins. Damaged tissue releases both chemicals signals and white blood cells, which activate the immune system to begin an inflammatory response. The purpose of the inflammatory response is to seal off the injury site to prevent the spread of infection or damage, to attack and neutralize toxins and invaders, and to remove damaged cells and products of inflammation. The goal of these processes is to allow healing to begin.

The four cardinal signs of acute inflammation are redness, heat, swelling, and pain. The redness occurs from local dilation of small blood vessels. The heat results from increased blood flow. Swelling occurs from local fluid accumulation and pain from tissue distortion.

Inflammation caused by infection also produces inflammatory exudates (pus) composed of white blood cells and cellular debris from destroyed cells and neutralized bacterial toxins.

The inflammatory response is part of our innate immune response and is essential to the healing process. Acute inflammation begins rapidly and resolves with repair of tissue damage. The inflammatory process is tightly controlled by the body. Inflammation itself can damage body tissues. Ocular tissues are particularly vulnerable, as they have a limited tolerance for even minor scarring.

Chronic inflammation can be a disease state. The cause may be unknown, and the inflammatory process may continue for prolonged periods. Many diseases, such as atherosclerosis and rheumatoid arthritis, are characterized by chronic inflammation.

Transmission of Infectious Disease

Infectious diseases are caused by an invading or infecting agent that can be transmitted to another individual. *Transmission* occurs by a series of events referred to as the *chain of infection*. Transmission cannot occur if any of the links in the chain are broken.

There are six links in the chain of infection (Figure 23-2).

1. The *pathogen* is the infectious agent, most commonly a bacteria, virus, fungus, or parasite.

2. The *reservoir* is the source of infection. It is the environment where the pathogen has been growing and multiplying. Reservoirs may be human, animal, plant, water, food, or inanimate surfaces. Human reservoirs that are colonized with a pathogen but not ill with the disease may be carriers and spread the disease to others.

3. The *portal of exit* is the route by which the pathogen leaves the reservoir. Pathogens may exit a human host reservoir in a variety of ways: in saliva, in respiratory secretions (sneezing), through breaks in the skin, and in blood, mucous membrane secretions, and feces.

4. The *mode of transmission* is the vehicle by which the pathogen travels from the reservoir to the next host.

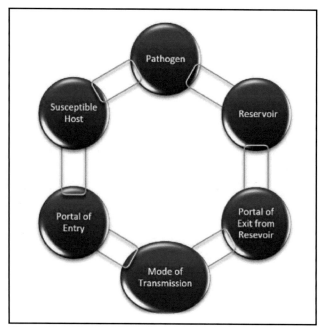

Figure 23-2. The chain of infection.

Direct transmission by physical contact is the most common mode of transmission, and hands are the most common vehicle of transmission. *Indirect transmission* of pathogens involves an intermediate host between reservoir and new host. A *vector* is a living animal or insect that carries the pathogen from the reservoir to the new host. A *fomite* is an inanimate object or surface that an infected person touches and contaminates. The contaminated surface transmits the pathogen to the next host. In a health care setting, contaminated medical equipment (such as a tonometer tip) can serve as a fomite and spread infection.

5. The *portal of entry* is the path for the infecting agents to enter the new host. This may occur through penetration of a body surface, through inhalation, or by ingestion.

6. The *new host* is the organism that next receives the pathogen. The new host may have a strong host defense system and may not develop the infectious disease but is a potential carrier of the pathogen, transmitting it to the next host.

The practice of *medical asepsis* refers to methods used to eliminate infectious agents, their reservoirs, and vehicles for transmission. Infection control experts agree that following standard precautions (covered in Chapter 37), using isolation guidelines (when required), and engaging in proper hand washing are essential to breaking the chain of infection. It is estimated that one-third of infections could be prevented by hand washing.

Nosocomial infections are infections acquired in a hospital or heath care setting. According to the Centers for Disease Control and Prevention (CDC), "Approximately 1.7 million hospital acquired infections occur in US hospitals each year, resulting in 99,000 deaths and an estimated $20 billion in health care costs."[3]

CLINICAL KNOWLEDGE

There are six major types of ocular infectious agents: bacteria, fungi, protozoa, helminths, viruses, and prions. With the exception of viruses and prions, infectious organisms are composed of cells. Cells are the smallest unit of life. A unicellular bacterium has all the properties that define a living organism: metabolism (chemical reactions that produce and use energy) and the ability to reproduce, respond to stimuli, grow, and mutate.

Two primary cell types have evolved in nature: prokaryotic cells and eukaryotic cells. Bacteria are *prokaryotic* cells; fungi, protozoa, and helminths are *eukaryotic* cell types. All higher life forms, plants, animals, and humans are eukaryotes.

Antibiotics are bacterial toxins. Antibiotics are toxic to (prokaryotic) bacterial cells, but are not highly toxic to (eukaryotic) human cells.

Fungi, protozoa, and helminths are eukaryotic cells. Diseases caused by these organisms are very difficult to treat because agents that kill these organisms are also highly toxic to (eukaryotic) human cells.

In the text that follows, some examples of infectious agents important in ophthalmology are presented. These are by no means comprehensive lists.

The Bacteria

Bacteria are small and remarkably efficient. Bacteria have a rapid method of reproduction called *binary fission*. The cell makes a copy of its genetic material and then divides into two identical cells, each carrying a complete copy of the genetic material. *Escherichia coli* cells can double every 20 minutes. A single *E. coli* can, under ideal conditions, become millions of cells in a few hours.

Bacteria have a variety of shapes, arrangements, and metabolic requirements. They have a unique rigid cell wall structure not seen in higher organisms. All these observable characteristics are used in the lab to help identify bacteria.

Bacteria are divided into two broad classes based on cell wall structure as determined by reaction to the Gram stain (discussed later). Gram-positive bacteria stain purple, gram-negative stain pink. The difference between gram-negative and gram-positive bacteria can be important when determining appropriate treatment for an infection.

Bacteria can form *biofilms* that assist their attachment to host cells and help them resist breakdown by host defenses, antibiotics, and surface disinfectants. Biofilms begin when bacteria produce a glue-like substance that

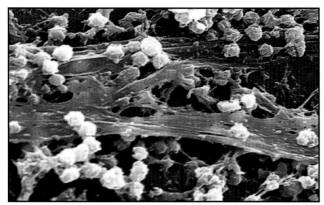

Figure 23-3. Biofilm of *Staphylococcus aureus*. (Reprinted with permission from the Centers for Disease Control and Prevention/Rodney M. Donlan, PhD, Janice Haney Carr.)

helps them stick to each other and to a substrate (Figure 23-3). The substrate to which they attach may be a living host cell or a moist surface of any kind. Dental plaque is an example of a biofilm. Biofilm-related infections are resistant to treatment and can form on many indwelling medical devices, such as central venous catheters and artificial heart valves. Biofilms can also form on contact lenses and in contact lens cases.

Cocci

Cocci (singular, coccus) are the most common bacterial form. Cocci are spherical microbes, generally about 1 micrometer (micron) in size. They appear in irregular clusters (Figure 23-4), chains, diplococci (pairs; Figure 23-5), and as sets of four (tetrads) or more.

Gram-Positive Cocci

Staphylococci are gram-positive spherical cocci grouped in irregular clusters. They are facultative anaerobes (meaning they can live with or without oxygen). *Staphylococcus aureus* is the most common staph species on the skin. *Staphylococcus epidermidis* is another common skin inhabitant. Staphylococci generally do not cause problems on the intact skin surface. When the epithelial barrier of the skin or mucous membrane is breached, staphylococci have a portal of entry. Infection can develop. Staphylococci are the most common cause of wound infections and the most common nosocomial infection (nosocomial means acquired in a health care setting). Common staphylococcal eye infections include blepharitis, chalazia, staph marginal ulcers, and meibomitis. Staph can live off the oil of the tear film layer and the meibomian glands.

A strain of *S. aureus*, called methicillin-resistant *Staphylococcus aureus* (MRSA) infection, has become resistant to many of the antibiotics used to treat staph infections. MRSA is a major public health concern.

Streptococci are gram-positive spherical cocci grouped in long chains. They are also facultative anaerobes.

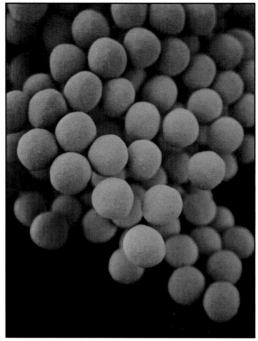

Figure 23-4. *Staphylococcus aureus* (artist's rendition). Note the round shape typical of cocci, but the clustered appearance. (Reprinted with permission from the Centers for Disease Control and Prevention/James Archer, Medical Illustrator.)

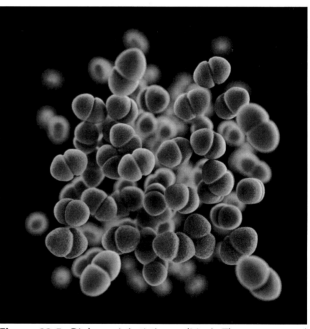

Figure 23-5. Diplococci (artist's rendition). These are round cocci that always occur in pairs. (Reprinted with permission from the Centers for Disease Control and Prevention/James Archer, Medical Illustrator.)

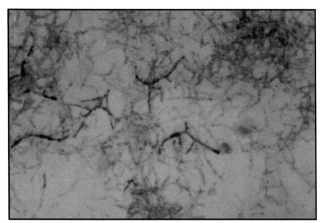

Figure 23-6. Acid-fast rod-shaped bacilli. (Reprinted with permission from the Centers for Disease Control and Prevention/Ronald W. Smithwick.)

Streptococci are less common as an ocular pathogen than staphylococci. They are well known to cause strep throat and skin infections like impetigo. Streptococcal eye infections can include acute or chronic dacryocystitis.

Gram-Negative Cocci

Neisseriaceae are bean-shaped gram-negative diplococci. *Neisseria* spp. have a preference for mucous membranes and can invade intact tissue. *Neisseria gonorrhoeae*, the causative agent for gonorrhea, can cause a severe and damaging conjunctivitis in newborns called gonococcal ophthalmia neonatorum. (There are other causes of neonatal conjunctivitis [*ophthalmia neonatorum*].) *N. gonorrhoeae* is either sexually transmitted or transmitted mother to child during birth.

Bacilli

Bacilli (singular, bacillus) are rod-shaped bacteria that may appear singly or in chains (Figure 23-6). Bacillus, like coccus, is a descriptor used to describe bacteria that share a specific shape.

There is a specific genus of rod-shaped bacteria called *Bacillus*. Just remember the rules of nomenclature: *Bacillus* in italics with initial capital refers to the genus *Bacillus*. Bacillus or bacillus, without italics, refers to any rod-shaped bacteria.

Gram-Positive Bacilli

Propionibacterium species are a common gram-positive inhabitant of the adult skin and conjunctiva, living off the sebum and oil produced in sebaceous glands. *Propionibacterium acnes* is a non–spore-forming anaerobe (an anaerobe does not require oxygen) that produces toxins, causing the inflammation of acne pimples.

Clostridium botulinum is a spore-forming (Sidebar 23-2) anaerobic gram-positive bacillus. It produces the well-known neurotoxin *botulinum*, used to treat spastic conditions of the face and periocular muscles.

Bacilli (singular *bacillus*) are gram-positive rod-shaped spore-forming bacteria. The most well known is *Bacillus*

anthracis, the causative agent of anthrax. Spores allow organisms to survive in hostile environmental conditions.

Gram-Negative Bacilli

Pseudomonas aeruginosa are gram-negative aerobic rods abundant in watery environments. Air conditioning systems, standing water, ventilators, and respiratory equipment are common reservoirs. Contact lens cases are also potential harborers.

Haemophilus influenza, a gram-negative rod, was a common pathogen in childhood eye infections, particularly orbital cellulitis. It is now less common in the United States due to use of the *Haemophilus influenza* type B (HIB) vaccine.

Serratia marcescens is a possible cause of contact lens-related keratitis. It is a mobile gram-negative rod. *S. marcescens* has also been known to cause nasolacrimal infections as well as conjunctivitis and wound contamination.

Spiral Bacteria

Spiral bacteria are motile, and their "corkscrew" shape facilitates their characteristic ability to penetrate into tissue (Figure 23-7).

Gram-Negative Spirochetes

Treponema pallidum is the causative agent of syphilis. It is gram negative but so thin that Gram staining is not useful. Dark field microscopy and serologic (blood serum) testing for antibodies are the diagnostic standards. *T. pallidum* is a true pathogen, and humans are the only host. *T. pallidum* is either sexually transmitted or transmitted from mother to unborn child.

Chlamydia trachomatis is a gram-negative spirochete with affinity for the mucous membranes of the genitourinary tract, lungs, and eyes. *Chlamydia* is the most frequently reported sexually transmitted disease in the United States. It is endemic in some developing countries and is the leading cause of preventable blindness worldwide. There are three types of Chlamydia presentations: neonatal conjunctivitis (chlamydia ophthalmia neonatorum), adult inclusion conjunctivitis, and trachoma (river blindness). *Chlamydia* is the most common infectious cause of neonatal conjunctivitis. Ocular trachoma and

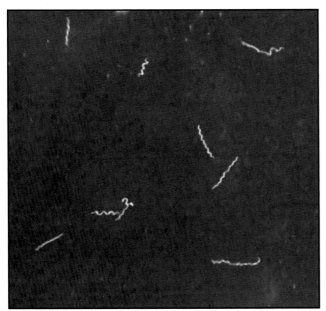

Figure 23-7. Spirochetes (note cork-screw shape) photographed via dark field microscopy. (Reprinted with permission from the Centers for Disease Control and Prevention, Bacterial Diseases Branch, Fort Collins, CO/Adam Replogle.)

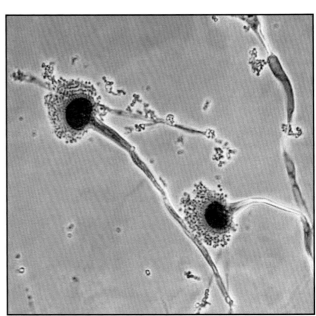

Figure 23-8. The fungus Aspergillus. Note the "stalk" and "bloom." (Reprinted with permission from the Centers for Disease Control and Prevention.)

inclusion conjunctivitis cause severe inflammation and scarring.

Most bacteria are independent and don't need host cells to reproduce; *Treponema* and *Chlamydia* are exceptions. They are obligate intracellular bacteria, meaning that they can only reproduce inside a host cell.

Borrelia burgdorferi is a gram-negative rod transmitted to human by ticks. It is the causative agent of Lyme disease.

The Fungi

Fungi (singular, fungus) are eukaryotic organisms that exist in a variety of forms: yeasts, molds, and macroscopic fungi (mushrooms). Yeasts are unicellular and spherical in shape, larger than bacteria (3 to 8 microns); the molds are multicellular and exist in many forms. Fungi generate and disperse spores to reproduce. Fungal infections are known as *mycoses*. Mycoses cause damage directly by invading host tissue and indirectly by instigating the inflammatory response.

Superficial fungal infections affecting the skin, hair follicles, or nails are fairly common, such as athlete's foot and ringworm (not a worm!). Systemic fungal infections are rarer. These are most often opportunistic, found in persons who are immunocompromised or have other risk factors.

Fungal eye infections in a healthy patient are usually exogenous (from the environment). These are associated with eye injury (especially injury from plant material), contact lens wear, or chronic ocular surface disease. Some fungal eye infections have been traced to contaminated medical products, such as contact lens solution or irrigation solutions used during eye surgery. Endogenous fungal eye infections can be caused by fungal bloodstream infections that spread to the eye.

Fusarium solani and *Aspergillus* (Figure 23-8) are often the causative agents of traumatic keratitis and corneal ulcer. These fungi are abundant in soil and plant material.

Keratitis caused by the yeast *Candida albicans* is more likely to be seen in the context of a preexisting ocular surface disorder or defect, especially in a diabetic or immune-impaired patient.

C. albicans from a bloodstream infection can cross into to the eye causing endogenous endophthalmitis.

Histoplasma capsulatum is caused by inhaled fungal spores that cause a pulmonary infection, which may progress to a systemic infection. *H. capsulatum* can travel through the bloodstream to the choroid where it causes inflammation and a chorioretinal scar. The disease is called *presumed ocular histoplasmosis* (POHS).

Mucormycosis is rare. It is an aggressive fungal infection associated with uncontrolled diabetes and a weak immune system. Ocular mucormycosis may be caused by a mucor sinus infection that has spread to the orbital and periorbital tissues.

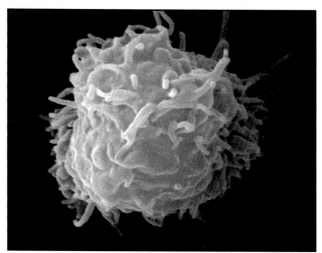

Figure 23-9. *Acanthamoeba*, taken with a scanning electron microscope. (Reprinted with permission from the Centers for Disease Control and Prevention/Catherine Armbruster, Margaret Williams, Janice Haney Carr.)

The Protozoa

Protozoa are eukaryotic unicellular organisms. The parasitic species are transmitted by contaminated food and water or by insect bites (eg, mosquito). There are 100,000 species of protozoans; only about 25 are important human pathogens. Malaria is a protozoan infection (*Plasmodium* spp.) transmitted only by the bite of a certain type of mosquito.

Several types of protozoans are of special ocular concern.

Acanthamoeba species are free-living amoebae found in soil and fresh water (Figure 23-9). Strains of the genus can infect the cornea causing Acanthamoebic keratitis, a very serious corneal infection that is difficult to treat and can result in blindness. *Acanthamoeba* is found in tap water, well water, lake water, and many other water sources. Contact lens wear is a risk factor. Contact lenses exposed to water carry the amoeba to the eye, where it has the potential to invade the cornea. Contact lenses should not be exposed to any type of water, including tap water, swimming pools, hot tubs, or shower.

Toxoplasma gondii, a single-celled parasite, is the causative agent for *toxoplasma chorioretinitis*, generally called *ocular toxoplasmosis*. The organism causes a large inflammatory response, which, if located in the macula, is blinding. *T. gondii* lives in the intestinal tract of cats. Transmission is via the fecal-oral route from infected meat, from contaminated water, or from exposure to cat feces. Persons with healthy immune systems may have this protozoan without developing disease. Pregnant women and immunocompromised persons are at risk for developing ocular toxoplasmosis. In the United States, most cases are acquired congenitally (infected mother to child during pregnancy).

The Helminths

Helminths are multicellular eukaryotic infectious agents. They are parasitic worms, larvae, and arthropods living either in the body (endoparasites) or on the body (ectoparasites). Transmission is from animals or insects. Parasitic helminths are difficult to treat because, like all eukaryotic pathogens, their cell physiology has similarities to human cell physiology.

Toxocara canis and *Toxocara cati* are transmitted by ingestion of larvae in dog or cat feces. Ocular toxocariasis is caused by the migration of the larvae into the eye, causing a severe inflammatory response. It is usually unilateral, most commonly seen in children.

Loa Loa (African eye worm) is a zoonosis, transmitted via the bite of deer flies. The worm migrates to ocular tissue at the surface of the body, typically under the conjunctiva.

Phthiris pubis (lice) is sometimes found at the lid margin between the cilia.

The Viruses

Viruses are not true cells but are classified as microbes. They are the most abundant microbes on the planet and are the most common cause of infectious disease. Even by microbial standards viruses are very small, about 10 to 300 nm (nanometers) in diameter. A virus particle is not a cell, but a strand of nucleic acid (either DNA or RNA) surrounded by a protein coat. Viruses can infect human cells, animal cells, plant cells, or even the cells of microorganisms (fungi, protozoa, algae, bacteria). They must infect a cell in order to reproduce, which makes them *obligate* (as in obligatory) intracellular pathogens.

Viruses are classified by a variety of criteria, including shape, size, type of genetic material, type of disease caused, and type of host required. The DNA viruses include the herpes viruses and the pox virus.

Herpes viruses are large DNA viruses and a common cause of ocular disease. Herpes simplex virus type 1 (HSV-1), herpes simplex virus type 2 (HSV-2), and varicella zoster virus (VZV) are the most common herpes viruses. Following the initial infection, the viruses remain latent in the dorsal root ganglia of the central nervous system. (The spinal nerves carrying sensory information back to the brain join the spinal cord at dorsal [or sensory] roots; the nerves sending motor impulses to the body join at ventral [or motor] roots. The root ganglia are bundles of the cell bodies of these nerves located near the root.)

There are a number of ocular viruses.

Molluscum contagiosum causes viral warts on the skin that are contagious and infectious.

HSV-1, nongenital herpes, is a causative agent for viral conjunctivitis and keratoconjunctivitis. Recurrences of HSV-1 can be in the form of a fever (or cold) sore and/

or skin rash, or as herpetic keratitis with a typical dendritic (branching) pattern (see Figure 33-12).

The first exposure to VZV can cause chicken pox (a disseminated virus). VZV reactivates less often than HSV, often after age 60 years as immunity declines. Varicella zoster reactivates as herpes zoster (shingles), which may cause vesicular lesions of the face along the distribution of a branch of the trigeminal nerve, as well as painful keratitis and uveitis. Nerve scarring may cause severe lasting pain called post-herpetic neuralgia.

Adenoviruses are typically upper respiratory viruses that may cause viral conjunctivitis and keratoconjunctivitis. One particular strain causes epidemic keratoconjunctivitis (EKC), which is highly contagious and easily transmitted via both direct and indirect contact. Swollen lymph nodes (especially just in front of the ear) are commonly seen with adenoviral conjunctivitis.

Picorna viruses are varied. The human polio virus and the coxsackie viruses are picorna viruses. Acute hemorrhagic conjunctivitis (AHC) is caused by a coxsackie virus. AHC is an epidemic form of highly contagious conjunctivitis that presents with painful red eyes, swelling, and conjunctival hemorrhaging. Epidemics are sporadic and large. A 2003 epidemic affected thousands of people. Treatment is symptomatic, and the disease is generally self-limited.

Prions (Proteinaceous Infectious Particles)

Proteinaceous infectious particles (*prions*) are a unique and relatively newly discovered pathogen, unique because they contain no genetic material and certainly don't fit into any known category of pathogens. Prions are an altered or misshapen form of a protein found in normal nerve cells. They appear to propagate by converting normal proteins to disease-forming proteins. The mechanism is unknown.

Fortunately, prion disease is rare. This degenerative disorder of the central nervous system may be acquired or familial. Alternatively, it may be the result of a random protein mutation. Acquired disease is transmitted by exposure to infected food or to infected brain or nervous system tissue, usually through certain medical procedures.

Creutzfeldt-Jakob disease is a human prion disease. Ophthalmology has been concerned about the possibility of transmission in corneal grafts. Eye banks have strict standards to ensure the safety of donor tissue. There have also been a few cases linked to contaminated instruments used in brain surgery. Neurosurgical instruments used for a patient with known or suspected Creutzfeldt-Jakob disease are isolated. Typical sterilization procedures do not destroy prions.

CLINICAL SKILLS

The role of the clinical microbiology laboratory is to identify disease-causing organisms from an infected site and, when appropriate, to determine antibiotic sensitivity for the organism. Today microbiologists use a combination of traditional microbial culture methods alongside newer diagnostic tools.

The clinical lab uses both direct and indirect testing methods. *Direct* methods demonstrate the presence of an infectious agent and utilize microscopy, culture and biochemical tests, and molecular methods. *Indirect* methods demonstrate that a host has antibodies to a particular infectious agent via immunologic tests. This section will mainly cover direct methods.

The Clinical Specimen: Care and Handling

We send diagnostic specimens to the clinical lab or sometimes generate them in-house to identify the cause of an infection. However, the process begins before the lab receives the specimen. It starts in the clinic or exam room; it begins with the specimen. The quality of the diagnostic information returned by the clinical laboratory is limited by the quality of specimen submitted (Sidebar 23-3). The ophthalmic technician who assists the physician in specimen handling has an important role in quality assurance.

The requisition is the doctor's communication to the clinical lab. It needs to be clear, complete, and legible (Sidebar 23-4).

Specimen Collection

When collecting a specimen, follow standard (universal) precautions (Sidebar 23-5). Standard precautions means that we treat all specimens as potentially hazardous.

The different anatomic structures of the eye are sampled using different techniques. The collection method also depends on the purpose of the specimen.

A *smear* is a thin film of microbes spread over a microscope slide. Stains are applied to the smear to assist in viewing and identification of the organism (Sidebar 23-6).

Swabs are samples of infectious material inoculated into a transport medium and sent to the lab for culture. Commercial collection and transport systems are routinely used. Bacterial swabs consist of a plastic tube containing a rayon-tipped applicator and a supply of bacterial transport medium. The applicator is removed from tube, wiped through the area of infection, and returned to the tube. Some types require that the bottom of the plastic tube be crushed to release the medium. If in-house culture plates are to be used, assemble the supplies for the swab in advance of the procedure (Sidebar 23-7).

SIDEBAR 23-3
SPECIMEN HANDLING

The overall attributes of a quality specimen include:

▶ Proper aseptic technique in collection to avoid contamination from other sites

▶ Proper labeling and identification of specimens

   • Label specimens at the time they are collected. An unmarked specimen is a potential lost or misidentified specimen.

   • Mark microscope slides with patient ID. Place dried slides in a slide carrier for protection during transport.

   • Specimens may be generated from one eye, from both eyes, or from different structures of one eye. Each site generates a separate specimen. Mark each specimen to indicate which site was sampled.

▶ A complete, legible requisition (see Sidebar 23-4)

▶ Appropriate selection of transport or culture media; a bacterial transport tube is not used for viral culture transport

▶ Adequate volume of specimen collected from the area most representative of the infection

▶ Expedited transport under controlled conditions, protected from excessive heat or cold

▶ If your office uses a specimen box, make a habit of checking it as you leave each day

---

SIDEBAR 23-4
SPECIMEN REQUISITION

Requirements for a complete specimen requisition:

▶ Complete (and correct) patient identification

▶ Specimen date and time

▶ Physician name and contact information

▶ Specific identification of each specimen site: which eye, which ocular structure

▶ Specific test(s) requested

▶ Brief clinical history (the clinical history can help guide the clinical microbiologist in assessment)

▶ Ensure that the diagnosis code and insurance information is attached—Don't let this be the reason processing is delayed

---

SIDEBAR 23-5
STANDARD PRECAUTIONS

Standard (universal) precautions for specimen collection include:

▶ The use of barrier precautions during collection (such as gloves)

▶ Aseptic technique is critical to avoid specimen contamination from other sites (eg, a conjunctival swab should not touch the lids or lashes)

▶ Avoidance of contaminating the external surfaces of collection containers or transport bag

▶ Don't contaminate paper lab requisition or place it in the same bag as the specimen—Place paperwork in the side pocket of the biohazard transport bag

▶ Disinfect the procedure area and any nondisposable supplies when finished

▶ Use proper biohazard labeling on lab specimens

A vitreous or aqueous *aspirate* may be generated in-office. Strict sterile technique is employed by the physician collecting the specimen and the technician involved in handling and transport. Avoiding contamination of an intraocular specimen is critical. Anything that grows out from a sterile site specimen must be considered as a source of the infection. A contaminate confounds appropriate diagnosis and effective treatment. The specimen is injected into a sterile microtube, or with approval of the clinical lab, it may be retained in the syringe (needle removed) during transport. Transport is expedited. The volume of a sample is generally very small, sometimes 1 mL or less. The lab can be consulted to ensure that the volume of sample will support all the requested tests.

Microscopy and Staining

Microscopy and staining can provide a presumptive diagnosis that can later be verified by culture. The most common microscopy technique is bright field microscopy used with a variety of simple or differential stains. Cell size, shape, arrangement, special structures, and staining characteristics can be determined.

Many stains are salts (with a positive and a negative ion) in which one of the ions contains color. *Simple stains* (using only one dye) bring out cell shape, size and morphology, and special structures. *Differential staining* techniques (using two or more stains) are used to categorize cell groups or types.

Simple and structural staining techniques use only one dye or stain to enhance contrast or to highlight structures, giving information about the size and shape

---

SIDEBAR 23-6

MAKING A SMEAR

To make a smear on a microscope slide, a moist cotton-tipped applicator is used to collect material (cells and exudates) from the infection site. Conjunctival smears are obtained by lowering the bottom lid and applying the applicator to the lower bulbar conjunctiva. The applicator tip should not touch lid margins or lashes. The applicator is then wiped across a clean glass slide in a thin, even layer. A *conjunctival scraping* is sometimes performed by the physician using a sterile spatula or blade. The scraping is then thinly applied to the glass slide. The slide is allowed to air dry before staining or placement in a slide transport tray.

SIDEBAR 23-7

SWABS

Supplies will be based on physician request, but a typical set-up may include:

▶ Sterile Kimura spatula, sterile knife blades, or sterile swabs.

▶ Microscopy slides and slide transport tray.

▶ Alcohol lamp: If a metal spatula is used, it must be flame sterilized between plate inoculations. Extreme care must be used to ensure that the spatula has cooled completely before reapplying it to the eye. When a disposable blade is used, an alcohol lamp is not needed.

▶ Culture plates and media (see Table 23-2): Store unused culture plates upside down in the refrigerator. Remove them about 30 minutes prior to use.

---

of bacteria. There are numerous simple stains. A common one, nigrosin (India ink), is a negative structural stain that outlines endospores and capsules.

Differential staining techniques use more than one stain to actually differentiate between organisms and aid in identification.

Differential Stains

There are several important differential stains. Note: The Clinical Lab Improvement Act (CLIA-88) defined three categories of laboratory tests: waived complexity (which are simple tests, including home-testing kits), moderate complexity, and high complexity.

The Gram Stain

Gram staining categorizes bacteria into two major groups based on their staining properties: gram negative and gram positive. Gram reaction is a key step in the process of microbial identification. Coupled with microscopic appearance, Gram staining can provide useful information within a very short time.

The Gram stain has been in use for more than 120 years. Many sophisticated tools are available to the clinical microbiologist today, but the Gram stain remains a key first step in the identification of unknown bacteria. Gram reaction is important in medicine because some antibiotics are effective against only gram-negative bacteria and some against only gram-positive ones.

Cells are stained with a primary stain (violet) and then decolorized with alcohol (Sidebar 23-8). Gram-positive bacteria retain the purple color. The cell walls of gram-positive bacteria have a thick structure that resists decolorization. Gram-negative cells are decolorized by the alcohol because their cell wall is much thinner. A red counterstain is finally applied. The gram-negative cells take up the counterstain and appear pink to red.

Gram stain is categorized as moderate complexity according to CLIA-88. There are extensive compliance requirements when moderate complexity tests are performed outside a certified laboratory setting.

Other Stains

Acid-fast staining is used to identify acid-fast bacteria, which includes *Mycobacterium* spp. and *Nocardia* spp. These bacteria cannot be Gram stained due to their cell walls, which are waxy.

Fluorescent dyes/stains such as direct fluorescent antibody are used in microscopy of a variety of organisms including *Chlamydia trachomatis* and *Herpes simplex virus*.

Giemsa-Wright staining (or the commercially available alternative kits) is used to examine conjunctival smears or scrapings for cytology (cell type) and microorganisms, particularly ocular *Chlamydia*. This is a differential stain technique that can suggest the type of infection or the type of inflammatory process present in a sample. The presence of specific cell types suggests the type of infection or inflammation present (Sidebar 23-9).

Calcofluor white is a special stain used to detect yeast cells and fungal elements. It is useful to evaluate corneal scrapings from a suspected fungal ulcer. Calcofluor white can be used with a potassium hydroxide wet preparation (KOH Prep) to visualize the fungal elements.

Culture

Microbial culturing increases the number of organisms in a sample with the goal of isolating a pure culture for definitive identification. The clinical specimen is taken from the infected tissue site and placed in a special

---

Sidebar 23-8
Gram Staining

Materials

▶ Crystal violet (primary stain)

▶ Iodine solution/Gram's iodine (fixes crystal violet to cell wall)

▶ Decolorizer (eg, 95% alcohol, acetone, or ethanol)

▶ Safranin (secondary stain)

▶ Water (preferably in a squirt bottle)

Procedure

▶ Fix smear to the slide with gentle heat

▶ Cover with primary stain (crystal violet) for 1 minute

▶ Gentle rinse with water (maximum 5 seconds)

▶ Cover with Gram's iodine for 1 minute and pour off solution

▶ Rinse with alcohol, acetone, or ethanol for 5 seconds to decolorize

▶ Gentle rinse with water

▶ Cover with counterstain (safranin) for 1 minute

▶ Rinse gently with water and gently blot dry

If the bacteria are gram positive, they will be purple/dark blue, having retained the primary stain. If the bacteria are gram negative, they will be pink/red, having lost the primary stain and taken up the counterstain.

Sidebar 23-9
Cell Types Seen in Infection

▶ Polymorphonuclear cells may indicate bacterial infection.

▶ Eosinophils suggest allergy.

▶ Inclusion bodies indicate Chlamydial infection.

▶ Mononuclear cells suggest viral infection.

▶ Giant cells may indicate Herpes virus.

Microbiological Culture Media

Culture media are gels and broths formulated to promote the growth of organisms from a clinical specimen, and to bring out characteristics that aid in their identification. *Selective media* are used to promote the growth of specific microorganisms and suppress the growth of others. *Differential media* are used to determine if a given organism does or does not carry out a specific biochemical process, such as oxygen requirement, the need for carbon dioxide, or carbohydrate fermentation.

Enriched media contain nutrients that support the growth of a wide range of organisms. These are used to attempt growth of whatever organism is present in the sample, including fastidious organisms that have specific nutritional requirements.

Transport media are intended only to keep the specimen viable during transport from the clinic/office to the clinical laboratory, where it will be inoculated into appropriate culture media for growth and testing. Bacterial and viral and chlamydial specimens use specific transport media. Viral and Chlamydia transport media contain antibiotics to suppress the growth of bacterial and fungal contaminants.

Many types of culture media are used in clinical micro labs. For example, non-nutrient agar with an *E.coli* overlay is used in the identification of *Acanthamoeba*. *Acanthamoeba* consumes the *E. coli*, leaving tracks in the plate. Other media might be used in the ophthalmic clinic or office setting. For example, it is not uncommon for ophthalmologists to directly inoculate corneal ulcer scrapings or smears into culture media. Some common media types used for this purpose are shown in Table 23-2.

Susceptibility testing is performed after a bacterial pathogen is identified. In general, it is known which antimicrobial drugs are effective against which bacteria. But bacteria constantly develop resistance to drugs that were previously effective. Susceptibility testing determines which antimicrobials work best against the particular bacteria isolated from this individual. In this test, the culture plate is inoculated with bacteria, then tiny disks (each impregnated with a different antibiotic) are added

specimen tube for transport to the lab as previously detailed. The material is then transferred onto a solid medium (agar [a gel made from seaweed] in a petri dish), and incubated for 24 hours. At that point, if any bacteria was present in the sample, the agar surface will show isolated bacterial colonies. A tiny, sterile loop of wire is used to pick up cells from an isolated colony and transfer them to fresh sterile media, both solid and liquid. The new plate and liquid media tube are now incubated for another 24 hours. These will then contain a pure culture of bacteria, which is observed for characteristics of shape, size, texture, color, and elevation.

The pure culture is now tested to confirm the identification of the bacteria using staining techniques, biochemical tests, and molecular tests. After isolation and identification, the sample undergoes susceptibility tests to determine the most effective antibiotic.

Cultures take time. Bacteria results are usually available in 48 to 72 hours, but viruses take days to weeks. Many fungi are slow growers and culture results can take several weeks.

TABLE 23-2
COMMON MICROBIOLOGIC MEDIA

Medium	Medium Type	Use
Blood agar	Enriched	Supports growth of most bacteria including fastidious organisms
	Differential	Distinguishes between hemolytic and nonhemolytic organisms
Sabouraud agar	Selective	Inhibits most bacteria; encourages growth of fungi
Chocolate agar	Enriched	Supports the growth of fastidious microorganisms, particularly *Haemophilus* and *Neisseria* spp
Thayer-Martin	Selective	This is a chocolate agar made selective by the addition of antibiotics; useful for isolating *Haemophilus* and *Neisseria* spp
Lowenstein-Jensen agar	Selective	Supports the growth of *Mycobacterium* sp
Thioglycollate broth	Enriched	Determines the oxygen requirements of an organism
	Differential	Differentiates between the various types of oxygen requirements (ie, strict vs facultative anaerobe)

to the medium's surface. If the bacteria is sensitive to an antibiotic, there will be a clear zone around that disk (Figure 23-10). The wider the clear zone, the more effective the antibiotic.

Bacteria exhibit a wide variety of biochemical properties that can also be used to help identify the organism. The microbiologist uses specific differential media to test the organism for biochemical properties such as production of enzymes, metabolism of carbohydrates, oxygen requirement, and carbon dioxide requirement.

Serologic Methods

Serology refers to the serum (basically the blood plasma) and other body fluids. The purpose of such testing is to evaluate immunity based on the antigen-antibody response. These tests are used for organisms that cannot grow in culture media. For example, it can be used when a specimen culture is negative (ie, no bacteria has grown from the sample) due to antibiotic therapy. It can also be used to determine how much antibody is present. The immune response takes time to develop, and an initial antibody test can be negative. The test may then be repeated in several weeks to see if antibody levels have become elevated.

Nucleic Acid-Based Tests

Genotypic methods analyze the genetic material of the organism. Polymerase chain reaction (PCR) is one widely used nucleic acid-based test. PCR is a technique sometimes referred to as "molecular photocopying." The test will be valid as soon as an organism is present; there is no waiting for antibodies to develop as with serologic methods.

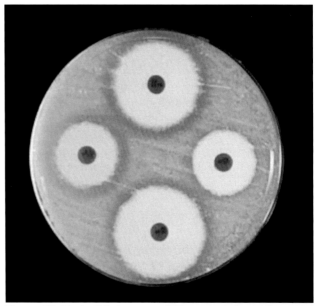

Figure 23-10. Antibiotic susceptibility test performed on agar plate. Each disk is impregnated with a different antibiotic. The disk with the widest clear zone around it will be the most effective against the bacteria on the plate. (Reprinted with permission from the Centers for Disease Control and Prevention/Gilda L. Jones.)

The nucleic acid amplification test (NAAT) is a commercially available assay that also amplifies and identifies the genetic material. (Amplification produces many exact copies of the genetic material, allowing accurate identification even if the sample is tiny.) This test is specific to a specific microorganism. For example, PCR for *Varicella zoster* tests only for that entity. A single specimen, however, can be analyzed for several suspected infectious agents.

Laboratory Testing for Ocular Infectious Disease

Some ocular infections have a characteristic presentation and can be diagnosed clinically on the basis of the patient history, symptoms, and the ophthalmic examination. Bacterial conjunctivitis is often diagnosed this way and treated empirically with a broad-spectrum antibiotic that is effective against both gram-negative and gram-positive bacteria. (*Empirical treatment* is treatment based on a clinical diagnosis.)

A laboratory diagnosis is indicated when the clinical history and exam suggest an unusual pathogen or when the infection is not responding to empirical treatment. Ocular infection following trauma or recent surgery, in a newborn, and in suspected intraocular infection require lab studies. A laboratory diagnosis is based largely on the laboratory identification of the pathogen.

The lab diagnosis of ocular infection has specific challenges. Prior empiric antibiotic treatment is common and complicates the diagnostic process. The very small specimen size of corneal scrapings and aqueous or vitreous samples also limits the extent of testing that can be performed.

Periocular and Conjunctival

Infectious orbital disease is often related to a sinus infection or a systemic infection in immunocompromised patients, and possibly to trauma in a healthy patient. Infections of the lids and other periocular structures are more likely to be caused by bacteria found on the skin.

Conjunctivitis is most commonly caused by bacteria of the upper respiratory tract. Bacterial conjunctivitis is typically not cultured unless it is severe. *Staphylococcus aureus, Streptococcus pneumoniae,* and *Haemophilus* are common causes of conjunctivitis. Severe purulent discharge and chemosis are suggestive of gonococcal conjunctivitis needing immediate Gram stain and culture. Chronic conjunctivitis might suggest *Chlamydia*. Viral conjunctivitis is most commonly caused by adenoviruses, and *Herpes simplex* virus may also be a causative agent. Viral conjunctivitis is typically not cultured.[4]

Possible microbiology studies for periocular infections and conjunctivitis may include a smear for microscopy as well as a swab for culture and detection of different types of organisms (Sidebar 23-10).

Corneal

Keratitis is an ocular surface infection of the cornea. Bacteria are the most common cause of keratitis; in fact, keratitis is generally assumed bacterial unless proven otherwise. Physicians generally culture keratitis ulcers that are larger than 1 mm, that are unresponsive to treatment, or that present with symptoms and history suspicious for unusual pathogens.[4]

Severe purulent discharge and chemosis is suggestive of keratitis caused by *Neisseria gonorrhoeae*. Fungal keratitis in a healthy individual is associated with trauma (especially from plants and vegetable material) and with contact lens wear. Fungal keratitis is an opportunistic infection in an immunocompromised patient. *Acanthamoeba* keratitis is characterized by acute pain and photophobia (in excess of what the slit lamp exam would seem to indicate) and is also associated with contact lens wear. *Herpes simplex* viral keratitis has a characteristic dendritic (branching) corneal staining pattern and is prone to recurrence.

Possible laboratory studies for the cornea may include more specialized techniques than other external infections (Sidebar 23-11).

Intraocular

Endophthalmitis is an intraocular infection that may be exogenous (ie, from the external environment) following ocular surgery or trauma. Postoperative infection is often due to *Staphylococcal* infection. Traumatic endophthalmitis may be caused by a variety of pathogens. Endogenous bacterial endophthalmitis occurs when bacteria from a systemic infection crosses the blood–eye barrier. Endophthalmitis carries a high risk of profound visual loss.

Vitreous aspirate for culture/detection of different types of organisms is sent directly to the clinical lab with no intermediate processing in the office or surgical suite. Laboratory studies requested may be very specific (Sidebar 23-12).

SIDEBAR 23-11
COMMON TESTS FOR CORNEAL INFECTIONS

► Culture of corneal scraping directly inoculated into culture plated media
   • Culture for bacteria, aerobic and anaerobic (blood agar)
   • Fungal culture (Sabouraud agar)
   • Culture for *Neisseria gonorrhoeae,* which may be seen in newborns (chocolate agar)
   • Culture for *Mycobacteria* and other bacteria (Lowenstein-Jensen agar) ulcer with history of LASIK
   • Non-nutrient agar with *Escherichia coli* overlay for suspected *Acanthamoeba*
   • Viral culture or viral detection for *Herpes simplex* virus by nucleic acid amplification test
► Smear of corneal ulcer cell scrapings for microscopy are spread thinly on glass microscope slide
   • Gram stain for bacteria
   • Calcofluor white-KOH stain for fungi, *Acanthamoeba*, and others
   • Acid-fast stain for *Mycobacteria* and others
   • Giemsa for bacteria, fungi, *Acanthamoeba*

SIDEBAR 23-13
ASK THE LAB...

► Does the lab perform this test?
► What transport or culture media is optimal?
► Are there special transport considerations (eg, transport on ice, at room temperature)?
► If transport is delayed, how can the specimen be stored?

After the specimen is sent out:

► Communicate with the lab to confirm receipt of the specimen.
► Ensure that the lab report returns to the practice and is viewed by the provider in a timely fashion.
► Ensure that appropriate follow-up for the patient is initiated.

SIDEBAR 23-12
COMMON TESTS FOR INTRAOCULAR INFECTIONS

► Direct microscopy with staining such as Gram stain, Calcofluor KOH
► Culture for aerobic and anaerobic bacteria
► Culture for fungi
► Molecular acid-based tests such as polymerase chain reaction for virus or mycobacterium

---

Communication With the Clinical Laboratory

Communicate with the lab before and after sending a specimen or culture. It is prudent to call the lab especially prior to generating a nonroutine specimen (Sidebar 23-13).

PATIENT SERVICES

Patient education and treatment of conjunctivitis and other common infections is covered in Chapter 26. Here are three vital applications of practical microbiology (more helpful hints are in Sidebar 23-14):

1. Break the chain of infection at every opportunity. Look at your work practices and ensure that they are compliant with standard (universal) precautions.
2. Use proper hand washing and hand hygiene techniques. An estimated one-third of infections could be prevented by hand washing.
3. Educate patients at every opportunity about safe contact lens care and handling. Explain the danger of water exposure. *Acanthamoeba* is commonly found in tap water, lake water, and well water. The keratitis it causes is painful, resistant to treatment, and potentially blinding. Water and contact lenses don't mix (Sidebar 23-15).

SIDEBAR 23-14
INFECTION CONTROL

▶ Follow disinfection and sterilization protocols for all your equipment. The adenovirus that causes epidemic keratoconjunctivitis is highly transmissible and can live on an environmental surface (like a tonometer) for days.

▶ Isolate infectious patients. That patient at the reception desk with "pink eye" should be escorted to a triage location without delay.

▶ Don't work when you are contagious. A single sneeze or a cough spreads a lot of viruses a long way.

CHAPTER QUIZ

1. A microorganism that is usually harmless but has caused an infectious disease because the host is weakened or immunocompromised, or because the microbes have gained entry to a normally sterile area of the body, is which type of pathogen?

    a. opportunistic
    b. virulent
    c. transient

2. Bacteria are divided into two broad classes based on cell wall structure as determined by their color reaction to the Gram stain. Gram-positive bacteria stain _____ (color), gram-negative bacteria stain _____ (color).

3. True/False: In the bacterium *Escherichia coli*, the first term, *Escherichia*, identifies the species.

4. In an infectious process, pathogens acquired from the external environment are called _____ . Pathogens that migrate from another site in the body to cause infection are called _____ .

5. Bacteria, fungi, and protozoa are measured in _____ . Viruses, the smallest microbes, are measured in _____ .

    a. nanometers
    b. micrometers (microns)

6. Culture media containing nutrients that support the growth of a wide range of organisms are referred to as _____ media. Media used to promote the growth of specific microorganisms and suppress the growth of other microorganisms are referred to as _____ media.

SIDEBAR 23-15
PATIENT EDUCATION WITH CONTACT LENS WEAR

The Centers for Disease Control and Prevention[5] and the American Academy of Ophthalmology[6] recommend:

▶ Keep contact lenses away from all water.

▶ Remove lenses before showering, swimming, or using a hot tub.

▶ Never rinse or store contact lenses in water.

▶ Wash and dry hands well before handling lenses.

▶ Throw away or disinfect contact lenses that touch water.

▶ If water touches contact lenses for any reason, take them out as soon as possible.[5]

▶ Rubbing lenses with lens solution prior to disinfection is considered by some experts to be a superior method of cleaning.

▶ Clean contact lens cases with solution to avoid contaminating the lenses with germs found in water. The current recommendation is to leave the empty case to air dry. However, some experts now suggest rubbing the lens case dry to discourage biofilm formation.

▶ Keep the contact lens case clean and replace it regularly, at least every 3 months. Lens cases can be a source of contamination and infection. Do not use cracked or damaged lens cases.

▶ Remove contact lenses at the first sign of irritation. If infection is suspected, call your eye care provider. Take the contact lens case and solutions to the visit.

Answers

1. a, An opportunistic pathogen is a microorganism that usually causes no harm. It requires a specific set of circumstances in order to cause disease. A virulent, or true, pathogen can cause disease in a healthy individual with a normal immune system.

2. Purple, pink

3. False, The first term is the genus, *Escherichia*. There are numerous species of *Escherichia*. Addition of the second term identifies the species *Escherichia coli*.

4. Pathogens acquired from the external environment are called *exogenous* pathogens. Pathogens that migrate from another site in the body to cause infection are called *endogenous* pathogens.

5. b, a

6. Culture media containing nutrients that support the growth of a wide range of organisms are referred to as *enriched* media. Media used to promote the growth of specific microorganisms and suppress the growth of other microorganisms are referred to as *selective* media.

REFERENCES

1. Reid A, Green S; American Academy of Microbiology. Human microbiome FAQ. http://academy.asm.org/index.php/faq-series/5122-humanmicrobiome. Accessed April 9, 2016.

2. Pollan M. Some of my best friends are germs. *The New York Times Magazine.* May 15, 2013. www.nytimes.com/2013/05/19/magazine/say-hello-to-the-100-trillion-bacteria-that-make-up-your-microbiome.html?_r=0. Accessed July 4, 2016.

3. Centers for Disease Control and Prevention. Preventing healthcare associated infections. *CDC at Work.* www.cdc.gov/washington/~cdcatWork/pdf/infections.pdf. Accessed July 4, 2016.

4. Gerstenblith AT, Rabinowitz MP, eds. *The Wills Eye Manual: Office and Emergency Room Diagnosis and Treatment of Eye Disease.* 6th ed. Philadelphia, PA: Lippincott Williams & Wilkins; 2012.

5. Water and contact lenses. Centers for Disease Control and Prevention website. www.cdc.gov/contactlenses/water-and-contact-lenses.html. Updated June 13, 2014. Accessed July 10, 2016.

6. Weiner G. Confronting corneal ulcers. *EyeNet Magazine.* American Academy of Ophthalmology website. www.aao.org/eyenet/article/confronting-corneal-ulcers?july-2012. Accessed July 10, 2016.

BIBLIOGRAPHY

Baron EJ, Miller JM, Weinstein MP, Richter SS, et al. A guide to utilization of the microbiology laboratory for diagnosis of infectious diseases: 2013 recommendations by the Infectious Diseases Society of America (IDSA) and the American Society for Microbiology (ASM)(a). *Clin Infect Dis.* 2013;57(4):e22-e121. doi:10.1093/cid/cit278.

Donlan RM. Biofilms: microbial life on surfaces. *Emerg Infect Dis.* 2002;8(9):881-890. doi:10.3201/eid0809.020063.

Engelkirk PG, Duben-Engelkirk J. *Burton's Microbiology for the Health Sciences.* 9th ed. Philadelphia, PA: Lippincott Williams & Wilkins; 2014.

Gerstenblith A, Rabinowitz MP, eds. *The Wills Eye Manual: Office and Emergency Room Diagnosis and Treatment of Eye Disease.* 6th ed. Philadelphia, PA: Lippincott Williams & Wilkins; 2012.

Hardy J. Nomenclature of microorganisms. www.hardydiagnostics.com/articles/nomenclature-of-microorganisms.pdf. Accessed July 10, 2016.

Leggett HC, Cornwallis CK, West SA. Mechanisms of pathogenesis, infective dose and virulence in human parasites. *PLoSPathog.* 2012;8(2):e1002512. doi:10.1371/journal.ppat.1002512.

Reid A, Greene S. FAQ: human microbiome. The American Society for Microbiology website. http://academy.asm.org/index.php/faq-series/5122-humanmicrobiome. Posted January 2014. Accessed July 10, 2016.

Rivera-Amill V. The human microbiome and the immune system: an ever evolving understanding. *J Clin Cell Immunol.* 2014;5:e114. doi:10.4172/2155-9899.1000e114.

Sack RA, Nunes I, Beaton A, Morris C. Host-defense mechanism of the ocular surfaces. *Bioscience Reports.* 2001;21(4):463-480. doi:10.1023/A:1017943826684.

Sharma S. Diagnosis of infectious diseases of the eye. *Eye (Lond).* 2012;26(2):177-184. doi:10.1038/eye.2011.275.

Stein HA, Stein RM, Freeman MI. *The Ophthalmic Assistant: A Text for Allied and Associated Ophthalmic Personnel.* 9th ed. Philadelphia, PA: Elsevier Saunders; 2013.

24

GENETICS

James Walsh, MD, PhD
Sandra Johnson, MD

BASIC SCIENCES

Genetics is a field that has held the promise to transform medicine for many years. Yet only in the past few decades has clinical practice quietly started to catch up to the possibilities that scientists have been envisioning for years. From the discovery of the first genetic diseases in the early 20th century, to the advent of the human genome project, to the vision therapies that can be directed to each individual's genetic make-up, there has been great progress. And yet for all the progress that has been made, it is a field that has the potential to continue to evolve at the same rapid pace for years to come. This chapter is a brief glimpse into where the field of genetics has come from, how it fits into a modern ophthalmology practice, and the potential it holds for future clinical practice.

A Brief History of Genetics

To understand how genetics affects clinical practice today, it is helpful to take a quick trip through history and put modern-day genetics into perspective. The origins of what we now know as genetics can be traced back to the mid-1800s to two very different scientists: Charles Darwin and Gregor Mendel.

The first of these two to publish his theories was Darwin, who postulated that traits were selected based on their utility to the organism. These traits underwent changes sporadically, and were only passed on if they were useful to the organism. Before this work, the predominant theory was that organisms had an innate "knowledge" about what would be beneficial, and by force of will each individual could adapt traits based on the environment. Darwin did not propose a basis for how this modification occurred, but through his observations deduced that the variations in the animals he saw on different islands were due to this change over time.

Not too long after Darwin's theory of evolution, Gregor Mendel, an Austrian monk, developed his theory of genetic inheritance through observation and rigorous scientific testing. By meticulously crossing pea plants with each other, he showed that traits were passed on in an orderly, predictable fashion from parents to offspring. Through his experiments, he developed several rules that can explain the appearance of the offspring based on the appearance of the two parents. Interestingly, these rules varied by trait: while some traits followed one set of rules for their inheritance, different traits could follow an entirely different pattern. Much of the theory of genetic inheritance now used follows the models that he described. Thus, genetic inheritance that follows these

Ledford JK, Lens A, eds.
Principles and Practice in Ophthalmic Assisting:
A Comprehensive Textbook (pp 459-472).
© 2018 Taylor & Francis Group.

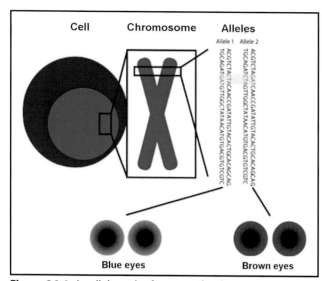

Figure 24-1. An allele codes for a specific phenotype.

rules is considered "Mendelian," and these rules govern the transmission of the majority of known genetic diseases. Because of the importance of these theories, he is now known as the "father of modern genetics."

The Molecular Basis of Genetic Inheritance

Before we get into the nitty-gritty specifics of genetic inheritance and how it relates to ophthalmic diseases, it is important to start with a few comments regarding terminology.

Deoxyribonucleic acid (a nucleic acid polymer), or DNA, is the primary way that genetic material is passed from one generation to the next (but not the only way, which we will get into later in detail). DNA has many advantages as a genetic material: it is redundant (genetic material is coded twice on each strand), and thus limited damage can be repaired without any loss of information. It can be selectively activated or repressed, which allows for a wide variety of cells to carry the same genetic material (eg, a brain and a liver cell). DNA can be packed tightly when it is not in use through structures called *nucleosomes*, which can be thought of as suitcases for DNA. When the DNA is stored in nucleosomes, it does not take up much space, but it is not available for use. The sections that are needed can be unpacked and used to make RNA and subsequently protein. Once the DNA is no longer necessary, it is repackaged in nucleosomes. Finally, and maybe most importantly, DNA can be copied and passed down to the next generation.

One distinction that is often confusing is the difference between the genetic material (which is a DNA sequence) that encodes a trait and the physical manifestation of the trait itself. We each have a predetermined set of genetic material, our *genotype*. This is fixed from

the time that fertilization takes place, and can influence anything from lifespan to height to eye color. In contrast to this genetic material, the actual appearance that results is called the *phenotype*. While the phenotype is generally thought of as a genetically stimulated construction, there are also environmental factors.

Consider the example of height. The genotype determines how tall someone has the potential to grow. However, someone with "tall" genetic information can still end up with a "short" phenotype if he/she is malnourished when young or has damage to the bones and growth is stunted.

It is also important to understand what an allele is. If you think of all the potential genetic combinations that encode for a particular trait (hair color, eye color, etc), an *allele* is one of those sequences of this genetic material (Figure 24-1). For simplicity's sake, an allele can be thought of the as the genetic material that codes for one possible phenotype. Therefore, for each trait that is described by a single genetic location, a person has two alleles (one from each parent).

Important Principles in Genetic Inheritance

There are a few specific principles regarding the genetic transmission of information that play an important part in the genetic basis of disease. The genetic material in humans is separated into 46 strands of information, our chromosomes. There are 22 pairs of chromosomes, the autosomal chromosomes (which account for 44 of our chromosomes, and are named 1 to 22 on the basis of their size), plus two for determining sex (the X and Y chromosomes), for the total 46. Because all of the genes are paired (except for the X and Y chromosome), there are two copies of each gene (except those on the X and Y chromosome). We receive one set of 23 chromosomes (one each of the autosomal chromosomes plus one X) from Mom, and one set (22 autosomal plus one X or Y) from Dad.

Patterns of Genetic Inheritance
Autosomal Dominant or Recessive

Perhaps the easiest type of inheritance to think about is dominant inheritance. As you would expect from the name, *dominant* alleles are those that produce their phenotype whenever they are present, regardless of what other alleles are also present. Simply put, if there's a dominant trait, that will "dominate" the phenotype. A *recessive* allele can be "hidden" by a dominant allele, and therefore the phenotype caused by recessive alleles is only seen in the absence of a dominant allele.

To conceptualize how dominant and recessive transmission works, suppose that the sky were a gene locus, and it could have either the "cloudy sky" or "blue sky" alleles. If there are only two "blue sky" alleles present, the sky would be blue; similarly, if only "cloudy sky" alleles are present, the sky would be cloudy. However, if there is one "cloudy sky" allele and one "blue sky" allele, and you could not see the blue sky due to the clouds, then the "cloudy sky" allele is dominant, the "blue sky" allele is recessive, and the phenotype would be cloudy.

The distinction between genotype and phenotype are particularly important when talking about the inheritance patterns of dominant and recessive traits. Just because one parent has the phenotype of a dominant trait doesn't mean that the offspring will necessarily have that phenotype. Therefore, in order to better understand the chances that a person will pass on a trait (or disease), it is important to understand the implications of a given phenotype.

Because of the principles of genetic inheritance discussed above, and specifically that of an independent assortment of chromosomes during reproduction, each combination of the alleles that could be contributed from the mother and father are equally likely. In a practical sense, this means that we can predict the probability of passing on a disease if we know the genotype of the parents and how that disease is inherited.

To understand how this works, it will help to be familiar with some labeling conventions that have developed in genetics. Because there are two alleles of most genes, a shorthand "code" was developed by Gregor Mendel that is still in use today. When writing about the passage of genetic material, dominant alleles are denoted by capital letters (eg, "A"), recessive alleles are denoted by lowercase letters (eg, "a"), and the sex chromosome denoted as "Y" and "X." If both alleles are identical, then the person is said to be *homozygous* at that gene, while if they have different alleles they are *heterozygous*. People who are heterozygous and have one recessive gene for a disease are considered *carriers* for that disease because they carry the potential to have an affected offspring, even though they do not have the disease themselves.

Doing the Math:
Inheritance of Dominant and Recessive Traits

The probability of a child inheriting a certain genotype depends on the genotype of the parents: each parent can either have two recessive alleles (aa, homozygous recessive), one dominant and one recessive allele (Aa, heterozygous), or two dominant alleles (AA, homozygous dominant).

The simplest situation is when both parents have either two dominant or two recessive alleles (they are homozygous), in which case the children will have the same genotype as that of the parents. However, in situations with more complex genetic inheritance, it becomes important to have a schematic that will help explain the possible outcomes. This is commonly done using a *Punnett square*, which is a technique to predict which alleles will be passed down from the parents. To make a

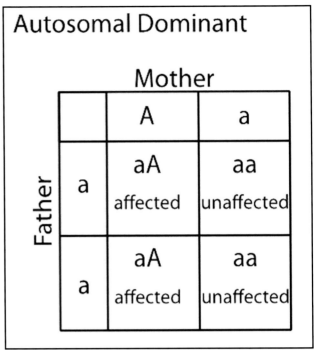

Figure 24-2. Punnett square showing autosomal dominant genotypes.

Punnett square, place the possible alleles of a locus that can be transmitted from the mother across the top and from the father down the left side (Figure 24-2). The possible genotypes of the offspring are the combination of the allele from the mother and that from the father where they intersect.

In an autosomal dominant diseases, one of the parents is usually homozygous recessive (does not have the disease) and the other is heterozygous (affected by the disease). In the monogenetic (consisting of only one gene) example (see Figure 24-2), two of the four possibilities will result in an affected offspring, for a 50% chance that each and every descendant could display the phenotype.

In an autosomal recessive disease, both of the parents are usually heterozygous and do not have the disease (ie, are carriers). In the monogenetic example of Figure 24-3, one of the four possible outcomes will result in an offspring that receives both recessive alleles, for a 25% chance of inheriting the disease.

Codominant Inheritance

Codominant traits are much less common than autosomal dominant or recessive traits, and are normally seen in situations where the immune system can recognize two different variants of a gene. The classical example of this is ABO blood type (Figure 24-4), which is determined by a gene that encodes a red blood cell protein. In this scheme, the blood type locus can be any combination of A, B, or neither A nor B antigens. In codominant inheritance, just because you have the A antigen doesn't prevent the B antigen on the other chromosome, and vice versa.

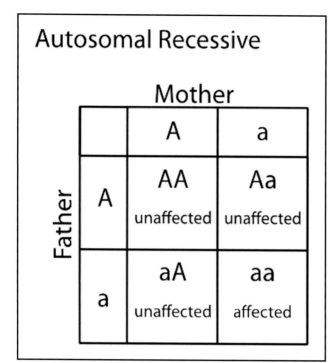

Figure 24-3. Punnett square showing autosomal recessive genotypes.

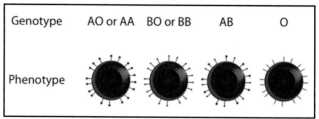

Figure 24-4. ABO bloodtyping is an example of a codominant trait.

This situation gives us the four blood types: O blood type, which has neither the A nor the B antigen present; the A or B blood type, which has only one antigen present; and the AB blood type, which has both antigens present.

Doing the Math: Codominant Inheritance

As with dominant and recessive inheritance, the genotype of codominant inheritance cannot always be determined by the phenotype. However, the genotype of the AB and O blood types are known just by phenotype: AB must have one copy of A and one copy of B, and O must have neither. The ambiguity lies in the A and B blood types, which can be either homozygous (AA or BB) or heterozygous (AO or BO). For this reason, a person can inherit the O blood type without having a parent that has the O blood type (if the genotypes of both parents were either AO or BO), but *not* if one of the parents has the AB blood type (where the parent would have to transmit either the A or B allele to the offspring).

X-Linked Disorders

X-Linked dominant and recessive genes are similar to autosomal dominant and recessive traits, but are thought of as a separate category because there are some special rules that apply to X-linked traits and how they are passed down.

Because there are 44 paired chromosomes that do *not* encode sex (the so-called autosomal chromosomes, numbered 1 to 22 with two copies of each), most genes are passed down in an autosomal manner, and the sex of the offspring does not affect the probability of inheriting

the genetic material. However, there are two special chromosomes, X and Y, which are integrally related to gender.

Since the Y chromosome contains very few genes, it does not play a major role in genetics other than determining sex. The X chromosome, however, is a normal-sized chromosome and contains the genes responsible for many diseases. Therefore, X-linked dominant diseases will always be passed from father to daughters (who have to receive the X from their father to become female) but never to sons (who must receive the Y chromosome from their father in order to become a male). Similarly, affected carrier mothers have a 50% chance of passing the affected gene on to both daughters and sons, since they will both receive one of the two X chromosomes from the mother.

X-linked recessive traits, on the other hand, are almost exclusively seen in males because males only have one X chromosome; by receiving an affected chromosome they will display the phenotype. In contrast, females would have to have two copies of the recessive gene in order to have the phenotype, which is a relatively rare occurrence.

Doing the Math: X-Linked Disorders

Using the same techniques we used for autosomal inheritance, we can determine the inheritance patterns of X-linked diseases by drawing a Punnett square with the maternal and paternal genes as the top and left side, respectively, with the special rule that the father has to have a Y chromosome, which can be thought of as a placeholder that does not contribute to the phenotype of interest. Any offspring who inherit the Y gene will be male, and those who receive two Xs will be female.

In one possible X-linked dominant situation (Figure 24-5), the mother is affected and the father is not. Because 50% of the offspring will receive the affected X from the mother, 50% of the daughters and 50% of the sons will inherit the trait.

In an X-linked recessive disease, the mother is usually heterozygous and the father carries a dominant allele. In the monogenetic example of Figure 24-6, none of the daughters will have the disease (but 50% will be carriers, like the mother), and 50% of the males will have the disease.

Other Forms of Inheritance

Mitochondria (the energy-producing structure in the cell) have their own genome, and mutations of the

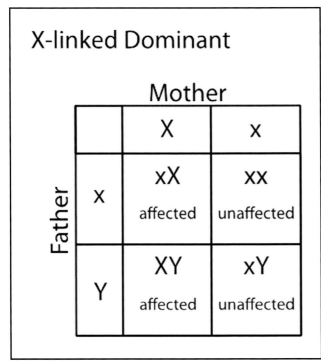

Figure 24-5. Punnett square showing an X-linked dominant trait. (Note lowercase x's representing a recessive gene.)

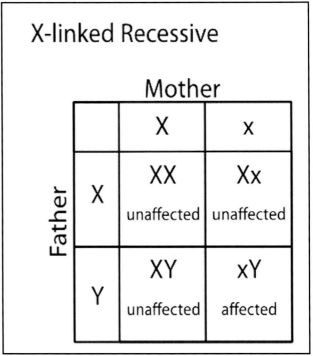

Figure 24-6. Punnett square showing an X-linked recessive trait. (Note lowercase x's representing a recessive gene.)

mitochondrial genome can cause disease just like mutations in the nuclear genome. Because mitochondria are derived exclusively from the egg (the sperm is streamlined to pass on just DNA, and does not contribute its mitochondria to the offspring), these diseases are passed down exclusively from the mother.

Another alternate form of genetic transmission that has been intensely studied recently is *epigenetic programming*. (Epigenetic refers to changes in how DNA is read, rather than changes in the DNA sequence itself.) These changes are frequently due to "tags" that are attached to the DNA to activate or silence certain regions of it. While much of this programming gets removed from generation to generation, there are certain epigenetic signatures that persist between generations. The classic example of epigenetic disease is Prader-Willi syndrome, which is due to aberrant epigenetic programming on chromosome 15. While there will surely be more diseases discovered where epigenetic programming plays an important role, it is not currently known to be a major factor in ophthalmic disease, and further discussion of this mechanism is deferred.

The Genetics of Disease: More Complex Inheritance

When it comes to figuring out the pattern of disease inheritance, there are several complexities that can occur even with Mendelian inheritance, two of which we will discuss here.

The first is *multigenetic inheritance*, where more than one gene contributes to a phenotype. While this makes the analysis of familial inheritance patterns more difficult, it is an easy concept if you understand the basics of monogenetic inheritance. When thinking about Mendelian genetics involving traits encoded by multiple genes, each gene is passed down independently of each other, and can be determined using a Punnett square as with single genes. An example is shown in Figure 24-7. The challenge in understanding this inheritance is figuring out how the genotype corresponds to the phenotype, because by definition there are more than two alleles in this situation.

The second common complexity is probably the best-studied modification of classical Mendelian inheritance: *incomplete penetrance*. When there is *complete penetrance*, everyone with the correct genotype will develop the disease, and the typical Mendelian ratios are seen when analyzing populations. However, there are often environmental factors and other genes that play an important role in how a disease presents, and in these cases not every individual who inherits the genes will end up developing the disease. This is incomplete penetrance.

Of course, many diseases are known to have a major genetic component (which can be determined by studying identical twins), but no clear-cut inheritance gene or pattern has been discovered to explain the genetic risk. This category of diseases includes some of the most common diseases in ophthalmology, such as age-related macular degeneration (AMD) and glaucoma. Because

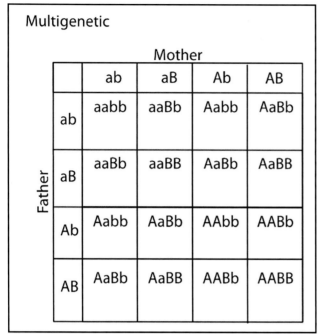

Figure 24-7. Punnett square showing multigenetic inheritance.

of the complex genetics of these diseases, new scientific techniques are being used to discover genetic risk factors. The most common method that scientists use involves sequencing the genes of patients and normal controls to determine if any small mutations might be overrepresented in patients with disease. These *genome-wide association studies* (GWAS) have begun to uncover many genetic associations with disease. While this tool is especially useful for identifying the genes associated with disease, it unfortunately does not give any information as to *how* the gene is involved. For example, in addition to directly causing disease due to loss of function in a protein, the mutations might also encode a protein that protects against the effects of other mutations or factors that modify the environmental risk of a disease. Or they could just be found more frequently in the disease purely by chance.

CLINICAL KNOWLEDGE
Genetics of Ophthalmic Diseases
Autosomal Dominant
Marfan Syndrome

Marfan syndrome is one of the most prevalent autosomal dominant diseases that cause ocular abnormalities, with a prevalence of 1-2:10,000. This disease is caused by mutation in the gene that codes for fibrillin formation, a protein that contributes to the elasticity of connective tissue. Marfan's is well known by its characteristic body shape, particularly that the person's arm span being greater than his/her height. The lifespan is often shortened due

to cardiovascular abnormalities. Ocular manifestations are high myopia, ectopia lentis (displacement of the lens from the visual axis), and glaucoma.

Retinoblastoma

Retinoblastoma is a tumor of undifferentiated cells in the retina that occurs early in childhood, usually by age 5. One-third of cases arise due to an inherited mutation in the tumor suppressor gene *Rb*, and the rest occur due to sporadic, nonfamilial mutations.[1] In addition to retinoblastoma, persons with hereditary Rb mutations are at risk for several other cancers including sarcoma, melanoma, and lung cancer.[2] Retinoblastoma is usually identified by the absence of a red reflex (either in photographs [see Figure 3-6] or upon examination by a doctor) or when the patient undergoes evaluation for strabismus, which commonly occurs in children who see poorly out of one or both eyes. While fatal if untreated, the treatment has greatly increased in the past 40 years, and now there is a 99% cure rate, though there are often visual complications (including blindness) from the treatment.

Dominant Optic Atrophy

Dominant optic atrophy is the most common hereditary optic neuropathy, leading to progressive loss of retinal ganglion cells. Loss of vision normally starts in the first or second decade and is slowly progressive, though there is rarely total vision loss. Family history of dominant optic atrophy is sometimes difficult to elicit due to the fact that complete visual loss is abnormal, so it is often unrecognized in previous generations. The disorder is due to a variety of mutations in an autosomal gene that encodes a mitochondrial protein important in the structural integrity of the mitochondria.[3]

Aniridia

As the name suggests, the most obvious manifestation of *aniridia* is lack of an iris, though there are additional ocular manifestations (including nystagmus and cataracts) as well as nonocular associations (such as tumors in the kidney). It is caused by mutations in the Pax6 gene, which encodes for a transcription factor that is important for proper development of the eyes in utero. Unlike many autosomal dominant diseases where the mutation induces aberrant function in the protein, aniridia is caused by deactivating mutations that decrease the "dose" of Pax6 present sufficient enough to cause the disease.[4] The lack of an iris has been linked to increased problems with glare and photosensitivity, so there have been several artificial irises developed that can decrease these symptoms and improve cosmesis. These include special contact lenses and surgically implanted irises.

Neurofibromatosis

There are two types of *neurofibromatosis* that can lead to a variety of tumors, including acoustic schwannomas (tumors affecting the nerves that conduct hearing), peripheral neurofibromas, and central nervous system gliomas. In particular, neurofibromatosis type 1 (NF1) is associated with important eye findings. *Lisch nodules* are benign nodules seen on the iris common to most NF1 patients, and are considered diagnostic for the disease. The primary clinically relevant ophthalmic concern of NF1 patients is tumors of the optic nerve, which can cause pain and affect vision. These tumors, called *optic nerve gliomas*, typically develop in the first 6 years of life. Typical clinical manifestations include proptosis from the tumor pushing on the orbit and optic disc edema from compression of the optic nerve, followed by degeneration secondary to the pressure. Though NF1 is a relatively common disease, affecting 1 in 3000 people, only a fraction of the patients will develop optic nerve gliomas.[5]

Autosomal Recessive

Homocystinuria

Homocystinuria is a disease that shares may clinical features of Marfan syndrome (discussed previously). It is caused by a deficit in the enzyme that catalyzes the breakdown of homocystine, a product of intracellular metabolism. Without this proper breakdown, there is an increase in blood homocystine levels and a decrease of molecules that are synthesized from homocystine. Because there are deficits in protein cross-linking (a process that stabilizes protein structure) in this disease, many of the manifestations are structural in nature, and include a Marfan-like body, dislocation of the lens inferiorly, and excess mobility in the joints. Unlike many inborn errors of metabolism, homocystinuria can be treated with supplementation of vitamins B_6, B_{12}, and folate, along with reduction in the dietary intake of homocystine. This treatment prevents further progression of the disease, but unfortunately does not reverse preexisting deficits.[6]

Oculocutaneous Albinism

Oculocutaneous albinism refers to a group of disorders that affect melanocytes, the cells responsible for pigmentation, most notably in the skin (*cutaneous*). Albinism, which also affects melanocytes in the hair, the iris, and the retinal pigment epithelium, can either be complete (where there is no pigmentation at all) or partial (where there is decreased pigmentation from normal). The most common types of oculocutaneous albinism are autosomal recessive, but there is a rare X-linked recessive form as well as several variants that have systemic associations. In the eye, the lack of pigmentation leads to several developmental abnormalities, including foveal hypoplasia (underdevelopment), nystagmus (rhythmic jerking of the eyes), and an abnormal crossing of nerve fibers at the optic chiasm. Though the exact mechanism for these abnormalities is not well understood, it is postulated that they could be related to the delayed visual maturation that is commonly seen in these disorders.

X-Linked Dominant

Incontinentia Pigmenti

Incontinentia pigmenti is best characterized by its dermatologic manifestations. The most obvious of these are patches of increased and decreased skin pigmentation. Ocular symptoms are mostly retinal, and include vascular anomalies, such as areas where there should be blood vessels but aren't, areas with abnormal growth of blood vessels, and the absence of a foveal pit. This aberrant vessel growth can then cause retinal hemorrhage similar to that seen in diabetes and retinopathy of prematurity. The treatment for the abnormal blood vessel growth seen in incontinentia pigmenti is panretinal photocoagulation (laser treatment of a broad area of the retina).

Alport Syndrome

Alport syndrome is a disease that causes hearing loss, decreased visual acuity, and kidney disease starting in childhood. It is caused by a mutation in the gene responsible for formation of a type of *collagen*, a major structural protein found throughout the body. Because of the resultant decrease in structural integrity, several structures of the eye show abnormalities. In the cornea, there is an outward bowing known as *keratoconus*, and in the lens there is a similar anterior bowing, called *lenticonus*. While anterior lenticonus only occurs in 22% of Alport's patients, it is a very specific sign of Alport's, and its presence is sufficient for diagnosis.[7]

X-Linked Recessive

Red/Green Color Blindness

Probably the best-known inheritance-linked phenomenon in ophthalmology is *red/green color blindness*, which is predominantly seen in men. This form of color blindness is caused by a mutation in the genes on the X chromosome that code for the pigment in the photoreceptors. Red/green color blindness (a term commonly used to describe a spectrum of disorders, Table 24-1) is seen in about 8% of males,[8] and is characterized by the inability to distinguish red from green due to mutations in the photoreceptor pigment. It should be noted that there are other more rare forms of color blindness, such as blue/yellow color blindness (the inability to differentiate blue from yellow) and complete color blindness (the inability to distinguish any difference in color).

Mitochondrial Inheritance

Leber Hereditary Optic Neuropathy

Leber hereditary optic neuropathy was the first disease shown to be due to mutations in mitochondrial DNA. Leber's is characterized by unilateral central visual loss with swelling at the optic nerve, followed weeks to months later by a similar loss of vision in the other eye. It typically affects patients in their 20s to 30s. In Leber's, the mutation leads to abnormal movement of mitochondria through axons. Retinal ganglion cells are especially

TABLE 24-1			
GENETICS OF COLOR BLINDNESS			
Disease	**Photoreceptor(s) Affected**	**Clinical Manifestations**	**Genetics**
Protanopia	Red	Inability to see red	X-linked recessive
Protanomaly	Red	Alteration in red	X-linked recessive
Deuteranopia	Green	Inability to see green	X-linked recessive
Deuteranomaly	Green	Alteration in green	X-linked recessive
Tritanopia	Blue	Inability to see blue	Autosomal dominant
Complete color blindness	Two or three types of cones	Inability to distinguish between colors	X-linked recessive or autosomal dominant

affected at the optic nerve head, where this deficit leads to swelling of the axons. Three mutations accounting for 97% of Leber's are commonly tested for clinically; however, Leber's displays incomplete penetrance, and only about 50% of males and 10% of females who harbor the genetic mutations go on to develop optic neuropathy.[9] Therefore, genetic testing for the mitochondrial mutation is useful for determining if a patient with symptoms has Leber's, but is not useful for determining if a patient with the mutations will develop Leber's in the future.

Multiple Types of Transmission

Retinitis Pigmentosa

Retinitis pigmentosa is degeneration of the retinal pigment epithelium layer, which clears the shed-off outer segments of the photoreceptors. Because there are more than 50 genes that can cause retinitis pigmentosa, the clinical phenotype and genetic inheritance has wide variability in both age of onset and visual acuity.[10,11] The classic symptom of retinitis pigmentosa is an inherited night blindness, followed by loss of peripheral vision and then central vision. Fundus exam shows a pale disc, pigmentary changes in the periphery, and attenuation (narrowing) of the arterioles. Despite the fact that there is a wide variety of clinical outcomes in retinitis pigmentosa, the disease is progressive and frequently reduces vision to less than 20/200 bilaterally, suggesting that referral to a low vision specialist would be beneficial for many of these patients.

Multigenetic

Despite the advances that have been made in molecular diagnosis and treatment of ocular diseases, many of the most common diseases in ophthalmology are known to have a strong genetic component, but the exact genetics of that inheritance is still not well understood. In most of these cases, it is presumed that there is no one gene that causes the disease, but rather an interaction of many different genes in conjunction with environmental factors. In these types of disease, the genome-wide association studies (described earlier) have been useful in determining the genetic underpinnings leading to the diseases. Here we will highlight some of the more experimental genetics associated with two common ophthalmic diseases: glaucoma and macular degeneration.

Glaucoma

Glaucoma is covered in detail in Chapter 29. It is not caused by a single factor, but is the manifestation of a complex disease process. While glaucoma has traditionally been thought of as a disease of increased intraocular pressure (IOP) causing the selective death of retinal ganglion cells, there are many other molecular pathways that converge to lead to the death of retinal ganglion cells. That is, not everyone with increased IOP will develop glaucoma, and not everyone who has glaucoma has increased IOP.

The most common form of glaucoma, primary open angle glaucoma, accounts for more than 75% of glaucoma cases, yet the genetics behind it are poorly understood.[12] GWAS has implicated a number of novel genes that contribute to this process. Not surprisingly, these genes encompass the spectrum of systems that contribute to glaucoma. Genes that have been implicated include those that affect neuroprotective factors and mitochondrial genes, factors that change IOP, and genes that influence anatomic development.

There are several familial cases of glaucoma caused by a single gene each that have helped us to understand some of the genetics behind the disorder. The discovery of these genes support the idea that this disease process is not due to a failure of just one pathway, but can be influenced by a network of systems that need to function together properly. Among the genes that can cause monogenetic glaucoma are myocilin (which regulates IOP), FOXC1 (which controls survival after oxidative stress [the accumulation of free radicals to the point where antioxidants can't neutralize them all]), LOXL1 (which is important in connective tissue production), and several different mitochondrial genes.

Age-Related Macular Degeneration

AMD is a leading cause of visual loss in patients over 60 years. The exact pathogenesis is still not completely understood, but the clinical hallmarks are deposits of waste material in the retina known as *drusen*. If this is followed by abnormal blood vessel growth, it is known as *wet* AMD. As with glaucoma, the exact cause of macular degeneration is most likely multifactorial, with many different processes playing a role. GWAS has also been useful in determining some of the genes that play a role in the disease. The strongest association has been with a protein that is commonly thought of as part of the immune response, called *complement factor H*, but other pathways (such as the one that regulates cholesterol) are also clearly involved in some way. While sibling studies have shown that genetics increases the risk of AMD about four-fold, the mutations that have been discovered only account for a small fraction of this risk. This suggests that there are other as-of-yet unknown genes that contribute as well.[13]

Genetic Testing

Use in Diagnosis/Prognosis

Probably the most common use of genetic testing is for the definitive diagnosis of diseases. While the clinical manifestations of certain disorders (such as aniridia) are sufficient for diagnosis, often there is an overlap in the clinical manifestations of diseases, and if there is a genetic test it can be used to clarify any ambiguity in clinical diagnosis.

While it might seem insignificant to know an exact diagnosis if it will not change medical treatment, there are still benefits to diagnostic genetic testing. And although diagnosis does not usually change the prognosis, it may be helpful to predict the course of a disease. For instance, there is quite a different prognosis for patients with Leber hereditary optic neuropathy vs dominant optic atrophy. These two diseases specifically affect the optic nerve and can be definitively differentiated based on genetic testing. By differentiating between the two, the patient can be prepared for progression of the disease and can plan accordingly. The psychological impact of having a diagnosis should also not be overlooked. And often just putting a name to the disorder is enough for patients to begin to feel like they have some control over what is happening to them.

Genetic Counseling

The clinical situation where genetic testing currently plays a prominent role is genetic counseling, both for patients who already have children and those who are planning a family. It is important to know the genetic inheritance patterns and to understand the risk of a disease being passed on. For instance, the chance of someone with a rare autosomal recessive disease passing on the disease would be low, since his/her partner would likely contribute a normal gene. But if one parent has an autosomal dominant disease, there is a 50% chance that it will be passed down.

Treatment

Unfortunately, there are currently few therapies that are directed by genetic testing. Treatment of genetic eye disease is still a field in its infancy, although possessing great promise. In pulmonology, the study of cystic fibrosis (CF) has led the way in developing genetically targeted therapies due to the well-described and relative simplicity of the genetics involved: CF is caused by mutations in a single gene. In 2015, a new drug was approved for patients with the most common mutation that causes CF, the $\Delta F508$ mutation. This success with genetically individualized therapy gives us hope that similar technology could eventually be applied to ophthalmic diseases. For instance, clinical trials regarding aniridia have been approved that may allow for treatment of certain genetic mutations. With continued research on the genetic causes of disease, this is likely only the tip of the iceberg as we begin to see individualized medicine go from fantasy to reality.

Methods of Testing

Chromosomal Analysis

The oldest form of genetic testing is *chromosomal analysis*. This technology takes advantage of the fact that the chromosomes are compacted and segregated during mitosis (the process by which cells divide), and that during this period they have the "x" appearance typically used to depict individual chromosomes. Using special stains on these compacted chromosomes, the architecture of individual chromosomes can be seen under the microscope, and the presence of the correct number of chromosomes can also be determined. This technique, known as *karyotyping*, is the most useful for determining significant changes in genetic structure, such as deletion of part of a chromosome or rearrangement of the genetic material. For example, this is the same method used after an amniocentesis to determine if there is an extra chromosome that would indicate Down syndrome in a fetus (Figure 24-8). Because the necessary growth of cells and the specialized techniques used to stain the DNA, this method tends to take several weeks before results are known.

Molecular Techniques: Polymerase Chain Reaction and Restriction Enzyme Digestion

To test for small changes in DNA, several molecular techniques can be utilized. These methods are not only more sensitive than karyotyping, but they also can be completed in a day. (Note: Some labs tend to batch them together so that results are still usually returned in a week

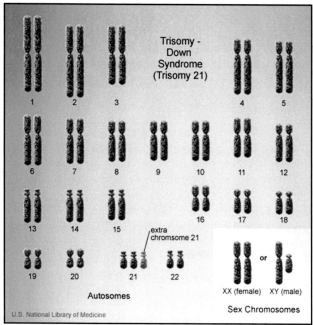

Figure 24-8. Karyotype of an individual with an extra chromosome 21 (Down syndrome). (This public domain image is reprinted from the US National Library of Medicine.)

or two.) *Polymerase chain reaction* (PCR) is a process that amplifies (makes copies of) a region of DNA using specific nucleic acid probes. A mutation might prevent the probes from binding and the DNA from amplifying, in which case the absence of amplified DNA would be diagnostic for a mutation in a specific region. Or, if the DNA is amplified, then the sample can be further evaluated via two ways: sequencing (discussed next) and *restriction digest analysis*. In the restriction test, the amplified DNA is mixed with enzymes that recognize and cut out (cleave) specific sequences of DNA, which releases certain chemicals. If the mutation either creates or deletes one of these specific sequences, then the presence (or absence) of DNA cleavage products can be used to indicate that a specific mutation is present.

Sequencing

While restriction digest analysis requires enzymes that recognize the specific DNA sequence of interest, *DNA sequencing* is a more powerful tool that determines the entire sequence of a given region of a chromosome. Sequencing uses PCR technology, so diagnostic sequencing can be directed to a gene of specific interest. One of the greatest advantages of DNA sequencing is that specific mutations do not have to be known ahead of time, but rather a gene can be tested for any mutation. This allows testing for multiple mutations at once, and can even find novel mutations that have not been described.

While entire-genome sequencing is not yet a technique that is clinically useful, the decreasing price of sequencing raises the question of whether it would be beneficial to sequence the whole genome of patients, rather than just selected genes. Current technology now allows for the sequencing of an entire genome for around $1000. (An amazing feat when you consider the first genome sequenced with current technology cost $1 million in 2007!) While this "shotgun" style testing (ie, not looking for one specific mutation) increases the sensitivity of detecting mutations, it also raises many ethical concerns. For example, do you treat a patient who has genes that suggest he/she will have a disease but currently has no manifestations of it? How will insurance companies use the sequence? How will privacy laws pertain to whole-genome sequences? These issues will have to be addressed before genome sequencing becomes a mainstream practice.

Gene Therapy

Gene therapy refers to the introduction of normal genes into malfunctioning cells, thus theoretically curing diseases by reintroducing the function whose absence caused the disorder.

Current State

At the time of publication, there is no gene therapy in clinical use. While there has been an explosion of knowledge about the genetic basis of diseases and how to best employ this knowledge clinically, there are many obstacles that have prevented its utilization.

Gene therapy using viral vectors (viral particles that are unable to replicate, but rather contain a therapeutic "payload") has been the best-explored avenue of research, not only because it introduces specific genes, but also because there is some selectivity to the cells that can be targeted. However, early trials using viral vectors were stopped because of several cases where leukemia was caused by damage to the host's DNA. This led to increased resistance by legislators and companies toward gene therapy trials. Other barriers preventing further development of gene therapies include allergic reactions to viral vectors, nonsustained response to therapy, and ineffective introduction of genetic material into the cells.

Despite the challenges, there are still clinical trials looking to harness gene therapy for diseases in ophthalmology. One disease that has been the focus of recent gene therapy trials is Leber congenital amaurosis (not to be confused with Leber hereditary optic neuropathy), a disease caused by mutations that lead to retinal dystrophy early in life. Preliminary trials using viral vectors to reintroduce one of the genes have shown promise in restoring some vision to these patients.

Clinical Skills

Sample Collection

Since our genetic material is transmitted to every cell in the body (and is only absent in hair, the outer keratinized layer of the skin, and red blood cells), sample collection for determination of genetic markers is relatively easy. For DNA testing via PCR or sequencing techniques, the simplest method is a cheek swab, which collects some of the mucosal cells that line the mouth. To do this, a sterile swab is rubbed against the mucosal surface in the cheek and immediately placed into a specimen container for transport to the lab. Because many of these genetic tests are sensitive to contamination by foreign DNA, it is important that the swab touch only the patient to avoid false results.

A simple blood draw is also commonly used in genetic testing. While red blood cells contain no nucleus (and thus no genetic material), white blood cells do contain genetic material and can be used for both PCR and sequencing. Additionally, because karyotyping relies on the ability of cells to be analyzed while they are dividing, a blood sample is required. White blood cells are easy to grow in culture and blood is relatively easy to obtain, so they are ideal cells for this technique. Patients may be understandably nervous about testing, but providing them with educational materials will help answer the most common questions (Sidebar 24-1).

Taking a Family History/ Establishing a Pedigree

One of the most useful techniques in determining the genetics of a particular disease is that of pedigree analysis, which is an evaluation of how genetic disease is passed down through multiple generations. While collecting an accurate history is the most important part of creating a pedigree, it is also vital that the data be documented in a way that is clear and concise, especially for complex family histories.

To document family histories and to help determine the inheritance of a disease, a graphic representation of who is and is not affected, called a *pedigree*, is used. By convention, each person is denoted by a square (for a male) or a circle (for a female). The circle/square of affected individuals is completely filled in, while those of nonaffected individuals are left open. Known *carriers* of a disease, who carry the gene that causes the disease but are not affected, are denoted by half-filled symbols. Genetic relationships are described by lines: horizontal lines denote pairings that have produced offspring together (Figure 24-9, arrow A), and vertical lines run from parents to children (Figure 24-9, arrow B). In this manner, each generation is recorded on a single row.

You can see in Figures 24-10 through 24-14 examples of pedigrees of autosomal and X-linked dominant and recessive, as well as mitochondrial inheritance. Note that 50% of the offspring of an individual with the disease also inherit the disease, that no generations are skipped, and that there is no bias for sex (see Figure 24-10).

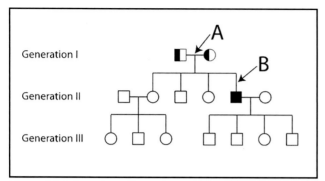

Figure 24-9. Sample pedigree. A square denotes a male; a circle denotes a female. Persons who exhibit a trait are noted with a filled-in symbol. A half-filled symbol indicates a carrier who does not exhibit the trait.

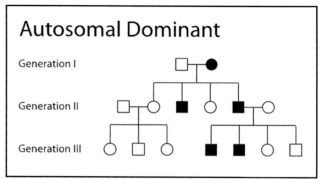

Figure 24-10. Pedigree showing an autosomal dominant pattern.

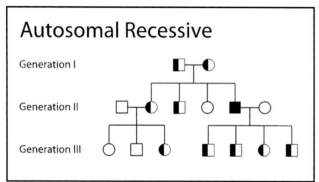

Figure 24-11. Pedigree with an autosomal recessive pattern.

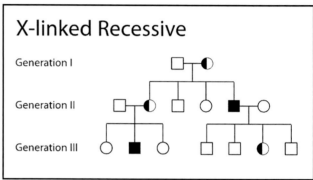

Figure 24-12. Pedigree with X-linked recessive pattern.

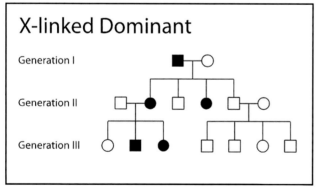

Figure 24-13. Pedigree with X-linked dominant pattern.

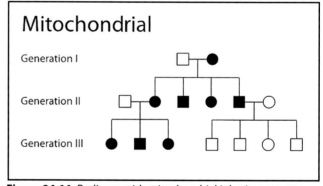

Figure 24-14. Pedigree with mitochondrial inheritance pattern.

Note that the disorder can result from two parents who do not display the phenotype, and that only one-quarter of the offspring from the two carriers are affected (see Figure 24-11).

Features that can clue you in to an X-linked recessive mode of inheritance is that only males are affected, that all daughters of affected males are carriers, and that that 50% of the sons of a carrier female are affected (see Figure 24-12).

Features that point toward an X-linked dominant form of inheritance is that all daughters of affected males will inherit the disease, but only half the children of the females (both the sons and daughters) inherit the disease (see Figure 24-13).

Mitochondrial inheritance might be the easiest mode of inheritance, because all the children of mothers with the disease will inherit the disease, but no offspring of affected males will (see Figure 24-14).

CONCLUSION

While the field of genetics is more than 150 years old, it is a still an area with the potential to drastically change ophthalmology in the future. Since we first understood the basics of genetics, great progress has been made in identifying genetic diseases, especially those due to a single mutation. While this has played an integral role in allowing us to understand the molecular basis of many eye disorders, the current clinical utility of genetics is in genetic counseling and diagnostic confirmation.

Despite the fact that there have been few translations of therapies directed to individual genotypes, there is currently much active research investigating the genetics of disease and how to best harness this information. With this emerging knowledge, it is likely we will soon be entering into the long-awaited world of personalized medicine, where genetics could occupy the heart of clinical practice. Even today, that promise seems to be coming closer to reality, with clinical trials that target patients with specific genetic mutations. With the exciting future of genetics, it is easy to forget that it has a place in ophthalmology practice already, and obtaining a deeper understanding is important for your patients even today.

CHAPTER QUIZ

1. Who is known as the father of modern genetics?
   a. Antoine Marfan
   b. Reginald Punnett
   c. Charles Darwin
   d. Gregor Mendel

2. How many chromosomes do humans have?
   a. 44
   b. 45
   c. 46
   d. 48

3. Which is an example of a phenotype?
   a. a mutation in the Pax6 gene
   b. a deletion of the X chromosome
   c. color blindness
   d. a set of three number 21 genes

4. Which of the following denotes a recessive phenotype?
   a. Aa
   b. xY
   c. AA
   d. aa

5. Which of the following chromosomes has less than two copies in each cell?
   a. Y
   b. 21
   c. V
   d. 18

6. Which ophthalmic disease is passed down in an autosomal dominant fashion?
   a. aniridia
   b. retinitis pigmentosa
   c. color blindness
   d. Alport syndrome

7. Which is *not* a use of genetic testing in clinical practice today?
   a. confirmation of the diagnosis
   b. for genetic counseling
   c. to guide treatment
   d. to determine insurance rates

8. Which cells are commonly used for genetic testing?
   a. buccal mucosa
   b. skin epithelial cells
   c. conjunctival mucosa
   d. hair

9. How are diseases with mitochondrial inheritance passed down?
   a. through the maternal line
   b. through the fraternal line
   c. from both the mother and the father
   d. this is not yet known

10. What is the inheritance pattern for red/green color blindness?
    a. autosomal recessive
    b. X-linked recessive
    c. mitochondrial
    d. autosomal dominant

11. What disorder is transmitted in an autosomal recessive fashion?
    a. homocystinuria
    b. Marfan syndrome
    c. aniridia
    d. Leber hereditary optic neuropathy

12. Which of the following is *not* an ophthalmic genetic disorder?
    a. oculocutaneous albinism
    b. central retinal artery occlusion
    c. aniridia
    d. retinitis pigmentosa

Answers

1. d
2. c
3. c
4. d
5. a
6. a
7. d
8. a
9. a
10. b
11. a
12. b

REFERENCES

1. MacCarthy A, Draper GJ, Steliarova-Foucher E, Kingston JE. Retinoblastoma incidence and survival in European children (1978-1997). Report from the Automated Childhood Cancer Information System project. *Eur J Cancer.* 2006;42(13):2092-2102.

2. Woo KI, Harbour JW. Review of 676 second primary tumors in patients with retinoblastoma: association between age at onset and tumor type. *Arch Ophthalmol.* 2010;128(7):865-870.

3. Burté F, Carelli V, Chinnery PF, Yu-Wai-Man P. Disturbed mitochondrial dynamics and neurodegenerative disorders. *Nat Rev Neurol.* 2015;11(1):11-24.

4. Lee HJ, Colby KA. A review of the clinical and genetic aspects of aniridia. *Semin Ophthalmol.* 2013;28(5-6):306-312.

5. Ferner RE, Gutmann DH. Neurofibromatosis type 1 (NF1): diagnosis and management. *Handb Clin Neurol.* 2013;115:939-955.

6. Walter JH, Wraith JE, White FJ, Bridge C, Till J. Strategies for the treatment of cystathionine beta-synthase deficiency: the experience of the Willink Biochemical Genetics Unit over the past 30 years. *Eur J Pediatr.* 1998;157(Suppl 2):S71-S76.

7. Amiraslanzadeh G. Is anterior lenticonus the most common ocular finding in Alport syndrome? *J Cataract Refract Surg.* 2008;34(1):5; author reply 5-6.

8. Delpero WT, O'Neill H, Casson E, Hovis J. Aviation-relevent epidemiology of color vision deficiency. *Aviat Space Environ Med.* 2005;76(2):127-133.

9. Kirkman MA, Yu-Wai-Man P, Korsten A, et al. Gene-environment interactions in Leber hereditary optic neuropathy. *Brain.* 2009;132(Pt 9):2317-2326.

10. Tsujikawa M, Wada Y, Sukegawa M, et al. Age at onset curves of retinitis pigmentosa. *Arch Ophthalmol.* 2008;126(3):337-340.

11. Grover S, Fishman GA, Anderson RJ, Tozatti MSV, et al. Visual acuity impairment in patients with retinitis pigmentosa at age 45 years or older. *Ophthalmology.* 1999;106(9):1780-1785.

12. Bankes JL, Perkins ES, Tsolakis S, Wright JE. Bedford glaucoma survey. *Br Med J.* 1968;1(5595):791-796.

13. Klaver CC, Wolfs RC, Assink JJ, van Duijn CM, Hofman A, de Jong PT. Genetic risk of age-related maculopathy. Population-based familial aggregation study. *Arch Ophthalmol.* 1998;116(12):1646-1651.

25

NEURO-OPHTHALMOLOGY

Beth Koch, COT, ROUB
Lisa Lystad, MD

BASIC SCIENCES

In this chapter, we will discuss many important areas in neuro-ophthalmology. A good understanding of ocular anatomy and physiology is essential. For a thorough discussion, see Chapters 2 and 3.

The Nervous System

The human nervous system is a network of structures and tissues with the job of transmitting information to and from the brain (Figure 25-1). It is generally divided into the central nervous system (CNS) and the peripheral nervous system (PNS).

The CNS consists of the brain and spinal cord; everything exterior to these two structures (with the important exception of the optic nerve) is part of the PNS. PNS nerves coming from the brain are *cranial nerves*; those arising from the spinal cord are sensibly called *spinal nerves*.

Neurons, or nerve cells, are very unique. The nerve body is the *soma*, and extending from this is a single *axon*. (The axon may branch many times *after* leaving the cell body; these branches are the same thickness as the original axon.) At the end of the axon's branches are *terminals*. Also arising from the soma are filaments called *dendrites*, which can be quite numerous and have additional branches. The dendrite branches get thinner and thinner. Impulses between nerve cells are sent from the terminals of one neuron to the dendrites of the next.

The terminals and dendrites must communicate with other cells (be it a nerve cell, a muscle cell, or other tissue), but there is a gap between them called a *synaptic gap*. In order for an impulse from the brain to reach the neuron (and vice versa), the gap must be breached by chemicals called *neurotransmitters*, which in turn must activate specific receptors either on the next nerve cell in line or on the target tissue. There are several neurotransmitters including epinephrine and histamine. Sometimes the release of one neurotransmitter will trigger the release of another.

Some nerve axons are encased by a sheath of a white, fatty substance called *myelin*. The myelin acts as an insulator. Axons that are thus myelinated are generically called *nerve fibers*. The "nerve fibers" of the retina, however, are usually not myelinated. (During embryonic development, myelination does not normally extend beyond the lamina cribrosa.)

A nerve that transmits signals from the brain is an *efferent* or *motor* nerve. A nerve that transmits signals to the brain is *afferent* or *sensory*. (You'll see these two terms a lot when studying pupillary responses.) Some nerves are one or the other, but most are both (*mixed*).

Ledford JK, Lens A, eds.
Principles and Practice in Ophthalmic Assisting:
A Comprehensive Textbook (pp 473-484).
© 2018 Taylor & Francis Group.

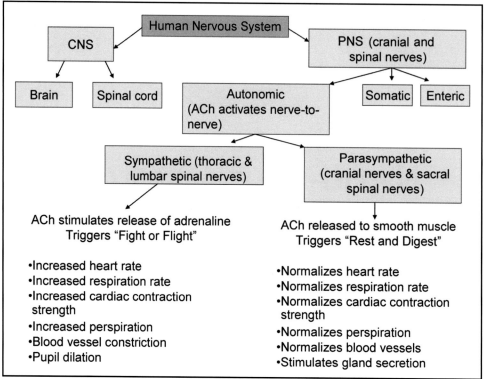

Figure 25-1. Divisions of the human nervous system. ACh=acetylcholine, CNS=central nervous system, PNS=peripheral nervous system.

The PNS is mainly made up of nerve cells and can be further divided into three branches: the somatic, enteric, and autonomic, each with its specific function and nerve cells. *Somatic* nerves supply muscles for voluntary movement, including that of the eye. The *enteric* is involved in digestion and other gastrointestinal functions. The *autonomic* supplies involuntary functions, such as heart beat, breathing, and pupil size.

The autonomic system consists of two parts, each with their own nerves: the sympathetic and parasympathetic systems. The *sympathetic* system is mediated (ie, controlled/activated) by the neurotransmitter *acetylcholine,* which in turn triggers the release of *adrenaline* (*epinephrine*). Adrenaline activates the "fight or flight" or "adrenaline rush" response when a person feels threatened. The heart and respiration rates increase, blood vessels constrict, perspiration increases, and the pupils dilate. In an emergency, adrenaline is released, crosses the synaptic gap, and activates the sympathetic reaction.

The *parasympathetic* system maintains homeostasis when the person is in a relaxed, nonthreatened state, dubbed "rest and digest." In this case the neurotransmitter acetylcholine stimulates the release of *noradrenaline* (*norepinephrine*). Noradrenaline affects the body in a way that "undoes" the sympathetic system's "panic" reaction. But rather than counteract each other, the more correct concept is that the two systems work in tandem to counterbalance each other.

These explanations are simplified, but provide enough basic information for this text.

Cranial Nerves

There are 12 cranial nerves (CN), each designated by a name and a Roman numeral:

▶ I—Olfactory

▶ II—Optic

▶ III—Oculomotor

▶ IV—Trochlear

▶ V—Trigeminal

▶ VI—Abducens

▶ VII—Facial

▶ VIII—Vestibulocochlear

▶ IX—Glossopharyngeal

▶ X—Vagus

▶ XI—Spinal accessory

▶ XII—Hypoglossal

The main cranial nerves we will be concerned with are the optic (II), oculomotor (III), trochlear (IV), trigeminal (V), and abducens (VI). Three of these (III, IV, and VI) control the extraocular muscles. The oculomotor (III) also plays a role in controlling the pupil. The trigeminal nerve (V) relays pain and touch from the eye, forehead, cheek, and sinuses.

The role of each cranial nerve involved in ocular movements (see Chapter 10) and pupil function (Chapter 9) is very important to determine what may be going on neurologically with the patient and to help narrow down the physician's list of possible diagnoses.

The Extraocular Muscles

Evaluating the extraocular muscles (EOMs) is another aspect of the technician work-up that helps the physician in assessing the patient. To check EOMs, the technician needs to know the action(s) of each muscle and which cranial nerve innervates it (Table 25-1). A formula to help you remember which nerve innervates which EOM is LR_6SO_4. This signifies that the lateral rectus (LR) is innervated by CN VI, the superior oblique (SO) is supplied by CN IV. (Some sources add "AO_3" to the mnemonic, signifying that "all others" [AO] are innervated by CN III.)

The LR and medial rectus (MR) each only perform one action—the LR only abducts while the MR only adducts. The rest of the EOMs each have primary, secondary, and tertiary movements. The EOM work-up is important not only in neuro-ophthalmology but in all ophthalmic evaluations. EOMs are discussed in great detail in Chapter 10.

Optic Nerve and Visual Pathways

The details of peripheral vision and visual field testing are covered in Chapter 14, but some discussion is warranted here.

Keep in mind that the retina and visual field have an inverted and reversed relationship. The upper visual field falls on the inferior retina (below the fovea), the lower visual field falls on the superior retina (above the fovea), the nasal visual field falls on the temporal retina, and the temporal visual field falls on the nasal retina. The visual field of each eye overlaps centrally. Normal visual field parameters for each eye are 60 degrees (°) superiorly, 70° to 75° inferiorly, 60° nasally, and 100° to 110° temporally.

The visual pathway can be evaluated by visual field testing (confrontation or formal/automated). It is important to be accurate to determine if there has been field loss. The practitioner uses this information to help pinpoint a diagnosis.

Visual field testing is an important part of the neurological exam because it can be used to detect and quantify visual field abnormalities and follow a patient's response to treatment. It can also confirm the presence of visual defects when other visual tests (ie, visual acuity) don't.

The pattern of visual field loss may pinpoint the location of the problem in the visual pathway (Figures 25-2 and 25-3). If the defect is one-sided (ie, manifests in only one eye), it generally has occurred between the optic nerve and the chiasm; if the defect shows up in both eyes but on opposite sides, it is most likely at the chiasm

TABLE 25-1
EXTRAOCULAR MUSCLES AND THEIR INNERVATION

Extraocular Muscle	Cranial Nerve
Lateral rectus	CN VI
Superior oblique	CN IV
Medial rectus	CN III
Inferior oblique	CN III
Superior rectus	CN III
Inferior rectus	CN III

where the nasal fibers cross. If the defect occurs after the chiasm, it will appear in both eyes but on the same side (*homonymous*) due to the nasal and temporal fibers of one eye traveling the same optic pathway.

CLINICAL KNOWLEDGE

In this section, we will discuss disorders of the optic nerve and intracranial visual pathway, ocular motility disorders, and pupil abnormalities. Patients with these types of problems may present with symptoms of vision loss, visual field loss, and diplopia. Various disorders have similar signs and symptoms, and it is part of the tech's job to do the detective work by taking a good history and performing the appropriate tests, which we will discuss later in this chapter.

Disorders of the Intracranial Visual Pathway

Note: The *intracranial* visual pathway refers to the visual pathway from where the optic nerve enters the optic canal and back to the occipital lobe. The *extracranial* portion of the pathway is the retina and optic nerve before it penetrates the skull.

Stroke

A *stroke* is a sudden loss of specific brain functions (eg, speech or movement) resulting from an interrupted blood supply. There may be a blockage from a thrombus (a clot that has formed at that location), an embolus (a clot that has broken lose and traveled the blood vessels until it encounters one too small to get through), or blood loss due to hemorrhage.

Patients who come to the office with indications of a possible stroke usually present with acute neurologic signs and symptoms (Sidebar 25-1). These signs and symptoms may include vision loss, visual field defect, double vision,

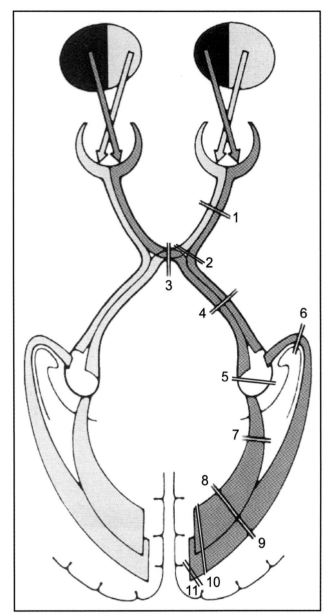

Figure 25-2. The visual pathway.

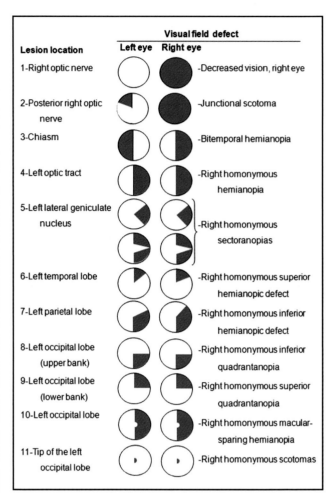

Figure 25-3. Visual field defects. The numbers coordinate with the numbered locations in Figure 25-2.

and oscillopsia (illusion that the environment is moving), as well as hemiparesis (incomplete or partial paralysis involving half the body) or hemiplegia (paralysis on one side of the body).

There are other conditions that can have similar symptoms. A *transient ischemic attack* (TIA, sometimes called a mini-stroke) occurs when the blood supply to the small blood vessels of the brain has been temporarily interrupted. It can produce a vision loss that usually recovers in less than 1 hour.[1] *Amaurosis fugax* is another vascular problem that is frightening but doesn't last long, this time involving decreased blood flow to the ophthalmic artery.[2] Symptoms may include not only a sudden

decrease of vision in one eye, but can vary from constricted peripheral vision to total loss of vision.

For these patients, it is important to check confrontation visual fields carefully (see Chapter 9), looking for *hemianopic* defects (ie, half of the field) due to stroke damage. The patient will usually notice temporal visual field loss on one side and not realize there is a nasal field loss in the other eye as well. This happens because the nasal fields of both eyes overlap to an extent, so the patient thinks there is only a temporal defect. There is, however, a small area in the nasal fields that does not overlap, leaving the patient with a small scotoma that may be mildly noticeable when scanning pages, leading to the complaint that words blank out while reading.

A stroke victim may have mild, moderate, or severe aphasia (difficulty in speaking), depending on the seriousness of the stroke. You may need to be creative to find ways that you and the patient can communicate to check vision and perform other subjective tests.

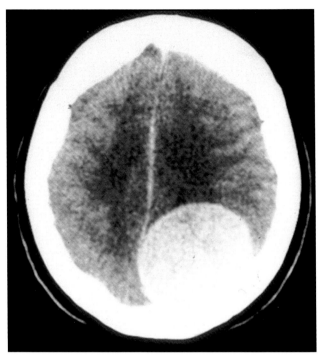

Figure 25-4. Post-chiasmal meningioma.

Tumors

Pituitary Tumors

Tumors can also create a visual pathway defect. In early phases, *pituitary tumors* can show signs of bitemporal field loss due to compression of the optic chiasm.

Patients with visual field loss from pituitary tumors are often unaware of the loss until it becomes advanced since the loss can be slow and symmetrical. By this time they have lost a considerable amount of the visual field. It is important to be accurate and carefully check confrontation visual fields and/or perform automated perimetry.

Meningioma

A *meningioma* is a tumor that forms from the tissue that covers the brain and spinal cord. It is usually slow-growing, but may put pressure on nearby structures. Thus it may cause problems with the optic nerve or chiasm, or grow into the orbit itself.[2] Meningiomas create unique visual field defects depending on where they are located in the visual pathway. A meningioma of the optic nerve sheath (pre-chiasmal) tends to affect only one eye and can cause peripheral field constriction. Peri-chiasmal lesions can affect both eyes, but are usually more prominent in one than the other. In this case, the constriction is peripheral but may be more temporal in the second eye. Post-chiasmal meningiomas (Figures 25-4 and 25-5) occur in the optic radiations, causing a right- or left-half (*hemifield*) field loss in both eyes. The defect may be on the same side in both eyes, or one on the left and the other eye on the right.

Multiple Sclerosis

Multiple sclerosis (MS) can cause an inflammatory response in the eye resulting in optic neuritis (inflammation of the optic nerve).[3] Optic neuritis will often cause a central scotoma with diffuse depression (overall decrease) in the visual field. There may also be subacute (ie, usually progresses rapidly over a few days), decreased visual acuity, and color vision problems. MS can also cause lesions in the optic tract that will result in a contralateral (opposite side) homonymous hemianopia (affects the same half of the visual field of each eye). Thus, if a lesion is in the left optic tract, the visual field defect will be a right homonymous hemianopia (ie, right temporal loss and left nasal loss).

Ocular Sarcoid

Ocular sarcoid can also result in optic neuritis, inflammation at the chiasm, and papilledema (swelling of the optic nerve head), causing associated visual field losses. Optic neuritis in sarcoid will elicit the same type of visual field loss as in MS. Chiasmal neuritis can cause a bitemporal hemianopia (ie, loss of temporal field in each eye) with or without a central scotoma. Papilledema tends to cause peripheral constriction in the visual field, which will be discussed in further detail under compressive disorders of the optic nerve.

Thyroid Eye Disease

Although thyroid-associated orbitopathy does not itself cause vision or visual field loss, it can cause exposure keratopathy (due to lid retraction) and diplopia (due to swelling or compression of EOMs). Visual field loss in thyroid eye disease is due to compressive optic

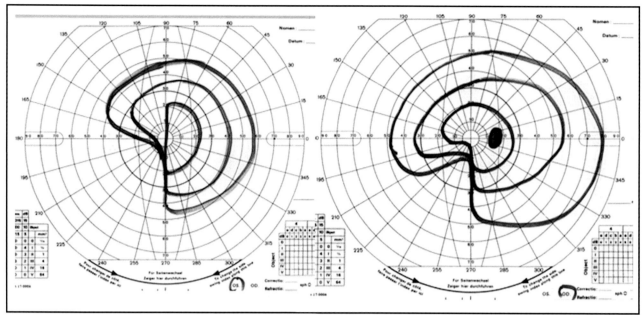

Figure 25-5. Visual field defect corresponding to scan in Figure 25-4.

neuropathy, where the optic nerve is being squeezed by muscles that are swollen.[4]

Compressive optic neuropathy generally has the hallmark of slow, progressive vision loss. Findings can also include dyschromatopsia (defects in color vision), relative afferent pupillary defect (RAPD), optic atrophy or edema, and visual field defects.[5]

Since compressive optic neuropathy affects mainly the optic nerve, and most of the nerve is linked to central vision, the associated visual field defect will be a central scotoma. There will also usually be some evidence of peripheral constriction. In some cases there may be altitudinal (upper or lower half of the visual field) or arcuate (arc-shaped defect near the blind spot) field defects that mimic glaucoma. Enlargement of the blindspot may be noted when disc edema is present.[5]

Pseudotumor Cerebri

Also known as *idiopathic intracranial hypertension*, patients with *pseudotumor cerebri* (PTC) will have symptoms and signs of raised intracranial pressure (ICP), such as headache, nausea, pulsatile tinnitus (pulsing ringing or rushing in the ears), papilledema (with vision loss), and diplopia (from unilateral or bilateral CN VI palsy). Management is based on the severity of the headache and presence of visual loss, specifically visual field deficits.[3]

Some of the visual field defects seen in PTC are an enlarged blind spot and nasal defects that can progress to involve the central 30°. If ICP is not treated promptly with a lumbar puncture (or cerebral shunts in severe cases), the field loss can become permanent. However, even with severe visual field loss, central vision can be preserved.

Optic Nerve Drusen

Optic nerve drusen are small, calcified concretions in the optic disc that occur in about 1% to 2% of the population.[3] They are usually bilateral, but may be asymmetrical, and can be seen in every age group. These drusen are generally asymptomatic, but some patients may have brief, transient episodes of vision loss. Drusen can also cause peripheral visual field constriction that may gradually worsen. Optic nerve drusen are generally discovered through funduscopic exam and can be imaged with photography, optical coherence tomography (OCT), and ultrasound. There is no treatment.

Ischemic Optic Neuropathy

Ischemic optic neuropathy refers to loss of optic nerve function due to an inadequate blood supply. There are several types.

Anterior ischemic optic neuropathy (AION) is always associated with disc edema and accounts for 90% of optic nerve ischemia.[1] It has two main classifications.

Arteritic AION (AAION) usually occurs in the presence of *giant cell arteritis* (GCA), which is an inflammation of the lining of the arteries. The arteries in the head (especially in the temples) are most often affected. For this reason, GCA is sometimes called *temporal arteritis* (TA). GCA frequently causes headaches, scalp tenderness, jaw pain, and vision problems (including double vision). Fatigue, weight loss, fever, and even death can occur. If left untreated, it can lead to stroke or blindness.[6] Smoking seems to be a risk factor. Blood tests and a biopsy may be needed to confirm the diagnosis.

GCA and ischemic optic neuropathy usually occur in the elderly (mostly 65 years of age and older) and can cause irreversible, bilateral, total blindness. But this devastating result can be prevented with prompt corticosteroid treatment. (This is another piece of evidence on the importance of promptly seeing a patient with sudden, painless loss of vision. See Chapter 33.)

The second classification is *nonarteritic AION* (NAION), which usually occurs in patients 50 years of age or older and is more common in White persons.[3] It is characterized by acute, painless vision loss that may progress over several hours or days. The involved eye may have an RAPD (see Chapter 9). The typical visual field defect can be altitudinal or arcuate (especially inferiorly).

NAION results from occlusive disease of the small vessels supplying the anterior optic nerve. Some of the signs for potentially developing NAION are a "disc at risk" (small, crowded disc), optic nerve drusen, severe papilledema, severely low blood pressure (104/58 mm Hg nocturnally), and hypercoagulation disorders (where the blood has an overtendency to clot).

Trauma

Traumatic optic neuropathy is not common but can be a complication of head injury. Any patient who has sustained a head injury (especially as a result of concussive blows to the head, particularly the forehead) or who may have optic nerve damage from either an orbital foreign body or bone fragments should be checked. This is especially true if there is unexplained vision loss, visual field loss, RAPD, or color vision loss. Any trauma to the head or eyes (gunshot wounds, history of intracranial surgery, paintball injuries, blunt trauma, etc) should be checked for possible neuro-ophthalmic problems.

Motility Disorders

Cranial Nerve Palsies

Cranial nerve palsies of CNs III, IV, and VI can have numerous causes and effects. In addition, there are other conditions that mimic these problems. In cases of a true palsy causing ocular muscle weakness and diplopia, prisms can often be used to help correct the tropia (discussed later in this chapter). In general, practitioners do not want to do surgery for double vision until at least 6 months after the palsy first appears, to give the condition time to resolve on its own.

Cranial Nerve III Palsy

A patient with a *CN III (oculomotor) palsy* may present with binocular vertical and horizontal diplopia, droopy lid, enlarged pupil, and/or blurred monocular vision at near. There are two classifications of a CN III palsy: *partial* (not all muscles innervated by the CN III are involved or there is only moderate paresis of the muscles) and complete (all muscles innervated by CN III are involved, with total paresis). A complete CN III palsy

has two further classifications: *pupil involvement* (there is anisocoria, where the larger pupil is on the side of the palsy and does not react well to light) and *pupil-sparing* (pupils are symmetric, and both react well to light).

Pupil involvement can indicate life-threatening disorders, such as an intracranial aneurysm or pituitary tumor causing compression of CN III. If it is isolated and pupil-sparing, it is thought to be caused by microvascular ischemia (insufficient supply of blood to the small blood vessels), usually associated with diabetes or other vascular risk factors. If the palsy is from a microvascular cause, there may be pain in the eye and/or headaches. Both types usually resolve after 3 to 4 months.[3]

Cranial Nerve IV Palsy

The two most common causes of a *CN IV (trochlear) palsy* are trauma (unilateral or bilateral) and break down (decompensation) of a congenital fourth nerve palsy. The congenital type is not often diagnosed during childhood because it is normally controlled in spite of the palsy. A patient with a trochlear palsy may present with diagonal double vision (a variant of vertical double vision) apparent at distance and near, and resolved by covering one eye or the other.

If a CN IV palsy occurs in a patient older than 50 years with vascular risk factors (specifically abnormal fatty deposits in an artery), it is most likely a microvascular CN IV palsy, which will usually completely resolve in 3 to 6 months.[3]

Cranial Nerve VI Palsy

Acquired

Patients with acquired *CN VI (abducens)* palsy will complain of horizontal diplopia that is worse when looking to the side of the palsy. Some of the causes of acquired CN VI palsy are infarction, infection (eg, meningitis), trauma, and microvascular disease (eg, diabetes). In microvascular disease, the palsy usually resolves in 3 to 6 months.[3]

Congenital

Congenital CN VI palsies can arise from conditions such as Duane syndrome and Mobius syndrome, as well as horizontal gaze paresis and progressive scoliosis (HGPPS).

A person with *Duane syndrome* (also called *Duane retraction syndrome*) exhibits marked limitation of abduction and variable limits on adduction. When trying to adduct the eye, the eyeball pulls back a little into the socket, and there is narrowing of palpebral fissure. This happens due to co-contraction of medial and lateral rectus muscles. The condition can be unilateral or bilateral, occurs more often in females, and more commonly in the left eye. Patients usually do not complain of diplopia and most do not have amblyopia.[3]

In *Mobius syndrome*, in addition to a sixth nerve palsy, the patient will also have a congenital paralysis of various muscles on both sides of the face. This palsy is very rare. In HGPPS, the CN VI palsy shows an absence of motor coordination of the eyes. Thus, there is a problem with bilateral fixation on a single object (ie, an absence of coordinated horizontal eye movements).

There are conditions that mimic CN VI palsies but really are not. For example, myasthenia can give an isolated abduction deficit. Also, in *convergence spasm* (spasm of the *near triad*—convergence, accommodation, and pupillary constriction), both eyes will turn toward the nose but cannot move laterally to either side, appearing to be a bilateral CN VI palsy. In this case, the patient can be checked for ductions (movement of one eye alone, with the other covered) and should be able to abduct and adduct each eye when tested individually. If dilating drops are instilled, the spasms will be disrupted.

Nystagmus

Nystagmus is an involuntary rhythmic side-to-side, up-and-down (oscillating), or "rotating" (torsional) eye movement. Nystagmus can be physiologic or pathologic.

Physiologic nystagmus is rapid and only present when the eyes are in extreme right or left gaze. The movement will "beat" in the direction of the gaze. It can diminish in seconds and completely resolves when the eyes are redirected closer to the midline. It is not visually disabling.

Pathologic nystagmus is characterized by jerk or pendulum-like movements. *Jerk nystagmus* is a rhythmic side-to-side movement that is faster in one direction than the other. *Pendular nystagmus* is a rhythmic eye movement where both eyes move together at about the same speed in each direction. This can cause poor vision and dizziness due to the constant eye movement. Many patients discover a *null point*—a head or gaze position that decreases or even stops the eye movement.

Other types of nystagmus include *infantile nystagmus,* which becomes apparent in first few months of life. *Latent nystagmus* is not evident during binocular fixation but is seen when either eye is covered. The uncovered eye beats away from the covered eye.

Pupil Abnormalities

There are different types of pupil abnormalities other than an afferent pupillary defect (see Table 9-1 in Chapter 9). *Anisocoria* is when the pupils are of unequal size. *Physiologic anisocoria* is the normal, benign inequality in the pupils that can occur from time to time and may even switch sides. The difference between the pupils is usually less than 0.5 mm.

Horner's syndrome is a pupil abnormality characterized by unilateral miosis (small pupil), lack of sweating (anhydrosis) on the same side, ipsilateral (same side) upper lid ptosis, and mild lower lid elevation (upside-down ptosis). In Horner's, pupil reaction to light is normal but pupillary dilation is not. A Horner's pupil has a dilation lag that is greatest 4 to 5 seconds after the lights

are turned off. The test to confirm this diagnosis is to instill topical apraclonidine 0.5% in both eyes. If the test is positive, the affected pupil dilates, and the lid elevates. The drops have no effect on the contralateral (opposite), unaffected eye.

Tonic pupils are enlarged pupils that respond very slowly to light and accommodation. It is associated with local processes affecting the nerve fibers that supply the iris sphincter and ciliary body. It can also occur after pan-retinal photocoagulation laser treatment.[3] Adie's tonic pupil is typically found in young adults, more commonly women. A patient with Adie's pupil may present with a larger pupil, blurred near vision (or possibly difficulty when focusing from near to distance), and photophobia. The test for Adie's pupil is to instill diluted pilocarpine (0.125%) into each eye. In a positive test, the pupil of the affected eye will constrict more than the fellow pupil. This is best assessed in dim light with the patient looking in the distance.

CN III palsy, discussed earlier, can elicit a pupillary mydriasis (dilation) if the pupil is involved. Acute CN III palsies involving the pupil affect the entire iris sphincter muscle. Most CN III mydriasis will respond within 3 to 7 days to treatment with a weak concentration of pilocarpine (ie, 0.125%, 0.25%, or 0.5%). Once the mydriasis resolves, the pilocarpine can be stopped.[7]

Headaches

Headaches are classified into three types (Sidebar 25-2). Of course, not all headaches are neurologic in nature. Some of the signs to look for are chronic headaches after age 50 years, dizziness, nausea, confusion, loss of consciousness, transient vision loss, increased frequency and intensity of headaches, and interruptions of daily life.

Migraine

Migraine headaches are notorious for their debilitating nature, although not all fall into that category.[3] Migraines can occur with and without auras. An *aura* may include visual and/or sensory and/or speech symptoms that develop gradually and last no longer than 1 hour. They often indicate the impending onset of a migraine headache, so the patient can use this as a signal to take medication to ward off the pain before it starts. Visual auras are the most common and often present as a zigzag figure near fixation, which may gradually spread right or left with a scintillating, shimmery edge and varying degrees of transient vision loss. A progressively increasing (*marching*) dark patch (*scotoma*) without other typical aura phenomena may also occur. Patients may see them with eyes open or closed.

Migraines with auras are defined as recurrent headaches where reversible neurologic symptoms develop gradually over 5 to 20 minutes (but can last up to 1 hour). These symptoms are usually followed by the headache on one side of the head, with a pulsating quality, that lasts 4 to 72 hours. The intensity can be moderate to severe in nature and may be aggravated by physical activity. There may also be periods of nausea and light sensitivity.

A migraine can occur without an aura, and an aura can occur without a headache. In the latter case, the patient may contact the eye clinic in a panic after experiencing the scintillating visual scotoma. In the absence of a subsequent headache, these benign but scary episodes are called *ocular* or *ophthalmic migraines*.

CLINICAL SKILLS

While the dilated fundus exam is usually done by the practitioner, the technician often performs tests that evaluate the function of the optic nerve and visual pathway.

History

Taking a good history is an important part of the screening process in any area of eye care, and is covered in detail in Chapter 7. This section will presuppose that the standard questions are covered. It is not only imperative to review the patient's ocular history but to ask questions about his/her medical history as well, since you may uncover clues as to what type of testing may need to be done to ascertain a diagnosis.

When asking about diabetes, ask if the patient has had a recent hemoglobin A1c test to see how controlled the condition is. If it is uncontrolled, this could be a factor in the problems he/she is experiencing. Another common condition to inquire about is hypertension; if it is uncontrolled, it can lead to optic neuropathy (disc edema), optic nerve pallor, and stroke. Ask about any autoimmune disorders such as Graves' disease (proptosis/exophthalmos, RAPD, and visual field defects), myasthenia gravis (diplopia and eyelid ptosis), sarcoid (cranial nerve palsies), MS (APD, visual field defects, and EOM irregularities), and giant cell arteritis (diplopia and vision loss).

When documenting vision loss, the key questions are when did it start, how fast (sudden or gradual), does it come and go or is it constant? Is there is any pain with eye movement or any headaches? Is there pain with jaw movement when chewing, or any scalp tenderness, unexpected weight loss, decreased appetite, or muscle pain (especially in the neck, upper arm, and thigh)?

In a patient with double vision, find out if is it vertical, horizontal, or diagonal; monocular or binocular; intermittent or constant; and was there any pain or trauma with onset.

While reviewing your patient's history, it is also important to be aware of past imaging history, both ocular and general (eg, computed tomography [CT], magnetic resonance imaging [MRI], OCT, fluorescein

angiogram, ultrasound, fundus photos). The neurological work-up should also mention any procedures involving the brain, spine, and nerves, such as lumbar puncture (being sure to document the opening and closing pressure if available).

Vision Assessment

Vision testing is covered in Chapter 8. Of special interest to neuro-ophthalmology is the discussion on functional and nonorganic vision loss.

Extraocular Muscle Testing

Diplopia (double vision) may indicate a defect in bilateral coordination of eye movements (eg, in neural pathways) or in CN III, CN IV, or CN VI. If diplopia persists when one eye is closed (monocular diplopia), the cause is probably a non-neurologic eye disorder. If the doubling goes away when either eye is closed (binocular diplopia), there is most likely a disorder of ocular motility. Testing EOMs is covered in great detail in Chapter 10. There you will also find even more information on CN palsies.

SIDEBAR 25-2
HEADACHES

Primary Headaches
- Migraines (with and without aura, see text)
- Tension-activated
- Cluster headaches
- Exertion-activated
- Other

Secondary Headaches
- Head and/or neck trauma
- Elevated blood pressure
- Side effect, reaction, or overuse of a substance (eg, hangover)
- Withdrawal of a substance (eg, caffeine withdrawal)
- Brain tumor
- Infection (including cold, flu, and sinusitis)
- Disorders of the head, neck, eyes (including strain and angle closure glaucoma), ears, nose, sinuses, teeth, mouth, or other facial/cranial structures
- Psychiatric disorders

Pupil Testing

Checking pupils is an important part of any eye exam and especially of the neurological exam. It is important to know how to evaluate pupils correctly. This is covered in Chapter 9. To briefly review, dim the lights and make sure the patient is looking at a distance target (so as not to stimulate miosis with accommodation). Check each pupil individually and then swing the light source from one eye to the other (*swinging flashlight test*) to check for the consensual response and rule out an afferent pupillary defect (APD). If you are going to use the documentation of PERRLA (Pupils Equal, Round, and Reactive to Light and Accommodation), then make sure to check the pupillary response to a near target as well.

If pupil testing picks up a possible but not definite APD, there are additional ways to try to verify it. In the *red saturation test*, the patient covers one eye and looks at a red object (the cap on a bottle of dilating drops, perhaps). Then the other eye is occluded. Normally, the red object would appear equally red to each eye. But in looking for pupillary defects, an eye seeing less red is usually the one with the APD. Be mindful, this is not a way to rule out an APD, but if there is one, there is usually a decrease in red saturation. If you suspect a defect, have your physician confirm it.

Alternately, there can also be a color deficiency related to the disease process in the suspect eye. A color vision test may show a color vision defect in the APD eye. (This would not apply if there is a congenital color deficiency.)

Visual Field Testing

Visual field testing is a vital part of a neurological work-up to help in making a diagnosis (especially if the patient has a number of problems). The modalities/methods available for visual field testing range from simple confrontation fields and Amsler grid to the formal Goldmann and computerized visual fields. These are discussed in detail in Chapter 9 (confrontation and Amsler grid) and Chapter 14 (formal/automated visual fields).

Imaging

The practitioner may order image tests based on the symptoms and suspected diagnoses of the patient (Table 25-2). Ultrasound (covered in Chapter 17) is a test using B-scans and standardized A-scans (eg, 30° test) to evaluate for increased fluid in the optic nerve sheath in cases such as pseudotumor cerebri or papilledema, or in ruling out optic nerve drusen. Disc photos (Chapter 15) and OCT (Chapter 16) scans are also used to document optic nerve and macular disorders, and may be necessary before starting medications for certain disorders (eg, MS and rheumatoid arthritis).

Other diagnostic imaging techniques that must be done outside the eye clinic can include CT, MRI, magnetic resonance angiogram (MRA), computed tomography angiogram (CTA), and lumbar puncture. The technician may be responsible for scheduling these tests for the patient as well as receiving the results.

PATIENT SERVICES

Patient services in neuro-ophthalmology centers mainly around education. While the practitioner makes the diagnosis, it may be the tech who explains things to the patient (and/or guardians). A thorough understanding of neuro-ocular disorders, testing, and treatment, as well as the physician's philosophy, is vital.

Some treatment options for patients may include surgical procedures such as temporal artery biopsy or optic nerve decompression. Educating the patient about the operation is part of the informed consent process required in such cases.

If the double vision is a temporary problem and may improve, the neuro-ophthalmologist may prescribe a temporary Fresnel press-on prism instead of a more permanent option like ground-in prism. This is covered in Chapter 10.

Some patients may need to see outside providers for low vision issues. It is a good idea to have a list of low vision centers in your area and to know the websites to check to locate a low vision center close to where the patient lives. Be aware of what a low vision center can offer your patients. Some patients may need an occupational therapist for driver rehabilitation due to stroke and other problems, for example. The more information you can provide patients, the more at ease they will feel.

ACKNOWLEDGMENTS

Author Beth Koch would like to thank Ann Pinter, CRA.

TABLE 25-2
IMAGING TECHNIQUES IN NEURO-OPHTHALMOLOGY

Technique	Uses
Ultrasound A-scan B-scan	Differentiate between exophthalmos and pseudoexophthalmos Disorders of the optic disc: Differentiate between papilledema and pseudopapilledema Optic nerve thickness Presence of intracranial pressure
Fundus photography	Document appearance of optic disc
Optical coherence tomography (OCT)	Thickening of retinal nerve fiber layer: Optic neuritis Thinning of retinal nerve fiber layer: Differentiate between papilledema and pseudopapilledema Prediction of visual field recovery after excision of pituitary adenoma[8]
Computed tomography (CT)	Orbital disorders (eg, trauma, infection, tumor, thyroid) Sinus disorders Lacrimal disorders Abnormailities in bone (fractures, calcification) Cases where MRI is contraindicated
Magnetic resonance imaging (MRI)	Soft-tissue evaluation: Hemorrhages Tumors Optic nerve imaging
Magnetic resonance angiogram (MRA) Computed tomography angiogram (CTA) Digital subtraction angiography (DSA)	Study of vascular system affecting the eye: Microaneurysms Stenosis (slow blood flow) Obstructions

CHAPTER QUIZ

1. What are the five main cranial nerves we are concerned about in the neuro-ophthalmic patient?

2. Which cranial nerves innervate which extraocular muscles?

3. Which two extraocular muscles only have a primary action?

4. Why is visual field testing important in the neuro-ophthalmic work-up?

5. What is the mnemonic for the signs of a stroke?

6. What two other conditions can mimic a stroke?

7. What are two types of tumors, discussed in this chapter, that can cause visual field defects?

8. Is pseudotumor cerebri caused by a tumor?

9. What are optic nerve drusen and can they cause visual field defects?

10. What are the two classifications of anterior ischemic optic neuropathy?

11. What are the three main cranial nerve palsies you may see in a neuro-ophthalmology clinic?

12. What is nystagmus?

13. Name three neuro-ophthalmic pupil abnormalities.

14. What is an aura and does it always occur with a migraine?

Answers

1. The cranial nerves of interest in neuro-ophthalmology are the optic (CN II), oculomotor (CN III), trochlear (CN IV), trigeminal (CN V), and abducens (CN VI) nerves.

2. EOM in nervation: lateral rectus (CN VI); superior oblique (CN IV); the inferior oblique, inferior rectus, superior rectus, and inferior rectus all are innervated by CN III.

3. The medial rectus (adduction) and lateral rectus (abduction) have only primary (ie, no secondary or tertiary) actions.

4. Visual field testing helps to determine field loss even if the vision is stable and where in the visual pathway the problem may be. It also gives the physician a way to follow the treatment course for the patient to see if the problem is progressing or improving.

5. The mnemonic for a stroke is *FAST*: Face droop, arm weakness, speech difficulty, time to call 911.

6. Transient ischemic attacks and amaurosis fugax can both mimic a stroke.

7. Pituitary tumor and meningioma are two types of tumors that can cause visual field defects.

8. No; pseudotumor cerebri is caused by increased intracranial pressure, which can cause optic nerve swelling (the appearance of tumor causing compression).

9. Optic nerve drusen are small, calcific concretions and can cause peripheral defects.

10. The two classifications of anterior ischemic optic neuropathy are arteritic (usually occurs with giant cell arteritis) and nonarteritic (which occurs in patients over 50 years).

11. CN III (oculomotor), CN IV (trochlear), and CN VI (abducens)

12. Nystagmus is an involuntary, rhythmic side-to-side or up-and-down (oscillating) eye movement.

13. Anisocoria (unequal pupils), Horner's syndrome (characterized by miosis, ptosis, and anhydrosis), and Adie's tonic pupil (enlarged pupils that respond slowly to light or accommodation).

14. An aura is a visual, sensory, or speech symptom that develops slowly and usually lasts no longer than 1 hour. Migraines can occur with and without an aura, and aura can occur without a headache.

REFERENCES

1. Cassin B, Rubin ML. *Dictionary of Eye Terminology.* 6th ed. Gainesville, FL: Triad Publishing Company; 2012.

2. Cassin B, Solomon SA. *Dictionary of Eye Terminology.* 3rd ed. Gainesville, FL: Triad Publishing; 1997.

3. Biousse V, Newman N. *Neuro-Ophthalmology Illustrated.* New York, NY: Thieme; 2009.

4. Ing E. Thyroid-associated orbitopathy. Medscape website. http://emedicine.medscape.com/article/1218444-overview. October 7, 2015. Accessed June 6, 2016.

5. Kim JW. Compressive optic neuropathy. Medscape website. http://emedicine.medscape.com/article/1217005-overview. Updated November 16, 2015. Accessed June 6, 2016.

6. Mayo Clinic Staff. Giant cell arteritis. Mayo Clinic website. www.mayoclinic.org/diseases-conditions/giant-cell-arteritis/basics/definition/con-20023109. Updated October 2, 2015. Accessed July 4, 2016.

7. Pupillary abnormalities. Patient website. http://patient.info/doctor/pupillary-abnormalities. Reviewed December 9, 2013. Accessed July 4, 2016.

8. Harak K, Rebane R. Optical coherence tomography in neuro-ophthalmology. EyeWikiWeb site of American Academy of Ophthalmology. http://eyewiki.org/Optical_Coherence_Tomography_in_Neuro-ophthalmology#The_most_useful_OCT_parameters_in_the_management_of_neuro-ophthalmologic_conditions. Posted May 30, 2016. Accessed July 10, 2016.

BIBLIOGRAPHY

Choplin N. *Visual Field Testing With the Humphrey Field Analyzer: A Text and Clinical Atlas.* 2nd ed. Thorofare, NJ: SLACK Incorporated; 1999.

Lyle TK, Clover P. Ocular symptoms and signs in pituitary tumours. *Proc R Soc Med.* 1961;54(7):611-619. www.ncbi.nlm.nih.gov/pmc/articles/PMC1870466/?page=2. Accessed July 4, 2016.

Singh P, Kaur R. A review of imaging techniques in neuro-ophthalmology. *Biological and Biomedical Reports.* 2012;2(2):99-107. www.biomedicalreports.org/index.php?journal=bbr&page=article&op=view&path%5B%5D=32.Accessed July 10, 2016.

Spot a stroke. American Heart Association website. www.strokeassociation.org/STROKEORG/WarningSigns/Stroke-Warning-Signs-and-Symptoms_UCM_308528_SubHomePage.jsp. Accessed July 10, 2016.

Suhr CL, DelGiodice M. Neuroimaging 101 for the optometrist. Review of Optometry website. https://www.reviewofoptometry.com/article/neuroimaging-101-for-the-optometrist. Published October 1, 2015. Accessed July 10, 2016.

Valerie BM, Newman N. *Neuro-Ophthalmology Illustrated.* New York, NY: Thieme; 2009.

What is the difference between primary and secondary headaches? Sharecare website. www.sharecare.com/health/headaches-migraines/what-difference-primary-secondary-headaches. Accessed July 10, 2016.

The figures in this chapter were contributed by the following, who are associated with this book as authors.
Beth Koch/Lisa Lystad: Figures 25-2 through 25-5
Jan Ledford: Figure 25-1

26

OCULAR DISORDERS AND CONDITIONS
EXTERNAL AND ANTERIOR SEGMENT

Jessica M. Barr, COMT, ROUB

In this chapter, we will review some common, and some not so common, disease and disorders of the external and anterior segment of the eye. These conditions can be caused by systemic disease, infection, foreign body, tumors, congenital conditions, or aging. Regardless of the cause, many maladies of the external eye and anterior segment can threaten the health of the eye and/or compromise vision. Before reading this material, it may be helpful to review ocular anatomy (Chapter 2).

PERIORBITAL SKIN

Cancerous Lesions

As a general term, *cancer* is a potentially invasive, abnormal growth of cells in the body. This can be caused by carcinogens such as ultraviolet and other radiation, chemical exposure, and smoking. The face and eyelids are especially susceptible to cancerous (*malignant*) lesions because of the amount of ultraviolet exposure this area receives throughout life. According to the American Cancer Society, skin cancer is the most common type of cancer.[1]

The most common type of skin cancer is *basal cell carcinoma* (BCC or BCCa), accounting for nearly 80% of cancerous skin lesions.[2] While BCC does not metastasize

(spread), it is destructive to surrounding issues. This type of lesion may present with its own abnormal blood supply (*telangectasias*), loss of lashes (*madarosis*), and/or an ulcerated center. Removal by frozen section margins, or Mohs technique, is generally preferred because the margins of the lesion may be difficult to assess in the office. (See Chapter 36 for more on Mohs surgery.)

The second most common form of skin cancer is *squamous cell carcinoma* (SCC or SCCa), accounting for 16% of skin cancers.[3] Squamous cell lesions typically begin as scabby or scaly premalignant lesions known as *actinic keratosis*. The presentation is similar to BCC, but when compared to basal cell lesions, the squamous cell type lesions are typically more aggressive and more invasive to surrounding tissues.

Nonmalignant Lesions

Papillomas are extremely common in the general population. They are round, smooth, and can be pigmented. They are benign in nature, and can be removed if the patient desires.

The two most common types of skin lesions caused by viruses are *verruca vulgaris* and *molluscum contagiosum*. The former is caused by the wart virus and the latter by a poxvirus. Verruca vulgaris appears similar to

Ledford JK, Lens A, eds.
*Principles and Practice in Ophthalmic Assisting:
A Comprehensive Textbook* (pp 485-498).
© 2018 Taylor & Francis Group.

a papilloma, but often with a rough surface. Molluscum contagiosum presents as a dome-shaped nodule, and can be very difficult to eradicate. It is most commonly seen in children.

Cutaneous horns are termed as such because of their horn-like appearance. Cutaneous horns represent compacted keratin from the skin, in an elevated and horn-like shape. Surgical excision and biopsy help rule out any malignant changes in the lesion.

Epidermal inclusion cysts are filled with cheesy looking keratin and debris. *Dermoid cysts* are congenital and are caused by hair follicles clogging sebaceous glands. *Hydrocystomas* are fluid-filled lesions caused by a blockage in the sweat gland.

A *hemangioma* is a red lesion, often described as a "strawberry mark." They are seen in infants from birth to 4 weeks, and are properly termed *infantile hemangiomas*. A child may present with a small red mark that can progress over a period of about 1 year. These growths regress over a period of 2 to 6 years. Treatment is warranted when the hemangioma causes a mechanical ptosis or closure of the eye, which can potentially result in amblyopia. The topical beta blocker timolol and, less frequently, systemic beta blockers are used to treat vision-threatening hemangiomas. Beta blockers work by inhibiting the growth of new blood vessels while constricting the existing blood vessels, thus stunting the growth and size of the lesion.

Xanthelasma is benign yellowish skin lesion that typically presents bilaterally on the upper eyelids. Although the lesion itself is benign in nature, it can be an indicator of elevated lipid levels in the blood. Correlative blood tests may be performed. Treatment options include observation or excision of the lesions for cosmesis.

Skin Conditions Affecting the Periocular Skin

Ocular rosacea is an ocular complication of the skin disorder acne rosacea. The skin is flaky, red, and inflamed. A staphylococcal blepharitis frequently occurs with this skin condition. The sloughing of skin from the eyelids can also cause significant ocular surface irritation and subsequent keratitis. It is most common in fair-skinned people of northern European descent. Rosacea of the skin is treated by oral doxycycline (an antibiotic), topical lubricants that usually include a steroid, and vitamin supplements to support healthy skin.

Psoriasis produces flaky, inflamed, and well-demarcated skin lesions that usually occur on parts of the body that are not exposed. In some cases, psoriatic lesions can occur on the face or around the eyes. Flaking of periocular skin can cause irritation, redness of the eye, and a potential for conjunctivitis. The most common treatment is topical steroids to reduce inflammation.

Contact dermatitis is as the name suggests: a skin inflammation caused by direct contact with an irritant or allergen. This is the most common type of inflammation affecting the periocular skin. A patient may present with redness, dryness, itching, burning, and irritation of the skin. It is important to ask patients about use of new lotions, perfumes, detergents, or fabric softeners.

Brow and Lids
Congenital Anomalies

Coloboma is a congenital condition where tissue failed to fuse in utero, and can affect different parts of the eye. Eyelid coloboma can be a partial- or full-thickness defect of the eyelids, causing a small, missing wedge to a complete lack of the eyelid structure. Upper eyelid defects are repaired in a timely manner to ensure adequate coverage of the eye and prevent exposure. Lower eyelid defects are less urgent and are typically repaired when associated with trichiasis that can damage the ocular surface.

A child born with drooping of an upper eyelid (*ptosis*) usually has poor development of the levator muscle. *Congenital* ptosis can also be caused by an oculomotor nerve palsy, heredity, or birth trauma. A serious consequence of uncorrected congenital ptosis is permanent vision loss from amblyopia. A full eye exam should be conducted, especially noting any abnormal head position, as well as pupil evaluation and motility measurements.

An *epicanthal fold* (see Figure 10-8) occurs in all infants and usually corrects itself as the nasal bridge develops. A *telecanthus*, or abnormal space between the eyes, may also be seen in a young child. A child may appear to have eyes that cross in, though the alignment is normal. This is termed *pseudoesotropia*. Persons of Asian descent tend to have prominent upper eyelids and epicanthal folds, which may also appear as a pseudostrabmismus.

Blepharophimosis is an eyelid condition that includes a shortening of the palpebral fissures and poor levator function, making it very difficult, if not impossible, to fully open the eyes. It is very common for the child to develop obstructive amblyopia (ie, amblyopia that develops because the eye is obstructed). Surgical correction to improve blepharophimosis is often necessary, and may need to be repeated as the child grows.

Lid Margin Malpositions

A patient with an inward-turning eyelid, termed *entropion*, often has severe ocular discomfort. This malposition of the eyelid causes the eyelashes to rub against the ocular surface, causing pain, irritation, and possibly corneal abrasions.

An eyelid that turns outward, or droops and exposes the palpebral conjunctiva, is an *ectropion*. Most commonly this is caused by a weakening of the muscles in the lower eyelid and can be associated with aging. An ectropion is termed *cicatricial* if fibrotic scar tissue in the area around the eyelid pulls the lid. A patient with a Bell's (or CN VII) palsy can experience a *paralytic* ectropion.

Ptosis

Defined as a drooping of the upper eyelid, *ptosis* (a general term referring to drooping of any part; Figure 26-1) can be caused by a number of factors. Most commonly, it is associated with a weakening of the levator muscle in the elderly, and is termed *aponeurotic* ptosis. Ocular surface disease or injury that causes the eyelid to droop is called a *protective* or *guarding* ptosis. This will generally return to normal when the causative agent is resolved. A tumor or lesion that causes the eyelid to droop is a *mechanical* ptosis. An injury to the upper eyelid or surrounding area that causes the upper eyelid to droop is a *traumatic* ptosis. A *neurogenic* ptosis is caused by nerve damage. Congenital ptosis has already been discussed.

A *neurofibroma* is a type of tumor associated with the systemic condition neurofibromatosis (specifically, type 1 neurofibromatosis). The lesions can be found throughout the body, though most commonly we see it in ophthalmology as a lid tumor, orbital tumor, or optic nerve glioma. The characteristic finding in upper lid tumors is an S-shaped curve to the lid. Ocular signs and symptoms include proptosis, Lisch nodules (elevated bumps, or nodules, protruding from the iris), and a potential for vision loss if an orbital lesion causes compression of the optic nerve or if the optic nerve itself is involved.

Sometimes redundant skin of the upper lid will push the entire lid down, resulting in a false or *pseudoptosis*. When contemplating surgical repair of the lids, it is important to differentiate between a true ptosis combined with dermatochalasis vs a pseudoptosis caused by the dermatochalasis itself.

Dermatochalasis

An excess of upper eyelid skin, or *dermatochalasis*, can give the appearance of droopy or tired eyes. (It is often mistakenly called *blepharochalasis*, see next section.) This is generally associated with loss of skin elasticity in the elderly. Dermatochalasis with *hooding* occurs when the eyelid skin hangs over the lashes or eyelid margin. Surgical correction via *blepharoplasty* (lid lift) is indicated when sagging skin impairs peripheral vision or the patient is seeking cosmetic correction. In order for most insurance to pay for a blepharoplasty, visual field testing and photographs must be done that show the impairment. (Visual field testing is covered in Chapter 14;

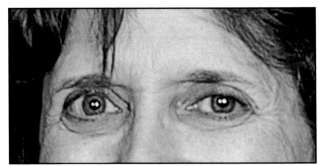

Figure 26-1. Ptosis of left upper lid.

photography is covered in Chapter 15.) Secondary payers (ie, insurance) generally won't cover procedures that are cosmetic only.

Blepharochalasis

Blepharochalasis is a spontaneous swelling of the upper eyelids that occurs in young people, usually around puberty. Prolonged or recurrent episodes of swelling can cause skin thinning, skin discoloration, or chronic ptosis. It is a definite, separate entity from dermatochalasis.

Eyelash Abnormalities

Trichiasis is the most common eyelash abnormality. It is an inward growth of the eyelashes that causes severe discomfort and potential damage to the ocular surface. Patients often call this a "wild hair." *Distichiasis* is a congenital abnormality where there is a double row of eyelashes. The innermost row tends to grow inward and irritate the ocular surface. These conditions can be treated by manual epilation with forceps, or electroepilation to prevent future lash growth. A cryoprobe may also be used to freeze the lash follicle.

Spasms

Blepharospasm (also called *benign essential blepharospasm* [BEB]) is an involuntary twitching of the orbicularis muscle, which may be severe enough to cause subsequent closure or blinking of the eyes. Mild presentations appear as an involuntary lid tic (*myokymia*), generally associated with stress, lack of sleep, and too much caffeine. Severe cases are related to abnormal neural function of the basal ganglion. They can be debilitating and impact daily activities. In some cases, the involuntary spasms can extend to the face and neck. The most troublesome cases are commonly treated with periodic Botox (onabotulinumtoxinA) injections to prevent the spasm (see Chapter 22, Pharmacology). Surgical intervention is much less common because of unpredictable outcomes and the risk of surgical complications.

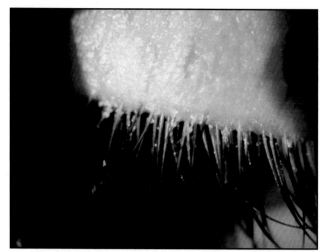

Figure 26-2. Anterior blepharitis. (Reprinted with permission from J. Kevin Quantaro, OD.)

Hemifacial spasm is a twitch that affects the left or right side of the face. It can be localized around the eye, or extend from the forehead to the jaw. It is most commonly caused by a blood vessel pulsing and compressing the seventh cranial nerve. Less commonly, it can be caused by a mass lesion in the brain. It is also treated with Botox.

Lagophthalmos

Lagophthalmos is an incomplete closure of the eyelids with the potential of drying the ocular surface and causing exposure keratitis. Any condition that affects the eyelid's ability to close can cause lagophthalmos. Common causes include surgical overcorrection of ptosis or dermatochalasis, proptosis (bulging of the eye), trauma, and nerve palsies (notably Bell's palsy).

Infections

A *chalazion* is a clogged and inflamed meibomian (oil) gland that presents as a lump on the upper or lower eyelid. It often starts as a sore, raised knot in the lid, and is usually treated with hot compresses and sometimes antibiotic ointment or drops. They will often resolve on their own, but sometimes a nonpainful lump remains that must be surgically excised. In such a case, once the lump is removed and sent for biopsy, the surrounding tissue is scrapped (a process called *curettage*) to remove any remaining inflammation and hopefully prevent recurrence. Occasionally, chronic chalazia will need to be injected with steroids. Lid hygiene is recommended to help keep the lid margins clean and the meibomian glands open.

Also called a *sty*, a *hordeolum* is an infection of a lash follicle. It presents as an external red and painful lump on the eyelid margin that often has a pimple-like "head." If this head is visible on the outer lid, it is called *pointing to*

the skin. If the head is on the inside of the lid, it is termed *pointing to the eye*. A hordeolum will often burst, drain, and resolve on its own. Like the chalazion, it is treated with warm compresses and sometimes topical antibiotics. Keeping the lid margins clean is key in preventing recurrence.

Blepharitis is an eyelid condition characterized by redness, swelling, and itching of the eyelid margins. There is often debris on the eyelashes. This debris can irritate the ocular surface and float around in the tear film. In *anterior blepharitis* (Figure 26-2) the cause is usually staphylococcal bacteria and may be remediated with antibiotics. In *posterior blepharitis*, there is a dysfunction of the meibomian gland secretions. Warm compresses and regular eyelid scrubs with tear-free baby shampoo or commercially available eyelid wipes will usually help to relieve symptoms.

Cellulitis is a general term referring to a skin infection. *Preseptal* cellulitis is a painful infection of the tissues that surround the eye, but does not affect the eyeball itself because it does not penetrate the orbital septum (a fibrous "sheet" that starts at the orbital rim and continues on into the tarsal plates of the lids). *Orbital* cellulitis refers to a deeper infection of the orbit that has penetrated the orbital septum. A large percentage of orbital cellulitis cases are caused by a sinus infection. It is treated most often with oral antibiotics. More severe cases may require intravenous antibiotics or surgery to drain the abscess. In rare cases, an orbital cellulitis can spread to the brain, causing a life-threatening infection.

LACRIMAL SYSTEM

Abnormalities of Tear Production

The absence of tearing is called *alacrima*. A human baby does not begin actually crying tears until several weeks of age. Congenital alacrima, known as Riley-Day syndrome, is an inherited disease found in people of Ashkenazi Jewish ancestry.[4] Less commonly it occurs in the presence of an acoustic neuroma or after surgery to the area where the cerebellum meets the pontine (part of the brainstem).[5] Reduced tear production may occur with any condition causing dysfunction of the lacrimal gland, such as tumors or trauma.

Epiphora refers to excessive tearing, specifically tears that spill over the eyelid and run down the cheek. This can be caused by either an excess of tears or inadequate drainage of the tears. Patients with dry eye often experience epiphora, which seems confusing to them. "How can I have dry eyes when they're watering all the time?" However, in this case the tearing is an overreaction of the tear gland to the dryness (see next section).

Dry Eye Syndrome

Also known as *keratoconjunctivitis sicca* (KCS or K sicca), *dry eye syndrome* (DES) is dehydration of the ocular surface due to lack of tear production or to tears evaporating too quickly. Common symptoms include burning, stinging, foreign body sensation, reflex tearing, light sensitivity, and redness. The condition can be exacerbated by external factors like extended near work, ceiling fans, air vents, and dry climates. Certain medical conditions can also contribute, including menopause, aging, diabetes, and Sjögrens syndrome. Certain medications add to the problems of dry eyes, including antihistamines, decongestants, and chemotherapeutic agents. Ophthalmological causes of dry eyes include meibomian insufficiency, lagophthalmos, exophthalmos, refractive surgery, and topical ocular medications (such as anti-glaucoma agents).

Normal blinking rate is 15 to 20 times per minute. Often a person will "forget" to blink when concentrating on something (TV, computer screen, book, driving, etc), causing the cornea to dry out. The result is usually the symptoms detailed above.

Treatment can range from topical lubricants, to dry eye vitamin supplements taken orally, to specially designed chamber goggles to retain moisture during the night, or even taping the eyelids closed while sleeping. An ophthalmologist may intervene and recommend that punctal plugs be placed, which helps keep the tears on the eye longer. If the plugs do not remain in place, laser or thermal cautery may be used to close the puncta. Topical lubricants ranging from low viscosity (drops) to high viscosity (ointments) will likely be recommended based on the severity of symptoms. Restasis (cyclosporine) is a topical ophthalmic medication for the treatment of dry eyes and is available by prescription only. This medication works by reducing the inflammation associated with chronic dry eyes. Chronic dryness of the ocular surface can cause inflammation, thinning or scarring of the cornea, and some vision loss.

Infections

Canaliculitis (Figure 26-3) is an inflammation of the canaliculus (tubules leading from the punctum, or tear drainage opening in the lid) usually caused by infection. Patients usually experience pain and redness in the corner of the eye, with mucoid discharge. Residual deposits may remain in the canaliculus after resolution of the acute infection, causing recurrent inflammation. Another cause of canaliculitis can be a punctal plug that has migrated into the canaliculus, blocking tear flow and causing stasis. The infection is usually treated with warm compresses and antibiotic drops or ointment. Persistent symptoms may require surgical intervention involving opening the canaliculus and removing any debris.

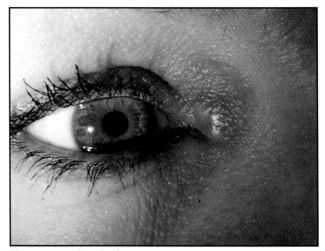

Figure 26-3. Canaliculitis.

Dacryoadenitis is an inflammation of the tear-producing lacrimal gland. Symptoms include pain, redness, swelling, tearing, and discharge. Acute cases are usually caused by infection. Chronic cases of dacryoadenitis are usually related to systemic medical conditions, such as sarcoidosis and thyroid eye disease, to orbital inflammatory syndrome, or to abnormal growths. Treatment may include antibiotics or anti-inflammatory drugs, depending on the underlying cause of the condition.

An inflammation in the lacrimal sac is termed *dacryocystitis*. (Note that dacryocystitis is found in the lacrimal drainage sac, while dacryoadenitis affects the tear gland.) It is usually related to infection and nasolacrimal duct obstruction (see next section). Symptoms include tearing, redness, swelling, and discharge.

Nasolacrimal Duct Obstruction

Nasolacrimal duct obstruction (NLDO) is a blockage in the nasolacrimal duct and can be congenital or acquired. The congenital condition is fairly common and usually related to a residual membrane covering the duct. The membrane forms as a normal part of fetal development, but usually opens just prior to birth. Symptoms include excessive tearing, crusting of the eyelid (most notable upon waking), and tenderness to palpation. Most resolve without intervention. Noninvasive treatment can include massaging the area as well as antibiotic drops if an infection has set up. Some cases may require probing and/or insertion of a stent (tube) to open the duct. Probing involves inserting a fine wire into the canaliculus and pushing it through the membrane, which may be done on an outpatient basis. Surgical insertion of a stent is intended to keep the opening patent.

Acquired NLDO may be related to an acute infection or a foreign body such as a displaced punctal plug. Common symptoms are pain, redness, swelling, discomfort, tearing, and mucous discharge. Probing and irrigation may help mitigate the obstruction, but surgical probing and a stent (a procedure known as a *dacryocystorhinostomy* [DCR]) may be required. Another less common cause of acquired NLDO is the anticancer drug docetaxel. This chemotherapeutic agent causes stenosis (narrowing) of the nasolacrimal system. Approximately half of the patients receiving this drug as a weekly anticancer therapy regimen will require some type of surgical intervention for the *epiphora* (constant tearing) related to narrowing of the nasolacrimal duct or canaliculus.[6]

Obstruction can occur anywhere in the drainage system. Chronic tearing that is not attributable to dry eye may be evaluated for blockages. There are several methods, including instilling fluorescein drops into the eyes then using a cobalt blue light to look in the patient's mouth to see if the drops have moved through the system and drained into the throat. Another method involves irrigating the system with saline via a syringe.

ORBITAL DISORDERS

A child can be born with an abnormally small and malformed eye known as *microphthalmia*. The condition can be unilateral or bilateral. It is sometimes assumed that the child has no eye(s) at all, given the appearance, but magnetic resonance imaging may sometimes reveal remnant eye tissue in the socket. These patients are frequently severely visually impaired or totally blind in the microphthalmic eye.

The absence of a normal-sized eye can impact facial growth and development as the child ages. To prevent facial deformity, an implant is usually placed into the socket. The implant is periodically changed out with one of increased size to promote normal orbital bone growth as the child ages. A dermis fat graft may also be harvested and implanted into the orbit for the same purpose. The child will eventually be fit with a prosthesis to achieve a better cosmetic appearance.

Buphthalmos is an unusually large eyeball, with a larger than average cornea. It is commonly seen in children with congenital glaucoma, as the elevated intraocular pressure causes structural changes in the eye. These structural changes can be an early indicator of infantile glaucoma in an otherwise asymptomatic patient.

Anophthalmos is the total absence of an eye within the orbit and can be congenital or acquired. Congenital anophthalmos is handled similarly to microphthalmia in that an implant is used to promote more normal facial growth. In acquired anophthalmos, the eyeball is intentionally removed (enucleated) due to trauma, cancer, or a blind and painful eye. A prosthesis is usually fit to match the fellow eye and achieve cosmesis.

Retraction of the globe and orbital contents is termed *enophthalmos*. The patient presents with a sunken appearance of the eye. Exophthalmometry measurements will confirm the globe's retroplacement, and radiological studies will probably be performed. This condition is most commonly caused by trauma and fractures of the bony orbit with a prolapse of orbital contents.

The normal eye protrudes some 12 to 21 mm beyond the temporal edge of the bony orbit. *Exophthalmos* describes an abnormal forward bulging or protrusion of the globe, also known as *proptosis*. Proptosis occurs when the contents of the bony orbit increase in size, forcing the globe forward. This can be related to a number of conditions including Graves' disease, sarcoidosis, neoplasms, and orbital inflammatory syndrome. Persons of African descent tend to have shallow orbits; therefore, the eyes naturally protrude on the upper end of average and perhaps several millimeters beyond.

Exophthalmos is measured using an exophthalmometer (see Chapter 9). The eyes should measure within 2 mm of each other. Exophthalmometry can be used to follow progression or regression of exophthalmos.

Eyelid retraction, including that due to exophthalmos, can leave the surface of the eye exposed, causing anything from a mild dry eye to significant ocular surface disease. Ocular surface exposure is treated with topical ocular lubricants, ranging from drops to more viscous ointments. In more severe cases, the increase in orbital contents can compress the optic nerve and cause permanent vision loss. Treatment is usually surgical debulking of the orbital contents and is usually delayed until the condition stabilizes. Emergent surgical intervention is indicated when optic nerve compression is present.

CONJUNCTIVA

Lesions and Growths

A *pinguecula* (plural, *pingueculae*) is a yellowish, fibrotic growth (Figure 26-4) that usually appears on the nasal side of the conjunctiva, often at the limbal edge. Sun exposure and chronic eye irritation may contribute to its growth. If irritation is present they can be treated by use of topical lubricants.

Conjunctival *nevi* (singular, *nevus*) are benign, hyperpigmented, and slightly elevated lesions. Careful examination to look for "feeder vessels" to the lesion should be performed to rule out potential for malignancy as a *melanoma* (aggressive cancerous tumor) may develop from a nevus. *Squamous cell* cancer of the conjunctiva appears as fleshy, pink, gelatinous, raised lumps with irregular edges (papillomatous), and may have "feeder" blood vessels. *Lymphoproliferative* lesions (caused by metastases from the lymphatic system) are described as "salmon patches" because of their fleshy pink appearance and smooth contour. All of these malignancies require excision and anticancer treatment, such as radiotherapy and chemotherapy.[7]

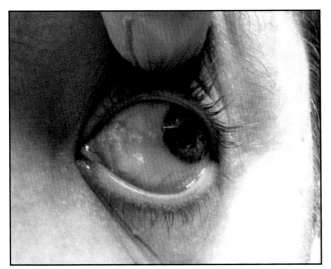

Figure 26-4. Pinguecula.

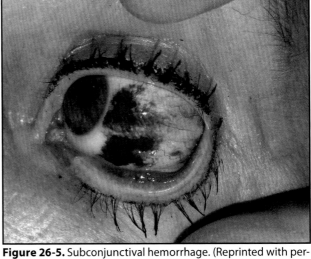

Figure 26-5. Subconjunctival hemorrhage. (Reprinted with permission from Stacy L. Green, COA, CCMA.)

Papillomas are lesions frequently associated with the human papillomavirus (HPV). They are raised, vascularized growths that typically occur near the limbus or fornix. They usually resolve on their own, but excision of large lesions may be indicated to alleviate discomfort.

The typical conjunctival dermoid is fleshy, whitish-yellowish, round, and raised. These are benign in nature, save for the discomfort that may be associated with the physical lesion. Since dermoids originate from dermal tissue, a small hair may sometimes be seen in these lesions.[7]

Also known as a *retention cyst*, cysts are fluid-filled lesions that can occur anywhere in the body, including the conjunctiva. They are benign in nature, and may occasionally cause irritation requiring treatment with topical medications. They commonly resolve on their own.

Infrequently, an orbital fat prolapse occurs where fat penetrates Tenon's capsule and intrudes into the subconjunctival space. This appears as a large, round, yellow, and globular lesion just under the conj. It can occur spontaneously, or from trauma or surgery.[8]

A build-up of epithelial debris on the bulbar conjunctiva is called a *concretion*. Occasionally, these can calcify and cause discomfort and irritation. They are very fine, nodular, and elevated lesions adherent to the conjunctiva. Concretions can usually be removed with a needle at the slit lamp.

Subconjunctival Hemorrhage

Although a *subconjunctival hemorrhage* (SCH) frightens most patients, it is a relatively benign condition. When a blood vessel in the conjunctiva ruptures, blood will pool under the mucous membrane. Against the white of the sclera, it looks like a blood-red "puddle" (Figure 26-5). Despite its alarming appearance, this is relatively common and is often "treated" by reassuring the patient.

These hemorrhages may initially spread further, then resolve gradually over 1 week or so. They can be caused by coughing, sneezing, straining, and heavy lifting, as well as spontaneously ("I got up this morning and my eye looked like this!"). People on blood thinning medications may be more prone to developing SCH, just as they are more prone to bruising. Less commonly, the hemorrhage can cause conjunctival *chemosis* (a fluid-filled swelling around the cornea) and *chalasis* (excess conjunctival tissue), which contributes to irritation of the ocular surface. If this occurs, topical lubricants are indicated. Ocular decongestants ("get the red out" drops) have little effect.

Conjunctivitis

The term *conjunctivitis* is very broad and simply describes inflammation of the conjunctiva. Since the conjunctiva is an exposed mucous membrane, it is especially prone to inflammation from external factors. From chemicals to allergens, infections, and irritations, conjunctivitis is common and has a multitude of possible causes.

Infectious Conjunctivitis

Starting around birth, *neonatal conjunctivitis*, also known as *ophthalmia neonatorum*, occurs within the first year of life. Common causes are staphylococcus bacteria, *Chlamydia trachomatis, Neisseria gonorrhoeae*, and the Herpes simplex virus (HSV). Transmission of infection usually occurs from contact with the mother during a vaginal birth.

An infection of the bartonella bacterium is called *cat scratch disease* (CSD) since it is commonly transmitted from felines to people. This infection can cause a myriad of ocular manifestations, including skin lesions, conjunctivitis, and retinitis. Conjunctivitis caused by CSD is hallmarked by large, red, granulomatous bumps (lesions composed of granulated tissue) on the inner eyelids.[9] These bumps may cause a foreign body sensation and tearing. The condition is usually self-limiting, and symptomatic relief with topical lubricants is indicated. In more severe cases, antibiotics may be prescribed.

Skin lesions associated with a *molluscum contagiosum* infection can also cause a secondary eye infection termed *molluscom contagiosum conjunctivitis*. This is due to sloughing of cells from the lesions into the eye. Symptoms include redness, tearing, and irritation. Treatment consists of addressing the primary lid lesion causing the irritation and symptomatic relief by using topical ophthalmic medication such as lubricants for comfort and steroids for related inflammation.

Bacterial conjunctivitis is a very common condition that occurs when bacteria enter the eye and cause an infection. *Staphylococcus*, *Streptococcus*, *Haemophilus influenzae*, and *Moraxella* are most often responsible.

A sudden and severe (hyperacute) bacterial conjunctivitis is usually related to *N. gonorrhoeae* (see Figure 31-1), while chronic bacterial infections are associated with chlamydia. Treatment usually consists of topical antibiotics, isolation for 24 to 48 hours, and follow-up in 5 to 7 days. In cases of hyperacute conjunctivitis, daily follow-up is recommended. Patients diagnosed with chlamydial conjunctivitis likely have a concurrent genital infection, and require oral antibiotics.

Trachoma is a type of conjunctivitis caused by the bacterium *C. trachomatis*. This aggressive form of granular conjunctivitis can eventually lead to ocular surface disease and scarring of the conjunctiva. Blindness usually occurs after multiple infections cause severe ocular surface scarring. It is most common in developing countries where access to clean water may be limited, sanitation is poor, and living conditions are crowded. Treatment aims to improve water quality, and may include the use of antibiotics. It is a common cause of vision loss in Africa.

The most common cause of *viral conjunctivitis* is the adenovirus, which accounts for 65% to 90% of all viral conjunctival infections.[10] Adenoviral conjunctivitis is highly contagious and easily spread, hence the term *epidemic keratoconjunctivitis* (EKC). Other viruses that may infect the conjunctiva include HSV, molluscum contagiosum, Varicella zoster virus (VZV), coxsackie, enterovirus, measles, etc. Patients should be counseled to wash hands frequently, to avoid rubbing the eyes, and not to share towels or bedding. Because the infection is self-limiting (usually clears up on its own in 10 to 14 days), treatment is usually for symptomatic relief and may include cool compresses and artificial tears. In more severe cases of viral conjunctivitis, the patient can develop preauricular lymphadenopathy (swelling of the lymph node just in front of the ear), fever, pseudomembranes (a thick band of mucoid discharge that appears attached to the bulbar or palpebral conjunctiva), subconjunctival hemorrhage, and

keratitis. Treatment may be escalated to topical steroids and systemic antiviral medications.

Fungal infections of the conjunctiva are much less common than viral or bacterial infections. The most common culprit is *Candida albicans*, and it usually occurs in patients who are immunocompromised or diabetic. Most fungal conjunctivitis cases appear granulomatous, and are treated with antifungal creams or drops. The main concern is that the infection will spread to the cornea, which can be quite serious. (See Cornea section.)

The best prevention for infectious conjunctivitis is a clean, healthy eye. There are natural mechanisms in place that act as barriers to infection. Physical barriers include the eyelids, eyelashes, tears, blinking, and the conjunctiva. When physical barriers to infection fail, the body's immune system kicks in and works to fight off infection by attacking the pathogen. Individuals that are immunocompromised, such as patients on chemotherapy, are at greater risk for infections because they lack the secondary barrier necessary to fight off infection.

Allergic Conjunctivitis

An allergy occurs when an individual is hypersensitive to a substance. When the conjunctiva encounters an antigen, it activates antibodies to target that antigen. Recurrent encounters with the same antigen cause a surplus of antibodies. The antibodies attach to mast cells and cause the mast cells to throw off biochemicals (like histamines) that trigger the allergic response.

Allergens are the most common cause of conjunctivitis. Allergies like hay fever can cause *seasonal allergic conjunctivitis*. More prolonged or *perennial allergic conjunctivitis* is caused by allergens like cat hair and dust mites. Associated signs and symptoms include red, itchy, and watery eyes. Treatment includes topical mast cell stabilizers and symptomatic relief with cool compresses and lubricating drops.

Vernal conjunctivitis is a more severe type of allergic conjunctivitis associated with grass and pollen. It is more common in warm climates and typically afflicts prepubescent children, boys more than girls, and can last up to 10 years.[5] The conjunctiva has large "cobblestone" papillae, and pseudomembranes are common.

Atopic conjunctivitis occurs in individuals who suffer from atopic dermatitis (eczema). The eyelids appear red, swollen, and dry. In mild cases, ocular symptoms include itching, burning, stinging, and mucous discharge. In severe cases, the patient may have large conjunctival papillae and ocular surface disease.

Giant papillary conjunctivitis (GPC; see Figure 21-20) is usually seen among individuals who wear contact lenses or artificial eyes (ocular prosthetics). Irritation arises from tissue exposure to the lens material, postulated to be an allergic response. The conjunctiva appears red and inflamed with large papillae. Remediation of symptoms is achieved by discontinuing the contact lens or prosthesis and applying topical lubricants. After the inflammation quiets, some patients may be able to resume contact lens or prosthesis wear, but a change of material or addition of topical lubrication may be necessary.

Chemical Conjunctivitis

Note: Any chemical splash is an ocular emergency, covered in Chapter 32. Prompt and extended irrigation with clean water for 20 minutes *before* coming to the eye care office is vital to minimize damage to the ocular surface.

Gouty Conjunctivitis

Gout is an inflammatory disease that causes acute and focal pain (often described as "hot") in the joints. The patient may report a "hot eye" and display signs of a mild conjunctivitis. Treatment is aimed at managing the systemic disease.

Other Inflammatory Conditions of the Conjunctiva

Stevens-Johnson Syndrome

A common syndrome affecting the skin and the mucous membranes is *Stevens-Johnson syndrome* (SJS). Ocular manifestations of SJS include blistering eruptions of the conjunctiva that cause secondary damage to the cornea. A hypersensitive immune response to a wide range of drugs, especially antibiotics, can cause a severe form of SJS called *toxic epidermal necrolysis* (TEN). Systemic manifestations of TEN include skin dryness, flaking, and blistering lesions throughout the body. Treatment usually includes discontinuing the causative medication and initiating steroid therapy. The ocular surface disease associated with SJS and TEN is managed on a case-by-case basis determined by the severity of eye disease. Topical lubricants are used for milder cases, but in more severe cases the patient may require a bandage contact lens to protect the cornea, or even mucous membrane grafts.

Sjögren's Syndrome

Sjögren's syndrome is an autoimmune disease that includes dry eye, dry mouth (*xerostomia*), and arthritis. Severe dry eye may present with conjunctival injection resembling a mild conjunctivitis. Treatment is often aimed at symptomatic relief with topical medications and/or punctal plugs to retain tears. In more severe cases, other therapies (including systemic) may be initiated. Dry eye syndrome is discussed in an earlier section of this chapter.

Folliculitis

In *folliculitis*, the follicles that line the conjunctiva become elevated and prominent. In contrast to papillae, which are larger and have a cobblestone appearance, follicles are smaller dome-shaped elevations with a central blood vessel. There is no associated inflammation. The condition can be chronic, is usually benign, and no treatment is needed.

Phlyctenulosis

A hypersensitivity to bacterial proteins such as staphylococcal or tuberculoprotein can cause *phlyctenules*. These are raised, whitish lesions that are surrounded by conjunctival injection (redness). They frequently occur in the limbal area and can involve the cornea. Phlyctenules can be treated with topical steroids and antibiotics.[5]

EPISCLERA/SCLERA

Episcleritis is a condition of localized inflammation of the episclera. It may present as an inflamed nodule, inflamed section, or diffuse inflammation of the white of (usually) one eye. Lack of palpebral conjunctival redness and no discharge indicate an episcleritis rather than conjunctivitis. Patients will present with redness and mild ocular discomfort. It is most common in middle-aged women, though men may also be affected. In the absence of systemic inflammatory disease, treatment usually includes topical ophthalmic medications, such as nonsteroidal anti-inflammatory drugs (NSAIDs), mild steroids, and/or topical lubricants.

Scleritis is an uncommon condition usually related to an underlying systemic problem, such as autoimmune disease, granulomatous disease (disorders that cause masses of immune cells in response to infection or inflammation), or infectious disease. Symptoms include redness as well as severe pain that usually wakens the patient at night. Scleritis may also include a reduction in vision. Scleritis can result in scleral thinning and necrosis (tissue death). NSAIDs are the first line of treatment, though severe cases may require oral or intravenous steroids and other immunosuppressants. Recurrence is common, which means diagnosis and treatment of underlying systemic disease is critical.

CORNEA

Disorders of Size

A large cornea associated with high myopia is a congenital condition termed *megalocornea*. The patient usually achieves normal levels of visual acuity. If both the cornea and globe are enlarged (*buphthalmos*, covered in an

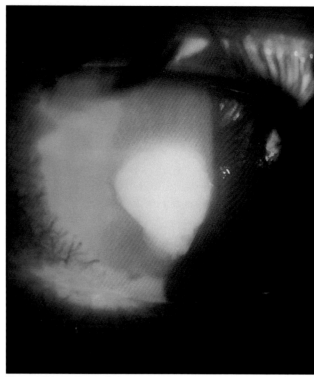

Figure 26-6. Corneal ulcer.

earlier section), the presence of elevated intraocular pressure signaling congenital glaucoma should be ruled out.

The opposite of megalocornea, *microcornea* is a cornea that is much smaller than average; usually less than 10 mm. There may be associated hyperopia or cataract. This condition can be an indication of an abnormally small globe, angle closure glaucoma, or microphthalmia.

Defects of the Corneal Surface

Corneal Ulcers

When the surface of the cornea is scratched or otherwise compromised and an infectious agent is introduced, a corneal ulcer (Figure 26-6) may occur. Necrosis of the corneal tissue from the infectious agent causes significant, and potentially permanent, damage to the cornea.

Sterile corneal ulcers can occur in the absence of an infectious agent when the ocular surface is compromised by exposure or *medicamentosa* (toxic effects of eye drops).

Patients usually present with severe pain (noted to be "worse than childbirth" in some cases), eye redness, extreme photophobia, mucous discharge, eyelid swelling, and guarding ptosis (ie, the lid naturally droops in an effort to protect the underlying cornea). In severe cases, corneal thinning may cause perforation. Corneal ulcers stain with fluorescein or rose bengal, and appear under the slit lamp as a pitted defect in the surface of the cornea.

Corneal ulcers are often cultured to determine the source of infection so that appropriate antibiotics may be prescribed, including fortified antibiotics. (See Chapters 22, Pharmacology, and 23, Microbiology.) Corneal haze or scarring may be present after resolution of the ulcer. In cases of severe corneal scarring or perforation, corneal transplantation may be necessary to regain functional vision.

Superficial Punctate Keratitis and Punctate Epithelial Erosions

Both superficial punctate keratitis (SPK) and punctate epithelial erosions (PEEs) refer to loss of epithelial cells on the surface of the cornea. The loss of epithelial cells is often associated with dry eye or ocular surface exposure and can be easily identified with slit lamp exam and fluorescein staining. Once the cornea is stained with fluorescein, SPK/PEEs will appear as small speckled spots the size of a pin head on the surface of the cornea. "Rare" SPK/PEEs would indicate only a couple of spots of staining, whereas with severe SPK/PEEs the spots would be so numerous that much of the cornea would appear stained. Localized defects can be associated with lagophthalmos and can be seen on the inferior cornea. Diffuse defects may indicate the presence of ocular surface drying from dry eye disease. In addition, some topical medications can be toxic to the cornea and also cause a breakdown or loss of epithelial cells after prolonged use. Chemical exposure can cause these defects as well.

There is some discussion regarding whether SPK and PEE refer to the same condition. Often times the terms are used interchangeably. Some argue that SPK refers to an inflammatory degradation of the epithelium, while PEE refers to epithelial loss from exposure.

Treatment options usually include topical lubricants, dry eye therapies, or surgical intervention to improve closure of the eyelids.

Recurrent Corneal Erosion

Any minor injury that causes disruption of the epithelium to its basement membrane may lead to *recurrent corneal erosion* or *recurrent erosion syndrome*. As the damaged epithelium heals, a weak attachment of the epithelium to the tissue beneath can allow the new cells to be stripped away, leaving a raw area of cornea exposed. This is frequently exacerbated during sleep, and a patient will report waking up in the middle of the night with pain and a foreign body sensation. This occurs because the eye has dried and the cells are peeled off by the lid when the eye is opened. Patients with recurrent erosion may additionally report stinging, burning, blurred vision, and sometimes redness. Treatment is aggressive surface lubrication, particularly before sleep. Recurrent erosion syndrome can even occur years after the initial injury, so a careful history of past ocular injury is important. (Note: Trauma is covered in Chapter 32.)

Keratitis

Keratitis is a general term meaning any inflammation of the cornea. Fluorescein dye is the go-to method for visualizing any irregularities in the corneal surface.

Exposure Keratitis

Exposure keratitis is an inflammation of the cornea that occurs when the ocular surface is exposed for longer than normal periods of time. Exposure occurs when the eye is not closing properly, completely, or frequently enough.

Causes can include ectropion, proptosis, incomplete blink, or eyelid retraction. Any damage or disruption in the function of the nerves controlling the eyelids can result in a *neurotrophic keratitis*. Bell's palsy (CN VII, the facial nerve) is a common example. A palsy of the trigeminal nerve (CN V) will reduce both corneal sensitivity and the blink reflex.

The patient may complain of tearing, discomfort, foreign body sensation, redness, or light sensitivity. If the symptoms are present on awakening, it is likely that the patient's eyes open during sleep. If oxygen is used during sleep (as for sleep apnea), a leaking mask can further dry an incompletely shut eye.

The use of diagnostic dye, such as fluorescein, can aid in identifying areas of drying and exposure. Since the dye stains the dry or exposed area, the more dense or diffuse the staining, the more severe the condition.

In milder cases, epithelial erosions can be managed with topical lubricating drops and ointments. In more severe cases where ulceration is present, more aggressive measures are taken such as Botox (to induce ptosis, thus covering more of the globe) or tarsorrhaphy (surgically sewing the eyelids together). Patients with incomplete blinking can be coached and trained to blink fully. In extreme cases, oculoplastic surgeons may implant a gold weight in the upper eyelid. The gold metal is inert inside of the body, and the weight helps the upper eyelid to close.

Viral Keratitis

HSV and VZV are the most common causes *viral keratitis*. If left untreated, these lesions can cause permanent corneal scarring and vision loss.

VZV is the virus that causes shingles, and the skin lesions will appear on one side of the face only. The eyelids on the affected side may become involved. If there is a lesion on the tip of the nose (Hutchinson's sign), then ocular involvement is more likely because the tip of the nose and the cornea share a nerve supply.

The patient experiences pain, red eye, blurred vision, and photophobia. Typical presentation of HSV includes a *dendritic lesion* on the cornea, which has a linear and branching contour (see Figure 33-12).

Both types are usually treated with systemic and/or topical antiviral medication. Since both viruses can remain dormant in the neural tissues of the cornea, repeated flare-ups may occur. These flare-ups may be triggered by illness, stress, or compromised immune status.

Acanthamoeba Keratitis

Acanthamoeba is a protozoan that can invade the cornea. It is present in soil and water (see Figure 23-9). *Acanthamoeba keratitis* is frequently associated with rinsing contact lenses in tap water and placing them in the eyes. Another common source is hot tubs. This is a serious vision-threatening condition. All contact lens patients should be counseled and advised against rinsing their lenses with tap water because of *Acanthamoeba* keratitis.

Patients will usually present with intense pain, redness, photophobia, blurred vision, and corneal defects such as epithelial erosion and stromal haze. Treatment includes debridement of the affected cornea, topical amebicides, and/or corneal transplant in severe cases.

Contact Lens Keratitis

Contact lens overwear syndrome (OWS) occurs when patients wear their contact lenses for extended periods of time. Patients who wear their contact lenses continuously without complication sometimes develop a false sense of security and eventually overwear their contact lenses. There are, however, patients who develop contact lens keratitis after just a day of overwear. "OWS" is an appropriate acronym, as pain may be intense. Signs and symptoms may also include photophobia and redness. A contact lens holiday (a period of time where contact lenses are not worn) usually resolves this condition. Patients should be counseled regarding healthy contact lens wearing habits.

Keratoconus

Keratoconus is a condition of progressive bulging and thinning of the corneal surface associated with high astigmatism (which can become irregular) and high myopia. Both eyes are usually affected, but can vary in severity. In some cases, frequent and prolonged eye rubbing can further exacerbate the condition by contributing to corneal thinning.

Upon examination, a patient with keratoconus will present with elevated (steep) keratometry measurements, irregular astigmatism, progressive myopia, very irregular corneal topography patterns, possible corneal thinning on anterior segment optical coherence tomography or pachymetry measurements, and a positive *Munson's sign* (protrusion of the cornea causing a v-shaped indention of the lower eyelid on downgaze).

In mild cases spectacle lenses will correct vision. In advancing cases, rigid contact lenses can be worn to help maintain a more normal corneal contour. Historically, a corneal transplant was the end consequence for keratoconus with severe progression. Over the past few years, the integration of corneal collagen cross-linking technology

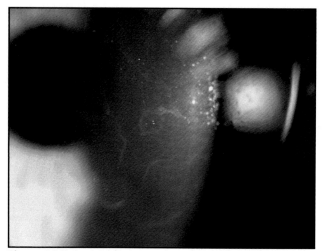

Figure 26-7. Anterior basement membrane dystrophy.

(discussed in Chapter 36) has shown promise in preventing progression of keratoconus. In the worst case scenario, the bulging and thinning of the cornea increase the potential for rupture, and will require corneal transplantation.

Corneal Dystrophies

Anterior Basement Membrane Dystrophy

Anterior basement membrane dystrophy (ABMD), also known as *map-dot-fingerprint dystrophy* (MDFD), produces cysts at the level of the epithelial basement membrane (Figure 26-7). There may be recurrent epithelial erosions associated with this condition. Vision is not usually affected in the absence of epithelial erosion.

Fuchs' Dystrophy

Fuchs' dystrophy (Figure 26-8) is a degenerative condition where there is a gradual and progressive loss of the endothelial cells. Since the endothelium is responsible for pumping water from the cornea and maintaining transparency, a gradual haze will develop if the endothelial cell density is inadequate. Unfortunately, the endothelium cells do not regenerate. Upon slit lamp exam, endothelial defects are noted to have a "beaten metal" appearance due to *guttata*. Guttata are fluid-filled lesions between the endothelium and basement membrane that cause endothelial cells to die off. In advanced disease, there is significant vision loss and the patient must undergo corneal transplantation. A partial transplant, called Descemet's stripping automated endothelial keratoplasty (DSAEK) has replaced the riskier penetrating keratoplasty (PK) as the favored surgical intervention. (See more about these surgical procedures in Chapter 36.) Because the endothelium is often "bumped" during routine cataract surgery, an eye with Fuchs' dystrophy may be further compromised as a result of the procedure. An endothelial

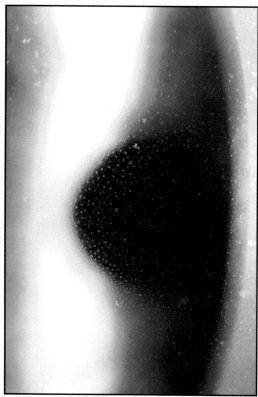

Figure 26-8. Fuchs' corneal dystrophy.

cell count may be ordered prior to intraocular surgery to ascertain that the endothelium is able to withstand the manipulation (see Chapter 16).

Growths and Deposits

A *pterygium* (plural, *pterygia*) grows over the limbus and onto the cornea (Figure 26-9). It is most common in equatorial populations because of the increased ultraviolet light exposure. Other causes include dryness and prolonged exposure to wind and debris. A pterygium can cause abnormal corneal astigmatism/distortion, irritation, and the potential for visual impairment. Since surgical intervention is risky, it is usually reserved for pterygia that extend toward the pupil and encroach on the visual axis.

Pannus describes an area of neovascularized and granulated tissue at the limbus. It has a semitranslucent, fan-shaped appearance, shot with fine blood vessels. Since new blood vessels grow in response to oxygen deprivation, it is often related to contact wear.

Arcus senilis describes a whitening of the cornea that arcs around parallel to the limbus. The arcus is composed of lipid deposits and may totally encircle the cornea. It is an extremely common, benign condition found in the elderly. Less commonly, the presence of a *nonsenile arcus* can indicate the presence of elevated blood cholesterol levels. Even in pronounced cases, vision is unaffected. No treatment is necessary.

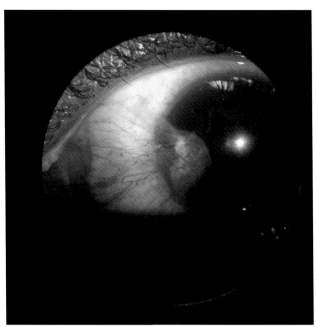

Figure 26-9. Pterygium.

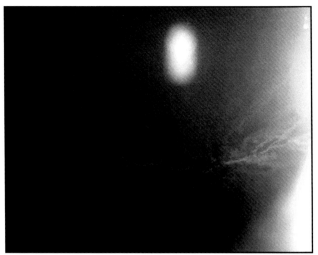

Figure 26-10. Verticillata (amiodarone swirls).

The drug amiodarone is used to treat irregular heart rate. It can cause small deposits below the corneal epithelium in a *verticillata* (vortex pattern; Figure 26-10), sometimes called *amiodarone swirls*. The condition is benign, rarely affects vision, and slowly resolves when the medication is discontinued.[5]

A *Kayser-Fleischer ring* is caused by copper deposits in Descemet's membrane just inside the limbus. The copper deposits are a strong indication of Wilson's disease (abnormally high levels of copper in the liver, brain, or other vital organs). The ring can vary in color from green to blue, or yellow and brown. They are benign to the cornea and vision, but Wilson's disease, if present, must be treated.

Krukenberg's spindle is a corneal finding that occurs in association with pigment dispersion syndrome. The sloughing of brown uveal pigments causes them to be carried by the flow of aqueous and deposited on the posterior corneal surface in a spindle-shaped pattern. Vision is not usually affected. There is an elevated risk for glaucoma since dispersed pigment can block the trabecular meshwork.

CHAPTER QUIZ

1. Identify three types of malignant skin lesions, and two types of nonmalignant skin lesions.

2. What is a xanthelasma?

3. What causes a congenital eyelid coloboma?

4. Describe dermatochalasis and the treatment for this condition.

5. Name the two types of involuntary facial spasms.

6. Identify at least five causes of dry eye syndrome.

7. What symptoms are associated with a nasolacrimal duct obstruction?

8. Buphthalmos is associated with what congenital eye disease?

9. How is exophthalmos (proptosis) monitored over time?

10. Why do subconjunctival hemorrhages occur? Why is this so alarming to patients?

11. List three different types of conjunctivitis.

12. Describe the process of recurrent corneal erosion.

Answers

1. Malignant lesions include basal cell carcinoma, squamous cell carcinoma, and melanoma. Nonmalignant lesions are papillomas, verruca vulgaris, molluscum contagiosum, cutaneous horns, epidermal inclusion cysts, hemangiomas, xanthelasma, and neurofibromas.

2. Xanthelasma is a skin lesion that is yellowish in nature, usually bilateral, and can be an indicator of elevated lipid levels. It can be waxy looking, and usually occurs on the upper lids, but can appear on the lower lids as well.

3. Coloboma describes a congenital condition where tissue failed to fuse during fetal development, and can affect different parts of the eye. Eyelid colobomas can be a partial- or full-thickness defect of the eyelids. The severity of the defects can range from a small missing wedge, to a total absence of the eyelid.

4. Dermatochalasis is excess skin of the upper eyelids. It causes a droopy, tired-looking appearance and can cause loss of superior peripheral vision. Treatment requires surgical intervention with a procedure called a blepharoplasty. The procedure is designed to remove the excess eyelid skin to reduce drooping and restore peripheral vision.

5. Two types of involuntary facial spasms are blepharospasm and hemifacial spasm.

6. Causes of dry eye syndrome can include:
   - External factors: Extended near work, ceiling fans, air vents, and dry climates.
   - Medical conditions: Menopause, aging, diabetes, and Sjögren's syndrome.
   - Medications: Antihistamines, decongestants, and chemotherapeutic agents.
   - Ophthalmic causes: Meibomian insufficiency, lagophthalmos, exophthalmos, refractive surgery, and some topical ocular medications.

7. Symptoms of nasolacrimal duct obstruction include excessive tearing, crusting of the eyelid, and tenderness to palpation.

8. Buphthalmos is associated with congenital glaucoma because the increased intraocular pressure causes structural changes of the globe.

9. Exophthalmometry can be used to follow progression or regression of exophthalmos.

10. Subconjunctival hemorrhages occur when a blood vessel ruptures. This can be caused by coughing, sneezing, straining, heavy lifting, or be totally spontaneous. It is very alarming to patients because of the prominent bloody appearance of the eye.

11. Possible answers: Infective, bacterial, viral, allergic, fungal, chemical.

12. A minor injury causing disruption to the epithelium may lead to recurrent corneal erosion. The damaged epithelium heals, but a weak attachment of the epithelium to the tissue beneath can allow the new cells to be stripped away again, exposing a raw area of cornea below.

REFERENCES

1. Skin cancer. American Cancer Society website. www.cancer.org/cancer/skincancer/index. Accessed July 4, 2016.

2. Bader RS. Basal cell carcinoma. http://emedicine.medscape.com/article/276624-overview. Updated September 15, 2015. Accessed July 4, 2016.

3. Jacobson AA. The two most common forms of skin cancer. *Clinical Advisor*. 2014;June:72-116. www.clinicaladvisor.com/features/the-two-most-common-forms-of-skin-cancer/article/354829/. Accessed July 4, 2016.

4. Albert D, Miller J. *Principles and Practice of Ophthalmology*. 3rd ed. Philadelphia, PA: Saunders Elsevier; 2008.

5. Riordan-Eva P, Whitcher JP. *Vaughan & Asbury's General Ophthalmology*. New York, NY: McGraw Hill; 2008.

6. Esmaeli B. Blockage of the lacrimal drainage apparatus as a side effect of docetaxel therapy. *Cancer*. 2003;98(3):504-507.

7. Kanski J, Bowling B. *Synopsis of Clinical Ophthalmology*. 3rd ed. Philadelphia, PA: Elsevier/Saunders; 2013.

8. Vislisel J. Subconjunctival prolapse of orbital fat. EyeRounds, a service of the University of Iowa Department of Ophthalmology and Visual Sciences website. http://webeye.ophth.uiowa.edu/eyeforum/atlas/pages/fat-prolapse/index.htm. Accessed June 6, 2016.

9. Accorinti M. Ocular bartonellosis. *Int J Med Sci*. 2009;6(3):131-132. doi:10.7150/ijms.6.131.

10. Maguire J, Murchison A, Jaeger E. *Wills Eye Institute 5-Minute Ophthalmology Consult*. Philadelphia, PA: Lippincott Williams & Wilkins; 2012.

27

OCULAR DISORDERS AND CONDITIONS
POSTERIOR SEGMENT

Jessica M. Barr, COMT, ROUB

AQUEOUS/ANTERIOR CHAMBER

Cells and Flare

Individual white blood *cells* can sometimes be seen floating in the anterior chamber. They are usually associated with inflammation of the eye. Careful examination with the slit lamp will reveal tiny, roundish particles circulating in the aqueous.

Flare is protein deposits throughout the aqueous. It can be view at the slit lamp and looks like dust or smoke in the aqueous. This usually occurs in tandem with inflammatory cells and is indicative of an inflammatory process within the eye. (See Chapter 12 for techniques on how to best view both of these entities.)

Hyphema

A *hyphema* occurs when there are red blood cells in the anterior chamber of the eye. This usually occurs with trauma, but may occur spontaneously with bleeding disorders. The red blood cells tend to settle to the bottom of the anterior chamber due to gravity. The hyphema is usually graded by how much of the chamber is filled with blood (1/4, 1/2, etc). If the entire chamber is filled with blood, it is called an *8-ball hyphema*. The larger a hyphema is, and the longer it persists, the more likely it is to cause increased intraocular pressure (IOP) due to a blockage of the anterior chamber angle. A hyphema will resolve over time without treatment, but frequent follow-up may be necessary to monitor IOP.

Hypopyon

A *hypopyon* is a collection of inflammatory cells (pus) in the anterior chamber indicating the presence of either an infectious agent within the eye or an inflammatory process such as uveitis. The whitish material can be seen pooling in the bottom of the anterior chamber. Treatment is targeted at the underlying cause or condition.

THE CRYSTALLINE LENS

The most common condition afflicting the crystalline lens is *cataract*, which refers to any opacity of the lens. At birth, the lens is crystal clear. Throughout life, the lens begins to change color and cloud, impairing the vision. See Chapter 28, Cataract, for a full discussion.

Ledford JK, Lens A, eds.
Principles and Practice in Ophthalmic Assisting:
A Comprehensive Textbook (pp 499-509).
© 2018 Taylor & Francis Group.

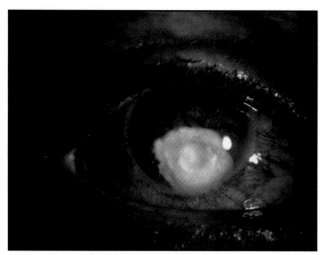

Figure 27-1. Subluxed lens/traumatic cataract.

Subluxation of the Lens

The natural crystalline lens may partially break loose from the zonules that keep it suspended centrally behind the cornea. This is known as *subluxation*. In a healthy individual, it may be related to trauma, and there is often an associated cataract (Figure 27-1). In patients with connective tissue disease, such as Marfan syndrome, the zonules are weak and may break, causing a subluxation of the lens. Thus, in the absence of trauma, a patient with subluxation should receive a thorough work-up for connective tissue disorders.

Luxation of the Lens

Luxation means that the lens has totally broken away from the zonules. This can be caused by trauma or a connection tissue disorder (such as Marfan's). The patient may present with a sudden onset of significantly blurred acuity, which may change with the patient's position. If the free-floating lens moves into the anterior chamber or sinks down into the posterior chamber, inflammation and glaucoma will result. It is corrected with surgery and should be treated immediately.

Mittendorf's Dot

Mittendorf's dot is a congenital opacity on the posterior lens. The opacity is a remnant from the hyaloid artery, part of the fetal ocular vascular system, which usually disappears during the 7th or 8th month of gestation. In some cases, however, the hyaloid artery does not completely regress and leaves this trace evidence where it connected anteriorly. Visual acuity is not usually affected.

UVEAL TRACT

Coloboma

A *coloboma* is an incomplete fusion of tissues during the embryonic stage of development. Colobomas in the uveal tract may affect the iris and ciliary body. Sometimes these defects can extend into the cornea, causing a "keyhole" defect. Uveal tract coloboma is also associated with the absence of zonules and may cause notching in the crystalline lens, though the lens itself is completely fused and whole. A mild coloboma may cause only an indentation in the iris without impacting vision.

Iris

Albinism

Albinism is an absence of pigment in various parts of the body and is a congenital condition. A person with albinism (*albino*) usually has very pale irides that transilluminate at the slit lamp. (This means that if you shine the slit lamp light onto the retina, the iris is lit from behind and has a translucent, almost see-through quality.) They also have fair skin, light hair, an underpigmented retina, and an underdeveloped fovea. These patients usually achieve low levels of visual acuity, and present with nystagmus and high myopia. Although the condition is not progressive, the visual impairments are not correctable.

Lisch Nodules

Lisch nodules are small, round, raised lesions on the iris associated with the systemic disorder neurofibromatosis. These nodules usually present in the first decade of life, and are only associated with neurofibromatosis type I. The nodules are benign and do not cause any ophthalmic complications.

Pigmentary Dispersion Syndrome

In *pigmentary dispersion syndrome* (PDS), pigment particles slough off of the iris, circulate through the anterior and posterior chambers, and deposit on the cornea and anterior lens surface. The pigment can adhere to the corneal endothelium, forming a vertical, spindle-shaped layer on the posterior cornea called *Krukenberg's spindle*. This does not impact visual acuity. The loss of pigment from the iris causes transillumination defects, which are notable on slit lamp examination. If pigment clogs the trabecular meshwork, then aqueous can't drain out of the eye properly, resulting in elevated IOP and leading to glaucoma.

Ciliary Body

Ciliary Body Melanoma

A *ciliary body melanoma* is a malignant tumor. The patient will often present with visual symptoms caused by the tumor pressing on the crystalline lens. Prominent "feeder vessels" on the conjunctiva warrant further investigation, as they may be related to an intraocular ciliary body melanoma. The tumor might be seen once the pupil is dilated. Depending on the size and location of the tumor, treatment modalities may include enucleation, tumor excision, radiation, or *plaque brachytherapy* (where a tiny radioactive plate is placed in or near the tumor itself).

Choroid

Choroidal Nevus

A *choroidal nevus* is a freckle in the eye, visible during ophthalmoscopy. It is a very common finding in the White population. There is no impact to vision, and it is usually an incidental finding. These lesions are generally monitored at regular intervals to evaluate for growth or changes that could indicate a melanoma, rather than a benign nevus.

Choroidal Melanoma

Choroidal melanoma is the most common type of malignant intraocular tumor in adults.[1] Early presentation of the melanoma may be mistaken for a choroidal nevus (see above). When clinical presentation does not differentiate between nevi or melanoma, careful observation is required. Nevi tend to have clearly defined margins and little to no elevation. Melanomas have steeply rising edges and irregular contour. Depending on the size of the tumor, it may be treated with brachytherapy, proton beam radiation, or enucleation.

Uveitis

Uveitis describes inflammation in any part of the uveal tract. Uveitis can occur in tandem with systemic inflammatory disease, such as rheumatoid arthritis, or it may occur only in the eye. The condition can be acute or chronic, and severity can range from mild to severe. In severe cases, inflammation causes damage to the ocular tissue and can induce glaucoma. Milder cases usually resolve with a course of topical ocular steroids. Uveitis is generally classified by what part or structure of the eye is inflamed.

Anterior Uveitis

Anterior uveitis is an inflammation of the iris (*iritis*) or of both the iris and ciliary body (*iridocyclitis*). The patient usually complains of aching eye pain (caused by any movement of the iris), redness (mainly around the limbus, as opposed to just generalized redness), photophobia, and blurred vision. Further examination of the eye reveals cell and flare in the anterior chamber. There are a variety of causes for anterior uveitis, including trauma, infection, and systemic inflammatory disease. In many cases, the etiology cannot be determined.

Intermediate Uveitis

Intermediate uveitis refers to inflammation more posteriorly within the eye, such as the ciliary body (*cyclitis*), peripheral retina (*retinitis*), or the pars plana (*pars planitis*). Signs and symptoms are pain, blurry vision, and floaters. Causes may include trauma, infection, or systemic inflammatory disease.

Posterior Uveitis

In the posterior aspect of the eye, inflammation of the retina (*retinitis*), choroid (*choroiditis*), retinal vasculature (*retinal vasculitis*), and optic disc (*papillitis*) are collectively termed *posterior uveitis*. Unlike anterior uveitis, trauma is an unlikely cause; systemic infection or inflammatory disease is more probable.

Causes of Uveitis

An injury or assault to the eye is a common cause of anterior uveitis. Any blunt force to the front of the eye is likely to cause inflammation. Treatment for traumatic anterior uveitis usually includes steroids for inflammation and cycloplegic agents to paralyze the ciliary muscle. Dilating the pupil prevents the iris from moving, greatly increasing the patient's comfort (rather like putting a splint on a sprained wrist).

Trauma, surgery, or a hypermature cataract may cause material to leak from the crystalline lens. This leakage can cause *lens-induced uveitis*. Symptoms and signs include severe light sensitivity, pain, tearing, and blurred vision. Surgical removal of the lens and lens material can resolve symptoms.

Sympathetic ophthalmia occurs when a penetrating injury to one eye results in uveitis and the fellow, uninjured eye also develops inflammation. (The injured eye is considered the *exciting* eye, while the fellow eye is the *sympathetic* eye.) It is also a dreaded (and fortunately rare) complication of any eye surgery that penetrates the globe. The patient presents with floaters and loss of accommodation, follow by uveitis and photophobia. Treatment usually requires enucleation of the injured eye before the inflammation in the uninjured eye destroys that eye as well.

In the absence of trauma, one must consider a systemic cause for uveitis. This can be infectious or inflammatory.

Infectious causes of inflammation can be viral, bacterial, fungal, or parasitic. Common culprits include Herpes simplex virus (HSV), Varicella zoster virus (VZV), cytomegalovirus, human immunodeficiency virus (HIV), Lyme disease, syphilis, toxoplasmosis, and histoplasmosis.

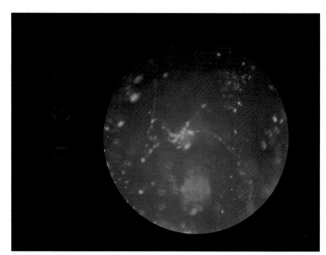

Figure 27-2. Asteroid hyalosis.

(Most of these microorganisms are covered in Chapter 23.) Careful diagnosis and management of the underlying infection is the most effective treatment. Ocular treatments may include topical steroids, intravitreal steroids, and systemic steroids.

Lastly, there may be an underlying systemic inflammatory disease. Rheumatoid arthritis (RA) and juvenile idiopathic arthritis (JIA) are diseases that cause inflammation of the joints. Ankylosing spondylitis is inflammation of the spine. Psoriasis is a condition that causes inflammation of the skin, and in some cases, inflammation of the joints. Sarcoidosis is a granulomatous disease that causes inflammation in many parts of the body. Crohn's disease and ulcerative colitis cause inflammation of the bowels. Each of these systemic disorders potentiates the risk for an ocular manifestation of inflammation. It is important that the eye care practitioner comanage ocular symptoms with the other specialists who follow the patient's systemic disease. Controlling and resolving the systemic inflammation can be a critical factor in resolving the inflammation of the eye.

VITREOUS
Posterior Vitreous Detachment

The vitreous humor gel liquefies as a natural consequence of aging. As this occurs, the vitreous can pull away from the retina, causing a *posterior vitreous detachment* (PVD). The prevalence of vitreous detachment increases with age. The most common symptoms of PVD include *flashes* of light (*photopsia*) and *floaters* in the vision. (Floaters may be described as bugs, hairs, and webs.) The flashes occur when a vitreous strand tugs at the retina or when loose vitreous bumps against the retina. Floaters occur when particles (clumps of cells and protein) in the vitreous cast shadows on the retina. (Some patients will describe seeing a "mouse" or "bug" moving on the floor

out of the corner of their eye, but when they look, the "mouse" isn't there. These are called *scoots*.)

In some cases, vitreous tugging at the retina can cause macular holes, epiretinal membranes, and retinal tears or detachments. If the patient is experiencing a curtain or veil over part of the vision, it may indicate the presence of a retinal tear or detachment. New onset of flashes and floaters should be evaluated (usually as an urgent case, see Chapter 33), and newly diagnosed PVDs should be followed at close intervals to check for the presence of retinal complications.

Asteroid Hyalosis

The presence of multiple, tiny deposits within the vitreous is termed *asteroid hyalosis* (Figure 27-2). The opacities are composed of calcium and phospholipids (as opposed to floaters, which are clumps of cells and protein). Although the exam findings may be impressive (the interior of the eye looks like a snow globe!), the patient is usually asymptomatic. This is a degenerative condition usually occurring in patients 60 years of age or older.

Vitritis

Inflammation within the vitreous is termed *vitritis*. It is manifest as clouding of the vitreous caused by the abnormal presence of inflammatory cells. It is often associated with uveitis.

OPTIC NERVE
Optic Nerve Cupping

The optic cup is a depression in the center of the optic disc. *Optic nerve cupping* is described by the *cup-to-disc ratio*, which is the size of the cup relative to the size of the whole disc. For example, a 0.5 cup-to-disc ratio describes a cup that takes up half the size of the disc. Normal, healthy eyes have some degree of optic nerve cupping. Cup-to-disc ratios higher than 0.6 are suspicious for glaucoma. Also, a cup-to-disc asymmetry between the two eyes of 0.2 or greater presents a concern for glaucoma. For more information, see Chapter 29, Glaucoma.

Physiologic Cupping

In *physiologic cupping* the nerve head has the appearance of glaucomatous cupping but the patient does not have glaucoma (ie, there is no elevated IOP, no visual field loss, and other parameters are likewise normal). It is important that anyone with optic nerve cupping has a thorough evaluation to rule out optic nerve disease. A person with physiologic cupping was "born with funny-looking nerves," but does not have optic nerve disease.

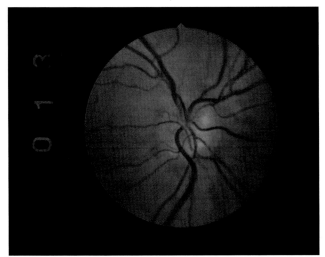

Figure 27-3. Optic nerve drusen.

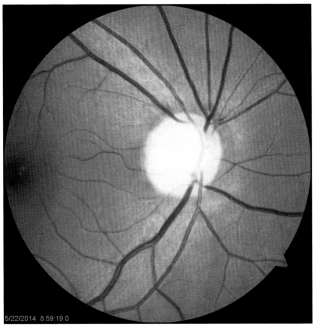

Figure 27-4. Optic nerve pallor.

Papilledema

Swelling of the optic nerve is called *papilledema*. This occurs when there is elevated intracranial pressure, which can be caused by a tumor crowding the intracranial space. Papilledema can also be caused by intracranial hypertension, which is called *pseudotumor cerebri*. Papilledema causes visual field defects. Treatment must address the underlying cause of optic nerve swelling. Additional studies, such as magnetic resonance imaging and lumbar punctures, can evaluate for an intracranial mass or elevated intracranial hypertension.

Pseudopapilledema

When the optic nerves appear swollen in the absence of intracranial pressure, it is termed *pseudopapilledema*. The optic nerves may seem to be elevated because they are tilted (a variation of normal). Hyperopia is also sometimes accompanied by pseudopapilledema. Since there is no underlying disease process, vision is unaffected and treatment is not necessary, but the condition must be evaluated to rule out true papilledema, which can indicate a more serious problem.

Optic Nerve Drusen

Optic nerve drusen can also give the appearance of papilledema if they are visible around the cup (Figure 27-3). Drusen are actually protein and calcium deposits in the optic nerve that look like yellowish spots. Their occurrence tends to increase with age. While they can cause visual field defects (ranging from unnoticeable to a sudden loss of vision), there is no treatment.

Optic Nerve Pallor

A pale appearance (*pallor*) of the optic nerve indicates the presence of *optic atrophy*, which is a loss of nerve fibers (Figure 27-4). Vision loss varies with the severity of atrophy, which can range from mild to severe. Ocular disorders associated with nerve pallor include glaucoma, ischemic optic neuropathy, and optic neuritis.

Optic Neuritis

Inflammation of the optic nerve, known as *optic neuritis* or *papillitis*, is most commonly associated with multiple sclerosis (Figure 27-5). Other causes of optic neuritis include sarcoidosis, lupus, anterior ischemic optic neuropathy, hereditary optic neuropathy, toxic amblyopia, and vitamin B_{12} deficiency.[2] The optic nerve head itself may swell. However, inflammation can also occur more posteriorly in the nerve, in which case it is called *retrobulbar optic neuritis*. The acute vision loss from papillitis differentiates this condition from papilledema.

Optic Nerve Coloboma

Optic nerve coloboma is a congenital defect where tissues fail to fuse during embryonic development. The pitting, or cupping, of the nerve appears similar to that seen with glaucomatous damage. There may be some visual field defects, but vision is otherwise normal. There can be an association with retinal detachments and other abnormalities.

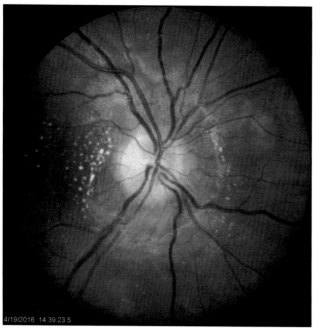

4/19/2016 14:39:23 5

Figure 27-5. Optic neuritis.

RETINA

Diabetic Retinopathy

For a full discussion of diabetic retinopathy, see Chapter 30, Diabetes.

Retinitis Pigmentosa

A hereditary retinal degeneration, *retinitis pigmentosa* (RP) is a progressive disease of the retina. RP is typically diagnosed in teenagers and young adults. The disease is gradually progressive, causing blindness by the age of 40 years. There is worsening function of the photoreceptors and cell loss that results in atrophy of the retina. Symptoms include progressive night blindness and continued loss of peripheral vision. It is possible to retain a small island of central vision with normal Snellen acuity while having severe and debilitating peripheral field loss. There is no treatment, but low vision aids such as telescopic lenses may help to restore some visual function. Recent successes with retinal implants are hopeful as well.

Albinism

The absence of melanin pigmentation throughout the body is termed *albinism* (also discussed earlier in the section on the iris). This is a genetic trait involving the X chromosome, making it more common in males because they only have one X chromosome. Individuals with albinism have hypopigmented (underpigmented, or abnormally pale) retinas and underdeveloped foveas, which results in poor visual acuity, nystagmus, and light sensitivity. *Oculocutaneous albinism* involves the skin and the eyes, and *ocular albinism* affects the eyes only. There is no treatment for albinism, but visual function can be optimized with refractive correction and special contact lenses and/or sunglasses for photophobia. For more information, see Chapter 24, Genetics.

Congenital Stationary Night Blindness

Infantile night blindness paired with retinal dysfunction is indicative of *congenital stationary night blindness*. The fundus may or may not appear abnormal. It is usually associated with reduced visual acuity, high myopia, nystagmus, and strabismus. Night blindness may be partial or complete. It is primarily a rod dystrophy, though the cones may be involved to a lesser extent. It is a hereditary retinal degeneration. The condition tends to remain stable over time, hence the term "stationary" night blindness. There is no treatment.

Leber Congenital Amaurosis

A heredity and congenital condition, *Leber congenital amaurosis* (LCA) is a genetic cause of vision loss in children. It is usually identified during infancy when the child exhibits poor visual interaction with environmental stimuli, as well as nystagmus. Further examination reveals sluggish pupillary response, pigmented retinas, and optic atrophy. The infant might also be observed pressing or poking the eyes to stimulate light flashes in the retina (*oculodigital syndrome*). This in turn may lead to *enophthalmos* (discussed previously). Electrophysiology testing (Chapter 18) is the only method for making an absolute diagnosis; a flat electroretinogram (ERG) is definitive. Genetic testing can reveal the gene mutation causing LCA, and there are currently several promising clinical trials for gene therapy.

Stargardt's Disease and Fundus Flavimaculatus

Stargardt's disease is a common hereditary macular dystrophy. It usually presents in the first or second decade of life.[3] Stargardt's disease is associated with fundus *flavimaculatus*, where there are yellow-whitish flecks in the retina at the level of the retinal pigment epithelium. The disease is progressive, eventually causing atrophy of the macula and severe loss of central vision. Although there is no established treatment, there is research in gene and stem cell therapies that show great promise.

Retinopathy of Prematurity

Retinopathy of prematurity (ROP; formerly called *retrolental fibroplasia,* or RLF) can occur in premature infants with underdeveloped retinal vasculature. Due to the immature body, there is an abnormal release of vascular growth factors into the avascular peripheral retina. This triggers the growth of abnormal, weak blood vessels, which can leak and bleed. The vessels can also tug on and potentially detach the retina. These children may face a life with compromised vision or blindness.

The increase in survival rate of premature infants has contributed to the increase in prevalence of ROP. In developed countries, widespread screening of premature infants for ROP is a standard of care. The most common treatment is laser photocoagulation of the abnormally vascularized retina. More recently, and with some controversy, anti-vascular endothelial growth factor (anti-VEGF) drugs such as Avastin (bevacizumab) are being used off-label for the treatment of ROP. These drugs work by reducing VEGF, a protein that promotes growth of new blood vessels.

Hypertensive Retinopathy

Individuals with systemic hypertension may be at risk for developing *hypertensive retinopathy.* When the blood pressure goes up, vasoconstriction of the retinal vessels occurs. Accelerated malignant hypertension (extremely high blood pressure) may cause hemorrhages (Figure 27-6), cotton wool spots (white patches in the retina), choroidal infarcts (localized area of damage to the choroid), and retinal detachment. Patients identified as having hypertensive retinopathy should be referred to their primary doctor or cardiologist for management of their systemic hypertension. Prolonged vasoconstriction causes arteriosclerosis ("hardening of the arteries"), which actually prevents elderly patients from developing pronounced retinopathy. However, arteriosclerosis also puts patients at risk for retinal blockages because the hardened arteries cross over and put pressure on underlying veins.

Presumed Ocular Histoplasmosis Syndrome

Histoplasmosis refers to a systemic infection by the *Histoplasma capsulatum* fungus. It is commonly found in the Ohio and Mississippi River valleys, and is transmitted by chickens, birds, and bats. Infection occurs when a person inhales the fungus. Systemic manifestation of this disease usually only occurs in the young, the elderly, and the immunocompromised.[4] The ocular condition is referred to as *presumed ocular histoplasmosis syndrome* (POHS). It is considered "presumed" because there have been no confirmatory studies demonstrating the presence

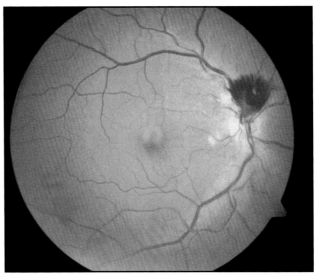

Figure 27-6. Hypertensive retinopathy.

of the fungus in the eye. Ocular findings include multiple "punched out" lesions in the retina, which may remain stable and innocuous. However, the disorder can "activate" and a vision-threatening choroidal neovascular membrane may develop. Active choroiditis can be treated with steroids, and retinal lesions may be treated with laser or intravitreal bevacizumab (an anti-VEGF drug that retards the growth of new blood vessels).[5]

Retinal Detachments and Tears

Retinal detachments and tears can occur spontaneously or be associated with other ocular disease processes. The information on traumatic detachments in Chapter 32, Trauma, is pertinent to nontraumatic situations as well.

Retinal Artery and Vein Occlusions

Occlusion of retinal arteries and veins are considered ocular emergencies, and are covered in more detail in Chapter 33.

Central retinal artery occlusions (CRAOs) cause a sudden, painless, severe, and irreversible loss of vision. Exam findings usually include a cherry-red spot (a tiny, bright red, circumscribed area) and subsequent optic nerve paleness. *Branch retinal artery occlusions* (BRAOs) usually cause peripheral vision loss, unless the fovea is involved.

Central retinal vein occlusions (CRVOs) also cause a sudden, painless loss of vision. Exam findings may reveal retinal hemorrhages, cotton wool spots, macular edema, and iris neovascularization. *Branch retinal vein occlusions* (BRVOs) usually occur where arteries and veins cross each other. When a BRVO occurs, the patient may experience a partial painless loss of vision and present with retinal hemorrhages, cotton wool spots, and retinal edema.

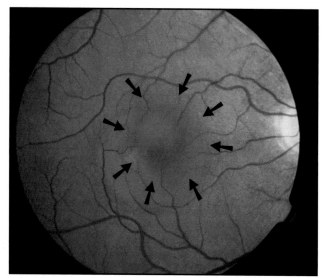

Figure 27-7. Central serous retinopathy.

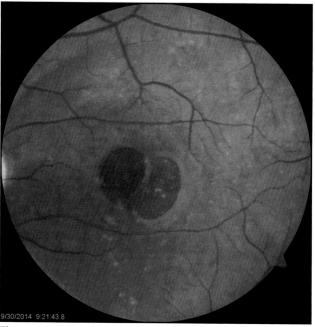

Figure 27-8. Macular hole.

Macular edema (covered next) may be effectively managed with anti-VEGF intravitreal injections. Neovascularization of the iris may cause blockage of the anterior chamber angle, elevated IOP, and glaucoma. Peripheral retinal neovascularization may occur and is usually treated with laser therapy. Anti-VEGF injections may be helpful if macular edema is present.

Macula

Macular Edema

Swelling in the macula (*macular edema*) may be caused by inflammatory disease, retinal disease, epiretinal membrane (ie, a fibrous membrane that covers the macula, reducing vision), intraocular surgery, and macular degeneration. Fluid leaks into the macular tissues in a localized or spread-out pattern, visible on optical coherence tomography (OCT). Patients usually experience distortion of central vision. Prolonged edema may cause permanent macular scarring and loss of central vision. Treatment is usually intravitreal injections of anti-VEGF drugs to quiet the swelling and thwart scarring.

Central Serous Chorioretinopathy

Central serous chorioretinopathy (CSR or CSCR) is a serous retinal detachment (ie, caused by fluid), usually seen in the macular region (Figure 27-7). The detachment occurs at the retinal pigment epithelium, and the space fills with subretinal fluid. It is much more likely to occur in men than women, and is associated with having a "type A" personality.[6]

Like macular edema, the patient will notice a distortion in the vision. Imaging the macula with OCT can reveal subclinical lesions in the retina. The fluid usually reabsorbs over several months, but persistent fluid can be treated with laser photocoagulation or intravitreal anti-VEGF drugs. (See more about these drugs in the section on macular degeneration.) Approximately one-third of patients with CSR will experience a recurrence.[5]

Vitreomacular Traction

When a posterior vitreous detachment occurs and the vitreous remains adherent to the macular surface, this causes *vitreomacular traction*. The vitreous tugging at the macula can cause macular edema, macular holes, or an epiretinal membrane.

Macular Hole

A partial- or full-thickness area of missing tissue in the central macula is called a *macular hole* (Figure 27-8). Vitreomacular traction may cause this, although some occur spontaneously. The patient may initially experience a gray spot or distortion of the central vision and subsequent degradation of central vision. Visual acuity loss usually ranges from 20/25 to 20/200, depending on the extent of the hole.[5] A dark, round spot in the foveal region typical of a macular hole can be well visualized with OCT. Surgery is the only treatment option; however, visual distortion in the central vision may persist.

Epiretinal Membrane

A thin, abnormal layer of tissue that forms on the surface of the retina, an *epiretinal membrane* (ERM), is also known as a *macular pucker* or *cellophane maculopathy* (Figure 27-9). It occurs most commonly in the elderly and is associated with vitreomacular traction. Patients may be asymptomatic or may experience a distortion

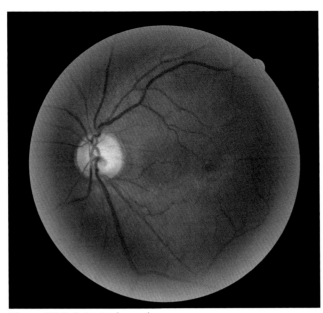

Figure 27-9. Epiretinal membrane.

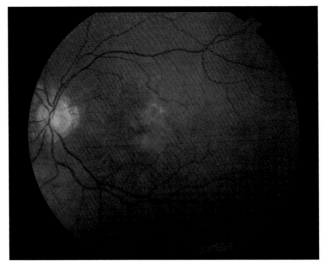

Figure 27-10. Macular degeneration.

of central vision, which can be correlated with Amsler grid evaluation and OCT imaging. If the ERM is severe and visual acuity is limited to 20/40 or worse, surgical intervention (where the membrane is peeled) may be indicated.

Age-Related Macular Degeneration

Age-related macular degeneration (AMD or ARMD) is the second leading cause of blindness in the developed world.[7] It usually occurs after the age of 60, and can have devastating effects on visual acuity. As the name suggests, the disease affects the macula, which is the most sensitive area of the retina and is responsible for central vision (Figure 27-10). Risk factors for ARMD include smoking, inadequate diet, race (White), ultraviolet exposure, and family history. ARMD is usually classified as dry or wet.

The *dry* form of ARMD is gradually progressive. In early macular degeneration, *drusen* (yellow deposits in Bruch's membrane), pigmentary changes, and retinal pigment epithelium atrophy may be present. Later, large areas of atrophy (known as *geographic atrophy* because of their map-like appearance) cause severe central vision impairment. While there is no treatment that can reverse or halt the progression of ARMD, specific formulations of vitamins may slow the progression of disease. It is important that patients monitor their vision at home on a regular basis using an Amsler grid (covered in Chapter 9). Any changes or new defects in the grid can indicate disease progression.

The *wet* form of macular degeneration occurs more acutely. It is characterized by choroidal neovascularization with material leaking from these abnormal and weak vessels into the retinal tissues. Swelling in the macula

occurs from this leakage, and persistent swelling causes macular scarring.

Historically, practitioners could only watch as wet ARMD caused vision loss. Over the past couple of decades, however, there have been several innovations in treatment. Most notably, the use of anti-VEGF drugs has revolutionized the treatment of wet macular degeneration. These must be injected directly into the vitreous. This treatment has been shown to slow or even prevent the vision loss associated with wet macular degeneration.

The primary drawback to anti-VEGF therapy is the need for regular and recurrent intravitreal injections. The injections are uncomfortable for the patient and carry a risk for endophthalmitis. Despite this, most people agree that the risk and discomfort are a small price to pay for preservation of vision. Some patients may require injections as frequently as every month, while others may only need them every 3 months. Some may need periodic injections for an indefinite period of time to stave off progression; others may have serial injections for several months, at which point the disease quiets. There is ongoing research to determine the most effective treatment patterns.

Patients are counseled to eat a healthy diet that includes lots of leafy green vegetables, take "eye vitamins," quit smoking, use ultraviolet protective lenses when outdoors, and monitor central vision with an Amsler grid.

Tumors

Retinoblastoma

Although rare (only a few hundred cases in the United States each year[8]) *retinoblastoma* is a life-threatening pediatric eye cancer. As the tumor grows, it causes an abnormal, white reflection from the retina (*leukocoria;*

see Figure 3-6), which is often the first sign of disease. This is sometimes noticed in photographs of the child, where one pupil reflects red and the other white. (Recently there was a reported case where an eye care professional noticed this in a photograph of a child on the Internet and alerted the family to the problem. The diagnosis was confirmed.) New onset of esotropia may also indicate the presence of retinoblastoma. Funduscopic examination reveals a bulbous, whitish tumor of the retina and sometimes *vitreous seeding* (small tumors in the vitreous). Ultrasound can identify the presence of calcium deposits within the retinoblastoma tumor, which helps differentiate the lesion from other abnormalities. Retinoblastoma is a very aggressive tumor, and can spread rapidly to the brain. Treatment may include radiation, chemotherapy, or enucleation.

Lymphoma

Systemic *lymphomas* (cancer that originates in the body's immune system's cells) can metastasize (spread) to the posterior segment. Presentation may be similar to retinitis, vitritis, or uveitis. Lymphoma should be considered when the cause of intraocular inflammation cannot be readily identified. Vitreous tap or retinal biopsy may be required to confirm the diagnosis.

Metastatic Tumors

Most *metastatic tumors* in the eye occur within the choroid. The most common primary cancer sites include the breast and lung. Less common primary sites are the gastrointestinal tract and kidney, as well as melanoma of the skin. Patients can present with new onset of strabismus, abnormal red reflex, intraocular tumor, or proptosis. Tumors can also metastasize from the area surrounding the eye and orbit, such as the sinuses or bony structures around the eye. Metastatic tumors in the eye usually indicate a high rate of mortality.[9]

CHAPTER QUIZ

1. Describe the difference between a hyphema and a hypopyon.

2. A coloboma occurs during which stage of development?

3. Identify five signs and symptoms associated with albinism.

4. What are the most common causes of uveitis?

5. Flashing flights and floaters in the vision can indicate the presence of ____ .

6. What controversial type of drug is being used to treat retinopathy of prematurity?

7. Describe the progression of vision loss associated with retinitis pigmentosa.

8. What key findings differentiate between wet and dry macular degeneration?

9. How can patients monitor and mitigate the progression of macular degeneration at home?

10. Identify three vascular events that cause a sudden and painless loss of vision.

Answers

1. A hyphema occurs when there are red blood cells in the anterior chamber of the eye. A hypopyon is a collection of inflammatory cells in the anterior chamber.

2. A coloboma is an incomplete fusion of the tissues during the embryonic stage of development.

3. Signs and symptoms associated with albinism include pale irides that transilluminate, fair skin, light hair, hypopigmented retinas, hypoplastic foveas, low vision, nystagmus, and myopia.

4. The most common cause of uveitis is systemic inflammatory disease such as rheumatoid arthritis, juvenile idiopathic arthritis, ankylosing spondylitis, psoriasis, sarcoidosis, and Crohn's disease.

5. Flashing flights and floaters in the vision can indicate the presence of a posterior vitreous detachment, retinal detachment, and/or retinal tear.

6. Anti-VEGF drugs, such as Avastin, are being used off-label to treat retinopathy of prematurity.

7. Retinitis pigmentosa is typically diagnosed in teenagers and young adults experiencing progressive night blindness and peripheral vision loss.

8. The dry form of macular degeneration is gradually progressive with areas of atrophy causing central vision impairment. The wet form of macular degeneration is more acute and is characterized by choroidal neovascularization with fluid leaking from these abnormal and weak blood vessels, resulting in macular edema.

9. Patients can monitor their central vision at home using an Amsler grid. Each eye should be checked individually, and checked daily. The patient can monitor existing defects for change and monitor for any new defects.

10. Vascular events that cause a sudden and painless loss of vision are central retinal artery occlusion, branch retinal artery occlusion, central retinal vein occlusion, and branch retinal vein occlusion.

REFERENCES

1. The Collaborative Ocular Melanoma Study. About choroidal melanoma. http://pages.jh.edu/wctb/coms/general/about-mm/coms1.htm. Accessed July 4, 2016.

2. Riordan-Eva P, Whitcher JP. *Vaughan & Asbury's General Ophthalmology.* New York, NY: McGraw Hill; 2008.

3. Rhee DJ. *The Wills Eye Manual: Office and Emergency Room Diagnoses and Treatment of Eye Disease.* 3rd ed. Philadelphia, PA: Lippincott Williams & Wilkins; 1999.

4. Mayo Clinic Staff. Histoplasmosis. Mayo Clinic website. www.mayoclinic.org/diseases-conditions/histoplasmosis/basics/symptoms/con-20026585. Accessed July 4, 2016.

5. Maguire J, Murchison A, Jaeger E. *Wills Eye Institute 5-Minute Ophthalmology Consult.* Philadelphia, PA: Lippincott Williams & Wilkins; 2012.

6. Yannuzzi LA. Type A behavior and central serous chorioretinopathy. *Trans Am Ophthalmol Soc.* 1966;84:799-845.

7. World Health Organization. Causes of blindness and visual impairment. WHO website. www.who.int/blindness/causes/en/. Accessed April 1, 2016.

8. National Institutes of Health. Retinoblastoma. NIH website. https://ghr.nlm.nih.gov/condition/retinoblastoma. Accessed April 1, 2016.

9. Kanski J, Bowling B. *Synopsis of Clinical Ophthalmology.* Philadelphia, PA: Elsevier Saunders; 2013.

The figures in this chapter were contributed by the following, who are associated with this book as authors:
Donna Bong: Figures 27-6, 27-7
Sergina M. Flaherty: Figures 27-2 through 27-5, 27-8, 27-9
Adeline Stone: Figures 27-1, 27-10

28

CATARACT

Roxanna Martin, BSc, OSC

BASIC SCIENCES

The human eye is a complex organ that converts light rays into electric signals that are sent via the optic nerve to the visual cortex. In order for the brain to register visual input, light must pass through numerous structures, including the lens. (See Light and Visual Pathways, Chapter 3.) If the lens is not clear, incoming light is not transmitted properly. One of the most common causes of gradual, painless blurring of vision, especially in the older population, is a *cataract*. A cataract is defined as any opacity in the crystalline lens. The only way to remove a cataract is to surgically remove the entire lens.

Cataracts usually develop gradually; surgery is not indicated in the early stages of formation. Initially, a change in spectacle correction will clear the blurring. In fact, a very common finding with early cataracts is that the glasses prescription will shift to be more myopic (or less hyperopic). As the cataract progresses, objects will gradually become more blurry to the point where changing the glasses won't help. Color vision is also affected, and objects often have a yellowish tinge. Glare and halos at night are other common, bothersome symptoms. When these symptoms start to interfere with the patient's day-to-day activities, it is time to consider surgical intervention.

In the United States, cataract surgery is one of the most common surgeries performed. It is generally safe and effective in restoring vision. With modern technology, including femtosecond-assisted cataract surgery and refractive intraocular lenses (IOLs), we can generally offer patients excellent, predictable visual outcomes. Recovery from cataract surgery is usually quick and straightforward.

CLINICAL KNOWLEDGE

The *crystalline lens* is located in the front part of the eye (anterior segment) behind the iris and pupil (and thus in the posterior chamber), and in front of the vitreous body (Figure 28-1). It is a biconvex, avascular, transparent structure enclosed in a membrane-like capsule. Thread-like fibers, known as *zonules*, hold the lens in place and allow it to change shape to adjust the focus from distance to near (*accommodation*). The primary function of the crystalline lens is to focus incoming light onto the retina, and its average power is 15 to 20 diopters (D) in its nonaccommodative state.

The lens is comprised of one-third protein and two-thirds water. It has three layers: the *capsule*, a thin, clear membrane that forms the outside layer; the *cortex*, the

Ledford JK, Lens A, eds.
*Principles and Practice in Ophthalmic Assisting:
A Comprehensive Textbook* (pp 511-522).
© 2018 Taylor & Francis Group.

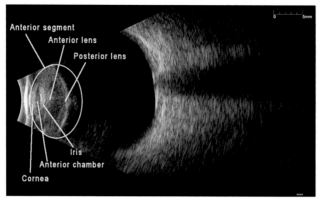

Figure 28-1. Ultrasound scan showing the lens of the eye.

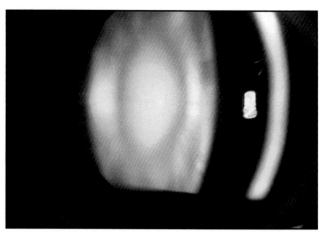

Figure 28-2. Nuclear cataract.

clear material just inside the capsule; and the *nucleus*, which is the core of the lens.

Classification of Cataracts

Categorization by Anatomic Location

The most common method of classifying cataracts is by their location in the crystalline lens.

Nuclear sclerotic cataracts (NSCs; Figure 28-2) are the most common type of cataract and are highly associated with advancing age. An NSC is caused by hardening and clouding of the central (nuclear) portion of the lens. The lens gradually becomes more and more opaque and yellowed, causing vision to slowly become more and more blurred. In its early stages, a nuclear cataract can cause a myopic shift in the patient's refraction, sometimes yielding better reading vision without glasses. This phenomenon is called "second sight" or the "honeymoon stage." As the cataract becomes more advanced, vision becomes more blurry and colors are not as vivid.

Cortical cataracts (Figure 28-3) involve the outer, softer layer of the lens. They usually start at the periphery (ie, not in the visual axis) and gradually grow toward the center of the lens. They often have the appearance of spokes pointing towards the center of the lens. This is called *cortical spoking*. Cortical cataracts are common in patients with diabetes. Because these cataracts start in the outer edges of the lens, the patient may initially have few, if any, symptoms. As the cortical cataract progresses toward the visual axis, it causes glare and loss of contrast, and degrades both the distance and near vision.

Posterior subcapsular cataracts (PSCs; Figure 28-4) are the fastest growing and tend to affect younger patients. These are granular opacities that grow on the back surface of the lens, just in front of the posterior capsule. This type of cataract commonly occurs as a complication of other conditions such as diabetes, chronic uveitis, steroid use, trauma, or retina surgery. It can also be age related. PSCs often occur centrally, therefore affecting the vision more when the pupil constricts (eg, when reading). They

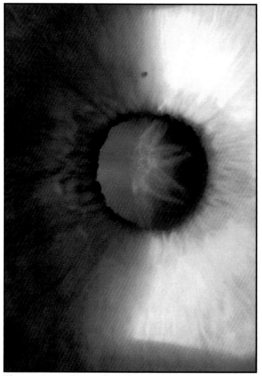

Figure 28-3. Cortical spoking.

also can cause glare, especially from car headlights while driving at night, as well as a loss of contrast.

Categorization by Age of Onset

Cataracts can also be classified by the patient's age at onset. Most cataracts are age related and occur in adults, usually after the age of 50 years. Early-onset lens opacities in children are usually related to a systemic disease or are genetic in origin, and can occur in infancy, early childhood, or adolescence. Many cataracts are mild, and if vision is not impacted they may go undetected without an eye examination. Other patients are less fortunate and can suffer severe vision loss. However, modern cataract

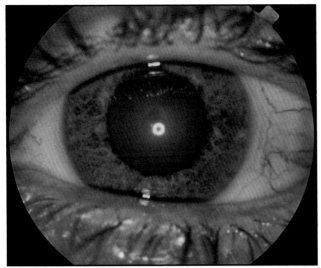

Figure 28-4. Posterior subcapsular cataract.

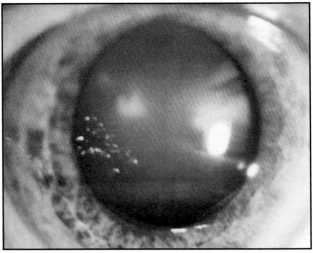

Figure 28-5. Christmas tree cataract. Note the tiny red and green "sparkles."

surgery is highly successful at all ages, and those with significant visual impairment can often have complete restoration of sight.

A *congenital* cataract is present at birth; *infantile* cataracts develop shortly after birth. The most common cause is genetic, usually autosomal dominant. If a cataract goes undiagnosed in an infant, permanent visual loss may occur due to amblyopia. Not all congenital cataracts are visually significant, and if the cataract is small, it may minimally impair visual development and not require any surgery. If surgical intervention is necessary, the decision to put an IOL in an infant's eye is controversial. If the surgeon opts to leave the infant aphakic (ie, without a crystalline lens or IOL), a contact lens will be required after surgery. Alternately, high-plus-powered spectacles may be used if both eyes are aphakic.

Juvenile cataracts can develop in a child or a young adult. If surgery is performed, an IOL is frequently utilized in a child after his/her first birthday.

Senile cataracts will usually develop after the age of 50 years with no obvious cause. Patients normally report a gradual, progressive deterioration in their vision.

Categorization by Cause

Multiple factors may contribute to cataract formation. The most common cause is advancing age. Several other causes are:

▶ Trauma—A traumatic cataract can develop after an injury, either immediately or several years after the event. Virtually any kind of traumatic injury can be associated with cataract development:
- Blunt trauma (eg, getting punched in the eye during a fight)
- Penetrating trauma (eg, metal or glass fragments that penetrate the eye during an auto accident)

▶ Corticosteroids—Both oral and systemic steroids are cataractogenic. The relationship among systemic dosing, duration of use, and cataract formation is unclear.

▶ Chemotherapy—Cataract formation can be accelerated after any cancer treatment. Blurred vision is a common symptom of chemotherapy, however, and it can be difficult to assess whether or not it is cataract related.

▶ High myopia—High myopia refers to a spherical equivalent of -6.0 D or more and/or an axial length of 26.0 mm or more. In a study published in 2011 of cataracts and cataract surgery outcomes among patients with high myopia, researchers found cataracts tended to develop sooner in highly myopic eyes compared with more average eyes.[1]

▶ Family history—Patients will be more likely to develop cataracts if they occurred in closely related family members at a younger age.

Categorization by Color/Appearance

Cataracts can be spoken of in terms of their color as well. In the common NSC, the color of the nucleus depends on the age of the cataract. It can vary from grey (1+ NS), grey-yellow (2+ NS), amber (3+ NS), to brown (4+ NS). A dense NSC will occupy most of the lens and will be the hardest. A black cataract is an age-related, vision-impairing cataract characterized by gradual, progressive thickening of the crystalline lens.

A *polychromatic* cataract, also known as a *Christmas tree* cataract, consists of highly reflective crystals of various colors (Figure 28-5). They are found with a higher prevalence in patients with myotonic dystrophy (the most common form of muscular dystrophy that begins in adulthood).

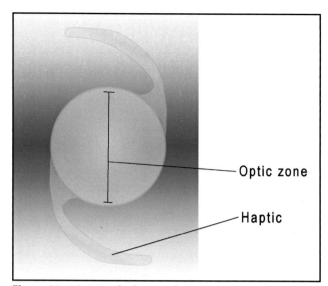

Figure 28-6. Intraocular lens implant.

The silvery *mother-of-pearl* cataract is also referred to as an *intumescent* or *white* cataract. Developmentally it falls between an early/incipient/immature cataract and a fully mature cataract. Its appearance is due to an infusion of fluid caused by the breakdown of lens proteins. This type of cataract is more commonly seen in third-world countries because in the West cataracts are removed before they get to this stage. A *morgagnian* cataract is a hypermature cataract in which the cortex has liquefied. This type of cataract will also have a white appearance.

A *sunflower* cataract is greenish in the center and has radiating spokes. It is actually a result of copper being deposited in the lens. This type of cataract is associated with Wilson's disease, where copper is not metabolized properly. (Copper will also deposit in the cornea, causing a Kayser-Fleischer ring.)

Basics of Cataract Surgery

During cataract surgery, the cataractous lens is replaced with an artificial lens to restore clear vision. Cataract surgery is usually performed at an outpatient surgery center.

You may hear patients talk about cataracts having to be "ripe" before they can be removed. This is a throwback to the days when cataracts were removed through an incision large enough to deliver the lens whole. The cataractous lens was easier to handle at a later stage when the lens was more rigid. (Cataract surgery may still be done by this method in some parts of the world.)

However, today's procedures typically involve the use of an ultrasound device called *phacoemulsification* or "phaco." This technique breaks up the cloudy lens into small pieces, which are then removed from the eye by vacuum. This procedure promotes faster healing and has a low rate of complications due to a smaller incision

than older techniques. It also means that a cataract can be removed at any stage without having to wait for it to "ripen."

Modern cataract surgery itself actually takes very little time. It is done on an outpatient basis, and most of the patient's time is spent in paperwork, preparations, and waiting. The pupil is dilated to allow easy access to the crystalline lens. Once in the operating room, the eye is draped and cleansed. Usually only a topical anesthetic is used, then a lid speculum is inserted to keep the eye opened during the procedure. Two tiny incisions are made in the cornea at the limbus, under the upper lid. A thick viscoelastic substance is injected to help keep the anterior chamber formed and to cushion the corneal endothelium, iris, and other structures. The anterior lens capsule is then opened in a procedure called a *capsulorhexis*. This exposes the lens/cataract, which is "teased" from the posterior face of the capsule with balanced salt solution. Once the lens is free, phacoemulsification (ultrasound) is used to break the lens into tiny pieces, which are then drawn from the eye via suction through a tiny tube. Additional viscoelastic is injected, and a foldable IOL (Figure 28-6) is inserted. The IOL is slipped behind the iris and onto the posterior capsule membrane, and allowed to unfold. The lens position is checked, viscoelastic is removed, eye drops instilled, a patch applied, and the procedure is complete. No sutures are usually needed.

In some cases, surgeons find that there is damage to the posterior capsule or lack of capsular support, so they implant an anterior IOL into the anterior chamber (an *AC IOL*, located in front of the iris; see Figure 12-17).

The Evolution of the Intraocular Lens

Artificial IOLs were developed in the early part of the 20th century, and the first was implanted by Dr. Harold Ridley in 1949 in London.[2] The first artifical IOL implanted in the United States was in 1952, at Wills Eye Hospital in Philadelphia, Pennsylvania.[2] Since that time, cataract surgery and IOLs have continued to evolve.

IOLs are made of inert materials such as plastic, silicone, or acrylic. Just like the eye's natural lens, IOLs have a refractive power, making it possible to correct nearsightedness, farsightedness, and astigmatism. With advancements in technology, patients have several options available when it comes to selecting an IOL that fits their lifestyle and visual goals.

Monofocal lenses (*mono* means one), in the absence of astigmatism, provide clear vision for either distance or near, but not both. Monofocal lenses are typically covered by a patient's health insurance and require no out-of-pocket expense.

A technique called *monovision* can provide clearer vision at distance and near after cataract surgery. In this option the patient's dominant eye would receive a full distance correction, and the nondominant eye would be left mildly nearsighted to allow for clearer near vision. Monovision works for some patients, while others don't tolerate it well. This option is usually recommended only to patients who have previously worn monovision contact lenses.

Toric IOLs are monofocal lenses that correct astigmatism, which also allows patients to be less dependent on distance glasses after cataract surgery. This is because the cylinder correction is in the IOL itself. Because the cylinder axis must be positioned precisely, intraoperative alignment of the IOL is critical. This IOL option is not completely covered by a patient's insurance.

Multifocal IOLs (*multi* means more than one) attempt to provide a patient with dual vision (ie, distance and near) simultaneously. Part of the lens is set to focus at distance, and the other part is set to focus at near. This lens option can significantly reduce dependency on glasses. Multifocal lenses are considered an upgraded option and are not a covered insurance benefit.

An *accommodating* IOL has a hinged design, which allows the lens to flex slightly. This enables the eye's natural focusing muscles to cause flexing and movement of the lens, allowing adjustable focus. A patient who opts for this type of IOL may still find that he/she needs over-the-counter reading glasses to help with fine print, although these are generally low powered. With this lens option there can be a substantial out-of-pocket fee.

The *accommodating toric* is the newest addition to the IOL family. It is designed to correct for preexisiting astigmatism along with imparting excellent distance and intermediate vision, as well as functional near vision, all through a single surgical procedure. Insurance coverage varies greatly from policy to policy. There is an additional fee to upgrade to a accommodating lens implant.

Laser-Assisted Cataract Surgery

Femtosecond laser is an exciting, ground-breaking technology that became available to cataract surgeons in the United States in 2011. The expectation is that the laser will create a safer, more precise surgical experience. Sophisticated scanning technology is used to carefully measure the eye at the time of the procedure. These images are used to plan the patient's customized laser surgery based on his/her real-time measurements. The laser is used to make small incisions in the cornea to access the cataract and reduce the patient's astigmatism. The capsulorhexis by the laser is perfectly centered and round. The lens nucleus is then divided and softened to prepare it for removal using phacoemulsification.

The three key patient benefits of laser cataract surgery vs traditional cataract surgery are:

1. The laser provides a more precise circular incision around the cataract and improves accuracy during placement of the IOL.

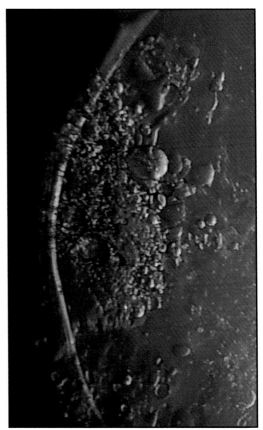

Figure 28-7. Posterior capsule opacity. This was photographed using retroillumination, which makes the details of the opacity obvious.

2. The laser presoftens the cataract, minimizing the use of ultrasound energy to remove the cataract lens. Decreased usage of ultrasound energy shortens recovery time.

3. Mild astigmatism correction can be done at the time of cataract surgery using the laser, as opposed to a manual incision using a surgical blade with traditional surgery.

Posterior Capsular Opacity ("Secondary Cataract")

When a cataract is removed, the back membrane of the crystalline lens's envelope is left in place to help stabilize the IOL and keep vitreous in its place. Although cataracts cannot return once they are removed, this membrane can get cloudy, producing a *posterior capsular opacity* (PCO; Figure 28-7), also known as a *secondary cataract*. (Secondary cataract is a misnomer, since once removed a cataract cannot "grow back." This term is confusing to patients.) PCO can occur within a few months to years after a successful cataract surgery in a relatively small percentage of patients. People who develop a PCO may notice symptoms similar to the initial cataract. These

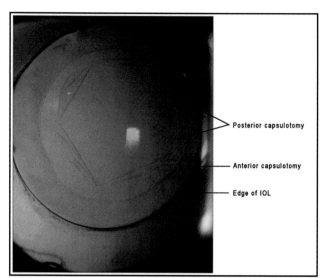

Figure 28-8. Posterior capsulotomy, where laser is used to create an opening in the cloudy capsule. (The anterior capsulotomy is performed at the time of surgery to remove the cataract and allow for insertion of the intraocular lens.)

symptoms may include blurry/hazy vision, double vision, decreased vision, increased glare, and photophobia.

PCO is treated with a procedure called *YAG laser capsulotomy* (YLC). (Laser is covered in Chapter 39.) In the YLC treatment, the ophthalmologist uses short pulses of laser energy to create a small opening in the cloudy posterior lens capsule (Figure 28-8). This creates a hole for the patient to look through, restoring vision. This in-office treatment is generally quick, painless, safe, and very effective.

After treatment, patients should contact their doctor's office immediately if they experience pain, redness, or irritation in the surgical eye; an increase in floaters; flashing lights in their vision; or a black shadow/curtain in the vision.

Adjuncts to Routine Cataract Surgery

Cataract surgery may be the most commonly performed procedure around the world, but not every case is routine. Many patients present with retinal or corneal conditions that require surgeons to take extra precautions before, during, and after surgery.

Cataracts and Glaucoma

For patients who have both cataracts and glaucoma, doing a combined procedure may be advised. (For a thorough review on glaucoma, see Chapter 29.) With advances in technology, surgeons have several options available. Each combined procedure is performed to not only improve the patient's vision, but to lower the intraocular pressure (IOP). By lowering the IOP, it is hoped that visual loss and optic nerve damage can be controlled.

Listed below are some of the glaucoma surgical options that are available, any of which might be combined with cataract extraction or can be performed independently of cataract surgery.

Trabeculectomy is a surgical procedure used in the treatment of glaucoma to relieve the IOP by removing a part of the eye's trabecular meshwork, increasing outflow of aqueous.

Canaloplasty is a minimally invasive glaucoma procedure that utilizes a microcatheter or tube that is placed in the canal of Schlemm to enlarge the drainage site. Canaloplasty can reduce IOP by 40%, hopefully allowing the patient to decrease or eliminate the use of glaucoma drops.

Shunts are devices implanted into the eye to provide an artificial drainage site for aqueous fluid to exit the eye. Aqueous is drained through the tube and absorbed by the surrounding tissue.

Endocyclophotocoagulation (ECP) is a procedure that lowers the IOP by ablating the ciliary processes (behind the iris), thereby slowing the production of aqueous humor. It is performed with a microendolaser that is inserted through the pupil, and is thus usually performed with cataract surgery since the eye is "opened" already.

Cataracts and Diabetes

Cataract surgery in patients with diabetes can range from routine to quite complex, depending on the level of any coexisting retinopathy and the extent of prior treatments. Optical coherence tomography (OCT) is useful in the preoperative assessment of patients with diabetes as an indicator for the potential development of *cystoid macular edema* (CME; swelling of the macula).

IOL selection is also an important issue for patients with diabetes since those with an increased risk for CME are not good candidates for multifocal IOLs. Swelling in the retina can affect the final visual result, and coupled with a multifocal IOL (which can also reduce best-corrected vision) can make for a dissatisfied patient.

Special Circumstances

In a patient with a high refractive error in both eyes and a cataract in only one eye, a decision must be made whether or not to correct the surgical eye to plano. The intention here is to prevent *aniseikonia* (the difference in image size between the two eyes) and diplopia (caused by the prismatic effect of spectacle lenses). If the patient wears contact lenses, he/she may elect to continue with the contact lens in the unoperated eye and fully correct the eye undergoing surgery. Another option is to insert an IOL that will correct the operative eye to a refractive error that is within a few diopters of the fellow eye (instead of plano). If only eyeglasses are worn, then undercorrecting the surgical eye may be a more prudent choice. Having refractive surgery later (including refractive lens exchange—removing the crystalline lens of the other eye even though it does not have a cataract; see Chapter 38, Refractive Surgery) is another option.

A patient who has previously undergone a successful cataract surgery but subsequently developed a retinal detachment and had silicone oil placed in the vitreous cavity would have a hyperopic shift. When the oil was later removed from the eye, there would be a myopic shift.

For complicated circumstances where a single IOL alone is not enough to achieve the desired correction, two IOLs may be implanted. This is known as *piggyback IOLs*, where a secondary lens is implanted in the ciliary sulcus over the existing IOL. This might also be performed if the IOL power selected for the primary lens was incorrect and the removal of that lens is not advisable for some reason.

CLINICAL SKILLS

Preoperative Evaluation of the Patient With Visually Significant Cataracts

History

The patient's visual complaints must have a functional component (ie, a negative effect on his/her activities of daily living) and a duration (how long the negative effect has continued) in order to qualify for cataract surgery. (See Chapter 7 for more on history taking.) A typical symptom is a reduced ability to see well when driving (eg, street signs), watching TV, or reading. Glare when driving at night is also a common symptom. The symptoms usually worsen slowly over a period of months to years. The patient's medical and ocular history should be thoroughly documented. Of particular importance to the surgeon are a history of diabetes, use of medications or supplements used to improve urinary flow (such as tamsulosin), and oral steroid use. Ocular conditions that can affect the outcome of cataract surgery include macular degeneration, glaucoma, and previous ocular surgery.

Examination

A complete eye examination is required for all cataract patients. Visual acuity with the patient's current spectacle correction as well as best-corrected acuity with manifest refraction should be documented. *Glare testing* may be performed to document how much the visual acuity declines when looking at a bright light that simulates night driving conditions. Glare testing is typically done when the patient is symptomatic, yet the visual acuity with best correction is 20/30 or better. (See Chapter 8 for specifics on glare testing.)

The crystalline lens can become thicker as cataracts develop and may push the iris forward, causing a shallow anterior chamber. This makes dilation more risky as it can cause an attack of acute angle closure glaucoma (see Chapter 29). Thus, evaluation of the depth of the anterior chamber is important before dilating the pupils (detailed in Chapters 9 and 12).

In patients with a history of ocular diseases causing reduced macular function, such as macular degeneration, the surgeon may ask you to perform a *Potential Acuity Meter* (PAM) or a *super pinhole* test. These tests (covered in detail in Chapter 8) help assess what the visual acuity would be if the cataract were removed. Surgery is not typically recommended if these tests do not predict improved vision.

Intraocular Lens Power and Calculation

The increased demand for improved visual outcomes in today's cataract patients heavily relies on the accuracy of preoperative biometry (measurement of axial length and corneal power). The gold standard for measuring the axial length is still considered to be ultrasonic immersion A-scan (see Chapter 17). However, this technique is cumbersome for both the patient and the A-scan operator, and requires a high level of expertise by the biometrist to obtain consistently accurate readings. When optical biometry (Lenstar and IOLMaster) became available, it was quickly adopted due to the easy configuration, the speed in acquisition of data, and the convenience to both the patient and the operator. However, while physicians and trained technicians favor optical biometric machines, these instruments are still limited in their ability to measure through very dense or mature cataracts.

There is definitely an art to biometry, and it requires a well-trained technician who is not only capable of taking consistent measurements but also able to correlate these measurements to a patient's history and examination. Biometrists should aim for consistency in their measurements and track their results. Mistakes are very easy to make, but much more difficult to rectify.

Biometry

Regardless of whether the axial length is measured by ultrasound or optical coherence biometry, there are a few simple steps that should be taken into consideration to achieve a more precise outcome (Sidebar 28-1).

The corneal power can be measured with a variety of instruments, including a manual keratometer, corneal topographer or tomographer, or an autokeratometer. There are some conditions that can interfere with the accuracy of preoperative corneal power measurements.

Dry eye syndrome (DES) can make corneal measurements a challenge. DES should be treated before cataract surgery with over-the-counter artificial tears, punctal plugs, and/or cyclosporine drops (Restasis). Also, have the patient blink frequently during the measurement.

Prior corneal refractive surgery renders all keratometric measurements inaccurate. Special formulas are needed to calculate corneal power in these patients.

SIDEBAR 28-1

HINTS FOR
BETTER AXIAL LENGTH MEASUREMENTS

▶ Make sure the machine is properly calibrated and set at the correct velocity (phakia, aphakia, pseudophakia).

▶ If using ultrasound, make sure that the echoes from the cornea, anterior lens, posterior lens, and retina are present and have good amplitude (see Chapter 17).

▶ If using ultrasound, the gain should be set at the lowest level at which you can obtain a good reading.

▶ Make sure that the patient blinks frequently or instill an artificial tear, as errors can arise from a poor tear film.

▶ Always measure both eyes and repeat if the difference between the eyes is greater than 0.3 mm.

▶ Pay attention to short eyes (< 22.0 mm) or long eyes (> 25.0 mm) as different IOL calculation formulas may be indicated.

Contact lenses of any type can alter corneal topography. Prior to preoperative cataract measurements, soft contact lens wearers should discontinue wear for at least 1 week (2 weeks for toric lenses) to allow the cornea to return to its natural shape. Rigid gas-permeable contact lens wearers will require several weeks without contacts for accurate corneal measurements.

Formulas

In order to select the best power of IOL for the patient, the measurements must be "plugged in" to a formula. While the surgeon is the one who selects the formula, it is important to understand the advantages and limitations of the current formulas. The following criteria are generally considered in selecting a formula:

▶ Usage—Most IOL power calculation formulas give a good outcome for axial lengths from 22.50 to 25.00 mm. However, for eyes outside these ranges, the Hoffer Q formula for short eyes and the SRK-T formula for average to long eyes may be considered.

▶ Generations—The latest generation of a formula should always be used.

▶ Personalization—Optimizing a physician's A-constant, anterior chamber depth, or "surgeon factor" (depending on the formula being using) should be a fundamental part of every cataract surgery practice. If surgeons want to optimize their lens constants, they can do so by using the software that comes with their biometer or they can use stand-alone software such as the www.doctor-hill.com/physicians/download. (This is a free service offered by Warren Hill, MD, FACS.) These data help to improve the accuracy of the postoperative refractive result.

Intraocular Lens Power Calculations After Refractive Surgery

Cataract surgery after any type of corneal refractive surgery is challenging because the true corneal power is difficult to measure and calculate even when the patient's previous records are available. The patient should be educated that even with all the most current techniques to estimate the corneal power accurately, there is a chance that the result will be either myopic or hyperopic. According to Dr. William Trattler, author, lecturer, teacher, and ophthalmic surgeon, "Perhaps the most common scenario...for residual refractive error following cataract surgery is related to patients who have previously undergone corneal refractive surgery..."[3]

Current techniques for calculating the corneal power include the history method (which requires the records prior to the refractive surgery) and the Shammas equation. The *history method* is one of the more popular methods for determining the post-refractive corneal curvature. The details needed for this method include the preoperative refractive error as a spherical equivalent, the preoperative average keratometry readings, and the postoperative spherical equivalent refractive error (Sidebar 28-2). The examiner should be cautious not to use the current refractive error due to a possible myopic shift related to the presence of cataracts.

Another popular method currently in use is the Shammas equation. This equation involves averaging the post-refractive K's into one number. It is not a complex formula and can be calculated by an experienced technician (Sidebar 28-3). The corrected K reading = 1.14 X the average K – 6.8.

Another resource for calculating corneal power is online calculators (eg, websites of the American Society of Cataract and Refractive Surgery [ASCRS], Alcon, Bausch + Lomb). These calculators are constantly being updated, and multiple methods are available that will provide instant results for comparison purposes.

Intraoperative biometry using devices such as the Optiwave Refractive Analysis (ORA) system has improved refractive accuracy in these challenging patients. The ORA is a wavefront aberrometer that attaches to the operating microscope and can be used for aphakic refractive measurements. This helps the surgeon choose the proper IOL, whether it's a standard cataract surgery or a more intricate case involving a patient who has had a previous refractive surgery.

Modern theoretical formulas may improve the accuracy of IOL power determination in post-refractive surgery patients.

SIDEBAR 28-2
THE HISTORY METHOD

If the patient had corneal refractive surgery for myopia:

Preoperative spherical equivalent refractive error (make sure to calculate vertex distance for high myopes), subtracting the preoperative average K.

Example 1

Pre-Rfx surgery: Average K of 44.00 and a refractive error of -3.00 D

Post-Rfx surgery: Plano

Calculate: There was a change of 3 D corneal flattening from pre- to postoperative Rfx surgery: 44.00 – 3.00 = 41.00

The K reading to use in the calculation is 41.00 D.

If the patient had corneal refractive surgery for hyperopia:

Preoperative spherical equivalent refractive error (make sure to calculate vertex distance for high hyperopes), adding the amount of correction due to the steeping of the cornea.

Example 2

Pre-Rfx surgery: Average K of 44.00 and a refractive error of +2.00 D

Post-Rfx surgery: Plano

Calculate: There was a change of 2 D corneal steeping from pre- to postoperative Rfx surgery: 44.00 + 2.00 = 46.00

The K reading to use in the calculation is 46.00 D.

SIDEBAR 28-3
THE SHAMMAS NO-HISTORY METHOD

The Shammas no-history method for the calculation of post-refractive PRK and LASIK eye is easy to use, and you only need biometry measurements from the Lenstar.

Shammas formula: Corrected K reading = averaged K x 1.14 – 6.8

Example

No pre-LASIK/PRK records are available

Take regular biometry readings with the Lenstar

Lenstar K reading: 44.00/46.00

Average the K reading values: 44.00 + 46.00 = 90/2 = 45.00

Now plug the average K into the formula: 45.00 x 1.14 – 6.8 = 44.5

The calculated K that you will plug into the Lenstar will be 44.50.

Avoiding Mistakes in Biometry

The preoperative measurements are critical in providing the desired postoperative refraction. Careful attention to details and repeating any questionable results is vital. An error in any of the following can cause an unanticipated myopic or hyperopic outcome (sometimes called a "postoperative surprise").

▶ Incorrect axial length—For every 1 mm of axial length inaccuracy you can anticipate a 3.0 D difference in the postoperative refractive error (even more for short eyes).

▶ Inaccurate keratometry readings—With increased use of toric IOLs and corneal relaxing incisions, it has become increasingly important to detect irregular corneal astigmatism. If the alignment of a toric IOL is off by 10 degrees, it loses 30% of its effect. That's not a big deal with low-power toric lenses, but in a large diopter lens like an Alcon SN6AT-9, that's almost 1.5 D of cylinder.

▶ Wrong formula used—Special formulas are used for long and short axial length and for those with previous refractive surgery. Using an incorrect formula can result in a residual refractive error.

▶ Wrong IOL implanted—The most common reason for removing an IOL, regardless of the type of lens, is an incorrect IOL power.[4] The surgeon will inform the patient immediately and then discuss options to resolve the problem.

Unanticipated refractive surprises can be corrected via glasses or contact lenses (usually not an attractive option to patients who have undergone refractive surgery), LASIK or PRK enhancement, piggyback IOLs, or IOL exchange.

PATIENT SERVICES

There are many ways to deliver patient education, and numerous ways that people learn. Some learn best by reading, others by seeing, and still others are hands-on. Thus, a mixed media approach works best. Methods and materials might include brochures, DVDs (played on small personal DVD players), company websites, Internet sites, PowerPoint presentations, one-on-one phone conversations, and educational talks.

Patient education starts in the office, but health care professionals today are providing care to an increasingly diverse patient population that is challenged with language barriers. Language barriers between physicians and patients are associated with:

▶ Problems in obtaining informed consent

▶ Higher risk of noncompliance with medical care

▶ Increased likelihood of missing follow-up appointments

▶ Increased need for repeat diagnostic testing due to translation errors between the translator, physician, and patient

Informed Consent

In order for a patient to make an intelligent, reasonable decision concerning treatment, he/she needs to have the appropriate information. This education can occur during discussions with medical staff, through discussions with friends who have previously undergone a similar procedure, or via the Internet. However, it normally occurs during the informed consent discussion with the surgeon, in which the risks and benefits of cataract surgery are explained. Only then can the patient sign the informed consent, a legal document stating the patient's intent to have the procedure.

The consent should begin with a brief description of the planned procedure, including the involvement of anesthesia. It is wise to describe what the patient may expect to experience during the surgery. Sufficient information to make an informed decision should include an explanation of risks and benefits involved with the planned procedure, alternative treatments avaliable, and the risks and benefits of doing nothing.

The consent is the opportunity to guide patients and help them make the best decision, and also to discuss any unrealistic expectations concerning the procedure. With advancements in technology and patients' elevated demands and expectation levels, a poorer-than-expected outcome may yield an upset patient. Quality patient education during the informed consent process is an opportunity to build a trusting relationship with the patient and make sure that his/her expectation levels are practical.

Complications of Cataract Surgery

Surgical candidates should be advised of all risks and benefits associated with cataract surgery. The vast majority of cataract cases are uncomplicated. In a small percentage of patients, a less-than-ideal outcome can occur for a variety of reasons. Patients should have a detailed conversation with their surgeon preoperatively about the common and serious risks of cataract surgery.

CME is one of the most common causes of decreased vision in patients following cataract surgery. It has already been mentioned as occurring more frequently in patients with diabetes. CME is painless, and affects the cental retina. When this condition is present, multiple cyst-like pockets of fluid appear in the macula causing retinal swelling. About 1% to 3% of patients who have uncomplicated cataract surgery will experience decreased vision due to CME, usually within a few weeks after surgery.[5] Most patients recover their vision with observation and treatment, which varies. CME is usually treated with corticosteroid eye drops. Ophthalmologists may also elect to inject the eye with an anti-vascular endothelial growth factor drug.

Retinal detachment occurs when there is a separation of the retina from the underlying tissue. A retinal detachment is very uncommon after modern cataract surgery, but the risk does exist. The patient should be cautioned to report any shower of floaters, curtain or veil over part of the vision, and/or flashing lights.

Endophthalmitis is a very serious intraocular infection. Signs and symptoms are redness, pain, photophobia, and decreased vision. This situation constitutes an ophthalmic emergency, and patients should be instructed to contact the physician immediately if these symptoms occur.

Instructions on Pre- and Postoperative Care

Prior to cataract surgery, the surgeon may have the patient begin taking eye drops. Typically, three different classes of medications are used in cataract surgery: antibiotics, nonsterodial anti-inflammatory drugs (NSAIDs), and steroids. Antibiotics are used to prevent infection of the eye. NSAIDs are used to treat inflammation and to help decrease the development of swelling in the retina. Steroids are used to treat inflammation.

Most surgeons have a drop protocol tailored to their experience and the needs of their patients. This protocol could involve the use of an antibiotic and NSAID drops a few days prior to surgery. This regimen is continued post-surgery along with the addition of a steroid drop. The current treatment regimen typically includes 3 to 4 weeks of self-administered drops, which requires strict compliance on the patient's part.

In recent years, the use of injectable drugs for delivering antibiotics and steroids to the eye after cataract surgery has gained popularity. These drugs are changing the management of cataract patients, simplifying the process while providing safeguards against infection and inflammation. The benefits of this method include lowering costs, reducing risks of adverse side effects from the eye drops, and increasing patient compliance.

After cataract surgery the patient will be asked to refrain from strenuous activities (heavy lifting or continuous bending) for a short period of time, but most normal activities can be resumed immediately.

Managing the Unhappy Patient

The best way to avoid an unhappy patient is a thorough discussion prior to the procedure about what to expect during the process. However, even when the patient had an uncomplicated surgery and received excellent pre- and postoperative care, he/she may still be dissatisfied. Some keys to handling these patients are:

▶ Always remain calm and professional

▶ Be empathetic

▶ Keep good clinical notes

▶ Make no judgmental comments, no matter who the surgeon was

▶ Always defer and refer to the eye care practitioner

Cataract surgery is generally a safe and effective procedure to restore vision in symptomatic patients. Continuous advances in the methods used to remove the cataract, and in the types of IOLs available to correct vision, make this an exciting time to be involved in the field of ophthalmology.

ACKNOWLEDGMENTS

The author would like to thank Michelle E. Akler, MD.

CHAPTER QUIZ

1. What is a cataract?

2. How many common types of cataracts are there? What are they?

3. Can a patient have more than one type of cataract in the same eye?

4. If a cataract goes untreated, can it cause blindness?

5. What are some commonly reported symptoms of cataracts?

6. Are there different intraocular lens options?

7. List some benefits to laser cataract surgery.

8. Can a cataract grow back after it has been removed?

9. What is the typical recovery time after cataract surgery?

10. Are the intraocular lens calculations more difficult in a post-refractive surgery patient?

Answers

1. A cataract is the clouding or opacity that develops in the crystalline lens.

2. There are three common types of cataracts. They are nuclear, cortical, and posterior subcapsular.

3. Yes, it is possible for a patient to have more than one type of cataract in the same eye.

4. Yes. If left untreated, most cataracts will eventually cause blindness.

5. Blurred vision, colors appearing faded, poor night vision, frequent changes in prescription lenses, and increase in glare and light sensitivity are common symptoms reported by persons with cataracts.

6. Yes, there are several options available: the standard IOL set at distance, the standard IOL with one eye for near and the other for distance, a multifocal or accommodative IOL, and a toric IOL.

7. The three key patient benefits of laser cataract surgery vs traditional cataract surgery are improved accuracy of IOL placement, minimized use of ultrasound, and laser correction of mild astigmatism (done at the same time).

8. Once a cataract is removed, it does not grow back. However, a clear membrane is left behind the IOL at the time of surgery. Over time, this membrane can get hazy, causing decreased vision and increased glare. When the haze is significant, a laser procedure can be performed (YAG capsulotomy) to clear it.

9. Blurry vision can last a few days or weeks postoperatively. Restrictions depend in part on the surgeon's preferences. The patient will need to put eye drops in the operative eye for a short period post-surgery.

10. Yes, as more individuals have refractive surgery, the number of cataract patients with refractive surgery in their history continues to increase. Calculating IOL power in these eyes can be quite problematic because of the altered corneal curvature.

REFERENCES

1. Yu L, Li ZK, Gao JR, Liu JR, Xu CT. Epidemiology, genetics and treatments for myopia. *Int J Ophthalmol.* 2011;4(6):658-669. doi:10.3980/j.issn.2222-3959.2011.06.17.

2. Apple DJ, Trivedi RH. Sir Nicholas Harold Ridley, Kt, MD, FRCS, FRS. *Arch Ophthalmol.* 2002;120(9):1198-1202. doi:10.1001/archopht.120.9.1198.

3. Trattler W. Complicated cataract cases: moderate postoperative refractive error in the first eye. ASCRS EyeWorld website. www.eyeworld.org/article-moderate-postoperative-refractive-error-in-the-first-eye. Published April 2013. Accessed July 5, 2016.

4. Mamalis N, Brubaker J. Complications of foldable intraocular lenses requiring explantation. *J Cataract Refract Surg.* 2008;34(9):1584-1591. doi:10.1016/j.jcrs.2008.05.046.

5. Schmier JK, Halpern MT, Covert DW, et al. Evaluation of costs for cystoid macular edema among patients after cataract surgery. *Retina.* 2007;27:621-628. www.reviewofophthalmology.com/content/d/retinal_insider/c/46967/#sthash.7jj8WhzV.dpuf. Accessed July 4, 2016.

The figures in this chapter were contributed by the following, who are associated with this book as authors:
Sergina M. Flaherty: Figures 28-2 through 28-5, 28-7, 28-8
Al Lens: Figure 28-6
Monique Rinke: Figure 28-1

29

GLAUCOMA

Sandra Johnson, MD
Eric Areiter, MD

Glaucoma is a commonly encountered ophthalmic condition that can have devastating effects if not properly treated. At its most basic, glaucoma is a build-up of pressure inside the eye that can cause irreversible optic nerve damage and blindness.

The World Health Organization has estimated that glaucoma causes 2% of visual impairment and 12% of global blindness.[1,2] It is the leading cause of irreversible blindness in the world, and the number of years an affected person spends being disabled by glaucoma doubled between 1990 and 2010. This increase can be blamed on the increase of the older population worldwide, and due to medical advancements and increases in standards of living across the planet. Glaucoma will only continue to escalate in prevalence. Estimates suggest that the number of patients with glaucoma will increase worldwide to 111.8 million by 2040, with significant proliferation expected in Asia and Africa.[3] Yet in 2013 the United States Preventive Services Task Force determined that current evidence is insufficient to assess the benefits of screening (eg, at a health fair) for primary open-angle glaucoma in adults.[4] Thus, how to detect cases in the community remains a challenge.

BASIC SCIENCES

A thorough discussion of ocular anatomy is found in Chapter 2, and of ocular physiology in Chapter 3. A quick review is appropriate here. Intraocular pressure (IOP) occurs as a result of the production of aqueous humor by the ciliary processes, which are found behind the iris in the posterior segment. The aqueous is a clear ultrafiltrate from the blood circulating through the ciliary processes.

Aqueous maintains the eye pressure and also provides nutrition to the anterior surface of the crystalline lens and the posterior surface of the cornea, neither of which have blood vessels to bring them sustenance. It flows from the ciliary processes where it is secreted, into the posterior chamber. It then courses through the pupil and into the anterior chamber. Between the iris and cornea an anatomical "angle" exists, which includes the trabecular meshwork, where the aqueous drains out of the eye. When aqueous does not drain properly, pressure can build up in the eye. It is this pressure that damages the optic nerve and causes defects in the visual field, the combination of which is identified as glaucoma.

Ledford JK, Lens A, eds.
Principles and Practice in Ophthalmic Assisting:
A Comprehensive Textbook (pp 523-536).
© 2018 Taylor & Francis Group.

TABLE 29-1
SYMPTOMS AND SIGNS ASSOCIATED WITH TYPES OF GLAUCOMA

Acute Angle Closure	Congenital	Open-Angle Glaucoma

Blurry vision
Eye pain
Nausea
Vomiting
Headache
High IOP
Redness
Corneal edema
Shallow anterior chamber
Mid-dilated pupil
	Large eyes
	Cloudy-appearing eyes
	Tearing
	Photophobia
	Horizontal ruptures in Descemet's membrane
	High IOP
	Redness
	Corneal edema
	Large corneal diameter
	Iris atrophy
	Long eyes
	Myopia
		Gradual peripheral vision loss
		Tunnel vision
		Optic nerve asymmetry
		Optic nerve cupping
		Visual field defects:
		    Enlarged blind spot
		    Bjerrum's scotoma
		    Nasal step
		Thinning of retinal nerve fiber layer

TABLE 29-2
TYPES OF OPEN-ANGLE GLAUCOMA

Primary open-angle glaucoma	Open anterior chamber angle with raised IOP and no identified secondary cause
Normal-tension glaucoma	Open-angle glaucoma with optic nerve damage or visual field deficits featuring IOP within normal limits
Pseudoexfoliation glaucoma	Deposition of exfoliation material in the anterior segment and trabecular meshwork resulting in obstructed aqueous outflow
Uveitis	Inflammation of uvea resulting in physical obstruction of the trabecular meshwork causing increased IOP
Steroid-induced glaucoma	Increased IOP due to increased outflow resistance in a person actively taking steroids
Traumatic glaucoma	Elevated IOP due to accumulated blood, debris, or scarring in the trabecular meshwork

Eye pressure is measured by tonometry, discussed later. Like many physiologic processes, there is fluctuation in eye pressure. The normal range is taken as 10 to 22 mm Hg, and eyes with glaucoma will fluctuate much more than normal eyes.[5] Unlike disorders such as diabetes, there is no exact number that means a person has glaucoma, and some patients have eye pressure in the 20s with no nerve damage or field loss. Elevated eye pressure is a significant and modifiable risk factor for glaucoma, just as high cholesterol is for heart disease. Many practitioners will treat eyes with IOP in the 30s, for concern that this level of IOP is too high for the ongoing health of the eye.

CLINICAL KNOWLEDGE

Glaucoma refers to a variety of ophthalmic disorders with characteristic changes in the optic nerve that result in distinctive visual field changes, usually associated with increased IOP (Table 29-1). Permanent changes in visual field and ultimate blindness are both associated with untreated glaucoma.

Open-angle (Table 29-2) and closed (or narrow) angle glaucoma (Table 29-3) are the two primary classifications used to distinguish different types of glaucoma, depending on whether the trabecular meshwork/angle appears open or closed on examination with gonioscopy.

As you would expect, in open-angle glaucoma (OAG, also called chronic open-angle glaucoma, or COAG) the angle appears to be accessible to the aqueous. The damage in OAG progresses gradually over time with few or no symptoms, earning glaucoma the nickname "sneak thief of sight," and a patient may present for eye care only after significant damage has already occurred. It is more commonly encountered in North America and accounts for about 90% of glaucoma cases in the United States.[6] OAG is referred to as primary (POAG) when there is no specific cause and the angle appears normal on exam. Secondary open angle occurs when the function of an open angle is jeopardized by prior trauma, inflammatory debris, or excess pigment. Another cause of secondary glaucoma occurs when the angle metabolism is altered by steroid medications and the IOP rises. In this case, the patient is said to be a steroid responder.

TABLE 29-3	
TYPES OF ANGLE-CLOSURE GLAUCOMA	
Primary	Patient has an anatomically narrow angle identified on gonioscopy, with iris and trabecular meshwork contact resulting in glaucoma with no identified secondary cause
Neovascular	Newly formed blood vessels from the iris typically seen with diabetes or ischemia branching over the trabecular meshwork
Iridocorneal endothelial syndrome	Typically unilateral and seen in females with varying degrees of corneal endothelial changes and iris defects resulting in glaucoma; variations include Chandler's syndrome, essential iris atrophy, and Cogan Reese syndrome
Axenfeld-Rieger syndrome	Autosomal dominant bilateral condition consisting of anterior chamber angle, trabecular meshwork, and iris abnormalities, with 50% associated with early childhood glaucoma due to neural crest cells being retained in the anterior chamber angle
Nanophthalmos	Small eye due to compromised growth with a short axial length, small cornea, large lens, and thick sclera, which results in narrow angle
Aqueous misdirection	Angle-closure eye that is postoperative; the anterior chamber is diffusely shallow with very high eye pressure

Closed-angle glaucoma is the term used when the angle between the iris and cornea becomes blocked or closes, inhibiting drainage of aqueous (Figure 29-1). It accounts for fewer glaucoma cases in the United States (10%), though in other countries that figure may be quite high.[7] In particular, people of East Asian descent are prone to closed-angle glaucoma due to having shallower anterior chambers.[8] Women are also more likely to have shallower anterior chambers, predisposing them to closed-angle glaucoma to a greater degree than men, due to a tendency toward having smaller eyes. The same holds true for hyperopic patients, who typically have "short" eyes.

The term *primary angle closure* applies to a patient with angle closure on exam but no glaucoma damage. The nomenclature changes to angle-closure glaucoma once there is damage.

Acute angle closure or *angle-closure attack* presents with very high IOP and a "rock hard eye" that is very firm to the touch. The patient presents in acute pain (may describe this as a headache), and the attack may occur suddenly without precipitating events. Other symptoms can include nausea, vomiting, blurred vision, and eye redness. Due to the severity of the symptoms, a patient will often seek medical attention soon after a closed-angle glaucoma attack begins.

The attack results from a block of aqueous flow drainage. Signs include very high IOP, conjunctival redness, a cloudy cornea, and a mid-dilated/fixed pupil. Since the eye pressure is so high in these cases, it is deemed an emergency as damage to the eye can occur quickly (see Chapter 33). Thus, an acute angle-closure attack must be ruled out when triaging any patient who complains of a painful red eye with blurred vision.

Closed or narrow angle glaucoma most commonly results from *pupillary* block where the flow of aqueous

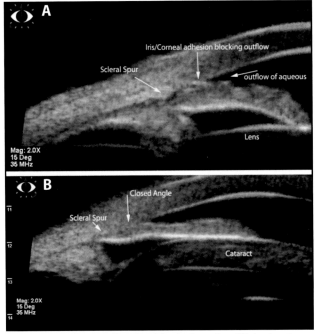

Figure 29-1. B-scan showing blocked angles. (A) is due to an adhesion between the iris and cornea. (B) is caused by a lens enlarged due to a cataract.

from the posterior to anterior chamber is impeded by the natural lens (which continually enlarges through life). A build-up of aqueous (and thus IOP) occurs in the posterior chamber, pushing the iris forward over the angle. This cuts off aqueous drainage from the eye. There can also be *secondary angle closure* from entities such as tumors, choroidal effusions (leakage of fluid from the choroid, which can collect under the retina), and iris cysts, which also can push the iris forward. Angle closure can occur from inflammation or membranes that can create synechiae

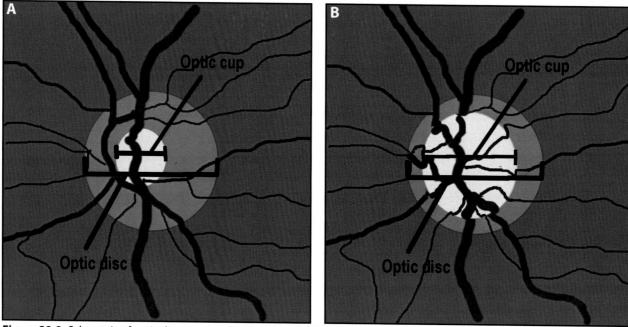

Figure 29-2. Schematic of optic disc cupping. (A) Normal optic disc and cup. (B) Glaucomatous disc. Note enlargement of cup and "dipping" blood vessels.

(adhesions) at the pupil between the iris and the lens (*posterior synechiae*) or in the angle between the iris and the cornea (*peripheral anterior synechiae* [PAS]). Uveitis and neovascular glaucoma are examples of diseases that can cause this type of closure.

A rare form of angle closure is *malignant glaucoma* (also called *aqueous misdirection* or *ciliary block*). In this type of glaucoma, the ciliary body secretes aqueous into the vitreous, and the build-up of fluid pushes the anterior segment structures forward. There is shallowing across the entire anterior chamber, and the eye pressure is very high. This condition most commonly occurs in eyes that have had laser or surgery for acute angle closure. It may be treated with cycloplegic drops, laser to the anterior hyaloid face, or anterior vitrectomy.[9] The intent of the surgical procedure is to release the aqueous that is "trapped" in the vitreous gel.

Glaucoma can be further classified into *high* or *normal/low tension*. High tension glaucoma involves visual field changes and optic nerve damage in association with increased ocular pressure, while *normal/low tension* glaucoma can have those changes, despite normal IOP. Not all people develop nerve damage at a particular pressure, and there is significant variation depending on the patient. Treatment (discussed later) is aimed at preventing further vision loss; once vision is lost it normally cannot be recovered. If a person has a persistently high IOP yet does not have any apparent changes in visual fields or damage to the optic nerve, this is termed *ocular hypertension* (OHT).

Congenital glaucoma refers to abnormal embryonic development of the eye resulting in glaucoma. It can present as early as birth and may simply be failure of the trabecular meshwork to form properly. It may also be associated with other anomalies of eye development, such as congenital cataract, or with syndromes like aniridia (absence of an iris) or Axenfeld-Rieger (which is characterized by deformities in the iris/pupil and cornea). Parents may notice something unusual about their young child's eye(s) and mention this to the pediatrician (see Table 29-1). From there they are likely referred to a pediatric ophthalmologist who would diagnose the condition.

Glaucoma and the Optic Nerve

The hallmark of glaucoma is optic nerve damage. As pressure builds up inside the eye, the force is transferred back; the optic nerve is the "weak spot." Examination of the optic nerve is critical in assessing a patient for glaucoma.

The round or slightly oval nerve head is the *optic disc.* At its center is a small, white area called the *cup.* The tissue between the disc and the cup is the *rim.* In evaluation of the optic disc, the question is how much of the entire disc is taken up by the cup? This is called the *cup-to-disc ratio.* In a normal, healthy eye the cup takes up 20% to 30% of the disc; this is translated to a cup-to-disc ratio of 0.2 or 0.3, respectively (Figure 29-2A). As the nerve fibers are damaged from elevated IOP, the cup gets larger. A cup-to-disc ratio over 0.5 (some say 0.3) is thus suspicious for glaucoma (Figure 29-2B).

In general, a person's body is symmetrical, so the cup-to-disc ratio of the two eyes is usually about the same. *Disc asymmetry*, where the cup-to-disc ratio of one disc is larger than the other, can signal glaucoma as well.

TABLE 29-4

CLASSES OF MEDICATIONS USED TO TREAT GLAUCOMA

Medication Class	Function	Generic Examples	Cap Color
Beta blockers	Decrease intraocular aqueous humor production	Timolol, betaxolol, levobetaxolol	Yellow (nonselective) Light blue (selective)
Prostaglandin analogues	Increase drainage of aqueous humor from the eye	Latanoprost, travoprost, bimatoprost, unoprostone	Turquoise (many patients call it green)
Miotics	Increase drainage of aqueous humor from the eye	Pilocarpine, carbachol, echothiophate iodide	Dark green
Carbonic anhydrase inhibitors	Decrease intraocular aqueous humor production	Dorzolamide, brinzolamide	Orange
Alpha agonists	Decrease intraocular aqueous humor production and increase drainage	Brimonidine, apraclonidine	Purple (Note: Brimonidine cap has a more bluish tone)
Combination drops	Decrease IOP by mechanism of ingredients	Brimonidine/timolol Dorzolamide/timolol Brinzolamide/brimonidine	Dark blue Dark blue Light green

If you look at a normal disc, you may notice that some areas of the rim are thicker than others. The Inferior part of the disc is thickest, then the Superior, Nasal, and finally the Temporal rim is the thinnest. This pattern is often called the *ISNT rule*, and it is used to assess a disc for its normal proportions.[10]

It has been suggested that glaucoma follows a progressive thinning of the disc from the inferior temporal rim to the superior temporal to the temporal then inferior nasal and then superior nasal.[11,12] This means that the disc may become vertically elongated in early glaucoma. In other cases cupping is overall enlargement or may be just in certain areas (*notching*). As the cup becomes evacuated, the blood vessels may be seen dipping down over the rim or even suspended over the cup without any supporting tissue beneath.

Deciding that a disc looks glaucomatous is not a simple process. There are many variations of normal. For example, a person might have disc asymmetry but this is just the way his/her body is and no disease is present. Myopic discs are particularly difficult to diagnose. In this case it has been suggested to look for a discontinuity in the inner margin of the optic rim between the superior or inferior quadrant and the temporal quadrant.[13] This is called the *crescent moon sign*.

Stereo disc photographs have long been a manner of documenting the baseline of patients for ongoing review. With the advent of optical coherence tomography (OCT), we can now evaluate the disc and surrounding area in greater detail than ever before. Photography and other imaging modalities offer us beneficial data in diagnosing as well as a visual record for following changes over time.

Treatment

Treatment for glaucoma can be with medications, laser therapy, or incisional surgery, depending on the type of glaucoma and/or the stage of the disease. For congenital glaucoma, medications are usually used until the incisional surgery can be done as the medications do not control the disease and the surgical success is high. Chronic angle closure, such as develops with neovascular glaucoma, is another type of glaucoma that usually cannot be controlled without incisional surgery.

Medication

Glaucoma medical management is usually attempted prior to surgical intervention in most patients who exhibit signs and symptoms suggesting glaucoma. Different classes of medical treatment function by different mechanisms, which vary in efficacy depending on the patient's ocular anatomy as well as the type of glaucoma he/she has. Most medications function to either increase outflow or decrease aqueous production (or both), and are given in eye drop form with colored-coded bottle caps to avoid patient confusion (Table 29-4). They may be used in combination therapy or individually. Patients are instructed to wait 10 minutes between administrations of eye drops when taking several at similar times.

Prostaglandin analogues decrease IOP by increasing the outward flow of aqueous humor from the eye. They are often the first glaucoma medication utilized in treatment of increased IOP, and exhibit fewer side effects than other topical glaucoma medications. Muscle and joint pain and headaches have very rarely occurred in some patients. Patients commonly note elongation and thickening of their lashes, and may develop mild redness of the eye and periorbital puffiness. Prolonged usage has been found to darken iris coloration in mixed-color irides through pigment increase. These drops typically lower IOP by 25% to 30% and are oftentimes more effective at lower IOP than beta blockers (discussed next).[14] Compliance is good due to once a day dosing. Examples include bimatoprost, latanoprost, and travoprost, all of which usually have a teal-colored cap.

Beta blockers are frequently used in the treatment of high IOP and function by blocking nerve receptors. (There are three beta [ß] receptors, but only ß1 and ß2 are of interest in this case.) This has the effect of decreasing aqueous humor production in the eye. They are believed to lower IOP by roughly 25%, and may take several weeks to reach an ophthalmic drug level sufficient to achieve maximum efficacy.[15]

Timolol has been the *nonselective* beta blocker standard (ie, will block ß1 and ß2) for years and is generally well tolerated. This class typically has a yellow cap. It is available in a gel form that is used once a day in the morning with less systemic absorption. But for patients with asthma, a selective ß1 blocker would be a better choice if a beta blocker has to be used. These have fewer adverse pulmonary effects and include betaxolol (with a light blue cap). Timolol is more effective at lowering IOP than the selective ß1 adrenoceptor blockers, though.

Miotics function by stimulation of the parasympathetic nervous system (the opposite of the "fight or flight" sympathetic nervous system response), resulting in pupillary constriction. This constriction results in the iris being pulled from the trabecular meshwork. These medications thus decrease IOP by increasing drainage of aqueous humor from the eye. Side effects can include miosis-related decrease in vision, increased tear production, and rarely an increased likelihood of developing cataracts and retinal detachment. While miotics have been frequently used in the treatment of glaucoma for more than 100 years, their usage has been decreasing as newer glaucoma medications have fewer side effects and greater efficacy. Pilocarpine, which typically has a green cap, is one example.

Carbonic anhydrase inhibitors (CAIs), which are sulfonamides, decrease the amount of aqueous humor by decreasing production. CAIs typically lower IOP by 15% to 50%.[16] Eye drop formulations include dorzolamide and brinzolamide, both with orange caps. Due to its pH, dorzolamide may sting upon instillation. Because brinzolamide is a suspension, it may cause a brief blurring of vision, and patients should be educated to shake the bottle prior to use.

An oral formulation of CAIs is available for patients whose IOP is not sufficiently managed through eye drop usage alone; however, oral CAIs are much more likely to have side effects. Commonly, they cause benign tingling in the fingers, and carbonated drinks taste "flat." Other oral CAI side effects include depression, fatigue, weight loss, increased risk of renal stone formation, and rarely a severe anemia. Oral CAIs decrease IOP rapidly and are often used in more urgent situations where IOP is very high (as in acute angle-closure glaucoma). The common oral formulations include acetazolamide and methazolamide.

Alpha agonists reduce IOP by decreasing aqueous production as well as by increasing aqueous drainage. Side effects include fatigue and dry mouth. There can also be an allergic reaction, which is typically delayed onset and usually involves redness of the lids. Examples include brimonidine and apraclonidine. Brimonidine (bluish-purple cap) is typically used for long-term treatment, and apraclonidine (purple cap) is more for short-term management.

Combination drops offer a mix of drugs that lower IOP in different ways. For example, the drop that combines dorzolamide (CAI) and timolol (nonselective beta blocker) has the action of both. There is also the convenience of using a single drop instead of two. Side effects could include those of either drug. The brimonidine/timolol and dorzolamide/timolol combinations have dark blue caps. Brinzolamide/brimonidine drops have a light green cap.

Laser

Laser can be used in the office to treat both narrow and open-angle glaucoma.

Laser peripheral iridotomy (LPI) is the procedure utilized for acute angle closure as well as to avoid angle closure in eyes with narrow anatomic angles. LPI is usually done in both eyes, since narrow angles are a structural variant and most eyes are symmetric (and thus carry similar risks). The procedure involves using the laser to "cut" a hole in the iris so that aqueous can more easily reach the anterior chamber (see Figure 39-2). The aqueous itself then helps push the iris back, away from the angle. Pretreatment with 1% or 2% pilocarpine (see above) is often used to stretch the iris by constricting it so that the laser can penetrate more easily. An alpha-adrenergic agent is also given to help blunt any post-laser IOP elevation. Patients are asked to have an IOP check 30 minutes to 1 hour post procedure to rule out an IOP spike that needs to be treated. Patients are prescribed topical steroid drops following the procedure in order to quell any inflammation.

Laser trabeculoplasty (LTP) is the most common laser procedure for open-angle glaucoma. The laser is used to stimulate the trabecular meshwork, which increases outflow of aqueous in the majority of treated patients. Historically, an argon laser is most commonly used (*argon laser trabeculoplasty* [ALT]). Often, one-half of the 360 degrees of trabecular meshwork is treated in a session and the other half later.

Selective laser trabeculoplasty (SLT) is a low wavelength YAG laser used for LTP, and it can be repeated on trabecular meshwork that was previously treated with argon or YAG, permitting more laser treatments per eye.

Surgical Treatment

Trabeculectomy is the most common glaucoma filter surgery currently performed, and is generally recommended for glaucoma patients when IOP continues to remain elevated despite medical and/or laser treatment. Trabeculectomy is performed to relieve IOP by the removal of a small piece of angle tissue. This creates a new drainage site and enhances flow of aqueous humor from the eye. The fluid is drained into a new space called a *bleb*, a sort of pouch created under the superior conjunctiva where aqueous absorption can occur. If a patient also has a cataract, trabeculectomy can be combined with cataract removal in the same procedure. The number of trabeculectomies being performed has been decreasing during the 2000s.[17] This may be due to increased efficacy of medical treatment and the use of antimetabolites (discussed next) for greater surgical success with an initial procedure, as well as earlier diagnosing of glaucoma. There are also other procedures coming into the market place that are alternatives to the trabeculectomy.

The most common reason for trabeculectomy failure is scar development. *Antimetabolites* are drugs that prevent scarring by targeting fast-growing cells, including the Tenon's fibroblasts that play a role in wound healing. 5-fluorouracil (5-FU) and mitomycin C are two antimetabolites often used during trabeculectomy. 5-FU, however, can also be administered postoperatively as an intraocular injection. However, their use can increase the risk of postoperative complications, including critically low IOP (*hypotony*), which can lead to flat (collapsed) anterior chamber and/or suprachoroidal hemorrhage. A lifelong risk for bleb leak and blebitis (infection in the bleb) is also induced, and post trabeculectomy patients with a red eye need prompt assessment.

Tube implants or *shunts* are often used as an alternative or if trabeculectomies fail. These tubes function as shunts that bypass the trabecular meshwork and redirect aqueous humor into an implant and into a sub-Tenon's bleb (Figure 29-3). Common indications for tube implantation include complicated glaucomas, such as uveitic, traumatic, and neovascular. Possible complications more specific to this type of glaucoma surgery include tube erosion as well as diplopia, as the plates of the implant are near the eye muscles.

CLINICAL SKILLS

History Taking

Careful history taking is an essential part of glaucoma care. Like many diseases, glaucoma can be inherited and thus family history is relevant. In fact, patients who have siblings with open-angle glaucoma are two to four times as likely to have it themselves.[18] It is also important to determine if patients exhibit certain risk factors that would predispose them to developing glaucoma.

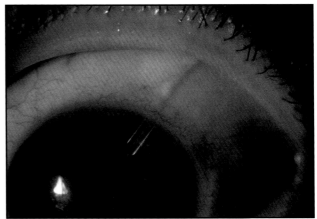

Figure 29-3. A drainage tube has been placed to increase aqueous outflow.

The Ocular Hypertension Treatment Study was a randomized trial that evaluated the efficacy of topical glaucoma medication in patients who exhibited elevated IOP. It also found several predictors that a patient may develop primary open-angle glaucoma (Sidebar 29-1). These included advanced age (60+ years), larger baseline cup-to-disc ratio, and thin central corneal thickness. Larger cup-to-disc and thinner central corneas have been found to be more prevalent in Black Americans, correlating with their increased risk for glaucoma.[19,20] The Baltimore Eye Study compared the prevalence of primary open-angle glaucoma (POAG) between Black Americans and White Americans. It defined primary open-angle glaucoma based on observation of optic nerve damage, significant optic disc cupping, and abnormal visual fields without consideration of measured IOP. The study found that rates of POAG among Black Americans were 1.23% for those aged 40 to 49 years, and 11.26% in those over 80, compared with 0.92% for White Americans aged 40 to 49 years and 2.16% in those over 80.[21] The study did not find a significant difference between men and women.

These risk factors should be kept in mind when examining patients, and increased vigilance for changes in IOP as well as other signs of glaucoma should be the rule for patients who have or exhibit risk factors.

A patient's systemic history is of particular interest to the physician as it relates to low tension glaucoma. Entities such as collagen vascular disease, Raynaud's phenomenon, migraines, systemic hemorrhages and transfusions, hypotension, prior infections (such as Lyme disease or syphilis), and sleep apnea can all be relevant.

History of systemic medication use is also important, especially beta blockers and steroids, both of which can affect IOP. Any allergies to medications can be pertinent. (For example, CAIs contain sulfa, and are sometimes used to treat glaucoma.) Past medical history of asthma or heart disease can also be relevant to the doctor prescribing glaucoma medications.

SIDEBAR 29-1
CASE STUDY
(PRIMARY OPEN-ANGLE GLAUCOMA)

History
Exam dated 2014. 70-year-old patient with a history of ocular hypertension; IOP by applanation ranges to 29 mm Hg in both eyes since 2012.

Findings/Testing Results
Central corneal thickness (CCT) 582 microns in both eyes.

Gonioscopy normal and open angles in both eyes.

Spectralis (Heidelberg Engineering) retinal nerve fiber layer (see figure to the right) demonstrates borderline thinning in both superior quadrants that represent a change from the baseline in 2012 and 2013 scan. Images of the discs are also visible on the scan.

Humphrey Visual Field (Zeiss) of the right eye and left eye (see figures below) demonstrate early inferior defects that correspond with the changes on the retinal nerve fiber layer.

Ocular Hypertension Treatment Trial calculator predicts 28% chance of change to glaucoma over 5 years.

Plan
Medication started.

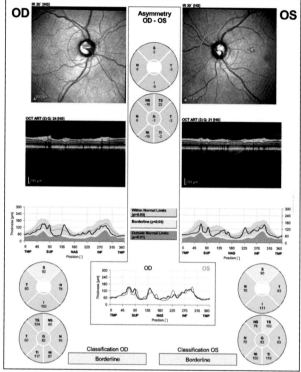

Retinal nerve fiber layer in case study.

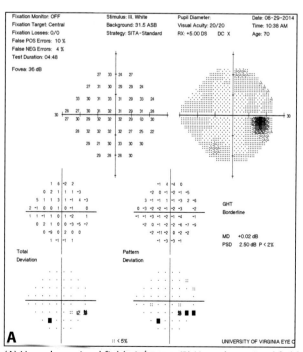

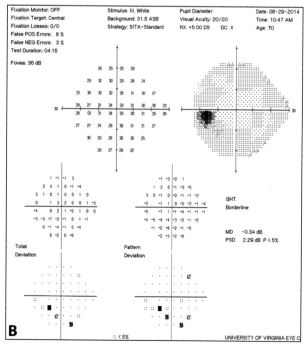

(A) Humphrey visual field, right eye. (B) Humphrey visual field, left eye.

The importance of the history is not limited to the patient's initial visit. A patient's health history may change. Additionally, once a patient has been put on medication for glaucoma, proper recording of its use is vital. Coaching patients to bring their eye medications and/or their written schedule to every visit can be very helpful. The patient must be carefully questioned regarding each medication used, specifically what the medication is (it might help if you refer to the eye drop by cap color), how often it is used, which eye (or both), and when the last dose was taken and at what time. This allows you to evaluate the patient's compliance and understanding of instructions. In addition, noting the last time the drops were used can help explain a "surprise" eye pressure. Each medication has a *peak effect*, after which its pressure-lowering attributes begin to wane. The peak effect of prostaglandin analogues, for example, is 10 to 14 hours after use.[22]

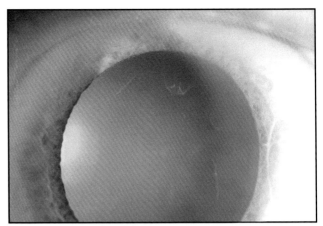

Figure 29-4. Pseudoexfoliation.

Pupil Evaluation

A pupil reactivity exam should be performed with all ophthalmologic testing. Pupil size should be observed as well as shape using an indirect light source such as a penlight. A mid-dilated, nonreactive pupil can be seen in acute angle-closure glaucoma. Pupil reactivity should be checked in each eye, followed by the swinging light test to evaluate for any afferent pupillary defect, which can indicate an eye with more severe glaucoma. A thorough discussion of pupil testing is in Chapter 9.

Slit Lamp Evaluation

A full slit lamp exam should be done in all ophthalmology patients, with special focus on particular areas depending on the patient's personal ocular history and risk factors. An undilated pupil is also best for observing transillumination defects of the iris, which are associated with pigmentary glaucoma, as well as rubeosis, which is associated with neovascular glaucoma. The *Van Herick test* is estimation of the narrowness or deepness of the temporal angle depth performed during a slit lamp exam. This test is covered in detail in Chapter 12, and is important because dilating a narrow angle could trigger an acute angle-closure glaucoma attack. A suspected narrow angle might also indicate the need for the doctor to perform a gonioscopy examination (a technique that allows the physician to view the characteristics of the angle) before dilation.

Slit lamp evaluation after dilation allows a more thorough examination of the lens, where pseudoexfoliation material may be more easily seen (Figure 29-4).

Tonometry

Tonometry (covered in detail in Chapter 13) is one of the primary methods of glaucoma evaluation. It is a measurement of the patient's IOP using an instrument called a *tonometer* to apply pressure using a probe or puff of air. It should always be done before any other test that compresses the cornea, such as gonioscopy or corneal pachymetry, which may massage aqueous out of the eye and thus give a falsely lowered reading. Any testing requiring a clear cornea without prior applanation (vision assessment, refractometry, imaging, etc) should ideally be done prior to tonometry.

Two of the most commonly used tonometers are the Goldmann applanation tonometer and the Icare PRO rebound tonometer, with the Goldmann more widely utilized in standard practice. The Icare is useful in children and other patients with positioning problems as it is hand held and has minimal contact with the cornea. The Tono-pen is another commonly used device for obtaining IOP and is a compact, portable instrument. It is known to slightly overestimate low IOP and underestimate high, and has a lower accuracy of measuring IOP compared to Goldmann tonometry.[23]

Fundus Examination

Evaluation of the optic disc is generally done by the physician as part of the fundus exam. The ratio of the cup vs the disc size, any thinning of the disc rim, and hemorrhages (Figure 29-5) are noted.

Visual Field Testing

A visual field test should be performed, starting with a *confrontational visual field*, as part of a standard ophthalmic exam. Confrontation fields are covered in detail in Chapter 9. Although it is an unsophisticated test, dense glaucomatous visual field defects can be detected in this fashion.

Formally documenting the visual field of a patient with suspected or known glaucoma is the standard of care. This is generally done using either a Goldmann manual perimeter or an automated perimeter (such as

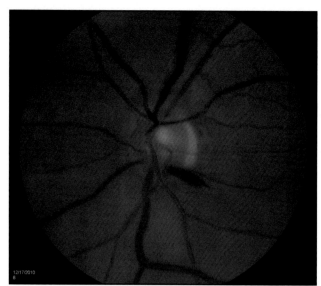

Figure 29-5. Disc hemorrhage (Bjerrum's hemorrhage) classic of glaucoma.

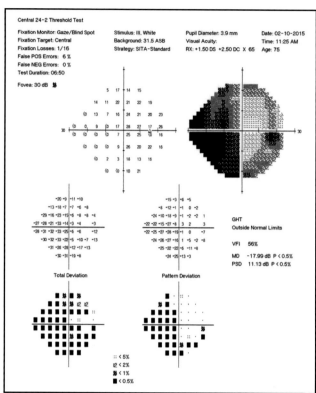

Figure 29-6. This Humphrey visual field shows a nasal defect, which is consistent with temporal thinning of the optic disc.

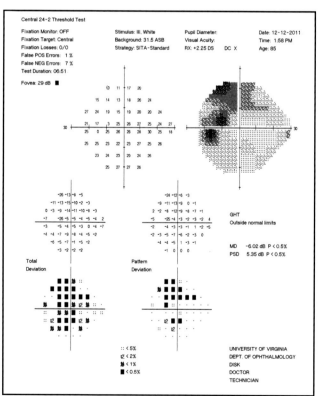

Figure 29-7. This Humphrey visual field depicts a superior arcuate that would be consistent with inferior disc thinning and the retinal nerve fiber layer analysis in Figure 29-8.

the Humphrey). Both of these are covered in detail in Chapter 14. The *SITA* program is a Swedish Interactive Testing Algorithm, part of the Zeiss Humphrey software, which allows the computer to determine which points should be retested based on the patient's responses rather than a random selection. This reduces testing time and patient fatigue, and thus yields better test results.

A frequency doubling technology (FDT) perimeter is a portable instrument with high sensitivity and specificity in detecting visual field loss, such as due to glaucomatous damage at an early stage.[24] The low test-retest variability of FDT makes it an excellent way to monitor progressive field loss, and this technology is incorporated into Matrix programs by Zeiss Humphrey, which are expanded and resemble the conventional white-on-white perimetry that doctors and patients are used to. FDT uses a combination of low spatial frequency and high temporal frequency to specifically target *magnocellular cells*. These are visual system neurons responsible for sensing motion, depth, and differences in brightness (vs precise detail), and are lost earlier in glaucoma.

Short-wavelength automated perimetry (SWAP), in contrast to FDT, targets *koniocellular cells,* visual system cells that receive information from short wavelength blue cones. SWAP can detect visual field deficits up to 5 years earlier than standard automated perimetry (SAP).[25] The test is performed with a blue light projected on a yellow background. Limitations of SWAP include high test-retest variability and long testing time.

Usually visual field defects are not detectable in glaucomatous patients until more than 30% of retinal ganglion cell axons of the optic nerve have been lost.[26] Visual field defects typically associated with glaucoma include a nasal step defect (Figure 29-6), a superior arcuate defect (with or without peripheral breakthrough; Figure 29-7),

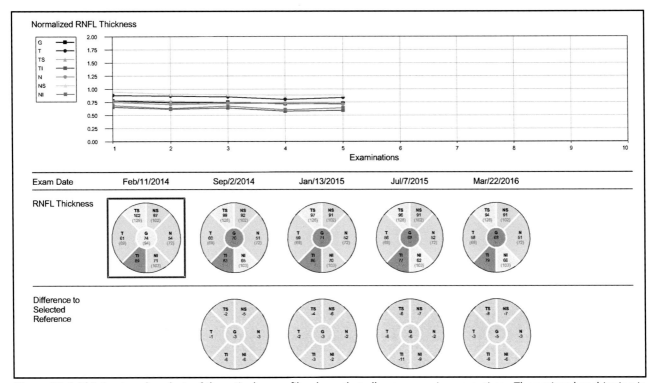

Figure 29-8. This is a trend analysis of the retinal nerve fiber layer that allows comparison over time. The patient has thinning in the inferior aspect, which is a classic area for thinning in a glaucomatous disc.

and a severe visual field loss that is temporal sparing (ie, there is an area of vision remaining in the temporal field). Some glaucoma-associated visual field defects, though, are nonspecific.

Imaging and Scans

Central Corneal Thickness

Thicker or thinner than average corneas are thought to cause inaccurate IOP measurements. The average cornea is 0.5 mm thick. Thinner corneas may show artificially low IOP, while corneas that are thicker than average read as artificially elevated. A thinner central cornea measurement is also associated with a propensity for glaucomatous change. *Pachymetry*, which uses ultrasound waves, should be performed to measure corneal thickness in patients believed to be at risk for glaucoma (see Figure 5-6).

Optical Coherence Tomography

The *retinal nerve fiber layer* (RNFL) is the innermost layer of the retina and consists of a collection of thinly-spread retinal ganglion cell axons. (Axons are the extensions of a nerve cell.) In the healthy eye, the RNFL thickness increases closer to the optic disc. In glaucoma patients, however, RNFL thinning is seen to occur. This can be evaluated with *optical coherence tomography* (OCT). The OCT parameters most associated with early

glaucomatous changes are RNFL thinning in the inferior and superior sections and the cup area (Figure 29-8).

Fundus Photography

Physicians often obtain photos of the optic discs for ongoing comparison and to document any asymmetry or disc hemorrhages. The photos may be taken on an annual basis or just repeated for a new baseline should change occur. Photography is covered in Chapter 15.

Corneal Hysteresis

The Ocular Response Analyzer (ORA) is a device that evaluates corneal biomechanics by emitting a puff of air onto the cornea while an infrared beam tracks resulting changes in corneal shape. *Corneal hysteresis*, the difference in air pressure between inward and outward deviation in response to this puff of air, is influenced by corneal rigidity, corneal thickness, hydration, and IOP. Corneal hysteresis is significantly lower in glaucoma patients, and may be a useful measurement in early glaucoma detection.[27] Some practices utilize this technology for care of their glaucoma patients.

Assisting With In-Office Glaucoma Procedures

Preparation for incisional procedures and injections includes topical proparacaine with antibiotic as well as

You are being placed on medication for glaucoma. The purpose of the medication is to lower the pressure inside your eye.

► Take the drops exactly as directed—No more and no less.

- If you are using more than one eye drop, wait at least 5 minutes in between so you don't wash out the first drop with the second.
- Use the drops on schedule even if you are coming in for an appointment.
- Please bring all eye medications to every visit.

► Do not allow yourself to run out of drops. Call our office if you need a refill.

► The purpose of these drops is to lower your eye's pressure.

- They are not meant to make your eyes feel good.
- They are not meant to help you see better.
- High eye pressure is not something you can feel. The only way to know if the drops are working is for you to come to our office and let us measure the pressure. Please keep all appointments.

► If you do not use the drops as directed, over time you may:

- Have irreversible optic nerve damage (this is not something you can sense or feel).
- Develop tunnel vision (this develops in such a way that you're not aware of it until it's too late).
- Lose your driver's license.
- Go blind.

We want to assist you in every way possible to preserve your precious eye sight. But we need your help. Let us know if you are having problems of any kind with your drops.

topical 4% lidocaine applied to the procedure site with a sterile cotton swab. This is followed by a Betadine (povidone-iodine) swab to the site and lids as needed, or a drop of Betadine 5% can be applied to the eye after numbing is complete. For anterior segment procedures at the slit lamp, the assistant may hold the lid up with a sterile cotton swab or a lid speculum maybe employed. To minimize the potential for germ-laden aerosols, talking is avoided while the procedure is being done or masks can be worn.

Therapeutic paracentesis is performed to lower IOP. It is done with a #15 blade, which touches nothing but the limbus as it creates a slit incision. Fluid is released as the blade is removed from the eye. This paracentesis can be depressed and opened by the physician with the needle of a tuberculin syringe to lower IOP, and can easily be depressed again within 48 hours as needed. A *diagnostic paracentesis* is performed to analyze aqueous fluid. The physician uses a tuberculin syringe, observing the needle's position in the anterior chamber, while an assistant pulls the plunger to extract the fluid. Alternately, a syringe without a plunger may be used, and aqueous flows into the syringe by capillary action.

An *anterior chamber reformation* may be required in the postoperative period after a filtration surgery if hypotony occurs. If the anterior chamber is too shallow, it may induce damage to the cornea and promote cataract formation. A #15 blade may be needed to create a new paracentesis. The surgeon slowly injects viscoelastic (a gel-like substance) between the iris and cornea while watching the chamber and the cannula. An IOP check should be done 10 minutes postoperatively.

For a failing bleb, *laser suture lysis* with an argon green laser may be performed even if the IOP of the eye is low. Phenylephrine drops are instilled to assist in viewing the sutures by whitening the conjunctival vessels overlying them. Red laser wavelength can be used if there is subconjunctival hemorrhaging associated with the sutures. The patient may be put on topical steroids after the procedure. 5-FU may be injected postoperatively with up to three to five doses based on the cornea's appearance, as this drug causes epitheliopathy (disruption to the epithelial layer). A 30-gauge needle is used to deliver the drug, often 180 degrees away from the surgical site.

A bleb may need to have a "*needling*" procedure where a 25-gauge needle is introduced near the bleb capsule and used to break adhesions, allowing better filtration. The flap of the trabeculectomy can even be elevated with this procedure. The syringe may be filled with preservative-free 1% lidocaine so that additional anesthesia can be delivered during the procedure if needed.

PATIENT SERVICES

Patient Education

Patient compliance with the use of topical and oral glaucoma medications can be the difference between retaining vision and blindness. From simple reinstruction to "tough love," don't underestimate the role of the technician in this matter. Educating the patient when these medications are first introduced is key (Sidebar 29-2).

As discussed above, even topical glaucoma medications can have systemic side effects. It is important to ask returning patients whether or not they have experienced anything unusual or different since beginning the medication. This can include problems such as shortness of breath, heart palpitations, erectile dysfunction, and tingling in hands or feet. Patients may not report these (or even associate them with the eye meds) unless you ask. In addition, some clinics routinely check the blood pressure or pulse of patients on certain glaucoma medications, such as beta blockers.

Systemic side effects of topical glaucoma medications can be reduced or avoided by instructing patients to close the eyes following administration. Some practitioners also recommend that patients gently press the fingertips into the nasal corners of the eyes to block off the puncta (*punctal occlusion*). These maneuvers act to prevent the drop from entering first the tear duct then the nasal blood vessels and thereby accessing the systemic circulation. Blotting the surface of the eye while the lids are closed can help avoid exposure of the lashes to prostaglandins, as well as decrease the risk of dermatitis from this type of eye drop.

Medicinal eye drops have been associated with increasing the severity of dry eye syndrome (DES). Ophthalmologists monitor for worsening of DES and may recommend preservative-free drops whenever possible to decrease the overall amount of preservatives in the tear film. Laser therapies may also be used instead, to minimize the need for glaucoma drops.

Patient education should be documented in the patient's chart. Topics might include explanations regarding the disorder itself; medications, side effects, and reactions; practical hints such as how to instill drops; and conversations regarding compliance. This information is useful in reviewing previous discussions with the patient, as well as for potential legal protection for the practice.

CHAPTER QUIZ

1. What percentage of total glaucoma cases does open-angle glaucoma account for in the United States?

   a. 1%
   b. 10%
   c. 35%
   d. 90%

2. What percentage of total glaucoma cases does closed-angle glaucoma account for in the United States?

   a. 1%
   b. 10%
   c. 35%
   d. 90%

3. Which of the following is *not* a classic sign of acute angle closure?

   a. high IOP
   b. clouded cornea
   c. mid-dilated pupil
   d. conjunctival discharge

4. Which of the following is *not* a clinical risk factor for glaucoma, as seen in the Ocular Hypertension Study?

   a. greater Humphrey visual field pattern deviation
   b. thinner central cornea measurement
   c. smaller cup to disc ratio
   d. elevated IOP

5. Which is considered to be a central corneal thickness within the normal range in a White man?

   a. 485
   b. 500
   c. 545
   d. 605

6. What is the mechanism by which prostaglandin analogues decrease IOP?

   a. decrease aqueous humor production in the eye
   b. increase the outward flow of aqueous humor from the eye
   c. increase aqueous humor production in the eye
   d. decrease the outward flow of aqueous humor from the eye

7. What is the mechanism by which carbonic anhydrase inhibitors decrease IOP?

   a. decrease aqueous humor production in the eye
   b. increase the outward flow of aqueous humor from the eye
   c. increase aqueous humor production in the eye
   d. decrease the outward flow of aqueous humor from the eye

8. What is the major mechanism by which alpha agonists decrease IOP?

   a. decrease aqueous humor production in the eye
   b. increase the outward flow of aqueous humor from the eye
   c. increase aqueous humor production in the eye
   d. decrease the outward flow of aqueous humor from the eye

9. Which in-office procedure is commonly performed for treatment of acute angle-closure glaucoma?

   a. laser trabeculoplasty
   b. laser peripheral iridotomy
   c. trabeculectomy
   d. glaucoma drainage device placement

Answers

1. d
2. b
3. d
4. c
5. c
6. b
7. a
8. a
9. b

REFERENCES

1. Visual impairment and blindness. World Health Organization Fact Sheet #282. www.who.int/mediacentre/factsheets/fs282/en/. Updated August 2014. Accessed July 4, 2016.

2. Global pattern of blindness changes with success in tackling infectious disease and as population ages. World Health Organization Media Centre website. www.who.int/mediacentre/news/notes/2004/np27/en/. December 16, 2004. Accessed July 4, 2016.

3. Tham YC, Li X, Wong TY, et al. Global prevalence of glaucoma and projections of glaucoma burden through 2040: a systematic review and meta-analysis. *Ophthalmology*. 2014;121(11):2081-2090.

4. Moyer V. Screening for glaucoma: US Preventive Services Task Force recommendation statement. *Ann Intern Med*. 2013;159(7):484-489.

5. Drance SM. The significance of the diurnal phase variation of intraocular pressure in normal and glaucomatous eyes. *Trans Can Ophthalmolog Soc*. 1960;23:131-140.

6. Eye Diseases Prevalence Research Group. Prevalence of open-angle glaucoma among adults in the United States. *Arch Ophthalmol*. 2004;122:532-538.

7. Quigley HA. The number of people with glaucoma worldwide. *Br J Ophthalmol*. 1996;80:389-393.

8. Wang N, Wu H, Fan Z. Primary angle closure glaucoma in Chinese and Western populations. *Chin Med J*. 2002;115(11):1706-1715.

9. Kaplowitz K, Yung Edward, Flynn R, Tsai JC. Current concepts in the treatment of vitreous block, also known as aqueous misdirection. *Surv Ophthalmol*. 2015;60:229-241.

10. Morgan JE, Bourtsoukli I, Rajkumar KN, et al. The accuracy of the inferior>superior>nasal>temporal neuroretinal rim area rule for diagnosing glaucomatous optic disc damage. *Ophthalmology*. 2012;119:723-730.

11. Jonas JB, Gusek GC, Naumann GO. Optic disc morphometry in chronic primary open-angle glaucoma: I. morphometric intra-papillary characteristics. *Graefes Arch Clin Exp Ophthalmol*. 1988;226:522-530.

12. Jonas JB, Fernandez MC, Sturmer J. Pattern of glaucomatous neuroretinal rim loss. *Ophthalmology*. 1993;100(1):63-68.

13. Kim MJ, Kim SH, Hwang YH, et al. Novel screening method for glaucomatous eyes with myopic tilted discs. *JAMA Ophthalmol*. 2014;132:1407-1413.

14. Bateman DN, Clark R, Azuara-Blanco A, Bain M. The impact of new drugs on management of glaucoma in Scotland: observational study. *BMJ*. 2001;323:1401-1402.

15. Abramowicz M. Drugs for some common eye disorders. *The Medical Letter*. 2010;9(99):1-8.

16. Schmidl D, Schmetterer L, Garhofer G, Popa-Cherecheanu A. Pharmacotherapy of glaucoma. *J Ocul Pharmacol Ther*. 2015;31(2):63-77. doi:10.1089/jop.2014.0067.

17. Whittaker KW, Gillow JT, Cunliffe IA. Is the role of trabeculectomy in glaucoma management changing? *Eye*. 2001;15:449-452.

18. Mabuchi F, Sakurada Y, Kashiwagi K, et al. Involvement of genetic variants associated with primary open angle glaucoma in pathogenic mechanisms and family history of glaucoma. *Am J Ophthalmol*. 2015;159:437-444.

19. Gordon MO, Beiser JA, Brandt JD, et al; Ocular Hypertension Treatment Study Group. Baseline factors that predict the onset of primary open-angle glaucoma. *Arch Ophthalmol*. 2002;120:714-720.

20. Ocular Hypertension Treatment Study Group, European Glaucoma Prevention Study Group. Validated prediction model for the development of primary open-angle glaucoma in individuals with ocular hypertension. *Ophthalmology*. 2007;114:10-19.

21. Tielsch JM, Sommer A, Katz J, et al; The Baltimore Eye Survey. Racial variations in the prevalence of primary open-angle glaucoma. *JAMA*. 1991;266(3):369-374.

22. Flanary WE, Meyers LA, Alward WLM. Medical management of glaucoma: a primer. EyeRounds.org website. www.eyerounds.org/tutorials/Glaucoma-Medical-treatment/index.htm. Posted September 1, 2015. Accessed July 23, 2017.

23. Kurtz S, Soiberman U, Shemesh G. Comparison of dynamic contour tonometry, Goldmann applanation tonometry and Tonopen for measuring intraocular pressure in normal tension glaucoma. *Harefuah*. 2013;152(11):643-646, 688-689.

24. Johnson CA, Wall M, Fingeret M, Lalle P. *A Primer for Frequency Doubling Technology Perimetry*. Skaneateles, NY: Welch Allyn; 1998.

25. Johnson CA, Adams AJ, Casson EJ, Brandt JD. Progression of early glaucomatous visual field loss for blue-on-yellow and standard white-on-white automated perimetry. *Arch Ophthalmol*. 1993;111:651-656.

26. Broadway D. Visual field testing for glaucoma—a practical guide. *Community Eye Health*. 2012;25(79-80):66-70.

27. Abitbol O, Bouden J, Doan S, et al. Corneal hysteresis measured with the Ocular Response Analyzer in normal and glaucomatous eyes. *Acta Ophthalmol*. 2010;88(1):116.

The figures in this chapter were contributed by the following, who are associated with this book as authors:
Sandra Johnson/Eric Areiter: Figures 29-3 through 29-8
Al Lens: Figure 29-2
Monique Rinke: Figure 29-1

30

DIABETES

Christine McDonald, COE, COA, ROUB, OSC

BASIC SCIENCES

The Pancreas and Insulin

The pancreas is a leaf-shaped organ approximately 6 inches long, located in the abdomen at the bottom of the rib cage. It is part of the digestive system and has two principle functions: to create insulin and produce digestive juices.

Insulin is a hormone that converts carbohydrates from food into sugar (glucose). Your body will either use the glucose for energy or store it for future use. Insulin helps keep your glucose at the right levels. If glucose levels get too high, it is called *hyperglycemia*. If they are too low, it is called *hypoglycemia*.

The cells in our bodies need glucose for energy, but glucose cannot go directly into the cells. After eating food the blood sugar levels rise, causing the pancreas to release insulin into the bloodstream. Insulin then attaches to cells of the body, which signals the cells to absorb the glucose from the bloodstream. With the help of insulin, excess glucose in the body is stored in the liver and muscles as *glycogen* for later use. The body releases the stored glycogen when needed for energy during physical activities or between meals. This stops the body from using fat and muscle as a source of energy, a process that causes the formation of ketones (also known as fatty acids). Ketones enter the bloodstream, causing a life-threatening chemical imbalance called *ketoacidosis*. Insulin also acts as a control signal for other body systems (eg, it signals amino acid uptake in the cells).

Diabetes

Diabetes mellitus, or diabetes, is a metabolic disease in which blood sugar (glucose) levels are too high in the body, either from inadequate insulin production, the body's faulty response to insulin, or both. According to the International Diabetes Federation, diabetes affects over 371 million people worldwide.[1] There are three main types of diabetes: Type 1, Type 2, and gestational. Other types include secondary and prediabetes. Although there is no cure for diabetes, it can usually be controlled and the damage to vital organs minimized. Uncontrolled diabetes will, over time, cause more rapid damage.

Type 1

Type 1 diabetes is an autoimmune disease where the body itself destroys its own pancreatic beta cells, which produce insulin. With the beta cells gone, the person must take insulin in order to process carbohydrates into a form that the body can use. In the past, it was known as

Ledford JK, Lens A, eds.
Principles and Practice in Ophthalmic Assisting:
A Comprehensive Textbook (pp 537-547).
© 2018 Taylor & Francis Group.

juvenile diabetes, because it is usually diagnosed in children and young adults. Other names for it have included early-onset diabetes and insulin-dependent diabetes. These terms are falling out of use, however, as Type 1 can be found at any age. This type of diabetes accounts for 5% to 10% of all people with diabetes and can be managed by insulin therapy, exercise, and diet.[2]

Type 2

Ninety percent of diabetic cases worldwide are *Type 2*, making it the most common type of diabetes.[3] Type 2 diabetes is a progressive disease where the body does not use insulin properly (*insulin resistance*). The pancreas then overreacts and creates too much insulin to make up for it, but then over time cannot keep up the increased production needed to normalize the glucose levels.

People with Type 2 diabetes are treated first with oral medications, and if the disease progresses, insulin may also be required. Proper diet and exercise also pay a role in managing Type 2 diabetes. People who are overweight have a higher risk of developing Type 2. Type 2 diabetes can be prevented by eating healthy foods, getting regular exercise or physical activity, and weight loss.

Gestational Diabetes

Gestational diabetes develops during pregnancy around the 24th week. The cause of gestational diabetes is unknown and may occur in women who have never had diabetes. One theory is that hormones from the placenta, which help the fetus develop, block the mother's insulin in her body. Gestational diabetes is treated with diet plans and insulin injections. If left untreated, gestational diabetes can cause fetal *macrosomia* or "fat baby," infants with a birth weight of more than 8 pounds 13 ounces. This is due to extra glucose going through the placenta, causing

the baby's pancreas to make extra insulin. This surplus insulin gives the baby more "energy" than is needed for development, causing the excess calories to be stored as fat.

Secondary Diabetes

As the term implies, *secondary diabetes* is the result of some other condition or situation. Genetic conditions, surgery, medications, infections, pancreatic disease, and other illness account for less than 5% of all diagnosed cases of diabetes in the United States.[4]

Prediabetes

Often patients will tell you that they are "prediabetic" or they have "borderline" diabetes. You may also see the terms *impaired fasting glucose* (IFG) and *impaired glucose tolerance* (IGT). These mean that they have blood sugar levels that are higher than normal, but not high enough to meet the diagnosis criteria of diabetes. These patients do, however, have a higher risk for developing Type 2 diabetes. Some health care professionals contend that there is no such thing as prediabetes. They believe that prediabetes is the first stage of diabetes, and patients who have had one test result of high blood glucose levels should be considered diabetic.

Who Is at Risk for Diabetes?

Type 1 diabetes is an autoimmune disease. (An autoimmune disease is where the body cannot tell the difference between what is a part of itself and what is foreign to it, causing the body to produce antibodies that attack normal cells by mistake.) There is no way to prevent Type 1 diabetes. It is estimated that 1 out of every 500 children has Type 1 diabetes (more often found in girls age 10 to 12 and boys age 12 to 14).[5] Of course it may also develop in adults, and occurs more in the White population than any other racial group.[6]

Type 2 diabetes is found more frequently in people with the risk factors shown in Sidebar 30-1.

Symptoms of Diabetes

For patients with Type 1 diabetes, symptoms can develop quickly. Those with Type 2 will notice a more gradual development. Yet, some patients never show any signs of diabetes. People with both types of diabetes experience common symptoms, such as those detailed in Sidebar 30-2.

Diagnosing and Testing for Diabetes

There are four tests used for diagnosing diabetes.

The *hemoglobin A1c* (*A1c* or *HbA1c*) is a test measuring glycated hemoglobin, a combination of red blood cells (hemoglobin) and glucose (sugar) in the blood. Since red blood cells live approximately 3 months, doctors can measure how much glucose is in the body over a 3-month period by measuring the glycated hemoglobin in the blood. This test does not require fasting and can be done any time of day. It is used to determine a diagnosis of Type 2 diabetes. A test result of 6.5% or higher means the patient is considered diabetic. If the results are between 5.7% and 6.4%, the patient may be termed prediabetic. Any result less than 5.7% is considered normal.[7]

The *fasting plasma glucose test* (FPG; also known as the *fasting blood sugar test,* or FBS) measures the body's blood sugar and exposes problems with insulin function. This is an inexpensive test performed in early morning after the patient has gone without eating for a minimum of 8 hours, with 12 to 14 hours being ideal. Prolonged fasting triggers the pancreas to produce glucagon—a hormone that causes the liver to create insulin. If the fasting body does produce insulin, then diabetes is ruled out. If the body does not produce insulin or does not respond properly, glucose levels will stay high and a positive diagnosis of diabetes is made. If the FPG test is performed later in the day, the result can be a false low.

With an FPG test, blood sugar levels are measured in milligrams per deciliter (mg/dL) in the United States and millimoles per liter (mmol/L) in metric countries. Readings between 70 and 99 mg/dL (3.9 and 5.5 mmol/L) are considered normal. Readings between 100 and 126 mg/dL (5.6 and 7.0 mmol/L) are positive for diabetes. Blood sugar levels between 126 mg/dL and 140 mg/dL (7.0 and 7.8 mmol/L) were once considered normal; however, the American Diabetes Association lowered the accepted amount of blood sugar levels after studies had shown that patients with levels between 126 and 140 mg/dL (7.0 and 7.8 mmol/L) tend to develop the medical complications of diabetes.[8]

An *oral glucose tolerance test* (OGTT, or simply GTT) measures the body's ability to use glucose. The test begins by measuring the glucose levels after fasting 8 hours and abstaining from any type of sweetened beverage for at least 2 hours, to achieve a baseline glucose reading for comparison with the rest of the test. The patient next drinks a sweet liquid drink containing between 75 and 100 grams of glucose. The patient's blood sugar levels are then measured at 30 minutes, followed by three 60-minute intervals for up to 3 hours, to see how the body processes the sugar. This test can also be used to identify gestational diabetes during pregnancy.

There are other situations that may affect the OGTT outcomes (false positives or negatives). These include smoking, alcohol consumption, recent surgery, infectious diseases, long periods of bed rest, and weight loss through dieting.

In the *random plasma glucose test* (RPG) a small amount of blood is drawn at any time of day, regardless of whether the patient has had anything to eat or drink.

SIDEBAR 30-2
POSSIBLE SYMPTOMS OF DIABETES

- ▶ Frequent urination (polyuria)
- ▶ Intense, increased thirst (polydipsia)
- ▶ Increased hunger (polyphagia)
- ▶ Weight gain
- ▶ Unusual weight loss
- ▶ Blurred vision
- ▶ Fatigue
- ▶ Slow-healing sores or wounds
- ▶ Dry, itchy skin
- ▶ Tingling or loss of feeling in the feet
- ▶ Acetone-smelling breath
- ▶ Nausea/vomiting
- ▶ Hyperventilation
- ▶ Abdominal pain

The plasma, or blood, is sent to a lab for measurement of glucose levels. A blood glucose reading of 200 mg/dL or higher along with any diabetes-related symptoms results in a positive diagnosis.

Effects on the Body

Diabetes is a serious disease and, if left uncontrolled, can affect nearly every organ in the body resulting in cardiovascular disease, stroke, kidney disease, nerve damage, problems with gums and teeth, problems with skin, and vision problems.

Cardiovascular disease is one of the most common complications of diabetes. It is estimated that 71% of adults with diabetes have hypertension (high blood pressure) and 65% have high cholesterol.[9] People who have Type 1 or Type 2 diabetes can develop *diabetic heart disease* (DHD). The higher the person's blood sugar level, the higher the risk of DHD.[10] Coronary heart disease, where plaque build-up in the arteries (atherosclerosis) increases the chance of blood clots and restricts the flow of oxygen-rich blood to the heart, can lead to angina (chest pain), arrhythmia (irregular heartbeat), heart attack, or death. Congestive heart failure (CHF) is a condition where the heart fails to pump enough blood to other vital organs, such as the brain, liver, and kidneys. Diabetic cardiomyopathy is a disease that damages the structure and function of the heart. This disease can lead to heart failure and arrhythmias, even in people with diabetes who don't have chronic heart disease.[10]

Stroke victims with diabetes fare far worse than non-diabetics. When a nondiabetic has a stroke, where the brain's oxygen supply is cut off, other arteries can usually deliver oxygen by bypassing the blockage. In people with diabetes, many of the bypass arteries are affected by atherosclerosis, impairing blood flow to the brain.

Too much glucose in the blood causes the vessels to thicken or narrow, restricting blood flow to limbs, most notably the feet. When this causes damage to the nerves, it is known as *diabetic neuropathy*. Diabetic neuropathy symptoms are pain, tingling, and numbness or loss of feeling. These problems occur in 60% to 70% of people with diabetes, with the highest rate among those having diabetes for 25 years or more and often in those who do not control their glucose levels.[11] Some symptoms of diabetic neuropathy can be relieved to a degree with oral antidepressants.

There are four types of neuropathy: peripheral, autonomic, proximal, and focal.

Peripheral neuropathy is the most common neuropathy found in people with diabetes, causing loss of feeling in toes, feet, legs, hands, and arms. Patients who have peripheral neuropathy are more prone to problems with their feet. Lack of sensation or feeling in the feet may cause cuts or sores to go unnoticed, resulting in infections or ulcers that, left untreated, can necessitate amputation. More than 60% of leg and foot amputations not related to injury are due to diabetes.[9]

Autonomic neuropathy causes changes in the digestive system, as well as changes in bowel and bladder function. It may also affect perspiration as well as the nerves that serve the lungs, eyes, and heart, and regulate blood pressure. Autonomic neuropathy may also cause *hypoglycemic unawareness*, where the patient is no longer aware of the symptoms associated with low blood sugar. This is dangerous because if the sugar level becomes too low, the patient can lose consciousness.

Proximal neuropathy causes hip, thigh, or buttock pain, usually on one side of the body and leads to leg weakness.

Focal neuropathy appears suddenly in one nerve or a group of nerves, causing muscle weakness or pain. Any nerve in the body may be affected, but most often this occurs in the head, torso, or leg. Focal neuropathy usually improves on its own over a period of weeks or months.

Diabetes is a leading cause of kidney disease and failure. The kidneys are responsible for filtering blood, removing waste, and controlling fluid in the body. Diabetes damages the small blood vessels in the kidney. When these blood vessels are injured, the kidney cannot filter blood properly.

Each kidney is made up of approximately 1.25 million nephrons, which can thicken and scar over time in patients with diabetes. When this happens, the kidneys leak and cannot filter blood properly, causing waste material to enter the bloodstream and protein to seep into the

urine (*proteinuria*). Over time, uncontrolled proteinuria will cause kidney failure and the need for dialysis or eventually a kidney transplant.

When blood is filtered by the kidneys, some sugar remains in the fluid that will eventually become urine. When blood sugar is normal, the body is able to reabsorb the small amount of sugar that remains before it leaves the kidneys. If blood sugar levels are high, there is too much sugar in the fluid for the body to reabsorb so it passes into the urine. Since diabetes can damage nerves, the nerve damage can alter the bladder muscles' ability to contract or cause a loss of sensation where patients may experience difficulty in emptying the bladder. Pressure from a full bladder can cause urine to back up into the kidneys. Urine that stays in the bladder too long will allow bacteria to grow. When urine contains high levels of sugar, bacteria can grow more rapidly, precipitating infections in the bladder and kidneys.

Kidney damage begins 5 to 10 years before the patient starts to notice symptoms. These symptoms can include fatigue, malaise (general feeling of not being well), headache, leg swelling, poor appetite, and itchy skin.

Approximately 30% of patients with Type 1 and up to 40% of patients with Type 2 diabetes will develop kidney failure.[12] Kidney failure may be treated to help slow the loss of kidney function. End-stage renal failure (kidney failure) occurs when kidney function is less than 10% to 15%, at which point the patient will need dialysis and/or a kidney transplant.

Diabetes affects the skin in several ways. People with diabetes are more prone to dry skin, boils, and staph infections, as well as infection of the hair follicles (folliculitis) and nails. Fungal or yeast infections can occur in folds of skin, between toes and fingers, in the groin area, in the armpits, and in the corners of the mouth. Another skin problem that can be found with patients with diabetes is *diabetic dermatology*, brown oval-shaped or round patches on the skin that look like age spots. A rare skin condition that can occur with people with diabetes is *scleredema diabeticorum*, a thickening of skin on the upper back and neck.

Diabetes also affects the teeth and gums. Decreased function of the salivary gland causes dry mouth, which can result in bad breath, tooth decay, and mouth sores. Lack of blood supply to the gums can cause infections and periodontal (gum) disease.

Treatment

Experts and doctors agree that the best way to prevent disorders resulting from diabetes is to keep glucose levels under control. Diet and exercise play an important role in treating diabetes. Processed foods should be avoided because they contain more sugar and refined carbohydrates, which can cause higher glucose levels. Foods that are lower in fat in addition to plant foods are better

TABLE 30-1

TYPES OF INSULIN AND THEIR ACTIONS

Type of Insulin	Name of Insulin	What It Does	How Used	Duration
Rapid-acting	Lispro (Humalog), aspart (Novolog), glulisine (Apidra)	Covers insulin needs for the meal being eaten, often used in conjunction with longer-lasting insulin	10 to 30 minutes prior to meal	1 to 5 hours depending on the insulin
Short-acting	Human insulin— Regular (Humulin R, Novolin R)	Covers insulin needs for the meal being eaten	30 minutes to 1 hour prior to meal	5 to 8 hours
Intermediate-acting	Neutral protamine Hagedorn (NPH), Humulin N, Novolin N	Provides background insulin needs for half a day or overnight, often used with rapid- or short-acting insulins	Usually taken twice a day	18 to 24 hours
Long-acting	Insulin glargine (Lantus), insulin detemir (Levemir)	Provides a steady level of insulin for the whole day; if needed, may be combined with rapid- or short-acting insulin	Every 24 hours	20 to 24 hours
Premixed	Combination of short- and intermediate-acting insulins in one bottle or pen (Humulin 70/30, Novolin 70/30)	Premeasured bottles and pens are helpful for patients with poor eyesight and dexterity	Usually taken two to three times a day prior to meals	14 to 24 hours

Adapted from Types of insulin for diabetes treatment. WebMD website. www.webmd.com/diabetes/guide/diabetes-types-insulin#1.

because they are rich in vitamins, minerals, and fiber, which help to promote better health and stabilize glucose levels throughout the day.

When patients exercise, they not only lose weight, they can increase muscle mass. During exercise, the muscles pull sugar from the blood, replacing the muscles' reserved sugar used during physical activity and naturally lowering blood sugar levels. Blood sugar levels should be monitored before and after exercise to avoid hypoglycemia.

There are several oral medications used to treat diabetes. *Insulin secretagogues* or *sulfonylureas* work by making the pancreas release more insulin. The medication is usually taken before eating meals, in consideration of the amount of food to be eaten. There is a risk of low blood sugar, however, if one takes too much medicine. This group of medications includes glyburide, glipizide, glimepiride, repaglinide, and nateglinide.

Insulin sensitizers (thiazolidinediones) work by making cells more sensitive to insulin. This group of medications includes metformin (Glucophage) and glitazones containing pioglitazone (Actos) or rosiglitazone (Avandia). These medications can be very expensive.

Other medications for treating diabetes are *glucose absorption inhibitors* or alpha-glucose inhibitors acarbose (Precose) or miglitol (Glyset), which keep blood sugar levels from spiking after meals by slowing the digestive process of complex carbohydrates and their absorption. These need to be taken with the first bite of a meal for maximum effectiveness. Pramlintide (Symlin) is an injectable medication that mimics the hormone amylin and helps slow the absorption of glucose by decreasing how quickly food leaves the stomach.

Insulin is yet another treatment for diabetes. Insulin must be injected by syringe, insulin pen (premeasured), or by an insulin pump (worn on the body and injects insulin through a catheter into the skin and fatty tissue). Insulin is used in amounts based on the patient's needs throughout the day. Insulin itself comes in different varieties: rapid-acting, short-acting, intermediate-acting, long-acting, and premixed. The insulin's duration can last from 1 to 24 hours and manages blood sugar levels based on which type is used (Table 30-1).

CLINICAL KNOWLEDGE

Effects of Diabetes on the Eye

Diabetes is the leading cause of new blindness in US adults ages 20 to 74 years.[13] Ocular complications

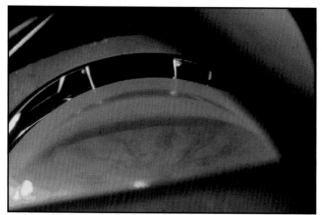

Figure 30-1. Abnormal growth of blood vessels on the iris (rubeosis iridis) as seen through a gonio lens. (Reprinted with permission from the Cogan Collection, National Eye Institute/ National Institutes of Health.)

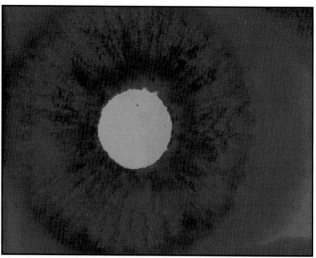

Figure 30-2. Transillumination defect in diabetes. Note how the red reflex from the retina is visible through areas of the iris. (Reprinted with permission from the Cogan Collection, National Eye Institute/National Institutes of Health.)

generally occur by 20 years after onset, despite apparently adequate diabetic control.[14] The term *diabetic eye disease* can include a number of disorders, as diabetes affects the entire eye from the cornea to the retina.

Lids, Lashes, and Lacrimal[15]

Since people with diabetes are often more prone to infections, they are more at risk for developing blepharitis and cellulitis. It is also more common for people with diabetes to have xanthelasma, yellowish deposits of cholesterol under the skin of the inner eyelids. Recurrent hordeola (painful infections of the eyelid margin and lash follicles) and blepharitis may be early signs of diabetes.

Dry eye may be more increased in patients with diabetes as tear film abnormalities are common due to the reduction of goblet cell density. A severe reduction in tear film has been noted in patients with nonproliferative diabetic retinopathy as compared to patients without retinopathy.

Cornea

Keratopathy (any abnormality of the cornea) can be more severe and more common in people with diabetes. Corneal endothelial damage or dysfunction may lead to increased thickness of the central cornea. Thickening of the cornea is one of the first symptoms of diabetic corneal changes and is associated with a higher A1c. Another problem in people with diabetes is a decrease in corneal sensitivity, leading to decreased tear flow. This can result in persistent epithelial defects from dry eye disease. Patients with diabetes have a higher risk of developing superficial punctate keratitis (small superficial corneal lesions), full-thickness breaks in the cornea, and recurrent corneal erosion. People with diabetes are also prone to corneal ulcers and delayed healing of the corneal surface. (Check the Index for more on specific disorders/ problems.)

Iris and Angle

Diabetes can affect the iris by changing its structure. The iris (which normally has a tissue paper-like consistency) can become leather-like, and vascular changes may occur (usually around the pupil margin). In patients with advanced diabetes, these new blood vessels can involve the entire iris, including the angles. These changes in the iris structure can result in poor pupil dilation or a miotic (small) pupil. *Rubeosis iridis*, numerous small intertwining blood vessels, may develop on the anterior surface of the iris (Figure 30-1). These can rupture and bleed into the anterior chamber (*hyphema*).

If abnormal iris blood vessels reach the trabecular meshwork, they can block aqueous flow, resulting in *neovascular glaucoma* (NVG). NVG can be difficult to control and manage. It is considered a form of secondary glaucoma, leading to high intraocular pressure, pain, and corneal swelling. NVG often coincides with proliferative diabetic retinopathy (discussed momentarily), so the underlying condition is treated with laser to the retina.

Trabeculectomy has shown limited success as a treatment due to excessive bleeding during surgery and the continuation of vessel growth postoperatively. Aqueous drainage implants have also had some success, but their effectiveness can decrease over time. (See Chapter 36 for more regarding glaucoma surgery.)

Diabetes can also cause pigment loss on the back of the iris, resulting in *transillumination defects*, or areas of the iris through which the red reflex from the retina can be seen on slit lamp examination (Figure 30-2). This pigment loss may be associated with *pigment dispersion glaucoma*. Pigmentary glaucoma, a type of open-angle glaucoma, occurs when pigment granules break free from the iris or ciliary epithelium and deposit in the trabecular meshwork, blocking aqueous flow and raising intraocular pressure. The incidence of iris depigmentation has been reported to be three times more likely in people with diabetes.[15]

Crystalline Lens

Exactly how the concentration of glucose in the blood causes changes in the crystalline lens of people with diabetes is not completely understood. But certainly the phenomenon is well-known and believed to be due to osmotic force between the crystalline lens and aqueous humor. The result may be a change in the thickness of the lens, the surface curvature of the lens, and/or the refractive index of the lens (this last seems most accepted in literature).

Studies have generally shown (although some dispute) that high glucose levels cause a myopic shift in a person with diabetes' refractive error.[16] Then a hyperopic shift occurs as the glucose levels revert back to normal. Changes in refractive power by as much as 2 to 3 diopters can occur when blood sugar levels are uncontrolled.[17]

Another cause of refractive changes from diabetes is cataracts. Although a true diabetic cataract (rapid onset in juveniles with diabetes where the lens becomes completely opaque within several weeks) is rare; early onset of senile cataracts is common. Posterior subcapsular cataracts and cortical opacities occur earlier and more frequently in patients with diabetes.

Cataract surgery can be more complicated for patients with diabetes, and the outcome will vary according to the presence and severity of retinopathy or macular edema. To prevent postoperative cystoid macular edema (CME) or diabetic macular edema (DME), doctors often prescribe nonsteroidal anti-inflammatory drops (NSAIDs) prior to and for up to 3 months following cataract surgery. Patients with diabetes having cataract surgery might also have a consultation with a retina specialist pre- or postoperatively for anti-vascular endothelial growth factor (anti-VEGF) injections to slow the growth of abnormal blood vessels.

The use of presbyopia-correcting or multifocal intraocular lenses (IOLs) may be used for patients with diabetes with controlled blood sugar levels and not showing any signs of diabetic retinopathy. However, these specialty IOLs should be discouraged in patients who have uncontrolled diabetes or diabetic complications involving the retina.

Vitreous and Retina

Changes may also occur in the vitreous humor, including posterior vitreous detachment. Vitreous hemorrhage (blood in the vitreous) can cause a painless, temporary, sudden vision loss, and is known to occur in patients with diabetic retinopathy, which will be discussed next.

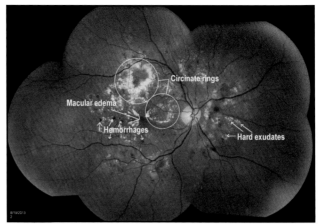

Figure 30-3. Montage showing various types of diabetic retinal disease. Circinate rings are where hard exudates have formed in a circular pattern. (Reprinted with permission from Retina Gallery and Mayo Clinic, Jacksonville, Florida.)

One of the biggest complications involving the diabetic eye is damage to the retina. *Diabetic retinopathy* (DR; Figure 30-3) is a common cause of blindness, affecting approximately one-third of people over the age of 40 years with diabetes. Early retinopathy may not cause any changes noticed by the patient. Symptoms of advancing diabetic retinopathy can include vision loss, decreased/blurry vision, fluctuating vision, empty areas in the vision, floaters, and decreased color discrimination.

Almost all patients with Type 1 diabetes and 58% of patients with Type 2 show signs of retinopathy.[18] DR can be broken down into four stages.

Mild nonproliferative retinopathy, or *background retinopathy* (BDR), is the early stage of retinopathy where small areas of bubble-like swellings, called *microaneurysms*, start to appear on the blood vessels. *Dot and blot hemorrhages* (tiny round hemorrhages) and *hard exudates* develop. (*Exudates* consist of blood-cell-free fluid that leaks from the blood vessels into the retina. *Hard exudates* have less fluid and more fat and protein.)

Moderate nonproliferative retinopathy exists when blockage of some retina-nourishing blood vessels begins.

Severe nonproliferative retinopathy (Figure 30-4) commences with the appearance of *cotton wool spots*. These are soft exudates within the retinal nerve fiber layer caused by small patches of retina that have lost their blood supply from vessel obstruction and resemble tufts of cotton. There is also further blockage of the retinal blood vessels, which disrupts blood flow and nourishment to the retina. This damage, in turn, signals the body to start producing more blood vessels in the retina.

Proliferative diabetic retinopathy (PDR) is the advanced, fourth stage of retinopathy where the lack of blood supply to the retina has caused ischemia (damage due to a lack of oxygen). This, in turn, causes abnormal new blood vessels to grow in the retina. These vessels are

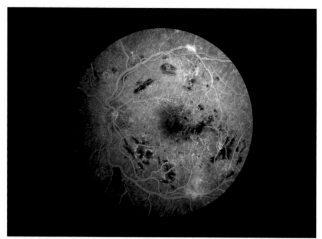

Figure 30-4. Fluorescein angiogram of severe nonproliferative diabetic retinopathy. (Reprinted with permission from Jarrod Wehmeier and The Retina Institute, St. Louis, Missouri.)

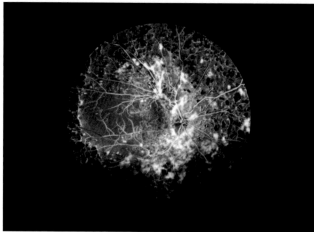

Figure 30-5. Fluorescein angiogram showing proliferative diabetic retinopathy. The many bright spots indicate leakage into the retinal tissue. (Reprinted with permission from Jarrod Wehmeier and The Retina Institute, St. Louis, Missouri.)

weak, and can rupture and bleed, causing hemorrhages in the retina and vitreous (Figure 30-5). Scar tissue can develop and pull on the retina, which can cause more damage, including retinal detachment.

Any type of DR can also cause macular edema (swelling), the most common cause of vision loss in people with diabetes.[1] DME is caused by fluid leaking from blood vessels within the macula and comes in two forms: *focal*, occurring from abnormalities in ocular blood vessels, and *diffuse*, where there is widening or swelling of retinal capillaries. As macular edema progresses, patients develop blurred central vision making it impossible to focus clearly. Other symptoms of DME include floaters, double vision, and (if left untreated) blindness.

The stage of retinopathy a person has is more closely related to the duration of the disease than the severity of it, although controlling diabetes does help delay its development. People with Type 1 diabetes are more prone to develop an advanced form of retinopathy, usually proliferative.[18] People with Type 2 diabetes often develop nonproliferative retinopathy with a risk of central vision loss from *maculopathy* (abnormality of the macula).[19]

Treatment

Control of blood sugar levels is key in preventing DR and DME from occurring. Once retinopathy begins, there are treatments ranging from laser, injections, and sometimes eye drops to help slow the disease's progress.

Laser photocoagulation, which targets specific blood vessels, remains the standard in treating diabetic retinal complications. Although laser procedures do not improve the patient's vision, they help prevent further vision loss from diabetic eye disease. There are two types of laser procedures commonly used to treat diabetic eye disease.

With *focal laser photocoagulation*, laser energy is aimed directly to the area being treated. In *grid laser photocoagulation*, the laser is applied in a contained grid-type pattern. Both of these methods destroy the tissue and cause scarring. Unfortunately, this also creates blind spots in the vision.

With *panretinal (scatter) laser photocoagulation* (PRP), between 1200 and 1800 tiny spots of laser energy are applied to the retinal periphery, leaving the central retina untouched (Figure 30-6). This destruction of the peripheral retina, which does not interfere with functional vision, improves blood supply to the central portion of the retina, allowing it to retain its visual function.

Injection with *anti-VEGF therapy*, such as bevacizumab (Avastin), ranibizumab (Lucentis), and aflibercept (Eylea), either as a first choice or in conjunction with laser treatment, has shown success in treating DME. It has also been successful in stopping the leakage of damaged blood vessels and slowing new vessel growth.

Corticosteroid drops can be used in the treatment of DME by reducing swelling and inflammation of the retinal tissue. Another treatment is steroid implants, such as dexamethasone intravitreal implant (Ozurdex) and fluocinolone acetonide (Iluvien, Retisert), which are surgically inserted or injected into the vitreous and held in place by suture or pressure, depending on which type is used. The inserts release sustained amounts of steroid over extended periods of time, some up to 36 months. Side effects from prolonged steroid use in the eye include the formation of cataracts and elevated intraocular pressure or glaucoma.

Patients who have PDR and bleeding into the vitreous can be poor candidates for laser treatment when blood from the hemorrhage blocks the laser beam. If the blood does not reabsorb, the doctor may perform a *vitrectomy* (removal of the vitreous) and a diabetic laser procedure at the same time or shortly following the vitrectomy.

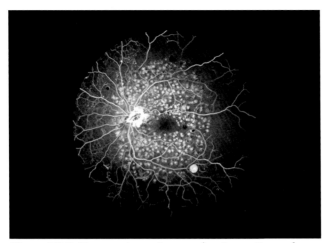

Figure 30-6. Fluorescein angiogram showing pattern of pan-retinal laser photocoagulation. Note that tiny laser dots are spread out over the retina, sparing the macula. (Reprinted with permission from Jarrod Wehmeier and The Retina Institute, St. Louis, Missouri.)

Retinal and vitreous hemorrhages can form bands of scar tissue. When these scar tissue bands are attached to the retina and begin to shrink, they can cause the retina to pull away, creating traction, which may result in retinal tears or detachment. The treatment for these is discussed in Chapter 36.

Neuropathy and the Eye

Diabetic neuropathy can affect any of the three cranial nerves responsible for eye movement (CN III, IV, and VII). Surprisingly, patients with diabetes with cranial nerve palsies were reported to have significantly less diabetic retinopathy.[15]

CN III, the oculomotor nerve, supplies four of the six extraocular muscles (EOMs). *Cranial mononeuropathy III*—diabetic type—is one of the most common cranial nerve disorders in patients with diabetes. Symptoms can include diplopia (double vision) and ptosis (drooping eyelid) of the affected eye, as well as pain in the head or behind the eye. The pupil is usually normal, but unequal pupil size (*anisocoria*) may occur. Ocular motor function will start to recuperate without treatment after about 3 months, and recovery is usually complete.

CN IV (trochlear) palsy is often idiopathic, but one known cause is small blood vessel disease from diabetes. This creates a loss of oxygen and tissue damage to the fourth nerve, causing the nerve to function improperly due to the blocked blood flow. This impairs the superior oblique muscle, which is supplied by CN IV. A palsy of this muscle causes vertical and slightly oblique diplopia, as well as problems looking down and inward.

The sixth nerve (CN VI, abducens nerve) controls the lateral rectus muscle. The paralysis may be temporary or permanent. The patient generally complains of horizontal diplopia.

In general, physicians like to give the patient at least 6 months to see if a palsy will resolve on its own. A prism may be applied to the glasses during this time for relief from diplopia. If no improvement is seen in 6 months, surgery to straighten the eye(s) may be considered. (See Chapter 36 for more on EOM surgery.)

Diabetic papillopathy is a unilateral or bilateral swelling of the optic nerve (CN II) caused by vascular leaking. Visual symptoms range from no visual disturbances to mild blurring or distortion. This condition is rare, usually occurring in younger persons with Type 1 diabetes, but can also occur in persons with Type 2. No treatment is required, and there is no known association between diabetic papillopathy and either the control level of diabetes or the stage of any diabetic retinopathy.

CLINICAL SKILLS

Patients with diabetes should have an annual exam with dilation. Here are some things to consider when these patients come to your clinic.

When taking a patient's history and chief complaint, both the past and present general medical history are important (Sidebar 30-3).

Fluctuating sugar levels can play havoc with the patient's glasses prescription, as mentioned earlier. Before performing refractometry on a patient with diabetes, ask if the blood sugar level is stable, and for how long. (Consistent A1c levels at 7 or below are considered stable, at which point it is acceptable to write an eyeglass prescription.) You may need to caution the patient that any glasses resulting from that day's refractometric measurement will be optimal only when the blood sugar is at the same level.

Since diabetic neuropathy may cause third, sixth, and (in rare circumstances) fourth nerve palsies, it is important to evaluate EOM movement during examination. Signs that the patient may have a third nerve palsy are difficulty moving the eye and deviation out (exotropia) and down (hypotropia). In patients showing signs of sixth nerve palsy, the affected eye will turn inward (esotropia) and cannot turn beyond the midline. With fourth nerve palsy, the patient's eye or eyes may turn upward (hypertropia). There may be a head tilt to the side, opposite the direction of the palsy, in order to reduce or eliminate the double image.

The slit lamp (biomicroscope) exam should include careful evaluation of the iris, making note of any abnormal blood vessels and pigmentary changes. Pigment dropout can sometimes cause an area to thin, which is visible on retroillumination (where the light beam is directed through the pupil at the retina, causing the iris to be back-lit; see Chapter 12).

Fundus photography and/or fluorescein angiography may be ordered to document macular edema and other signs of diabetic retinopathy, along with responses to treatment.

Optical coherence tomography (OCT) is a valuable advance in retinal imaging and the diagnosis of diabetic retinopathy and macular edema. OCT uses low coherence interferometry (light waves) to generate cross-sectional images of retinal tissue showing the different layers of the retina and its thickness, including any fluid that may have leaked into the retina. (See Chapter 16 for more.) OCT images are of high resolution and easy to repeat over time, making it a good method of tracking the disease's progression and whether medications or surgical treatments are effective.

PATIENT SERVICES

Many communities provide patient services to help treat the disease and its side effects (Sidebar 30-4). It is important for ophthalmologists and staff to be aware of services for those patients who have been diagnosed with diabetic retinopathy and are losing their vision. These patients need to know where they can go to find support groups, receive diabetic services, find low vision specialists, and connect with local resources that help patients who are going blind from the disease.

ACKNOWLEDGMENTS

The author would like to thank the following: Jarrod Wehmeier, Lauren McDonald, and Dave Yates.

CHAPTER QUIZ

1. What is the pancreas and what does it do?

2. Name the three main types of diabetes.

3. Describe Type 1 diabetes.

4. What is the most common type of diabetes?

5. What is hemoglobin A1c?

6. How is diabetes treated?

7. What parts of the eye can diabetes affect?

8. Name the four types of diabetic retinopathy.

9. What may be used to treat diabetic retinopathy and diabetic macular edema?

Answers

1. The pancreas is a leaf-shaped organ of the digestive system that produces digestive juices and insulin.

2. Type 1, Type 2, and gestational are the three main types of diabetes.

3. Diabetes is an autoimmune disease where the body does not produce enough insulin.

4. Ninety percent of diabetic cases worldwide are Type 2.

5. The A1c is a test measuring the glycated hemoglobin that does not require fasting and is used to determine Type 2 diabetes and monitor patients' blood glucose over a period of 8 to 12 weeks.

6. Diet, exercise, oral medications, and insulin are the standard treatments for diabetes.

7. Diabetes affects the cornea, lens, iris, retina, and cranial nerves III, IV, and VI.

8. The four types of diabetic retinopathy are mild nonproliferative, moderate nonproliferative, severe nonproliferative, and proliferative.

9. Treatment for DR can include focal and panretinal photocoagulation. DME may be treated with corticosteroids in the form of topical drops or intraocular injections or implants. Anti-VEGF intraocular injections may be used for either DR or DME.

REFERENCES

1. Castillo M. 371 million people have diabetes globally, about half undiagnosed. CBS News website. www.cbsnews.com/news/371-million-people-have-diabetes-globally-about-half-undiagnosed/. Accessed March 12, 2016.

2. What is diabetes? NIH Senior Health website. http://nihseniorhealth.gov/diabetes/diabetesdefined/01.html. Accessed March 12, 2016.

3. Santos-Longhurst A. Type 2 diabetes statistics and facts. Healthline website. www.healthline.com/health/type-2-diabetes/statistics. Reviewed September 8, 2015. Accessed March 12, 2016.

4. Centers for Disease Control and Prevention. National diabetes statistics report. www.cdc.gov/diabetes/data/statistics/2014StatisticsReport.html. Published 2014. Accessed March 12, 2016.

5. Healthwise Staff. Who is affected by type 1 diabetes. Health system University of Michigan Health System website. www.uofmhealth.org/health-library/hw127678/. Last revised September 18, 2010. Accessed March 12, 2016.

6. Type 1 diabetes. dLife website. www.dlife.com//diabetes/type-1. Accessed March 12, 2016.

7. The hemoglobin A1c (HbA1c) test for diabetes. WebMD website. www.webmd.com/diabetes/guide/glycated-hemoglobin-test-hba1c. Accessed March 12, 2016.

8. Pape J. Diagnosing diabetes. Diabetes Self-Management website. www.diabetesselfmanagement.com/about-diabetes/diabetes-basics/diagnosing-diabetes/. Updated March 10, 2011. Accessed March 12, 2016.

9. High cholesterol, high blood pressure often neglected in diabetics. WebMD News Archive website. http://www.webmd.com/diabetes/news/20000616/high-cholesterol-high-blood-pressure-often-neglected-in-diabetics. Accessed March 12, 2016.

10. What is diabetic heart disease? National Heart Lung and Blood Institute website. www.nhlbi.nih.gov/health/health-topics/topics/dhd/. Accessed March 12, 2016.

11. Diabetic neuropathies: the nerve damage of diabetes. National Institute of Diabetes and Digestive and Kidney Disease website. www.niddk.nih.gov/health-information/health-topics/Diabetes/diabetic-neuropathies-nerve-damage-diabetes/Pages/diabetic-neuropathies-nerve-damage.aspx/. Accessed March 12, 2016.

12. Diabetes—a major risk factor for kidney disease. National Kidney Foundation website. www.kidney.org/atoz/content/diabetes/. Accessed March 12, 2016.

13. Eye problems and diabetes. WebMD website. www.webmd.com/eye-health/eye-problems/. Accessed March 12, 2016.

14. Riordan-Eva P, Whitcher JP. *Vaughan & Asbury's General Ophthalmology*. 17th ed. New York, NY: McGraw-Hill Companies; 2008.

15. Skarbez K, Priestley Y, Hoepf M, Koevary SB. Comprehensive review of the effects of diabetes on ocular health. *Expert Review of Ophthalmology*. 2010;5(4):557-577. doi:10.1586/eop.10.44.

16. Yarbag A, Yazar H, Akdogan M, Pekgör A, Kaleli S. Refractive errors in patients with newly diagnosed diabetes mellitus. *Pak J Med Sci*. 2015;31(6):1481-1484. doi:http://dx.doi.org/10.12669/pjms.316.8204.

17. Watkins PJ, Amiel SA, Howell SL, Turner E. *Diabetes and Its Management*. 6th ed. Hoboken, NJ: Wiley-Blackwell; 2003:150.

18. Hietala K, Harjutsalo V, Forsblom C, Summanen P, Groop P-H, on behalf of the FinnDiane Study Group. Age at onset and the risk of proliferative retinopathy in type 1 diabetes. *Diabetes Care*. 2010;33(6):1315-1319. doi:10.2337/dc09-2278.

19. Zander E, Herfurth S, Bohl B, et al. Maculopathy in patients with diabetes mellitus type 1 and type 2: associations with risk factors. *Br J Ophthalmol*. 2000;84(8):871-876. doi:10.1136/bjo.84.8.871.20.

The figures in this chapter were contributed as noted in the figure captions.

31

OTHER SYSTEMIC DISORDERS/ CONDITIONS AFFECTING THE EYES

Al Lens, COMT

BASIC SCIENCES

The body consists of numerous systems: muscular, skeletal, digestive, excretory, reproductive, digestive, nervous, respiratory, circulatory, and endocrine. For the purpose of this chapter, we will go into a little more detail for the nervous, respiratory, circulatory, and endocrine systems. If you need a refresher on cells, organs, and systems, please refer to Appendix A.

Nervous System

The nervous system controls body movements, respiration, circulation, digestion, hormone secretion, and body temperature. Efferent (motor) neurons carry impulses away from the central nervous system to muscles and glands. The afferent (sensory) neurons bring stimuli from the sensors (eyes, ears, skin, etc) to the central nervous system.

The central nervous system consists of the brain and spinal cord. The human brain is like a super computer that perceives and translates information, then creates a response. The spinal cord is a two-way conduction pathway between the brain and the peripheral nervous system.

The peripheral nervous system consists of all the nerves and ganglia outside of the brain and spinal cord.

It is responsible for sending information to the brain and carrying out its decisions. There are 12 pairs of cranial nerves (originating from the brain) and 31 pairs of spinal nerves (arising from the spinal cord).

There are functions of the body that we can't "forget" to do, like breathing, heartbeat, and digestion. That's what the autonomic (involuntary) nervous system is for. It runs in the auto-mode 24 hours a day to keep us alive.

Respiratory System

The body cannot survive without oxygen. In addition, as the cells use the oxygen, they emit carbon dioxide that the body has to get rid of. The nose, throat, larynx, trachea, and lungs are all part of the respiratory system that supplies the body with oxygen and disposes of the carbon dioxide. It also purifies blood and allows coughing, sneezing, and talking.

Circulatory System

Blood carries oxygen and nutrients to the body's cells. The heart pumps the oxygenated blood through the body via arteries that branch off repeatedly and end as capillaries. There are about 5 to 6 liters (just over a gallon) of blood in the male human body, and 4 to 5 liters for a female.

Ledford JK, Lens A, eds.
Principles and Practice in Ophthalmic Assisting:
A Comprehensive Textbook (pp 549-555).
© 2018 Taylor & Francis Group.

On the way back to the heart, the blood travels through veins. The oxygen-deficient blood flows from the heart to the lungs where it picks up oxygen, then back to the heart before going through the body again.

Blood is 55% to 60% plasma and 40% to 45% blood cells. Plasma contains mostly water, but also has proteins, nutrients, hormones, and cellular waste products in it. There are three main types of blood cells. Erythrocytes (red blood cells) are the bulk of blood cells, with leukocytes (white blood cells) and platelets making up just 1% of the blood volume. The function of red blood cells is primarily to transport oxygen to the body's cells. White blood cells protect us from bacteria, viruses, parasites, and toxins. When the body needs white blood cells, it increases their production. A high white blood cell count (leukocytosis) typically means there is an infection present. Platelets (or thrombocytes) function to plug injured blood vessels.

Endocrine System

Our body relies on hormones (chemical messengers) to influence the metabolic activities of the cells. The glands that secrete hormones make up the endocrine system. Endocrine glands include the thymus, thyroid, parathyroid, pituitary, pineal, and adrenal glands. Exocrine glands secrete their products onto body surfaces or into body cavities. The exocrine glands include the liver, pancreas, salivary glands, sweat and oil glands, mucous glands, mammary glands, and various others. There are some organs that are dual-purpose (part endocrine and part exocrine), such as the pancreas and gonads (ovaries/testes).

CLINICAL KNOWLEDGE

Systemic diseases affect tissue, organs, or the body as a whole. There are many that have an impact on the eyes. It is those systemic diseases that we will focus on in this chapter (in alphabetical order). There are numerous diseases that can affect the eyes that are not listed here, but they tend not to be common.

Ankylosing Spondylitis

A type of arthritis, ankylosing spondylitis can cause parts of the spine to fuse together. It is more common in men than women, and usually first appears in adolescence. The inflammation can affect other parts of the body, including the eyes. Uveitis can be a complication of ankylosing spondylitis, causing painful red eyes and light sensitivity.

Arteriosclerosis/Atherosclerosis

Hardening of the arteries, or arteriosclerosis, causes thickening of the blood vessels and a loss of elasticity. It can reduce the blood flow to tissue and organs, including the eyes. Atherosclerosis also reduces blood flow, but the narrowing of the blood vessels is due to a build-up of plaque on the walls of the blood vessels. Both conditions can cause a blockage of the blood flow, which can cause ischemic optic neuropathy and retinal artery or vein occlusion, resulting in partial or complete loss of vision that may be irreversible.

Asthma

Asthma causes difficulties with breathing when the muscles in the bronchi contract, usually as a response to antigens. Stress, overexertion, irritants (smoke, perfume, etc), and infections can also trigger an asthma attack. Like other atopic (hyperallergic) diseases such as eczema and hay fever, asthma is associated with keratoconjunctivitis, blepharitis, and (in long-standing cases) cataracts.

Diabetes

Diabetes is covered in detail in Chapter 30.

Eczema

Like asthma, eczema is an atopic disease. It is an inflammatory skin disorder that is caused by a hypersensitivity to any number of agents or to stress. It causes red, itchy skin, which can include the eyelids. Individuals with eczema are more likely to develop dry eyes. For those suffering from eczema for more than 10 years, atopic cataracts may develop.

Gonorrhea

Gonorrhea is caused by a bacterium (*Neisseria gonorrhoeae*) that is sexually transmitted. It typically affects the genital tract, causing painful urination and pus-like discharge. Ocular involvement includes pain, photophobia, and purulent discharge of one or both eyes (Figure 31-1). An infant born to a mother who has gonorrhea is also at risk for the disease, mostly affecting the eyes.

Hypertension

High blood pressure, or hypertension, increases the risk of having a heart attack, kidney failure, and stroke. Hypertension is caused by blood vessels that have lost elasticity and/or have become narrowed by plaque build-up on the vessel walls. (See Arteriosclerosis/Atherosclerosis above.)

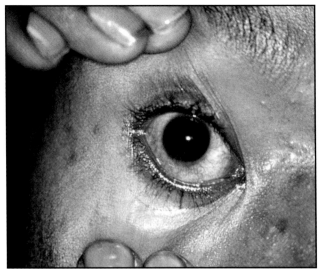

Figure 31-1. Gonorrheal conjunctivitis. (Reprinted with permission from the Centers for Disease Control and Prevention/Joe Miller.)

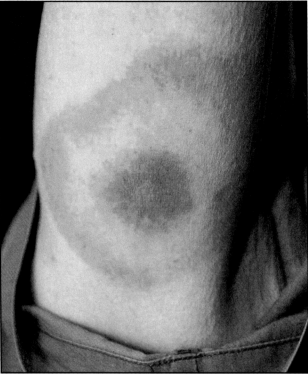

Figure 31-2. Typical bullseye rash seen in Lyme disease. (Reprinted with permission from the Centers for Disease Control and Prevention/James Gathany.)

When the blood pressure is measured, there are two numbers to be noted: The first number is the systolic pressure, which is when the heart contracts, and the second number is the diastolic pressure, representing the blood pressure when the heart relaxes. The systolic number is expected to rise somewhat as we age. Normal blood pressure of a younger person is 120/80 mm Hg or less.

The consequences of high blood pressure in the eyes are caused by cerebral edema, resulting in disc edema, and vasculopathy (changes in the blood vessels causing hemorrhages and damage to nerve fibers; see Figure 27-6).

Leukemia

Leukemia refers to a group of cancers that start in the stem cells of the blood. It can cause tumors in various structures of the eye. Relapses of leukemia can sometimes be first identified by presentation in the eye. The eye can also suffer an increased risk of infection as a result of immunosuppression treatment.

Lyme Disease

Getting bitten by a tick is never a good thing, but it is made worse if the tick transmits Lyme disease. The disease is named after the small town of Lyme, Connecticut, where it was first identified in the 1970s. The early symptoms often mimic those of the flu, making it difficult to diagnose, especially if the victim does not recall being bitten by a tick. Presence of a bullseye rash at the site of the bite is typical (Figure 31-2).

In the early stages of Lyme disease, ocular involvement may include conjunctivitis or episcleritis. In more involved stages, uveitis, endophthalmitis, keratitis, cystoid macular edema, optic neuropathy, and cranial nerve damage (causing Bell's palsy or Horner's syndrome) are possible.

Marfan Syndrome

Marfan syndrome is an inherited connective tissue disorder. People with Marfan syndrome are typically tall and thin with long fingers and toes. The syndrome can affect the eyes, skeleton, heart, and blood vessels. In many cases, Marfan syndrome is first suspected when an ophthalmologist observes a subluxated (dislocated) crystalline lens. Other ocular manifestations include high myopia, retinal detachment, premature cataracts, strabismus, glaucoma, and myopia.

Psoriasis

Psoriasis is a skin condition characterized by red, scaly, thickened skin. It is an autoimmune disease that can also cause dryness of eyes and the skin around the eyes. Persons with psoriasis have a greater-than-average risk of developing uveitis, especially in the case of psoriatic arthritis.

Rheumatoid Arthritis

Rheumatoid arthritis (RA) is an autoimmune disease that causes painful swelling and erosion of joints in the body. It is more likely to present itself after the age of 40 years, and is more common in women than men. Ocular manifestations include keratoconjunctivitis sicca, keratitis, episcleritis, and scleritis. Medications used to treat RA, such as chloroquine and hydroxychloroquine, can cause retinopathy and corneal deposits. Those who take corticosteroids may experience an increase in intraocular pressure (known as being a *steroid responder*). Prolonged use of corticosteroids may also cause cataracts, often of the faster-developing posterior subcapsular type.

Rosacea

Rosacea (sometimes called acne rosacea or adult acne) is a chronic condition that causes redness, mostly in the face. In moderate cases, it can lead to bumps in the skin that appear similar to acne. Severe cases can cause thickening of the skin of the nose and make it appear bumpy. Rosacea usually develops between the ages of 30 and 50 years and is treatable, but not curable.

It is quite common for people with rosacea to experience dryness of the eyes and/or redness of the eyelids. Ocular rosacea can sometimes precede the skin symptoms. Treatment is usually artificial tears, but sometimes oral antibiotics may be required. There may be periods of remission, but dry eye symptoms usually recur. Rosacea can also lead to a more serious condition called keratoconjunctivitis (inflammation of the cornea and conjunctiva) that may cause a painful eye, photophobia, and blurred vision.

Sickle Cell Disease

Sickle cell disease is a group of inherited conditions that affect hemoglobin (a protein in red blood cells). The cells become crescent (or sickle) shaped, rather than the normal disc shaped. These cells are not as flexible as normal blood cells and can stick to the walls of blood vessels, leading to occlusion of the vessel. Eye involvement, like any other organ affected by sickle cell disease, is based on vascular occlusion. Ocular manifestations include iris atrophy, retinal hemorrhages, vitreous hemorrhages, and retinal detachment. The disorders are most commonly seen in those of African and Mediterranean descent.[1]

Sleep Apnea

Sleep apnea is the interruption of breathing while sleeping. This decreases the oxygen available to the body and can cause heart problems, high blood pressure, stroke, and diabetes. Once sleep apnea has been diagnosed, the use of a continuous positive airway pressure (CPAP) machine may be advised. The CPAP involves wearing a mask that provides a continuous flow of air. This treatment can lead to dry eyes caused by the air escaping around the mask. Sleep apnea is also considered a risk factor for glaucoma.

Stevens-Johnson Syndrome

This rare, potentially lethal skin disease is usually caused by a reaction to medications. It begins with flu-like symptoms, and then a rash develops on the face and trunk of the body. The rash may develop into blisters and involve mucous membranes, including the eyes. It can cause dry eye, conjunctivitis, anterior uveitis, panophthalmitis (inflammation of all parts of the eye), and corneal ulcers. If the person survives, there may be long-term ocular problems such as entropion (inward turning of the eyelid), synechiae (adhesion of the iris to either the lens or cornea, or both), xerophthalmia (abnormal dryness of the eye), symblepharon (adhesion of the bulbar conjunctiva to the palpebral conjunctiva), and blindness.

Syphilis

Syphilis is a bacterial infection (caused by *Treponema pallidum*) that is sexually transmitted. It is sometimes asymptomatic or mimics symptoms of other conditions, allowing for the spread of the disease by unknowingly engaging in sex with an infected partner. It is very contagious in the primary stage of the disease when an ulcer appears in the infected area. While this can resolve without treatment, failure to treat the disease can allow the bacteria to enter the bloodstream, carrying the bacteria to other parts of the body and causing a rash in the secondary stage. This can also clear without treatment, but the bacteria may remain in a latent stage. Those who do not receive treatment for syphilis can suffer from tertiary syphilis, which can cause severe damage to organs, possibly including death. The disorder has so many possible symptoms, in fact, that it is known as "the great imitator," being confused for other diseases. Syphilis can affect the eyes at any stage, but it is more likely when it is in the tertiary stage. Ocular manifestations include uveitis, keratitis, retinitis, retinal vasculitis (inflammation of the retinal artery branches), and neuropathies involving the cranial and optic nerves.

Systemic Lupus Erythematosus

Lupus is an autoimmune disease that causes the body to attack its own healthy tissue. The most serious and most common type of lupus is systemic lupus erythematosus (SLE). It has various symptoms and there is no single test that provides a diagnosis. Ocular involvement includes keratoconjunctivitis sicca, episcleritis, scleritis, and retinopathy.

Systemic Viral Infections

While some viruses confine themselves to one area of the body, there are many that can impact the eye along with other body parts. We will discuss the more common viruses here.

Adenovirus

There are numerous types of adenoviruses. The majority of viral conjunctivitis is caused by an adenovirus; signs and symptoms of viral conjunctivitis include watery discharge and a burning sensation. An enlarged, painful lymph node in front of the ear occurs in roughly half of the cases.

Epidemic keratoconjunctivitis (EKC) is a highly contagious infection involving the adenovirus. If a patient is identified with EKC, anything the patient would have come into contact with (including doorknobs) should be thoroughly cleaned with a disinfectant. It can be unilateral or bilateral. Numerous infiltrates may develop on the cornea, causing light sensitivity and decreased vision in some cases. Treatment is aimed at reducing symptoms because there is no cure for the infection itself. If the patient wears contact lenses, they should not be worn again until the infection resolves. At that point, lenses, cases, and solutions should all be replaced.

Pharyngoconjunctival fever is also highly contagious and is most commonly found in children. As the name implies, a fever accompanies the ocular manifestation. Punctate keratitis and corneal infiltrates may develop. It is usually bilateral and resolves on its own in a few weeks.

Herpes Simplex

Herpes simplex can be divided into Type 1 and Type 2. In most cases, it is Type 1 that affects the eyes (and is also associated with cold sores). It usually causes acute but often recurring episodes. Reactivation can be triggered by ultraviolet exposure, wind, fever, stress, or trauma (including surgical). The patient may complain of a red, painful eye that is sensitive to light, tearing, and perhaps decreased vision. Upon slit lamp examination, dendritic (branch-like) ulcers are the tell-tale sign of *Herpes simplex* (see Figure 33-12). Iritis may also be seen. Treatment with topical and/or oral antiviral medication is targeted to prevent permanent corneal scarring that may cause reduced visual acuity or even blindness. Corticosteroid drops or oral steroid therapy is contraindicated in patients with a recent history of Herpes simplex keratitis, as the drugs may trigger a recurrence due to the suppression of the immune system. In cases of active keratitis, corticosteroid drops are sometimes used in conjunction with antiviral therapy when the keratitis is causing unbearable discomfort or corneal damage.

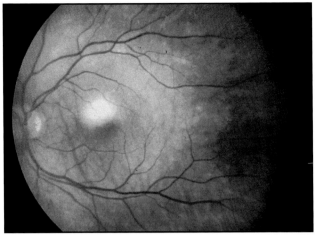

Figure 31-3. Chorioretinitis as seen in AIDS, caused by HIV. (Reprinted with permission from the Cogan Collection, National Eye Institute/National Institutes of Health.)

Herpes Zoster

Herpes zoster (shingles) is caused by the *Varicella zoster* virus, the same one that is responsible for chicken pox. The virus takes up residence on a nerve, and the nerve that feeds the forehead and end of the nose also involves the eye. The majority of herpes zoster patients who present with a rash on their forehead and on the tip of the nose will also have ocular involvement. Conversely, the eye can be a victim of the virus even if the nose is free of any rash. Signs and symptoms can include a red, painful eye; photophobia; lid swelling; and corneal edema. The patient is contagious while the blisters are open.

Human Immunodeficiency Virus

The human immunodeficiency virus (HIV) leads to ocular manifestations in the majority of cases, either directly or through opportunistic infections. Dry eye is common among HIV patients; there are several causes ranging from blepharitis to damage of the lacrimal glands. Retinal microvasculitis (inflammation of small blood vessels) is another common finding of HIV patients, but is often asymptomatic. Chorioretinitis (Figure 31-3) can also occur. More serious retinal involvement can be caused by cytomegalovirus or varicella zoster virus. Highly Active Antiretroviral Therapy (HAART) is a multiple-drug therapy used in an effort to suppress HIV and fortunately has decreased serious ocular manifestations of the disease.

Rubella

Rubella, aka German measles, is a fairly mild infection caused by the rubella virus. While it has a red rash like rubeola (measles), it is not the same. Rubella has been virtually eliminated from North America due to vaccines. Ocular manifestations are typically limited to infants born to mothers who had rubella during the

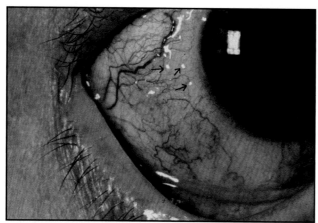

Figure 31-4. Nodular granuloma seen in sarcoidosis. (Reprinted with permission from the Cogan Collection, National Eye Institute/National Institutes of Health.)

first trimester. In this case, pigmentary retinopathy, cataracts, glaucoma, corneal clouding, strabismus, and microphthalmia (small eyeball) are possible. For adults with acquired rubella, conjunctivitis is the primary complication.

Rubeola

Rubeola, aka measles, usually affects children and is highly contagious. Ocular redness, tearing, and photophobia are often experienced. The involvement of the eyes could also include corneal clouding, macular edema, disc edema, choroiditis (inflammation of the choroid), and retinal pigment epithelial defects.

Temporal Arteritis

Temporal arteritis is an inflammation of the arteries that lead to the head and brain. The patient may come to the ophthalmologist's office complaining of double vision or a sudden loss of vision in one eye. He/She may also report a throbbing headache in the temple region, or tenderness in this area. Blood tests and/or a biopsy of the artery are used to confirm the diagnosis. Left untreated, temporal arteritis can lead to aneurysms and strokes, possibly causing death. The treatment of temporal arteritis with corticosteroids can cause secondary cataracts and glaucoma.

Thyroid Disease

The thyroid gland, located at the base of the neck, secretes hormones that regulate growth and metabolism. It can become underactive (hypothyroid) or overactive (hyperthyroid). It is the latter that is most likely to affect the eyes. The most common cause of a hyperthyroid is Graves' disease. This has ocular implications, which include protrusion of the eyes (exophthalmos or proptosis; see Figure 10-15), eyelid retraction, dry eye, double vision, and decreased vision.

Sarcoidosis

Sarcoidosis is an autoimmune disease that causes inflammatory cells to collect in various organs, most commonly the lungs and lymph nodes. The cause is unknown. Most cases occur between the ages of 20 and 40 years, with women affected more often than men. Cough, fatigue, and shortness of breath are the most common symptoms, but many people with sarcoidosis have no symptoms. Ocular symptoms can include red, sore eyes (Figure 31-4); photophobia; and blurred vision. Those who have been diagnosed with sarcoidosis should have regular eye exams, even when symptoms do not exist. Uveitis can occur, as well as posterior synechiae, glaucoma, and cataracts. Vitritis, retinal vasculitis, cystoid macular edema, and retinal detachment are also associated with sarcoidosis.

Wilson's Disease

Wilson's disease is linked to copper deposits throughout the body, but especially the brain, liver, cornea, and kidneys. It can be fatal if not treated. One of the findings used to diagnose the disease is a Kayser-Fleischer ring (copper deposits on the peripheral endothelium of the cornea); this is present in about half of cases without neurologic symptoms. Almost all patients with neurologic symptoms will have a Kayser-Fleischer ring. Copper may also deposit onto the crystalline lens, creating a sunflower cataract. The patient is usually asymptomatic from an ophthalmic point of view.

PATIENT SERVICES

History Taking

For more detailed information, please read Chapter 7, History Taking. Taking a history is a complex task. There is no quick reference guide that makes it a simple exercise. The interviewer has to know what part of the information the patient offers should be included in the written history. A broad knowledge of the systemic diseases that may affect the eyes is required to understand the pertinent details. And like any good interview, there needs to be follow-up questions to get all the information that will complete the history.

Since many of the ocular manifestations of systemic diseases are related to the duration of the disease, it is good to record when the diagnosis was first made. It should also be noted how well the disease is being controlled. If the patient is symptomatic, the onset of the symptoms should be recorded, along with whether they are getting better, worse, or stable. Sometimes systemic diseases are diagnosed after the patient begins to suffer ocular symptoms. Another important piece of information to include is any medications that are being used, and (in the case of medications that can have a lasting effect on the eyes) any that were used in the past.

Patient Education

The patient should be made aware of symptoms to watch for with respect to his/her systemic disease. Such cautions may relate to distortion in the vision, decreased vision, darkness of vision, or double vision, to name a few (refer to the ocular manifestations of each systemic disease). The prognosis is best left to the doctor to discuss with the patient.

If treatment is advised, the patient will benefit from a conversation about the frequency of the treatment, any possible side effects and when to be concerned about them, and what outcome is expected. In some cases, the treatment is aimed at preventing or limiting damage, rather than improving the situation. If the patient is wrongly expecting things to improve, he/she may discontinue treatment when no progress is experienced.

CHAPTER QUIZ

1. Which of the following carries blood back to the heart?
   a. arteries
   b. veins
   c. capillaries
   d. lymph nodes

2. All of the following is *true* about *Herpes zoster except*:
   a. it is caused by the same virus as measles
   b. can cause a red, painful eye
   c. it is contagious while blisters are open
   d. most cases that involve the forehead and tip of the nose will affect the eye

3. Epidemic keratoconjunctivitis is caused by:
   a. trauma
   b. Herpes simplex virus
   c. adenovirus
   d. bacterial infection

4. Hydroxychloroquine, used to treat rheumatoid arthritis, can cause:
   a. glaucoma
   b. cataracts
   c. increased pigment in iris
   d. retinopathy

5. Which of the following is *not* part of the respiratory system?
   a. heart
   b. lungs
   c. trachea
   d. nose

6. Lyme disease is caused by:
   a. eating a contaminated lime
   b. tick bite
   c. liver cirrhosis
   d. HIV

7. What is the most likely eye condition associated with eczema?
   a. conjunctivitis
   b. iritis
   c. keratitis
   d. dry eye

Answers

1. b, The arteries carry blood away from the heart; veins carry it back to the heart.
2. a, *Herpes zoster* causes both shingles and chicken pox.
3. c
4. d
5. a
6. b
7. d

REFERENCE

1. Maakaraon JE, Taher AT. Sickle cell anemia. Medscape website. http://emedicine.medscape.com/article/205926-overview. Updated October 3, 2016. Accessed February 5, 2017.

The figures in this chapter were contributed as noted in the figure captions.

32

OCULAR TRAUMA

Adel Ebraheem, MD, MS

Ocular trauma is a significant cause of decreased vision, disfigurement, disability, and blindness. Complications as a result of eye injuries depend on the nature and severity of the injury, ranging from a corneal abrasion with complete healing within 24 hours to a more serious injury causing irreversible, complete loss of vision and/or of the eye itself. Eye care personnel should have knowledge and skills regarding basic assessment, first aid management, and methods of injury prevention.

The United States Eye Injury Registry (USEIR) is an organization that was established in 1988 and acts as an epidemiologic data source of eye injuries. It helps us get a better understanding of eye injury types, their frequency, preventative measures, and treatment outcomes.

BASIC SCIENCES

Epidemiology and Eye Trauma

Epidemiology is the science of studying the distribution, frequency, and risk factors of health-related events. It also involves subsequent prevention and correcting measures (Sidebar 32-1).

Incidence is the measurement of new cases of a disease or injury, in a particular population (eg, specific age groups or gender), over a specific period of time. The incidence rate is the number of new cases of a disease or condition divided by the number of persons at risk for that disease or condition. For example, if over the period of a year seven children are diagnosed with retinoblastoma out of the total 300 children included in the study, the incidence of retinoblastoma would be 7/300, or 0.023. (If you want a percentage, multiply by 100 and the answer in this case becomes 2.3%).

Prevalence is the total number of people affected by a particular health-related problem or injury at a specific time. The prevalence rate is the total number of cases of a disease existing in a population divided by the total population. Thus, if we want to know the prevalence of diabetic retinopathy in a total diabetic population of 60,000, and 800 of them have retinopathy, the prevalence is 0.013 (800/60,000, or 1.3%).

Morbidity is another term for illness or disease. The morbidity rate is the number of all cases of a particular disorder in a given group. *Mortality* is another term for death. The mortality rate is the number of deaths due to a health-related problem divided by the total population.

Classification of Ocular Injuries

Standardized definitions of eye trauma help ophthalmologists and ophthalmic personnel to accurately

557

Ledford JK, Lens A, eds.
Principles and Practice in Ophthalmic Assisting:
A Comprehensive Textbook (pp 557-572).
© 2018 Taylor & Francis Group.

SIDEBAR 32-1
EPIDEMIOLOGY OF OCULAR INJURIES

▶ There are approximately 2.5 million eye trauma cases annually in the United States.[1]

▶ The hospital admission incidence rate as a result of eye injuries is 13.2 annually.[1]

▶ Most chemicals and thermal eye injuries occur in workers of age range from 20 to 44 years.[1]

▶ The cost of eye injuries related to sports ranges from $175 to $200 million (US) per year.[2]

▶ Eye trauma is responsible for 5% of all blindness in children.[1]

SIDEBAR 32-2
BIRMINGHAM EYE TRAUMA TERMINOLOGY DEFINITIONS INVOLVING OCULAR INJURIES

▶ Eyewall: Includes sclera and cornea only

▶ Closed-globe injury: A non–full-thickness eye wall injury

▶ Open-globe injury: Full-thickness eye wall injury

▶ Penetrating eye injury has entrance wound only

▶ Perforating eye injury has entrance and exit wounds caused by the same object

▶ Rupture: Full-thickness wound caused by blunt trauma

▶ Laceration: Full-thickness wound as a result of injury by a sharp object

describe and record patient clinical data. Currently, there are two systems used in eye injury classification.

The *Birmingham Eye Trauma Terminology* (BETT) provides a standard terminology of ocular trauma and has been recognized by international organizations such as the American Academy of Ophthalmology and the International Society of Ocular Trauma. Based on BETT, eye trauma is divided into open- or closed-globe injury depending on the existence of a full-thickness eye wall wound (Sidebar 32-2).

The *Ocular Trauma Score* (OTS) provides a numerical value, which is translated into a prediction of visual outcome following injury. First, the patient is given a raw score based on visual acuity following the trauma. The better the vision, the higher the score. Points are then deducted if there is rupture of the globe, evidence of endophthalmitis, a perforating injury, a retinal detachment, and/or a relative afferent pupillary defect. This final score is then looked up on a chart that gives a predicted visual recovery in 6 months following the trauma.

Tissue Reactions to Injury
Early Reactions and Complications

Eye injuries are similar to other tissue injuries in regard to specific pathophysiological response to trauma. The initial reaction to injury is acute inflammation, which is characterized by constriction of blood vessels (vasoconstriction) as a response to the stress-induced hormone catecholamine. This is a compensatory mechanism to prevent blood loss. Vasoconstriction is followed by dilation (vasodilation). There are also other cellular events, such as the release of inflammatory mediators by the damaged cells, which attract white blood cells (leukocytes) to start the infection defense mechanism. Other chemical mediators are released that initiate the blood clotting system. This draws even more leukocytes to the area.

During the acute inflammatory stage, there is an increased possibility of infection because the cell membranes have lost integrity. This is what attracts the leukocytes to the tissue injury site as the first line of defense against disease-causing germs.

In cases where a foreign body is involved, it is critical to determine the nature of the substance, because some materials can lead to a particular tissue reaction. There is no tissue reaction if the foreign body is glass, plastic, gold, silver, or platinum. Other materials, such as wood and aluminum, produce local irritation. Mercury, nickel, zinc, and pure copper can cause festering wounds. Iron can cause *siderosis bulbi*, a set of degenerative changes that occur because the iron molecules bind to the cell proteins.

Late Complications

Endophthalmitis is an inflammatory condition of the intraocular structures, usually caused by infection. Post-traumatic bacterial or fungal endophthalmitis can occur following eye injury (including the "intentional injury" of surgery). Studies have attributed the highest incidence of endophthalmitis to *Bacillus cereus*, which is a gram-positive bacterium.[3] Other studies show that *Staphylococcus aureus* and *Streptococci* (also gram positive) are the most frequent causes of post-traumatic endophthalmitis.[4] Despite early treatment, about 50% of eyes become blind after an acute bacterial endophthalmitis infection.[5]

The clinical manifestations of endophthalmitis include eye pain, marked visual loss, pus in the anterior chamber (hypopyon), and the absence of a red reflex. (The *red reflex* is the orange-reddish light reflection from the retina visible during photography, pupil evaluation, retinoscopy, etc.)

Management of endophthalmitis is very challenging. First, there is an attempt to identify the causative microorganism by vitreous sampling and cultures. Intravitreal injection of broad-spectrum antibiotics as well as topical antibiotics and steroids are usually administered. Vitrectomy may be performed in severe cases.

Sympathetic ophthalmia is a much-dreaded complication where there is the threat of losing both eyes, even though only one eye was injured. It is a bilateral inflammation of the uveal tract (iris, ciliary body, and choroid) and occurs mostly after penetrating eye trauma with uveal prolapse. It almost always appears within the first year following the injury. The injured eye shows the first signs of inflammation, followed by the other eye. The patient will complain of blurred vision, redness, and severe light sensitivity of both the injured and noninjured eye.

Immediate intervention is essential. The management plan depends on the severity of the original trauma. Treatment of the sympathizing (noninjured) eye with high doses of systemic and topical steroids can be started in less severe cases. Enucleation of a severely damaged, sightless eye is recommended within 2 weeks of the injury.

CLINICAL KNOWLEDGE

Types of Ocular Injuries

Note: This section gives some general information about various types of eye injuries. For details on specific trauma, see the section entitled Review of Injuries.

Blunt Trauma

Blunt eye trauma, as by a fist or tennis ball, generally causes a temporary decrease in the eyeball's anterior-posterior diameter (length) with an increase in the equatorial diameter (width). This may cause a brief but dramatic elevation of the intraocular pressure. One of the most severe complications of this type of injury is globe rupture. The most common site of rupture is where the rectus muscles attach to the globe, because the sclera is thinnest at these locations and the insertions are close to the limbus.

Penetrating Trauma

This type of injury occurs when a sharp-ended foreign body impacts the eye at a high velocity (eg, from hammering, drilling, or gunshot). If the penetrating injury is severe enough, it can cause a puncture with protrusion of intraocular contents.

Penetrating eye injuries can be categorized into two divisions based on whether or not the foreign body is retained in the eye. However, *penetrating* eye injuries, with or without foreign body retention, have a better prognosis than *perforating* eye injuries (where there is both an entrance and exit wound).

Chemical Injuries

Ocular complications after chemical eye injuries depend on:

▶ The total surface area of the eye that comes into contact with the chemical agent

▶ The degree of the chemical's penetration into the tissues

▶ The severity of damage to corneal stem cells (which are located in the limbal area and are responsible for corneal epithelial cell regeneration)

▶ Any heat-causing effect of the chemical

Alkali burns, such as caustic soda (NaOH), ammonia, and lime (concrete, mortar, etc), are twice as common as acid burns. This is unfortunate because alkaline chemicals (also known as bases) cause more ocular damage than acids. Once the alkali binds with the lipid component of the corneal tissue, it carries damaging effects to the corneal matrix, which leads to further penetration.

If the chemical penetrates into the anterior chamber, the intraocular structures undergo necrosis (cell death). The dying cells release enzymes that further promote the inflammatory reaction and causes even more damage.

Acidic compounds include sulfuric, acetic, chromic, and hydrochloric acids. Sulfuric acid exposure may be complicated by thermal damage and high-velocity impact (eg, after a car battery explosion). Acid burns cause less severe damage than alkali because the acid coagulates the surface tissue, which then acts as a barrier to limit further penetration.

Poisonous gases include lachrymatory agents ("tear gas," such as pepper spray and phenacyl chloride), mustard gas, and arsenic. Tear gas (categorized as a nonlethal) works by irritating the mucous membranes of the eyes and respiratory tract. It can lead to eye pain and temporary blindness. Mustard gas can cause blindness up to 10 days after severe exposure. With mild to moderate exposure, the patient will complain of irritation, pain, swelling, and tearing. Arsenic gas can cause conjunctival congestion, eye pain, and sticky discharge.

Radiation Injuries

Infrared rays are invisible, with a wavelength between 700 nm and 1 mm, which is longer than the visible light spectrum. Exposure to these rays can lead to cataractous changes over time. This risk is very common among glass and steel workers who are continuously exposed to infrared radiation.

Risk of infrared radiation injury also exists any time a person looks directly at the sun, although the bright light causes pupil constriction, which limits the amount of infrared waves reaching the retina. Also, the discomfort caused by the intense light reduces the amount of time a person can look at the sun. Focal retinitis with a macular burn is often caused by a person looking directly at a partial or total eclipse of the sun without any filter. While the observer may believe it is safe, a percentage of the sun's rays are still entering the eyes, causing retinal damage. This is exacerbated by the fact that an eclipsed sun is not as bright and daylight decreases, allowing a larger pupil, which increases exposure.

Ultraviolet (UV) rays are characterized by a wavelength shorter than 300 nm. The primary source of UV rays is sunlight, as they make up 1% to 2% of the total radiation. Its harmful effects can be a result of exposure to sunlight at high altitude as well as in areas where shorter wavelengths are reflected from bright surfaces such as sand, water, and snow. The hazards of UV radiation are always present, even on a cloudy day, because the invisible UV rays penetrate the clouds. Welding or glass blowing as well as commercial tanning without using proper eye protection are other sources of UV wave injury. Exposure to UV radiation can lead to *photophthalmia* (essentially a sunburn of the eye) with resultant pain, light sensitivity, and tearing.

UV rays have also been implicated in ocular disorders such as macular degeneration. A high percentage of UV radiation is absorbed by the crystalline lens as well, which can later manifest as cataract formation.

Low voltage *X-rays* can cause superficial skin lesions such as dermatitis (skin inflammation) and eyelid scarring, which may result in entropion (turning in of the eyelid) or ectropion (turning out of the eyelid). Loss of eyelashes and keratoconjunctivitis (inflammation of both the cornea and conjunctiva) with dry eye symptoms may also occur. High-voltage X-rays can cause cataracts several months to years after exposure if radiation reaches a dose of 500 to 800 rad. (A *rad* is the unit used to measure the absorbed dose.) Adverse effects of X-rays can occur after a single high-dose exposure or after multiple exposures of smaller doses over a period of time. The damaging effect of X-rays is cumulative.

Ocular complications resulting from *electrical* injuries include corneal perforation, iritis, cataract, retinal pigment epithelium damage, macular edema, retinal detachment, macular hole, optic neuritis, and choroidal atrophy. These effects are due to cell death that occurs because of compromised blood supply to tissues.

In general, *ultrasonic* waves do not have adverse effects on the human body or the eye, so no negative effects occur from using A-scan, B-scan, or biometry. However, during cataract surgery, the ultrasonic waves of the phacoemulsification tip can have a deleterious effect on the corneal endothelium.

Laser is used in many sectors, including medicine, military, and entertainment. Laser radiation's harmful effects are linked to the laser's wavelength, thus the type of injury varies. Surface trauma to the cornea and sclera may cause discomfort. Retinal injuries (photochemical damage) can lead to a sudden loss of vision and scotomas (blind spots).

Thermal Injuries

Thermal injuries can be caused by any source of heat, such as hot ashes, splashes of molten metal, exploding powder, hot liquids, and steam. Any hot object that comes into contact with the eye will cause a burn (curling irons come to mind). Electricity and lasers of certain wavelengths and some chemical agents can also cause thermal injuries.

External burns are divided into three groups depending on the severity of the burn. *First-degree* burns involve only the outer layer of skin (epidermis), evidenced by redness. *Second-degree* burns involve the epidermis and the dermis. If this type of burn is more superficial, it is manifest by pain, swelling, redness, and blistering. A deeper second-degree burn may look pale and wet. *Third-degree* burns involve the full thickness of the skin and can include muscle and bone. These classifications apply to thermal injury of the eyelids/skin in determining the management protocol and prognosis, but cannot be applied to the globe itself because of its complexity.

Review of Injuries

Eyelid Trauma

Eyelid Laceration

Eyelid lacerations (Figure 32-1) can be divided into several types.

A superficial laceration does not reach the eyelid's deep skin layers. If the injury occurs to the upper eyelid, it may extend into the muscle that opens the lid (levator palpebrae superioris) and can cause a permanent post-traumatic lid droop (ptosis).

A lid margin cut can cause irregular healing and/or scarring. This can lead to malformations of the lid, including entropion, ectropion, notched lid margin, and/or trichiasis (misdirection of eyelashes).

If the injury involves the inner corner of the lower eyelid and the canalicula is lacerated, the tear drainage system can be damaged. This can result in long-term tearing where tears run down the cheek (epiphora) because the normal drainage route has been disrupted.

Presentation and Management

The patient should be seen immediately by an eye doctor as the outcome is much better if surgical repair is done early. This is especially true in the case of canalicular laceration because the tissues must be properly aligned in order to restore the tear drainage system. In addition, initial consultation may help prevent wound contamination and infection. Broad-spectrum antibiotic and tetanus toxoid vaccine are usually recommended.

Hematoma ("Black Eye")

A black eye (Figure 32-2) is the most common type of blunt eyelid injury, usually caused by objects such as a tennis ball or fist. The black color is bruising due to

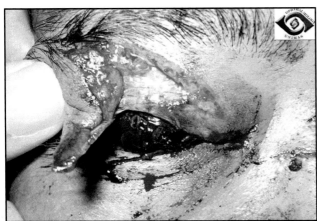

Figure 32-1. Eyelid laceration of the upper lid. Lower lid lacerations can be problematic if the lacrimal drainage system is involved. (Reprinted with permission from Ophthalmology Unit, Universiti Malaysia Sarawak [UNIMAS], Kuching, Sarawak; Adrian Koay.)

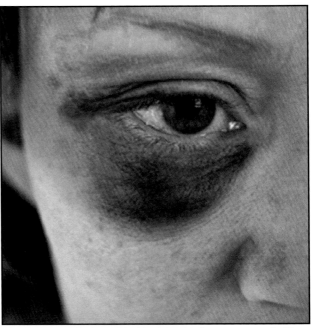

Figure 32-2. "Black eye." Lid bruising is often accompanied by a subconjunctival hemorrhage, but the real concern is concussive damage to the globe itself, such as retinal detachment.

the leakage of blood from the damaged blood capillaries underneath the skin.

It is important to exclude other conditions that might be associated with the eyelid trauma:

► Globe trauma causing a hyphema (an accumulation of blood in the anterior chamber), dislocated lens, vitreous hemorrhage, and/or choroidal or retinal tears/detachments

► Frontal fracture of the skull, the characteristic feature of which is subconjunctival hemorrhage that extends beyond the visible white of the eye

► Basal skull fracture characterized by bilateral ring hematoma (also known as "raccoon eyes" or "panda eyes/sign")

► Blowout fracture of the orbital floor (discussed later)

► Blowout fracture of the orbital medial wall (broken nose), which can lead to more eyelid swelling if the patient blows his/her nose (discussed later)

Presentation and Management

It is much easier to examine the eye before the lids become swollen shut, so this patient should be seen by an eye doctor as soon as possible. First aid includes application of cold compresses to reduce swelling and oral analgesics to relieve pain. The bruising usually fades away within 1 week as the blood decomposes and is absorbed.

Conjunctival and Corneal Foreign Bodies

This type of injury mostly occurs from high-velocity foreign bodies during activities such as hammering, sanding, or lathing. The damage ranges from a simple corneal scratch with embedded foreign body in the corneal epithelial layer (Figure 32-3) to corneal perforation. A corneal scar (Figure 32-4) can occur after wound healing, especially if the foreign body damages the deeper

layers of the cornea. Blinking and tearing can sometimes be sufficient to dislodge a superficial foreign body without intervention.

The patient may complain of eye irritation, a foreign body sensation, eye ache, tearing, blurred vision, and sometimes photophobia.

Presentation and Management

The patient should be instructed not to rub the eye. It is important to ascertain whether or not the foreign body has penetrated the eye. Any leakage of aqueous fluid may be detected by instilling a drop of fluorescein onto the eye and observing with the slit lamp. If aqueous is leaking, it will be seen as a tiny, clear "stream" flowing through the dye (positive Seidel sign).

A superficial foreign body might be dislodged by irrigation with saline solution. A more deeply embedded foreign body may require the use of a corneal spud or a drill (after topical anesthetic has been applied). Certain types of metal can sometimes be extracted more easily with a magnet than with forceps. In addition, some metallic foreign bodies will begin to rust directly on the corneal tissue, creating a rusted ring that must be drilled out. Finally, the lids must be inverted in order to check for retained foreign matter either loose in the cul-de-sac or embedded into the palpebral conjunctiva.

Once the foreign body has been removed, the patient should be warned that the eye will probably feel as if there is still something in it once the topical anesthetic wears off. This is usually resolved within 24 hours.

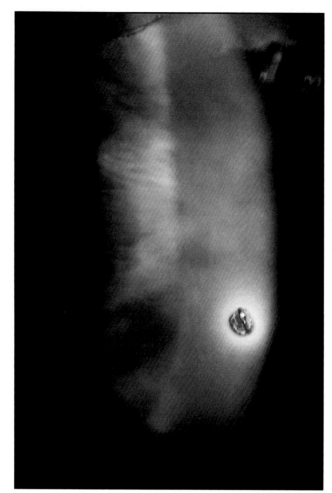

Figure 32-3. Corneal foreign body. A rust ring often forms after metallic fragments embed into the cornea.

The physician may recommend topical antibiotics and/or lubrication for home use. Topical anesthetic is never given to the patient for personal use as this can retard healing. (The use of several drops of anesthetic in the office is not enough to cause problems.)

Penetrating Eye Injuries

Statistics shows that men are more prone to penetrating eye trauma than women by a 3:1 ratio.[5] It is more common in the younger age group and is often the result of sports or assault. The severity of the injury and its prognosis are determined by the nature of the foreign body, its size, and its speed (Figures 32-5 through 32-7).

Determination of the type of foreign body is critical because certain materials can lead to specific tissue reactions. There is no tissue reaction if the foreign body is glass, plastic, gold, silver, or platinum. Aluminum can produce a local irritation. Mercury, nickel, zinc, and pure copper can cause festering wounds. Some particular tissue reactions are linked to specific metals. For example, *siderosis bulbi* is caused by retained iron as it deposits on the intraocular structures and reacts

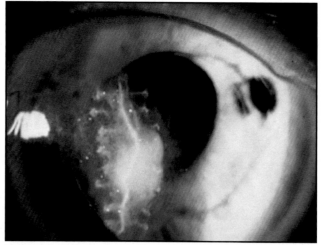

Figure 32-4. Corneal scar. Corneal scarring can result in a haze that impairs vision. (Reprinted with permission from George Harocopos, MD.)

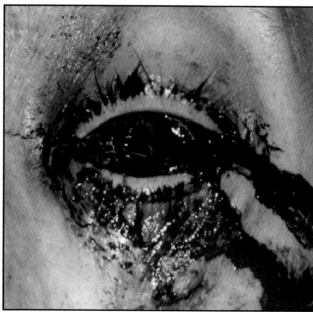

Figure 32-5. Penetrating injury. (Reprinted with permission from George Harocopos, MD.)

chemically with them. *Chalcosis bulbi* is a tissue reaction to copper alloys.

The speed of a flying foreign body also affects the extent of damage. For example, an air gun bullet can cause more eye damage than shrapnel fragments because the former has more kinetic injury.

Presentation and Management

The role of the ophthalmic assistant in these types of injury is to record a full detailed history. In the case of eye trauma involving a fast-moving object, the patient may not complain of eye pain or even have gross visible signs. If a patient reports of having a "little black blob on the white of the eye," this may be a prolapse of uveal tissue

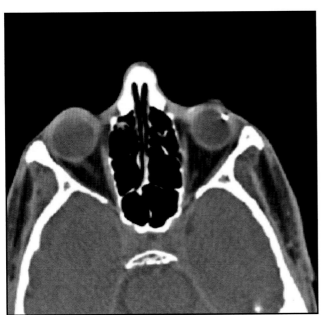

Figure 32-6. Metal intraocular foreign body located in the left temporal pars plana region as seen on axial CT scan. (Reprinted with permission from George Harocopos, MD.)

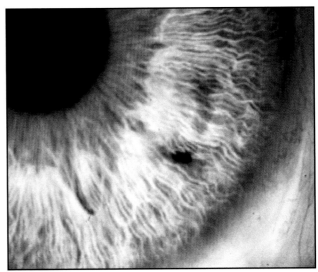

Figure 32-7. A hole in the iris can occur from a penetrating eye injury with a small foreign body. (Reprinted with permission from George Harocopos, MD.)

through the laceration. The longer this tissue is exposed to the air, the poorer the prognosis for recovery.

If squinting is severe, do not try to separate the eyelids. Pressing on the globe can extrude intraocular contents. A slit lamp exam may reveal a collapsed anterior chamber, irregular pupil, or iris tear/hole. Prolapsed uveal tissue may also be visible. Administration of eye drops or ointment is prohibited unless instructions are given by an ophthalmologist.

Defining the type of the foreign body is also important in management. For example, the health care provider would not order magnetic resonance imaging (MRI) if the foreign body is iron because the magnetic nature of the MRI will attract the metal foreign body, perhaps traumatically pulling it out of the eye. If the eye was penetrated by organic material such as plant or wood (with or without intraocular retention), there is a much higher risk of developing an infection (including fungal) and treatment would be directed toward preventing this.

Special tests maybe ordered as appropriate, such as orbital X-rays, computed tomography (CT) scan, or B-scan, to determine the foreign body's location and the extent of damage. Surgical removal of a retained intraocular foreign body and repair decisions depend upon the doctor's clinical judgment and risk management. Home care will include anti-infectives, perhaps both topical and oral.

Orbital and Globe Injuries

Blunt Trauma

Blunt trauma, or closed-globe contusion, can be caused by objects such as a tennis ball or by concussive forces such as air bags. Blunt trauma results in an initial compression of the globe in the direction of the force, and then an associated recovery in the opposite direction, which briefly overshoots the tissue's original position. This phenomenon explains the nature of the complications associated with this type of injury (Sidebar 32-3 and Figures 32-8 and 32-9). Not only can the orbital bones break (see next section), but there can be soft tissue damage and retinal damage as well. If the vision following the injury is light perception or less, hypotony (low intraocular pressure) or a vitreous hemorrhage may be present. Hypotony can cause problems with the macula, which is accompanied by vision loss.

Bony Orbit Fracture

An orbital fracture can result from a high-velocity object that is more than 2.5 inches in diameter, such as a tennis ball (Figure 32-10). This impact leads to a rapid pressure on the bony orbit and fracture of the orbital wall.

The most common orbital wall fracture sites are the orbital floor and the medial wall because they are adjacent to sinuses. Some bones of the sinuses are nearly paper-thin, so as the pressure of the blow is transferred back, these are the bones that most commonly break. On the other hand, the orbital roof and the lateral wall, being of thicker bone, are usually able to withstand the sudden force.

There are two types of fractures of the orbital floor (or *blowout fractures*). A pure fracture does not involve the orbital rim, and an impure fracture does involve the orbital rim.

Presentation and Management

It is not always obvious by just looking that a fracture has occurred. The patient presenting with an orbital fracture may be experiencing numbness involving the lower lid, side of the nose, and cheek because of damage

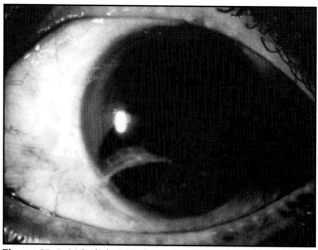

Figure 32-8. Iridodialysis is the result of a tear in the iris root. It may be repaired surgically or concealed with a cosmetic contact lens. (Reprinted with permission from George Harocopos, MD.)

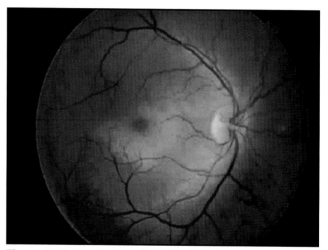

Figure 32-9. Commotio retinae usually follows blunt eye trauma. When a blunt object strikes the eye, shock waves traverse the eye to the posterior pole. The retinal blood vessels are clearly seen in this photo because the outer retinal layers have blanched (whitened). (Reprinted with permission from Sarah Gardner, CRA.)

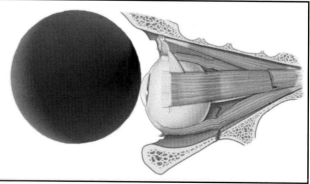

Figure 32-10. Schematic of orbital fracture caused by blunt trauma.

to the infraorbital nerve (a branch of the maxillary division of trigeminal nerve, cranial nerve V), which runs along the orbital floor. If the inferior rectus and inferior oblique muscles have protruded through a fracture of the orbital floor and become entrapped, the patient will have binocular diplopia (double vision when looking with both eyes). The whole eyeball itself may be displaced posteriorly and downward if the globe has sunk into the maxillary sinus.

Both external and slit lamp examination may reveal typical blunt trauma signs. The range of motion test in the case of entrapped extraocular muscles will be abnormal (ie, the eyes will not fix on the muscle light together in certain positions of gaze). Intraocular pressure and pupils should be checked as well. An afferent pupillary defect may indicate damage to the optic nerve. A dilated fundus exam is done to check for intraocular injury.

The physician will likely order X-rays and/or a CT scan or other testing to validate the existence of a fracture. Surgical management depends on the displacement of the globe and the degree of diplopia. It may involve the insertion of a metal plate over the orbital floor. Oral antibiotics are commonly prescribed because of sinus involvement and the proximity and connection of the eye to the brain.

The patient with an orbital floor fracture should be instructed not to blow the nose. Doing so may force air from the sinuses through the break and into the orbital cavity, causing orbital inflation (*periorbital subcutaneous emphysema*) and a very strange "crackling" noise (*crepitus*). It can also push bacterial-laden material from the sinuses into the orbital area.

Chemical Eye Injuries

Chemical eye injuries (Figure 32-11) are more common in the workplace; only one-third of such eye injuries occur at home.[5] If a patient phones in about a chemical splash, the very first thing is to tell him/her to immediately irrigate the eye for 20 minutes (if this hasn't already been done), then come into the office for further attention.

Presentation and Management

When the patient reaches the eye care facility, irrigation should begin at once if it has not already been done in the field. The ophthalmic assistant can then instill topical anesthetic to relieve eye discomfort and lid spasm, and further irrigate the eye with normal saline for 15 to 30 minutes as necessary. (See Patient Services section for instructions on how to irrigate.)

The assistant should obtain a detailed history concerning the nature of the injury (chemical involved), its concentration, duration of exposure, and when first aid was initiated and for how long. Material Safety Data Sheet (MSDS) information may be accessed online for more information on the chemical/solution. (The MSDS is information required by law on every chemical, solvent, and compound and must be supplied by the manufacturer. It includes the nature of the compound and other information, including what to do if the product is ingested or comes into contact with the skin, eye, mucous membranes, etc.)

If the irrigation has effectively neutralized the chemical, the eye's pH should range from 7.3 to 7.7. Ocular pH can be obtained by placing a testing strip in the lower fornix. (pH is a way of identifying the strength of an acid or base, and is explained in Appendix A.) If the pH is not

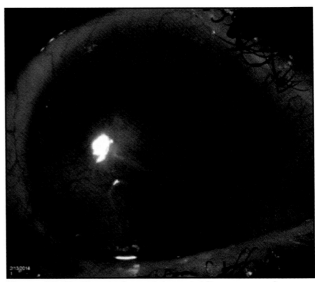

Figure 32-11. Chemical eye injury. Acidic compounds cause surface burns, while basic compounds penetrate the tissues. (Reprinted with permission from Sarah Gardner, CRA.)

satisfactory, further irrigation should be done. (Note: Do NOT attempt to "counteract" a harmful pH by instilling any chemical of the "opposite" pH.)

The physician will carefully examine the inner surfaces of the eyelids to check for any trapped material. In some cases, hospital admission may be in order so that the eye can be continuously irrigated. Home treatment depends on the severity of the injury.

Radiation and Thermal Injury

Ultraviolet Radiation

The nature of UV radiation injury was discussed earlier in this chapter. It is the most common type of radiation injury, but can be prevented by wearing proper UV-filtering eye protection.

Presentation and Management

A few hours after UV exposure, the patient will experience a foreign body sensation, tearing, moderate to severe eye pain, eye redness, and light sensitivity. These symptoms are due to a sunburn of the eye (*photophthalmia*). Placing anesthetic eye drops to relieve pain and distress will facilitate the examination. Slit lamp evaluation using fluorescein dye will reveal tiny, pinpoint spots (punctate keratitis) in the corneal epithelium over the corneal surface.

The practitioner will send the patient home with lubricating eye drops and/or gel as well as antibiotic ointment to prevent infection and promote the healing process. Topical anesthetics are never sent home with the patient as prolonged use is toxic to the corneal tissue.

The patient should be warned that the foreign body sensation and eye ache will likely return once the topical anesthetic wears off. The patient can use oral painkillers as directed by a physician.

SIDEBAR 32-4
RISK OF EYE INJURIES IN SPORTS[6]

High Risk
- Small, fast projectiles
  - Air rifle/BB gun
  - Paintball
- Hard projectiles, sticks, close contact
  - Basketball
  - Baseball, softball
  - Hockey
  - Squash
  - Racquetball
  - Fencing
  - Wrestling
  - Intentional injury
    - Boxing
    - Full-contact martial arts

Moderate Risk
- Tennis/badminton
- Soccer
- Volleyball
- Water polo
- Football
- Fishing
- Golf
- Cycling

Low Risk
- Swimming
- Diving

SIDEBAR 32-5
EYE INJURIES AND MOST COMMONLY ASSOCIATED SPORTS[7]

Blunt Eye Trauma
- Golf
- Racquetball
- Tennis
- Cycling

Open Eye Injury
- Squash
- Paintball
- Fishing

Perforated Eye Injury
- Skiing
- Hockey
- Shooting sports

Infrared Radiation

Infrared light rays have already been discussed. The ocular hazard of infrared radiation is restricted to a macular burn manifested by permanent visual impairment.

Presentation and Management

After exposure to infrared radiation, the patient complains of blurred vision. The best protocol of management is prevention, because the damaging effect on the retina is irreversible. Patients should be taught that Polaroid lenses and UV filters do not offer any protection against this type of radiation.

X-Ray Radiation

X-rays were discussed earlier in this chapter. They carry a high amount of energy, and health care personnel who work around X-rays are required to wear a special indicator badge that warns if exposure has reached an unacceptable level. Since this is a trauma that occurs over time, most cases do not present with acute symptoms with the possible exception of uveitis. The long-term complications can include cataract, glaucoma, skin cell death, and loss of eyelashes. Prevention is key.

Sports Eye Injuries

Sports eye injuries can be multifaceted with severe vision-threatening complications. Some types of sports, such as hockey, golf, and racquet sports, carry a higher risk of eye injury (Sidebar 32-4). These injuries can be minimized by using approved eye protection. (Almost all sports organizations, like the National Football League, focus on player safety by encouraging or requiring the player to wear approved eye protection.) However, other sports can also be risky because the player doesn't typically wear protective eye glasses, as in boxing and wrestling. Some types of injury are associated more with specific sports (Sidebar 32-5). This type of trauma is handled in the eye clinic on a case-by-case basis.

Injuries Related to Abuse

Eye trauma related to physical abuse crosses all age groups and socioeconomic categories, and may be associated with other bodily injuries. However, one of the challenges that investigators face is that other signs of violence may not be evident. For example, ocular injury without head trauma is common among children. Bilateral intraocular bleeding could point to shaking as the source of eye injury (discussed next).

Adults are not immune to abuse-related eye injuries, of course. Blunt trauma, with or without a blowout fracture and its associated complications, can occur as a result of a closed-fist blow to the eye. A unilateral black eye is a sign of this type of injury. A penetrating eye injury from a fingernail or sharp object is also common.

Shaken Baby Syndrome

Shaken baby syndrome (SBS) is a specific type of child abuse where a baby or toddler is shaken violently, perhaps because a frustrated caregiver thinks this will stop the child from crying. Three-quarters of cases are committed by a male on a child during its first year of life.[8]

In addition to the fragility of a baby's brain tissue, an infant's neck muscles are not fully developed. During the action of shaking, the brain moves back and forth in the skull cavity. This can lead to swelling, bruises, and bleeding of the brain (subdural hemorrhage), as well as retinal hemorrhages. The complications of SBS can be permanent brain and spinal cord damage leading to paralysis, vision loss, hearing loss, speech and learning disorders, and death.

Presentation (Sidebar 32-6) and Management

A child with SBS will probably present for ocular evaluation as a consultative exam from the emergency room or other clinic, rather than an initial urgent visit directly related to the trauma. It is likely that tests such as an MRI or CT scan have already been performed and documented.

As always, a complete history should be taken. Be sure to document who brought the child to your clinic and who gave the child's history. If abuse has been determined, it is likely that a guardian or social worker has brought the child in and his/her knowledge of events may be limited.

Your evaluation should include a vision assessment, pupil evaluation, and motility testing as neurological injury may show up in any of these tests. External findings should be noted (subconjunctival hemorrhage, tiny "dot" conjunctival hemorrhages [petechiae], bruising, etc), but it is more likely that any ocular damage will be internal, so the dilated exam is key.

Reporting Suspected Abuse

Specific eye injuries among children could be a sign of physical abuse and needs further investigation. Cues that may signal child abuse include:

▶ Injuries to infants who are not mobile

▶ Injuries that routine, age-appropriate supervision of the child should have prevented

---

> ## SIDEBAR 32-6
> ## PRESENTATION OF SHAKEN BABY SYNDROME
>
> ▶ Lethargy
>
> ▶ Seizures
>
> ▶ Soft tissue bulging in the forehead
>
> ▶ Decreased appetite
>
> ▶ Vomiting
>
> ▶ Breathing difficulties
>
> ▶ Convulsions
>
> ▶ Bruising on arms or chest
>
> ▶ Inability to lift the head
>
> ▶ Tremors
>
> ▶ Inability to focus or follow movement
>
> ▶ Unequal size of pupils
>
> ▶ Unconsciousness
>
> ▶ Coma

▶ A significant injury with no explanation or reasonable cause

▶ Multiple injuries in various stages of healing

Around 30% of SBS cases end in a fatality. Many of the survivors will develop mental retardation or learning disabilities. Due diligence in reporting suspected cases can be vital. The regulations that determine who should report child abuse are different among the 50 states, but most states require members of the health care professions to report suspected abuse. Proof, however, does *not* rest with the person(s) making the report.

It is the responsibility of the investigator to determine if the injury occurred intentionally by the caregiver or happened accidentally. Inappropriate actions by parents or a caregiver can sometimes be due to a lack of parenting skills, a situation that needs to be rectified.

Motor Vehicle-Related Eye Injuries

According to one study, approximately 5% of motor vehicle accident-related injuries involve the eye.[9] The mechanism of eye injuries in these types of accidents ranges from blunt trauma (eg, being struck by the airbag, steering wheel, or dashboard) to penetration from sharp debris (eg, glass splinters from the windshield). If any injuries are potentially severe, the patient will first be taken to the emergency room and admitted if appropriate. It is more likely that the eye clinic will become involved after initial emergency care has been completed.

Sidebar 32-7
History Taking in Ocular Trauma

▶ What is the nature of the eye injury? Were there any witnesses?

▶ Describe in detail the mechanism of injury.

▶ Where did it happen?

▶ What was the time of injury?

▶ Was any first aid management received? When? By whom?

▶ Were you wearing eye protection?

▶ Does the injury involve one eye or both eyes?

▶ Were you wearing contact lenses when the injury occurred?

▶ Have you noticed any changes in vision? Sudden or gradual?

▶ Do you have any double vision?

▶ Was your vision OK before the injury?

▶ Is the eye red/sore/itchy?

▶ Do you have any flashes and floaters/headaches?

▶ Have you had a recent eye trauma or eye surgery?

▶ Do you have any systemic medical conditions (especially vascular disorders, hypertension, diabetes, etc)?

▶ Do you currently take any anticoagulants, medications for high blood pressure, or any type of eye drops?

▶ Do you have any allergies to medications?

▶ Do you have a family history of any eye conditions?

Another study of persons presenting to emergency rooms in the United States estimated that about 10,000 eye injuries associated with motor vehicle accidents occur annually.[10] During 2001 through 2008, some 59.6% of these were male and 62.2% were the driver.[10] Incidence of injury was highest in the 15-to-19 age bracket.[10] The most common ocular trauma was contusion/abrasion (61.5%) followed by foreign body, hemorrhage, and laceration.[10]

Home Eye Injuries

The American Academy of Ophthalmology has conducted public surveys about eye injuries at home. The studies show that nearly 50% of the most severe eye injuries occur in the garage or the yard, and around one-third of eye trauma cases occurred in the kitchen and living room.[11] There are numerous, common household materials that carry the risk for eye injuries, such as solvents, cleaning chemicals, and hot liquids or oil. Any maintenance task that produces fragments is considered a risk for eye injuries, not only to people doing the work, but also to bystanders (perhaps children who are watching). Even pleasant tasks, such as opening a champagne bottle or using fireworks, can be a source of sight-threatening incidents.

Occupational Injuries

Due to the potentially severe impact of occupational accidents, there are numerous organizations that have developed strict safety standards and provide direct supervision over certain industries For example, the Occupational Safety and Health Administration (OSHA) ensures that manufacturers comply with the safety measures it has put into place. Despite rigid safety precautions, however, eye accidents continue to occur.

One such safety measure is the use of personal protective equipment (PPE) for the face and eyes. Protective safety glasses are made of impact-resistant polycarbonate and provide a barrier against chemical splashes, flying debris, and UV radiation.

Safety data sheets (SDS, formerly known as material safety data sheets) are OSHA-required documents with information about the physical and chemical properties and toxicity of every chemical used at a worksite. They also include first aid management and the recommended PPE to be used when handling a product. These sheets should be available to the worker as well as the health care team guiding them, providing the proper safety procedures of handling particular materials. However, this information varies from one manufacturer to another, and even among different countries.

The American National Standards Institute (ANSI) is a private, nonprofit organization that establishes testing methods and performance specifications for safety issues such as PPE. Standards are given for protective eyewear used for work hazards including splashes, impact, radiation, and dust. These standards vary depending on the type of hazard. For example, eyewear should have side protection if the activity involves chipping or grinding.[12]

Clinical Skills

History Taking

One of the most important tasks of ophthalmic medical personnel is to get a full, detailed history, especially in cases of eye trauma. Include the nature of the injury, when and where it happened, and any other pertinent details (Sidebar 32-7). Make a note whether or not the injury took place on the job, as worker's compensation claims would need this information.

Note the symptoms that the patient is currently experiencing. (Ocular symptoms can be categorized into three types: vision problems, abnormalities of ocular appearance, and abnormalities of ocular sensation/pain.) Current or previous eye problems, surgeries, and any eye medications in use should also be recorded. In cases where the patient is a child, list any attendant witnesses.

The history should also include the standard systemic medical history, which reflects the patient's general health. Finally, a list of medications that includes over-the-counter remedies (eg, aspirin thins the blood and can inhibit clotting) and any known allergies to medications should be compiled. See Chapter 7 for a detailed review of ocular history taking.

Basic Eye Examination

The primary eye examination is important in determining what further tests may be needed. However, if there is obviously a penetrating wound or extrusion of ocular contents, the physician should be alerted at once. If there has been a chemical splash, then irrigation should be started right away.

In some cases, the patient may not be able to open the eye(s) because of eye pain, light sensitivity, or swelling. Never press on the globe when trying to separate the eyelids. While numbing eye drops can ease the pain, it is not recommended in cases of penetrating eye injuries. In those cases, the ophthalmic technician should ask for the doctor's recommendation.

Visual acuity is performed with correction, if any, and with pinhole if vision is not 20/20. If possible, record pupil size, shape, reaction to light, and the presence/absence of an afferent pupillary defect. Examination of eye movements and restrictions should be done, along with notes about pain or diplopia in any gaze. Evaluation of extraocular muscle function can help detect an entrapment of muscles within an orbital bone fracture. Visual field assessment may suggest an underlying retinal detachment. Checking eye pressure is important, but whether it can be done varies from case to case. It is important to obtain the practitioner's permission in questionable cases.

Precautions

The ophthalmic tech should keep in mind the following precautions:

► Only sterile eye drops should be used on an injured eye. Tetracaine and fluorescein strips are available in sterile, individual dose units. Use these instead of anesthetic drops combined with fluorescein.

► Do not place miotic or mydriatic eye drops in an injured eye unless directed to do so.

► Be very careful when trying to separate the eyelids of an injured eye, as putting pressure on the globe can lead to protrusion of ocular contents.

► Do not give a prognosis of the injury based on the external appearance.

► Do not assure the patient of a good (and possibly wrong) prognosis.

► Lightly cover the eye and ask for the practitioner's opinion if you are not sure about the case's severity, how to proceed, or both.

PATIENT SERVICES

Triage

Triage is evaluating and prioritizing patient emergencies according to their level of urgency. This topic is covered in more detail in Chapter 33. However, in the case of known or suspected injury, triage may divide into three categories (Sidebar 32-8).

Eye trauma will be categorized as an emergency or urgent case. While not all injuries have permanent effects, most produce significant pain. However, the severity of an eye injury can't be determined by depending on the patient's description on the phone, nor on the patient's external appearance, vision, or level of discomfort.

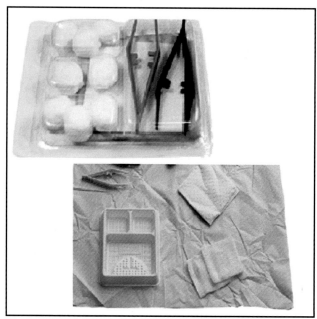

Figure 32-12. Intravenous set for irrigation.

Irrigation

Eye irrigation is always performed after a chemical eye injury, and sometimes in the case of a conjunctival or corneal foreign body.

Materials needed for eye irrigation:

► Waterproof cape to protect patient's clothes

► Towel

► Irrigation solution/sodium chloride 0.9% in a stream bottle

► Emesis basin

► Administration set (an intravenous set that can be used for eye irrigation [Figure 32-12]; a 10-cc syringe can be a good alternative)

► Sterile swabs to remove any solid particles from the fornices

► Gloves

► Sterile dressing pack, if needed

► pH check strips, if available

Procedure:

► Explain the procedure to the patient.

► Wash hands, put on gloves. Drape the patient with the cape.

► If using pH strips and it is possible to do so quickly, check the pH of the eye. But don't delay the irrigation itself to search for the strips, etc.

► Ask the patient to rotate his/her head in the direction of the affected eye.

► Place the emesis basin close to the cheek on the side of the affected eye.

► Pull down the lower eyelid and hold the upper eyelid to keep the eye widely opened, making sure that you don't exert any pressure on the globe. Note: Some patients are not able to open their eyes because of pain. Do not try to instill numbing eye drops to relieve pain without asking the doctor, and do not try to open their eyes forcefully.

► Hold the irrigator about an inch from the eye, and irrigate from the nasal canthus side. If the eye has not been numbed, it will be more comfortable for the patient if you can direct the stream into the nasal canthus vs directly on the cornea.

► If using pH strips, continue irrigating until the pH is 7.3 to 7.7.

Patient Education

Prevention

Patient education about safety measures is one of the tasks of all eye care personnel. Patient awareness includes determination of eye injury risks and hazards, and about the possible complications after eye injuries. Educating people about eye safety measures (such as using ANSI-approved eyewear during maintenance work) is crucial to prevent the types of trauma we have been discussing in this chapter. In the clinic, this information can be provided through posters and brochures. These are often available free of charge from various organizations involved in ocular health.

Eye safety education can also be provided at the workplace, where the worker is exposed to the risk of eye injury. Eye safety awareness can be accomplished through offering eye safety programs in schools and colleges, providing brochures about eye safety, and televised safety programs sponsored by nonprofit organizations such as the Red Cross.

Prognosis

Ophthalmic medical personnel should not provide the patient or relatives with a prognosis of a traumatic situation. The eye care provider is the one to determine this. While it is tempting to reassure the patient, we should not say "everything will be all right." If everything does not turn out "all right," your words could later be brought up in court as evidence of a guarantee of a better outcome. Supportive comments such as "We will do everything we can to help" are still comforting, and more appropriate.

Rehabilitation Issues and Psychological Support

Ocular trauma can lead to vision loss and have a significant impact on a patient's lifestyle. Referral to a social worker will help these patients find and access the help and resources they need for rehabilitation and support. (See Chapter 1 for descriptions of various professionals in the health care field who work in rehabilitation.)

Patients with a severe eye injury may have cosmetic issues, which can have a deep effect on them psychologically. A low vision specialist, contact lens specialist, and ocularist, as well as mental health professionals, may be called on to help these patients. The whole health care team is needed to provide support for these patients and their families.

CHAPTER QUIZ

1. True/False: Double vision can occur after blunt eye trauma.

2. True/False: A hyphema is an intravitreal hemorrhage.

3. True/False: Infraorbital nerve damage can cause numbness on the cheek area.

4. True/False: The ophthalmic assistant may put numbing eye drops to relieve eye pain after suspected penetrating eye injury.

5. True/False: The eye care technician should not assure the patient about his/her condition and prognosis.

6. True/False: Acid burns of the cornea are more dangerous than alkali burns.

7. True/False: Endophthalmitis is a bilateral uveal tract inflammation.

8. True/False: Blowing the nose should be discouraged after a blowout orbital fracture.

9. True/False: Either hypotony or high intraocular pressure is a possible complication after chemical eye injury.

10. True/False: Eye irrigation should be done immediately after a chemical eye injury.

11. True/False: Lid laceration is categorized as an emergency case.

12. True/False: Post-traumatic acute bacterial endophthalmitis carries an excellent prognosis of full recovery.

13. True/False: Exposure to ultraviolet, infrared, and X-radiation can be harmful to the eye.

14. True/False: It is recommended to use single-dose eye drop bottles after eye injury.

Answers

1. True, Muscle entrapment after a blowout fracture will limit extraocular muscle movement and cause diplopia.

2. False, Hyphema is blood accumulation in the anterior chamber.

3. True, The infraorbital nerve supplies the lower lid, side of the nose, and cheek.

4. False, Instilling eye drops in the case is contraindicated because it carries the risk of introducing infection to the eyeball.

5. True, This is the doctor's responsibility.

6. False, Alkaline (basic) chemicals penetrate more deeply than acid and lead to more damage.

7. False, Bilateral uveal tract inflammation is sympathetic ophthalmia.

8. True, Doing so may force air and bacteria into the orbit.

9. True

10. True, Irrigation should be done as quickly as possible after a chemical exposure and continued for at least 20 minutes.

11. False, It is categorized as an urgent case.

12. False, 50% of these cases result in blindness.

13. True

14. True, In contrast, multiple-dose bottles are not considered sterile.

REFERENCES

1. Kuhn F, Pieramici DJ. *Ocular Trauma: Principles and Practice.* New York, NY: Thime Medical Publisher; 2002:14,15,19.

2. National Eye Health Education Program. Sports-related eye injuries: what you need to know and tips for prevention. www.gsa-nutley.org/gsa/Athletics/Archives/Sports%20Related%20Eye%20Injuries.pdf?1444758099. Accessed July 4, 2016.

3. Durland ML. Endophthalmitis. *Clin Microbiol Infect.* 2013;19(3):227-234. doi:10.1111/1469-0691.12118.

4. Long C, Liu B, Xu C, Jing Y, et al. Causative organisms of post-traumatic endophthalmitis: a 20-year retrospective. *BMC Ophthalmology.* 2014;34. doi:10.1186/14712415-14-34.

5. Kanski JJ. *Clinical Ophthalmology.* 4th ed. Oxford, England: Butterworth-Heinemann; 1999.

6. Mishra A, Verma AK. Sports related ocular injuries. *Med J Armed Forces India.* 2012;68(3):260-266. doi:10.1016/j.mjafi.2011.12.004.

7. Vinger PF. The mechanisms and prevention of sports eye injuries. www.lexeye.com/UserFiles/The-Mech-and-Prev-of-Sports-Eye-Injuries.pdf. Accessed July 4, 2016.

8. Palmer S. Shaken baby syndrome. The Arc website. www.thearc.org/what-we-do/resources/fact-sheets/shaken-baby-syndrome. Revised 2009. Accessed July 4, 2016.

9. Yulish M, Pikkel J. Motor vehicle accident eye injuries in northern Israel. *Int J Environ Res Public Health*. 2014:11(4);4311-4315. doi:10.3390/ijerph110404311<.

10. Armstrong GW, Chen AJ, Linakis JG, et al. Motor vehicle crash-associated eye injuries presenting to U.S. emergency departments. *West J Emerg Med*. 2014;15(6):693-700.

11. Eye injuries at home. *EyeSmart Newsletter*. American Academy of Ophthalmology website. www.aao.org/eye-health/tips-prevention/injuries-in-home. Accessed July 4, 2016.

12. ANSI/ISEA Z87.1-2015. https://safetyequipment.org/standard/ansiisea-z87-1-2015/. Posted June 22, 2015. Accessed July 4, 2016.

13. Stein HA, Slatt BJ, Stein RM. *The Ophthalmic Assistant: A Guide for Ophthalmic Medical Personnel*. 7th ed. St Louis, MO: Mosby; 2000:432.

BIBLIOGRAPHY

Levin LA, Nilsson SFE. *Adler's Physiology of the Eye*. 11th ed. Philadelphia, PA: Mosby Elsevier; 2011.

Scott R. The ocular trauma score. *Comm Eye Health*. 2015;28(91):44-45.

Unver YB, Kapran Z, Acar N, Altan T. Ocular trauma score in open-globe injuries. *J Trauma*. 2009;66(4):1030-1032. doi:10.1097/TA.0b013e3181883d83.

Yaniv B, Belkin M. Laser eye injuries. *Surv Ophthalmol*. 2000;44(6):459-478. doi:10.1016/S0039-6257(00)00112-0.

Unless otherwise noted, the figures in this chapter were contributed by the following, who are associated with this book as authors:
Adel Ebraheem: Figure 32-12
Sergina M. Flaherty: Figure 32-3
Al Lens: Figure 32-10

33

NONTRAUMATIC OCULAR EMERGENT AND URGENT SITUATIONS

Gayle Roberts, COMT, BHS

When emergencies present to an eye care office, it is often the responsibility of the auxiliary staff to gauge the severity of the patient's problems. Techs who are comfortable with screening these types of situations may be assigned to triage as a regular rotation in their duties. Triage, according to the *Merriam-Webster Dictionary*, is defined as "the sorting of patients (as in an emergency room) according to the urgency of their need for care."[1]

All allied ophthalmic personnel (AOP) should be familiar with handling emergencies in a variety of ways. Often, the more acute, or recent, the onset of symptoms, the more urgent the situation. Red flags include pain, loss of vision, and systemic symptoms (ie, vomiting, fever, chills). In the case of trauma, the triage process is probably easy: come to the office or go to the emergency room *now* (see Chapter 32).

But not all ocular emergencies involve trauma. Such cases may not be so clear cut as, say, a lid laceration. Yet they may be even more sight-threatening. Many of the symptoms patients describe can implicate a number of possible causes. To complicate matters, patients tolerate levels of discomfort differently and what one may brush off as a slight irritation may totally incapacitate another. As AOP it is not our job to diagnose the problem when triaging these calls, but rather to weigh which problems need evaluation sooner than others. Possessing a working understanding of the origins of potential problems greatly assists in efficiently scrutinizing these situations.

When in doubt regarding whether or not to bring a patient in for an evaluation, you might have the doctor speak directly with the patient. This will allow the practitioner to make the determination and alert him/her to the situation. If the doctor is not available, err on the side of caution and fit the patient into the day's schedule. In the grand scheme of things, seeing that "one more patient" may result in a vision-saving outcome.

BASIC SCIENCES

A strong background in ocular anatomy (Chapter 2) and physiology (Chapter 3) is needed for understanding nontraumatic emergencies, so please review this material as necessary. In addition, knowledge of various ocular disorders and conditions will be invaluable in discerning what is an emergency...and what isn't.

CLINICAL KNOWLEDGE

The urgency of any situation may be broken down into three basic categories. The first is *emergent*. As the

Ledford JK, Lens A, eds.
*Principles and Practice in Ophthalmic Assisting:
A Comprehensive Textbook* (pp 573-591).
© 2018 Taylor & Francis Group.

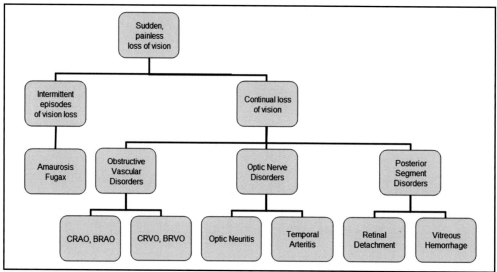

Figure 33-1. Differential diagnosis of sudden painless vision loss.

name implies, these are emergency cases requiring immediate attention. The second is *urgent*. These are problems that should be seen within a day. The final group is *routine*. They are longer-standing problems that may be attended to at the next available appointment. The focus of this chapter is the first two groups.

Emergent situations may be traumatic or nontraumatic. Traumatic ocular injuries are discussed in depth in Chapter 32.

Emergent referrals to the eye care practitioner come from many sources including other physicians, urgent care clinics, and hospital emergency rooms. These are cases that require immediate attention, probably on arrival, to avoid compromising the patient's vision or well-being.

The next level of severity in screening ocular emergencies is referred to as the *urgent* situation. The danger of imminent ocular damage or vision loss is not as high as the emergent classification, but should still be considered serious. The symptoms of an urgent case can share common elements with those of an emergent condition, sometimes making it difficult to distinguish between the two. Under these circumstances, it is wise to consult with the physician to make the determination. Erring on the side of caution is always good policy. The urgent case is one that should be seen in the office within 24 hours.

Eye problems can be roughly categorized into three categories: abnormalities in vision, abnormal appearance, and abnormal sensation/pain. This chapter will be divided using these headings with two exceptions: the painful red eye and the postoperative eye. These topics each have a section all their own.

Changes in Vision

Sudden, Painless Loss of Vision (Figure 33-1)

Of particular concern are those situations that produce a sudden, painless loss of vision. This usually occurs in one eye, but rarely does occur in both. Determining whether or not the visual deficit is intermittent or constant will help in forming a differential diagnosis of the problem. It may also help gauge the urgency in seeing the patient.

In such cases, the possibility of a *central retinal artery occlusion* (CRAO) must be in the back of your mind. This ocular emergency is analogous to a cerebral stroke. The same systemic diseases that create risk factors for atherosclerotic heart disease (diabetes, high blood pressure, high cholesterol, temporal arteritis, etc) are also culprits in causing CRAOs. A blood clot or fatty deposit blocks the essential blood supply in the central retinal artery, depriving the retina of oxygen-rich blood, causing ischemia (tissue deprivation) and paleness. The classic clinical finding is a "cherry-red spot" in the macula upon funduscopic evaluation (Figure 33-2). This area remains a rich red color from the choroidal circulation showing through from below. The result is a monocular, complete loss of vision if the central retinal artery is obstructed, or a partial loss of vision if it is a *branch retinal artery occlusion* (BRAO).

Time is of the essence in providing treatment. Optimistically, it should be administered within a very narrow window of 2 to 4 hours of onset. Even with prompt intervention, the prognosis for regaining sight following a CRAO is very poor. Permanent damage occurs to the retina after only 90 minutes of blood deprivation. Patients often do not recognize they are in trouble. Since

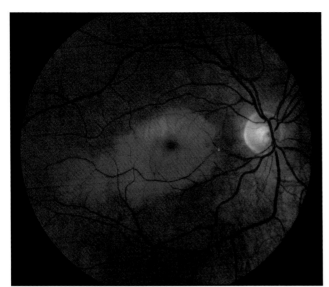

Figure 33-2. Branch retinal artery occlusion with cherry-red spot and Hollenhorst plaque. (Used with permission from the University of Iowa and EyeRounds.org.)

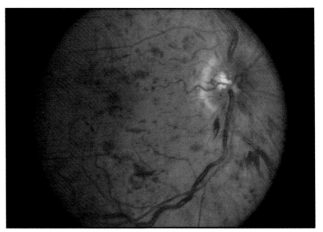

Figure 33-3. Central retinal vein occlusion.

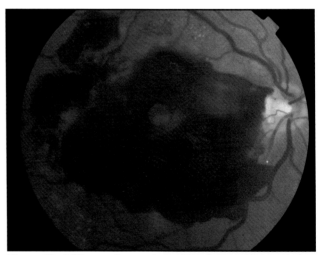

Figure 33-4. Vitreous hemorrhage. (Reprinted with permission from Retina Gallery, http://retinagallery.com.)

they experience no pain and their opposite eye continues to provide vision, the devastating loss in the affected eye may be masked. By the time they do seek attention, the window of opportunity has often passed.

Ophthalmologists will attempt treatment if too much time has not elapsed. The hope is that these measures will dilate the blood vessels, dislodge any clots, and perhaps reestablish blood flow. Treatments include administering certain glaucoma medications or performing a paracentesis (withdrawing fluid from the anterior chamber) in an effort to lower the intraocular pressure (IOP). They may have the patient inhale 5% carbon dioxide gas, followed by massaging the globe. The patient may also be given medication to disintegrate the clot. If these treatments are not delivered expeditiously, there is usually little success in restoring vision loss. However, having a CRAO may alert the patient's medical team to address systemic atherosclerosis, with its increased risk of cerebral stroke and ischemic heart disease.[2]

The central retinal vein is the main vein that carries blood away from the retina. It, too, can become blocked, producing a *central retinal vein occlusion* (CRVO; Figure 33-3). Blockage of smaller retinal veins produce *branch retinal vein occlusions* (BRVOs). The same health modalities that cause CRAOs also contribute to CRVOs—high blood pressure, diabetes, and high cholesterol. In fact, researchers in Denmark have associated an increase in mortality rate in such patients. They recommend referring patients found to have CRVO if they are not already under the watch of a primary care physician for treatment of their systemic disease.[3]

Acute vision loss occurs in CRVOs due to macular edema caused by fluid build-up from a blockage in the vein, preventing the blood from exiting the eye. The long-term outcome varies per patient. Some spontaneously regain most of their vision. Others require intervention with focal laser or vitreal injections of steroids or a vascular endothelial growth factor inhibitor (anti-VEGF), such as Lucentis (ranibizumab) or Eylea (aflibercept). These therapies stabilize leaking blood vessels.

Macular edema and neovascular glaucoma can be persistent complications to the health of the eye following a CRVO. They may not present, though, until months after the initial episode and require continued follow-up care to monitor.

Another cause of sudden vision loss is a *vitreous hemorrhage* (Figure 33-4). The vitreous is a clear, avascular, gelatinous substance that fills the vitreous cavity in the back of the eye. It is separated from the retina by a layer of cells called the internal limiting membrane. Some causes of vitreous hemorrhages are retinal neovascular bleeds due to proliferative diabetes, retinal vein occlusion,

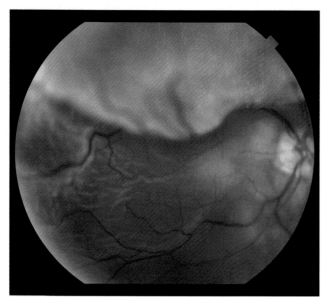

Figure 33-5. Retinal detachment. (Reprinted with permission from Retina Gallery, http://retinagallery.com.)

retinal tears or detachments, sickle cell retinopathy, macular degeneration, and trauma. The symptoms that patients describe when having a vitreous hemorrhage include an onset of floaters, cob web or lace curtain, blurry vision, darkened areas in the visual field, and a reddish hue to the vision.

Upon dilated exam, the view of the retina and the origin of the hemorrhage can be obscured by the blood. To help improve the visibility, patients may be asked to limit activity, avoid using anticoagulants (eg, aspirin), and stay in an upright position even while sleeping until the blood settles and allows for a thorough exam. An ultrasound can help determine if there is a retinal detachment. Depending on the extent of damage, a surgical vitrectomy may be performed to remove the vitreous and repair the retina. Ideally, the body will spontaneously absorb the blood. If not, once visibility improves, treatment is focused on the primary source of the bleed. Laser or cryotherapy may be used to treat retinal tears and holes. Neovascularization is usually treated with laser and/or a VEGF blocker such as Lucentis (ranibizumab). Prognosis depends on how well the underlying cause is managed. If the retina is attached, the patient may be observed in follow-up.

A *retinal detachment* (RD) occurs when the retina pulls away from the back of the eye. The retina adheres to the eye in two places: the ora serrata (behind the iris) and the optic nerve. Fluid can infiltrate the layers of the retina, causing them to separate. It is also possible for the full thickness of the retina to detach. Quadrants of the retina can pull away or it can totally detach (Figure 33-5). Patients often experience floaters or peripheral light flashes prior to the event. Triaging calls from patients with these symptoms can be tricky, as these symptoms

are similar to those describing a vitreous hemorrhage or a posterior vitreous detachment (PVD). In this scenario, it is best to err on the side of caution. Postponing evaluation of patients with these symptoms puts them at risk for a potentially serious vision problem. These types of triage calls are often at 4:00 PM on Friday afternoon. As tempting as it may be to put the patient off until Monday, the patient may permanently lose vision if not treated. Patients should be evaluated as soon as possible in case they need to be referred to see a retinal specialist.

The classic, textbook complaint a patient with an RD describes is an area of vision that is missing, as if a dark curtain has been pulled down, up, or sideways, obscuring part of the vision. The patient may not be aware of any visual impairment since the opposite eye compensates. RDs can happen spontaneously, from traction due to high myopia or retinal disease and by trauma. Detachments that do not involve the macula tend to have better visual outcomes.

Sudden, Painless Blurring of Vision

A sudden blurring of unknown etiology requires further investigation even if there is no pain. Work-up should include thorough history, visual acuities, color vision, meticulous pupil evaluation, and dilation. Visual fields may be ordered as well as a blood work-up to rule out certain autoimmune disorders.

Patients with *subacute angle-closure glaucoma* from narrow angles may have no indications at all, or symptoms including intermittent episodes of blurred vision, ocular pain, and seeing haloes in one or both of their eyes. Corneal edema due to periods of elevated IOP causes these symptoms. The symptoms come and go as the angles alternately open or become shallow but do not completely close. Activities that dilate their pupils, such as driving at night or going to a movie, may exacerbate the symptoms. These patients should be evaluated urgently even though they are not in pain, because they are at risk for going into a full angle-closure attack. In addition to measuring visual acuity, attention should be given to the depth of the anterior chamber and any corneal edema present on slit lamp examination as well as measuring IOPs. Dilation should be deferred until the angles are evaluated by the doctor using gonioscopy.

Patients who suffer with *dry eye* can experience intermittent or continual visual changes. Patients may describe that vision gets blurry when watching television, working on the computer, or reading for long periods. Often they will notice if they look away from the object of interest and blink a few times that their vision is restored. But the cycle keeps repeating itself as they continue these activities. In severe cases, areas of inflammation may occur in the cornea, called *keratitis*, which contribute to distorted or blurred vision. Patients who describe a more continual visual disturbance should be seen sooner to evaluate the corneal surface for damage due to dryness.

Clinical evaluation of vision and the cornea surface, especially by instilling a diagnostic dye (fluorescein, rose bengal, or lissamine green), may help accentuate corneal surface disease.

Curtain Over Part of Vision

Patients who present complaining of seeing a curtain over part of their vision should be evaluated immediately. Their description may range from an opaque, black shade that has been drawn down, up, or side to side. It may appear more as a lace curtain or cob web. Testing should include a thorough history, visual acuity, careful pupil evaluation, careful confrontational fields, measurement of IOPs, and dilation. Several different problems can produce this symptom (PVD, RD, stroke, vitreous heme, or brain tumor). Further clinical evaluation will help determine the underlying cause.

Missing Area of Vision

Patients may discover an area in their vision that is blacked out or missing. The nonaffected eye usually compensates, and the deficit goes undetected until the patient accidentally occludes one eye. Often the patient cannot pinpoint the exact time of onset. It is best for the patient to be seen immediately, with thorough history, visual acuity, meticulous pupil evaluation, and careful confrontational fields as well as an Amsler grid, measurement of IOPs, and dilation. Possible causes of these symptoms include RD, vitreous heme, macular edema, and optic neuritis.

Transient Loss of Vision

Transient loss of vision can be a symptom of a serious process. In cerebrovascular ischemia, blood cannot reach the brain, depriving the brain of adequate nutrients and oxygen. Temporary loss of vision in one or both eyes may be one of several symptoms patients describe.

Small retinal arteriolar emboli may interfere with the proper blood flow to the eye itself, resulting in intermittent vision loss. These episodes are often precursors to permanent retinal arteriolar strokes. Often referred to as *amaurosis fugax*, the blood flow to the retina of one eye is blocked, indicating the presence of a plaque in the carotid artery. Amaurosis fugax is an early warning sign of an impending stroke.[4] Although it does not cause permanent vision loss, continued observation and treating the carotid artery disease is recommended. Patients who call with these complaints warrant emergent attention.

The *ocular aura* of an *ophthalmic migraine* may produce temporary, bilateral loss of vision. Patients may see a scintillating scotoma, or swirls of colorful light as if looking through a kaleidoscope, which is seen with eyes opened or closed. They may also report areas of vision missing. Usually the episodes last for 20 to 30 minutes

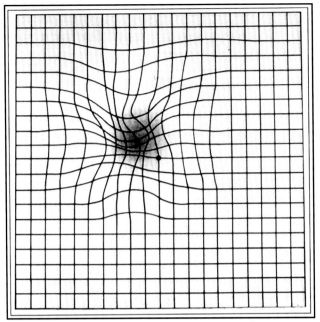

Figure 33-6. Distorted Amsler grid. (Reprinted with permission from the National Eye Institute/National Institutes of Health.)

before spontaneously resolving. Treating patients urgently, within 24 hours, is appropriate.

Amsler Change in Patients With Macular Degneration

Patients with macular degeneration are usually given an Amsler grid so they can monitor their vision at home. At some point, they may detect sudden distortion when testing their central field with the grid (Figure 33-6). This urgent situation may potentially indicate a worsening retinal problem. Patients may not show much distress since they have become accustomed to these persistent symptoms. Regardless of their demeanor, however, further investigation is required to rule out new pathology or progression of the primary diagnosis by checking visual acuity, performing a confrontational field evaluation (in addition to an Amsler grid), checking the pupils, measuring the IOPs, and dilating.

Floaters/Flashes

A fairly common complaint patients will seek attention for is the onset of *floaters* and *peripheral light flashes*. Usually these occur in one eye, with patients describing various shapes of floaters, including spots, bugs, hairs, worms, and webs. Sometimes they are black, while others see them as translucent. The peripheral light flashes appear as lightening streaks or as an arc. They are often more apparent at night or if the patient changes body position.

Although seeing a few floaters is usually benign, a shower of floaters with peripheral light flashes could be symptoms of a posterior vitreous separation/detachment or possible RD. Patients should have an urgent evaluation of their visual acuity, careful confrontational fields, meticulous check of pupils, measurement of IOPs, and dilation to rule out retinal problems.

Patients may have difficulty describing their symptoms. They may complain of seeing flashing lights, but upon further investigation you learn that they actually see brightly colored, diffracted lights as if looking through broken glass or a kaleidoscope. The lights occur in both eyes and appear whether their eyes are opened or closed. The flickering lights may begin small, in one area of their vision, and expand and move over the course of a 20- to 30-minute period. This is a typical description of the *aura of an ocular migraine* and may occur independently, precede, or accompany a migraine headache.

In contrast, a *retinal migraine* has similar symptoms, but occurs in only one eye. The transient visual disturbance may be fleeting or prolonged. The retinal migraine headache usually begins within 1 hour of the onset of visual symptoms and develops on the side of the head where the visual changes occur.[5] When encountering either of these situations, patients often believe they are experiencing a stroke. In this instance it is best to bring the patient in for evaluation on an emergent basis to alleviate his/her fears, as well as rule out any serious pathology, with a complete ocular examination.

Haloes Around Lights

Patients may call complaining of seeing haloes around lights. Key questions include asking how long they have been experiencing this, does it occur with their glasses on or off, are they aware of it only at night or is it present during the day, and whether they wear contact lenses.

If the haloes appear as rainbows, it can signify the presence of *corneal edema*. When the cornea swells, light is diffracted into its color components, thus the appearance of rainbows. Some conditions that cause corneal edema include angle-closure glaucoma, contact lens overwear, corneal endothelial dystrophies, inflammatory processes such as herpetic keratitis, toxic reaction to the preservative benzalkonium chloride (BLK) found in many eye drops, or trauma from injury or surgery. Symptoms such as these prompt emergent evaluation.

If inquiry finds that the haloes occur around lights only at night and are without color, it is more indicative of a *media opacity*. Haloes around car headlights after dark are a common finding when cataracts are present. Performing a glare test (Chapter 8) quantifies this symptom and plays a key role in diagnosing a clinically significant cataract or posterior capsular opacity. Usually a complaint of this nature has a more gradual onset and presents more of an urgent assessment vs emergent.

In addition to haloes, patients may also describe a "starburst" effect around lights, especially at night. As with haloes, a glare evaluation may indicate a heightened sensitivity to light in patients with cataracts. Starbursts

may also be a symptom described by patients who have uncorrected astigmatism. The aspherical shape of an astigmatic cornea causes incoming light to be unequally refracted to two different focal points, usually 90 degrees away from each other. If left uncorrected, images appear distorted and are exacerbated by lights at night.

Diplopia

Persistent or sudden onset of *diplopia* (double vision) should be checked within 24 hours. It can indicate the presence of a viral infection, tumor, stroke or aneurysm, or a diabetic event affecting the function of one of the six extraocular muscles or the nerves that supply them (Table 33-1; see also Chapter 10). Patients suffering with myasthenia gravis, multiple sclerosis, Parkinson's disease, and thyroid conditions can also experience diplopia.

Patients (usually adults) will complain of seeing two distinct images, either side by side or one above the other. They may also feel nauseated and off balance. Clarify that indeed the doubling occurs binocularly and thus goes away if the patient closes one eye. Patients may be sent for a CT scan or MRI to identify the problem's source. Treating the underlying cause may alleviate symptoms. Otherwise, patients are observed for 6 months for improvement. Prism incorporated into the patient's glasses may temporarily relieve the diplopia. Strabismus surgery may eventually be indicated to restore ocular alignment if it does not resolve spontaneously. See Chapter 10 for more on palsies and diplopia.

Loss of Glasses/Contact Lenses

While patients consider losing or breaking their glasses or running out of contact lenses an emergency, the eye clinic may not hold the same belief. If there is a prescription for glasses or contact lenses under 1 year old on record, with good vision documented, this can be given to the patient. However, when a prescription is older than 1 year, or if the patient has cataracts or other medical conditions that could affect vision, it is best to bring the patient in for a new refraction.

Depending on the policy of the office, the time frame for scheduling can range from fitting the patient in within a day to setting an appointment a few weeks out. The urgency of this appointment can depend on the severity of the patient's refractive error and how reliant he/she is on the glasses.

Presbyopes who have lost their reading glasses may be appeased by suggesting they purchase some over-the-counter readers to tide them over until they can be seen. Unfortunately, some contact lens patients do not have an up-to-date pair of glasses to fall back on and will often complain adamantly if they cannot be seen immediately. Those with high refractive errors will truly be incapacitated without proper correction.

		TABLE 33-1		
		CHARACTERISTICS OF OCULAR NERVE PALSIES		
Type of Palsy	**Image**	**Muscle(s) Involved**	**Findings**	**Etiology**
Third		All except LR and SO	4 D's: Diplopia, droopy eyelid, down and out position of eye, dilated pupil	Diabetes mellitus, hypertension (vascular disorders), aneurysm (especially with pupil involvement)
Fourth		SO	Vertical diplopia, patient often assumes head posture to compensate	Trauma (known as the "trauma" nerve) Rare: Stroke, tumor, aneurysm
Sixth		LR	Horizontal diplopia, eye turned in, cannot ABduct (move eye outward)	Stroke, diabetes mellitus, inflammation, viral illness, trauma, increased intracranial pressure, migraine headache, brain tumor

Painful Red Eye

There are numerous causes of a red eye (Figure 33-7). Some are more serious than others. When pain is also a factor, the decision between emergent and urgent becomes even more important. Asking specific triage questions helps differentiate between more emergent causes with those less pressing and tapers down the broad etiology.

The onset of ocular pain and redness may be symptoms of an *angle-closure glaucoma* attack. This is considered the "granddaddy" of painful, red eyes. It is a true ocular emergency, and is the reason that *any* painful red eye is taken seriously. Did the pain and redness occur suddenly? Is there loss of vision? Does the patient have nausea and stomach upset? In acute angle-closure glaucoma, the aqueous is unable to exit the eye as it normally should through the trabecular meshwork. Fluid accumulates within the eye, quickly causing the IOP to spike, placing the patient in a medical emergency. Symptoms often include ocular pain, loss of vision, haloes around lights, a mid-dilated pupil, a red eye, a headache, nausea, and vomiting. Upon presentation, the patient will be visibly ill, the cornea hazy, and the pupil mid-dilated. The vision will be poor and the IOPs will be elevated above 21 mm Hg, reaching as high as 60 mm Hg.[6] If the IOP is not lowered, permanent damage to the optic nerve will result, with loss of peripheral vision.

Pain and redness along with photophobia (light sensitivity) may indicate a form of *uveitis*, an internal inflammation of the eye. *Iritis* is the most common presentation of uveitis. Symptoms can develop acutely or gradually and are the result of iris spasms that accompany the inflammatory process. Patients with iritis typically complain of ocular pain and photophobia, and have a salmon-pink flush around the limbus. The pupil may be irregularly shaped or small due to iris spasms. Inflammatory cells are usually visible in the anterior chamber. Iritis can occur spontaneously as an isolated incident or as a result of injury to the eye. It may recur if it is associated with an autoimmune disorder such as rheumatoid arthritis or lupus.

The redness seen with scleritis or episcleritis is more spread out across the sclera than that seen in iritis, with pronounced blood vessels. While some patients may only complain of the redness, others may describe fullness and tenderness (as if the globe is "tight" in the socket), especially upon ocular movement. Both inflammations involve the outer protective layers of the eye. Although the cause is unknown, episcleritis and scleritis often emerge with active systemic autoimmune disorders. The appearance may mimic an early onset of conjunctivitis.

Pain, redness, and light sensitivity are symptoms of *keratitis*, or inflammation of the cornea. Possible causes of corneal inflammation include severe dry eyes, ocular infections, allergic reactions, and contact lens misuse. If only one eye is affected, the problem could be an infection, such as Herpes or cellulitis. If both eyes are symptomatic, it can indicate an allergic response. If the patient wears contact lenses and slept in them, a corneal ulcer or abrasion may be suspected.

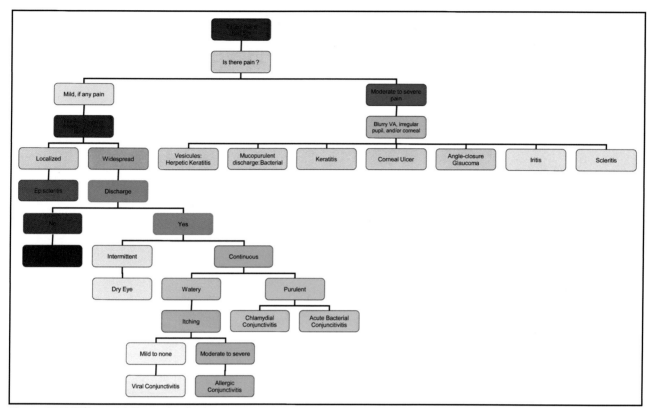

Figure 33-7. Differential diagnosis of red eye.

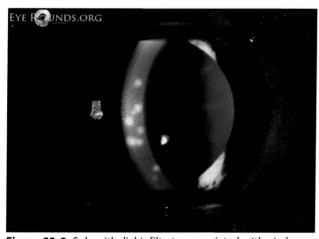

Figure 33-8. Subepithelial infiltrates associated with viral conjunctivitis. (Used with permission from the University of Iowa and EyeRounds.org.)

Several ocular infections can cause redness and discomfort. *Periorbital* and *orbital cellulitis* present as redness around the eye, with lid swelling and pain. While periorbital redness may be related to the presence of a sty, orbital cellulitis is more serious and can be indicative of a sinus infection or abscess. Because of the proximity of the eye and sinuses to the brain, cellulitis can be potentially dangerous.

The various types of *conjunctivitis* can also produce redness. Bacterial conjunctivitis can affect one or both eyes and is accompanied by a purulent discharge. Viral conjunctivitis (Figure 33-8), as with *Herpes zoster*, affects one eye. However, if caused by the adenovirus or *Herpes simplex*, both eyes can be affected. Allergic conjunctivitis also affects both eyes, with the additional symptoms of itching, burning, and tearing. (See Chapter 26.)

Abnormal Sensations/Pain

Painful Eye

Everyone has different tolerance levels for pain. Ocular pain is no different. If the patient includes pain as one of the symptoms, it is usually best to bring him/her in for evaluation to rule out a serious problem and possibly prevent the condition from worsening (Table 33-2).

When questioning patients, try to have them rank the discomfort they're experiencing on a scale of 1 to 10, where 1 is hardly noticeable and 10 is most severe. This will gauge how much distress the patient is in. Try to determine if the pain is constant or intermittent, a dull ache, or sharp/shooting, and whether it is the globe itself that hurts or just around the eye. (See also the previous section on the red painful eye.)

TABLE 33-2

PAINFUL OCULAR EMERGENCIES

Problem	Pain	Blurred Vision	Light Sensitive	Redness	Swelling	Physical Signs	Causes	How It Is Treated
Acute iritis	√	√	√	√ Ciliary flush		Cells in anterior chamber, small or irregular-shaped pupil	Imflammation due to trauma or surgery, infection or autoimmune process	Topical steroids, treat underlying cause
Episcleritis	√ Especially with eye movement	√	√	√		Redness, tortuous conjunctival vessels	Possible autoimmune process	Topical corticosteroids, nonsteroidal anti-inflammatories, treat underlying cause
Optic neuritis	√ Periorbital	√ Decreased visual acuity, decreased color visual acuity				Relative afferent pupillary defect	Inflammatory response in central nervous system, can be idiopathic, multiple sclerosis	Oral and intravenous corticosteroids
Corneal ulcer	√ With foreign body sensation	√ Depends on corneal location	√ Possibly	√ Possibly	√ Possibly	Visible upon slit lamp exam, if large can see with naked eye	Erosion of cornea due to infection, complication of severe dry eyes, contact lens use, autoimmune disorder	Aggressive use of topical antibiotics, possible intravenous antibiotics, debride ulcer, corneal transplant
Angle-closure glaucoma attack	√	√	√	√		Hot, steamy cornea; mid-dilated pupil; shallow anterior chamber; nausea; vomiting; headache	Channels for aqueous to exit eye blocked, ophthalmic emergency	Pilocarpine 2%, timolol 0.5%, Diamox (acetazolamide), glycerin, or isosorbide all to lower IOP; peripheral iridotomy
Orbital cellulitis	√ Especially with eye movement	√	√	√	√ May extend to eyebrow and cheek	Proptosis, purplish eyelid, fever, malaise	Bacteria from sinus infection	Hospitalized with intravenous antibiotics, drain abscess
Suspected endophthalmitis	√	√		√	√	Greater than usual postoperative inflammation, hypopyon	Bacterial or fungal infection of vitreous following surgery, vitreal injection, trauma	Intravitreal antibiotics, if visual acuity is light perception, then pars plana vitrectomy

Optic neuritis produces periorbital pain and sudden vision loss (Figure 33-9). An acute onset is typically seen with demyelinating disorders (which attack the sheath around the nerve fibers), inflammation, inadequate blood flow, and trauma.[7] Patients with autoimmune disorders such as multiple sclerosis, sarcoidosis, and systemic lupus are also vulnerable for developing optic neuritis. Certain infections such as Lyme disease or herpes also place patients at higher risk.[8] AOP should be meticulous when checking the patient's pupils to look for a relative afferent pupillary defect (RAPD). Color vision should also be evaluated.

Similarly, *retrobulbar neuritis* is an inflammation of the optic nerve fibers where they leave the eye and enter the visual pathway in the brain. This swelling disrupts the transmission of signals to the visual cortex, causing impaired vision. Patients with these symptoms should be evaluated immediately. Intravenous steroid therapy may be used to treat both optic and retrobulbar neuritis.

Giant cell or *temporal arteritis* is an inflammatory vascular disorder often affecting the temporal artery, thus the name. It is considered a neuro-ophthalmic emergency, requiring immediate attention. It usually affects patients over age 50 years, with onset of a severe headache located over the temple, an elevated erythrocyte sedimentation rate (aka sed rate, a blood test used to monitor inflammation), and a positive finding of inflamed or damaged tissue from a temporal artery biopsy. Blindness occurs when the blood vessels swell and cut off blood to the optic nerve, producing *arteritic anterior ischemic optic neuropathy* (AAION; Figure 33-10). If caught early, high-dose steroid treatment may restore vision in the affected eye and prevent the process from occurring in the second eye, which may become involved within 24 hours if treatment is delayed.[9]

Possible causes of ocular pain include nontrauma-induced *foreign body sensation*. Insult to the anterior segment from dry eyes, ocular allergies, blepharitis, pterygium or pinguecula, or meibomian gland dysfunction can all produce an uncomfortable, scratchy sensation in the eyes ("grit in the eyes"). Contact lens wearers may state that their eyes feel fine while their contacts are on, but become painful once the lenses are removed. In this case, the contact lenses may be acting as a bandage that masks a corneal surface problem.

Patients may describe their discomfort as *pressure* in or around their eyes. Since the eyes are surrounded by the sinuses, environmental changes in barometric pressure can contribute to the sinuses filling or draining. This can create a pressure sensation that may feel like it originates from the eyes. Sinus or migraine headaches may be the underlying cause. Patients with open-angle glaucoma usually are *not* aware of the elevated IOP in their eyes. However, some are sensitive to fluctuations or prolonged elevations, and report periorbital pressure. In addition, patients who have subconjunctival hemorrhages may express they feel a "fullness" around the eye. Swelling of the ocular adnexa can also result in pressure on the globe.

Heightened sensitivity to light, or *photophobia*, also produces ocular pain. Patients often present wearing dark sunglasses or holding a cloth over their eyes to shield them from light. Possible causes of photophobia include iritis, keratitis, and a plethora of ocular infections.

Both forms of *herpetic eye disease*, zoster and simplex, are viral infections that produce ocular pain, redness, and corneal lesions. Herpetic inflammation of the nerve sheath triggers intense pain along the nerve fibers.[10] Reactivation of the dormant varicella zoster virus produces a red rash or outbreak of blister-like lesions occurring on one side of the face and around the eye. A lesion appearing on the tip of the nose, called *Hutchinson's sign*, predicts a greater incidence of ocular involvement (Figure 33-11). While herpes zoster is unilateral, herpes simplex can affect one or both eyes. Excessive tearing and dendritic ulcers are hallmark findings with herpes simplex keratitis (Figure 33-12).

In addition to herpes, eye infections frequently emerge from the adenovirus, which causes the common cold. Not only does it produce ocular discomfort, but may also blur patients' vision and produce a watery discharge. Patients will often have had a recent upper respiratory infection with congestion and a runny nose. The infection usually begins in one eye and then affects the second eye within a week. Commonly referred to as "pink eye," it is highly contagious. Patients should be encouraged to practice precautions of frequent hand washing and not sharing towels or pillow cases in an attempt to limit contamination.

Other ocular infections also elicit pain and usually present with accompanying symptoms. Patients with bacterial infections complain of pain, decreased vision, and a purulent discharge, often crusting their eyelids closed. These infections are often caused by normal flora of the skin, like *Staphyloccocus aureus*. Rarely, the eye can be attacked by virulent bacteria, such as *Pseudomonas aeruginosa*, which can destroy an eye within days. *Pseudomonas* can be found in contaminated mascara and contact lens solutions. The moist containers are the perfect environment for this bacterium to grow.

Rare infections that produce pain in the eye are those caused by fungi and *Acanthamoeba*. Patients contract a fungal infection by an injury involving plant material (Figure 33-13). Their history is usually an account of doing yard work and getting whacked in the eye by a branch. Along with pain, there is decreased vision, photophobia, and excessive tearing. Fungal infections are resistant to treatment, and failure to respond to antifungal therapy often results in a need for a later corneal transplant surgery.[11]

Acanthamoeba keratitis is a parasitic infection seen mostly in contact lens wearers. This amoeba naturally

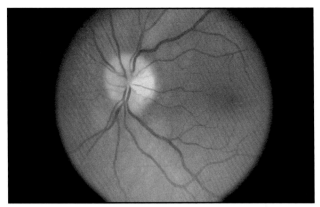

Figure 33-9. Optic neuritis.

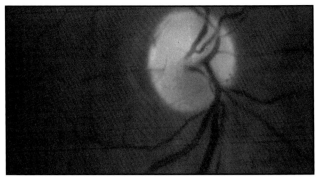

Figure 33-10. Arteritic anterior ischemic optic neuropathy. (Reprinted with permission from Duncan Anderson, Jason Barton, and www.neuroophthalmology.ca.)

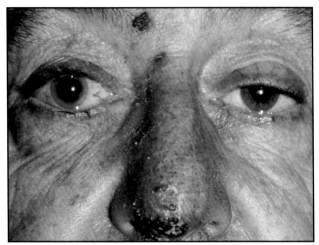

Figure 33-11. Herpes zoster ophthalmicus with Hutchinson's sign. (Reprinted with permission from Piotr Brzezinski, MD, PhD.)

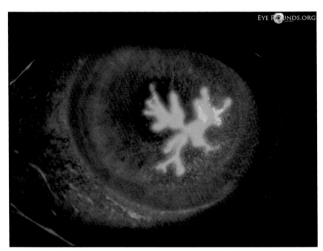

Figure 33-12. Herpes simplex virus dendrite. (Used with permission from the University of Iowa and EyeRounds.org.)

seeks out wet places to live: pools, showers, hot tubs, tap water, and unpreserved contact lens solutions. Contact lens patients who do not remove their lenses prior to exposure to any of these environments, who use tap water to rinse their lenses, or who make their own saline solution are at risk. Ask questions regarding the patients' contact lens hygiene habits as well as if they swim or use a hot tub while wearing the lenses. Teaching proper contact lens handling and disinfection methods helps reduce the likelihood of contracting this infection.

Photophobia

Photophobia is an abnormal intolerance to light. Patients will complain that light elicits extreme discomfort, excessive tearing, and the inability to keep their eyes open. Photophobia may be the result of a long list of inflammatory processes affecting the anterior segment. Infection, extreme dryness, or edema may disrupt the corneal integrity, creating surface irregularity that diffracts incoming light, scattering it and possibly

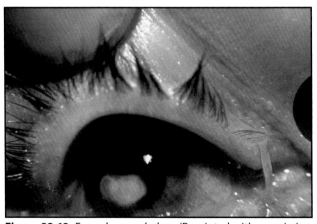

Figure 33-13. Fungal corneal ulcer. (Reprinted with permission from the Centers for Disease Control and Prevention/Brinkman.)

magnifying it. The corneal nerve stimulation relays distressed impulses in the form of photosensitivity. The internal inflammatory cells seen with iritis create a similar state of diffraction, along with ciliary spasm, making the eye photophobic and painful.

In addition, albinism and certain retinal dystrophies can affect the normal ocular pigmentation that protects against excessive bright light. Patients suffering with certain medical conditions, such as migraine headaches, pituitary tumors, head trauma, or meningitis, exhibit photophobia due to the insult to the brain. Although there is no actual ocular involvement, patients attribute the light sensitivity as originating from their eyes and often first seek attention from an eye care physician in their quest for relief.

Pain on Movement

Patients may describe discomfort upon moving their eyes. Looking in extreme gazes or using their eyes for prolonged periods may aggravate the aching. Eye movement worsens the pain due to inflammation of the extraocular muscle insertions into the sclera.[12] Patients may state that their eye actually feels swollen and seems "tight" when moving within the socket. Possible explanations include scleritis or episcleritis, orbital cellulitis, and optic neuritis. The discomfort stems from the inflammatory process precipitating the condition.

Foreign Body Sensation

Patients will often describe feeling as if their eyes have sand or gravel in them. The discomfort may be chronic or intermittent and vary in severity. Periodic bouts of foreign body sensation can occur with *blepharitis*, an inflammation of the eyelids. The inflammation may be caused by seborrheic dermatitis (causing dandruff of the eyelashes), acne rosacea, a bacterial infection, meibomian gland dysfunction, allergies, or lice. Prophylactic warm compresses and regular lid hygiene, or lid scrubs, will help reduce accumulation of dandruff and bacteria on the eyelids.

Patients who suffer with *dry eye* may also experience sporadic grittiness. Dry eye syndrome causes the tear film to lack the proper balance of mucus, lipid, and aqueous layers necessary to lubricate and cleanse the ocular surface. Instead of adequately flushing away any microscopic debris, each blink scrapes these particles across the surface of the eye. The result is irritated, scratchy-feeling eyes. Regular use of over-the-counter lubricating eye drops can help alleviate symptoms.

Environmental pollens or sensitivity to certain foods, pet dander, or skin products may elicit an ocular *allergic reaction*. Symptoms may occur seasonally or throughout the year. The allergen provokes an autoimmune, inflammatory response in the conjunctiva. The angry tissue feels rough and irritated, as if something is in the eye. However, the more the eye is rubbed in an attempt to ease

the symptoms, the more irritated it becomes. Patients may find relief by using ocular (in the form of eye drops) as well as oral antihistamines.

Possible causes of sustained foreign body sensation include corneal ulcers, corneal erosions, an actual foreign body in the eye, or a herpes infection. Disruption to the corneal epithelium creates the impression that there is a foreign object in the eye. The cornea has more nerve endings than any other tissue in the body; corneal sensation is a highly sensitive, protective defense mechanism. Patients may localize the origin of the defect to either the nasal or temporal canthal areas, when in fact the actual lesion may be present more centrally in the cornea.

Abnormal Appearance

Swelling

Swelling of the ocular adnexa can be painful, cause redness, and elicit great anxiety for patients because the problem is so visible and cosmetically difficult to conceal. Possible causes include the following.

Orbital cellulitis is a sudden onset of infection in the tissues around the eye (Figure 33-14). It can extend from the brow to the ear and down the cheek. Both upper and lower eyelids swell with fluid-filled abscesses, often to the degree of closing the eye. The lids become red, warm to the touch, and very painful. Patients report feeling physically ill with a fever, lack of energy, and/or malaise. There is also decreased vision and discomfort upon ocular movement. The infection can be the result of *Staphylococcus aureus* or *Streptococcus pneumoniae*. Children may contract it from a sinus infection. It is considered a medical emergency as serious complications can result not only in permanent loss of vision, but also loss of hearing, and the occurrence of meningitis and systemic sepsis.[13]

An *allergic reaction* may precipitate swelling of the ocular tissue. It may be the result of exposure to an ingredient found in cosmetics, lotions, or even laundry detergent. Reactions can occur at any point in a patient's life—even when they have used certain products for years. Other triggers can be environmental, such as pollen, dust, or dander from animals. Patients may also experience adverse reactions to foods (such as shellfish) or medications (certain antibiotics or pain relievers).

The eyes usually itch, which prompts the patient to rub them and exacerbate the swelling. In addition, the eyes may tear excessively, along with a burning sensation and redness.

Patients who are prone to *water retention* can experience swelling in the face and around the eyes. There is usually no pain involved, but the eyes may feel "full" or "heavy." Common causes of fluid retention include diets high in salt and leading a sedentary lifestyle. Medical conditions such as hypothyroidism, hypertension, kidney or liver disease, and diabetes can also produce edema.[14] Swelling can be a side effect of certain medications like steroids, blood pressure or diabetic medications, and birth control pills. Women may suffer with water retention during their menstrual cycles and pregnancy. The edema is not a disease in itself, but a symptom of an underlying condition.

Two fairly common causes of eyelid swelling are *chalazia* and *hordeola*. A chalazion results from inflammation caused when a meibomian gland (oil gland) in the eyelid becomes blocked. If an acute infection of a lash follicle occurs, with redness and pain, it is referred to as a hordeolum or sty. Patients with conditions such as excessively oily skin, blepharitis, meibomian gland dysfunction (MGD), and acne rosacea are more prone to develop chalazia.

Chalazia usually resolve spontaneously within a few weeks, but most patients are alarmed by their appearance and want a fast fix. Application of warm compresses for 10 minutes up to four times a day for several days is a first course of action. Topical antibiotic or steroid ointments may be prescribed, as well as oral antibiotics, to alter the viscosity of the oil produced by the glands. If there is no improvement, surgical removal and/or steroid injection may be recommended to reduce the inflammation and prevent the formation of a granuloma (an inflamed nodular lesion) or scar tissue. Once resolved, incorporating warm compresses and lid scrubs into a daily hygiene regimen is advised to prevent recurrence.

Painless Red Eye

A red eye prompts patients to seek medical attention quickly. When determining how urgently the patient needs to be evaluated, consider whether there is pain or not, as well as the presence of other signs and symptoms (see Table 33-2). There is a lot of overlap of complaints, of which redness is one, in many ocular problems. Some are more serious than others. (Please refer to the section on the painful red eye, earlier in this chapter.)

Probably the most disconcerting cause of redness is a *subconjunctival hemorrhage* (SCH). The source is blood vessels just under the conjunctiva that have leaked. Part, or all, of the white of the eye turns a brilliant red, in an alarming, almost horror-movie appearance (see Figure 26-5). There is no associated pain or loss of vision. Patients may describe a sense of fullness in the orbit. SCH occur spontaneously or from exertion when the patient coughed, sneezed, lifted something heavy, or bent down to pick something up. Patients who use blood thinners, such as aspirin, are more susceptible. The location of the redness may migrate if the patient changes from a reclining to an upright position. As the body reabsorbs the blood, the red may vary in color to green or yellow. Subconjunctival hemorrhages are benign and similar to a bruise, usually resolving within 1 week to 10 days without treatment. Patients usually will insist upon being

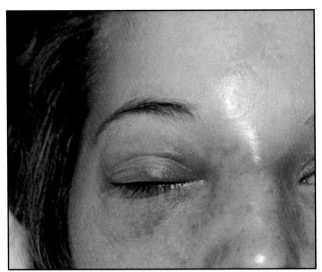

Figure 33-14. Orbital cellulitis. (Reprinted with permission from the Centers for Disease Control and Prevention/Thomas F. Sellers, MD, Emory University.)

evaluated out of fear. In this instance, your clinic may see the patient and reassure him/her it is not as serious as it looks.

Discharge

Discharge from the eyes often prompts patients to seek attention. It may affect one or both eyes and occur chronically or intermittently. Patients may describe waking in the morning with the eyelid crusted closed by debris that has collected overnight. The skin around the eye may become raw, scaly, and irritated from the constant leaking and wiping away of fluid. The consistency of the discharge may shed some light on what the problem is, and help in making triage decisions. These disorders have been described before in this chapter, so we will only present a few notes here.

▶ Iritis: Patients with iritis have light sensitivity, which can trigger reflex tearing.

▶ Infection: Different ocular infections produce a characteristic discharge that distinguishes one type of contaminant from another.

   • Viral: Produces a clear discharge with a watery consistency from one or both eyes. Early in the process, it may be hard to differentiate between an adenovirus (cold virus) or herpes simplex infection, as the tearing will appear similar. *Herpes simplex* can induce decreased corneal sensitivity, or hypoesthesia, which can be tested as long as the cornea has not been anesthetized.

   • Bacterial: Generates a yellow to greenish, purulent (pus-like) and goopy discharge in one or both eyes.

- Allergies: Usually affects both eyes with watery tears, itching, burning, and white mucous strands.

▶ Dry eye: Excessive epiphora, or watery tearing, usually in both eyes. Tears well up and spill onto the cheeks. Patients may also complain of foreign body sensation and intermittent episodes of blurred vision and ocular fatigue, especially after long periods of reading or computer work. They may report that vision clears if they look away and blink several times.

Ptosis

A suddenly droopy eyelid (*ptosis*) can be a sign of a *Bell's palsy*. A Bell's palsy usually is a temporary paralysis to the VII cranial nerve (the facial nerve), which controls blinking, eyelid closure, and facial expression (ie, smiling or frowning). The palsy is caused by an unknown process that results in swelling or compression of CN VII. Not only does the upper eyelid droop, but the cheek and mouth may sag on the affected side as well. Treatment includes antibiotics if there is a suspected infection, prednisone to reduce inflammation, and topical artificial tears or ointment to keep the cornea lubricated. In some cases, the eye must be taped closed at night. In most incidences, patients notice improvement after 2 weeks and most spontaneously resolve in 3 to 6 months. Rarely, the paralysis persists, requiring surgical intervention to improve eyelid closure on the affected side.

A drooping eyelid may also result from a *diabetic third nerve palsy*. An easy way to remember the symptoms is the 4 D's of a diabetic third: droopy eyelid (ptosis), double vision (diplopia), down and out (position of patient's eye), and dilated pupil. As with a Bell's palsy, the patient is usually observed for improvement over 6 months. In the interim, the patient may wear an eye patch or prism glasses to alleviate the double vision. If the problem continues after this period, strabismic surgery to bring single vision in straight-ahead gaze, as well as a ptosis repair to lift the eyelid, may be recommended.

Anisocoria

Anisocoria (difference in size between the pupils) also raises suspicion for a neurologic problem. It may be physiologic, or a normal developmental variant that occurs in 20% of the population, with size disparity being no greater than 1 mm.[15] If the difference exceeds 1 mm, a more serious condition could be the culprit. Tumors, strokes, infections, and aneurysms may manifest with anisocoria. Pupil size should be carefully evaluated in light and dark, as well as looking for constriction with accommodation when the patient views a near target. The smaller pupil is suspect if the discrepancy is greatest in the dark. If the pupil does not enlarge after instilling a dilating agent (cocaine 10%), Horner's syndrome may be the cause. In contrast, the pupil that is larger in bright light is abnormal. If it does not narrow with instillation of

a constricting drop (pilocarpine 1%), then an Adie's tonic pupil, pharmacologically induced mydriasis (dilation), and damage to the iris are possible reasons.

Postoperative Problems

Surgical procedures are considered controlled trauma. Problems such as corneal edema, floaters, or elevated IOP can occur. Other, more serious, conditions such as intraocular hemorrhage, RD, and macular edema can also be present. Despite good clinical practice, complications can arise that AOP should recognize as outside of the usual postoperative course.

Postoperative *endophthalmitis* is a rare bacterial infection that can arise as a complication of intraocular surgery (Figure 33-15). It occurs when microbes from the normal flora of the patient's skin or conjunctiva, or contaminated surgical instruments, enter the eye. Symptoms usually occur within 6 weeks of surgery, but rarely can present months, even years after.[16] Patients present with severe ocular pain, decreased vision, and a red, inflamed eye. The cornea is usually edematous, and a hypopyon, or collection of white blood cells (pus), is visible in the anterior chamber.

A vitreous tap may be performed to identify which organism is responsible for the infection and help decide which treatment modality to follow. Treatment may include a vitrectomy, with the intent of reducing both the bacterial count and inflammatory products inside the eye. Intravitreal, topical, and systemic antibiotics may be administered to fight the infection, as well as corticosteroids to reduce inflammation.

A procedure with a relatively high risk of complication is corneal transplantation. The incidence of graft rejection is greatest during the first year following surgery, with failure seen as early as 2 weeks postoperatively and as long as 20 years post-transplantation. Thirty-five percent of corneal grafts fail within the first 5 years.[17] The symptoms of rejection range from the patient being completely asymptomatic to displaying a decrease in vision, redness, light sensitivity, ocular pain, and irritation. These patients should be seen on an urgent basis.

Rejection can occur in any of the three main layers of the donor tissue, with the stromal layer usually being affected by an endothelial malfunction. In *epithelial failure*, a rejection line may be seen with the slit lamp. This line forms from host epithelium growing into the graft. Presence of subepithelial infiltrates may also indicate an epithelial rejection. *Endothelial rejection* is characterized by an endothelial rejection line, *keratitic precipitates* (deposits of cells on the corneal endothelium), and edema. The edema is caused by the endothelial cells being unable to adequately pump out fluid. There may also be inflammatory cells in the anterior chamber. Treatment of suspected graft failure consists of frequent instillation of

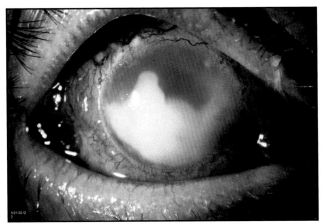

Figure 33-15. Endophthalmitis. (Reprinted with permission from Retina Gallery, http://retinagallery.com.)

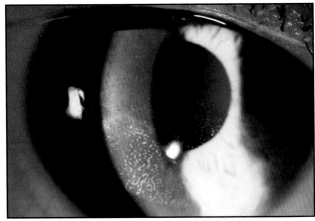

Figure 33-16. Epithelial ingrowth from LASIK. (Used with permission from the University of Iowa and EyeRounds.org.)

corticosteroids. Care must be taken to check the patient's IOP as it may become elevated due to the steroid use.

As of 2011, more than 11 million LASIK procedures had been performed in the United States.[18] LASIK is done by using a *microkeratome* (a special blade) to create a flap of epithelium that is folded back so the corneal tissues underneath can be reshaped with a laser. The epithelium is then returned to its original position. Potential problems associated with this procedure include under- and overcorrection, induced astigmatism, fluctuating vision, glare, and dry eyes.

A rare complication is epithelial in-growth, where the epithelium grows under the flap during the healing process (Figure 33-16). This usually occurs within the first 3 months following surgery. Patients with epithelial in-growth may be asymptomatic but the problem can be observed with the slit lamp during a postoperative visit. As the underlying cells change the corneal topography, patients will complain of decreased vision (due to the increased astigmatism), foreign body sensation, dryness, and light sensitivity.[19] Treatment differs depending on the severity of the problem. Patients may be observed to see if the condition will spontaneously resolve. Topical antibiotics and corticosteroids may be prescribed. In severe cases, surgery involving relifting the flap and scraping away the offending epithelial cells is performed.

CLINICAL SKILLS

It takes experience to effectively and confidently assess emergencies. AOP benefit not only from exposure to different types of pathology they see in the office, but learn by taking continuing education courses as well. Classes offer up-to-date training for common and unusual situations. AOP can acquire pearls of wisdom from other professionals in the field. One such gem is developing an office triage flow sheet to act as a step-by-step

guide (Figure 33-17). It alleviates some of the pressure related to screening emergencies.

Probably the most valuable skill is learning to ask specific questions in a concise manner to determine the nature of the patient's complaint. Extracting key information expedites the entire process. It is a true art, guiding patients to stay focused on relevant information without going off on tangents. The signs and symptoms of specific eye problems tend to follow predictable patterns that AOP learn with experience. A few examples of this include:

▶ People with autoimmune disorders are more prone to iritis or scleritis. Recognizing the symptoms associated with these disorders (redness, photophobia, blurred vision, and discomfort) may efficiently lead AOP to ask patients whether they suffer from one of these conditions. Alternately, the physician may suggest other testing to verify such disorders.

▶ Floaters, peripheral light flashes, cob webs, a lace curtain, or a dark shade occluding the patient's vision typically indicates a retinal problem or vitreous detachment. Asking the patient if he/she is near- or far-sighted is informative since RDs occur more frequently in high myopes. Regardless, the patient needs evaluation to determine the underlying issue.

▶ When triaging a red eye, it is pertinent to ask whether the patient is experiencing other symptoms such as pain, photophobia, or discharge. Also ask if the patient wears contact lenses, or if the patient (or anyone in the household) has had a cold or upper respiratory infection. This is valuable information the physician can use to begin formulating a differential diagnosis.

History Taking

Obtaining a thorough history is fundamental in helping the practitioner focus on the problem at hand. (History

Date: _____   Time: _____
Patient: _____
Date of Birth: _____
Phone Number: _____
Last office visit: _____

Triage done by: _____

Patient's Chief Complaint: _____
_____
_____
_____

Date of onset: _____   Gradual or Sudden
One or both eyes: OD OS OU
Pain: Yes / No   _____/10 on pain scale
Loss of Vision: Yes / No
Other Symptoms: Redness   Yes / No
                     Discharge   Watery / Purulent
                     Other: _____

Injury / Recent Post-op   Date of surgery: _____

Current Eye-related Medications: _____
_____
_____
_____

Plan: _____
_____
_____
_____

Patient Given Appointment: Yes / No   Date: _____

Consulted w/ Dr. _____

Figure 33-17. Example of telephone triage form.

taking is covered in detail in Chapter 7.) According to the Health Care Financing Administration (HCFA) and the American Medical Association (AMA) guidelines, the history should contain four elements: chief complaint (CC), history of present illness (HPI), review of systems (ROS), and past family and/or social history (PFSH).[20]

Emergent situations fall under the category of a problem-focused examination, with attention centered on whatever is pertinent to the problem. The history should include the signs and symptoms of the complaint, the location (which eye), the duration (onset), level of pain (on a scale of 1 to 10, with 10 being the worst), description of the pain (dull ache, sharp, shooting, etc), anything that improves the discomfort, and whether it is getting any better or worse.[21]

An example of a usable medical history is: "Patient walked into office today, complaining of the right eye suddenly becoming blurry at both distance and near since last evening. The right eye has severe, aching 10/10 ocular pain. Patient also has a headache and is nauseated." There is enough information in this example to tailor the patient's examination to address the complaints and help the doctor to formulate a differential diagnosis based

upon the history. (It may ultimately be the physician's responsibility to make certain all the necessary elements are present in the documentation, but providing a good history will expedite that duty.)

Examination

The patient's history will guide the tech in how to approach the emergent/urgent exam. Keep in mind that it is more important for the practitioner to see any pathology than it is for the tech. If the patient is in great distress, attempt to perform only the necessary tests the patient will allow and defer the remainder of the exam to the doctor.

Follow office protocol as far as administering topical anesthetics prior to examining suspected corneal defects. Although these drops will relieve the patient's pain and allow for a more comfortable examination, some practitioners prefer to see the patient first to make that determination. Whenever in doubt, always confirm using any medication or performing any tests with the doctor. If there is a suspicion that the globe has been ruptured, avoid using any eye drops or applying any pressure to the eye.

Certain diagnostic tests are relevant to emergent ocular evaluation. There are "cookbook" protocols that become part of a repertoire to follow depending on the problem (Figure 33-18).

▶ All examinations should include an assessment of visual acuity. If the vision is diminished, a pinhole can distinguish whether the problem is caused by an optical/refractive problem vs an organic disorder. The vision will improve using a pinhole with an optical/refractive defect, but not with an underlying organic problem.

▶ Check the ocular motility when there is any complaint of double vision.

▶ Perform confrontation fields or an Amsler grid as well as pupillary reactions if the suspected problem affects the retina or the visual pathway.

▶ A slit lamp exam, using a fluorescent dye, will help evaluate for suspected surface problems such as corneal abrasions and ulcers. Inflammatory cells, as seen with iritis, and depth of anterior angles can be visualized as well.

▶ Applanation IOPs may need to be deferred until the practitioner evaluates a corneal abnormality, or in the case of a potentially contagious infection. Otherwise, pressures can be taken as usual, especially in cases of suspected elevated IOP as seen with acute angle-closure glaucoma attacks or iritis.

▶ Any problems involving the posterior segment of the eye (vitreous, retina, or optic nerve) should be evaluated by a dilated exam.

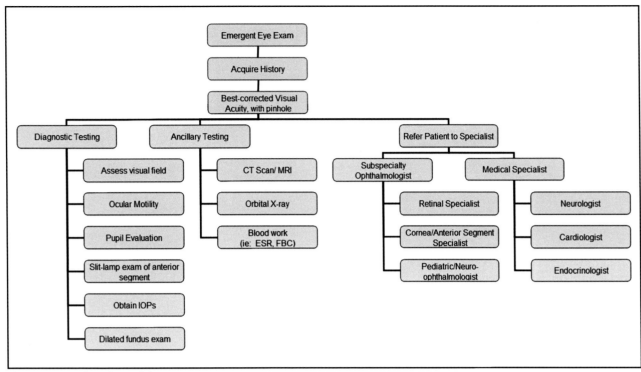

Figure 33-18. Flow chart of the emergent eye exam.

Clinic Preparedness

Being prepared helps reduce the stress associated with the often critical, fast-paced thinking involved in dealing with emergencies. It is always better to be proactive than reactive. Sustaining an up-to-date inventory of emergency supplies is vital. Essential items include an assortment of bandage contact lenses, eye pads and dressings, and access to a well-maintained laser. (The YAG laser is used to perform a peripheral iridotomy in the presence of angle closure glaucoma, while argon laser is employed to coagulate vitreous hemorrhages and repair retinal tears.) Rotating items and watching expiration dates help to prevent unexpected shortages.

The inventory should include easily accessible surgical instruments. Make certain instruments are properly sterilized and package them together by procedure. Kits can be created by labeling 1-gallon plastic storage bags with the names of the various procedures performed in the office. The package can contain 3-x-5 cards listing on one side the contents, including instruments, syringes, needles, alcohol swabs, gauze pads, cotton-tipped applicators, etc. The opposite side lists the step-by-step instructions for the particular procedure. This allows AOP to quickly set up for an emergency procedure and easily refill the kit in preparation for the next.

Preparedness includes a well-stocked medicine cabinet. It should contain appropriate pharmaceuticals to quickly reduce the IOP during an acute angle-closure glaucoma attack, such as acetazolamide tablets, oral glycerin or isosorbide, pilocarpine 2% eye drops, and timolol 0.5% drops.[22] An assortment of antibiotic drops and ointments and anesthetics, as well as nonsteroidal and steroid medications, should also be included. Having both topical and injectable versions of these medications covers even more bases. Although it has not been proven successful, some physicians wish to have certain medications on hand to treat CRAOs. These may include carbachol inhalant gas, IV mannitol or acetazolamide, and clot-busting drugs.[23]

PATIENT SERVICES

No one enjoys spending any more time in a doctor's office than necessary. When emergencies are added into an already-busy clinic schedule, delays are inevitable. Patients become irritated when they have to wait and will often vent their frustration at office staff. If the addition of emergency cases puts the schedule behind, make it a practice to inform patients of the delay as they check in. Patients tend to be more understanding if they are made aware of the wait when they arrive. This empowers the patients to decide whether to stay or to reschedule. Thank the patients for their patience and understanding.

If the emergent patient is forced to wait, try to make him/her as comfortable as possible. Often times they are frightened and look to AOP for reassurance. Ways to calm them may include offering to get a magazine to read or a glass of water (as long as their problem is nonsurgical). If they are nauseous, bring a waste basket or emesis basin and a damp, cool cloth. Dim the room lights if there is photosensitivity. Check in every so often until the doctor sees him/her.

One of the most rewarding, as well as important, duties of being an AOP is educating patients. Patients appreciate hearing instructions while they are in the office and have the chance to ask questions directly. This is a perfect opportunity for techs to demonstrate their eye care knowledge. Techs can teach patients preventative measures such as wearing protective safety goggles or face shields in industry or sports. AOP also instruct patients on the proper handling and cleaning of contact lenses. (This includes explaining circumstances when contacts should be avoided.)

Techs also answer questions regarding the use of medications. They must stay on top of the dosages, possible side effects, and duration of therapy of a barrage of currently prescribed and over-the-counter ocular drugs. Finally, they demonstrate how to perform self-administered treatments such as eyelid scrubs, eye drop instillation, and other after care regimens.

ACKNOWLEDGMENTS

The author would like to thank the following: Barbara Cassin, MEd, CO, COMT (deceased); Diana Shamis, MEd, CO, COMT; Ella Rosamont-Morgan, COMT (deceased); and Dave Taylor, Senior Manager, Medical Marketing at Reichert, Inc.

CHAPTER QUIZ

1. Symptoms are considered more urgent when:
   a. the onset is more recent
   b. they are long-standing
   c. the patient calls to complain frequently
   d. the patient is irate

2. All are examples of true ocular emergencies *except*:
   a. penetrating ocular injury
   b. chemical burn
   c. sudden, painless loss of vision
   d. excessive tearing

3. Treatment must be initiated within hours of onset with which type of painless vision loss?
   a. iritis
   b. chalazion
   c. central retinal artery occlusion
   d. subconjunctival hemorrhage

4. The purpose of triage is:
   a. to schedule routine appointments
   b. to update a patient's medical history
   c. to gauge the urgency of patient's chief complaint
   d. give patients over-the-phone advice

5. Situations considered urgent should be seen within:
   a. 24 hours
   b. 3 to 6 hours
   c. 1 to 2 weeks
   d. 5 days

6. AOP can help prepare for office emergencies by which of the following?
   a. keep an up-to-date inventory of necessary medications
   b. develop an office protocol in dealing with emergencies
   c. take continuing education courses to learn the latest advances
   d. all of the above

7. Which should *not* be scheduled as a routine appointment?
   a. difficulty seeing fine print
   b. intermittent eye strain
   c. occasional headaches
   d. sudden onset of diplopia

8. The elements of a medical history should include all *except*:
   a. location of problem
   b. chief complaint
   c. has no ocular problems at this time
   d. duration of problem

9. What should an AOP do if uncertain whether an emergency patient needs to be seen by the practitioner?
   a. ask the practitioner to speak to the patient
   b. give the patient medical advice over the phone
   c. have the receptionist make a routine appointment
   d. use an opened bottle of eye drops

10. All are common causes of a red eye *except*:
    a. conjunctivitis
    b. iritis
    c. optic neuritis
    d. subconjunctival hemorrhage

Answers

1. a, The more recent the onset of symptoms, usually the more urgent the situation.

2. d, Excessive tearing is not considered a true ocular emergency.

3. c, Treatment for central retinal artery occlusions should be started within hours of when the symptoms begin.

4. c, Gauge the urgency of the patient's problem and determine how quickly the patient needs to be seen.

5. a, Although the immediate risk for loss of vision or damage to the eye is less, urgent situations are still considered serious and should be evaluated within 24 hours.

6. d, All activities listed are helpful in preparing for office emergencies.

7. d, The sudden onset of diplopia can indicate a more serious problem like a stroke, and should be addressed more urgently.

8. c, If the patient has no ocular problems at this time, then what is the reason for the appointment?

9. a, Whenever in doubt, the AOP should ask the practitioner to screen the urgency of a patient's problem.

10. c, Optic neuritis is swelling of the optic nerve and does not cause the exterior of the eye to become red.

REFERENCES

1. Definition of triage. Merriam-Webster website. www.merriam-webster.com/dictionary/triage. Accessed June 11, 2016.

2. Varma DD, Cugati S, Lee AW, Chen CS. A review of central retinal artery occlusion: clinical presentation and management. *Eye.* 2013;27:699-697.

3. Bertelsen M, Linneberg A, Christoffersen N, et al. Mortality in patients with central retinal vein occlusion. *Ophthalmology.* 2014;121(3):637-642.

4. Amaurosis fugax. MedlinePlus website. www.nlm.nih.gov/medlineplus/ency/article/000784.htm. Updated June 7, 2016. Accessed June 11, 2016.

5. Carson-Dewitt R. Retinal (ocular) migraines. About.com website. http://headaches.about.com/lw/Health-Medicine/Conditions-and-diseases/Retinal-Ocular-Migraines.htm. Updated February 28, 2016. Accessed June 11, 2016.

6. Freedman J, Aherne A, Sinert RH. Acute angle-closure glaucoma treatment and management. Medscape website. http://emedicine.medscape.com/article/798811-treatment. Updated October 27, 2015. Accessed June 11, 2016.

7. Behbehani R. Clinical approach to optic neuropathies. *Clin Ophthalmology.* 2007;1(3):233-246.

8. Mayo Clinic Staff. Optic neuritis. Mayo Clinic website. www.mayoclinic.org/diseases-conditions/optic-neuritis/basics/causes/con-20029723. Updated February 18, 2014. Accessed June 11, 2016.

9. Roque MR, Barb Roque BL, Miserocchi E, Foster S. Ophthalmic manifestations of giant cell arteritis. Medscape website. http://emedicine.medscape.com/article/1201429-overview#showall. Updated November 4, 2015. Accessed June 11, 2016.

10. Cason JB. Herpes zoster ophthalmicus. EyeWiki website. http://eyewiki.aao.org/Herpes_Zoster_Ophthalmicus. Modified September 30, 2014. Accessed June 11, 2016.

11. Corneal ulcers and infections. MedlinePlus website. www.nlm.nih.gov/medlineplus/ency/article/001032.htm. Updated September 2, 2015. Accessed June 11, 2016.

12. Hung J, Tai J. Scleritis. EyeWiki website. http://eyewiki.aao.org/Scleritis. Modified December 17, 2015. Accessed June 11, 2016.

13. Orbital cellulitis. Medline Plus website. www.nlm.nih.gov/medlineplus/ency/article/001012.htm. Updated September 2, 2014. Accessed June 11, 2016.

14. Water retention. Healthgrades website. www.healthgrades.com/symptoms/fluid-retention. Reviewed August 9, 2013. Accessed June 11, 2016.

15. Anisorcoria and Horner's syndrome. American Association for Pediatric Ophthalmology and Strabismus website. www.aapos.org/terms/conditions/27. Updated May 2015. Accessed June 11, 2016.

16. Clark WL. Postoperative endophthalmitis. Medscape website. http://emedicine.medscape.com/article/1201260-clinical#showall. Updated January 5, 2016. Accessed June 11, 2016.

17. Jacobs J. Corneal graft rejection. Medscape website. http://emedicine.medscape.com/article/1193505-overview#showall. Updated February 18, 2016. Accessed June 11, 2016.

18. Lindfield D, Poole T. Nd: YAG treatment of epithelial ingrowth. *Cataract and Refractive Surgery Today Europe.* 2013;February:26-27.

19. Santaella R. Post LASIK epithelial ingrowth management. EyeWiki website. http://eyewiki.aao.org/Post_LASIK_Epithelial_Ingrowth_Management. Updated January 20, 2015. Accessed June 11, 2016.

20. Centers for Medicare & Medicaid Services. CMS website. www.cms.gov/Outreach-and-Education/Medicare-Learning-Network-MLN/MLNEdWebGuide/Downloads/97Docguidelines.pdf. Accessed June 11, 2016.

21. Vicchrilli SJ. E & M documentation requirements, part 3: the chief complaint and elements to the history of the present illness. AAO website. www.aao.org/young-ophthalmologists/yo-info/article/em-documentation-requirements-part-3-chief-complai. Accessed June 12, 2016.

22. Pokhrel PK, Loftus SA. Ocular emergencies. *Am Fam Physician.* 2007;76(6):829-836.

23. Retinal artery occlusion. MedlinePlus website. www.nlm.nih.gov/medlineplus/ency/article/001028.htm. Updated May 8, 2014. Accessed June 11, 2016.

34

SUBSPECIALTIES IN OPHTHALMOLOGY AND OPTOMETRY

Donna Bong, COMT

In this chapter we will discuss different subspecialties in eye care. Each subspecialty is unique, and treats and manages different conditions or situations. There is definitely some overlap of subspecialties (such as cornea and cataracts, both of which deal with the anterior segment), so some practitioners will specialize in more than one area. In addition, there are specialties unique to optometry or ophthalmology, and several that are found in both.

As ophthalmic and optometric technicians, we should be aware of the different subspecialties that exist. There are distinctive tests that we do for each subspecialty, and practitioners also perform different treatments in each area. You may find a certain subspecialty to be more interesting than others. You can further explore that subspecialty to become a more valuable technician by understanding and having the skills to perform the special diagnostic tests required.

Prerequisite to reading this chapter, it might be helpful to review ocular anatomy (Chapter 2). Other useful information might include text regarding specific ocular diseases, disorders, and injuries, as well as surgical procedures. These can be found using the Index.

COMPREHENSIVE EYE CARE PRACTITIONERS

Ophthalmologists obtain their medical degree after successfully completing their 5 years' residency program after 4 years of medical school. After completing medical school, graduates undergo varying terms as interns and then residents. These residents become a general (or comprehensive) ophthalmologist. They can also choose to spend additional years as a fellow and train with experienced specialists to become an expert in a certain area. (An *osteopath* can also specialize in ophthalmology. After 4 years of osteopathic training, these doctors spend another 3 to 8 years focusing on eye care.)

Comprehensive ophthalmologists are an important part of the community because they are able to provide care for common eye diseases. Patients are referred by family physicians, optometrists, and other specialists such as cardiologists, endocrinologists, or rheumatologists to have an ocular assessment performed pertinent to that specific patient's health and medical needs.

Ledford JK, Lens A, eds.
Principles and Practice in Ophthalmic Assisting:
A Comprehensive Textbook (pp 593-609).
© 2018 Taylor & Francis Group.

Comprehensive ophthalmologists may further refer these patients to specialists to provide better management and treatment. In addition, there are unique diagnostic tests and instrumentation that a comprehensive ophthalmologist may not have in the office. Referring patients to a specialist with proper diagnostic tools helps to diagnose and treat the patient in a timely manner. General ophthalmologists are medical doctors who can prescribe glasses and medications as well as perform eye surgeries. They can detect and treat eye diseases.

Optometrists obtain a doctor of optometry degree after successfully completing 4 years of optometry school. After obtaining their optometry degree, optometrists can choose to do a 1- to 2-year residency in certain subspecialties as their special interest. Optometrists prescribe glasses and are trained to detect eye diseases. In most countries and states, they do not perform surgery.

Optometrists are primary eye care providers to many patients. Patients do not require a referral to see optometrists. Optometrists can perform an ocular assessment, prescribe glasses, and detect eye abnormalities and diseases. They can start treatment for certain eye diseases and can also comanage a patient with ophthalmologists. This is very important as there are more optometrists than ophthalmologists, providing access to more patients in rural areas. They also refer patients to an ophthalmologist if the patient requires further evaluation.

THE SPECIALTIES

Oculoplastics (Lids, Lacrimal Gland, and Orbit)

Oculoplastics encompasses everything that protects and cushions the eyeball. This includes the skin, eyebrows, eyelids, lashes, lacrimal glands, orbital wall, and tissue within the orbital cavity.

Where They Work

Ophthalmologists specializing in oculoplastics (oculoplastic surgeons) are usually found in hospitals, universities, or private group practices. They require access to a small procedure area (usually in the office) to perform minor procedures, such as removing lumps and growths or performing biopsies. They also require surgical suite access to perform major procedures as well as combined cases with other specialists (such as an ear/nose/throat surgeon, neurosurgeon, or oncology surgeon). These specialists work with a team of technicians, clerks, nurses, anesthesiologists, and consultants. Oculoplastics is a unique subspecialty in that medical doctors (ie, non-ophthalmologists) can take a residency in plastics and then a fellowship in ophthalmology, and vice versa. They can also choose to perform cosmetic or elective surgery, medically required surgery, or both.

What They See and Do

Oculoplastic surgeons will offer treatment options to repair and/or restore any anatomical abnormality. This could arise from congenital issues such as ptosis, benign lesions such as chalazia, or malignant growths such as basal cell carcinoma. Diseases that they manage include infections or inflammatory conditions affecting the orbit and which could cause swelling of tissue leading to exposure and dryness of the cornea, double vision, restriction of extraocular muscles, and optic nerve compression. Other orbital issues such as trauma or lesions affecting the lids, lacrimal glands, or orbit require a consultation and assessment by an oculoplastic surgeon.

Patients are usually referred to oculoplastic surgeons for a consult or second opinion. These patients could be seen for atypical lumps and bumps on the eyelid area and to have them surgically removed and biopsied.

Procedures on drooping brows and lids, as well as removing redundant skin of the eyelid, are commonly performed. Repairs for malpositions of the lower lid are done to help restore normal anatomy to the eyelid structures to reduce tearing and discomfort, as well as potential damage to the globe. The lacrimal pathway can be assessed, and patients with a nasolacrimal duct occlusion may require surgical intervention to help restore the tear pathway. Botox (onabotulinumtoxinA) injection may be offered as a treatment for patients with spasms of the eyelid or face.

Some patients with thyroid eye disease may require orbital decompression surgery to help reduce bulging as well as optic nerve compression. Oculoplastic surgeons perform delicate surgery such as optic nerve fenestration (creating incisions around the optic nerve to relieve intracranial pressure) and skin grafts.

On the other end of the spectrum, they are called upon to perform extensive surgeries such as orbitotomy, evisceration, enucleation, and exenteration of the eye (see Chapter 36). They often assist other specialists during surgery when lesions close to the eye are removed. Patients requiring reconstructive surgery after trauma or lesion removal are also treated by oculoplastic surgeons.

This subspecialty is considered more "blood and gore" compared to all other subspecialties in eye care. Technicians who assist in this field can expect to perform basic testing in addition to tasks as shown in Table 34-1.

Cornea

The cornea and tear film are the first refractive layers that allow people to see clearly. Most corneal issues are manageable and treatable if diagnosed early.

Where They Work

Ophthalmologists and optometrists specializing in cornea (corneal specialists) usually work in hospitals

TABLE 34-1
SPECIAL TESTING/SKILLS IN OCULOPLASTICS

Test/Skills	Rationale
Color vision testing	Evaluate for compression of optic nerve
Exophthalmometry	Monitor exophthalmos/enophthalmos/proptosis
External measurements	Documentation of lid position pre- and postoperatively
Orthoptic analysis	Restriction or paralysis of extraocular muscles due to trauma Differentiation of congenital vs acquired misalignments Preoperative lid surgery
Photography—External/slit lamp	Documentation of condition pretreatment Documentation of surgical/treatment results "Before-and-after" photos for patient/legal
Tear testing	Lacrimal disorders
Ultrasound	Evaluation of the eye through the eyelids (eg, post-trauma, post-tarsorraphy) Measuring the thickness of eye muscles Imaging of the orbit (evaluation of lacrimal gland, lacrimal sac, globe) Measuring length of eye for enucleation
Visual field testing	Documentation of visual field loss (eg, due to drooping lids) Estimation of surgical benefit (eg, taped visual field to simulate surgical results) Documentation of binocular diplopia field (eg, due to trauma)
Order ancillary testing	Coordination of out-of-office testing (eg, MRI, CT scans, blood work)
Minor surgery skills	Set up for in-office procedures Assist surgeon during in-office procedures Care and handling of surgical instruments Educate patients on procedure and postoperative care
Surgical assisting	Assist with procedures (eg, blepharoplasty, entropion repair) Care of patients pre- and postoperative procedure

or private group practices. Ophthalmologists are often involved in teaching and training residents and medical students. Part of this specialty may include external disorders of the eye as well as anterior segment problems. (The external disorders could involve the eyelid, eyelashes, and eyelid margin; anterior segment includes the conjunctiva, cornea, sclera, iris, and anterior chamber.) Some corneal diseases can affect the anterior chamber and some anterior chamber problems can affect the cornea. Thus, corneal specialists look at the entire anterior segment when seeing a patient. Optometrists often comanage patients with corneal issues or work with patients requiring special contact lenses.

What They See and Do

Corneal specialists receive referrals from other physicians and see patients with external and anterior segment concerns or complications. Chapter 26 has details on various common entities.

These specialists provide diagnosis and management of ocular issues such as corneal erosions, corneal abrasions, corneal infections and inflammations, as well as keratoconus and other corneal degenerations and dystrophies. Patients with any compromise of their tear film or tear production caused by issues such as dry eye, meibomian gland dysfunction, and ocular rosacea may require an evaluation.

Patients who have lesions on the conjunctiva, sclera, cornea, or eyelids often need to have them surgically removed, and suspicious lesions may require a biopsy. Complicated traumatic injuries to the cornea will require emergent care by a corneal specialist. Common injuries might include corneal penetrations, corneal lacerations, and trauma caused by foreign bodies. These patients frequently require surgical repair to the anterior segment in order to restore comfort and vision.

Other interventions that they offer are laser or surgical procedures of the conjunctiva, cornea, iris, and anterior chamber. This includes excisions of pterygia and pingueculae, as well as other lesions or tissue on the cornea or the conjunctiva, such as keratopathy, dense stromal scars, and melanoma. Corneal transplants or any repair from corneal lacerations or penetrating injuries (with or without foreign body) will also require surgical intervention.

	TABLE 34-2
SPECIAL TESTING/SKILLS IN CORNEA SUBSPECIALTY	
Test/Skills	**Rationale**
Contact lens fitting	Special contact lens fitting (eg, bandage contact lens, scleral contact lens, rigid gas-permeable lenses for keratoconus patients)
Corneal pachymetry	Corneal thickness evaluation
Corneal topography	Corneal contour evaluation Pre- and postoperative evaluation Rule out corneal irregularities
External measurements	Corneal diameter ("white-to-white") Size of pterygium, pinguecula, scars
Intraocular lens measurements and calculation	Preoperative for cataract evaluation Selection of intraocular lens strength for proper postoperative results
Keratometry	Corneal curvature measurements
Photography— External/slit lamp	Document of condition pretreatment Document of surgical/treatment results
Photography— Gonioscopy photos	Documentation of the angles (eg, elevation, pigment, lesion)
Photography— OCT	Anterior segment OCT to evaluate the cornea, conjunctiva, sclera, angles, and anterior chamber Posterior segment OCT to evaluate the macula for postoperative prognosis
Photography— Specular microscopy	Evaluation of the endothelial cell layer (eg, pre-surgery and post-surgery, Fuchs' dystrophy)
Tear testing	Lacrimal disorders and corneal evaluation
Ultrasound	Evaluation of the ciliary body and iris (eg, iris nevus, iris cyst, ciliary body cyst, ciliary body mass)
Order ancillary testing	Coordination of out-of-office testing (eg, MRI, CT scans, blood work)
Minor surgery skills	Set up for in-office procedures Assist surgeon during in-office procedures Care and handling of surgical instruments Educate patients on procedure and postoperative care
Surgical assisting	Assist with procedures (eg, corneal debridement) Care of patients pre- and postoperative procedure

Depending where their fellowship is obtained, corneal specialists can also perform cataract and refractive surgery as well. Other surgical cases might include reconstruction of the iris after iridocyclectomy or insertion of an aniridia lens to help reduce glare. They also care for patients with ocular issues caused by systemic health problems and/or medications such as Stevens-Johnson syndrome or Sjögren's syndrome.

When working for a corneal specialist, special equipment is used to help evaluate and treat the anterior segment (Table 34-2).

Uveitis and Ocular Immunology

Where They Work

Ophthalmologists specializing in uveitis and ocular immunology are usually found in hospitals, universities, or private group practices. They are also often involved in teaching and training of residents in ophthalmology and medical students from affiliated universities. These ophthalmologists may be called uveitis specialists. Some residents from immunology, rheumatology, and internal medicine will also learn from uveitis specialists as there are many ocular manifestations of systemic diseases and/or medications that can trigger an inflammatory response.

Test/Skills	Rationale
TABLE 34-3	
SPECIAL TESTING/SKILLS IN UVEITIS AND OCULAR IMMUNOLOGY SUBSPECIALTY	
Color vision testing	Rule out optic nerve involvement
Photography—Disc photos	Documentation of the optic nerve appearance
Photography—External/slit lamp	Documentation of the eye pre- and postoperative treatment
Photography—Fluorescein angiography	Evaluation of blood circulation and integrity of vessels of retina
Photography—OCT	Rule out macular involvement and optic nerve changes
Ultrasound	Rule out ciliary body involvement (eg, ciliary body swelling) Rule out orbital inflammation (eg, choroidal thickening, scleritis, episcleritis)
Order ancillary testing	Coordination of out-of-office testing (eg, MRI, CT scans, blood work)
Minor surgery skills	Set up for in-office procedures Assist surgeon during in-office procedures (eg, injections) Care and handling of surgical instruments Educate patients on procedure and postoperative care

What They See and Do

The uvea consists of the vascular system of the eye including the iris, ciliary body, and choroid. Any inflammation in these structures requires management to help reduce the discomfort and any visual disturbances. Occasionally, inflammation could spread to the sclera, episcleral layers, or the ocular muscles. Uveitis specialists receive referrals from other physicians and see patients with ocular inflammation or any kind of systemic inflammation that requires an ophthalmic examination.

Patients with a preexisting systemic inflammatory condition would benefit from seeing a uveitis specialist for a baseline eye exam. The ophthalmologist will evaluate these patients for risks of inflammation or manage them if they are showing inflammatory signs in the eye. Uveitis specialists usually see patients with certain types of arthritis, tuberculosis, sarcoidosis, and other inflammatory conditions.

Patients who see uveitis specialists are usually under the management of a rheumatologist as well. Signs of ocular involvement may necessitate treatment with eye drops and/or ointment, intraocular injections, and subconjunctival injections to help reduce inflammation.

Patients with any kind of ocular inflammation such as episcleritis, scleritis, myositis, iritis, pars planitis, uveitis, or vitritis might be managed with steroidal drops to help minimize the inflammation. This requires careful follow-up to monitor intraocular pressure (IOP), which can rise in some people as a response to the steroid. Prolonged elevated IOP can permanently damage the optic nerve. (See Chapter 29, Glaucoma.)

If ocular inflammation causes adhesions (*synechiae*) between the iris and cornea and/or lens, surgical intervention may be required. In cases of complicated uveitis, patients often develop secondary issues that may require surgical intervention from other subspecialties.

Special diagnostic equipment is used to help evaluate and monitor inflammation (Table 34-3). The tech who can operate these various modalities will be invaluable to this type of practice.

Cataract Surgeons

With an increase of the aging population, cataracts are going to be more and more common. This subspecialty helps to restore preventable vision loss. Patients have their eyes assessed thoroughly during a cataract consultation, and other pathology may be detected.

Where They Work

Cataract surgery is one of the most common ophthalmic procedures. Vision is impeded as the lens opacifies and hardens into a cataract. Extraction is required to restore functional vision. Ophthalmologists specializing in cataract surgery are usually found working in hospitals, teaching institutions, or private offices, and require access to surgical suites. They are often involved in teaching and training of residents in ophthalmology and medical students. These ophthalmologists are called cataract specialists. Some cataract specialists work with pharmaceutical companies to develop better intraocular lenses or perform research on lens performance.

TABLE 34-4	
SPECIAL TESTING/SKILLS IN CATARACT SUBSPECIALTY	
Test/Skills	**Rationale**
Biometry testing	Biometry by optical light or ultrasound to measure precise axial length
Corneal topography	Corneal contour evaluation—To find astigmatism and meridian Rule out corneal irregularities
Intraocular lens calculations	Selection of intraocular lens strength for proper postoperative results
Keratometry	Corneal curvature evaluation
Photography—OCT	Posterior segment OCT to evaluate macula for postoperative prognosis
Photography—Specular microscopy	Corneal endothelium evaluation for any abnormalities
Ultrasound	Evaluation of the posterior segment when there is no view secondary to dense cataracts Measure axial length when biometry is not used
Order ancillary testing	Coordination of out-of-office testing (eg, MRI, CT scans, blood work)
Minor surgery skills	Set up for in-office procedures Assist surgeon during in-office procedures (eg, suture removal) Care and handling of surgical instruments Educate patients on procedure and postoperative care

What They See and Do

Cataract specialists receive referrals from other physicians and see patients with cataract development that require surgical intervention. Cataract surgeons can see all kinds of cataracts ranging from congenital, medication-induced, and traumatic, to the "standard" age-related type.

Patients are typically in the older age group as aging is the most common cause of cataracts. Nevertheless, cataracts can also occur from trauma. Pediatric ophthalmologists usually perform cataract procedures on children. Other complicated procedures might include performing surgery in patients with a narrow anterior chamber, with increased risk of active inflammation, and with stretched or absent zonules.

This specialty involves the team effort of technicians, ophthalmologists, nurses, and optometrists throughout the entire process from preoperative assessments to postoperative care. A complete cataract work-up is necessary so physicians can determine how much the vision is impeded by the cataract. A reliable prognosis can then be given to the patient.

Technicians and physicians need to have good communication skills and knowledge about monovision, distance correction only, and other options such as different accommodative lenses for presbyopia. Discussions must include information about the newest intraocular lenses available. In cases where only one eye has a cataract, some patients might choose to have a refractive lens extraction in the other eye to equalize the vision in the two eyes or to completely eliminate the need for glasses. Clinical personnel need to be prepared to provide accurate information so that the patient can understand the surgeon's recommendations and make informed decisions. Special testing might include those shown in Table 34-4.

Refractive Surgery

Refractive surgery is an elective procedure, so attracting patients can be quite competitive. The field is ever-evolving with continuing, new advances in technology.

Where They Work

Ophthalmologists who perform refractive surgery are usually found in private clinics that are collaboratively owned by several physicians or in a corporation, as the diagnostic machines and lasers are quite expensive. These ophthalmologists are called refractive surgeons. Most undergo training while obtaining their cornea or cataract fellowship, and some train with experienced surgeons while working at a refractive center. They work with a team of technicians, consultants, laser technicians, and surgical assistants to provide care to patients who choose refractive surgery. Optometrists are found commonly working in refractive surgery centers to help with pre- and post-surgery care. Some states in the United States allow optometrists to perform refractive surgery. Refractive surgery is discussed in detail in Chapter 38.

	TABLE 34-5
	SPECIAL TESTING/SKILLS IN REFRACTIVE SURGERY SUBSPECIALTY

Test/Skills	Rationale
Biometry testing	Biometry by optical light or ultrasound waves to measure precise axial length (refractive lens exchange)
Corneal pachymetry	Evaluation of corneal thickness
Corneal topography	Rule out any corneal irregularities Corneal contour evaluation—To find astigmatism and meridian Evaluate spherical aberration
Intraocular lens calculation	Determine accurate intraocular lens strength for accurate postoperative results
Keratometry	Corneal contour evaluation
Orthoptic analysis	Rule out any intermittent or accommodative misalignments
Photography—External/slit lamp	Documentation of appearance of eye pre- and postoperatively
Photography—OCT	Anterior segment OCT to evaluate cornea and angles Posterior segment OCT to rule out macular irregularities
Photography—Specular microscopy	Examination of the corneal endothelial layer
Tear testing	Lacrimal testing
Ultrasound	Measurement of sulcus to sulcus Evaluation of pre- and postoperative lens placement Measurement of axial length when biometry is not used
Order ancillary testing	Coordination of out-of-office testing (eg, blood work)
Minor surgery skills	Set up for in-office procedures (eg, laser refractive surgery) Assist surgeon during in-office procedures Care and handling of surgical instruments Educate patients on procedure and postoperative care
Surgical assisting	Assist with procedures Care of patients pre- and post-procedure Set up and calibration of laser machines

What They See and Do

Patients who see refractive surgeons want to eliminate or reduce their need for glasses. This includes myopia, hyperopia, astigmatism, and presbyopia. Refractive surgery is becoming better known to the public, and consequently, other eye issues that require attention are detected during the routine exam. More keratoconus patients are diagnosed and receiving treatment since the introduction of refractive surgery because surgery candidates have their corneas carefully analyzed. Since keratoconus is an underdiagnosed condition until its late stages, earlier screening is occurring as more people are interested in eliminating their glasses. Other patients who see refractive surgeons seek laser treatment to remove scars on the cornea.

Corneal refractive surgery has evolved from radial keratotomy (requiring physical cutting with a blade) to the well-known laser-assisted in situ keratomileusis (LASIK). The application of lasers has also evolved to helping reduce postoperative aberrations significantly with the new advanced custom wavefront lasers. Corneal cross-linking is also performed in refractive surgery centers to help patients with keratoconus and similar issues.

Other, more invasive refractive surgery involves an implantable lens that sits between the posterior iris and the anterior crystalline lens, known as an intraocular contact lens. Refractive lens exchange (RLE) is also being offered as a treatment for patients who are not good candidates for corneal refractive surgery. Some patients who have a cataract in one eye choose to have RLE performed in the noncataractous eye in order to equalize the prescription in each eye. New procedures and lenses (such as the KAMRA inlay [AcuFocus]) have been developed to help eliminate the need for reading glasses in presbyopic patients.

A lot of special equipment is needed in a refractive surgery practice, most of which evaluate corneal curvature (Table 34-5). Skills to operate and understand the use of each machine is important as this will help the ophthalmologist review the candidacy of potential surgical patients. Strong social and communication skills are also very important as patients will have a lot of questions and need proper understanding before having the procedure.

Glaucoma

Glaucoma can be a silent vision thief; hence, screening is important to ensure that prevention is available to patients who are at risk. For patients with sudden glaucoma attacks, urgent care must be provided to relieve discomfort and treat uncontrolled pressures. Management of glaucoma can be stressful for patients as routine follow-ups are required. Glaucoma specialists and their technicians must be empathetic and patient to explain the progression of the disease.

Where They Work

Ophthalmologists specializing in glaucoma are typically found in private offices, group practices, hospitals, and research institutions. They require both special laser machines and surgical suite access to perform glaucoma surgery. These ophthalmologists are known as glaucoma specialists. They typically have training as fellows to learn surgical skills and clinical management. Optometrists are also active in glaucoma care, including screening, detection, topical treatment, and comanagement.

What They See and Do

Glaucoma is a subspecialty that involves clinical, pharmaceutical, laser, and surgical management of the disorder in all ages (see Chapter 29).

Glaucoma specialists receive referrals from optometrists, family physicians, emergency physicians, and other ophthalmologists for consultations and possibly surgical or laser intervention. If there is a family history of glaucoma, high intraocular pressure, angles are narrow, or optic nerve cup-to-disc ratio appears enlarged, then patients are sent in to evaluate their risk of glaucoma. Narrowing of the angles, changes to the iris (such as bowing, elevations, transillumination), pseudoexfoliation to the lens, or any changes or suspicious appearance of the optic nerve usually benefit from a consultation. Commonly seen entities include primary open-angle glaucoma, juvenile open-angle glaucoma, congenital glaucoma, ocular hypertension, and chronic angle-closure glaucoma. Glaucoma can also develop secondarily to trauma, cataract formation, and acute angle closure. Other secondary causes include inflammatory conditions causing uveitic glaucoma, poorly controlled diabetic retinopathy causing neovascular glaucoma, or late-stage ocular diseases causing certain forms of neovascular glaucoma.

Patients include those who need their IOP monitored, annual visits to ensure there are no glaucoma changes, or those who require treatment. Treatment can range from medications (such as eye drops or oral medications) to laser or surgical procedures.

Patients whose glaucoma is controlled are often comanaged by optometrists. In other circumstances, patients who have poor compliance or poor control with medications may require laser treatment.

With more complicated cases, glaucoma surgeons can offer surgery as an alternative to lasers and eye drops. Minimally invasive or micro-invasive glaucoma surgery (MIGS) has been introduced as a new approach to controlling glaucoma. MIGS makes use of surgical instruments such as the Trabectome (NeoMedix, Inc), iStent (Glaukos), or Ex-PRESS mini glaucoma shunt (Alcon), all of which help with the outflow of aqueous humor.

The gold standard of surgical treatment is still the trabeculectomy, which is more invasive and requires more intensive postoperative management. It is not uncommon for glaucoma surgeons to perform cataract surgery or combined glaucoma and cataract procedures. Cataract surgery also helps enlarge the anterior chamber depth, increasing outflow and decreasing the chances of angle closure.

Goldmann applanation tonometry is the gold standard for checking IOP, so every technician must be fluent with its use. Other tonometers can be used to obtain the IOP as well, but are not considered as reliable as the Goldmann tonometer in most cases. Other instruments and tests are covered in Table 34-6. Physicians perform laser treatments to help increase the outflow of the aqueous humor or reduce the production of aqueous humor, so a technician must be able to assist in these procedures.

Perhaps more than any other, this field requires technicians to provide accurate and continuing patient education. Because "glaucoma drops" don't make the patient's eye "feel better," the patient can find it difficult to believe that the medication is necessary and/or working. Compliance must be evaluated at every single visit, and encouraged at every single visit. The importance and method of drop use must be enforced frequently.

Ocular Oncology

Oncology is a high-stress subspecialty that yields big rewards when patients' lives are being saved. The order of priority is 1) save the life, 2) save the eye, 3) save the vision, and 4) preserve what vision there is.

Where They Work

Ophthalmologists specializing in oncology are usually found working in hospitals, universities, academic institutions, and private practices in major cities. They are involved in teaching and training ophthalmology and medical residents from affiliated universities. These

TABLE 34-6
SPECIAL TESTING/SKILLS IN GLAUCOMA SUBSPECIALTY

Test/Skills	Rationale
Color vision testing	Rule out optic neuropathy
Corneal pachymetry	Measurement of corneal thickness for true intraocular pressure
Photography—Disc photos	Documentation of appearance for future comparison
Photography—External/slit lamp	Documentation pre- and postoperatively
Photography—Gonioscopy	Angle assessment
Photography—HRT/GDx	Optic nerve assessment
Photography—OCT	Retinal nerve fiber layer assessment and macular assessment
Tonometry	Diurnal tension curve measurement to determine intraocular pressure fluctuation Single tonometry reading by applanation for accurate intraocular pressure measurements
Slit lamp/gonioscopy evaluation	Assessment of angles Assessment of the cause of narrow angles (eg, iris plateau, iris cysts, iris lesion, pupillary block, iris bombe)
Visual field testing	Central visual field assessment, peripheral visual field assessment, follow-up of glaucoma progression
Order ancillary testing	Coordination of out-of-office testing (eg, MRI, CT scans, blood work)
Minor surgery skills	Set up for in-office procedures (eg, laser procedures) Assist surgeon during in-office procedures Care and handling of surgical instruments Educate patients on procedure and postoperative care

ophthalmologists are called ocular oncologists. Some residents from oncology or plastics will also spend time with an ocular oncologist, as neoplasms in the eye can originate from another part of the body. Ocular oncologists require surgical suite access in hospitals to perform removal of suspicious lesions, as well as in cancer institutes to perform radiation to lesions.

What They See and Do

Ocular oncologists receive referrals from other physicians and see patients with any suspicious lumps and bumps around and in the eye. A biopsy is usually done to verify whether the lesion is benign or malignant. Patients can also be managed by an oculoplastic surgeon. If there is a pigmentation or lesion inside the eye, a clinical diagnosis is usually given based on the appearance of the lesion as well as patient risk factors. Other diagnostic testing may be required to help the ocular oncologist arrive at a diagnosis.

Patients referred to an ocular oncologist might also have cancer elsewhere in the body and require an ophthalmic exam to ensure the eye is not involved.

An oculoplastic surgeon will often work with the ocular oncologist. Patients with basal or squamous cell carcinoma require care from an oncologist for management or an ear/nose/throat (ENT) specialist for further removal if the tumor extends beyond the eye.

For patients with an intraocular lesion, a thorough examination of the eye along with a proper clinical history is important. Special imaging, usually done by technicians, may be required before the ocular oncologist is able to provide a clinical diagnosis. If the lesion is diagnosed as benign, patients are required to be evaluated once or twice a year to ensure no changes occur. If a lesion appears suspicious, the ocular oncologist will classify it into low, medium, or high risk and appropriate follow-up times are done to evaluate for any change. If the lesion is malignant and aggressive (eg, melanoma, retinoblastoma), the ocular oncologist may recommend treatment such as *brachytherapy*, which involves an insertion of a radiation plaque onto the eye for a duration of time. This slowly kills the tumor and reduces radiation side effects to the surrounding tissues. Other treatments might include external beam radiation or removal of the eye to completely excise the tumor. All options are carefully reviewed.

If the lesion appears to be metastatic, the patient is sent for more testing and a general oncologist will take over. Generally, the patient will then visit the ocular oncologist after treatment.

	TABLE 34-7
	SPECIAL TESTING/SKILLS IN OCULAR ONCOLOGY SUBSPECIALTY
Test/Skills	**Rationale**
Color vision testing	Rule out optic nerve involvement/compression
External measurements	Size of lesions on the lid, conjunctiva, or cornea
Orthoptic analysis	Evaluation of eye misalignments caused by extensive eye lesions
Photography—Autofluorescence	Presence/absence of orange pigment
Photography—External/slit lamp	Documentation of lesions apparent during external or slit lamp exam on the eyelid, conjunctival, sclera, cornea, and iris Documentation of pre- and post-treatment/radiation/removal
Photography—Gonioscopy photos	Documentation of lesions in the angle
Photography—Fluorescein angiography	Evaluation of presence/absence of circulation in a lesion
Photography—Indocyanine green	Evaluation of the choroidal circulation
Photography—OCT	Presence/absence of subretinal fluid within a lesion
Ultrasound	Standardized A-scan—Internal reflectivity evaluation B-scan—Evaluation of the lesion and globe B-scan—Evaluation of position of radiation plaque Ultrasound biomicroscopy—Evaluation of iris, angle, or ciliary body lesions
Visual field testing	Documentation of visual field pre- and post-treatment
Order ancillary testing	Coordination of out-of-office testing (eg, MRI, CT scans, PET scans, ultrasounds, blood work)
Minor surgery skills	Set up for in-office procedures (eg, fine needle aspiration biopsy) Assist surgeon during in-office procedures (eg, excision, biopsy) Care and handling of surgical instruments Educate patients on procedure and postoperative care

Typical entities seen are choroidal ephelis (freckle), choroidal hemangioma, choroidal osteoma (deposit of bony material), choroidal granuloma, choroidal nevus, choroidal malignant melanoma, choroidal metastasis, iris nevus, iris malignant melanoma, ciliary body melanoma, uveal melanoma, and retinoblastoma.

The ocular oncologist works with a large team consisting of technicians, a medical physicist, radiation therapists, and nurses, as well as an anesthesiologist and a radiation oncologist. Special testing a technician might be called upon to perform are summarized in Table 34-7.

Patients undergo a lot of tension and emotions while waiting for and receiving a diagnosis. Those practicing in this field need to work well together and have empathy and patience.

Vitreous and Retina

The vitreous and retina are the last two media through which light must travel prior to accessing the optic nerve. Because both entities are inside the eye, there are special challenges when testing, diagnosing, and treating their disorders.

Where They Work

Ophthalmologists specializing in vitreous and retina are usually found working in hospitals, universities, academic institutions, or individual/group private practices in major cities. They are also involved in teaching and training residents from affiliated universities. These ophthalmologists are called retinal specialists.

What They See and Do

Retinal specialists receive referrals from other physicians and see patients who require a retinal evaluation. This could be for screening for ocular manifestations of systemic diseases, retinal health baseline prior to starting certain medications, or consultation regarding the vitreous, retina, and choroid.

TABLE 34-8
SPECIAL TESTING/SKILLS IN VITREOUS AND RETINA SUBSPECIALTY

Test/Skills	Rationale
Electrophysiology testing	Retinal function investigation
Photography—Autofluorescence	To document areas that autofluoresce (eg, optic nerve drusen)
Photography—Fluorescein angiography	Evaluate retinal circulation and vessel integrity
Photography—Indocyanine green	Evaluate choroidal circulation
Photography—OCT	High-resolution evaluation of retinal layers
Photography—Red-free	Examination of retinal blood vessels, drusen, and subtle defects
Ultrasound	Examination of the vitreous cavity, orbit and globe contour for tears, detachments, elevations, vitreous hemorrhage, or vitritis
Visual field testing	Patients who are taking medications that could cause retinal or visual field problems Retinal degeneration or retinal diseases
Order ancillary testing	Coordination of out-of-office testing (eg, MRI, CT scans, blood work)
Minor surgery skills	Set up for in-office procedures (eg, injections) Assist surgeon during in-office procedures (eg, anterior chamber tap) Care and handling of surgical instruments Educate patients on procedure and postoperative care

The most commonly seen patients are those with diabetes, macular degeneration, or abnormalities noted by general eye care practitioners during routine exams. Optometrists and family physicians are primary sources of referrals. The retinal specialist may refer patients to other specialists such as a geneticist, ocular oncologist, or neuro-ophthalmologist.

As the population ages, the prevalence of macular degeneration is on the rise. Diabetes is also widespread, associated in part with the high occurrence of obesity. These patients require ongoing care and close follow-up. Patients with vascular occlusive events, degenerative retinal conditions, and strokes need to be monitored. Urgent care is required for patients who have sudden vision loss due to retinal detachments and choroidal lesions. Retinal specialists can choose to care for all patients requiring retinal assessments or to further specialize in pediatric retinal, medical retinal, or surgical retinal cases.

In pediatric retina care, patients requiring consults and diagnosis are usually those with congenital issues, such as retinopathy of prematurity, uveitis, retinoblastoma, and developmental malformations, as well as hereditary macular dystrophy and retinal blood vessel disorders. Cases of trauma such as shaken baby syndrome, blunt trauma, or globe ruptures may also be evaluated.

In medical retinal care, patients who require follow-up for diagnoses such as diabetic retinopathy, retinal toxicity, retinal tears, posterior vitreous detachment, or macular degeneration are typical.

In surgical retinal care, procedures would encompass treating retinal detachment, vitrectomy (for vitreous hemorrhage), internal limiting membrane peel (for epiretinal membranes), macular hole repair, or a combination of surgery and laser for diabetic retinopathy. More invasive treatments might include lasers or intravitreal injections for treating cases of wet macular degeneration and persistent macular edema, as well as prevention of neovascularization in patients with blood vessel-blocking events in the retina.

All patients requiring retinal evaluations must be dilated in order to properly examine the fundus. Ancillary testing includes most imaging modalities as well as other techniques (Table 34-8).

Technicians in this field would be expected to assist with laser procedures as well as intraocular injections. Expertise in low vision testing and aids is also helpful.

Neuro-Ophthalmology

Neuro-ophthalmology involves the relationship of the brain and the eye and how each affects the other. Some neurologic conditions cause an ocular manifestation before the true neurologic condition is obvious, and vice versa. The study of neuro-ophthalmology looks at the visual pathway from the eye to the brain.

TABLE 34-9		
SPECIAL TESTING/SKILLS IN NEURO-OPHTHALMOLOGY SUBSPECIALTY		
Test/Skills	**Rationale**	
Color vision testing	Rule out optic nerve involvement/compression	
Electrophysiology testing	Optic nerve and pathway function investigation (eg, visual evoked potential) Discern between organic and nonorganic vision loss	
Orthoptic analysis	Evaluation of eye motility problems or misalignments	
Photography—Retinal	To document appearance of optic nerve for follow-ups	
Photography—Fluorescein angiography	Evaluation of fluorescein delivery through vascular structures in the eye (eg, evaluating circulation or looking for blockage)	
Retinoscopy/refractometry	Document best-corrected visual acuity as accurately as possible	
Visual field testing	Visual field defects could be caused by optic nerve problems or brain lesions (eg, Humphrey visual fields, Goldmann visual fields, Octopus visual fields)	
Order ancillary testing	Coordination of out-of-office testing (eg, MRI, CT scans, blood work)	
Minor surgery skills	Set up for in-office procedures (eg, temporal artery biopsy) Assist surgeon during in-office procedures Care and handling of surgical instruments Educate patients on procedure and postoperative care	

Where They Work

Ophthalmologists specializing in neuro-ophthalmology typically work in hospital settings or universities. Neuro-ophthalmologists can be trained as neurology residents undergoing a fellowship in ophthalmology or as ophthalmology residents undergoing a fellowship in neurology. This subspecialty is generally nonsurgical. However, some practitioners choose to do a fellowship in oculoplastics so they can perform orbital surgery.

What They See and Do

Any disruption to the visual pathway can cause a visual or ocular problem. These visual problems could manifest as double vision, blurry vision, or difficulty focusing. Ocular manifestation could involve eye motility problems, eyelid issues, pupillary dysfunctions, or nystagmus.

Neuro-ophthalmologists tend to spend more time with each patient to understand or figure out the diagnosis. They are also very good at identifying organic vision loss vs nonorganic vision loss based on the variety of testing modalities often not found in the typical, general eye practice.

Appointments with a neuro-ophthalmologist are generally on referral. Diagnosing ocular manifestations of neurological syndromes can be very complex. Most neuro-ophthalmologists require consultation with other specialties when attempting to determine the problem(s).

Disruption of the visual pathway can cause changes to pupil size and/or reaction. Eye movement can be compromised by a nerve palsy, restricted extraocular motility

due to chronic progressive paralysis of the extraocular muscles and lid muscles, or something more sinister, such as nystagmus from a brain tumor. Some patients could have a combination of neurological symptoms that require further investigation.

Patients with a brain tumor may require a neuro-ophthalmology assessment. Some patients with signs of ocular or brain stroke might also be seen at the clinic. Additionally, the neuro-ophthalmologist is concerned about the optic nerve and sees patients with signs of optic atrophy, papilledema, underdeveloped optic disc, and elevated optic nerve head.

Technicians who work with neuro-ophthalmologists have to be good listeners, as patient history is very important to the diagnosis. In addition, having acute observation skills for evaluating pupils and other tasks will make a technician very useful (Table 34-9).

Neuro-ophthalmologists sometimes need other special test modalities to diagnose the patient. For example, magnifiers may be needed to measure the amount of nystagmus the patient exhibits. Special filters can be used to measure the degree of relative afferent pupillary defect.

Ocular Genetics

The study of genetics and the ocular manifestations of inherited anomalies is slowly evolving. If a gene is defective or absent, the patient may experience systemic and/or ocular disorders, depending on the problem. This is a rare subspecialty, but it is very helpful with the advancement of research in gene therapy. Once pathologies are classified according to the defective gene(s),

TABLE 34-10
SPECIAL TESTING/SKILLS IN OCULAR GENETICS SUBSPECIALTY

Test/Skills	Rationale
Electrophysiology testing	Retinal function investigation (eg, full field electroretinogram to visualize the severity of defects to the rods, cones, or other layers of the retina)
Photography—Autofluorescence	To document areas that autofluoresce (eg, the retinal pigment epithelium is easily seen, the "sick or dying" areas tend to glow/hyperfluoresce, and areas that are dead appear dark/hypofluoresce)
Photography—Fluorescein angiography	To evaluate the retina and the vascular structures
Photography—OCT	High-resolution evaluation of retinal layers
Photography	Slit lamp images, external images, and fundus images for documentation
Visual field testing	Certain genetic disorders cause visual field defects (eg, retinitis pigmentosa)
Order ancillary testing	Coordination of out-of-office testing (eg, MRI, CT scans, blood work, gene testing)

patients with the issue may qualify to have gene therapy to help with visual preservation.

Where They Work

Ocular genetics is a subspecialty that involves the study of heredity and its effects on the eye and body (see Chapter 24). Ophthalmologists who work in this subspecialty have special interest in the research and cure of ocular expressions of genetic disorders. Ophthalmologists involved with ocular genetics generally work in large institutions such as universities and hospitals. Working in an institution also allows for more grants and funding toward genetic research. Optometrists are involved with ocular genetics indirectly as being knowledgeable in genetic diseases helps them counsel and refer patients.

What They See and Do

Eye problems that are commonly seen by an ocular geneticist are choroideremia (where the retinal and choroidal tissues degenerate over time), retinitis pigmentosa, ocular albinism (where ocular pigment is lacking), oculocutaneous albinism (where skin pigment is also lacking), hereditary retinal dystrophies, macular dystrophies, and iris anomalies causing glaucoma (such as aniridia). Other genetic diagnoses could be any form of cone-rod dystrophy, rod dystrophy, or cone dystrophy.

An ocular geneticist receives referrals from pediatricians and doctors who suspect their patients have genetic conditions. Most of these patients require an eye exam to ensure that there are no ocular manifestations, but some of them may be affected by the systemic issue(s) and require other subspecialists to see them.

Patients who require an ocular genetic evaluation usually see a genetic counselor. These professionals are educated and knowledgeable regarding how a specific genetic defect causes the systemic and ocular problems.

Some patients with intraocular malignant melanomas might undergo genetic testing of the tumor to discover the nature of the lesion. Other patients, such as those with choroideremia or certain forms of retinitis pigmentosa, may have an opportunity to undergo trial genetic modifications to help preserve vision.

Technicians who understand genetics are helpful in explaining how blood work and other samples are needed to trace and map out specific genes. The knowledge of mapping a family tree related to the disease can also be very helpful to the ocular geneticist. Experience in low vision testing and training is also an asset, as patients may require some form of low vision aid. Other special diagnostics may be required as well (Table 34-10).

Strabismus

The majority of patients seen in the eye clinic for "crossed eyes" are children. This is fortunate, because in terms of visual development the earlier treatment is begun, the better the chances are for the patient to develop and maintain binocular single vision, as well as avoid amblyopia. In addition, eye muscle imbalances are often cosmetically obvious. This can lead to self-consciousness and embarrassment, which can be alleviated and prevented by straightening the eyes with surgery. Strabismus is covered in Chapter 10, where you can read a thorough discussion on strabismus, amblyopia, and binocular vision. Strabismus surgery is explained in Chapter 36.

Where They Work

Ophthalmologists who see patients with eye muscle imbalances and treat them surgically or nonsurgically are also known as strabismologists. They usually work in clinics with access to surgical suites, as many patients require surgery. Ophthalmologists who work in this field

Test/Skills	Rationale
	TABLE 34-11
	SPECIAL TESTING/SKILLS IN STRABISMUS SUBSPECIALTY
Amplitude measurements	To evaluate fusion
Extraocular motility	To measure eye misalignments (eg, Bielschowsky head tilt test, vergence testing, range of motion testing)
Hess/Lees screen	Isolate motility issues and isolate which muscle is under- or overacting
Maddox rod testing	To measure the amount of torsion
Photography—External	Nine positions of gaze is performed to document appearance of the eye looking into different areas (eg, pre- and post-surgery documentation)
Stereo acuity	To measure depth perception
Synoptophore	Subjectively measures vertical, horizontal, and torsional deviation and tests for fusion (eg, to see if patient can see single after surgery)
Ultrasound	Identifying the location of horizontal muscles for surgical planning
Order ancillary testing	Coordination of out-of-office testing (eg, MRI, CT scans)
Minor surgery skills	Set up for in-office procedures (eg, suture removal) Assist surgeon during in-office procedures (eg, adjustable sutures) Care and handling of surgical instruments Educate patients on procedure and postoperative care

have special interest in binocular vision and extraocular muscles. It is common for strabismologists to train in pediatric ophthalmology as well, as there are many congenital forms of strabismus.

Optometrists with special interest in binocular vision also see patients with eye misalignments. They do not perform surgery on these patients but are able to provide corrections such as prescribing prisms or bifocals for these patients. Optometrists can monitor patients and refer them if needed, or offer eye exercises to reduce straining of the eyes due to weak muscles.

What They See and Do

The strabismus surgeon will typically receive referrals from other physicians. The most common diagnosis seen in children is congenital misalignment. Other patients could be referred for nystagmus or a disorder such as Duane syndrome, Brown syndrome, or accommodative esotropia (all discussed in Chapter 10). Some deviations are the same in all gazes and some are not. In cases such as these, the surgeon must have experience and knowledge on how to handle these complex issues.

Strabismus in children can have a direct correlation to their best-corrected visual acuity, because an eye that is habitually crossed may develop amblyopia. In these cases, the strabismologists will manage amblyopia with patching and other treatment strategies.

The strabismus surgeon prefers to perform procedures to align the eyes while the patient is young and

the visual system is still developing to achieve alignment when the patient looks straight ahead. In children, the hope is to encourage the two eyes to "lock together" and thus develop binocular vision. In other cases the procedure's only goal may be cosmetic so that the patient doesn't look "cross-eyed."

Most patients who first experience eye deviations after childhood suffer symptomatic diplopia, which can be quite debilitating. Common adult misalignment issues include thyroid eye disease, trauma, tumors, inflammatory conditions, and neurological changes (including nerve palsies). Consultation with a strabismologist will provide better decisions on how to manage these, whether surgically or optically. However, there is usually a waiting period of at least 6 months to see how much the condition will resolve on its own before surgery is considered. In the meantime, these patients are generally counseled on options to reduce or eliminate the troublesome second image.

Strabismus surgeons rely heavily on a proper and thorough orthoptic evaluation. Besides obtaining accurate visual acuity and basic orthoptic measurements, technicians can expect to perform or order other special tests as well (Table 34-11).

In children with amblyopia, technicians help educate parents and patients about the importance of patching or other treatment. If an orthoptist works in the same clinic, he/she will often help to comanage the patching therapy with the ophthalmologist.

TABLE 34-12
SPECIAL TESTING/SKILLS IN PEDIATRIC SUBSPECIALTY

Test/Skills	Rationale
Pediatric vision tests (eg, fix/follow/steady/ maintained, preferential looking, pediatric optotypes)	Detection of amblyopia
Extraocular motility (eg, Krimsky, Hirschberg, cover tests, prism and cover tests, Worth 4 dot, range of motion)	Detection and measurement of strabismus
Stereo acuity	To measure depth perception, evaluation of strabismus and amblyopia
Photography—External	Nine positions of gaze to document appearance of the eyes looking in different directions (eg, pre- and post-surgery documentation)
Color vision	Detection of hereditary color vision abnormalities
Retinoscopy	Evaluation of refractive errors

Pediatrics

Pediatric eye care is a subspecialty that is full of fun and challenges. Doctors and technicians need to be creative and on their toes to keep their patients engaged and attentive. A quick look at the eye may sometimes be all you're going to get.

Where They Work

The subspecialty of pediatric eye care involves both medical and surgical management of congenital and acquired eye problems in children. Pediatric ophthalmologists and optometrists can work in children's hospitals, universities, and their own private practices just like other eye care practitioners.

What They See and Do

Pediatric specialists manage all aspects of ocular abnormalities including strabismus, amblyopia, glaucoma, retina, and cornea. Other ocular conditions such as trauma, inflammation, infections, and lesions require careful treatment and management as well. Within pediatrics are a number of subspecialties including pediatric neuro-ophthalmology, pediatric retina, pediatric glaucoma, and pediatric surgery.

Pediatric patients are often referred with specific problems such as strabismus/amblyopia, congenital ptosis, congenital cataracts, congenital glaucoma, nasolacrimal duct obstruction, or retinopathy of prematurity. Pediatricians may request an appointment for ocular screening if the patient has any systemic issues such as neurofibromatosis, Down syndrome, or other genetic conditions. Pediatric patients with trauma or acute inflammations/infections may require urgent care and treatment. Any neoplastic growth in the brain or along the visual pathway will need a proper ophthalmic assessment as well.

An ability to perform retinoscopy and refractometry...quickly, and on a wiggly subject...is very important in order to provide children with glasses. Cycloplegic drops for a proper refraction may present a challenge depending on the tech's creativity in eliciting patient cooperation. Performing accurate ocular assessments and visual acuity testing is key; hence, it is necessary to have a variety of visual acuity charts and interesting fixation targets. Technicians need to be able to perform IOP checks on children using different devices. Other diagnostic testing is similar to other subspecialties, depending on the focus of the practitioner (Table 34-12).

Most children are able to undergo diagnostic testing in the eye clinic. In certain cases, however, patients must undergo examination under anesthesia for a better evaluation as well as diagnostic testing. This might include measuring and imaging with ultrasound, performing electrophysiology tests, and measuring IOP.

Electrophysiology

By using electrophysiology, physicians are able to test retinal function without subjective responses from the patient. This is useful for assessing visual potential of nonverbal and potentially malingering patients, as well as classifying and evaluating pathology.

Where They Work

Ophthalmologists and optometrists who have an interest in electrophysiology typically work closely with technicians who perform the testing. Electrophysiology specialists are usually found working in universities or hospitals. It is common for a retinal specialist, neuro-ophthalmologist, or an ocular geneticist to interpret electrophysiology test results, as there are numerous ocular disorders that arise from the retina, the brain, and heredity. Some departments have electrophysiology scientists who interpret the data. Optometrists who work in this field are involved with teaching optometry students about electrophysiology. They could also work in hospitals and perform testing on patients.

What They See and Do

Electrophysiology testing (see Chapter 18) evaluates the function of the retinal layer, optic nerve pathway, and visual cortex. This type of evaluation is very useful as it assesses the function objectively, hence being especially valuable in nonverbal patients. Because the subjective factor is thus removed from the testing, it can also be invaluable when malingering is suspected.

Referrals typically come from other physicians and ophthalmologists who want to assess the retinal function layer or explain the cause of decreased vision. Evaluation can also be done to rule out ocular toxicity due to systemic medications or radiation. Common situations that are assessed in this manner include hydroxychloroquine toxicity, Best's disease (a genetic macular dystrophy), retinitis pigmentosa, forms of rod-cone dystrophy, and cone dystrophy. These patients often have ocular pathology that is of genetic origin.

The expertise of an electrophysiologist is usually requested by a neurologist or ophthalmologist. They sometimes work closely with researchers investigating the function of a gene. Clinical electrophysiologists perform tests on patients with existing ocular issues. Research electrophysiologists perform testing on animals or humans with or without ocular issues. Patients referred for electrophysiology testing may present with an abnormal fundus with no visual symptoms, an abnormal fundus with visual symptoms, or a normal fundus with visual symptoms that an ophthalmologist needs more information about in order to complete the investigation and diagnose.

The set-up for electrophysiology testing is quite complex. It usually requires a dark room with a way to reduce the light, including that emitted by the examiner's computer. Depending on the kind of testing to be done, the technician who performs the test needs to know how to interact with patients of all ages. Standard electrophysiology tests are based on the International Society for Clinical Electrophysiology of Vision (ISCEV) protocols for testing, and consist of eletroretinography, electro-oculography, visual evoked potential, and other testing such as dark adaptometry, electromyography, and electronystagmography (see Chapter 18).

Research

Research is vital and allows for advancement in every aspect of eye care. This exciting field helps find new treatments for genetic disorders, new surgical techniques for better prognoses, and new medications for better efficacy. The end result is better patient care.

Where They Work

Ophthalmologists and optometrists who are involved with research typically work for research institutions, pharmaceutical companies, hospitals, and labs. Some may perform studies in their own practices. Most continue performing research and studies while in practice, as they are able to recruit study patients and perform treatment to evaluate the efficacy of the research.

What They Do

The application of research is done with the goals of improving surgical techniques and tools, the diagnosis and management of specific disorders, studying how drugs move through the body, and evaluating innovations such as new diagnostic equipment or lasers that can advance patient care.

Research varies depending on what is being studied, so the equipment and testing modalities used would differ from one subject to another. For example, in research regarding the effects of a systemic medication on the posterior pole, diagnostic imaging would be required to document changes.

CHAPTER QUIZ

1. Name five different subspecialties in eye care.

2. What are the education background differences between an ophthalmologist and an optometrist?

3. What kind of patients are referred to an ocular oncologist?

4. Which of the following is *not* a diagnostic tool used by a refractive surgeon?
   a. corneal topography
   b. tear testing
   c. ultrasound
   d. color vision testing

5. Some ophthalmologists subspecialize in two or more different subspecialties. Which of these combinations is most likely?
   a. cataract and refractive surgery
   b. oculoplastics and ocular oncology
   c. cataract and glaucoma
   d. retina and electrophysiology
   e. all of the above

Answers

1. Possible answers: Surgery, glaucoma, ocular oncology, vitreous and retina, neuro-ophthalmology, ocular genetics, strabismus, pediatrics, electrophysiology, research.

2. An ophthalmologist has to have a medical degree, a 5-year ophthalmology residency, and an optional fellowship to become a specialist. An ophthalmologist is a medical doctor. An optometrist has to possess an optometry degree and an optional residency to subspecialize. An optometrist is a doctor of optometry.

3. Patients with suspicious lumps and bumps around and in their eye get referred to an ocular oncologist. These patients could have benign or malignant lesions. Patients with cancer may be evaluated for any spread of cancer to the eye.

4. d

5. e

35

LOW VISION

Beth Koch, COT, ROUB

BASIC SCIENCES

Low vision patients require the patience and skills of qualified technicians. These patients are becoming a bigger part of our practices due to increasing life span. People are now living longer; they have to deal with more irreversible vision losses. Additionally, technicians in developed countries are reaching out to the people in third-world countries where cataracts, corneal issues, and other vision-debilitating ocular diseases still create low vision issues due to lack of good medical care and treatment.

CLINICAL KNOWLEDGE

Terminology

The term *low vision* can encompass a wide range of visual impairment. Vision loss means that part or all of the vision has decreased, whether this occurs suddenly or gradually.[1] Low vision or *visually impaired* describes people with significant vision loss that can't be corrected with glasses or contacts, medication, treatment, or surgery. The problems encountered by patients with vision loss are many, and impact every facet of their lives.

The World Health Organization (WHO) uses these classifications of visual impairment: *moderate* visual impairment is defined as best-corrected visual acuity of 20/70 to 20/160; *severe* visual impairment (or *legally blind* in the United States) is a best-corrected visual acuity of 20/200 to 20/400 or a visual field of 20 degrees or less. *Profound* visual impairment is best-corrected visual acuity of 20/500 to 20/1000 or a visual field of 10 degrees or less. *Near total* visual impairment is defined as best-corrected visual acuity of less than 20/1000 or a visual field of 5 degrees or less, and total visual impairment is NLP (no light perception).[2]

Functional vision loss is when an individual is unable to see well enough to perform the *activities of daily living* (ADLs) needed to survive, as defined by WHO. Functional vision loss can be disorder related (ie, with an organic cause) or hysterical (usually without an organic cause) in nature.

Common Disorders Associated With Low Vision

Any part of the eye involved in creating a visual image can play a role in causing low vision. The cornea is

Ledford JK, Lens A, eds.
Principles and Practice in Ophthalmic Assisting:
A Comprehensive Textbook (pp 611-619).
© 2018 Taylor & Francis Group.

responsible for two-thirds of the focusing power in the eye, and if it is damaged in any way that distorts or clouds the tissue, there will be a decrease in image clarity. Disorders of the crystalline lens (responsible for one-third of focusing power) can also cause low vision issues. In the back of the eye, disorders of the retina, macula, and optic nerve can all affect visual acuity as well. Vascular diseases and glaucoma can damage the retina and optic nerve, causing visual field loss all the way to total visual impairment. The macula is responsible for central vision, and if compromised, results in blurred to very poor vision.

While there are many causes for low vision, the five leading causes are macular degeneration, cataracts, glaucoma, retinal dystrophies, and diabetes. Each of these is discussed in detail in other chapters (please check the Contents and Index) but bear mentioning here.

Macular degeneration is the leading cause of legal blindness in people over 55 years in the United States, and affects more than 1.75 million.[3] This number is expected to rise. The two forms of macular degeneration are *dry* (nonexudative) and *wet* (exudative).

In the dry form, key early identifiers are *drusen*, which are tiny yellow or white deposits in Bruch's membrane of the retina. Drusen are made up of lipids and may result from the eye's inability to dispose of waste products. There are different types. Drusen can be hard, small, and scattered from each other (this type may not cause vision loss for a long time and may not even be indicative of macular degeneration). Or they can become larger, softer, and closer together (which prove to be a greater risk factor for severe vision loss in wet macular degeneration). Drusen are sometimes associated with pigment epithelial detachments due to their propensity to disrupt the layers of the retina.[4] The main cause of vision loss in dry macular degeneration is *geographic atrophy*.

The wet form affects only 10% to 15% of people who have age-related macular degeneration (AMD).[3] Vision loss, in this case, is due to bleeding and leaking of abnormal blood vessels as well as scarring, all of which cause distortion and destruction of central vision. It is frequently treated using intravitreal injections that inhibit the growth of new, abnormal blood vessels.

Age-related *cataracts* remain one of the most common causes of blindness in the world due to the lack of appropriate surgical services in third-world countries. However, any type of cataract can cause low vision. Vision loss with cataracts is usually a slow, gradually progressive process. Cataracts become denser and cloudier as we age, creating a decrease in vision and problems with glare (this is the most common type of cataract). Treatment is surgical removal of the cataract and insertion of a lens implant. Prior to surgery, a change in glasses prescription may be helpful up to a point, when surgery is required for further improvement.

Glaucoma is the second most common cause of blindness worldwide, and in the United States, half the

people with glaucoma are probably not aware they have it.[5] The hallmarks of glaucoma are loss of peripheral vision (which is not distinguishable by the patient in its early stages), high intraocular pressure (which cannot be felt by the patient), and optic nerve damage (which cannot be discerned by the patient). Thus, glaucoma is called the "sneak thief of sight." Left untreated, irreversible damage and drastic visual field loss can result.

There are a number of hereditary, progressive retinal degenerations/dystrophies. Of these, *retinitis pigmentosa* (RP) is the most common, affecting about 1.5 million people across the globe.[6] It specifically affects the light receptor cells: rods (responsible for vision in low lighting) are involved early in the disease, and cones (responsible for central vision) are affected later.

The loss of vision in RP begins in the periphery because the rod cells are affected; this also causes problems with night vision. The patient's visual field shrinks slowly. Central vision, mediated by the cone cells, is usually retained until late in the disease. At that point, color vision and central (reading) vision are affected. Low vision and legal blindness occur from as early as childhood to as late as the fourth decade of life. Disease progression varies from patient to patient.[7]

At this time, there is no specific cure or treatment for RP. Optical field expanders are one way for making use of the remaining sight. Research is being done with the Argus II Retinal Prosthesis System (Second Sight Medical Products, Inc), which is a retinal implant designed to bypass the damaged light receptor cells. The patient wears a headset that includes a video camera and a wireless computer. The unit sends information to the brain "creating the perception of patterns of light."[8] The device is intended for patients with bare light or NLP in both eyes due to RP.

Diabetic retinopathy is the most common eye disease in diabetics and a significant cause of blindness in adults of working age.[9] Diabetic retinopathy can be progressive and usually affects both eyes. It occurs in identifiable stages and can worsen if blood sugars are left uncontrolled. The most severe stage is proliferative retinopathy, where vitreous hemorrhages lead to severe vision loss or blindness. Collection of fluid in the macula (*macular edema*) can occur in every stage. It causes blurred and/or distorted central vision, resulting in difficulty with reading and daily activities.

CLINICAL SKILLS

When greeting patients with low vision, remember to introduce yourself and speak directly to them, making eye contact. Many people with vision loss can see some things, so it helps to make eye contact with them and include them in the orchestration of their care. When escorting an individual with low/impaired vision anywhere in your office, remember to *ask* if they need assistance. These individuals like to retain their independence and will ask for help when needed. If they do ask for guidance, offer them your elbow and give clear verbal directions on turns, doorways, and obstacles. Don't assume that since they can see some things that they can see everything. Finally, if the patient is accompanied by a service dog, do not grab the harness or touch the animal.

Low vision not only affects adults but children as well. Both have similar needs, but these are addressed differently. Children can be difficult to work with at times, even for the experienced technician. This challenge is even more evident when a visual disability is present, and you need to be creative in your work-up to try to assess their problems.

History Taking

History taking is covered in depth in Chapter 7, and taking the history of a low vision patient is similar to most patients. But there are some differences to keep in mind. A low vision patient history will likely be more extensive. Start by documenting the ocular health history and note what caused the vision impairment (eg, systemic disease, ocular disease, trauma, congenital disorder, stroke). Also, record how long the patient has had low vision and how he/she is coping with it in daily life. Some of the activities to focus on are safety around the home and neighborhood, performing self-care, and remaining an active part of society.

Inquire if the patient is still able to perform job duties, and talk over what hobbies he/she has enjoyed and if they are still possible. For many people, being able to do the activities that help them relax is very important, and when they can't enjoy them, it can create anxiety and depression.

You also want to find out more about general medical health, such as diabetes, hypertension, neurological issues, etc. This information is important to better help the patient determine low vision needs, such as identifying medication bottles or being able to use a glucose meter to test blood sugars.

Review family history as usual; this may be particularly important when dealing with children and young adults since there may be a genetic component.

Document any previous low vision assessments and their outcome. Also, ask the patient if he/she has tried any low vision devices and what success was attained.

Vision Testing

Visual acuity testing is covered in detail in Chapter 8. Getting the most accurate visual acuity is a very important part of the low vision assessment. Measuring the patient's distance and near visual acuity, including best corrected, may take more time than usual, especially for those with severe visual loss.

Low vision acuity testing is usually done using charts such as the Early Treatment Diabetic Retinopathy Study (ETDRS), Bailey-Lovie, or Feinbloom. These charts (especially the ETDRS) are preferred over Snellen because they were found to have better accuracy across the board.

The ETDRS is considered the best due to its standardization. The ETDRS design criteria includes:

▶ Equal spacing of letters per row (five letters per row)

▶ Equal spacing of the rows on a log scale (rows are separated by 0.1 log unit)

▶ Equal spacing of the letters

▶ Individual rows balance for letter difficulty

Bailey-Lovie charts integrate the European design of LogMAR (where the letters are arranged in an inverted triangle). Some practitioners prefer the LogMAR and Bailey-Lovie charts due to their standardization and the fact that each has five letters per row, so it is easier to see if a patient got half the row correct. This is especially true in the rows denoted for poorer visual acuity. Snellen does not have this feature; in the larger letters there are only one to three letters, which can make it difficult to interpret when a patient got half the line correct. Therefore, the more standardized log charts are better for individuals with low vision.[10]

Obtaining best-corrected visual acuity may require refractometry (Chapter 11). This can, at times, prove to be a task that needs extra patience by the technician (Sidebar 35-1). Some patients with low vision might not see the largest letter on the screen yet still have some correctable visual acuity.

Other tests may need to be done. Knowing the extent of a patient's visual loss, including how much visual field is present, is very important so the doctor can establish clear goals as well as levels of low vision for Medicare. Detailed visual field testing (covered in Chapter 14) by computerized or Goldmann perimeter may be necessary. When testing confrontation visual fields, make sure the patient looks in the center of your face. Even if the patient can't see centrally, tell him/her to continue to focus straight ahead so you can plot your confrontations accurately.

Contrast sensitivity (see Chapter 8) is tested using a special contrast chart (available on many of the computerized visual acuity screens). *Glare testing* (see Chapter 8) shows if the patient's level of visual acuity changes significantly under various lighting conditions.

Color vision testing (Chapter 9) may be helpful in determining reasons for the patient's current level of vision loss, and what treatment might be beneficial. Some disorders are associated with specific color vision changes. Historically it has been noted that retinal disease is manifest by blue/yellow discrimination loss and optic nerve disease by red/green discrimination loss.[11] There

---

SIDEBAR 35-1

HINTS FOR REFRACTOMETRY IN LOW VISION

▶ Allow the patient to adopt any head position that helps him/her see better.

▶ Encourage the patient to use eccentric fixation, if that helps.

▶ When changing lenses, use large steps (1 whole diopter or more).

▶ If distant vision is extremely poor but the patient retains some near vision, perform the entire refractometric measurement at near.

▶ Start with retinoscopy. This will give you an idea of the refractive error, even if there is no improvement in vision. You can also use the appearance of the reflex as a rough indicator of media clarity.

▶ If there is nystagmus, use +3 over the eye you are not testing instead of occluding it.

▶ Use a higher-powered Jackson cross cylinder.

▶ Hold trial lenses over the patient's current correction, and see if you can get any improvement.

▶ Use full-aperture trial lenses (borrow from the set used for visual field testing).

---

are exceptions, however. Early changes in glaucoma occur in the blue/yellow range, with advanced disease moving into the red/green area.[11]

If vision is so poor that the patient cannot fixate for cover testing, the extraocular muscle evaluation may be limited to Hirschberg and Krimsky tests. These are covered in Chapter 10.

Pupil evaluation must be meticulous as afferent pupillary defects can be subtle (see Chapter 9). Be sure to use a very bright light source in a dark or semi-dark room.

Low Vision Aids

Low vision aids come in the form of optical and nonoptical. Optical aids include magnifiers, bioptics (eyeglasses with a miniature telescope mounted toward the top of the eyeglass lens), and telescopes. Nonoptical aids include special lighting, talking devices, and audio books. It is the intent of these sections to familiarize you with the basic options available to patients with low vision and blindness.

Optical Low Vision Aids (Table 35-1)

The technician's role in low vision aids is often more toward teaching and instructing the patient about what aids would be most helpful depending on the patient's

lifestyle. A technician who works in a practice with an optical shop that sells magnifiers might work with the patient to find the magnifier most suited for him/her.

When determining what power of magnifier will be helpful for the patient, first ask what near activities he/she enjoys, such as reading, computer, sewing, needlepoint, puzzles, etc. Measure the patient's comfortable working distance(s) and remember the more plus (magnification) given, the shorter the working distance will become. Adapting to low vision devices such as magnifiers can be challenging, but may enable a patient to return to some activities previously abandoned due to declining vision.

Measuring for advanced devices such as bioptics and telescopic lenses would be done by a practitioner who specializes in low vision or works at a low vision center.

One of the newest optical aids available is the OrCam MyEye. It consists of a camera that is affixed to glasses; this head unit weighs less than 1 ounce. The camera works with a small computer base unit that clips on a waistband or belt and contains a rechargeable battery. The OrCam MyEye has three main functions: reading text, product recognition (ie, will describe objects), and facial recognition. The OrCam MyReader is only for reading and costs a bit less. Neither of these devices is meant for driving, but can still give the individual with low vision a greater independence.[12]

Nonoptical Low Vision Aids (Table 35-2)

There are many nonoptical aids available to help make life easier for the low vision patient, but they sometimes come with a steep price, making it difficult for patients to obtain them. Other aids are inexpensive. For example, keyboard labels are stickers with enlarged letters designed to help the low vision patient see the keys for typing on a computer (Figure 35-1). Stick-on foam dots of various sizes and shapes (Figure 35-2) can be used in different areas of the home to help the patient with everyday activities (eg, applied to stove/oven dials to identify heat levels).

Don't be afraid to be innovative! Wide, bright orange tape is inexpensive and effective if the patient retains some vision (Figure 35-3). Three-dimensional paint (such as fabric paint, which comes in small squeeze bottles) can be applied to surfaces for a tactile signal.

There are low vision apps for smart phones and computer tablets, which may also be an affordable option for some low vision patients. Most cell phones have magnifying apps, and many phones can read text messages and emails aloud. Cell phones and computers have text-to-talk as part of their functions as well. Apple has developed a free app for the iPhone called Visual-Access (TCS Associates, LLC). This app is designed to increase the self-sufficiency of the blind and low vision community by providing real-time assistance on-demand. Patients can simply call a "visual agent" from the app on their phone to have a live video or audio session for help in identifying

TABLE 35-1 EXAMPLES OF OPTICAL LOW VISION AIDS		
Optical Aid/Device	**Purpose/Use***	**Notes**
Magnifier (hand-held)	Reading/near	User must maintain proper focal distance Magnifier is moved as user reads/observes
Magnifier (stand)	Reading/near	Magnifier rests on page and is moved across reading material
Magnifier (page)	Reading/near	Magnifier lies flat on page, enabling hands-free use
Magnifier (bar)	Reading/near	Magnifier lies flat on page, but must be moved from one line to the next
Magnifier (illuminated)	Reading/near	User must maintain proper focal distance Adds light to magnified image
Magnified mirror	Shaving, makeup	Also comes in illuminated styles
Strong reading glasses	Reading/near	User must maintain proper focal distance Hands-free
Loupes	Reading/near	Usually affixed to glasses Patient can look under or over loupes as desired Hands-free
Microscopic glasses	Reading	For extremely fine near tasks; not intended for long work periods
Video magnifier system/ closed-circuit television	Reading/near	Tabletop unit magnifies objects/text
Absorptive sunglasses	All-purpose wear as patient finds helpful	Reduces glare Enhances contrast Blocks harmful ultraviolet rays
Telescope (hand-held)	Spotting at distance	Not for use when moving
Telescope (clip-on, mounted, bioptics)	Distance viewing	Not advisable to wear when walking about States vary regarding driving with bioptics
OrCam MyReader	Reads text	Head-worn camera with tiny computer that reads text
OrCam MyEye	Reads text, product identification, facial recognition	Head-worn camera with tiny computer that reads text, identifies products and faces
*The power (strength) of many near vision aids can be adjusted for intermediate tasks.		

their surroundings, reading mail, checking food labels, or any task for which they may need sighted assistance. There is even a color app to identify colors.

PATIENT SERVICES

Part of our job as technicians is to assist patients in determining their low vision needs and formulate a management plan to get them pointed in the right direction. When determining a patient's needs, it helps to place yourself mentally in his/her shoes so you can better understand the challenges. Look at the society in which they live and how it views individuals with such impairments. Our primary goal is to aid our patients, but we must make sure to honor their cultural differences as well.

When a patient loses vision, it often has a devastating impact on his/her life. The prospect of doing ordinary tasks, such as cooking meals, check writing, and reading mail, can be very scary and stressful. It can also be difficult for patients to rely on family and friends who can't comprehend their vision loss and often don't know how to help.

Part of the management plan is to help the patient get a support system in place, be it family, friends, church group, or a low vision support group. Support is very important for a low vision patient, especially those who have recently lost their sight. Individuals who experience

TABLE 35-2 EXAMPLES OF NONOPTICAL LOW VISION AIDS	
Nonoptical Aid/Device	**Comments**
Lighting	
Reading stand	
Reading guide (Typoscope)	Opaque cardboard with a cut-out area that corresponds to a line of type, lies directly on page, eliminates glare and improves contrast
Large print	
Colored/tinted acetate sheets	Lays directly on page, reduces glare, enhances contrast
Writing guides	Templates with cut-out areas that correspond to blank areas on checks, etc
Talking books	Many libraries have a collection, some e-readers have apps that will read aloud, Library of Congress offers books on tape to those with vision impairments
Talking watch	
Talking calculator	
Talking bill reader	Identifies denomination of paper money
Braille	
Phone/tablet apps	

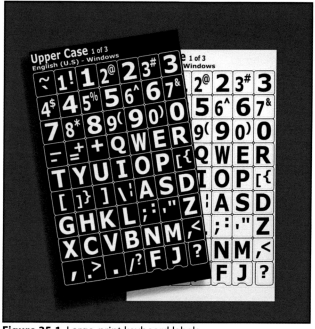

Figure 35-1. Large-print keyboard labels.

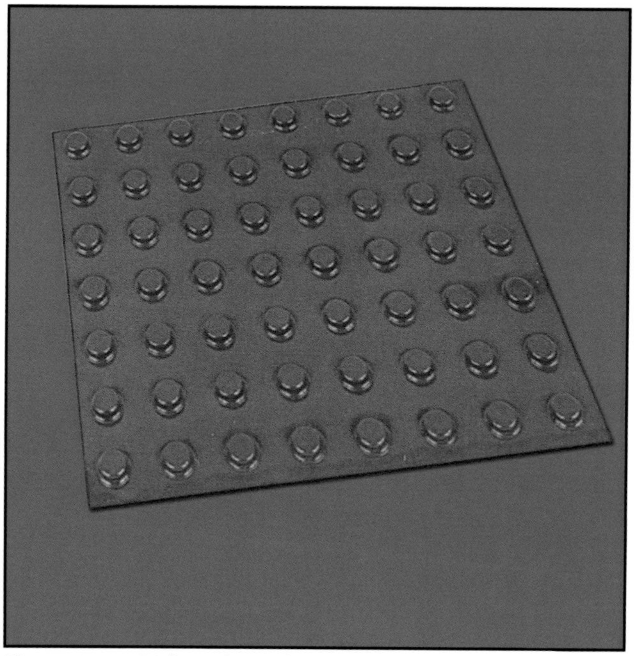

Figure 35-2. Stick-on foam dots can be attached to most anywhere.

vision loss can become depressed and isolated very easily. It is a good idea to talk to the patient's family (as long as you have patient consent), so they can better understand what their family member may be going through, and the role they can play in assisting.

Many low vision centers (discussed momentarily) offer support groups at their facility or in a grassroots fashion out of an individual's home. These support groups are generally run by people with vision problems who desire to reach out and help others with similar situations. Some centers utilize buddy programs where mentors help the newly impaired patient learn how to cope with this "new world."

Low Vision Resources

Adults often have a hard time changing old habits and adapting to new ones to cope with low vision. Older individuals have probably lived a good portion of their life independently with good vision and now find themselves in a new situation. Also, they may have other health issues that they have to cope with, making learning to use vision aids more challenging. They may have problems with arthritis or neurological issues, making it hard for them to use hand-held devices. Some may have hearing issues as well, making explanations difficult and causing them to feel more isolated. They may also experience denial regarding their vision. There are many resources available to assist the patient at every level, from ADLs to psychological issues.

Become familiar with the people and services at the nearest low vision center so you can better educate your patients. These resources can be found on the Internet (such as Lighthouse International at www.lighthouse-guild.org) or by word of mouth.

Most low vision centers dispense optical aids and offer in-home training to help patients adapt their ADLs, from in-home tasks to getting to the nearest bus stop. Some centers have their own radio station that reads books and newspapers. (A special receiver may be required.) Others have social outings and support groups.

One of the biggest hurdles for a low vision patient is the cost of getting help. There are organizations lobbying for better coverage for low vision and to get insurance companies to cover more in this area. Each state has different types of grants or loans to offer patients. Have printouts featuring the financial assistance available in your area. Also advise the patient to check with the low vision center itself, as some may have private grants.

Career rehabilitation and employment is another service offered at some low vision centers. Many patients have had to leave their careers due to their disability. Some low vision centers offer job aptitude tests to help place clients in new jobs so they can continue to lead productive lives. Some centers even employ the patients themselves. This helps monetarily and also creates a comfortable environment for those who are just entering the world of visual impairment.

Occupational therapists can help patients regain and maintain an independent lifestyle. When a patient sees an occupational therapist, the services are billable through Medicare. This is a great help for the patient since most low vision services are paid out of pocket. An occupational therapist treats the patient as a whole, finding ways for him/her to cope with visual and other disabilities. The occupational therapist will assess the patient's visual impairments and help him/her find and learn to use

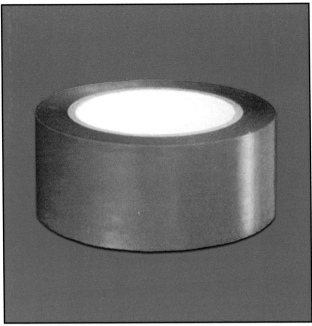

Figure 35-3. Brightly colored, wide tape can be used to mark items, steps, and walkways for those who retain some vision.

adaptive equipment. Occupational therapists can also teach patients ways to compensate for their visual deficit so they can return to a functional and more independent lifestyle.

Children tend to be more adaptable to low vision, especially if the condition was present early in life. Involve and educate the parents and teachers of children with vision problems. Help them understand that using glasses and devices will help the child see better and use any remaining vision to its fullest potential. One of the areas that children need more help with is the support of teachers and peers so they understand why children with vision issues may need magnifiers, telescopes, or other visual aids. Helping teachers and parents better understand the needs of the child will ensure better success for him/her in coping with the visual challenges.

Some low vision centers may have nursery schools that allow for mainstreaming with sighted children. This is beneficial for both groups of children. The children with visual disabilities are given the opportunity to blend in and be part of the big group, and to adapt to a sighted world. The children without disabilities are exposed to others who are different from themselves and learn that, after all, they are not really that different.

ACKNOWLEDGMENT

The author would like to thank Lisa Lystad, MD.

CHAPTER QUIZ

1. What is the definition of low vision or visually impaired?

2. What is functional vision loss as defined by the World Health Organization?

3. What are the two categories of functional vision loss?

4. What are the five leading causes of low vision?

5. What are the two forms of macular degeneration, and what is the main cause of vision loss in each form?

6. Why are cataracts still one of the most common causes of blindness in the world?

7. What is the second leading cause of blindness worldwide?

8. What is the leading cause of inherited blindness in the developed world?

9. Should you bother to make eye contact with a patient with low vision and why?

10. What are some key questions to ask a low vision patient in the history portion of the exam?

11. Name several reasons that Snellen charts are not used when evaluating acuity in low vision patients.

12. Name some optical and nonoptical aids.

13. Why is it important to set up a management plan for a patient with low vision (ie, a support system)?

14. Are low vision aids covered by insurance?

15. Should children with low vision be mainstreamed with sighted children?

Answers

1. Low vision/visually impaired is defined as significant vision loss that can't be corrected medically (including glasses) or surgically.

2. WHO defines functional vision loss as when an individual is unable to see to perform the tasks of daily life needed to survive.

3. Functional vision loss is divided into organic (due to an ocular disorder of some kind) and nonorganic (hysterical).

4. The five leading causes of low vision are macular degeneration, cataracts, glaucoma, retinal dystrophies, and diabetes.

5. The two forms of macular degeneration are dry (vision loss due to geographic atrophy) and wet (vision loss due to bleeding and leaking of abnormal blood vessels and scarring).

6. Cataracts are still causing blindness in the world due to lack of appropriate surgical services in third-world countries.

7. Glaucoma is the second most common cause of blindness in the world.

8. Retinitis pigmentosa is the leading cause of inherited blindness in the developed world.

9. Yes, you should make eye contact with the low vision patient. Many of these patients do retain some vision, although it may not be central (and thus they never appear to be looking at you). It is important to include him/her in the orchestration of care and to foster a feeling of independence.

10. Some key questions for the low vision history include cause of impairment, length of impairment, and coping with daily life (safety at home and neighborhood, self-care, active in society, etc).

11. Snellen acuity charts often do not have large enough optotypes for practical use in low vision patients. In addition, some lines have only one or two optotypes, making it impossible to quantify vision in a standardized way. ETDRS and Bailey-Lovie charts have five optotypes per line and a calculated decrease in size.

12. Optical aids include magnifiers, bioptics, and telescopes. Nonoptical aids incude talking devices, audiobooks, and special lighting.

13. A management plan is necessary because patients can become depressed and isolated, and it's important to let them know they are not alone. It's also important to educate family members on how to help their low vision relative keep safe and active.

14. Most low vision aids are an out-of-pocket expense for patients, making it difficult if they are on fixed incomes.

15. Children with low vision should be mainstreamed because it helps them learn and adapt to the real world. It benefits sighted children because they learn that peers with disabilities are really no different from themselves.

REFERENCES

1. Blindness and vision loss. Medline Plus website. www.nlm.nih. gov/medlineplus/ency/article/003040.htm. Accessed July 2, 2016.

2. Low vision. American Optometric Academy website. www. aoa.org/patients-and-public/caring-for-your-vision/low-vision?sso=y. Accessed July 2, 2016.

3. Haddrill M. Understanding age-related macular degeneration (AMD). All About Vision website. www.allaboutvision.com/conditions/amd.htm. Updated March 21, 2016. Accessed July 2, 2016.

4. What are drusen? Dry AMD symptoms. Macular Degeneration Partnership website. www.amd.org/what-are-drusen/. Accessed July 2, 2016.

5. Glaucoma facts and stats. Glaucoma Research Foundation website. www.glaucoma.org/glaucoma/glaucoma-facts-and-stats.php. Reviewed May 5, 2015. Accessed July 2, 2016.

6. Marazova K. Retinitis pigmentosa: prevalence. Institut De La Vision website. www.institut-vision.org/health/eye-diseases/28-diseases/97-retinitis-pigmentosa.html?showall=&start=1. Published May 12, 2015. Updated October 6, 2015. Accessed July 2, 2016.

7. Retinitis pigmentosa. Foundation Fighting Blindness website. www.blindness.org/retinitis-pigmentosa. Accessed July 2, 2016.

8. Argus II retinal prosthesis system. Second Sight website. www. secondsight.com/argus-ii-retinal-prosthesis-system-en.html. Accessed July 2, 2016.

9. Facts about diabetic eye disease. nei.nih.gov/health/diabetic/retinopathy. Reviewed September 2015. Accessed July 2, 2016.

10. Colenbrander A. Introduction to visual acuity measurement: letter chart measurements. Precision Vision University, Precision Vision website. http://precision-vision.com/b-letter-chart-measurements/. Accessed July 2, 2016.

11. Pacheco-Cutillas M, Sahraie A, Edgar DF. Acquired colour vision defects in glaucoma—their detection and clinical significance. *Br J Ophthalmol.* 1999;83:1396-1402. doi:10.1136/bjo.83.12.1396.

12. OrCam MyReader. OrCam website. www.orcam.com. Accessed July 10, 2016.

The figures in this chapter were contributed by the author, Beth Koch. The tables were contributed by Jan Ledford.

V

SURGICAL SERVICES AND SKILLS

36

OVERVIEW OF OPHTHALMIC SURGERY

Cynthia Matossian, MD, FACS
Henry Lee, MD
Sebastian Lesniak, MD

Ophthalmic surgery encompasses a very wide array of procedures, starting with eyelid surgery at the front of the eye and extending to orbital surgery at the back of the eye. Most major eye procedures are done in the operating room under sedation, ranging from topical to general anesthesia. Minor procedures, on the other hand, are performed in the examination room or in a room/suite designated for minor surgical procedures within an office setting (see Chapter 37).

A solid understanding of ocular anatomy and physiology is necessary when learning about ocular surgery (Chapters 2 and 3). A background of pharmacology (Chapter 22), operating room procedure (Chapter 40), ocular trauma (Chapter 32), and ocular disorders (Chapters 26 and 27) is also essential.

EYELID AND BROW SURGERY

Procedures of the eyelid vary from medically necessary to cosmetic.

Entropion repair is done to correct an eyelid that has turned inward toward the cornea. Patients will often complain of irritation, foreign body sensation, eye redness, and tearing. Surgery is performed to correct the underlying pathology responsible for the entropion. Typically,

this includes tightening of the eyelid, reattachment of ruptured lower eyelid muscles, and excision of a portion of the orbicularis oculi muscle. An alternative and less invasive procedure can be undertaken in the office with the two or three absorbable sutures, called the *Quickert procedure*. However, the success rate with the Quickert procedure is lower than that of traditional surgery.

Ectropion repair corrects the malposition of an eyelid that has turned outward toward the cheek. For patients with an ectropion, the typical symptoms include irritation, tearing, and eye redness. This malposition is most commonly due to laxity of the eyelid. In these cases, surgical tightening of the eyelid is undertaken, which results in a very high success rate.

Blepharoplasty is usually performed to correct redundant upper eyelid skin or to correct bags under the eyes. Surgery involving the upper eyelids can be functional or cosmetic in nature, whereas surgery for the lower eyelids is almost always cosmetic. For the upper eyelids, excess eyelid skin with or without underlying orbicularis oculi muscle is excised. Occasionally, excess orbital fat is excised, trimmed, or repositioned. The incision is closed with absorbable or nonabsorbable sutures.

Lower eyelid blepharoplasty can be complex in nature, and individualization of the surgery is essential to ensure optimal outcomes. Surgery can involve one or more of the

Ledford JK, Lens A, eds.
Principles and Practice in Ophthalmic Assisting:
A Comprehensive Textbook (pp 623-630).
© 2018 Taylor & Francis Group.

following steps: excision or repositioning of orbital fat, excision of lower eyelid skin, tightening of the orbicularis oculi muscle, tightening of the lower eyelid in patients with eyelid laxity, and lifting of the suborbicularis oculi or midface fat, among other procedures. (The suborbicularis oculi fat pad is an anatomic structure in the cheek and midface that is sometimes lifted during a lower eyelid blepharoplasty.)

Ptosis repair is performed when either one or both upper lids droop down, either causing a cosmetic problem or a medical problem by encroaching on the pupil. This is especially important in children, as an eye that is occluded by a lid will develop amblyopia. While ptosis can occur for many different reasons, the most common causes are age-related stretching or dehiscence (splitting open) of the levator superioris muscle, the main eyelid levator. Surgery to reattached or strengthen the muscle is performed, usually through an upper eyelid skin incision or from the inner surface of the eyelid.

Excision of tumors is performed for the removal of growths that may be cosmetically unappealing, interruptive of function, and either benign or malignant in nature. Small tumors are generally removed as a minor procedure. Larger growths, however, will be taken to the operating room. Excised tissue is sent for pathology evaluation.

If the tumor is determined to be malignant based on pathology reports, the margins of the tumor have to be very carefully examined, making sure that all the cancer was completely removed. This is usually accomplished by *Mohs surgery*, which involves the precise and complete excision of common skin malignancies. While the patient is still on the surgery table, tissue is sent to pathology and examined slide by slide to make sure all margins are clear (tumor-free). This process continues until clear tissue is reached.

Mohs surgeons are dermatologists who undergo additional fellowship training. This surgical technique has helped to increase the success rate for surgical excision of malignant eyelid lesions. Following the excision by a Mohs surgeon, patients typically have surgery with an ophthalmologist or oculoplastic surgeon for reconstruction of the eyelid.

Repair of traumatic eyelid lacerations can be minor to very extensive depending on the type of injury and the causative agent. The repair may require a staged approach with multiple procedures. Patients should be reminded that healing can take 6 months or longer. Therefore, if multiple surgeries are required, it may be 1 year or more before the final result is achieved.

A *brow lift* can be done for cosmetic or functional issues. When the brows droop, they can cause a mechanical ptosis because of the added weight of the brow tissues pushing on the eyelid. The brow drop also increases the ptotic appearance of upper eyelid dermatochalasis (where there is extra skin on the upper lid).

There are numerous methods for lifting the brow. In a *direct brow lift*, tissue above the brow is excised. When the incision is closed, the brow is pulled up. Excision of greater amounts of tissue leads to greater elevation of the brow. Unfortunately, the direct brow lift results in a visible scar, which may be undesirable to some patients. In an *internal browpexy*, the subcutaneous brow tissues are addressed via a standard, upper eyelid crease incision. An internal browpexy is considered more of a brow stabilizing procedure as opposed to a brow lift, since significant brow elevation is not possible with the internal browpexy.

Other methods of brow lifting include a *pre-trichial* (in front of the hairline) brow lift, a *post-trichial* (behind the hairline) brow lift, a *coronal* (incision all the way across the scalp) brow lift, and an *endoscopic* brow lift (where a tiny camera in a tube is used to guide the surgery, which is done with very fine instruments). The procedure is chosen based on the patient's individual needs and expectations, the height of the forehead, the presence or absence of significant forehead *rhytids* (wrinkles), the hairline, and the presence or absence of hair, among other factors.

Reconstructive Surgery

Eyelid reconstruction is performed for a variety of reasons, such as trauma or excision of tumors or eyelid lesions. Depending on the size and location of the eyelid defect, the wound may be left to heal by *secondary intention* (allowing the wound to scab and heal itself). If the edges of a wound can be reapproximated (ie, pulled together and matched up) with minimal tension, then a primary closure with absorbable or nonabsorbable sutures can be performed. If there appears to be moderate tension, absorbable sutures can be placed to reapproximate the deeper tissues, thereby reducing the tension at the skin edges.

If the wound is too large to be closed via primary closure, then additional techniques may need to be employed, such as flaps or skin grafts. *Flaps* typically involve rotating or advancing adjacent skin and/or subcutaneous tissues into the area of the defect. This requires significant dissection of the adjacent skin and/or subcutaneous tissues in order to provide enough tissue to cover the wound. *Skin grafts* involve removing skin from a donor site, which most commonly is from another eyelid, the preauricular region (in front of the ear), the postauricular region (behind the ear), or the supraclavicular region (above the collarbone). These are all non–hair-bearing regions, which is useful for reconstruction of the non–hair-bearing periocular area.

LACRIMAL SURGERY

Surgery of the lacrimal system can involve the punctum, canaliculi, lacrimal sac, and lacrimal gland.

The most common procedure involving the puncta is a *punctoplasty* for punctal stenosis (ie, the puncta is stopped up). Punctal stenosis can result in excessive tearing due to obstruction of the tear outflow. The punctoplasty procedure can be performed in the office with local anesthetic and involves dilating the punctum with a punctal dilator, followed by three small incisions into the posterior wall of the punctum and vertical portion of the canaliculus. This results in enlargement of the punctum, which improves tear outflow.

Canalicular surgery is most commonly performed for stenosis or infection (canaliculitis). For stenosis, excision of scar tissue with subsequent *stenting* (insertion of a tube to keep it open) of the canaliculus can be undertaken, though success rates can vary for this procedure. For canaliculitis, an incision is made through the canaliculus. Purulent material is typically encountered and removed with a curette. Occasionally, foreign bodies (such as a displaced punctal plug) are discovered and removed. The canaliculus is usually carefully sutured closed with or without a stent following this procedure.

An infection of the lacrimal sac (dacryocystitis) is a common indication for surgery involving the lacrimal sac or duct. Dacryocystitis usually results from obstruction of the nasolacrimal duct. In these cases, a *dacryocystorhinostomy* (DCR) is performed, which creates a new outflow path for the lacrimal system, thereby bypassing the obstruction. Surgery can be done via an external incision through the eyelid or via an endoscopic approach through the nose. Success rates for both approaches are high. A stent may be inserted at the end of the surgery, which will need to be removed in the office, usually anywhere from 4 to 12 weeks later.

Lacrimal gland surgery is rarely done, but might be undertaken for infections, inflammatory conditions, age-related changes, and tumors, among other reasons. The details of the surgery vary greatly depending on the cause for surgery.

ANTERIOR SEGMENT PROCEDURES

Conjunctiva

Excision of conjunctival tumors is similar to removal of a pterygium (discussed later). The suspicious conjunctival lesion is dissected from the underlying sclera and excised. In addition, absolute alcohol, mitomycin C, or cryotherapy (freezing) of surrounding tissues may be utilized. These additional procedures decrease the rate of tumor recurrence.

Nonrefractive Corneal Surgery

Procedures of the cornea vary from medically necessary for scars, edema, or severe deformation, to elective refractive options for the correction of myopia, hyperopia, astigmatism, and/or presbyopia. Refractive surgery is covered in Chapter 38.

A *corneal transplant* involves removing the central portion of a scarred or diseased cornea and replacing it with clear donor tissue. This replacement tissue comes from a deceased person, is harvested by trained personnel, and is then evaluated carefully by an eye bank. Blood type matching is not necessary and does not improve the outcome. The tissue is commercially shipped from the eye bank, on ice.

Full-thickness corneal transplant or *penetrating keratoplasty* (PKP) is indicated for visually significant corneal scars, perforations (which can result from trauma, infection, or disintegration [melt]), keratoconus, corneal edema and haze not amenable to partial-thickness transplantation (covered momentarily), or failed prior corneal transplant. The procedure involves creating a full-thickness, circular incision in the patient's cornea using a "cookie cutter" instrument called a trephine. This diseased corneal button is then removed, and an identically shaped section of donor cornea is sutured to the host bed. Typically, 16 interrupted sutures are used, but in corneas without peripheral vascularization and with good visual potential, a continuous running suture can be used along with a lesser number of interrupted sutures. (Running sutures are thought to decrease postoperative irregular astigmatism.) Recovery is typically up to 1 year, and patients often require spectacle correction (or rigid contact lenses in cases of irregular astigmatism). The sutures are selectively removed starting at 3 to 6 months postoperatively, generally at the location of the steep axis of astigmatism.

Patients require long-term use of topical steroid drops to prevent rejection, an occurrence that eye care personnel must always be alert for. Signs and symptoms of rejection include pain, photophobia, redness, and decreased vision.

Deep anterior lamellar keratoplasty (DALK) is typically performed in keratoconus patients or in patients with superficial corneal scars where endothelial function is good. The procedure is similar to PKP, but the corneal incision is not full thickness and an attempt is made to transplant all layers of the cornea except the endothelium. Preserving the patient's own endothelium is thought to decrease the rate of transplant rejection.

Keratoplasty that involves insertion of a *keratoprosthesis* (such as the Boston KPro) is also similar to PKP, but is typically offered to patients with multiple prior failures of corneal transplants. The device consists of both artificial components and traditional corneal donor tissue. A small opening is created in the center of the donor cornea, and an artificial polymer front plate with an optical stem is inserted. Additionally, a titanium or polymer plate is inserted on the back surface of the donor cornea. This assembly is sutured to the host bed with interrupted sutures similar to PKP. Patients with KPro's require long-term use of a large soft contact lens over the transplant, as well as long-term use of antibiotic, antifungal, and steroid eye drops.

Descemet's stripping endothelial keratoplasty (DSEK) has become the standard of care for patients with endothelial dysfunction resulting in corneal edema and decreased vision. The most common causes of endothelial dysfunction are Fuchs' dystrophy and pseudophakic bullous keratopathy. The procedure involves stripping and removing only Descemet's membrane and the endothelial corneal layer, while leaving the patient's own stroma and other layers in place. The donor tissue consists of a very thin layer of donor stroma, Descemet's membrane, and endothelium. This donor tissue is inserted into the eye and placed against the inner surface of the patient's cornea. It is then held in place by an air bubble injected into the eye at the end of the surgery. The air bubble is absorbed and disappears after about 2 days. The patient has to maintain a face-down position for approximately 2 days after surgery to maximize tissue adherence. In some cases more air has to be added if the inner donor layer detaches. This is called rebubbling. DSEK has a much shorter recovery of up to 3 months (vs PKP), requires a few small incisions, and typically requires just one suture. Irregular astigmatism is much less common and rejection rates are lower than PKP.

Descemet's membrane endothelial keratoplasty (DMEK) is a further refinement of DSEK. The host Descemet's membrane and endothelial layer are stripped the same way as in DSEK. The difference is that the donor tissue is much thinner and consists of only donor Descemet's membrane and endothelial layer (ie, without any stroma as in DSEK). The procedure is much more difficult technically, but the rejection rate is lower and final visual acuity is better compared to DSEK.

Phototherapeutic keratectomy (PTK) is typically used for treatment of corneal scars or opacities. It is similar to photorefractive keratectomy (PRK) in that corneal epithelium is removed by scraping after application of alcohol. The underlying corneal tissue is reshaped by excimer laser. Because the epithelium has to regenerate, recovery can be painful and can take about 1 week. Mitomycin C is typically used to prevent corneal haze.

Superficial keratectomy is indicated for visually significant scarring under the epithelial layer (subepithelial fibrosis), scarring, or Salzmann nodules (subepithelial nodular scars). The procedure involves removal of the epithelium and the underlying corneal lesions manually with a blade. Postoperatively, a bandage contact lens is applied until the surface is reepithelialized.

Sodium EDTA chelation is indicated for removal of calcium deposits at the level of the Bowman's layer in band keratopathy (BK). Epithelium is first removed by scrapping with a blade. The underlying calcium deposits are then removed by cotton applicators or sponges saturated with sodium EDTA. Postoperatively, a bandage contact lens is applied until the surface is reepithelialized.

Corneal collagen cross-linking is indicated for conditions that result in significant corneal deformation and decreased vision. These disorders include keratoconus, pellucid marginal degeneration, and post-LASIK ectasia, which are similar conditions resulting in significant distortion of the corneal surface and formation of a cone-like bulge on the corneal surface. In the most common approach, the corneal epithelium is removed with alcohol and scrapping. Riboflavin (vitamin B_2) is applied to the corneal surface until the cornea is adequately saturated. Subsequently, ultraviolet radiation is applied to the corneal surface for several minutes. This process increases bonding between corneal fibers and strengthens the cornea. The main purpose of this treatment is to halt progression of corneal deformation; however, studies indicate that cross-linking can decrease corneal steepness and improve vision in some patients.[1]

Corneal gluing is indicated for small corneal perforations and melts that can occur in neurotrophic corneas (which have decreased or absent corneal sensation), in patients with connective tissue diseases, or after trauma. A small amount of cyanoacrylate glue is applied over the perforated area. Once the glue dries, a bandage contact lens is placed on top. This procedure can allow the underlying perforation to heal or can serve as a temporary seal until a corneal transplant can be performed.

Surgical repair of traumatic corneal lacerations is required when there is penetrating full-thickness laceration of the cornea. The surgery involves placement of corneal sutures to seal the eye. These injuries are traumatic and surgery may also involve removal of corneal foreign bodies. It is very important to rule out a possibility of intraocular foreign body in the vitreous cavity with a CT scan. If present, intraocular foreign bodies must be promptly removed by a retinal surgeon.

Pterygium surgery entails the removal of this vascular growth that encroaches on the cornea and interferes with vision due to the astigmatism it causes (see Figure 26-9). Moreover, the pterygium can have an unappealing cosmetic appearance or cause constant irritation and redness. A conjunctival autograft (meaning the tissue comes from the patient him-/herself) is typically used to prevent recurrence. The graft is usually harvested from the bulbar conjunctiva under the upper lid and is attached to the sclera with tissue glue or sutures at the site where the pterygium was removed. A small percentage of these lesions can be cancerous, and the excised tissue is sent for pathological evaluation.

Anterior Chamber Reconstructive Surgery

Iridoplasty involves surgical repair of iris defects typically caused by trauma, prior surgery, or chronic inflammatory conditions. Nondissolvable sutures are placed in the iris tissue to close the defect. Iridodialysis (separation of iris from the angle structures) is repaired by suturing the separated iris tissue to the sclera.

Pupilloplasty involves surgical repair of a large or irregularly shaped pupil. This can also be caused by trauma, prior surgery, or chronic inflammatory conditions. Large pupils can result in photophobia and decreased vision, while irregularly shaped pupils can have an unappealing cosmetic appearance. A circular suture is placed in the iris tissue around the pupil and tightened to the desired pupillary diameter.

Artificial iris implants are used in cases of traumatic or post-surgical iris tissue loss, or in cases of congenital aniridia (absence of iris). These patients can experience photophobia and decreased vision. The iris implant is color-matched to the other eye and either placed in the capsular bag in front of the intraocular lens (IOL) or sutured to the sclera.

Anterior Vitrectomy

Lens-based surgery for the removal of a cataract and its replacement with an implant is the most common type of surgery performed in ophthalmology. It is covered in Chapter 28.

Sometimes during cataract surgery the vitreous may prolapse out of the vitreous cavity into the supracapsular space. In this case the vitreous must be meticulously removed via a procedure called an *anterior vitrectomy*. This procedure might be planned because of preexisting disorders of the zonules (*zonulopathy*) or history of ocular trauma, as these situations have an increased risk of vitreous prolapse around the missing or damaged zonules. At other times, an anterior vitrectomy is unplanned, as when the posterior capsule becomes torn or ruptured during cataract surgery and the vitreous prolapses through the opening. The vitrectomy has to be performed thoroughly to avoid any residual vitreous strands to the wound; these can be associated with an increased risk of cystoid macular edema (CME) as well as infection.

Cataract and Intraocular Lens Implant Procedures

Cataract surgery is discussed in Chapter 28.

IOL repositioning is performed when an IOL becomes dislocated. This can occur after trauma or as a postoperative complication of cataract surgery. IOLs can also dislocate spontaneously as in cases of pseudoexfoliation or Marfan syndrome, conditions in which the capsular bag or zonules that hold the IOL become weak or break. Repositioning may simply involve rotating the IOL to a more stable position. If the capsular bag or zonules are not structurally sound, the IOL may have to be sutured either to the iris or exchanged.

IOL exchange is performed for a variety of reasons including complete dislocation, malposition with zonular loss or capsular breaks, incorrect IOL power, glare or halos from multifocal IOLs, inflammation caused by an IOL rubbing against the iris, and corneal decompensation caused by an anterior chamber IOL. If after IOL removal the capsular bag and zonules remain intact, the new IOL may simply be placed in the capsular bag. However, a large percentage of these cases require anterior vitrectomy and suturing of the IOL to the iris or sclera due to lack of adequate support structures.

Secondary IOL implantation is performed in aphakic eyes (where the natural crystalline lens has been dislocated or removed). Patients can become aphakic after trauma, after retinal surgery that requires lens removal, or after childhood cataract surgery (since IOL implants are not recommended for very young children). These cases typically require anterior vitrectomy and suturing of the IOL to the iris or sclera due to lack of adequate support structures.

Glaucoma Surgery

Glaucoma is covered in Chapter 29. Glaucoma surgery entails a wide variety of procedures all designed to lower the intraocular pressure.

Trabeculectomy is a filtering surgery where an opening is created into the anterior chamber through a partial-thickness scleral flap to allow the aqueous to flow out of the eye. The aqueous flows into the subconjunctival space, usually leading to an elevation of the conjunctiva, referred to as a filtering bleb.

Glaucoma drainage devices are designed to divert aqueous humor from the anterior chamber to a reservoir that is placed under the conjunctiva. These devices are used in eyes with previously failed trabeculectomy or in eyes with insufficient conjunctiva because of scarring from prior surgical procedures or injuries. The devices are available in different sizes, materials, and designs with the presence or absence of an IOP regulating valve.

The iStent Trabecular Micro-Bypass Stent (Glaukos) is a heparin-coated titanium stent with a snorkel shape. (The heparin helps prevent blood from clotting inside the stent.) The device is placed into Schlemm's canal in the angle of the eye at the time of cataract surgery for patients who do not have advanced glaucoma. The iStent is the smallest Food and Drug Administration-approved device, measuring at 0.3 mm in height and 1 mm in length.

Goniotomy is one of the major surgical options for primary congenital glaucoma. This procedure is preferred when the cornea is clear enough to permit visualization of anterior segment structures. An incision is made across the trabecular meshwork under direct gonioscopic visualization to establish aqueous outflow.

Trabectome is a surgical system that allows a trabeculotomy to be performed via an internal approach. The procedure works by removing a strip of trabecular meshwork and the inner wall of Schlemm's canal in order to create a path for the drainage of aqueous humor.

Endocyclophotocoagulation (ECP) is a method of destroying the ciliary body to treat glaucoma. The goal of each laser application is to whiten and shrink the ciliary processes, which are responsible for excreting aqueous. ECP can be performed in phakic, pseudophakic, or aphakic eyes with an endolaser probe through the limbus or pars plana. ECP can be combined with phacoemulsification to treat cataract and glaucoma at the same time.

Eye Muscle (Strabismus) Surgery

Eye muscle surgery is performed to reposition one or multiple muscles of the eye to correct misalignment (strabismus). The misalignment can be congenital, so surgery is often performed on children. However, strabismus can also be acquired, that is, caused by trauma, a stroke, a palsy of one of the nerves that innervate the eye muscles, or from other medical conditions such as thyroid eye disease.

The eye muscles are attached to the sclera (white wall of the eye). The surgeon incises the conjunctiva to access the eye muscle(s), and uses a delicate hook to isolate the muscle, cut it, and either loosen (*recession*) or tighten (*resection*) it to improve ocular alignment. A single muscle or multiple eye muscles can be operated on during a single surgery depending on the type and severity of strabismus. Adjustable sutures can be utilized that allow for small corrections after the surgery. No skin incisions are made. The eyeball is NOT removed from the eye socket during strabismus surgery.

Retinal and Vitreous Surgery

Retinal surgery encompasses a broad spectrum of procedures from retinal detachment repair to excision or treatment of choroidal tumors.

Vitrectomy is the surgical removal of the vitreous gel from the middle of the eye. (This is called an *anterior vitrectomy* if the vitreous comes forward into the anterior chamber, discussed earlier.) This can be challenging because the vitreous has the consistency of an egg white, and is very sticky. A vitrectomy may be necessary when there is a retinal detachment in order to gain better access to the back of the eye, or it may be performed to remove blood from the vitreous gel (vitreous hemorrhage) that is not clearing on its own. During a vitrectomy, the surgeon inserts small instruments into the eye, cuts the vitreous gel, and suctions it out. After removing the vitreous gel, the surgeon may treat the retina with a laser (photocoagulation), cut or remove fibrous or scar tissue from the retina, flatten areas where the retina has become detached, or repair tears or holes in the retina or macula. At the end of the surgery, silicone oil or a gas bubble may be injected into the eye to lightly press the retina against the wall of the eye. Oil cannot be absorbed by the body, so if an oil bubble is used, a second procedure to remove the oil after the retinal detachment has healed will be required. If a gas bubble is used, patients typically have to lie face-down for several weeks. Silicone oil has less strict postoperative positioning requirements and is more suitable for patients who are unable to maintain face-down positioning.

Retinal detachment repair can only be achieved through surgery. The goals of surgery are to reattach the retina and to prevent or reverse vision loss.

Almost all retinal detachments can be repaired with scleral buckle surgery, pneumatic retinopexy, or laser. (See Chapter 39 for information on lasers.) *Scleral buckle surgery* involves suturing a silicone belt around the eye, under the conjunctiva. It is performed in the operating room and does not require removal of the vitreous. The scleral buckle compresses the eye, and the external pressure allows the retina to reattach. Not all forms of retinal detachment can be repaired with scleral buckles. *Pneumatic retinopexy* involves injecting an air bubble into the posterior chamber of the eye to flatten the retina and allow it to reattach. It can be performed in the office for certain types of retinal detachment.

Time is of the essence for repair of retinal detachments. How soon surgery is required usually depends on whether the retinal detachment has or could spread far enough to affect central vision. When the macula loses contact with the retinal layer beneath it, it quickly loses its ability to process images. Having surgery while the macula is still attached will usually save most vision. If the macula has become detached, surgery may be delayed for a few days because the outcome is not as sensitive to timing as in cases when the macula is still attached. Good vision after surgery is still possible but less likely.

Scar tissue or epiretinal membranes may form on the surface of the retina in many situations, including macular pucker, macular hole, and complicated retinal detachment. This tissue can be removed via a *membrane peel*. After completion of a vitrectomy, the epiretinal membranes are delicately peeled from the surface of the retina and removed from the eye using micro-forceps. If the membrane is particularly dense, micro-scissors may be used to release it from the retina. The purpose of this surgery is to restore normal retinal anatomy and improve vision that may be distorted by the membrane.

Orbital Surgery

Orbital surgery is usually performed by ophthalmologists who have completed additional training in oculofacial and reconstructive surgery. The procedures span a large spectrum from orbital fracture repair to enucleation of the eye.

In cases of periocular trauma, the orbital bones surrounding the globe and orbital contents can fracture. Surgical repair varies depending on the type and extent of the injury. The most common orbital fracture is an orbital floor blowout fracture (see Figure 32-10). Most orbital floor fractures can be repaired 1 or 2 weeks following the injury. However, in certain cases, such as impingement and entrapment of the inferior rectus muscle, repair should be undertaken as soon as possible to decrease the risk of permanent injury to the muscle.

In *orbital floor fracture repairs*, an incision is most commonly made through the conjunctiva of the lower eyelid. The fracture site is identified and any herniated orbital contents are released. Then an orbital implant is inserted to cover the fracture site. This implant can be made of a variety of materials, including nylon sheet, porous polyethylene, titanium mesh, and autogenous (ie, the donor is the patient him-/herself) bone grafts. Following the repair, the conjunctival incision may or may not be closed with sutures. Patients are typically asked to avoid blowing the nose and any physical activity until approximately 2 weeks following the repair.

Thyroid ophthalmopathy (also referred to as thyroid eye disease or thyroid orbitopathy) is a complex disease. In some patients with thyroid eye disease, enlargement of the extraocular muscles, the orbital fat, or both can cause exophthalmos (forward displacement of the globe). This in turn can result in eye irritation and dryness, lagophthalmos (inability to completely close the eyelids), corneal abrasions and ulcers, and in rare cases, optic neuropathy (which can lead to blindness). Patients with significant exophthalmos or optic neuropathy are treated with *orbital decompression*. Orbital decompression surgery creates more space in the orbit by thinning or removing of one or more of the orbital bones. After this expansion of the bony orbit, the orbital contents (including the globe, extraocular muscles, and fat) have more room, decreasing the proptosis of the globe.

Fortunately, orbital tumors are rare. Surgery to biopsy and/or excise these tumors depends on the size and location of the orbital tumor. For malignant tumors, additional therapy, including chemotherapy or radiation therapy, may be indicated.

Enucleation involves the removal of the eye, whereas *evisceration* involves the removal of the intraocular contents. Both surgeries are typically performed for patients who have blind, painful eyes or advanced ocular infection. Enucleation is also performed for patients with intraocular malignancies. Following the removal of the eye or the intraocular contents, an orbital implant is inserted. The implant can be made of a variety of materials, including silicone, polymethylmethacrylate, porous polyethylene, hydroxyapatite, and autogenous skin-fat grafts. For enucleations, the extraocular muscles are typically sutured to the implant, whereas in eviscerations, the implant is inserted and covered by the remaining sclera. Several weeks following surgery, patients are evaluated by an ocularist, a specially trained professional who will make the patient an artificial eye.

Exenteration surgery involves the removal of the eye as well as some or all of the surrounding structures, which may include the extraocular muscles, orbital fat and bones, and eyelids. This extensive surgery is reserved for potentially life-threatening conditions, such as malignancies or aggressive infectious diseases. There can be significant postoperative deformity following an exenteration. Patients can be referred to an ocularist who has had experience making orbital prostheses, which is an essential step in the rehabilitation of these patients.

CHAPTER QUIZ

1. True/False: A lid tightening procedure can be used to repair both entropion and ectropion.

2. True/False: Lower eyelid blepharoplasty is almost always cosmetic as opposed to functional.

3. True/False: Mohs surgery involves examining tumor margins by a pathologist while the patient is still on the operating table until clear margins are reached.

4. True/False: Punctoplasty is performed in patients with severe dry eye who underproduce tears.

5. True/False: The most common indication for canalicular surgery is stenosis or canaliculitis.

6. True/False: During excision of conjunctival tumors, absolute alcohol, mitomycin C, and cryotherapy all decrease the recurrence of the tumor.

7. True/False: Corneal transplant tissue comes from a live donor similar to a kidney transplant.

8. True/False: Penetrating keratoplasty is typically performed to eliminate the need for glasses.

9. True/False: Recovery after penetrating keratoplasty is typically 1 month.

10. True/False: Patients require long-term use of steroid drops after corneal transplant.

11. True/False: Deep anterior lamellar keratoplasty is thought to have a lower rejection rate than penetrating keratoplasty.

12. True/False: The patient has to maintain face-up position for 2 weeks after DSEK or DMEK surgery.

13. True/False: PTK is an alternative to LASIK and treats refractive errors.

14. True/False: Collagen cross-linking eliminates corneal deformation and can cure keratoconus.

15. True/False: Corneal gluing permanently seals corneal perforations.

16. True/False: Conjunctival autograft for pterygium excision surgery is typically harvested from under the lower eyelid.

17. True/False: Iridoplasty is a cosmetic procedure that alters the color of the iris.

18. True/False: Trabeculectomy is performed by inserting a tube into the anterior chamber and redirecting the aqueous outflow.

19. True/False: Goniotomy is primarily performed in primary open-angle glaucoma.

20. True/False: Eye muscle surgery is performed by complete excision of malpositioned extraocular muscles.

21. True/False: Vitrectomy involves surgical removal of detached retina to prevent further detachment.

22. True/False: Silicone oil cannot be absorbed by the eye and has to be removed after the retina has healed.

23. True/False: Retinal detachment repair may be delayed by several weeks without significant consequences.

24. True/False: All orbital floor fractures must be repaired immediately.

25. True/False: Orbital decompression surgery is typically indicated for optic neuropathy or significant exophthalmos.

26. True/False: Enucleation involves removal of the entire eye from the eye socket.

Answers

1. True
2. True
3. True
4. False
5. True
6. True
7. False
8. False
9. False
10. True
11. True
12. False
13. False
14. False
15. False
16. False
17. False
18. False
19. False
20. False
21. False
22. True
23. False
24. False
25. True
26. True

REFERENCE

1. Greenstein SA, Shah VP, Fry KL, Hersh PS. Corneal thickness changes after corneal collagen crosslinking for keratoconus and corneal ectasia: one-year results. *J Cataract Refract Surg.* 2011;37(4):691-700.

37

IN-OFFICE MINOR SURGERY

Kesha Hyde, COT
Jan Ledford, COMT

BASIC SCIENCES

In order to have the knowledge base needed for this chapter, please review Chapters 2 (Anatomy), 3 (Physiology), and 26 (Anterior Disorders) as necessary.

CLINICAL KNOWLEDGE AND SKILLS

Blood-Borne Pathogens, Other Potential Contaminants, and Standard (Universal) Precautions

Blood-borne pathogens are microbes that can cause human disease and can be transmitted by coming into contact with the blood of an infected person. (See Chapter 23 for a review of microbiology.) The most notable of these are the hepatitis B virus (HBV) and the human immunodeficiency virus (HIV, which causes acquired immunodeficiency syndrome [AIDS]). Other potentially infectious materials (OPIM) that might transmit disease include semen, vaginal secretions, cerebrospinal fluid, saliva, unfixed (ie, unpreserved by any chemicals) tissue, and any body fluid in which blood is visible. Notably missing from this list are tears, sweat, urine, and feces, unless blood is visible. While the HIV virus has been isolated from human tears, there are no cases where HIV was transmitted by contact with nonbloody tears.[1]

In 1987, the Centers for Disease Control and Prevention (CDC) published the document *Recommendations for Prevention of HIV Transmission in Health-Care Settings,* which set forth precautions to be used to protect health care workers from exposure to HIV, HBV, and other blood-borne pathogens.[2] These *standard precautions* (previously known as *universal precautions*) are a method of reducing and preventing exposure to blood-borne pathogens and OPIM. It means that we must consider *all* blood and OPIM from every source as being contaminated with HBV and HIV. It includes use of *personal protective equipment* (PPE) and methods of disposing of and/ or decontaminating items that may have blood or OPIM on them. In addition, reusable materials and instruments that potentially come into contact with more than one patient must be sterilized after each use (see Chapter 40).

PPE is one of the most important necessities in a surgical procedure. PPE includes gloves, masks, gowns, and eye protection. Which items are used depends on the type of procedure and the likelihood of exposure to blood-borne pathogens. By law, your clinic must provide this equipment for you without charge.

Ledford JK, Lens A, eds.
Principles and Practice in Ophthalmic Assisting:
A Comprehensive Textbook (pp 631-644).
© 2018 Taylor & Francis Group.

Common Surgical Supplies and Instruments

When assisting with a procedure, no matter what the setting, preparation is vital to keep the flow steady. Having all the necessary instruments and supplies at hand, as well as knowledge about the procedure to be performed, will help the surgery run more efficiently. For example, even the most minor procedure, such as a suture removal, can easily be prolonged if the supplies and instruments needed are not present.

Whether your physician performs procedures in the office surgical suite or the exam chair, keeping a log of supplies will help when it is time to reorder, as well as for setting a budget. This section should help you create a list of your own surgical supplies (always refer to your office surgeon for any preferences), as well as give you an overview of commonly performed minor surgery procedures.

Sutures

One of the most important supplies needed in a surgical setting are sutures. These are thread-like materials of various kinds (Sidebar 37-1) attached to a delicate needle and used to close wounds.

Sutures that perform best are durable, nonirritating, sterile, noncarcinogenic, absorbable, and resistant to knotting. Unfortunately, there are not many sutures on the market that meet all of the criteria.

Sutures are manufactured in two main types: absorbable and nonabsorbable. With absorbable sutures, the thread-like part of a suture is usually broken down by the body in somewhere between 7 to 10 days. Additionally, absorbable sutures can be purchased as either natural or synthetic. The body cannot degrade nonabsorbable sutures; these must be removed after the wound has healed.

Suture material comes in varying thickness, or diameter, measured in millimeters. A smaller diameter suture is more delicate and is usually the suture of choice in ophthalmic procedures. There are several ways of designating suture size, which also depends on the material of the suture itself. (Thus, a 4-0 collagen has a diameter of 0.2 mm and a 4-0 nonabsorbable is 0.15.) In the United States, the US Pharmacopeia (USP) designation runs from 11-0 (the very finest) to 0 and from there, up to 7 (the thickest). The smallest diameter suture that will adequately hold and mend a wound should be used in order to minimize trauma as the suture passes through the tissue. A suture should not be stronger than the tissue on which it is being used.

The characteristics of an ideal needle are high-quality stainless steel, sterile, corrosion-resistant, and stable in the grasp while held by the needle holder. The best needles are sharp enough to penetrate tissue with minimal resistance.

There are three parts to a suture needle: the swage (where there the suture cord connects), the body, and the point (Figure 37-1). The delicate suture needles are offered in different shapes, sizes, and diameters. The most commonly used needle body shapes are straight, half-curved ski, and curved (Figure 37-2).

The smallest diameter needle possible for any particular surgical site involved is generally recommended.

Needle Holders

Needle holders (also called needle drivers) are designed for grasping and controlling needles during suturing. They are composed of jaws, a joint, and a grip (Figure 37-3). Many have a "lock" mechanism. Selecting the correct size needle holder is essential to avoid damage to the needle and the surrounding tissue during the procedure. In ophthalmology, there are typically two sizes of needle holders: micro and standard. The micro needle holder is used for 8-0 needles or smaller, and the standard needle holder is for anything larger than 8-0.

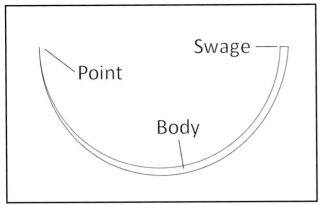

Figure 37-1. Parts of a suture needle.

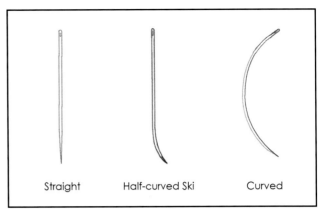

Figure 37-2. Types of suture needles.

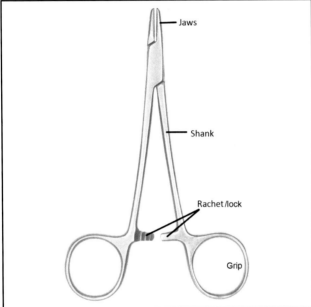

Figure 37-3. Needle holder/driver.

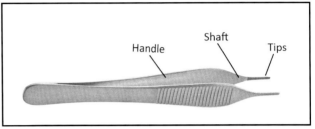

Figure 37-4. Parts of a forceps.

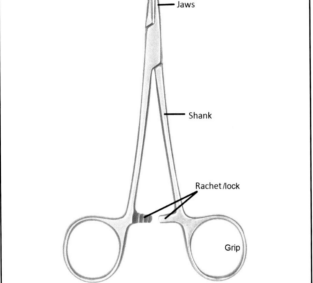

Figure 37-5. Blade holder.

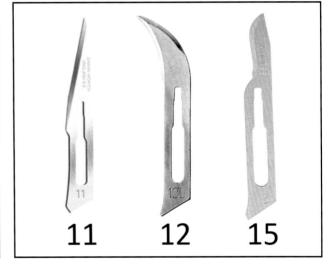

Figure 37-6. Types of blades.

Forceps

Forceps are designed for seizing or holding tissues or sutures. Many different designs of forceps are available in ophthalmic surgery, but they can be broadly divided into two types. In general, toothed forceps are used for holding tissues, whereas smooth forceps are more practical for tying sutures. Some forceps are designed for both purposes. Ophthalmic forceps have three parts (Figure 37-4): the working ends (tips), the shaft, and the handle.

Blade Holder and Blades

A *blade holder* is essentially a handle to which a surgical blade is attached (Figure 37-5). It allows the surgeon to firmly grip the instrument and have control of the blade while making incisions.

Surgical *blades* are often used for excisions and removal of lesions. There are many different blade shapes and sizes, used for an array of purposes. In ophthalmic procedures the blades most commonly used are the No. 11, No. 12, and No. 15 (Figure 37-6).

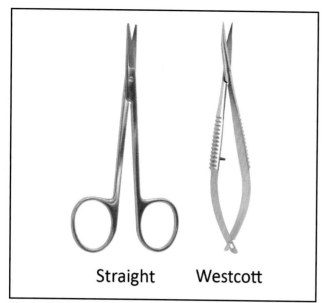

Figure 37-7. Types of surgical scissors.

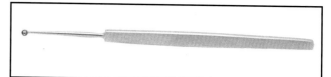

Figure 37-8. Curette.

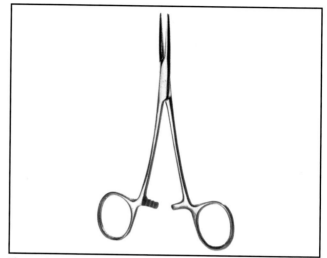

Figure 37-9. Hemostat/clamp.

Scissors

Surgical scissors play an important role in ophthalmology and their uses are nearly endless. They are manufactured in different shapes (straight and curved in various ways) and sizes for specific purposes (Figure 37-7). Spring scissors are often used for small-sized tasks.

Curettes

A *curette* is a small hand tool used for scraping or debriding tissue, which is helpful in the removal of inflamed tissue (eg, chalazion incision and drainage). The handle is often similar in shape to a knitting needle. At the working end of the curette is a small scoop, hook, or gouge (Figure 37-8). They come in various sizes.

Hemostats and Clamps

A *hemostat* (clamp) is a surgical tool used to clamp a ruptured blood vessel to decrease bleeding, improve visibility, and allow the surgeon to continue the procedure (Figure 37-9). In the office, they might be used for grabbing orbital fat during a blepharoplasty.

A chalazion clamp is two-sided (Figure 37-10). One side is a small oval or round plate. The other side, which clamps down over the plate, is an open ring. A screw in the handle tightens the two sides together like a vise. When used, the lid is slipped between the ring and the plate, and the chalazion is centered in the ring. The clamp is then tightened down. The clamp isolates the surgical site, helps mobilize the tissue, and acts as a hemostat to control bleeding.

Speculums

Speculums are instruments used to hold something open. In the case of eye surgery, we use a lid speculum (Figure 37-11). It is more commonly used in major eye surgery, but it might be needed in the office during corneal scraping, foreign body removal, and intraocular injections.

Lacrimal Kits

Lacrimal kits (Figure 37-12) can be prepacked and are composed of a lacrimal dilator, probe, sterile cannula, syringe, and sterile saline.

A *lacrimal dilator* is a small metallic or plastic rod with pointed ends; one end is usually a little smaller than the other. The smaller point is inserted into the punctum and gently twisted and pushed to make the punctum opening a little wider. Then the larger point is used in the same manner to dilate the punctum further.

Lacrimal probes are double-ended and come in a variety of sizes. Once the punctum is dilated, the probe wire is inserted into the punctum then turned vertically so it will pass down through the nasolacrimal duct. The purpose is for the wire to puncture and open a blocked nasolacrimal duct.

Cannulas are stainless steel needle-like tubes with a blunt or pointed (not sharp) end. They come in various shapes and gauge sizes and fit on the end of a syringe. In lacrimal procedures, a syringe is filled with saline and the cannula is inserted into the punctum. The solution is

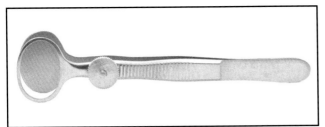

Figure 37-10. Chalazion clamp.

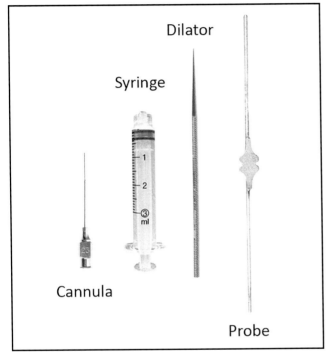

Figure 37-12. Lacrimal kit.

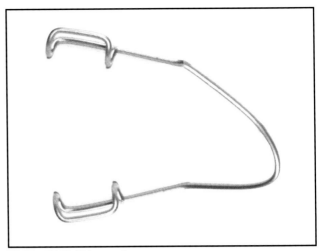

Figure 37-11. Lid speculum.

ejected into the lacrimal drainage system to wash out any debris. If the saline does not go through (into the patient's throat), then the lacrimal system is still blocked.

Other Surgical Materials and Supplies

A sterile *drape* is a towel-like cover (usually disposable) placed over a tray on which all sterile instruments and equipment are placed. Only sterile items should be placed on this sterile field. Do not place specimen bottles, nonsterile syringes, nonsterile packages, etc, on the sterile drape, as such items will contaminate the field. (See Tray Set-Up for how-to's.)

Sterile *fenestrated drapes* are a pertinent part of most in-office procedures. They offer a localized sterile field with a small opening (the fenestration) for the surgeon to perform the procedure through. Some fenestrated drapes are manufactured with an adhesive around the edges of the hole so they can be "stuck" to the surrounding area to keep the drape from moving during the procedure.

Disposable sterile items such as gauze, cotton-tipped applicators, and absorptive sponges are generally part

of the set-up for minor procedures as well. These can be placed on the sterile-draped tray prior to use. PPE is selected depending on the likelihood of exposure to blood-borne pathogens during the procedure.

CLINICAL SKILLS

Hand Washing/Gloving

Most minor procedures require the surgeon and assistant to be gloved. Surgical gloves are manufactured in various types of material to suit the needs of both patient and physician, as well as the type of procedure being performed. These gloves are produced in sizes such 6, 6½, 7, 7½, and up, with 6 being the smallest. Some minor surgery procedures do not require sterile technique, so nonsterile gloves may be used.

A full scrub is not generally needed for in-office minor procedures. (Scrubbing is covered in Chapter 40.) The hands and up over the wrists should be thoroughly washed with soap and warm water and dried with a clean or disposable towel. If sterile gloves are required for the procedure, once you've put them on you should not touch any nonsterile items. If you make a mistake and touch something nonsterile, remove the contaminated gloves and replace them with a fresh pair. Hands should be washed again after the gloves are removed after the procedure.

Patient/Site Prep

If any incision is to be made, the skin of and around the surgical site must be properly cleansed. An antiseptic solution, like povidone or chlorhexidine, is applied with gentle friction using a sterile applicator on the area where the incision will be made. Start at the incision site and work outward. Never go back to rewipe the incision site unless a fresh applicator is used.

Tray Set-Up

If the surgery is going to involve cutting or penetration into the skin, a sterile tray should be set up. First, using sterile gloves, a sterile drape is placed on the surgery tray. The area of the drape that will have instruments on it should not be touched.

Sterile instruments and sterile disposable items can be added to the tray with clean, ungloved hands if the no-touch method is used. In this technique, only the outer packages are touched. Once the package is opened, the item is carefully and gently "dumped" onto the sterile tray. The item and the drape are not touched. If anything is touched by accident, the entire tray is considered contaminated and you must start all over.

Two assistants working together make tray set-up much easier. An assistant with clean hands can open the packages without touching the contents, and a gloved assistant can place the items on the tray without touching the packages.

Clean-Up

When the procedure is over, the area is cleansed if appropriate. If needed the area is bandaged; in some cases this might mean the application of a bandage contact lens or a pressure patch (Sidebar 37-2).

Any unopened, sterile materials or instruments that were not used can be returned to storage as long as the wrappings have not been soiled or punctured.

Used instruments must be first cleaned then sterilized according to clinic protocol. (See Chapter 40 for instructions on cleaning, using an autoclave, and other methods to sterilize reusable instruments.)

Any used, disposable sharps (ie, blades, needles) must be handled carefully and disposed of properly as soon as possible. If a used needle is to be recapped, never hold the cap in one hand. Leave it on the tray and "scoop" the needle into it. Contaminated blades can be picked up with forceps or tongs.

All used or opened disposable sharps must be discarded in an approved sharps container. Such a container must be strong and rigid (so that sharp items cannot poke through), leak-proof, and red in color. There must be plenty of room in the container; never fill one full. Finally, before disposing the container itself, it must be closed. If there is fluid inside that could possibly leak out, the container must be placed into yet another container that is properly marked. The way to properly discard a full sharps container is regulated by each state.

Any tissue that has been removed must either be sent for biopsy or properly disposed of. The clinic should have a specimen disposal protocol in place. Tissue sent for biopsy is placed in a leak-proof specimen container filled with a *fixative* (a liquid preservative). This will maintain the tissue until it reaches the pathologist's lab for evaluation. Careful attention must be paid to labeling the container, which generally must include patient's name and identifying numbers, date of removal, and where the specimen came from (eg, "left lower lid").

Common In-Office Surgical Procedures (Table 37-1)

Removing Cutaneous Sutures

Removal of stitches in the skin often falls to technicians. Wash your hands and put on gloves. Clean the area with an eye-safe cleanser. Use sterile forceps to pick up one suture end. Using fine-point scissors, cut one side as close to the skin as possible. (This is done so that when you pull the suture out, you don't drag an exposed end of suture through the healing tissue.) Grasp the other side and gently pull the suture through.

TABLE 37-1

ASSISTING WITH COMMON IN-OFFICE SURGICAL PROCEDURES

Procedure	Purpose/Intent	Patient Preparation	Supplies Needed for Procedure	Steps of Procedure
Anterior chamber tap	To obtain a sample of fluid (aqueous humor) from the anterior chamber or To remove aqueous in order to quickly lower the intraocular pressure	Patient seated in upright position	Eyelid speculum Topical anesthetic Syringe and needle of appropriate size (consult with physician on preferences), 4 × 4 gauze, large cotton swab, sterile drape, specimen container Loupes or slit lamp	1. Administer oral sedative such as Valium (diazepam) to patient 20 to 30 minutes prior to procedure if needed. 2. Prepare the patient by cleansing the surgical area with topical povidone-iodine or other cleansing solution safe for eyes with a large cotton swab, gently using a circular motion. 3. Apply 1 to 2 drops of topical anesthetic to the globe, then repeat Step 2 to ensure sterility. 4. The patient should be ready for the surgeon, and can be draped with a fenestrated drape. 5. The surgeon aspirates the fluid with the syringe and needle to obtain the specimen. 6. The specimen is placed in the container and sent for culture processing.
Chalazion removal	To remove a chalazion by incision and drainage when other treatment (eg, warm compresses and antibiotic ointment) fails; curettage helps prevent recurrence	Patient in supine position	Sterile chalazion set which includes 1 curette #1, 1 curette #2, 1 curette #3, 1 curette #4, 1 curved eye scissors, 2 chalazion clamps, 1 No. 11 blade, 1 blade holder Other supplies: 4 × 4 gauze, cotton-tipped applicators, sterile eye patches, surgical tape, 5% povidone-iodine swabs, topical anesthetic, syringe and needle of appropriate size, local anesthetic (1% lidocaine with epinephrine preferred) If sutures are anticipated: Suture forceps, absorbable or nonabsorbable sutures (depending on site of chalazion), needle holder, curved hemostat, toothed chuck-handle forceps	1. Apply 1 to 2 drops of topical anesthetic to the globe for comfort. 2. The surgeon will inject local anesthetic and allow a few minutes for numbing to take effect. 3. The chalazion clamp is put on and tightened to secure the area and reduce bleeding. 4. The lid is everted (depending on the site of the chalazion). 5. The incision is made with No. 11 blade into the tarsal area of the conjunctiva. (Chalazion may drain at this point.) 6. A curette is used to remove the inflamed tissue. 7. The chalazion clamp is removed. Mild pressure may be applied with gauze if there is any bleeding. 8. Gently clean the wound with balanced salt solution (BSS) or normal saline on a saturated gauze pad, then apply an antibiotic ointment of the surgeon's choice to the area. 9. Fold one eye pad and place a second eye pad on top for mild pressure and firmly affix with about three strips of tape to keep the globe from moving.

(continued)

TABLE 37-1 (CONTINUED)

ASSISTING WITH COMMON IN-OFFICE SURGICAL PROCEDURES

Procedure	Purpose/Intent	Patient Preparation	Supplies Needed for Procedure	Steps of Procedure
Excision of lesion on eyelid or palpebral conjunctiva	To remove a lesion for biopsy and/or cosmesis	Patient in supine position	Sterile excision kit: Needle holder, forceps (toothed and smooth), scissors for cutting skin/tissue, blade holder, No. 15 blade, cautery unit, scissors for cutting sutures Topical and/or local anesthetic, 5% povidone-iodine for conjunctiva, 10% povidone-iodine swab for skin Sutures of appropriate size for area (possibly absorbable and nonabsorbable) Sterile gauze, sterile cotton-tipped applicators, fenestrated drape Antibiotic ointment, eye patch or bandage, surgical tape	1. 1 to 2 drops of topical anesthetic are instilled for comfort. Local anesthetic is then injected by the doctor into the desired area on the lid. 2. Bulbar and palpebral conjunctiva can be disinfected with 5% povidone-iodine gently squeezed into the cul-de-sac. Outer lids can be cleaned with a 10% povidone-iodine swab in a circular motion (start in the center going outward like a swirl). 3. Drape with a sterile fenestrated drape. 4. The surgeon removes the lesion. 5. If there is a specimen, the surgeon may leave the sample on the side of the tray for you to get later. Alternately he/she will drop the specimen inside the bottle at the time of removal. 6. If sutures are needed for the procedure, you may have to assist the surgeon (if you are gloved). 7. If there is constant bleeding, the area may need to be cauterized by the surgeon before the closure is finished. 8. Once the wound is closed, gently clean the area with BSS or normal saline on a saturated gauze pad, then apply an antibiotic ointment of the surgeon's choice to the area. 9. A pressure bandage may be needed depending on the amount of bleeding.

(continued)

TABLE 37-1 (CONTINUED)

ASSISTING WITH COMMON IN-OFFICE SURGICAL PROCEDURES

Procedure	Purpose/Intent	Patient Preparation	Supplies Needed for Procedure	Steps of Procedure
Epilation	By forceps: A nonpermanent method of eyelash removal that temporally relieves the irritation of turned eyelashes rubbing on the cornea By electroepilation: A more permanent method of treatment that destroys abnormally growing eyelashes by applying a small electric current into the hair follicle, thus destroying the hair bulb	Patient seated in upright or in supine position (surgeon's preference)	For forceps epilation: Smooth forceps For electroepilation: Cautery machine with cord (cord must not have a sterile cover), electrode needle for cautery Topical and/or local anesthetic 4 x 4 gauze, antibiotic ointment	Forceps epilation: 1. Apply 1 to 2 drops of topical anesthetic to the globe for comfort. 2. The surgeon examines the abnormal eyelash(es) under the slit lamp. 3. For forceps epilation the surgeon gently pulls out abnormal lashes with the smooth forceps. Electroepilation: 1. 1 to 2 drops of topical anesthetic is applied to the cul-de-sac. Local anesthesia is injected by the doctor into the areas to be treated. 2. The electrode needle is injected into hair shaft and electric current applied to damage the hair follicle and the bulb. 3. The burnt hair is removed with smooth forceps. Repeat Steps 2 and 3 as needed. 4. Antibiotic ointment of choice may be placed on the patient's eyelid.
Foreign body removal	To remove an object or foreign body from the external eye	Patient seated in upright position	Smooth forceps, foreign body spud, 30-gauge needle or Beaver blade (for removing embedded objects), drill and burr (for removing rust), slit lamp Topical anesthetic (if needed to decrease sensation) Cotton-tipped applicators, saline for flushing the eye	1. Place patient in front of the slit lamp. If patient is unable to open the eye due to irritation, apply 1 to 2 drops of topical anesthetic for comfort. 2. Examine eye under slit lamp with medium to low illumination to find the foreign body. 3. If unable to find the object, flip the upper lid (a cotton-tipped applicator can aid with this) to exam the upper tarsal area. 4. Depending on its location, a foreign body embedded in the lid/palpebral conjunctiva might be removed gently with a pair of smooth forceps. If the foreign body is located under the upper tarsal area, flush the eye with saline while lifting the upper eyelid. Reexamine patient after flushing to ensure the foreign body is gone. If not, repeat Step 4. 5. If the foreign body is embedded in the sclera or cornea, the physician will remove the foreign body gently with a 30-gauge needle or Beaver blade by gently plucking it out. 6. If there is a corneal rust ring, the physician will use the drill and burr to buff it out.

(continued)

TABLE 37-1 (CONTINUED)

ASSISTING WITH COMMON IN-OFFICE SURGICAL PROCEDURES

Procedure	Purpose/Intent	Patient Preparation	Supplies Needed for Procedure	Steps of Procedure
Punctal plug insertion	To insert absorbable or nonabsorbable plugs into the puncta to help correct dry eye by keeping tears from draining off the eye	Patient seated in upright position	Smooth forceps, collagen or silicone plugs (with preloaded applicator when possible), punctum measuring gauge, slit lamp Topical anesthetic	1. Apply 1 to 2 drops of topical anesthetic in the patient's cul-de-sac. 2. Use the punctum measuring gauge to find correct plug size. 3. The physician will insert appropriate-sized plugs into upper and lower puncta. (Collagen plugs will be inserted with forceps, silicone are inserted with preloaded inserter.)
Intravitreal injection	To place medication in the vitreous to treat various ocular disorders	Patient seated in Fowler's position (upright, back at 90 degrees)	Eyelid speculum TB syringe and needle, appropriate injectable intraocular medication Topical and/or local anesthetic, 5% povidone-iodine Cotton-tipped applicators	1. Apply 1 to 2 drops of topical anesthetic in the patient's cul-de-sac. 2. Prep the eye with 5% povidone-iodine by generously applying it to the lids and lashes. 3. The physician inserts the lid speculum and positions the eye by instructing the patient. 4. Injection is administered and speculum is removed. 5. If there is any initial bleeding, a cotton-tipped applicator is placed on the area for pressure. 6. The patient's intraocular pressure is checked 15 to 20 minutes after injection; consult with the physician to see if patient can leave.
Nasolacrimal duct (NLD) probe and irrigation	To open an occluded NLD	Patient seated upright or in Fowler's position (surgeon's preference)	Topical and/or local anesthetic, sterile saline, several sterile 4 x 4 gauze pads, NLD probe (may need various sizes), punctum dilator, sterile cannula with syringe, magnification loops or slit lamp (depending on surgeon's preference)	1. Place patient in the preferred position. 2. Apply 1 to 2 drops of topical anesthetic to the cul-de-sac. If necessary, the surgeon will inject local anesthetic, depending on the status of the duct occlusion. 3. Punctal dilator is inserted into the punctum to stretch it open a little more. 4. Probe is inserted into the occluded duct to open for irrigation. 5. The cannula with sterile saline is inserted into the obstructed NLD and gently flushed. If procedure is successful, the patient will taste mild salt water. If not, repeat Step 4.

(continued)

TABLE 37-1 (CONTINUED)

ASSISTING WITH COMMON IN-OFFICE SURGICAL PROCEDURES

Procedure	Purpose/Intent	Patient Preparation	Supplies Needed for Procedure	Steps of Procedure
Laceration repair	To close an open wound	Patient in supine position	Sterile laceration kit: Needle holder, toothed forceps, scissors for cutting tissue, blade holder, No. 15 blade, cautery unit, scissors for cutting sutures Sutures of appropriate size for area (possibly absorbable and nonabsorbable) Topical and/or local anesthetic, 5% povidone-iodine for conjunctiva, 10% povidone-iodine swab for skin Sterile cotton-tipped applicators, sterile gauze, sterile fenestrated drape Antibiotic ointment, eye patch or bandage, surgical tape	1. Apply 1 to 2 drops of topical anesthetic for comfort. The surgeon will inject the area with local anesthetic. 2. The bulbar and palpebral conjunctiva can be disinfected with 5% povidone-iodine gently squeezed into the cul-de-sac area. Outer lids can be cleaned with a 10% povidone-iodine swab in a circular motion (start in the center going outward like a swirl). 3. Drape the patient with a sterile fenestrated drape. 4. If sutures are needed, you may have to assist the surgeon if you are gloved. 5. If there is constant bleeding, the area may need to be cauterized by the surgeon before the closure is completed. 6. Once the wound is closed, gently clean the area with BSS or normal saline on a saturated gauze pad. Apply antibiotic ointment of the surgeon's choice to the area. 7. A pressure bandage may be needed after this procedure, depending on the amount of bleeding.
Corneal/globe suture removal	To remove nonabsorbable sutures	Patient seated upright	Forceps (smooth or toothed), pointed scissors or ophthalmic Beaver blade (surgeon's preference), eyelid speculum (if needed), slit lamp or loupes Topical anesthetic if needed	1. Apply 1 to 2 drops of topical anesthetic if needed. 2. Surgeon uses forceps to hold suture, then cuts it with either scissors or Beaver blade depending on site. Note: For corneal sutures, the surgeon may not remove all sutures in one visit.
Corneal scraping	To create a smooth surface for rehealing	Patient seated upright at slit lamp	No. 15 blade or sterile needle or loop (surgeon's preference) Topical anesthetic Bandage contact lens	1. Apply 1 to 2 drops of topical anesthetic. 2. Surgeon uses blade to scrape and smooth away damaged tissue. 3. Apply antibiotic and/or nonsteroidal anti-inflammatory drops at surgeon's request. 4. Apply bandage contact lens at surgeon's request.

(continued)

TABLE 37-1 (CONTINUED)

ASSISTING WITH COMMON IN-OFFICE SURGICAL PROCEDURES

Procedure	Purpose/Intent	Patient Preparation	Supplies Needed for Procedure	Steps of Procedure
Corneal gluing	To seal corneal perforations and wound leaks	Patient seated upright or in supine position (surgeon's preference)	Items for corneal scraping may be needed Forceps (jewellers, .12's), ophthalmic Beaver blade (surgeon's preference), eyelid speculum (if needed), drape (surgeon's preference), slit lamp or loupes Topical anesthetic, 5% povidone-iodine Sterile cotton-tipped applicators, Weck sponge, tissue glue Bandage contact lens (surgeon's preference)	1. Corneal scraping/debridement may be done first. 2. Apply 1 to 2 drops of topical anesthetic. 3. Eye can be disinfected with 5% povidone-iodine gently squeezed into the cul-de-sac. 4. Surgeon applies drape and speculum if desired. 5. Surgeon dries area with sponge. 6. Surgeon applies thin layer of glue with back of sponge. 7. Apply bandage contact lens as directed.

Returning the Patient to the Referring Practitioner

Sometimes the surgeon is not the patient's routine eye care provider. Ophthalmic surgeons often work from referrals. Patients are usually seen and evaluated by the surgeon, and if necessary, a procedure is scheduled then performed. A 90-day postoperative period where the surgeon will see the patient as necessary is customary for most procedures. During that time, the surgeon will write progress reports to the referring physician to keep him/her in the loop about the patient's progress. Once the 90-day period is over and the patient's healing is successful, then the patient can be sent back to the original, referring physician.

PATIENT SERVICES

Preoperative Patient Education

Informed consent is required prior to any type of procedure. We often think of informed consent as a piece of signed paper, but it is actually a process. The patient is given an overview of the condition, treatment options, benefits, and risk factors. The patient must also have the opportunity to ask and receive answers to any questions. After that, the piece of paper can be signed. Informed consent is covered in several places in the text; kindly consult the Index.

It is also important to advise the patient of any preparatory needs such as discontinuing blood thinners or other medications beforehand. The patient will also need to know if he/she can drive afterward, or will need a driver for the trip home. Any medications and supplies that the patient will need following the procedure are best obtained prior to the surgery, before any swelling and/or discomfort become a factor.

Post-Surgical Patient Education

Post-surgery education lets the patient know what to expect after the procedure. It is always a good idea to have written literature for the patient to refer to. Taking a few minutes to go over the written material and answer any questions will help put the patient and family members at ease for the days after the procedure. This information should include instructions for the at-home regimen of care they will need to adhere to. It is always a good idea to write customized instructions clearly in order for the patient to understand. A "what to do" and "things to avoid" feature should be included, as well as details about situations where the patient should contact the office.

CHAPTER QUIZ

1. What is the proper way to dispose of tissue that was removed during a procedure?

2. List surgical instruments needed for a chalazion excision.

3. True/False: The largest suture material that a tissue can support is the one that should be used.

4. True/False: The smallest diameter needle possible for any particular surgical site involved is generally recommended.

5. True/False: Surgical scrubbing is required of the assistant for every type of eye surgery including minor procedures.

6. Which of the following is the smallest suture size?
   a. 4-0
   b. 11-0
   c. 0
   d. 4

7. The purpose of a cannula is to:
   a. debride dead tissue
   b. inject local anesthetic
   c. introduce irrigating solution
   d. hold the eyelid open

8. When removing sutures, one should:
   a. cut off the knot and then pull the stitch out
   b. cut one side as close to the skin as possible and then pull the stitch out
   c. cut the middle of the suture and then pull the stitch out
   d. cut both sides as close to the skin as possible and discard

Answers

1. Any tissue that is not sent for biopsy must be disposed of properly as a biohazard.

2. Instruments for a chalazion excision would include a chalazion clamp, blade holder and blade, and a curette. One might also want forceps, plus sutures and a needle holder.

3. False, A suture material should not be stronger than the tissue on which it is being used.

4. True

5. False

6. b, Think of 11-0 as 11 zeros and 4-0 as four zeros. 11-0 is the finest suture material. 4-0 would be the largest.

7. c

8. b

REFERENCES

1. How do you get HIV or AIDS? AIDS.gov website. www.aids.gov/hiv-aids-basics/hiv-aids-101/how-you-get-hiv-aids/. Accessed June 12, 2016.

2. Perspectives in disease prevention and health promotion update: universal precautions for prevention of transmission of human immunodeficiency virus, hepatitis B virus, and other blood-borne pathogens in health-care settings. CDC website. http://wonder.cdc.gov/wonder/prevguid/p0000255/p0000255.asp. Reviewed January 27, 2016. Accessed June 12, 2016.

BIBLIOGRAPHY

Ethicon Wound Closure Manual. Ethicon, Inc. www.sutureonline.com/wound-closure-manual. Accessed July 4, 2016.

OSHA FactSheet: protecting yourself when handling contaminated sharps. OSHA website. www.osha.gov/OshDoc/data_BloodborneFacts/bbfact02.pdf. Accessed June 12, 2016.

Plus Antibacterial Suture Portfolio. www.ethicon.com/healthcare-professionals/products/wound-closure/absorbable-sutures/plus-antibacterial-suture-portfolio. Accessed July 4, 2016.

Stein HA, Stein RM, Freeman MI. *The Ophthalmic Assistant: A Text for Allied and Associated Ophthalmic Personnel.* 8th ed. Philadelphia, PA: Mosby; 2006.

Stein RM, Slatt BL, Stein HA. *The Ophthalmic Assistant: A Guide for Ophthalmic Medical Personnel.* 7th ed. Philadelphia, PA: Mosby; 2000.

The figures in this chapter were contributed by Al Lens.

38

REFRACTIVE SURGERY

Paul M. Larson, MBA, MMSc, COMT, COE, CPC, CPMA

BACKGROUND KNOWLEDGE

One of the most exciting things to come along in eye care is the ability to alter or eliminate the need for corrective lenses while maintaining, or even improving, best-corrected acuity. The goal in refractive surgery, however, is not always full elimination of contact lenses or glasses—some patients may still require one or both—and even when this may be possible for certain distances, it is not always desirable due to lifestyle or other considerations. In short, while some may be served best with a "plano" postoperative goal, this is not the most desirable result for all.

The technician's task, in addition to having an active role as part of the team caring for patients before, during, and after refractive surgery, is to understand the basic science of ocular anatomy, optics, and refractive errors (Chapters 2 and 4) and to provide surgeons and patients with the best measurements possible. This may entail learning new skills or knowledge. Remember too, that some test results make the patient less suitable for some procedures. This might mean, for instance, that a patient with a thin cornea might be a candidate for lens replacement but not for procedures requiring a minimum thickness (eg, LASIK). It is not the place of the technician to make recommendations for any type of surgery. This is solely the job of the surgeon after careful review

of the usual measurements (most commonly included are keratometry, topography, refraction, pachymetry, and aberrometry) and a discussion with the patient. However, a tech should be conversant regarding the relative pros and cons of one refractive procedure over another based on measurements.

CLINICAL KNOWLEDGE

There are a large number of surgical options to correct refractive errors, and this is a field replete with acronyms. Please refer to Sidebar 38-1 as you read this chapter.

It's important for technicians to be knowledgeable about the myriad of options. In addition, the ocular structures that can be altered to correct refractive error have greatly expanded since the old days of *radial keratotomy* (RK) in the 1970s and 1980s, when only the exterior cornea was treated via a blade. Modern refractive procedures still overwhelmingly involve the cornea and lens, but other ocular structures or tissues may be involved as well.

In the past, the refractive errors we heard about as most frequently being correctable with surgery were myopia and astigmatism, but it's common today for hyperopia, presbyopia, and even higher optical aberrations to be corrected as well. It's an exciting area for technicians to be involved in—and often life-changing for the patients.

Ledford JK, Lens A, eds.
Principles and Practice in Ophthalmic Assisting:
A Comprehensive Textbook (pp 645-654).
© 2018 Taylor & Francis Group.

Corneal Procedures

In terms of refracting the light entering the eye, the cornea and tear film are the most anterior entities. They also generally have the greatest effect on image quality. Moreover, about two-thirds of the total refractive power of the eye comes from the cornea. Because of this, the most common structure to consider modifying in order to reduce refractive errors is the cornea. Corneal procedures seek to change the corneal power by altering its shape. In photorefractive procedures, ablating (removing) some of the central cornea would generally remove plus power and correct myopia. (Remember that another way to think about myopia is as a refractive condition where the eye has "too much plus." Correcting it requires neutralizing [or removing, in the case of refractive surgery] the appropriate amount of "over-plus.")

There are two basic types of corneal refractive surgery. *Laser-based* surgeries use a laser to adjust the corneal shape by removing tissue or creating incisions. These procedures will be discussed in more detail. (Information about the lasers themselves is found in Chapter 39.) In *blade-based* surgeries, a blade is used to "relax" the cornea. This allows the eye's inner pressure to make the cornea bulge into the new desired shape, where it will presumably heal. Blades are now mostly used to correct astigmatism. In the past, RK was a blade-based method used for both spherical and astigmatic errors. It was largely abandoned when the results did not provide refractive stability.

Far less common, but no less exciting, are procedures that involve a *corneal inlay* (covered later in this chapter). The appeal of these procedures is that tissue is not removed and they may have greater reversibility (if that's a relevant issue). Artificial material such as specially shaped plastics as well as corneal donor tissue may be involved.

Laser-Based Surgery

These procedures involve the use of the laser to *photoablate* or *photodisrupt* the corneal tissue at the microscopic level. Both photoablation and photodisruption cause formation of a microscopic plasma bubble and then very small shock waves, which result in tissue separation or vaporization. The difference between ablation and disruption lies in how short the laser's "pulse" is (microseconds to nanoseconds) and other complex laser and tissue factors that the surgeon takes into account. The excimer laser wavelength for tissue vaporization is in the far ultraviolet spectrum at 193 nm. The amount of energy is significant, but the exposure time is exceedingly short. Short exposure times are very important as they help to minimize collateral tissue damage.

Laser-assisted in situ keratomileusis (LASIK) treatment (Figures 38-1 and 38-2) is done by sculpting the corneal stroma. A thin anterior corneal flap is created with a femtosecond (FS) laser or mechanical keratome (blade). The flap remains attached by a "hinge" of tissue, usually located superiorly. The flap is then lifted, exposing the intrastromal tissue. The underlying corneal stroma is treated by the excimer laser in the amount and location desired. The excimer laser allows for precise tissue ablation, and the adjacent corneal tissue is almost completely unaffected. The corneal flap is then moved back into position. The central corneal epithelium is largely undisturbed in uncomplicated LASIK, so the acuity and comfort may be better in the first few postoperative days vs other techniques; only the small circular epithelial defect needs to heal. Sutures are not generally required to hold the flap down. Because of this, LASIK seems to have a bigger initial "wow" factor than other cornea-only refractive surgeries.

Sub-Bowman's keratectomy (SBK) is very much like LASIK but in this situation, an FS laser creates a very thin anterior corneal flap and then the desired power treatment is applied to the exposed corneal bed. It is sometimes known as "FS-assisted" LASIK.

Photorefractive keratectomy (PRK) treatment is similar to LASIK and SBK, but no corneal flap is created (Figure 38-3). The excimer laser treatment is done on the anterior stromal surface after the epithelium is removed (typically with a rotating brush or alcohol). Postoperatively, there is an initial epithelial defect, so comfort is commonly delayed for a few days to a week.

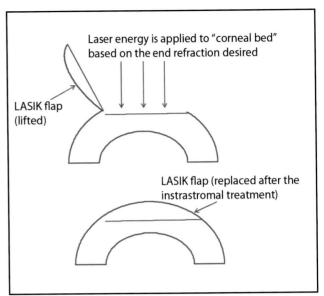

Figure 38-2. Schematic of LASIK procedure.

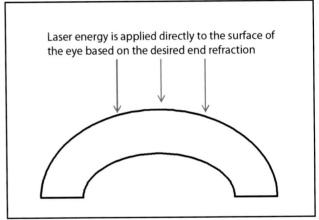

Figure 38-3. PRK schematic.

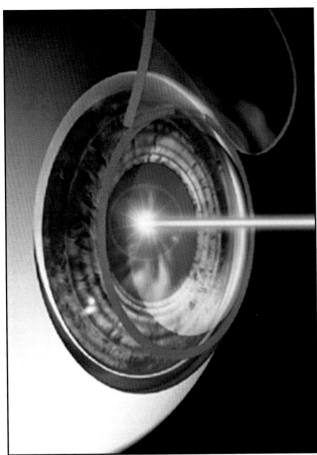

Figure 38-1. Schematic of intraoperative LASIK procedure showing flap and laser location.

Best vision generally takes a bit longer to recover than the epithelial healing.

LASIK, SBK, and PRK can be performed for all types of refractive errors, although there are practical limits in terms of the amount of correction realistically obtainable. When these lasers were introduced, one manufacturer's laser might have been approved for different correction types and amounts, but those concerns are less relevant today than in the past (although it remains an important fact for the surgeon to know). Some surgeons may feel that hyperopic correction is best done with LASIK or SBK as opposed to PRK, so you should know your surgeon's preferences in this regard.

Limbal Relaxing Incisions and Corneal Relaxing Incisions

These two procedures (LRI and CRI, respectively) are sometimes referred to as separate entities but they are not different and the goal is the same: treating corneal astigmatism (Figure 38-4). They are generally done on the peripheral or mid-peripheral cornea for altering the corneal power *in specific axes*. This is done by making relatively deep incisions, typically in an arc shape, at specified segments of a circle centered on the desired axis

(in degrees). The effect in CRI/LRI is gained by weakening the corneal tissue in the selected axes. This results in flattening the cornea, thereby reducing the plus power only in the treated axes, reducing or eliminating the corneal cylinder power. CRI and LRI can be made with blades or via an FS laser.

Prior to the actual procedure, the corneal axis is marked if a blade is to be used (usually with gentian or similar blue or violet dye) for the previously determined position, length of arc, and diameter of the planned cuts. (Some surgeons may remeasure corneal thickness intraoperatively at these locations.) Before the actual incision(s), the depth of the blade is set to the desired depth.

When blades are used, they are typically made from a metal or gem (such as a diamond or sapphire). The blade is set within a handle for the surgeon to hold, but on the patient end of the knife, there is a "foot" on the blade assembly that creates a "stop" so the blade can penetrate

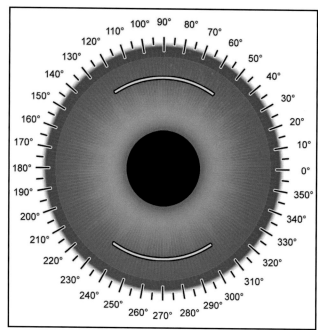

Figure 38-4. Schematic of corneal relaxing incisions for the correction of astigmatism.

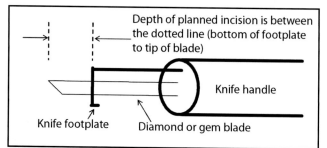

Figure 38-5. Schematic showing blade depth for limbal and corneal relaxing incision surgery.

no further into the cornea than the desired depth (Figure 38-5). On most blades, there is a dial or some other indication of depth; the location may vary dependent on the blade manufacturer. The incision depth is thus determined by how far the blade itself extends *beyond* the foot. The blade's extension can be checked under a microscope with a micron-marked ruler for verification.

During the surgery, the surgeon presses the extended blade into the cornea up to the instrument's foot to achieve the desired depth. The surgeon then follows the previously made markings, moving the blade slowly while carefully holding it perpendicular to the corneal surface to ensure maintenance of the desired depth.

If the CRI/LRI surgery is done using FS laser technology, the cornea and anterior segment are imaged with optical coherence tomography (OCT) technology first. (The OCT is part of the imaging/guidance systems on FS lasers.) The surgeon then analyzes the OCT results. Finally, the surgeon chooses the desired depth and location for the incisions by programming the FS laser's computer template before actuating the laser.

Corneal Inlay Procedures

Certain types of correction can be achieved without tissue removal. A plastic device might be placed between the layers of the cornea to flatten or steepen it. (Note here that *flattening* means *decreasing* the plus power of the cornea.) None of these procedures is currently common, but they may be used for small amounts of myopia and astigmatism, to bolster a weak cornea, or even for presbyopia correction.

As of this writing, only the INTACS (Addition Technology, Inc) and KAMRA (AcuFocus) products have US Food and Drug Administration (FDA) approval. This is an area of intense research in both the United States and other countries worldwide because the number of potential candidates is so large. The variety of choices is many, and the product names may change over time or differ between countries.

INTACS

This intrastromal insert (Figure 38-6) has two possible and separate effects, each FDA approved. One is to flatten the corneal surface in cases of mild myopia associated with keratoconus. The other provides flattening in certain meridians by acting as a bolster to the corneal tissue to help correct astigmatism associated with keratoconus.

The thickness of these optically clear, 150-degree arc-shaped devices varies; actual use is determined by the surgeon. The pocket for the insert can be created surgically with specially designed instruments or via FS laser.

KAMRA

The KAMRA[1] is a small opaque device implanted centrally via an FS laser-created pocket. The device is pigmented with carbon nanoparticles in order to block peripheral light rays, allowing only central light through. By this means the depth of focus is increased (like a pinhole), with the intent to eliminate the need for reading glasses. The device is manufactured from a material that allows necessary passage of corneal nutrients. The FDA restricts KAMRA to one eye in patients who have not had cataract surgery.

Other Corneal Procedures

While not often thought of as strictly refractive procedures, there are corneal surgeries that usually have a secondary refractive effect. They are not the subject of this chapter, but are mentioned here (Sidebar 38-2) so you are aware of the possibility of refractive changes (both major and minor) when seeing them in clinical settings.

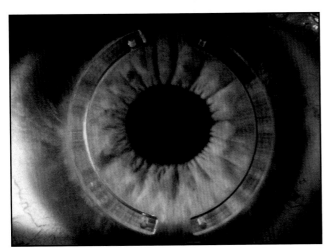

Figure 38-6. INTACS (Addition Technology, Inc) intrastromal insert.

Lens-Based Correction

Some patients are not candidates for corneal surgery due to the curve, thickness, past history, or other factors. Since the lens has the next greatest refractive effect, surgeons may decide to remove, supplement, or replace a patient's natural lens to achieve the desired refractive goal. This can be done alone or in combination with corneal surgery. Postoperative care is similar to standard lens-based surgery.

Refractive Lens Exchange

In refractive lens exchange (RLE), the natural lens is removed and replaced with an intraocular lens (IOL). (See Chapter 28, which has more information on various types of IOLs.) This surgery is like cataract extraction with IOL implantation for the patient, the surgeon, and the ophthalmic technician, but in this case there is little if any cataract, and the surgery is done mainly or solely for refractive purposes. The patient base is generally skewed toward a younger demographic as well. The RLE designation is used to connote that lens opacity (if any) is not the primary indication for surgery. In this regard, the lens removal procedure is a *clear lensectomy*.

As in standard cataract surgery, corneal curvature and axial length measurements are obtained. A few other anterior or posterior segment measurements might be done as well. These might include:

▶ Contact lens overrefraction (when previous corneal surgery has been done)

▶ Anterior segment OCT (for anterior chamber depth and configuration, looking for anomalies)

▶ Corneal topography (for corneal and total astigmatism)

▶ Retinal OCT (to ensure that there are no retinal or vitreoretinal interface issues and to ensure the desired postoperative result)

SIDEBAR 38-2

OTHER CORNEAL PROCEDURES WITH SECONDARY REFRACTIVE EFFECT

▶ Keratoplasty—The refractive effects here can range from small amounts to quite large and may include high amounts of astigmatism.

• Penetrating keratoplasty (PK) is a full-thickness removal of the patient's own cornea and replacement with a donor cornea from a human host.

• Deep anterior lamellar keratoplasty (DALK) differs from full-thickness PK described above in that the recipient's own Descemet's and corneal endothelium are retained rather than removed.

• Descemet's stripping endothelial keratoplasty (DSEK) is almost the opposite of DALK. In this case, a thin layer of far posterior stroma, Descemet's, and endothelium are the only parts of the cornea transplanted.

• Descemet's membrane endothelial keratoplasty (DMEK) is much like DSEK but only Descemet's and endothelium are transplanted.

▶ Corneal (collagen) cross-linking (CXL)—In CXL, a special concentration of sterile riboflavin (Vitamin B$_2$) eye drops are applied at specified intervals, generally over 30 minutes, before a strictly timed ultraviolet exposure. It is done to strengthen the chemical bonds within the cornea in order to halt progressive and irregular changes in corneal shape due to conditions such as keratoconus. The procedure can be done with the epithelium intact or removed. Refractive changes are mostly minor.

Note that it is possible that a zero-power or a negative-power IOL will be needed depending on the amount and power of the desired correction. Simultaneous or subsequent corneal procedures may be indicated to reach the final desired result.

Toric- and Presbyopic-Correcting Intraocular Lenses

This procedure is performed identically to RLE, but instead of a standard spherical IOL, the implant chosen has one or both of the following characteristics:

▶ Both spherical- and cylinder-correcting functions within a single IOL (for astigmatism)

▶ A spherical IOL that has two different powers simultaneously (used for distance and near corrections)

Careful power selection for both distance and near is key when an IOL can function in this way.

Astigmatism-correcting IOLs come in a wide selection of spherical and astigmatic corrections; these may vary slightly by IOL manufacturer. Likewise, presbyopia-correcting IOLs come in many different powers for the distance spherical power. The add power for near has fewer options, differing from one manufacturer to another. Corneal surgery may be indicated concurrently or subsequently to achieve the desired net refractive result.

Phakic Intraocular Lens

Some patients are not candidates or do not desire cornea-based refractive surgery. Additionally, they may not desire removal of their natural lens. If young enough, they may still have usable accommodation and, with a distance correction in place, have minimal or no need for reading glasses. In this surgery, the natural crystalline lens remains in place and an IOL is placed in front of it. The IOL is inserted into one of two anatomical locations: the anterior chamber (iris- or angle-fixated) or behind the iris (in the posterior chamber but in front of the natural lens).

Piggyback Intraocular Lens

In this setting, the patient already has an IOL after lens surgery (cataract/IOL or RLE), but the refractive result is not as desired. A second IOL is added to compensate—hence, the "piggyback" terminology. These lenses typically are placed in the posterior chamber behind the iris and into the capsular bag if possible—but anterior to the original IOL. They can also be placed in the anterior chamber with either angle-fixation or iris-fixation. While less common, toric- or presbyopic-correcting IOLs could be used in piggyback configuration.

Intraocular Lens Exchange

When an implanted IOL creates refractive issues and piggybacking (see above) is not an attractive option for the surgeon or patient, the current IOL can be removed and replaced with one of different power. This is most often done early in a postoperative course of the original surgery since the original IOL is more easily removed (and likely with fewer complications) at this point.

CLINICAL SKILLS
History Taking Considerations

Basic history taking is covered in Chapter 7. While your routine patient work-up (including the review of systems and patient questionnaire) is still critically important, the patient who is considering refractive surgery is different. First, this is an elective procedure. These patients also tend to be very demanding, so the history

involves some additional concerns such as impending or current presbyopia. It's not enough, for example, to note how a patient is employed. You've got to know what tasks the patient actually does and the working distances required for each. The surgeon must understand these things when considering the most appropriate approach. Remember that not every patient wants or is best served by a "plano" final result (ie, fully corrected for distance).

Lifestyle concerns are also important when the goal is changing someone's refraction. How he/she uses his/her eyes in his/her hobbies and outside-of-work activities is critical. A particular refractive goal may arise more from these activities than from work.

Another item of importance when taking the history is to listen carefully for suggestions of symptoms that might suggest ocular pathology, such as glare (cornea or cataract) or distortion with reading (macular disorders).

The patient's expectations should also be deliberated, and patients whose motivations for surgery are unclear should be identified. Be on the lookout for the patient who makes statements that suggest an unwillingness to accept anything less than a perfect result. Most patients do understand that perfection cannot be guaranteed, although it may be achieved. In this case, it is mandatory that the technician inform the surgeon if the patient seems unwilling or unable to accept less than his/her ideal.

Pretesting and Measurements

Two of the major considerations in refractive surgery are the potential acuity and the refractive error(s). It's important to know the best-corrected acuity preoperatively since it will also likely be the maximum possible after surgery and healing. The refraction entails the sphere, cylinder, and axis, but may also involve consideration of the patient's accommodative needs.

Low-order aberrations include refractive error and presbyopia. Higher-order aberrations might also be an important consideration for both patient and surgeon. Refractive surgery with a laser may be able to correct these aberrations. Correction requires knowing what all these "errors" are, so accuracy in these measurements by the technical staff is critical.

There are many ways to measure the patient's lower-order aberrations; we are familiar with sphere, cylinder, axis, and add. Higher-order aberrations are more complex, and measuring them requires special instrumentation. When measuring higher-order aberrations via specialized instrumentation, don't take short cuts. Centration is critical. If the results cannot be regarded as completely reliable, the test should be repeated. If the repeat measurements show variability or an uncertain endpoint, repeat it again or have the patient return to try again another day. Remember that the surgical result is planned for a lifetime, and a delay of a few days or a week to achieve it is inconsequential. While the patient and surgeon may have planned a date, it's only tentative until everything is ready.

Some other measurements also require centration to be accurate. Topography that is off-center may lead the surgeon to cancel a viable case, or to plan correction that is unnecessary (in either lens- or corneal-based surgeries). In some cases, the wavefront (higher-order) aberrometry measurements might be directly transferred to the laser in corneal surgery, so any off-center results will be translated directly onto the cornea.

In lens-based surgery, aberrometry is important in guiding the surgeon's selection of IOL types. There are some IOLs that have various configurations in terms of certain higher-order aberrations. Most surgeons want their patients to have a small amount of net positive spherical aberration postoperatively if possible (the "average" in most populations), because a high overall net spherical aberration may reduce the postoperative acuity and affect contrast sensitivity.[2,3] Choosing a negative-spherical aberration IOL when the patient already has the same (negative) corneal condition may leave the patient with a "plano" lower-order aberration result but intolerably high spherical aberrations that could have been avoided by selecting a different IOL model.

When the patient has had prior corneal surgery, regular "spectacle-only" correction may not yield the best-corrected acuity that is possible. Because of this, it may be important to place a rigid contact lens of known power on the cornea and perform refractometry over the top of the lens to see if the acuity improves compared to that without the contact lens. Improvement with the contact lens does not become exclusively diagnostic for irregular astigmatism (which might be a disqualifier for refractive corneal surgery), but since that is a possibility, it is an important consideration for the surgeon in the preoperative work-up.

When astigmatism procedures are contemplated, in addition to corneal topography noted previously, other tests have importance for the surgical work-up. Corneal thickness via ultrasonic or optical pachymetry is essential; thin corneas are generally more pliant. Pachymetry also assists the surgeon in setting incision depth for CRIs. If not done as part of a "whole cornea" optical scan of the front and back surfaces (as with certain instruments), the technician should provide central, mid-peripheral, and peripheral corneal thickness measurements at various "clock hours." That many measurements would be confusing if documented as a long list; it is more helpful to use a preprinted "map" of each cornea and place the thickness values in the appropriate locations (Figure 38-7). Get your surgeon's input on the measurement locations desired and format the template to his/her specifications.

When the refractive surgery is lens based, other measurements are important, such as horizontal corneal diameter (also known as "white to white") and A-scan/

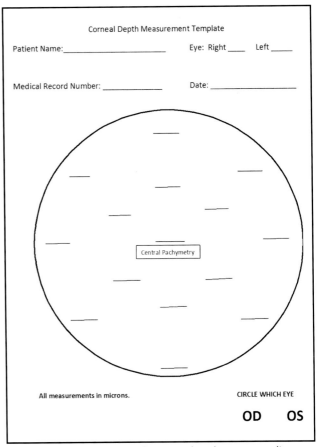

Figure 38-7. Map/template for corneal pachymetry readings.

optical coherence biometry. Horizontal corneal diameter is important because a larger or smaller than normal (11.5 to 12 mm) measurement might mean a larger or smaller anterior segment. This can make a difference in the "effective lens position" number in IOL formulas. Remember that there are multiple instruments for both ultrasonic and optical coherence methods for measuring axial length, so proper calibration and adherence to manufacturer's guidelines is key to providing proper numbers to input into the IOL formula.

There are various formulas available for calculating IOL power—and for vastly different indications. So be sure to use the formula(s) preferred by your surgeon for any given situation. Many surgeons use a variety of formulas depending on the patient's prior ocular history and refractive error. Surgeons may also want to view multiple formulas for the same patient and same eye in order to determine an appropriate IOL power. IOL calculations are also discussed in Chapters 17 and 28.

When there is a history of globe injury or congenital condition, or when there is a highly hyperopic eye, some surgeons may perform gonioscopy or have the technician perform anterior segment OCT to determine the anterior segment morphology and anterior chamber depth at the angle. This can be an important factor in the choice of IOL power and size.

Other testing may be ordered before determining patient suitability for refractive surgery. This testing is to ensure that any pathology that might affect the result is accounted for and explained to the patient. For example, the technician may be asked to perform OCT of the macula to verify the absence of any vitreomacular issues, such as undiagnosed early epiretinal membranes. In this way, although no assurances of a result can be guaranteed, the surgeon may have a higher chance of avoiding a poor acuity result.

Sometimes the surgeon considers a result where one eye is set for distance (a "net" result near plano) and the other set for mild myopia (to read or do intermediate tasks with less dependence on spectacles). This may be referred to as *monovision*, *blended vision*, or other similar terminology. (Some practices have very specific terminology and you should be careful to use it consistently.) A simulation can give the patient and surgeon an idea of a possible outcome by assessing the patient's tolerance for such an anisometropic result. In this case, the technician may be asked to demonstrate this arrangement to the patient via contact lenses worn in the office. Based on feedback from this test, the surgeon might adjust the near-eye result with the "net result" in mind. If the patient and surgeon feel there is a chance of success with this option, the technician may be asked to instruct the patient on contact lens use so that the temporary trial can be taken into the patient's work/life use for input before a final refractive plan is made.

Intraoperative Considerations

As with any surgery, the protocol for identifying the patient and the eye(s) being operated on should be verified at each conversation with the patient and before moving to the surgical room. Once in the room, the surgeon performs a *call to order* (also called a *time out*) and all the information (patient, eye[s], and procedure) is verified with the patient. Typically, at this point, the nurse or laser technician will ask the surgeon to confirm the information regarding refractive power selection (IOL if lens based and the programmed correction values if laser based).

Once the surgeon is completely satisfied with the result of the call to order and data verification, the patient is then prepped for surgery. Each surgeon or surgical facility likely has a personalized protocol, which must be followed to the letter. No variability is allowed in the prep without approval from both surgeon and circulating nurse. Following this, the draping is completed and the procedure commences.

Some instrumentation requires special care and handling, such as the diamond or sapphire blades used in surgery, and ophthalmic technicians should have training in this area. For instance, saline is typically used for rinsing delicate eye instruments, but diamond blades require distilled or deionized water as a final rinse. An additional consideration is the temperature of the autoclave, which will need to match the diamond blade manufacturer's requirements. "Hotter is not better" when it comes to the sterilizing process for these gem-quality blades. While diamond and sapphire blades are very hard, hardness comes with brittleness; damaging one of these blades is something to be avoided. They are neither easy nor inexpensive to repair. Initial purchase costs can be in the thousands of dollars (US). Repairs involving the gem are likely half (or more) of the original price.

Other instruments may be equally as fragile or just plain expensive. (Refractive lasers cost in excess of $500,000.) Additionally, being able to operate one laser does not guarantee familiarity with all software versions, models, or lasers produced by other manufacturers. Technicians should ask for and receive training on the lasers used before assisting with these cases.

PATIENT SERVICES
Postoperative Considerations

Once the case is finished, postoperative care begins. Technicians may be involved in reviewing the take-home instructions for the refractive surgery patient. Typically there will be a set of written instructions provided, with the patient's name and date of surgery. There may be prescriptions for medications attached, although in some cases these may have previously been phoned in to the desired pharmacy. Yet other patients already have the medications and can begin using them without delay. This is also a good time to review proper technique of eye drop instillation.

In any case, the technician or nurse will usually begin reviewing the instructions once the patient is settled after surgery, away from the operating suite. In the case of a patient who has been mildly sedated, you may be instructing the caregiver. Be sure you know what the instructions clearly state the patient CAN DO as well as what he/she CANNOT DO; patients sometimes hear only what they wish.

Since you do not want to be explaining these instructions in a way that contradicts or casts doubt on the written instructions they will take home, you must anticipate questions. If the instructions seem unclear to you, check with the provider before sitting down with patients. In no case should you allow the patient to depart the facility until the instructions are absolutely clear (to the patient and/or caregiver).

Other considerations are to review who to call if there are questions/problems, and the possible schedule of postoperative visits. Most surgeons have a planned series of postoperative visits anticipated in advance and based on the patient responding as planned. These future appointments may or may not already be on the office schedule. Each surgeon and/or surgical procedure may have different schedules; you should know each surgeon's preferences before beginning the review of the postoperative instructions.

If other eye care providers are involved (eg, a referring practitioner), be sure appropriate appointments are scheduled and that they receive notification from the surgeon, including the expected postoperative medication regimen.

Facilities always have a blanket policy to which patients agree beforehand, which likely specifies that the patient must have a method of transportation home, typically via a friend or family member. Even though acuity can be remarkably good immediately following some of these surgeries—even to the point of meeting driving standards—remember that other factors are involved. For example, sedatives of some sort might have been given. It's also not advisable for technical staff to drive patients home because of liability concerns.

Finally, be sure the patient is aware of what is appropriate activity at each stage of recovery. Refractive surgery patients often will try to do more because they are otherwise healthy, so it's important to outline what their surgeon regards as the boundaries.

Handling Phone Calls in the Postoperative Period

While the expectation is that the vast majority of patients will do exceedingly well with modern refractive surgery, occasionally someone has a bumpier postoperative course. When these calls come in, do not minimize the patient's concerns. If a problem sounds in any way suspicious, inform the surgeon.

It's important not to overpromise a result once surgery has been done; some problems may not manifest themselves for a period of weeks. Don't be dragged or trapped into saying more than you should, which is quite easy as you learn more. Knowing something does not mean it is your role to explain it. Defer to the surgeon or a more senior person in the office as needed.

There are a few situations where it is quite clear you should ask the patient to come in. The most common among these are pain and blurry vision. You must tactfully ask the patient if these are new or worsening. After speaking with the patient, if you are unsure about the urgency of the problem, request help from either another person in the office or the surgeon.

CHAPTER QUIZ

1. Why is the cornea most often considered when refractive surgery is contemplated?
   a. it accounts for the majority of the total refractive power of the eye
   b. it's at the front of the eye and is therefore easily accessible
   c. both a and b
   d. that's a false statement; lens surgery is far more common

2. It is part of the technician's role to explain the best surgery options to the patient before the surgeon has seen them to save time.
   a. True: The surgeon's time is so valuable it makes sense to do that.
   b. False: It is not appropriate for the technician to do this.

3. What are the main differences between LASIK/SBK and PRK?
   a. LASIK/SBK involve flap creation and intrastromal treatment.
   b. LASIK/SBK are done on the surface of the cornea.
   c. They are the same.
   d. LASIK/SBK patients are generally less comfortable for the initial postoperative period compared to PRK patients.

4. Which of the following are done for cylinder correction?
   a. myopic LASIK
   b. LRI, CRI, or toric IOL
   c. monovision or blended vision
   d. hyperopic SBK or PRK

5. True/False: Flattening the cornea in only one meridian means correcting for presbyopia.

6. How does PK differ from DMEK/DSEK?
   a. DMEK and DSEK both involve full-thickness corneal surgery
   b. PK involves using full-thickness corneal graft tissue.
   c. all three are appropriate for use when anterior corneal scarring is the main pathology issue
   d. none of the above

7. True/False: It's possible to do refractive surgery by removing the crystalline lens and replacing it with an IOL of appropriate power.

8. True/False: History taking on a possible refractive surgery patient involves asking about hobbies, outside activities, workplace needs, as well as other visual and eye problems.

9. True/False: Centration for diagnostic testing is an important consideration when refractive surgical planning is undertaken.

10. What is the purpose of the surgical call to order/time out?

    a. it ensures the correct patient is in the room
    b. it ensures the correct surgery type is planned
    c. it ensures the proper amount of surgical correction is checked
    d. it ensures the proper eye(s) are scheduled
    e. all of the above

11. True/False: Proper postoperative instructions must explain both what the patient CAN and CANNOT do.

Answers

1. c
2. b
3. a
4. b
5. False, It is astigmatism that is corrected in this situation.
6. b
7. True
8. True
9. True
10. e
11. True

REFERENCES

1. FDA approves first-of-its-kind corneal implant to improve near vision in certain patients. FDA website. www.fda.gov/NewsEvents/Newsroom/PressAnnouncements/ucm443471.htm. Released April 17, 2015. Accessed July 4, 2016.
2. Yamaguchi T, Dogru M, Yamaguchi K, et al. Effect of spherical aberration on visual function under photopic and mesopic conditions after cataract surgery [abstract taken from PubMed website]. *J Cataract Refract Surg.* 2009;35:57-63. www.ncbi.nlm.nih.gov/pubmed/19101425. Accessed July 4, 2016.
3. Kim SW, Ahn H, Kim EK, Kim T-I. Comparison of higher order aberrations in eyes with aspherical or spherical intraocular lenses. *Eye.* 2008;22:1493-1498. www.nature.com/eye/journal/v22/n12/full/eye2008302a.html. Accessed July 4, 2016.

The figures in this chapter were contributed by the following, who are associated with this book as authors:
Paul M. Larson: Figures 38-1 through 38-3, 38-5 through 38-7
Al Lens: Figure 38-4

39

OPHTHALMIC LASER SURGERY

Adeline Stone, COT, CRA, CDOS

BASIC SCIENCES

History of Lasers

The very first documented change to eye tissue by light was described by Plato, who documented solar retinopathy—a thermal reaction in the retina caused by staring at a solar eclipse.[1] Lasers have been a functioning reality since the 1960s, and a majority of medical lasers are used for ophthalmic procedures. LASER is an acronym for light amplification by stimulated emission of radiation, which describes the properties of how light waves react when placed between two mirrors: the energy of light (or photons) becomes amplified energy. This amplified energy continues in the same direction as a wavelength, and when released is in the form of a laser.[1,2]

One of the first commercially used lasers, the argon laser (available in 1970), was introduced for the treatment of retinal tumors and leaking blood vessels. The argon laser uses argon gas reacting with electricity to form the laser beam. Other lasers to treat glaucoma were also trialed in the 1970s, such as the neodymium: yttrium aluminum garnet (Nd:YAG) laser. Use of laser to treat lens membrane opacification ("after cataract") began in 1983.[2]

In 1999, the Food and Drug Administration approved two refractive surgeries for correction of myopia, hyperopia, and astigmatism: photorefractive keratectomy (PRK) and LASIK.[2] The original LASIK procedure has since undergone changes to use the laser to create a flap rather than using the blade of a microkeratome. Sub-Bowman's keratomileusis (SBK) also uses a femtosecond laser to create the flap, and has been shown to aid in healing and to yield better visual results.[2-4]

Laser Principles

Lasers are used in everyday items to take measurements, read CDs, print on paper, and scan barcodes. Lasers are categorized into different classes, or levels, that require special use and precautions. Class I is nondamaging to tissues. Printers as well as DVD and CD players are everyday items that are Class I lasers. Many instruments in ophthalmology that use laser to image or measure tissues are Class I, such as optical coherence tomography (OCT) units (see Chapter 16) and optical biometers.

Class II, IIa, IIIa, IIIb lasers can cause damage to the eye if viewed either too long or with some sort of magnification device. All Class II and above must have warning labels (Figure 39-1) posted in the vicinity. Lastly, Class IV "diffuse reflections" off a surface can cause tissue or eye damage. Safety glasses that block the wavelength of the specific laser in use should be worn with this class.[5,6]

655

Ledford JK, Lens A, eds.
Principles and Practice in Ophthalmic Assisting:
A Comprehensive Textbook (pp 655-663).
© 2018 Taylor & Francis Group.

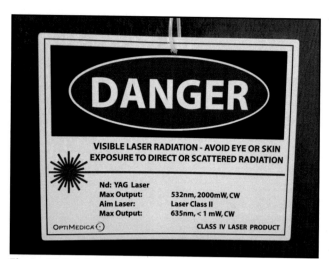

Figure 39-1. Safety sign placed on closed doors to notify that a laser is in use.

Lasers are monochromatic (ie, a single wavelength of color) and can vary from red, yellow, blue, green, and infrared dependent on the lasing material. The color of the laser is determined by the frequency of the wavelength emitted, as well as the charged particle material that is used to create the laser.

Medical class lasers can alter tissue by photocoagulation (a thermal reaction), photodisruption (a reaction to light), photoablation (removal of tissue), or photochemical reaction (chemical reaction from laser activation).

The laser beam used within the different subspecialties of ophthalmology may be pulsed or continuous. Pulsed lasers use a Q-switch mechanism that interrupts the laser beam with a shutter; these lasers use short bursts of energy. Femtosecond and picosecond lasers are examples of pulsed lasers. Continuous lasers discharge a constant wavelength of energy that is emitted in the same direction, creating a coherent wavelength. Examples of continuous lasers are Class I lasers, such as a CD/DVD player or laser printer.

Utilizing laser technologies either surgically or for imaging will continue to become more technologically advanced, aiding in patient care.

Clinical Knowledge

The same type of laser can be used to treat both glaucoma and retinal diseases. The action of the laser is determined by how the laser will transmit its wavelength to focus on or absorb the ocular tissue, and which structure is being focused on for treatment.

An example is the argon laser, which is used for retinal treatments including retinopathy, diabetic macular edema, tumors, vein occlusions, and retinal tears. It is also used on the trabecular meshwork for glaucoma. An argon laser typically has a wavelength of 488 to 514 nm,

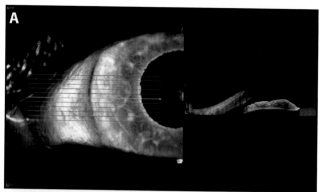

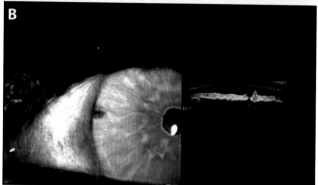

Figure 39-2. (A) Anterior OCT of narrow angle, before laser peripheral iridotomy. (B) Anterior OCT after laser peripheral iridotomy.

and is green or blue. The argon laser uses photocoagulation to seal leaky vessels, especially in diabetic retinopathy, or to bind tissue as in repairing retinal tears.

Photodynamic therapy (PDT) laser is used to treat neovascular lesions of the choroid. This type of laser requires an infusion of verteporfin, which is an injected photosensitive dye that binds to abnormal vessels and is activated by a laser wave length of 630 to 700 nm.[7] The spot size of the laser is adjusted based on the size of the localized leakage as shown via fluorescein angiogram (FA) or indocyanine green angiogram (ICG). (Testing such as FA, ICG, or fundus photography may be necessary before the patient has a laser procedure to help document the areas of leakage as in diabetic retinopathy or central serous retinopathy [CSR]. These techniques are covered in Chapter 15.)

Glaucoma (covered in Chapter 29) is known as the "silent thief of sight," but luckily there are more options than just drops to help reduce intraocular pressure (IOP). The Nd:YAG (or simply YAG) is a doubling frequency laser with a wavelength of 532 nm. In cases of narrow angles it can be used to create a small hole in the iris (iridotomy), providing a new path for aqueous to move from the anterior to posterior chamber even if the angles should become blocked (Figure 39-2).

Another tool for a glaucoma specialist is the red diode laser with a wavelength of 810 nm. Cyclodiode photocoagulation with the diode laser is used as a last resort in

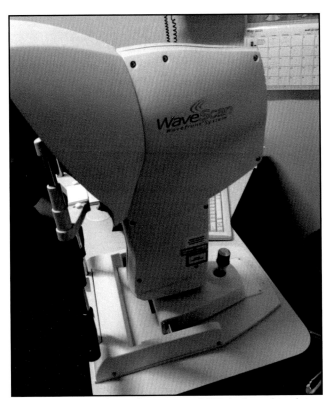

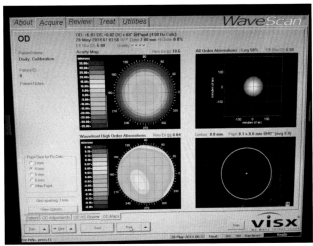

Figure 39-4. Customized display that gives wavefront parameters and the treatment report (VISX, Inc).

Figure 39-3. Wavefront aberrometer (VISX, Inc) used to determine refractive error and measure higher-order aberrations.

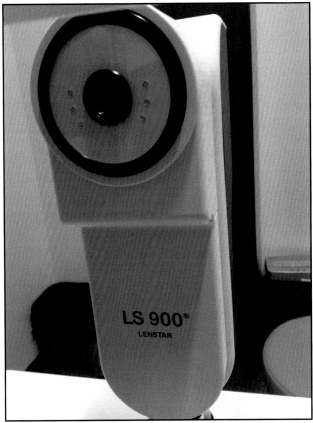

Figure 39-5. Lenstar (Haag-Streit USA) is an optical biometer that measures the structures of the eye. These values go into formulae to determine the IOL power for cataract surgery.

cases with uncontrolled pressure or traumatic glaucoma. In this case, the ciliary body is targeted in an effort to stop aqueous production and thus prevent high pressures.

Two of the best-known refractive laser surgeries are LASIK and PRK. (See Chapter 38, Refractive Surgery.) The excited dimer laser (known as the excimer) has a wavelength of 193 nm and is used to treat the stromal layer after the epithelial flap is lifted in LASIK. (PRK abrades the epithelial layer with either an alcohol solution or brush.) The excimer laser uses a premix of fluorine (argon and halogen) gases for the medium that creates the laser. In the operating suite there must be special venting systems in the event of a gas leak, as well as controlled temperature and humidity. SBK uses the femtosecond laser to create the flap.

One of the most exciting advances using laser has been the development of technology that uses principles of laser to image the eye. Using noncontact methods of imaging has improved the quality of care in ophthalmology, as well as our understanding of pathology. Some of the most useful and popular devices include the wavefront aberrometer, optical biometer (Lenstar and IOLMaster), and the optical coherence tomographer. These instruments are covered in Chapter 16.

A wavefront aberrometer (Figure 39-3) is a Class I laser that measures how light is focused on the retina and creates a customized "fingerprint" of the eye. These measurements are used to formulate a personalized treatment

plan that is loaded into the excimer laser for LASIK, PRK, and SBK (Figure 39-4).

Optical biometers use coherent light waves that either image the eye or take measurements. IOLMaster and Lenstar are Class I lasers in popular use (Figure 39-5). These devices are known as interferometers, which use

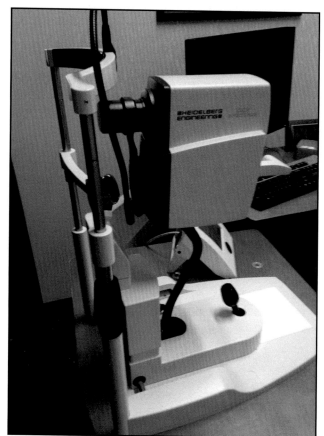

Figure 39-6. The Heidelberg Spectralis OCT (Heidelberg Engineering) is a spectral domain instrument.

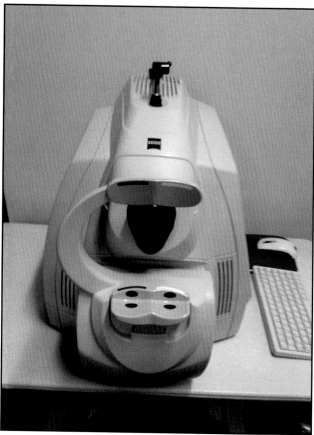

Figure 39-7. The Zeiss Cirrus OCT (Carl Zeiss Meditec) is a spectral domain laser.

coherent waves that reflect from biological tissues back to the instrument. The amount of time this takes is converted into the measurement, usually in microns (μm) or millimeters (mm). The possible measurements include corneal curvature (K-readings), anterior chamber depth (ACD), axial length (AL), lens thickness, and white-to-white (corneal) diameter. These readings are plugged into formulas for intraocular lens (IOL) power calculations prior to cataract surgery (see Chapter 28).

Using OCT for retina and glaucoma subspecialties has greatly transformed clinical decisions and care for vision-threatening diseases. OCT allows quick and comfortable imaging for the patient and a wealth of information for the doctor. This technology is one of the most useful tools in diagnosing and treating macular degeneration. Distinguishing whether macular degeneration is wet or dry can be determined from a cross-section image.

Glaucoma can also be tracked with OCT by using retinal nerve fiber layer (RNFL) scanning protocols that measure the thinning of the nerve fiber layer surrounding the optic disc. Older examples of OCT technologies include Glaucoma Diagnostics (GDx) and Heidelberg Retinal Tracking (HRT). Progression reports are used in conjunction with visual fields to help watch for changes.

OCT can also be used to monitor the retina after intraocular injections, laser treatment, and retinal surgery (to track swelling of the macula), or to document a baseline before a procedure.

There are currently two versions of the OCT: time domain and spectral domain. Time domain refers to an internal reference mirror that moves with a delay while imaging each section. Many practices have moved away from time domain to the higher-resolution spectral domain (Figures 39-6 and 39-7), which does not have a moving reference mirror and can capture many more scans at one time. This allows for a higher-definition image with more detail and the ability to create a three-dimensional model (Figure 39-8).

Types of Laser Surgery

There are numerous lasers used in eye surgery of various kinds (Table 39-1). For information on any particular disorder, consult the Index.

To treat weak, leaking vessels from diabetic retinopathy, panretinal photocoagulation (PRP) with the argon laser is commonly used in the periphery. The leaking vessels are "cauterized" when the laser reacts with the pigmentation of the retina. Treating the peripheral retina is safer for the patient's vision, and will help prevent further leaking, swelling, and damage within the tissue (Figure 39-9).

Retinal tears in the periphery are also treated with the argon laser.[8] The photothermal properties of the argon help seal the peripheral retinal tear and prevent more damage from occurring, such as retinal detachment.

Focal treatment using argon laser photocoagulation (ALP) can be used to treat macular edema, but must avoid the foveal avascular zone (FAZ; Figure 39-10). The FAZ is the area closest to the macula that has a high concentration of cones. These cones are nourished by the underlying choroid, and are responsible for central vision. If laser treatment is done too close to the macula, permanent central vision loss can result. In the case of branch retinal vein occlusion, ALP may be used to help treat the macular edema that can result (Figure 39-11).

PDT treats actively leaking choroidal neovascular (CNV) lesions. Central serous retinopathy (as an off-label treatment) and macular degeneration are also sometimes treated with PDT, which causes a photochemical reaction with the drug verteporfin (Visudyne).[7,9,10] An IV is used to inject the verteporfin, which takes approximately 10 minutes for infusion. (Which personnel are allowed to place an IV varies by state. Before assuming that technicians are legally allowed to perform an invasive IV placement, the state's laws should be reviewed.) Once the infusion is complete, there is a 10- to 15-minute window for laser treatment. The actual laser treatment lasts about 83 seconds.[9,10] The wavelength of the PDT laser activates the verteporfin, causing a lack of oxygen in the abnormal neovascular lesions, which in 1 to 2 months can cease to actively leak.[7] It is important to note that OCT should not be performed after an infusion of verteporfin, since it can inadvertently activate the chemical reaction.

The Nd:YAG laser with a wavelength of 323 nm is used during laser capsulotomy. This procedure is used to open the opacified membrane that sometimes develops after cataract surgery (Figure 39-12). Some patients refer

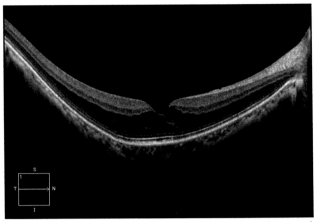
Figure 39-8. High-definition OCT of cystic macular edema and lamella macular hole.

to this as a "second cataract," but it is not a true cataract since the crystalline lens has been completely removed and replaced with an IOL. A "YAG" is a quick procedure where the patient is seated into a slit lamp headrest, and the surgeon directs the laser to the center of the opacified capsule. The action of the laser cuts a hole of approximately 3 to 4 mm in the opacified posterior lens capsule.

Glaucoma specialists use laser to target specific structures of the eye to help decrease IOP. The Nd:YAG laser can be used to make an opening or peripheral iridotomy (PI) in the iris. The patient is seated into the headrest. The surgeon places a special lens directly on the eye that focuses the laser on the iris. A tiny area of the iris is disrupted and opened to allow aqueous flow from the anterior to the posterior part of the eye, which helps lower IOP. Some cases require immediate PIs if the patient's angle is closed or very narrow. Laser peripheral iridotomy can be placed at the superior lid margin, but some surgeons prefer 3 or 9 o'clock position because the tear fluid at the upper lid can cause visual aberrations if the PI is at 12 o'clock.[8]

Another glaucoma procedure is to target the trabecular meshwork with a selective laser trabeculoplasty (SLT)

TABLE 39-1
TYPES OF OPHTHALMIC LASER SURGERY AND CORRELATING LASERS

Laser	Laser Surgery	Ocular Structure	Notes
Argon	PRP, ALP	Retina	Gas
Nd:YAG	LPI, OC	Iris, capsule	Solid state, double frequency
Excimer	LASIK, PRK	Cornea, stromal	Gas
Diode	CP	Ciliary body	Decrease aqueous formation
Femtosecond	SBK, cataract	Cornea stroma, crystalline lens capsule	Photodissection
Photodynamic therapy	PDT	Retina	Photochemical reaction
Argon	ALP, SLT	Trabecular meshwork	Gas

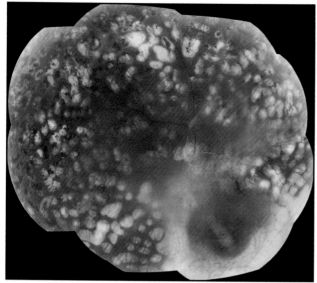

Figure 39-9. Severe retinopathy and choroidal lesion. Patient has had multiple laser spot treatments and has very low vision.

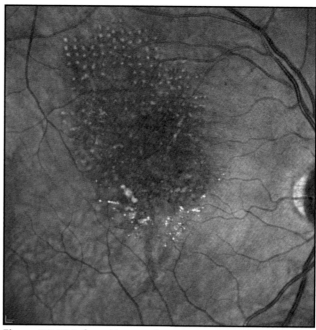

Figure 39-10. Infrared image of past argon laser photocoagulation treatment, avoiding the foveal avascular zone.

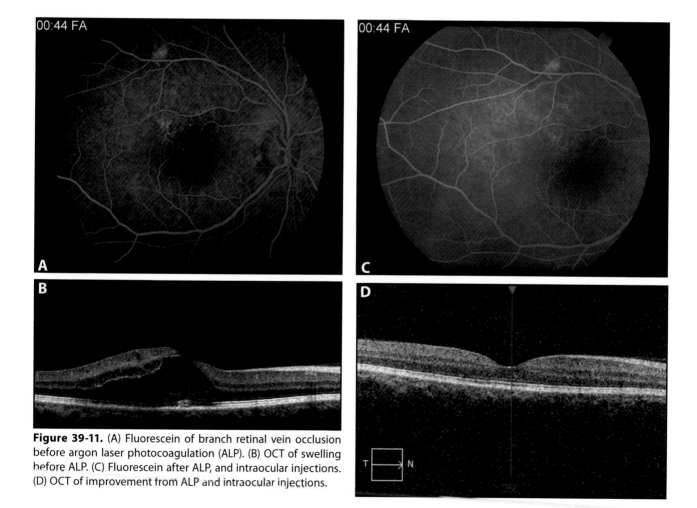

Figure 39-11. (A) Fluorescein of branch retinal vein occlusion before argon laser photocoagulation (ALP). (B) OCT of swelling before ALP. (C) Fluorescein after ALP, and intraocular injections. (D) OCT of improvement from ALP and intraocular injections.

with the Nd:YAG laser, which helps improve aqueous drainage in primary open-angle glaucoma (POAG). A gonio lens (which has mirrors in it) is placed directly on the patient's eye, and the laser is focused on the trabecular meshwork. The action of the laser in this case is photodisruption, creating a better opening for drainage.[11,12]

There are several refractive laser procedures that can greatly reduce a patient's need to wear contact lenses or glasses. (See Chapter 38 for more details.) LASIK stands for *laser-assisted in situ keratomileusis*, in which a corneal epithelial flap is made and lifted, and then the excimer laser is used to ablate the underlying stroma. The flap is then replaced and allowed to heal. The action of ablation works by removing corneal stromal tissue to focus incoming light onto the correct focal point of the retina.

Photorefractive keratectomy (PRK) involves abrading the surface of cornea, and then using the excimer laser to change the cornea's shape. A dilution of mitomycin C (an anti-cancer antibiotic drug) may be applied for 2 minutes using a Weck sponge, followed by irrigation with normal saline to prevent corneal hazing. A bandage contact lens is then applied.

LASEK is *laser-assisted subepithelial keratomileusis*. In this procedure about 50 microns of the cornea's epithelial layer is removed. This refractive procedure can be used for patients with thinner corneas. The flap can be created by alcohol solution or a circular trephine blade.

Phototherapeutic keratectomy (PTK) may be used when recurrent corneal erosion is affecting vision. Using a noncustomized treatment plan, PTK is therapeutic (vs correcting a refractive error). Risks can involve poor healing and induced astigmatism.

Pre-/postoperative LASIK, PRK, and SBK instructions are very specific to ensure a smooth procedure and good outcome. Patients are instructed to not wear makeup or strong perfumes the day of the surgery. (Molecules from scents can cause an unexpected fluctuation in the excimer laser during the laser treatment.) Generally, patients will take a pain reliever and anti-anxiety medication 40 minutes prior to the procedure. (The combination prescribed will depend on the surgeon's preference.) The patient is given a list of instructions for any oral antibiotics, antibiotic drops, and anti-inflammatory drops to be used after the surgery.

CLINICAL SKILLS

Once it has been determined that a patient will benefit from laser treatment, an informed consent form must be signed. The procedure itself is explained prior to signing, as well as the expected benefits, potential risks, and alternative treatments. (See the Index to find more on informed consent.)

The benefits of having laser surgery greatly outweigh the risks involved in most cases. That being said, however,

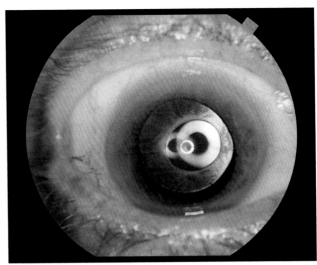
Figure 39-12. Anterior opacified membrane after YAG laser.

a laser treatment can have unintended consequences. These risks can involve blood clots, damage to other ocular structures, continued loss of vision from the underlying disease, and the need for laser surgery or other eye surgeries in the future.

Many clinics have surgical schedulers or technicians who make the arrangements for the procedure. This includes obtaining preapproval from the patient's insurance and discussing surgical costs. Also, any medications that need to be prescribed prior to the procedure must be submitted to the patient's pharmacy, along with instructions on how to use eye drops. Any necessary testing will generally be done prior to or on the day of treatment.

Getting the laser suite prepped for a day of treatment is important to ensure a smooth process. Check the patient schedule for various laser procedures beforehand. The time and scheduling of the laser procedure will depend on the urgency of the case. Patients with high IOPs may require a same-day treatment, as may patients with retinal tears. Be sure to stock supplies: drops, antiseptic wipes, Goniosol gel (hydroxypropyl methylcellulose), sterile saline, gauze, laser contact lenses, and any other items preferred by the clinic and physician.

Turn the laser on by priming the key prior to treatment. There is usually a setting that will allow the laser to switch to live mode. The excimer laser requires calibration and a warm-up sequence, as well as the patient's treatment card, which contains data from the aberrometer.

Place elbow rests on the right or left side of the laser table for physician comfort if a lens must be held on the patient's eye during the procedure. Any such lenses that are to be used must be filled with a coupling solution. Squeeze enough Goniosol or Gonak gel (hypromellose ophthalmic demulcent solution) in a steady stream without air bubbles to the edge of the lens cup. (Storing the bottle upside down helps reduce bubbles.)

Anesthetic drops are instilled into the eye(s) that will undergo laser treatment. A skin marker or a sticker is used to designate the eye(s) to be treated. A *time out* check is called before performing the laser procedure. At this point the physician and all other staff must stop everything they are doing, and check and agree that the correct patient is present, which eye is being treated, and what procedure is to be done. Only after this should you position the patient into the headrest of the laser.

Although the patient's eye is numb during a laser treatment, it can still be a little uncomfortable if a lens is placed on the cornea. There also may be a slight stinging sensation, almost as if a rubber band is snapping inside the eye. This discomfort may last a few seconds.

Wearing safety glasses that are correct for the wavelength of the laser is important to prevent any accidental injury to those in the room. Maintaining the lasers for accuracy and functionality is also important. Consult the user's manual for specifics on your instrument.

Review postoperative instructions and the time of the postoperative appointment before the patient leaves the office. Keep infection control processes in place by sanitizing anything that came into contact with the patient.

PATIENT SERVICES

A patient may have questions after the treatment. Have a set of standard answers that your physician is comfortable with, but always refer patients to the physician if they are experiencing out-of-the-ordinary symptoms. Some of these could be vision-threatening if not triaged correctly.

Patients are often concerned that they will continue to see "light spots," which appear in the peripheral vision after laser treatment on the retina. Recovery from seeing these after-images of the laser treatment varies, but most patients will find that the spots will be less noticeable by about 2 weeks after the procedure.

LASIK/LASEK/SBK/PRK patients will need to follow their after care instructions very specifically to ensure proper healing. They are monitored very closely to ensure that the flap heals with LASIK/LASEK/SBK. PRK patients will wear a bandage contact lens while the epithelial layer heals. Patients who have had refractive laser surgery may experience dryness, grittiness, and irritation for a time after surgery. These symptoms may be relieved by having them use preservative-free artificial tears frequently and wearing moisture goggles.

Patients undergoing PDT are advised to avoid direct sunlight and bright artificial lights for at least 72 hours after treatment. They will need to wear sunglasses, gloves, long sleeves, and long pants on the day of the procedure. If they do not, towels can be draped over any exposed skin, especially on a very sunny day.

ACKNOWLEDGMENTS

The author would like to thank the following: the Spokane Eye Clinic; Nicole Brandt, MD; Kandon Kamae, MD; and Eric Guglielmo, MD.

CHAPTER QUIZ

1. True/False: LASIK stands for laser-assisted in situ keratomileusis.

2. True/False: The photochemical process used in photodynamic therapy uses ablation to remove neovascular tissue.

3. Selective laser trabeculoplasty is used to help which structure of the eye and what condition?
   a. retina, diabetic retinopathy
   b. trabecular meshwork, primary open-angle glaucoma
   c. iris, closed angle
   d. cornea, refractive errors

4. True/False: Photodynamic therapy patients should avoid the dark after infusion of verteporfin.

5. What does the acronym LASER stand for?

6. What is required during the time out, before proceeding with a laser procedure?

7. What laser is performed when a patient experiences an opacified capsule following cataract removal?

8. Name other equipment used in ophthalmic imaging that uses coherent laser technology.

9. When and what kind of safety glasses should be worn during laser procedures?

10. True/False: PRK creates a flap, then the stromal tissue is ablated with an argon laser.

Answers

1. True, LASIK is a refractive procedure that uses the excimer laser to ablate the stromal layer to correct the cornea's curvature.

2. False, photodynamic therapy uses the activation of verteporfin to stop neovascularization.

3. b

4. False, Patients must stay out of direct light for minimum 72 hours.

5. LASER is an acronym for light amplification by stimulated emission of radiation.

6. Stop for a time out to confirm the correct patient, correct eye/location, and correct type of laser procedure is about to be performed.

7. YAG laser capsulotomy

8. OCT, GDx, HRT, optical biometry, and aberrometry

9. Glasses specific to the laser wavelength are worn when laser waves are directed parallel to the floor. When directed perpendicular to the floor, glasses are not needed.

10. False, PRK does not have a flap. The cornea is mechanically or chemically abraded, then ablated with the excimer laser.

REFERENCES

1. Marmor M, Palanker D, Blumenkranz M. Fifty years of ophthalmic laser therapy. *Arch Ophthalmol.* 2001;129(12):1613-1619.

2. Azoulay K, Pianka P, Loewenstein A. The evolution of retinal laser technology and retinal photocoagulation as therapeutic modality. *European Ophthalmic Review.* 2012;6(3):185-189.

3. iFS Advanced Femtosecond Laser. Abbott Medical Optics website. www.abbottmedicaloptics.com/products/refractive/ilasik/ifs-advanced-femtosecond-laser. Accessed July 4, 2016.

4. Manche EE, Carr JD, Haw WW, Hersh PS. Excimer laser refractive surgery. *West J Med.* 1998;169(1):30-38.

5. Classes of lasers. Environmental Hazard Safety Columbia University website. www.ehs.columbia.edu/LaserClass.html. Accessed July 4, 2016.

6. Zdybel M, Pilawa B, Krzeszewska-Zareba A. Lasers in ophthalmology. In: Rumelt S, ed. *Advances in Ophthalmology.* Published March 7, 2012. Intechopen website (open access publisher). doi:10.5772/29433.

7. Bausch + Lomb: Visudyne (Verteporfin for injection). www.bausch.com/ecp/our-products/rx-pharmaceuticals/rx-pharmaceuticals/visudyne-verteporfin-for-injection. Accessed July 4, 2016.

8. Gerstenberth A, Rabinowitz M. *The Wills Eye Manual: Office and Emergency Room Diagnosis and Treatment of Eye Disease.* 6th ed. Philadelphia, PA: Lippincott Williams & Wilkins; 2012:106-107,209,425,444-445.

9. Lim HS. Development and optimization of a diode laser for photodynamic therapy. *Laser Therapy.* 2011;20(3):195-203. doi:10.5978/islsm.20.195.

10. Bressler NM, Bressler SB. Photodynamic therapy with verteporfin (Visudyne): impact on ophthalmology and visual sciences. *Invest Ophthalmol Vis Sci.* 2000;41(3):624-628. http://iovs.arvojournals.org/article.aspx?articleid=2199926. Accessed July 4, 2016.

11. Lumenis SLT: how and why it works? Lumenis Energy to Healthcare website. www.lumenis.com/Solutions/Ophthalmology/Products/SLT-Laser-Therapy-for-Glaucoma. Accessed July 4, 2016.

12. Palanker D, Blumertranz M, Weiter J. Retinal laser therapy: biophysical basics and applications. In: Ryan SJ, Hinton DR, Schachat AP, Wilkinson P, eds. *Retina.* 4th ed. Philadelphia, PA: Mosby; 2006:539-553.

BIBLIOGRAPHY

About lasers. Laser Fest website. www.laserfest.org/lasers/index.cfm. Accessed July 4, 2016.

Alderich R. Laser fundamentals: laser theory and operation. www.fas.org/man/dod-101/navy/docs/laser/fundamentals.htm. Accessed July 4, 2016.

American Academy of Ophthalmology. Clinical education: laser surgery education center. www.aao.org/clinical-education/laser-surgery-education-center. Accessed July 4, 2016.

Basic laser principles. In: *Introduction to Laser Technology.* CVI Melles Griot website. www.bgu.ac.il/~glevi/website/Guides/Lasers.pdf. Accessed June 8, 2016.

Definitions of classes of laser. *Stanford University Laser Safety Manual.* www.stanford.edu/dept/EHS/prod/researchlab/laser/procedures/classes.html. Accessed July 4, 2016.

Lasers for dummies. Wicked Lasers website. www.wickedlasers.com/laser-tech/dummies.html. Accessed July 4, 2016.

LASIK vs. LASEK comparison chart. The LASIK Directory website. www.the-lasik-directory.com/lasik_lasek_chart.html. Accessed July 4, 2016.

Optical coherence tomography. Heidelberg Engineering website. www.heidelbergengineering.com/us/company/company-technology/optical-coherence-tomography/. Accessed July 4, 2016.

Renk KF. Basics of laser physics. In: *Graduate Texts in Physics.* Published 2012. doi:10.1007/978-3-642-23565-8.

Rose M. A history of the laser: A trip through the light fantastic. Photonics Spectra website. www.photonics.com/Article.aspx?AID=42279. Published May 2010. Accessed July 4, 2016.

Silfvast W. *Laser Fundementals.* 2nd ed. New York, NY: Cambridge University Press; 2004. www.creol.ucf.edu/Research/Publications/3613.pdf. Accessed July 4, 2016.

Southwest Innovative Solutions, Inc. Educational tool for medical laser programs: laser safety. www.sislasered.com/resources/docs/BasicLaserSafety.pdf. Accessed July 4, 2016.

The figures in this chapter were contributed by the author, Adeline Stone.

40

SURGICAL ASSISTING

Robert M. Kershner, MD, MS, FACS
Jacob P. McGinnis, BA, COT

BASIC SCIENCES

The goal of ocular surgery is to improve and preserve vision. In rare cases, such as ocular malignancies, eye surgery may even save a life. No matter what the purpose of the surgery, assisting the surgeon during ophthalmic procedures can be both challenging and rewarding.

Prior to studying the material in this chapter, review ocular anatomy (Chapter 2), physiology (Chapter 3), microbiology (Chapter 23), disorders (Chapters 26, 27, and others), and types of surgical procedures (Chapter 36). Minor in-office surgery is covered in Chapter 37.

CLINICAL KNOWLEDGE

Informed Consent

Before the patient enters the operating room, extensive consulting, evaluating, educating, and instructing must take place. The surgical patient must be adequately informed as to the diagnosis, treatment options, risks, alternatives, and expected benefits of the surgical procedure. The patient must then make an informed decision.

This informed decision has two parts: the personal one-on-one discussion between the operating surgeon and the patient and the written document. If surgery is elected, the patient (and/or guardian) must sign the surgical consent form documenting that he/she has had questions and concerns addressed, has received and understood information regarding the treatment, and wishes to proceed with the operation. This process is referred to as *informed consent* and is necessary both in establishing the physician-patient relationship as a matter of practice, as well as a legally binding agreement between the patient and physician. No surgical procedure, regardless how "minor," can be performed without it. (Find more on informed consent, via the Index.)

The ophthalmic assistant may play an important role in explaining the document and its purpose to the patient, answering questions, and witnessing the process. However, the discussion of surgery remains the sole responsibility of the operating surgeon. Informed consent cannot be delegated to anyone else. Many a malpractice litigation has been lost by a physician who failed to properly obtain and document informed consent prior to undertaking the patient's surgery.

Operating Room Personnel

Surgery is not a solo exercise undertaken lightly no matter how "simple" or "quick" the procedure. It is made

Ledford JK, Lens A, eds.
Principles and Practice in Ophthalmic Assisting:
A Comprehensive Textbook (pp 665-679).
© 2018 Taylor & Francis Group.

possible by a coordinated, highly trained, experienced, and dedicated team whose mutual goal is to ensure that the patient receives the best possible outcome in the most efficient and expedient manner. This means that the responsibility of the assisting anesthesiologists, nurses, and technicians (who each play an important role to the operating surgeon) is never to be taken lightly. If you are fortunate enough to assist an ophthalmologist in a vision-saving surgical procedure, you have to accept the obligation that goes with the role; namely, to be motivated, trained, and dedicated to the patient's well being.

It is important to know what type of surgery you will be assisting with in advance, and to have reviewed and trained in that procedure. If you are not prepared, poor outcomes can be the result. It is always best policy to inform the surgeon if you are unsure of anything or if the procedure is new to you.

Surgeon

In the United States, no one can perform surgery on another human being without being licensed as a medical doctor and have credentials demonstrating additional specialty training in surgery. In other words, surgery can and should only be performed by a surgeon. The surgeon has undergone a minimum of 12 years of additional medical education, and more years after that to become a specialist in diseases and surgery of the eye.

The surgeon is in charge. It is the role of the surgical assistants to carry out the physician's orders. That is not to say that you have to tolerate someone yelling at you; that is never acceptable behavior under any conditions. But you have an obligation to do precisely as instructed. After all, it is the surgeon's license that is on the line, not yours. If you do not agree with what the surgeon is doing, only after the procedure is complete and the patient is out of risk can you discuss your concerns with the surgeon or your supervisor. Remember, just because one surgeon does something different than another, does not imply that either way is wrong. Always give the surgeon the benefit of the doubt and be respectful at all times.

Anesthesiologist/Anesthetist

Anesthesia is an induced, temporary state of one of the following: analgesia (relief from or the prevention of pain), paralysis (extreme muscle relaxation preventing movement), amnesia (no memory of the procedure), and unconsciousness. Types of anesthetics are discussed in Chapter 22, Pharmacology, and vary according to the type of procedure as well as the patient. In the majority of ophthalmic procedures, topical or local anesthesia is the method of choice, and the patient is usually awake. In a procedure that is expected to be lengthy or painful, or in a patient who is young or unable to respond to instructions, general anesthesia can be employed.

The *anesthesiologist* is a physician who is specialized in the safe administration of anesthetics and the monitoring of a patient in the process of undergoing anesthesia. An *anesthetist* can be a registered nurse or physician assistant specially trained in the art and practice of anesthesia.

The person administering the anesthesia often sits by the patient's head, establishes an intravenous line to administer anesthetic agents, monitors vital signs, and adjusts fluids, breathing, and cardiac support as necessary. An anesthesiologist is often present but not necessarily administering the anesthesia. With the increasing shortage of MD anesthesiologists, the role of ancillary anesthesia personnel is expanding.

Surgical Assistant

The surgical assistant (SA) does just what the name implies, assisting the surgeon during the procedure (Sidebar 40-1). The SA can be a registered nurse, surgical technician, or ophthalmic tech (possibly subcertified in surgical assisting). The SA has an important role in setting up the surgical room before the procedure begins, obtaining the sterile surgical instruments and supplies. He/she must scrub and wear a clean, fresh scrub outfit with proper head and shoe coverings and a surgical mask. The SA must also see to it that the surgeon has all the instruments that are required, and pass them safely and efficiently as needed. A good SA is not only well-trained and experienced in numerous procedures, but is adaptable in working with different surgeons and personalities in a variety of settings.

SAs are expected to practice proper surgical technique, maintain absolute sterility at all times and adhere to aseptic technique, standard precautions (see Chapter 37, In-Office Minor Surgery), and infection control measures in the proper handling and disposing of all surgical materials. They must be up-to-date on all policies, protocols, standards, and best practices in every aspect of the surgical procedure. SAs execute their responsibilities with patient safety and well-being as the foremost concern. The SA's credibility, honesty, and integrity in the operating room should be above reproach. The SA is expected to do what is right whether or not someone is observing or monitoring his/her actions. SAs will occasionally make mistakes (everyone does). When they do, they must recognize and acknowledge the mistake immediately, report it appropriately, and take full responsibility for their own actions.

Circulator

The circulator is most commonly a nurse who is responsible for making sure that the operating room is set up correctly. The circulator is not scrubbed in for the case, and is therefore free to move within the room and exiting as necessary to obtain supplies. This includes checking inventory and restocking. The circulating nurse also ensures that all of the sterilized instruments are available. The circulator and scrub tech set up the surgical suite together in advance of the surgeon's arrival, laying out instruments and supplies according to the surgeon's preferences. The circulator also checks that all equipment required during the procedure is in the room and functioning normally. In the case of a prosthetic (such as an intraocular lens, glaucoma valve, or scleral band), the circulator makes sure that what is required for the particular procedure is in the room prior to the surgery.

When the patient arrives, the circulator verifies the patient's identity and the operative eye, and confirms that the proper consent forms are in the chart. The circulator will ask the surgeon if there is anything that may be required prior to the procedure. With the anesthetist, the circulator will assist in moving the patient onto the operating table and positioning him/her for surgery. The circulator connects electrical cords, cautery, IVs, tubing, and any nonsterile cassettes and equipment that will be used during the procedure. He/She may be called upon to assist the anesthesiologist with intubation, if necessary.

During the operation, the circulator provides the surgical team with sterile fluids and medications as needed, and also replenishes the supplies if additional disposables or instruments are needed. Due to the patient's inability to respond for him-/herself during the procedure, the circulator also advocates on the patient's behalf, monitoring the overall condition of the patient during surgery.

Operating Room Set-Up

Most operating rooms have similarities in their set-up whether they are located in a hospital, ambulatory surgical center, or physician's office. The central feature is the operating table, which is situated beneath a surgical microscope. Adjacent to the head of the table is the phacoemulsification machine, laser, and other automated devices used for surgery. If anesthesia is required, there will be an anesthesia machine containing inhalational gases and drawers stocked with anesthetic and analgesic agents. There will be a back table that is draped and sterile for storing supplies such as sterile towels, surgical gowns, and gloves. A Mayo stand contains the surgical tray and instruments.

Preparation Table

The *prep table* contains all the necessary supplies and solutions needed for preparing the skin, as well as topical drops and local anesthetics. Included on the table are antiseptics, applicators, sponges, gauze, syringes with requisite needles, and irrigating solutions. Unless otherwise specified, this table should be removed after the eye is prepped.

SIDEBAR 40-1

IMPORTANT POINTS TO FOLLOW IN AND OUT OF THE OPERATING ROOM

▶ First, confirm that you have the correct patient and identify the surgeon's mark on the proper side for the scheduled procedure. Only the surgeon can identify and mark the surgical site using a marking pen or a nonremovable skin label; your job is to verify that it is correct by asking the patient and confirming it with the surgical consent and chart.

▶ Take the time to establish good rapport with the patient. The patient does not need to know that you have 30 procedures scheduled for that day; he/she just wants to know that you are paying attention to him/her. A patient who is comfortable with the staff, physician, and facility will be more cooperative, which increases the probability of a successful outcome.

▶ Inquire if the patient understands the procedure and if he/she has any questions or concerns. Do not "wing it" if you are not sure about the answer, check with the physician.

▶ All operative notes should be completed after surgery; if not immediately following the procedure, then at the conclusion of the day. Do not delay. Incomplete charts create problems for the postoperative nursing team, staff, and administration, and increase the likelihood of errors.

▶ Always maintain accurate office and hospital records. Make sure that any communication with the patient, no matter how trivial it may seem, is clearly documented in the electronic medical record, particularly any advice or information given over the phone. Be sure to document when a phone call is made, even if the patient was not available, and the plan for follow-up.

Back Table

The *back table* is located just out of reach of the operating sterile area, but is still included as a sterile surface as it is the launching area for all of the operative instruments and solutions. The back table is set up by the SA and is draped with a sterile drape. The items that are placed on the back table are all sterile, and strict sterile precautions must be maintained in and around this area. Items on the back table will make their way to the surgical instrument stand and should be arranged in the order of use. First will be sterile towels, gowns, and gloves for the SA and surgeon. Adjacent to this will be the surgical pack that contains the sterile eye drape and other drapes for the patient.

TABLE 40-1
COMMON INSTRUMENTS FOR EXTRAOCULAR PROCEDURES*

- ▶ 1 disposable stainless steel knife
- ▶ 1 pair Steven's tenotomy scissors
- ▶ 1 pair spring scissors
- ▶ 1 straight and 1 angled fixation forceps
- ▶ 1 double-pronged scleral forceps
- ▶ 2 muscle hooks
- ▶ 1 caliper
- ▶ 1 right and 1 left muscle clamp
- ▶ 2 straight and 2 curved fine hemostats
- ▶ 1 packet of suture
- ▶ 2 towel clips
- ▶ 2 skin hooks, fine
- ▶ 1 irrigating cannula, 19 gauge
- ▶ 1 eyelid speculum

*Always check with the operating surgeon for personal preferences and whether he/she will be using the facility's instrument trays or his/her own.

TABLE 40-2
COMMON INSTRUMENTS FOR INTRAOCULAR PROCEDURES*

- ▶ 1 pair spring scissors
- ▶ 1 stainless steel blade of appropriate size (2.2 mm) or diamond keratome
- ▶ 1 pair Vannas scissors
- ▶ 1 straight and 1 angled fixation forceps (0.12 teeth)
- ▶ 2 fine-tying forceps
- ▶ 1 anterior chamber irrigating cannula
- ▶ 1 Sinskey hook
- ▶ 1 lens chopper or manipulating probe
- ▶ 1 measuring caliper
- ▶ 1 eyelid speculum
- ▶ 2 straight and 2 fine hemostats
- ▶ 1 muscle hook
- ▶ 1 iris spatula
- ▶ 1 synechia spatula or cyclodialysis spatula
- ▶ 2 needle holders, finely curved
- ▶ 3 anterior chamber irrigating tips (19, 27, and 30 gauge)
- ▶ 1 irrigating cannula
- ▶ Irrigation-aspiration tip, handle, and tubing
- ▶ Phacoemulsification tips and handpieces
- ▶ Special keratomes for incisions
- ▶ Cautery cord and tip

*Always check with the operating surgeon for personal preferences and whether he/she will be using the facility's instrument trays or his/her own.

Instrument Stand

The *instrument* or *Mayo stand* is a small table that can be adjusted for height to accommodate the SA and the surgeon's operating level. Some SAs stand while assisting, others sit. Usually there will be two surgical stools present, one for the surgeon and one for the SA. The surgeon's will have added features to allow hands-free height adjustment, and it may also have a back- and armrests.

The Mayo stand is usually positioned temporally (ie, to the side) if the surgeon operates at the patient's head. If the surgeon operates temporally, then the SA and Mayo stand will be positioned at top of the patient's head. The job of the SA is to make sure all necessary instruments are arranged in order of use. (For example, in the case of cataract surgery, the order might be drape scissors followed by eye speculum, keratome knife, capsulorhexis forceps, and intraocular lens insertion syringe.) Strict attention must also be paid to protecting and keeping these instruments clean and sterile.

Usually instrument handles face the SA, and the action area of the tips face the surgeon. This is done so that passing the instrument to the surgeon's hand can be accomplished smoothly and efficiently without the surgeon having to move or reposition his/her grip. Once used, the instrument is returned to its position on the stand.

The phacoemulsification, irrigation-aspiration, or vitrectomy handpieces, as well as irrigating solutions, Weck-cell sponges, applicators, sutures, cannulas, and syringes, will each have a specific area on the stand as well.

There is really no such thing as a standard instruments list. Each surgeon has preferences based on experience and training. It is the SA's job to learn what instruments are used for what procedure and the differing needs of different surgeons. A standard list for extraocular procedures is outlined in Table 40-1 and intraocular surgery in Table 40-2. Surgeons will have a preference for instruments they require on the stand and those that only need be nearby on the back table.

When an instrument *may* become necessary but is not ordinarily used, it is left in its sterile envelope or tray until called for. Special instruments may be required for specific procedures (eg, canthotomy, enucleation, evisceration); often these are kept in the preoperative sterile storage area.

Remember: All microsurgical instruments are very delicate (some have tips that are invisible to the unaided eye) and are easily damaged during use, handling, cleaning, and sterilization. Microsurgical instruments are very costly both in loss of use and replacement, and should be treated with the utmost care. If you are not sure how to handle or properly clean an instrument, ask someone who knows or contact the manufacturer. This is always best policy rather than losing a month's salary to replace something due to your own mishandling or carelessness.

Ophthalmic Instruments

Microsurgical instruments are made from stainless steel or titanium. Titanium is more expensive and less durable, but due to its ability to maintain shape and edge (and the fact that it does not rust) has all but replaced stainless steel. Instruments can also be single-use and disposable or *resposable* (disposable but may be used more than once).

A complete discussion regarding the myriad of ophthalmic microsurgical instruments that are available for ocular use is well beyond the scope of this textbook. However, there are some important concepts you should keep in mind when viewing, identifying, and learning which instrument is which.

To add to the confusion regarding the identity of a microsurgical instrument, many common instruments have more than one name. They may be called one thing by one surgeon and another by someone else. Often there is a proprietary name (such as the Kershner capsulorhexis forceps), a generic name (capsule forceps), and/or a manufacturer's name (Rhein medical forceps). It can be difficult, if not impossible, to learn all the names of all of the instruments used in ocular surgery. In fact, even if you could, the entry of new instruments every single day (and by dozens of manufacturers) makes it a fruitless task. Fortunately, you will undoubtedly work with a small group of surgeons, and since most ophthalmologists use a small number of instruments for a given procedure, you will be able to learn and identify those that are used most frequently.

Instruments are always stored in covered instrument trays. These trays may be made of stainless steel, titanium (very expensive), or rigid polycarbonate that can withstand repeated use as well as the high temperatures and pressure of sterilization.

Prior to any procedure, remove the cover and set it aside on an adjacent sterile table. Then count the instruments and make note of the number (you can use a marker to jot it down on the Mayo stand). This way, if an instrument goes missing, you can identify whether it was in the tray from the beginning or misplaced during surgery.

Next, quickly scan the tray and make a mental note of the order and position of the instruments. The purpose of most instruments can be deduced by examining the handle, the shaft, and the tip. Is the handle smooth, is it covered with cross-hatching to improve grip, or holes to make it lighter? Is the shaft at the end of the handle straight, angled, or curved? Which ones are probes with smooth, round handles and a single shaft with a tip? Which are double-handled forceps and scissors?

Most instruments used for eye surgery have tips that are virtually invisible to the naked eye (eg, 100 micron forceps) and can only be seen clearly under a microscope. Ophthalmic SAs will usually have access to a microscope either in the operating room (ie, the surgical microscope) or a small portable microscope in the sterilization room.

CLINICAL SKILLS

An SA should always be familiar with both the operating suite and the procedure being performed. If at all possible, speak with the surgeon beforehand to determine preferences for the preoperative care of patients, topical agents, skin and eye prep, operating room set-up, specific instrumentation and location (eg, which side is preferred for microscope and phacoemulsification pedals), sutures, instrument set-up, and supplies. If the surgeon is not available, speak with other operating room personnel to determine if they are aware of any preferences specific to the doctor with whom you'll be working. Most multiuse surgical centers keep surgeon preference cards handy that can be referred to prior to setting up for a surgical procedure.

The more you know about the operating room and the surgical procedures that will be performed there, as well as the special needs of a particular surgeon, the more valuable you will be as a member of the surgical team.

Scrubbing

The purpose of scrubbing is to remove all surface debris and contaminants, and to disinfect the skin prior to donning surgical gloves and gown. Your skin has two distinct populations of microbiologic flora: *resident flora*, which pretty much lives with you throughout your life (and differs from person to person), and *transient flora*, which is that which you acquire from contact. Some of the transient flora could be pathogenic, but all microbial life can be a potential pathogen when it gets inside a sterile body cavity (such as the eye). Learn the proper technique (covered momentarily) and stick to the same protocol each and every time you scrub in. Never cut corners or rush the scrub. Scrubbing off surface debris and microbial flora takes time to do properly, and disinfecting soaps take time to work; if you hurry through the scrub, you may inadvertently carry contaminants into the operating room with you.

The first scrub of the day should take approximately 17 minutes. If you leave the operating room after a procedure, you must rescrub. If you remove your sterile gown and gloves and outer coverings and return to the operating room immediately after a procedure, an abbreviated scrub and application of antiseptic lotion may be acceptable. Check with your surgical center policy manual for the proper routine.

Remember to don your scrub suit, head covering or bonnet, shoe covers or operating room shoes, and mask *before* you begin your scrub. Once your hands are clean you cannot touch anything that is not sterile.

Before beginning the scrub, remove all jewelry (rings, watches, bracelets, etc). Fingernails should be neatly trimmed and clean; ensure that the area under the nails is cleaned by using the disposable nail file that comes in the brush packet.

The water should be as hot as can be comfortably tolerated. Cold water does not allow soap to lather properly, and warm water dissolves oils better, eliminating bacteria where they cling. Most operating room scrub sinks have faucet controls at your feet, knee, or elbow, and some are preset to the proper temperature and come on when you approach them.

Use the provided antiseptic and disposable brush to wash. Do not wash so vigorously that water is splashed onto operating clothing, or so roughly that the skin is abraded. Remember to keep your hands up and elbows down at all times.

Once you start washing, begin timing yourself. There is always a clock or timer nearby. Do not assume that you have scrubbed enough and be sure that you fill the requisite time each time you scrub. Some operating facilities issue a badge that times your scrub and prevents you from entering the operating room until you have done so adequately. Even if such an advanced system is not available in your facility, everyone has to trust that you have performed your scrub properly and for the adequate length of time. Methicillin-resistant *Staphylococcus aureus* (MRSA) and nosocomial (ie, spread at health care facilities) bacterial infections are on the rise. It is everyone's job to minimize the likelihood of introducing an organism into the operating room.

Start by scrubbing the tips of your fingers of one hand first. (Most people are right handed, so start your scrub on your left hand.) Treat your hand as if it were a four-sided box. Scrub each finger, first on the outside, then the top, then the inside until each finger on one hand has been scrubbed. Follow this with a scrub of the palm-side surface, always starting at the tip of the fingers and working down toward the wrist. Finish the hand by scrubbing the back surface from the tips of the fingers to the wrist.

The brush is then used to scrub the forearm to the level of the elbow by spiraling down from the wrist. Never go back up the arm with the scrub brush. Always scrub from the top to the bottom, holding your hands just below face level and keeping them upright until entering the operating room to towel off with a sterile towel.

When the left hand is complete you then repeat the process for the right hand. Some people prefer to drop the used sponge into the waste receptacle adjacent to the surgical scrub sink and begin with a fresh one on the other hand and arm. Remember to keep your keep your hands higher than your forearms at all times. This prevents the contaminated soap and water from dripping back onto the clean hands. If at any time during the procedure your

hand touches anything other than the brush, you must extend the washing time with attention to the contaminated area.

Rinse your arms by passing them through the water in one direction, allowing the water to run down from the fingertips to the elbows; do not pass your arms back and forth through the water and do not allow your hands to drop lower than your forearms and elbow.

At this point you should not touch anything, so if the sink handles are manual, you cannot turn off the water. Have someone else turn it off. Be careful when leaving the sink, it is always slippery and wet beneath your feet, even if there is a rubber floor mat.

Proceed to the gowning area by backing in through the doorway so that you do not touch anything with your scrubbed hands. Keep your hands and arms where you can see them and never below your waist or above your face. Pick up the sterile towel by its corner and dry one hand from fingertips to elbow, then turn the towel over and use the other (clean) side to dry the other hand, wrist, and arm.

Remember, it is your job to be meticulous about disinfection, antisepsis, and sterility. According to the Centers for Disease Control and Prevention (CDC), an estimated 1.7 million patients get a hospital-related infection every year, and 99,000 people die from the infection.[1] The World Health Organization (WHO) says that most of these can be prevented by proper hand hygiene.[2] Hand hygiene is critically important to safe, high-quality patient care. Do your part in slowing the growing rate of health care-associated infections (HAIs). It is literally in your hands to do so.

Gowning

If you are the scrub tech and therefore the first person to enter the operating suite, you will have to gown and glove yourself. If someone has already set it up for you, then he/she may provide you with a sterile towel and assist in your gowning and gloving.

Gowns are designed to create a sterile field on the front of the operator from mid-abdomen to chest, and to minimize contamination of the sterile surgical field from the operator's sleeves, wrists, and shoulders. Once gowned and gloved, only the area within the surgical field is considered truly sterile. Therefore, the surgeon's and assistant's hands should never migrate from the mid-chest area and should always be kept in view. Breaching of the sterile barrier can, and will, occur. The important thing is that it is recognized, identified, and remedial countermeasures applied. The worst situation would be the contamination of the surgical field without the operator's or assistant's knowledge.

After scrubbing and toweling dry, the SA should approach the back table and retrieve the sterile gown by grasping the inside of the collar. Gently lift it from the table so contact with any surface (including the scrub suit) is avoided. The gown will gently unfold as the right hand is placed inside the right sleeve, followed by the left, until the gown covers the front. As you guide your hands and arms through the sleeves, slightly raise and spread your arms outward in front of you (but not skyward). Be especially careful NOT to expose the hands through the wrist cuff just yet. (The cuffs will be needed to pick up the sterile gloves, using the sterile sleeve as a barrier between skin and glove.)

A circulating nurse or scrub tech will then assist you by grasping the back of the neck and shoulders of the gown and tying it in the back. Each sleeve end has an elastic wristlet that seals around your wrist. Your hands should still be behind that wristlet. Once donned, the gown's back is no longer considered sterile.

Gloving

The sterile gloves will also be on the back table. Use the left sleeve cuff to grasp the inside collar of the glove with the thumb facing the opposite hand and pull it onto your right hand and over the sleeve. As you do so, extend your hand through the sleeve and into the glove. With your right hand covered, grasp the other glove and pull it onto the cuff and sleeve. Once both hands have extended through the sleeves and into the gloves, they can be adjusted. Be careful not to allow the inside of the glove collar to make contact with the outside of the opposite glove. It is much easier having this demonstrated, rather than following written directions. If you have a gowned and gloved assistant in the operating room, the process is much easier as he/she can assist you.

Once the gloving process is completed, pass the paper tab holding the gown's waist band to the circulator. This band will be rotated clockwise around your waist, completely covering your torso with the sterile gown. An assistant can either walk around you clockwise to accomplish this, or preferably, you can simply spin 360 degrees. (We call this the "surgical dance.") You can then tie the two sterile strings in front of you, securing the sterile gown at the waist.

One duty of a scrub assistant is to assist the surgeon with his/her gown and gloves. Offer a sterile towel to the incoming scrubbed surgeon. Then hold the gown by the outside front so the physician can placed his/her arms into the sleeves. Next grasp a sterile glove with both hands and spread it open 180 degrees as the surgeon pushes the right hand through the sleeve and into the glove. (Be careful to protect your own sterile gloves by holding the outside edges of the glove as his/her hand goes inside.) Don't let go until you have pulled the glove completely over the cuff and onto the sleeve. Repeat the process for the other hand. The surgeon will offer you the paper tab. Tightly grasp the waist band as he/she turns until he/she can take the two ends and tie them. You both are now ready for surgery.

Removing Personal Protective Equipment

Gloves and gown come off as one piece in the operating room (usually pulled off by circulator) to avoid making contact with any surface and to avoid bringing anything from the operating room outside. The gown is placed immediately in the biohazard bag. (Remember the nurse in Ethiopia who did not do this and contracted Ebola?)

Most operating rooms today avoid the need for excessive laundry and the added cost of reusable gowns, towels, and drapes by using disposable fiber, lint-free surgical gowns.

Mayo Stand Set-Up

On your back table should be a plastic bag to serve as the Mayo stand cover. Commonly one side is fiber and the other is blue plastic. It is preferable to place the plastic side up as the microfibers can contaminate the field as foreign bodies. If the instruments are covered with a fiber or two, it is not uncommon for the fibers to end up inside the eye. It is always distressing and undesirable to see blue filament floating inside the eye the next day, although they are usually harmless.

The scrub tech will have already set up the Mayo stand during room preparation. The final preparations and arrangement of instruments that will be used during the procedure (including the addition of any specially requested instruments) is done while the surgeon is positioning him-/herself at the surgical microscope.

It is always best to give yourself plenty of time to set up before the surgeon enters the room. In most cases, the circulator will deliver the sterile tray covered with a sterile towel. The tray is then either placed on the back table to retrieve the instruments, or (if it is small and has the correct instruments in it) placed directly onto the Mayo stand. It is usually much easier to pass instruments from the covered Mayo stand rather than from a surgical instrument tray, so instruments are most commonly removed from the tray and placed on the stand handle side toward the assistant and action tip/side toward the surgeon.

Time Out

Time can be a friend or foe. In the operating theater, rushing almost always leads to trouble. Surgeon and team must be time conscious, but mindful that every aspect of a procedure must be performed flawlessly and methodically in a timely fashion to ensure a successful outcome. Each stage of a surgical procedure hinges on the proper performance of the previous step.

Before any surgical procedure can be undertaken, a preprocedure checklist should be consulted much like a pilot would check off a preflight checklist. (The surgeon actually need not be a part of this protocol; it can be successfully carried out by the surgical team.) However, there must be one point prior to the procedure where everyone is required to participate. It is called the *time out*, and is designed to obligate the surgical team to step back from the bustle of activities to confirm together that this is the correct patient, the proper procedure, the right surgical site, and that everyone is on the same page *before* the surgery commences. The surgery cannot begin until this is done.

Sterile Fields

A sterile field is a work area considered completely free of microbial contamination and demarcated by either a blue or green cover. Once scrubbed, gowned, and gloved, a person's hands and arms and front of the gown are considered sterile from shoulders to table level. The back of the gown is not sterile. The drape on a patient is sterile on the outside, as is the cover on the Mayo stand. Instruments and sterile packaged items are sterile, but the packaging is not. Items that are below waist level are not sterile. (No bending over to look at something on the floor. This renders your carefully scrubbed and gowned self unsterile!) Always face the sterile field; don't turn your back on the operating room table. Keep movement and talking to a minimum.

It is best to consider any area within the operating room environment to be unsterile even if it is not. If any surface is touched or brushed by anything other than a sterile instrument, sterility is broken, everyone should be informed, and a new sterile area created. If the break is witnessed by someone and only a small area has been breached (an arm of a gown, or a corner of a table), then it is acceptable to drape out that area with a new sterile towel or cover. (An arm can be recovered with a disposable, sterile gown arm that is packaged separately for this specific occurrence.)

Passing Instruments

It is the SA's primary responsibility to "pass instruments," that is, to select the appropriate/requested instrument, place it safely and securely in the surgeon's hand, remove it when done, and place it back on the Mayo instrument stand. The SA also assembles and sets up the sterile end of automated devices, such as the phacoemulsification handpiece, irrigation and aspiration handpiece, vitrector, intraocular lens injector, cautery tip, light pipe (tiny light source that can be inserted into the eye), or irrigation cannula. In all instances, familiarity and efficiency in carrying out these responsibilities is important.

There is a specific and elegant method of passing instruments. I (RMK) train physicians, fellows, residents, and ophthalmic medical technologists in the same method. The best way to become the best SA is to observe, assist, and practice.

When learning how to hold and pass a specific surgical tool, first examine it, keeping in mind that form follows function. If a handle is flat, it will be held between the tips of the thumb and index finger of the dominant hand when used. If it is round, it will be rotated between the tips of the index finger and thumb. If it has two handles, such as a forceps (never call them tweezers; tweezers are used to pluck eyebrow hairs!), they will be squeezed. If the instrument is a probe, it will be pushed and therefore firmly grasped.

Try it. Hold the instrument, feel how it sits between your fingers, how light it is, and how gently you are holding it.

When working through a microscope, your field of view is limited. You would want the instrument handle to be placed exactly between your fingers just as you would want to use it, without having to look away from the scope. That is how you should position it in the surgeon's hand.

To become proficient, you first have to learn how an instrument is used. If the action of the tip points downward, that is the direction it needs to be positioned in the surgeon's hand. When the surgeon completes the maneuver for which the instrument was designed, you will need to remove it and replace it with the next instrument. Watch how a professional team executes these movements. A great SA not only knows what instrument the surgeon will need in advance of the step of the procedure, but the next one required after that, and so on. This only comes with experience, so expect the surgeon to ask for what he/she wants until you are comfortable with all the steps of the procedure.

To pass an instrument, grasp it at the proximal end of the handle. Avoid the tendency to move your hands up or down. Stay below the plane of the microscope and never, ever reach over the surgical field being viewed to deliver or remove one. The instrument being passed must always be gently, though firmly, held until the surgeon has it in perfect position. If in doubt, ask.

Ideally, a surgeon never reaches for an instrument; it is always placed in his/her hand. Nor does the physician put the instrument back on the tray; that is the SA's job. There has been more than one instance in my career where a crackerjack SA gently slapped my hand (not with an instrument in it, of course!) because I was either reaching for an instrument or attempting to put one back on the tray. An experienced SA not only gives me the correct instrument, but sometimes hands me what I need, not necessarily what I asked for!

The last important rule to remember is when passing sharps. You do not want to get stuck, nor do you want to stick anyone else. Especially with the risk of nosocomial and potentially fatal pathogens, the safe handling and passing of sharp objects requires training and skill.

Today's surgical blades, either steel or diamond, disposable or reusable, all come with a guard that must be retracted before using. In most cases, it is best to keep the guard on when passing the sharp, and allow the surgeon to retract it, use it, and then reposition the guard before allowing the SA to retrieve it. In some exclusive cases, the SA may retract the guard, place the handle in the surgeon's hand, and when taking it back, reposition the guard. This will only happen when the level of trust and understanding is at a very high level between surgical tech and surgeon.

Instrument Care

The composition of steel surgical tools is often modified by instrument manufacturers who use carbon to harden the steel or by adding nickel and chromium to decrease the tendency to magnetize. In either case, steel instruments are still more widely used in other surgical specialties. However, in ophthalmology, any corrosion, rust, and metal shavings on an instrument can pose serious problems. For this reason steel is much less desirable.

Today, nearly all microsurgical ophthalmic instruments are made from titanium. Titanium is brittle but very hard and can be fashioned into remarkably delicate shapes for every purpose imaginable. To distinguish titanium from steel, many microinstrument manufacturers dye their material bright blue.

Because the tips of microinstruments are extremely fragile, they must be handled with great care (Sidebar 40-2). To protect the handles and tips of these instruments, they have either a special storage case or silicone tip protectors. These should be used whenever the instruments are not on the Mayo stand. All instrument trays have a silicone pad with hundreds of upward projecting "fingers" to keep the instruments separate and to prevent them from touching other instruments.

Many facilities, surgeons, and manufacturers have strict protocols in place on how to handle and care for their instruments. Before you take an instrument out of a tray, handle it, inspect it, or attempt to clean it, make sure that you know exactly what you are doing. If in doubt, do some research, read the manufacturer's recommendations, or ask someone who is well-versed in proper care and handling before you dive into a tray of instruments whose total cost exceeds $35,000.

Cleaning

The purpose of instrument cleaning is to remove soil and debris from surfaces, prepare instruments for their next use, and to detoxify and disinfect them from becoming a source of contamination. Reusable instruments are the only items that are removed from the operating room after surgery and brought to the cleaning, disinfection, and sterilization room (which is usually adjacent to the

---

SIDEBAR 40-2
CARING FOR AND HANDLING SURGICAL INSTRUMENTS

Never store or carry instruments on your person nor leave them in your automobile. All instruments must be protected and stored in a visible, covered, clean, dry area. Avoid putting instruments in areas where they may come into contact with pathogens (eg, do not take them out of the surgical suite or operating area, never store instruments under sinks or near sources of water or waste). Discard single-use materials in biohazards containers after they are used.

Most common causes of instrument damage:

▸ Improper or rough handling

▸ Inadequate cleaning and drying prior to sterilization

▸ Leaving detergent residues

▸ Contact with corrosive chemicals or sterilizing solutions

▸ Use of water other than distilled or soft

▸ Carelessness when placing instruments into trays before closing the cover

---

operating room). Cleaning alone does not rid surfaces of microorganisms, but it does clear surfaces of blood and organic matter that would cover a surface, preventing the instrument from being thoroughly sterilized later.

Gloves must be worn during this process. A clean gown and facemask should also be worn. This is to protect you as well as to prevent the spread of disease. When handling any instrument that was opened or used in the operating room, strict adherence to standard precautions should be maintained (see Chapter 37).

Read the manufacturer's instructions before cleaning any instrument. Note: Ophthalmic instruments should never be lubricated. Lubrication adds a potential toxic film to the instrument that can lead to postoperative inflammation.

Ophthalmic instruments are unlike other surgical instruments, and treating them as if they are the same will result in damage. Wire baskets should be avoided, because the small holes allow delicate instrument tips to be exposed and slip through. Metal or plastic trays can be used during cleaning and decontamination as long as one instrument never touches another.

It is recommended that first the instruments be rinsed with distilled water. Some instruments must then be soaked in a solution bath. The solution should be close to a neutral pH level (7 to 8) such as sterile water, or a specialized cleaner designed for that purpose. If the solution is particularly acidic, it can cause pitting on the surface of the instruments, and an alkaline solution can cause staining. Note: Some cleaning solutions such as "instrument milk" and detergents leave a toxic film on the surface that can incite intraocular inflammation when used. In no case should any nonapproved solution be used for cleaning ophthalmic microsurgical instruments.

If an instrument's handles are hinged, they must be left open to ensure that the cleaning agents come into contact with all surfaces. If there are pointed or have sharp ends, it is best to orientate them all in the same direction.

Some instruments should be placed into an ultrasonic cleaner bath. Ultrasonic cleaners use acoustic vibrations at high frequencies through a liquid medium to clean surfaces. The vibration of the liquid is so rapid that it causes cavitation bubbles, which can adhere to the surface of the instruments, breaking down and dislodging debris and foreign matter. Ultrasonic cleaning gently completes the process in minutes without damaging delicate instrumentation. However, in most cases the instrument handle should be held outside the bath such that only the tip enters the bath. Under no instance should more than one instrument be placed into the bath at a time, as they would be damaged by vibrating against one another.

Once the instruments are properly and thoroughly cleaned, they should be inspected under the microscope to verify the cleansing and to identify any damage. (See the next section also.) Following this, each instrument is dried using pulsed air. Avoid blasting the tips; simply wave the air gun around the instrument to blow off excess water.

Each instrument is then carefully placed into the instrument tray with all of the handles facing one direction and the tips the other. Take care so that no instrument can come into contact with another. Angled probes and forceps should be laid on their sides between the silicone fingers of the tray so that no instrument tip is exposed above the surface of the tray. Be careful when placing the cover over the instruments; this is a common point when damage occurs.

Once the tray is ready for the sterilization process, it is wrapped with a sterile blue drape and a sterilization tape is placed on its surface. (After proper heat, temperature, and pressure is obtained, the tape turns dark and stripes or other indicators become visible, signifying that the product inside is sterile.) The wrapped tray is then covered with an additional blue disposable or reusable cloth that will be removed before the tray is placed upon the back table prior to sterilization.

Inspection

Before the sterilization process takes place it is important to inspect the instruments carefully. Check to ensure that all parts of a device are present and working appropriately. Verify that no instrument has been damaged. If an instrument is damaged, it can be sent to the manufacturer for repair, often at no cost. Never, ever, attempt to fix an instrument yourself. Bending it back or straightening it with another instrument will almost always render both pieces irreparable. Make sure everyone knows if a tray is missing an instrument, if an item has been damaged, or if one is sent out for repair, so that a replacement can be obtained. It is unacceptable to discover at surgery that a critical instrument is missing and the nearest available one is in Switzerland.

Hinged instruments should be inspected to ensure they are aligned appropriately and that no joints are cracked or stiff. If jaw misalignment occurs, then the instrument needs to be repaired.

Check scissors for the sharpness of the cutting edge by examination only. Never use a pair of scissors to cut anything but human tissue (unless they are large Mayo or bandage scissors designed to cut drapes). Inspect the blades for bending, pitting, and burs.

High temperatures and repeated sterilization can weaken stress points on instruments. Examine the instruments carefully, paying particular attention to the thinnest areas.

Sterilization

Sterilization is the process of eliminating all potentially pathogenic organisms, such as bacteria, viruses, fungi, protozoa, spores, endospores, and prions, on an inanimate surface. (See Chapter 23 for information on these.) This procedure is carried out either by physical or chemical means. Whereas *disinfection* only destroys vegetative (actively growing) organisms, sterilization is used in all surgical environments where even a single microorganism could prove disastrous or fatal (Table 40-3).

The most common methods used to sterilize or disinfect instruments include steam under pressure (autoclave), dry heat (hot oven), gas, chemical disinfectants, boiling, and radiation. Always read the labeling instructions provided by the manufacturer of any of these agents or methods.

Answers to questions concerning the proper cleaning, disinfection, and sterilization of medical surfaces can be found in the CDC's document *Guideline for Disinfection and Sterilization in Healthcare Facilities* (see Bibliography).

Steam Under Pressure (Autoclave)

The most common and effective type of sterilization is that obtained with a combination of high heat and steam under high pressure (the higher the pressure, the higher the heat), as produced by the autoclave. Moist heat has a far greater destructive power on bacteria and spores than heat alone.

Time required for sterilization in an autoclave differs based on temperature and pressure. Generally the higher the temperature and the pressure, the shorter the overall length of time it takes for sterilization. For example, 15 pounds per square inch (psi) of pressure (or 6.8 kg) at 250°F (121°C) will sterilize instruments in 15 minutes. (This is called "flash sterilization" and is only used when instruments are needed immediately.) If the pressure is kept the same and the temperature is raised to 270°F (132°C), sterilization time is decreased to 3 minutes. However, the higher the temperature, the greater the likelihood of damage to delicate instruments.

Accordingly, most autoclave methods utilize 15 psi at 250°F (121°C), making sure that the steam reaches all surfaces of the instrument or device and is sustained for 20 minutes or more. Proof that sterilization has taken place is facilitated by the use of sterilization tapes that change color when the product has been properly sterilized (mentioned earlier).

Floor model autoclaves record the pressure, temperature, and moisture to ensure proper sterilization before the instruments can be removed (and the pressure lowered to atmospheric levels).

When packaging instruments and putting them in the autoclave, it is important that they be arranged in such a fashion that the steam and heat can reach every package. Crowding may result in insufficient sterilization.

Ensure that the autoclave is in good working order. Regular maintenance of desktop sterilizers is important, and a record should be kept of the upkeep. If there is a water reservoir, drain it regularly in accordance with manufacturer's specifications. It is also important to only use distilled water, as the minerals in hard tap water can cause corrosion to the autoclave.

If a floor model sterilization unit is used (such as those found in hospital and ambulatory surgical centers), distilled water is supplied with a direct line.

Dry Heat (Hot Oven)

A small instrument oven provides a constant and controllable source of heat to sterilize instruments and other equipment that can withstand high temperature. A temperature of 340°F (170°C) should be maintained for 1 hour to adequately reach sterilization. The longer duration makes dry heat disadvantageous as a routine sterilization method. It is usually reserved for incineration of biological waste.

Gas

Gases are used to sterilize materials that cannot withstand other methods because they might be damaged by the high heat or pressure. This method is expensive compared to the alternatives, and therefore is reserved for extremely delicate instruments or those made of plastic (such as intraocular lenses, syringes, and plastic injectors). Ethylene oxide is the most commonly used gas but it is extremely toxic. Hence it can only be used in a specialized chamber that has a trap for gas evacuation and a door lock that will not open until all of the gas has been safely removed.

Gas is effective against all types of microorganisms and achieves excellent penetration as long as all surfaces are exposed to the gas. To be completely effective the item has to be in contact with the gas for hours to days.

Radiation

Ionizing radiation uses short-wavelength, high-intensity radiation (such as gamma or X-rays) to destroy microorganisms. It is used in industry to sterilize mass-produced, disposable items such as syringes, needles, IV sets, etc. It is not used to sterilize reusable instruments, and thus is not found in hospitals for routine use.

Disinfection

Disinfection methods are almost exclusively limited to in-office instruments that are frequently used for "clean" (ie, not sterile) procedures, and are not used in a sterile operating room setting.

Chemical Sterilization

Whereas heat may destroy plastics and the edges of finer instruments, chemicals usually will not. The process of using chemical germicides to sterilize instruments is called *cold sterilization*. This is somewhat of a misnomer because instruments would need to soak for hours in order to be completely sterile. The 20- to 30-minute immersion used in the office actually disinfects the instruments.

The ideal cold sterilization chemical agent would have rapid action in low concentration with broad-spectrum activity against a wide variety of organisms. It would also be inexpensive, noncorrosive, nonstaining, and penetrate well. Finally, it would be soluble, stable, and readily and widely available.

With all those requirements, it's easy to see that the ideal agent does not exist. Thus when using cold sterilization we have to make compromises and apply the technique only when better methods cannot be or are not used. In addition, it is vital to read and follow the manufacturer's instructions for each compound. (Some, for example, might need to be diluted prior to use.) Other precautions may include the need for gloves or proper ventilation.

There are three types of chemical disinfectants using low-, intermediate-, and high-level germicides (see Table 40-3).

Low-level disinfectants include *iodophors*. In ophthalmology, we commonly use these for surgical hand scrubs and disinfection iodides (ie, contains iodine) for skin preps. Brand names include Betadine. *Phenols*, such as Lysol, are effective surface low- to intermediate-level de-germers and are frequently used to clean surgical surfaces between cases.

Halogens are intermediate disinfectants often used because they are freely available and economical. Examples include chlorine, hypochlorite (chlorine

TABLE 40-3
DISINFECTION AND STERILIZATION

▶ Controlling microorganisms is accomplished by the use of one of the following:
- Antiseptics: Application of agents onto body surfaces (skin, conjunctiva) to destroy or slow the growth of microbes
- Disinfectants: Application of agents onto inanimate surfaces (counters, instruments) to destroy or slow the growth of microbes
- Sterilization: The complete removal and destruction of all microbes (including spores) on an inanimate surface

▶ The effectiveness of any given process is a function of the microbe's resistance to destruction
- Highest microbial resistance:
  Nonliving prions
  Dormant bacterial endospores
- Moderate microbial resistance:
  Pseudomonas
  Mycobacterium tuberculosis
  Staphylococcus aureus
  Protozoan cysts
- Least microbial resistance:
  Bacterial vegetative cells
  Fungal spores, hyphae, yeast
  Enveloped viruses
  Protozoa in active, feeding stage

bleach), and chloramine. *Alcohols* (ethyl and isopropyl) also decontaminate at this level.

Oxidizing agents such as hydrogen peroxide have an intermediate to high effect, and are especially effective against anaerobic bacteria. Hydrogen peroxide is usually reserved for disinfecting plastic tips in examination areas (such as tonometer tips).

The most potent of the high-level germicides are the *aldehydes*. Examples are glutaraldehyde and formaldehyde. They are highly effective against bacteria, but just as toxic to living tissue. In fact, 37% formaldehyde, known as Formalin, is used to preserve biopsy tissue and as an embalming agent. Glutaraldehyde 2% solution (Cidex) is used to sterilize heat-sensitive instruments.

Boiling

Boiling is effective in killing many microorganisms quickly, often in as little as 20 minutes. It takes much longer to kill more resistant organisms, such as bacterial endospores, so this method is considered disinfecting rather than sterilizing. Boiling should only be done with distilled water and is usually used only in a rural, nonmedical environment where more effective methods of sterilization are not readily available. A slow boil is

desired, as a rapid boil causes the instruments to be bumped around in the container. After 20 to 30 minutes, instruments are removed from the boiler with disinfected tongs and allowed to air dry.

Radiation

Nonionizing radiation uses long wavelengths and low energy, such as ultraviolet light. Because it has little penetrating power, ultraviolet radiation is reserved for disinfecting surfaces such as floors, walls, and counters. The units are often installed over doorways and turned on at night in the operating rooms to reduce germ count. There are also mobile units where the radiation is delivered by a robot.

Patient Services

Preoperative Considerations

Preoperatively, clearly state the procedure to be performed and which eye will be operated on.

Offer ample opportunity for any last minute questions. Involve the significant other, driver, or caregiver in the process. This lessens patient anxiety and allows the patient to be in control. Knowing "what is going to happen" is a collaborative effort.

Consideration should be given to the type of anesthesia the patient is going to undergo. (See Chapter 22.) Topical and local anesthetics allow the patient to remain alert in the operating room, and this may cause concern to some patients. ("Can't you just knock me out?") Be encouraging and explain that you'll "be right there" throughout the entire process.

Although it is important for the patient to remain still while the procedure is underway, many patients feel that they will be unable to keep their eyes open or their head still. Reassure them that the doctor will be in control of these matters during the procedure and all they have to do is relax or take a snooze. Explain the need for the patient not to squeeze the eyes, to keep the head still, and to keep the hands by his/her sides, but don't make a big deal of it.

Make sure the patient knows whether to eat and/or take usual medications prior to surgery. Instruct in the proper way to instill eye drops (if these are to be used pre- or postoperatively) and pre- and postoperative hygiene. Be sure to explain if there will be an eye patch following surgery (and/or an eye shield), demonstrate the proper way to place an eye shield and/or bandage, and explain what to do if the dressing becomes saturated or comes off. Tell how the eye will probably feel, and what his/her vision may be like.

Patients do not know what to expect, and if you leave it up to them to speculate (or worse yet, seek information on the Web), they may not adhere to the proper regimen. Let them know that although the procedure should be relatively pain free, they may feel pressure. If they are uncomfortable they should inform the surgeon and staff.

Most patients are amazed at how fast ophthalmic procedures are completed.

Intraoperative Considerations

During the surgery, part of your job is to ensure a quiet, calm environment. Often a surgeon may play music, or talk about anything and everything. Just be careful about what is said. Patients remember everything that happens in the operating room, especially if their senses are blocked (such as drapes to prevent them from seeing what is going on). We call the process of topical, local anesthesia, "vocal-local." This is because what you and the operating room personnel say and do during the procedure can make all the difference in a patient's comfort and outcome. Remember, it is still the surgeon's patient and not yours; the physician has the ultimate responsibility. If in doubt, it is always the best policy to keep your thoughts to yourself and only talk when asked. Pay attention to the anesthesiologist and circulator, as well as the patient. But if you are the primary SA, your obligation is first and foremost to the doctor performing the procedure, so keep your attention there.

Postoperative Considerations

The patient will be transported from the operating room to the post anesthesia care unit (PACU) to recover. Blood pressure, respirations, and heart rate will be monitored. Any dressings will be assessed and the eye(s) observed. In the immediate postoperative period the eye is watched for hemorrhage (hyphema), loss of chamber depth, excessive tearing, irregular pupil, or undue pain. Any of these adverse signs will be promptly reported to the surgeon. Patients are also given a snack and a drink.

The patient is told to call the office and provided with the number should there be any questions, pain not relieved by acetaminophen, loss of vision, flashes or floaters, or unusual or persistent discharge or swelling. Postoperative instructions including a handout, any prescriptions that need to be filled, and a follow-up appointment date will be given to the patient or driver.

In general, the patient should be instructed not to drive the day of surgery. Lifting should be avoided. The caregiver should be instructed to wash hands prior to tending the patient's eye as well as the proper way to instill any postoperative eye drops. Further instructions that apply to specific procedures should also be provided. For more information, read through your clinic's postoperative instruction sheet for patients (Sidebar 40-3).

Postoperative pain is unusual and most commonly is the result of an unexpected complication (excessive inflammation, increased intraocular pressure, or endophthalmitis). If the patient has pain that cannot be relieved by aspirin or acetaminophen, he/she should contact the doctor immediately.

SIDEBAR 40-3
SAMPLE PRE- AND POSTOPERATIVE INSTRUCTIONS FOR PATIENTS

- If you have pain that cannot be relieved by aspirin or acetaminophen, contact the doctor immediately.
- It is normal for the vision to be blurred following any ocular procedure.
- The eyes may also be sensitive to light, tear excessively, and feel scratchy or sore after surgery. This can persist for days to weeks depending upon the procedure.
- Wear sunglasses and/or a shield when outdoors.
- Refrain from drinking any alcohol.
- If in doubt, it is always best to check with your doctor as to what should and should not be expected.
- If you were provided with an eye shield, position it with three pieces of tape as instructed to protect the eye while up and about and especially while sleeping.
- If a bandage is present, bother it as little as possible. Keep it clean and dry, and do not remove until seen by the doctor (unless otherwise instructed).
- If there is no bandage, be very careful not to rub the eye or allow any water to touch the surface.
- Be careful not to get anything in the eye, especially while bathing or washing.
- Keep your hands clean at all times and especially before instilling any eye drops.
- It is okay to watch television or work on a computer.
- It is always best to minimize strenuous activity/straining in the first weeks after any ocular procedure. Lifting should be avoided. If you experience constipation, take a stool softener to avoid straining.
- Eat a regular diet.
- Call the office immediately if:
  - You experience pain not relieved with aspirin
  - You have excessive discharge from the eye
  - If the eye appears more red than after surgery
  - If your vision worsens
  - If you experience new floaters or flashing lights
- Our 24-hour phone line is: ( ) _____ .
- Your next appointment is: _____ .

Acknowledgment

Author Jacob P. McGinnis would like to thank Teresa Coffee, COA.

Chapter Quiz

1. The skin has two populations of microbiologic flora. Which one is the most affected by scrubbing? (In other words, what are we actually removing when we wash?)
   a. resident
   b. transient
   c. foreign
   d. inherited

2. True/False: Standard precautions need be applied only in an operative setting.

3. Which type of infection is acquired in a hospital or medical setting?
   a. zoonosis
   b. idiopathic
   c. transient
   d. nosocomial

4. If an ophthalmic surgical assistant is unsure of what instrument to select for a specific procedure, he/she should:
   a. follow your own good judgment
   b. trust that the surgeon will correct you if you get it wrong
   c. ask someone who is knowledgeable about the procedure
   d. pretend to know more than you actually do

5. When passing a surgical instrument to the surgeon, the surgical assistant should:
   a. push the instrument into the surgeon's hand
   b. keep the handle low and place it directly between the surgeon's index finger and thumb
   c. hold the instrument as the surgeon would
   d. in a manner that seems natural and comfortable

6. The ophthalmic surgical assistant plays an important role in explaining the informed consent document to the patient, its purpose, answering questions, witnessing, and documenting the process. What is the surgical assistant *not* allowed to do?
   a. discuss the actual surgery, risks, benefits, and alternatives
   b. sign the document in lieu of the surgeon if the surgeon is not available
   c. alter the document or remove items the patient does not agree with
   d. all of the above

7. Surgical assistants are expected to do all of the following *except*:
   a. practice proper surgical technique
   b. maintain absolute sterility at all times
   c. assist in moving the patient
   d. delegate the disposal of surgical materials

8. True/False: The prep table in the operating room contains all of the necessary supplies and solutions needed for preparing the skin, plus topical drops, local anesthetics, and all of the surgical instruments that will be used in the operative procedure.

9. Once gowned and gloved, only the area within the surgical field is considered truly sterile and therefore the surgeon's and assistant's hands should:
   a. never migrate from the mid-chest area
   b. be held behind the back to prevent contamination
   c. rest comfortably on either sleeve of the gown
   d. be kept at eye level at all times

10. Microsurgical instruments used in ophthalmic surgery are most commonly sterilized using:
    a. an ionizing source of radiation
    b. an autoclave steam sterilizer
    c. a potent high-level germicide
    d. boiling water

Answers

1. b
2. False, Standard (universal) precautions are applied in every setting where exposure is possible.
3. d
4. c
5. b
6. d
7. c, The circulator assists in moving the patient.
8. False, The prep table does not contain instruments. Those go on the Mayo stand.
9. a
10. b

REFERENCES

1. Preventing healthcare-associated infections. Centers for Disease Control and Prevention website. www.cdc.gov/HAI/prevent/prevention.html. Accessed May 28, 2016.

2. The evidence for clean hands. World Health Organization website. www.who.int/gpsc/country_work/en/. Accessed May 28, 2016.

BIBLIOGRAPHY

Rutala WA, Weber DJ; Healthcare Infection Control Practices Advisory Committee (HICPAC). Guideline for disinfection and sterilization in healthcare facilities, 2008. www.cdc.gov/hicpac/pdf/guidelines/Disinfection_Nov_2008.pdf. Accessed May 29, 2016.

Top 10 disinfectants to control HAIs. Hospital Management.Net website. www.hospitalmanagement.net/features/featureppc-disinfectants-hai-globaldata/. Published May 15, 2012. Accessed May 30, 2016.

VI

ADMINISTRATIVE SKILLS

41

AROUND THE OFFICE

Jane T. Shuman, MSM, COT, COE, OCS, CMSS, OSC

It may seem like all the credit in eye care goes to the "back office," aka the technicians. But without the "front office," aka clerical staff, there would be little to no order or organization in the clinic. The first section of this chapter covers some of the more common administrative duties needed to make every patient contact a smooth and efficient one. Medical personnel will benefit from this information as well, both to better understand (and appreciate!) their front office counterparts and to facilitate those times when the office requires a little cross-over of duties.

With the evolution of electronic media, a new vocabulary (and a plethora of acronyms) has sprung up and new terms continue to appear. The middle section of the chapter covers the terminology that both administrative and medical assistants need to understand so they can communicate with each other in a meaningful way.

Finally, the third part of the chapter discusses special patient populations, from children to pregnant women to people with disabilities, and some of their unique needs while in the clinic.

ADMINISTRATIVE DUTIES

Phone Calls

The person answering the phone is often the first contact a potential patient has with your practice. There should be a greeting used by all members of the staff, using the utmost professionalism and warmth. The patient wants to "hear the smile" that assures him/her that you are actively listening.

Examples:

▶ Vision Care of Cincinnati. This is Kathryn. How may I help you?

▶ Thank you for calling Outstanding Eyecare. This is Aaron. May I ask you to hold, please? There is one caller in front of you. [Wait for an answer.]

▶ This is Dr. Smith's office. Violet speaking. What may I help you with today?

Other suggestions that can't go wrong:

▶ Address the patient by name at least twice during the call.

▶ Ask permission to put the caller on hold, if necessary, and wait for the reply.

▶ Thank people for calling, and when applicable, let them know that you look forward to seeing them in the office soon.

▶ When telling the caller that you will follow up, do so in a timely manner. If more time is needed, let the patient know by calling at the end of the business day.

Telephone triage is the prioritization of appointment need; those with the most emergent situations are seen immediately. Those who are classified as urgent are to be seen within 24 hours, and most others at the next available slot. Many practices have classified the most common patient needs into one of these categories. There are situations, though, that may be unclear. These should be referred to the appropriate person familiar with clinical protocols and ocular disorders. Triage is discussed in Chapters 32 and 33.

Patients call for a variety of reasons other than to schedule an appointment. Often it is to relay a message to the doctor. Summarize the message as you record it, repeating it back to the patient. Before giving it to the doctor, include the date, time, caller's phone number, and your initials. If the patient has a paper chart, attach the message to this record. If electronic, there is often a feature that allows phone calls to be inserted into the record and sent forward to the person who can handle the matter; follow the instructions provided by your electronic medical record (EMR) vendor.

When the reason for the call is a medication refill, the doctor must authorize this refill. If the doctor is out of the office, explain to the patient that it may be a day or two before the refill is authorized, or that another doctor in the office will be asked to reissue the prescription. If the patient is requesting glaucoma drops, check that there is an upcoming appointment prior to giving the prescription request to the prescribing provider. If an appointment does not exist, make one during the initial patient call, explaining that glaucoma patients must be checked regularly to ensure that the medication is working.

Appointment Scheduling

Scheduling appointments in an eye care office is often more complex than in most other disciplines of medicine. This complexity is a result of the variety of exam types as well as specific eye problems and their work-ups. Another consideration is the approximate 15 minutes that some patients must spend dilating before being examined. Dilated exams include most new patient and comprehensive exams and retinal follow-ups, as well as others according to provider preferences. Postoperative exams and focused rechecks (ie, glaucoma follow-ups) are most often quick appointments.

Eye care providers order many diagnostic tests that are done in the office. When possible, these should be noted in the previous visit note and planned accordingly.

If surgery is performed in the clinic, there needs to be a list that details how long specific procedures usually take so that appropriate time can be assured.

A balanced schedule is one with a template that includes long and short appointments, with the goal of keeping the doctor(s) seeing patients with minimal wait time for doctor and patient.

Patient Flow

Patient flow is the term used to describe the patient's journey through the office from check-in through check-out. The goal is to minimize patient wait time at all touch points including reception, work-up, diagnostic testing, dilation, evaluation, counseling, optical, and check-out. Much of the flow relies on the master schedule. Other factors that influence patient flow are the layout of the office, staff competency and availability, and the amount of time the techs and doctors spend with each patient.

Time studies are often performed to determine where the bottlenecks are in order to reduce wait times and increase efficiency. These can be reported from the electronic scheduling and record system, stand-alone software programs, or manual documentation of each process. In analyzing the data, the person responsible for interpreting these reports can determine if there are gaps to allow for an additional patient, too many of the same appointment types grouped together, and even the productivity of the staff.

TERMINOLOGY

Both the administrative and medical sides of the practice must talk the same language in order to best help the patient. Many of these terms fall more under the administrative side of things, but should be understood by everyone involved in any aspect of caring for and assisting patients. (See also Appendix C, Medical Terminology.)

Charting and Coding

▶ New patient: For coding purposes, this is someone who has not been seen in your office or by one of your doctors (even in an unaffiliated location), in the past 3 years.

▶ Established patient: For coding purposes, this is a person who has received care by one of your doctors in the past 3 years. (This includes patients seen by one of your doctors elsewhere in that time period.)

▶ Practice management system: The software program used to schedule patients, enter and post claims, and run financial reports.

- Patient medical record: The chart that contains all documents related to a patient's medical care received at your office. This may include visit notes, diagnostic and lab tests, correspondence, etc. This information may be contained in a paper chart or an EMR.

- Centers for Medicare & Medicaid Services (CMS): The branch of the US Department of Health and Human Services that regulates the value of the procedural codes based on relative value units.

- Procedure codes: Current Procedural Terminology (CPT) is a medical code set that is used to report medical, surgical, and diagnostic procedures and services to entities such as physicians, health insurance companies, and accreditation organizations.[1]

- Relative value units (RVUs): A measure of value used by Medicare to determine the reimbursement for each procedure code based on geographical area.

- Superbill: The form used to document the procedural and diagnosis code(s) of services performed in order to submit a claim to the payer. It may also be called an encounter form or fee ticket.

Federal Incentives

- Patient portal: This is a secure method for patients to communicate with the office via an interface with the practice's website. Common functions include requesting or changing appointments, completing forms, communicating with the physician, ordering contact lenses, and paying bills.

- Meaningful use: The federal program that awards health care providers and facilities financial incentives for using certified EMR programs when providing care to Medicare and Medicaid subscribers. The goals of this program include improved safety and efficiency, as well as to engage patients and their families in their health care.

- Physician Quality Reporting System (PQRS): A federal reporting program that uses both financial incentives and penalties for reporting on predetermined quality measures. (Examples: Sending findings related to diabetic eye exams to the referring provider, or documentation that the optic nerve was examined for glaucoma patients.)

- Merit-Based Incentive Payment System (MIPS): The MIPS is a new program that combines parts of the PQRS, the Value Modifier (VM or Value-Based Payment Modifier), and the Medicare Electronic Health Record (EHR) incentive program into one single program based on:

- Quality
- Resource use
- Clinical practice improvement
- Meaningful use of certified EHR technology[2]

Regulatory

- Health Insurance Portability and Accountability Act (HIPAA): Initiated in 1996, this law allows citizens to maintain their health insurance, and protects the confidentiality and security of their personal information.

- Confidentiality: The principles of medical ethics that any information a patient shares with a health care provider (or the staff) remains private.

- Occupational Safety and Health Administration (OSHA): This is the federal body whose job it is to keep employees safe in the workplace. Its areas of interest include the proper disposal of sharps and biohazardous waste products and personal protective equipment (based on the risk of exposure to bloodborne pathogens).

- Hazardous waste: Hazardous waste is trash that is dangerous or potentially harmful to human health or to the environment. In a medical setting this includes, but is not limited to, blood-soaked bandages, excised tissue, and discarded needles and syringes.

- Compliance: An internal program designed to ensure quality care and accurate billing by means of checklists, reports, and inspections.

Insurance

- Medical coverage: The patient's insurance for exams that have medical necessity. This could be a symptom or being followed for an existing condition. This may or may not include annual or biannual routine vision exams.

- Vision coverage: Also known as routine eye exam, this coverage may be a rider to the patient's medical insurance plan. It covers an exam for eyeglasses or contacts, and may also cover a portion of the cost of eyeglasses or contact lenses.

SPECIAL PATIENT POPULATIONS

We naturally want every patient who comes to our clinics to receive the best care possible. This section discusses ways to assist and relate to those with special needs.

Low Vision/Blind

Approach these patients quietly and address them by name so they are not startled. Keep in mind that like others, they pride themselves on their independence. Offer to help them; if they accept ask what assistance they prefer. They may be proficient with the white cane; others may have a service dog at their side. (If this is the case, the dog is at work and should not be petted, although it may be tempting to do so.)

Explain what you are going to do at each step of the exam. Especially give warning if you are going to touch the patient. Be alert to ways you can help him/her feel at ease and participate in the exam. For example, the patient's hand can be placed on the slit lamp's chinrest so he/she knows where the head needs to be positioned.

Hearing Impaired/Deaf

Ask the patient (or his/her companion, if there is one) as to the preferred method of communication. This might be using a sign language interpreter, reading lips, or creating notes on paper. If an interpreter is contracted, keep in mind the burden of this expense falls to the practice, and when necessary, it is prudent to prioritize these patients during long wait times. Persons with hearing impairments may be able to hear if words are spoken clearly and loudly. It may also be helpful to lower your voice so it is deeper. If your office has an amplifying device available for these patients to use, be sure it is easily accessible.

Wheelchair Use

Not all patients who use a wheelchair are unable to ambulate, but use the chair because they have difficulty walking long distances. Just remember that the wheelchair doesn't necessarily mean he/she cannot transfer to the exam chair. There are several ways to transfer, if the patient is able.

▸ ALWAYS lock the wheelchair before the patient begins to move.

▸ Flip the exam chair footrest up, out of the way. Never allow any patient to get into the exam chair by climbing up onto the footrest.

▸ If there is enough space in the exam room, the arms of both the wheelchair and exam chair can be removed (or raised) with the wheelchair placed adjacent to the exam chair. The footrests on the wheelchair may be either removed or rotated out of the way. The patient can then slide from the wheelchair to the exam chair. (There are also special slide boards that can be used to "bridge" the gap between wheelchair and exam chair; the patient then slides across the board, which is then removed once he/she is in place.)

▸ The wheelchair can be brought in facing the exam chair. The patient can then stand up, grip the armrests on the exam chair, pivot, and sit.

For patients who are totally wheelchair bound and unable to transfer, use a wheelchair lane if the office is equipped with one. Such a set-up might include an exam chair that is on locking gliders. This way the exam chair can be rolled out of the way and the wheelchair positioned in its place. Most pieces of exam equipment (slit lamp, phoropter, etc) can be adjusted to accommodate. In some cases you might have to get a little creative or resort to less common practices (such as trial frames).

Aphasic

Patients with aphasia are unable to speak, or have great difficulty with speech, often as the result of a stroke. These patients understand what you say, but have little ability to respond verbally. Address the patient directly, making eye contact as you speak. Determine the patient's preferred way of communication by discussing this with the caregiver and noting it in the record for future visits. (For example, the patient may use hand signals to indicate positive or negative responses.)

Non-English Speaking

A family member may accompany the patient to act as an interpreter, or a professional interpreter may be scheduled to join the patient at the appointment time. Similar to the interpreters contracted for nonhearing patients, the practice is responsible for payment. In areas of the country populated by immigrants, it is not uncommon to have bilingual staff members who can converse with the patients in their native tongue. Not only does this put the patient at ease, but when translation is not required, the amount of time spent at each part of the encounter is greatly reduced. There are also translation services available on the Internet, apps for hand-held devices, and telephone services available.

Young Children

When children are the patients, it is important to address them directly, getting corroboration from the parent or guardian. The parent will necessarily provide the historical information, including the perinatal period, but include the child as much as possible.

Many young children have short attention spans and respond well to making a game of the work-up components. Positive reinforcement is also critical to the success of these visits. In addition to losing interest rapidly, children also accommodate very quickly, often making refractometry a challenge. A cycloplegic refraction will allow for measuring refractive errors without the interference of accommodation, and is often the preferred method of pediatric refractometry.

Children who have seen many doctors may be fearful of people wearing white lab coats (*white coat syndrome*). Once this has been determined to be a problem, have the doctor leave his/her lab coat outside the room, and note the situation in the record for future visits.

Pregnant Women

A woman's refractive error can change during pregnancy, largely due to the effects of hormones on the cornea. Thus, pregnancy is not a good time for a woman to be fit with contact lenses. In addition, depending on the patient's need for eyeglasses and the degree of the change, new glasses might not be a good idea either until a follow-up refraction is done several months after delivery. She may also find that contact lens wearing time is shortened during pregnancy. Follow clinic protocols regarding instilling eye drops in women who are pregnant or nursing.

Mentally Challenged

Include the patient as much as possible during every element of the exam. If the patient is able, obtain the history of present illness/chief complaint from the patient him-/herself, collaborating with the patient's guardian. You may need to obtain all of the patient's medical history from the accompanying guardian. It may not be possible to perform many elements of the standard workup, but an effort should be made to complete each test. If appropriate, it may be helpful to employ some of the same tactics used during a pediatric exam. Notate any special techniques that were effective. Any elements that are tried to no avail should be documented as "attempted." This will allow each element to count for billing purposes.

CHAPTER QUIZ

1. True/False: The clinical staff is more critical to the operation of the office than the clerical staff.

2. Which of the following is an appropriate way to answer the telephone?
   a. "Hello?"
   b. "Doctor's office, please hold."
   c. "Dr. Smith's office."
   d. "Hello, this is Dr. Smith's office. Cheryl speaking. How may I help you today?"

3. What is triage?
   a. booking appointments for patients who call
   b. unexpected situations that require technician or physician advice for proper appointment scheduling
   c. the prioritization of appointments according to need
   d. booking every appointment into the next available slot

4. An urgent appointment is one that must be seen:
   a. immediately
   b. within 24 hours
   c. the next business day
   d. the day the patient calls

5. True/False: It is always appropriate to refill medication for glaucoma patients.

6. Time studies are performed to determine:
   a. who works the fastest
   b. the cause of bottlenecks
   c. what changes can be made to the schedule
   d. where patient wait times can be reduced

7. True/False: An established patient is one who has been seen by any of the practice physicians at any of his/her offices in the past 3 years.

8. MIPS is an acronym for:
   a. Meaningful-Use Is Past System
   b. Merit-Based Income Payment System
   c. Maximum Incentive Payment System
   d. Merit-Based Incentive Payment System

9. Aphasic patients are those who:
   a. cannot hear
   b. cannot speak
   c. have no crystalline lens
   d. have a lens implant

10. The fear of doctors some children develop as the result of having multiple medical issues is called:
    a. white coat syndrome
    b. black tie syndrome
    c. doctorphobia
    d. none of the above

Answers

1. False
2. d
3. c
4. b
5. False
6. d
7. True
8. d
9. b
10. a

REFERENCES

1. Lee K. Current procedural terminology (CPT). SearchHealthIT website. http://searchhealthit.techtarget.com/definition/Current-Procedural-Terminology-CPT. Accessed July 4, 2016.
2. The merit-based incentive payment system (MIPS) and alternative payment models (APMs). Centers for Medicare & Medicaid Services website. www.cms.gov/Medicare/Quality-Initiatives-Patient-Assessment-Instruments/Value-Based-Programs/MACRA-MIPS-and-APMs/MACRA-MIPS-and-APMs.html. Accessed July 4, 2016.

42

RECORD KEEPING AND ELECTRONIC MEDICAL RECORDS

Jane T. Shuman, MSM, COT, COE, OCS, CMSS, OSC
Amanda J. Shuman, Esq

Maintaining confidential and thorough records, regardless of how tedious it seems, is one of the most important aspects of any medical practice. Proper record keeping allows patients to easily access their records as permitted by law. In addition, the practice is able to comply with the Centers for Medicare & Medicaid Services (CMS) guidelines, and liability is kept to a minimum.

Proper maintenance of records also requires proper storage. If a practice uses an electronic medical record (EMR) system, these concerns center primarily around the security of the network. A more thorough look at EMR security issues will appear later in this chapter. However, paper records lend themselves to other concerns, such as how to keep them out of patient view in order to maintain confidentiality, looking for misplaced or misfiled charts, or how to decide when to transfer records to off-site storage.

RECORD KEEPING

Registration and Billing Documents

The front desk is a practice's gatekeeper. It is imperative that front desk staff ensures that patient information is updated at every visit and that insurance information is up to date. The accuracy of patient information allows the practice to get reimbursed by insurers, paid by patients for out-of-pocket services, and to keep the practice's records current.

Many different documents are maintained by the practice. Some are mandatory (eg, assignment of benefits, the practice's financial policy), some are optional but generally recommended (such as patient demographics), and others are the clinical records from exams and procedures. All of these documents are important, and all must be confidentially maintained.

Mandatory Documents

Assignment of Benefits

The *assignment of benefits* (AOB) is an agreement between the health insurer and the beneficiary (ie, the patient) wherein the beneficiary assigns his/her health insurance benefits to a third party (ie, the practice). In other words, the patient uses the AOB to request that the health insurer pay the practice directly for the services received. In the event the patient is a minor or mentally incompetent, the form must be signed by the patient's parent or guardian.

Financial Policy

The *financial policy* is an internal form created by the practice that sets forth the practice's policy about the patient's financial responsibilities (eg, a copay or

Ledford JK, Lens A, eds.
Principles and Practice in Ophthalmic Assisting:
A Comprehensive Textbook (pp 689-694).
© 2018 Taylor & Francis Group.

deductible due at the time of service, billing the patient for any services that insurance won't cover). By signing this form, the patient is acknowledging his/her financial responsibility to the practice, and that the practice has given the patient notice of these responsibilities

Health Insurance Portability and Accountability Act Acknowledgment

In 1996, the *Health Insurance Portability and Accountability Act* (HIPAA) was passed, setting forth standards for transmitting health information in order to improve the health care system while also ensuring that patient privacy is protected. (For more on HIPAA, see Chapter 44.) All medical providers were then required to provide their patients with the opportunity to review the act and have their questions answered. How providers gave their patients that opportunity was left to the individual practice, but they must be able to prove that each patient has had such an opportunity. Therefore, having each patient sign an acknowledgment form is now required.

This acknowledgment form should set out how the patient is given the opportunity to review HIPAA (eg, whether the practice has copies of the act to give to all new patients, or whether a new patient is given a laminated copy to read and return to the front desk), and the patient must acknowledge receipt. This acknowledgment must then be kept in the patient's record.

Superbills

Superbills are the forms utilized by the practice to reflect services rendered. They set forth an itemized list of charges with the billing codes for those charges. These superbills are then submitted to the health insurer by the practice for reimbursement. In other words, the superbills ensure the practice gets paid for the services that the patient's health insurer covers. There are many EMR programs that provide coding modules that eliminate the need for paper superbills because the claims are transmitted electronically. In this case, the codes are maintained within the system. (See Chapter 43 for more on coding.)

Clinical Records

Clinical documents are what someone generally thinks of when thinking about a patient's medical record. While a more in-depth look at what a medical record contains will be discussed later in this chapter, a patient's medical record includes the doctor's exam notes from every appointment. The medical record also includes test results, phone messages (and notes on phone calls), and correspondence (both sent and received). Copies of prescriptions, records from other providers, and completed forms (as detailed above) are also kept in the chart.

Consent forms must also be maintained in the patient file. Before a patient undergoes any kind of invasive procedure, *informed consent* must be given.

Invasive procedures include injections, laser, and surgical procedures. Informed consent is given in writing by the patient after having received information from the doctor regarding the foreseeable and possible risks and benefits for a procedure. Informed consent must be given in writing, it must be given prior to the procedure being performed, and a copy of the form must be kept in the medical record. Prior to signing, the patient must be given an opportunity to ask questions about the proposed procedure. Informed consent laws vary from state to state and may include disclosure from physicians about any financial interest he/she may have in the practice, in devices used, and/or in any surgery center where the procedure is taking place.

Additional Documentation

Although some documents are not required to be maintained in patients' files, they can help the practice stay organized, especially if the practice is not using an EMR system. In addition, some of these documents can prevent potential problems for the practice down the road, as they require patients to acknowledge additional costs for which they may be responsible.

Demographic Face Sheet

The *demographic face sheet* consists of patient information such as name, address and other contact information, an emergency contact, insurance information, and employment information. While these data are now most likely to be captured in the practice's practice management software, keeping all of these details in one place in the file is convenient in the event that you need to return a phone call or verify an address. It is a good idea to have patients verify this information at every visit, either by asking them to state their address and phone number, or by providing them with a copy of the face sheet and asking them to make any necessary corrections. Double-checking patient information ensures that the practice is able to confirm upcoming appointments, ship contact lenses and other orders correctly, and make sure that any bills are being sent to the correct address (thereby ensuring the practice gets paid in a timely manner). Most importantly, the demographic information must be the same as what is on file with the insurance carrier in order to be paid promptly.

Benefit Election Form

If the patient has vision coverage, there is a difference between a patient's vision benefits and medical benefits in terms of what services the insurer will cover. Therefore, the practice may have the patient elect, in writing, which benefit they want the practice to use. This is known as a *benefit election form*. For example, a patient may only have vision benefits that allow him/her a routine eye exam every 2 years. But he/she may have a condition that qualifies as "medical" and not as "routine" (such as glaucoma), and the doctor may want to see the patient every 6 months. In that case, the patient is seeing the doctor not for routine vision checks, but rather for regular monitoring of a medical condition. Since the patient's *vision benefits* wouldn't cover such frequent visits, the patient should elect to use his/her *medical benefits* instead, and the benefit election form is the way to let the practice know to do so.

Refraction Statement

Medicare rules dictate that a refraction is not considered a medical service. Therefore, patients run the risk of not having this service be covered by their medical insurance. Because getting paid for services rendered is a major concern of every practice, many offices ask their patients to sign an acknowledgment that they understand that refraction may not be covered, and that they agree to be directly responsible for the fees. This form is known as a *refraction statement*. Having patients agree in advance to assume the responsibility to pay allows the practice to be assured that it will be paid for its services. This also gives the practice legal recourse if the patient fails to pay when billed. Many practices opt to collect for this service when it is rendered and then reimburse the patient if the carrier covers it.

THE MEDICAL RECORD

Although people often mistake a patient's entire file as their medical record, a medical record is actually a specific part of a patient's file. The *medical record* is the part of the patient's file that is a chronological account of examinations and treatments. It includes the patient's medical history, his/her complaints, the doctor's findings, results of any diagnostic tests performed, prescriptions, and any procedures performed. Basically, doctors are required to prove what services they provided to their patients.

The medical record will also contain all correspondence regarding the patient—letters between specialists, referring physicians, and the practice, and even correspondence from the patient him-/herself. It's important to keep this correspondence in the record because it may discuss other doctors' examinations or procedures performed on the patient.

The record also includes phone messages, prescription refills, and contact lens and glasses orders. All of these documents directly relate to the treatment of the patient, and must be maintained in the record in chronological order.

Because of confidentiality, access to patients' medical records must be limited. Practices should make sure to have a policy in place that restricts employees from accessing patient records unless they are working with the patient directly or doing something for the patient's

benefit (eg, calling a prescription in to a pharmacy). In addition, every effort must be taken to ensure that patients are not able to see charts of other patients. If a practice is using EMRs, this is easier. But for those practices still using paper charts, it is important to take preventative steps, such as keeping the day's charts facing away from the waiting room if at the front desk. If charts are left outside the exam room, the patient information should face the wall as opposed to the hallway.

Access to Medical Records

There will be times when someone outside the practice (other than the patient) requires access to patient records. It is important for the practice to understand when granting access is permitted and, in some cases, required.

First and foremost, a patient has nearly unlimited access to his/her own medical record. Included in that right to access is the right to authorize a third party to receive the records directly from the provider. *Records release* requests must be in writing, signed, and dated by the patient. Information pertaining to alcohol or drug abuse, HIV/AIDS, and mental health treatment must be specifically authorized by the patient or it cannot be provided. In addition, if the patient is a long-time patient of the doctor, he/she may permit or request that the doctor provide a summary of medical care.

Third parties may need access to a patient's record for a variety of reasons. These might include a patient transferring care to a new provider or visiting a specialist, the patient's insurance company disputing a claim that the patient has submitted, a patient's attorney needing records to put together the client's court case, or an opposing attorney seeking to prove the falsity of your patient's claims. In addition, a third party may hold your patient's power of attorney. A *power of attorney* (POA) is the written legal authority given for one person to act on another's behalf.

Requests from the patient to send records to a new provider are fairly common and easily understood by providers, as are requests to health insurers. But what about when lawyers, or those with POAs, get involved?

A letter from an attorney should include an authorization from the patient. So long as there is such a signed authorization, the request must be honored, as it is the same as the patient requesting his/her own records directly. If the practice has any questions about the request, they should call and discuss their concerns with the requestor.

When a case is in litigation (ie, in court), the attorneys handling the matter are permitted to serve a *subpoena*, which is a document that requires someone to appear as a witness. When the party serving the subpoena simply wants to obtain records, there will also be a list outlining the information requested. In almost all cases, after discussing with the party who sent the subpoena, the practice will be permitted to send the records and no one will have to personally appear on the date and time in the subpoena.

If your patient is one of the parties to the lawsuit (ie, actually named in the caption on the subpoena), more than likely the practice will have to comply with the records request. However, if the patient is not, it may not be necessary; doctor/patient confidentiality may overrule. If you receive a subpoena, especially if it is not apparent that your patient is one of the parties to the lawsuit, it's best to consult with your attorney.

If the request comes from an individual claiming to hold your patient's POA, you will first want to require a copy of the POA paperwork, and that it includes permission to speak to the patient's doctor(s). (Ask your attorney to look at the paperwork if you are uncertain.) But as long as the paperwork is provided along with the request and it does cover speaking with medical providers, the practice must comply with the request.

There is a major caveat with someone holding your patient's POA, however. If the physician, in his/her professional opinion, reasonably believes the patient may be suffering from domestic violence, abuse, or neglect at the hands of the individual holding the POA, the physician may choose to disregard that individual as the patient's POA, if doing so would be in the patient's best interest.

Although there are instances where third parties do have access to medical records, maintaining confidentiality is paramount for medical providers. In cases where doctors or hospitals have been sued for unauthorized disclosures and violations of HIPAA, the provider has usually been required to implement an extensive compliance plan that he/she must not only pay to implement, but also to develop, often with the use of attorneys and/or consultants who specialize in these programs. In addition, the provider is often fined (or the patient is awarded damages) for tens (or hundreds) of thousands of dollars.[1]

Charges for Medical Records

Practices may charge a fee for copies of medical records. However, they are not allowed to profit from this service. Providers may, but are not required to, charge reasonable costs for copying and mailing records, and the permitted costs are often dictated by state law. Many states allow a practice to charge the patient when the record is given to him/her directly. It is considered professional courtesy to send the record or a summarization of clinical care to another provider when the patient transfers care or is referred to a specialist. In addition, if a physician summarizes the medical records as opposed to providing a complete copy, the practice may reasonably charge for time spent preparing such a summary.

A practice should check with its attorney before establishing a policy on whether to charge for copies of medical records. Further, a practice may not deny a patient a copy of his/her records because payment for medical or other services has not been received by the practice.

Retention of Medical Records

Space is often at a premium in any doctor's office, especially if the practice still utilizes paper charts. However, patient records must still be maintained while the patient is under the doctor's care. Specific retention periods are determined by state law, with most being between 5 to 10 years for adult patients. For pediatric patients, the requirements are often 1 to 3 years after the patient reaches the age of majority. Be sure to check with your practice's attorney regarding your state's laws regarding record retention.

State laws are not the only governance of record retention, however. Under HIPAA, medical providers are required to maintain records for a minimum of 6 years from the date of its creation, or from the date when it was last in effect, whichever is later.[2] Additionally, because HIPAA is a federal law, it supersedes your state law if the state allows a shorter retention period.

Determining when to move inactive records from in the practice to off-site storage is a decision that is best left to individual practices based on their own needs. However, determining when a patient becomes "inactive" is difficult. A good rule of thumb is to keep patients' charts on-site for 3 to 5 years from the last contact with the practice, and then move it off-site. However, do take into consideration how easy it will be to obtain a record if needed unexpectedly (eg, if the patient calls with an emergency, or needs a call back within 24 hours).

ELECTRONIC MEDICAL RECORDS

EMRs are being utilized in more and more practices because of their many benefits. They are easily accessible from any computer terminal in the office, so if a call comes through, the triage person can bring up the patient's information immediately. EMRs are also legible (vs some written records), so the treatments performed and diagnoses made are clear to everyone involved. However, there are additional concerns when utilizing an EMR.

Security

As with paper charts, keeping the electronic record confidential is imperative. Permissions must be put in place. These allow limits to be set as to who can access a patient's chart and who is able to enter information into different parts of the record. These measures are put into place to prevent things like staff members digging around in patient records during their down time to see what the doctor diagnosed their next-door neighbor with.

These protective measures also prevent falsification of medical records, either intentionally or accidentally. By limiting who can enter information into certain sections of the record, the practice ensures that only the physician is making medical diagnoses, and that someone who is not trained to administer diagnostic tests is not reporting those results.

Finally, these permissions allow for an audit trail. In other words, they allow the practice to see who accessed which parts of a patient's chart, and at what time. With this trail, the practice is able to enforce its policy that no one should be looking at patient records that he/she has no reason to view. It allows confidentiality to be maintained.

Passwords are important for security and confidentiality of records. Passwords should be unique to each individual, including all receptionists, technicians, scribes, and doctors. This is partially so that the access trail discussed above is accurate as to which individual was accessing which record, and also to prevent one employee from entering information under another employee's identification and causing confusion. These passwords are generally set up through the software company, and the administrator should make sure that employees are not disclosing their passwords to anyone.

Passwords should be strong and difficult for someone to guess. Generally, this would be done with a combination of upper and lowercase letters, numbers, and symbols. Employees should be encouraged to be creative when setting their passwords, and to not rely on things like birthdays, anniversaries, or pets' names. To add extra security, the EMR should require passwords to be changed at regular intervals, and users should not be able to repeat past passwords.

Employees must be made aware that they cannot enter information for another employee on an EMR, because that is record falsification. An EMR username is unique just as handwriting is unique, and one employee would not write out information in a paper chart and sign a coworker's name. In short, EMRs must be treated as carefully as paper records, but the additional security measures outlined above must also be taken.

Whatever EMR product your practice goes with, the vendor should have a back-up storage system in case your practice loses power or data. This back-up system must be both remote and secure.

Transferring Information Into Electronic Medical Records

If your practice is just converting to an EMR from paper records, all the old records will need to be added to the EMR because they must still be retained, as discussed previously. In order to transfer them into the EMR, they will need to be scanned into the system. If the practice chooses to hire someone to come in and handle this project, that person should be aware of HIPAA and patient confidentiality before beginning work.

Keeping all forms and records easily accessible is important. An easy way to do this is to create a separate file within the patient's EMR for a copy of the paper record. Many practices choose to create files for copies of diagnostic tests, too.

Don't forget that even as your practice is established on an EMR system, you will still receive correspondence from outside physicians, or even the patient, that will need to be scanned and added manually to the EMR. Clearly labeling the information and keeping it stored in a logical place on the EMR is important to making sure your EMR is as well documented as your old paper charts.

If, after converting the practice to an EMR, every paper document has been scanned and saved, the paper records can be shredded. These documents must never be merely thrown away. It is worth it to engage a professional shredding service to handle the disposal in order to preserve confidentiality. However, if not everything has been scanned in (or there is the possibility that not everything has been scanned in), then the paper records must be retained and stored in keeping with the retention requirements discussed previously.

Diagnostic tests also have to be integrated into the EMR. This generally occurs in one of three ways: 1) via direct upload, where the tests are uploaded directly into the EMR; 2) via a portable document format (PDF) which is printed and then scanned into the EMR (and must then be shredded); or 3) via an imaging system. (An imaging system is managed by a third-party vendor who acts as the holding area for all diagnostic tests. This holding area might be online or via a cloud storage system.)

CHAPTER QUIZ

1. What is the assignment of benefits form?

2. What is the financial policy document?

3. What does the acronym HIPAA stand for?

4. Which of the following documents is *not* considered a mandatory part of the patient's medical record?
   a. visit notes
   b. insurance referrals
   c. consent forms
   d. HIPAA acknowledgment form

5. What constitutes the medical record?

6. When the patient signs a request for his/her medical records, which information is *not* included without explicit consent?

7. Is HIPAA a federal or state law?

8. True/False: Once a paper record is migrated to an electronic health record, the practice may discard the paper chart.

Answers

1. The assignment of benefits (AOB) is an agreement between the health insurer and the beneficiary (ie, the patient) wherein the beneficiary assigns his/her health insurance benefits to a third party (ie, the practice). In other words, the patient uses the AOB to request that the health insurer pay the practice directly for the services received.

2. The financial policy is an internal form created by the practice that sets forth the practice's policy about the patient's financial responsibilities (eg, a copay and deductible due at the time of service, billing the patient for any services that insurance won't cover). By signing this form, the patient is acknowledging his/her financial responsibility to the practice, and that the practice has given the patient notice of the same.

3. HIPAA stands for the Health Insurance Portability and Accountability Act.

4. b

5. The medical record is the part of the patient's file that is a chronological account of examinations and treatments. It includes the patient's medical history, complaints, the doctor's findings, results of any diagnostic tests performed, prescriptions, and any procedures performed. The medical record will also contain all correspondence regarding the patient—letters between specialists, referring physicians, and the practice, and even correspondence from the patient him-/herself. The record will also include phone messages, prescription refills, and contact lens and glasses orders.

6. Information pertaining to alcohol or drug abuse, HIV/AIDS, and mental health treatment must be specifically authorized by the patient, or it cannot be provided.

7. HIPAA is a federal law and thus supersedes state law.

8. False, The paper chart cannot be thrown away. Instead, it must be shredded by a certified documentation destruction company, provided the entire record has been scanned into the system.

REFERENCES

1. Health information privacy. US Department of Health and Human Services website. www.hhs.gov/ocr/privacy/hipaa/enforcement/examples/allcases.html. Accessed June 8, 2016.

2. Policies and procedures and documentation requirements. 164.316(b)(2). Fed Regist. 68 FR 8376, Feb. 20, 2003, as amended at 78 FR 5695, Jan. 25, 2013. CFR §164.316.

43

THE BASICS OF CODING IN AN OUTPATIENT SETTING

Jane T. Shuman, MSM, COT, COE, OCS, CMSS, OSC

Coding is the term used to create a claim for billing third-party payers; primarily, this is the subscriber's health insurance company that is responsible for covering medically necessary services. Coding must always accurately reflect what transpired during the patient visit, whether it is for an exam, a procedure, or both. This is accomplished using procedure codes to explain *what* was done and diagnosis codes explaining *why*. Add-on codes (modifiers) indicate special circumstances and affect the payment received for services. The number of self-pay procedures continues to grow as reimbursements from third-party payers decrease.

The *procedure code* is a numerical description of services performed, whether it is an exam, minor office procedure, diagnostic test, or major surgery. They are supported by also submitting *diagnosis codes* that explain the findings during the exam, or the reason for the procedure. These codes, used by all of medicine, are updated annually; practices are responsible for changing their fee schedules regularly to reflect the changes and to prevent denials for billing retired codes.

If coding is of special interest, there are certifications that can be pursued. The Ophthalmic Coding Specialist (OCS) is available through the American Academy of Ophthalmology, and the Certified Professional Coder (CPC) is offered through the American Academy of Professional Coders.

THE CARRIERS

The *Centers for Medicare & Medicaid Services* (CMS) is the US federal government's health care system. Both employees and employers pay into this system every pay period to fund the reimbursements to the doctors and hospitals that care for the patients entitled to these benefits. This group is comprised of retirees, those on disability, and the population that requires federal subsidy.

Medicare has three parts:

▶ Part A is hospital coverage

▶ Part B is outpatient coverage (including Part A)

▶ Part D is drug coverage

For our purposes, when referring to "Medicare benefits," we will be referring to Part B.

There are 10 regional Medicare Administrative Contractors (MACs) that are responsible for processing claims and reimbursing the provider or facility for services rendered to beneficiaries of traditional Medicare. Although the guidelines for each MAC are similar, there are occasional differences in how each procedural code is justified.

Every Medicare beneficiary has an annual deductible. (The *deductible* is the fixed amount that is the beneficiary's responsibility after which Medicare pays; the amount is subject to change every January 1st.) Part B pays 80% of

Ledford JK, Lens A, eds.
Principles and Practice in Ophthalmic Assisting:
A Comprehensive Textbook (pp 695-703).
© 2018 Taylor & Francis Group.

SIDEBAR 43-1
ACRONYMS

- CMS: Centers for Medicare & Medicaid Services
- CPT: Current Procedural Terminology
- E/M: Evaluation and Management Codes
- HCPCS: Healthcare Common Procedure Coding System
- HMOs: Health Maintenance Organizations
- ICD: International Classification of Diseases
- MAC: Medicare Administrative Contractors
- NCCI: National Correct Coding Initiative
- NPI: National Provider Identification Number
- PPOs: Preferred Provider Organizations
- TIN: Tax Identification Number

what they have deemed the "allowable" reimbursement for every procedure. The patient is responsible for either paying the remaining 20% or paying for a secondary insurance plan that will reimburse the rest of the allowable.

Medicaid is the term used for the federally subsidized insurance plan "for some low-income people, families and children, pregnant women, the elderly and people with disabilities. In some states the program covers all low-income adults below a certain income level."[1] Each state has its own term for Medicaid (eg, Mass Health in Massachusetts) and applicants must qualify with proof of income.

The *commercial payers* are those for-profit companies that insure employer groups. There are some not-for-profit commercial payers as well. Each of these third-party payers has multiple plan categories; within each category, the plans may be customized to the employer's specific preferences. There are often copayments of a fixed amount for every visit, or a deductible that is capped according to the policy specifics. Aetna, United Health Care, and Blue Cross Blue Shield are examples of commercial payers.

Common acronyms for organizations involved in health care provision are listed in Sidebar 43-1. *Preferred provider organizations* (PPOs) are a subset of the commercial carriers. Although the premium is high, the patient can have services provided by any doctor that is credentialed with that carrier. *Health maintenance organizations* (HMOs) offer the subscriber a lower premium, but with that comes restrictions as to which doctors he/she can see. Those specialists who are also contracted with the same insurer are considered to be *in network*. They must have a referral from their primary care physician (PCP) to see specialists, thus the PCPs have been

referred to as "gatekeepers." Very often, the specialists must be part of the same hospital group. *Point of service* (POS) is the mid-level offering; if a patient chooses to see a specialist outside the PCP's circle, he/she will bear responsibility for a contracted percentage of the claim. This is called an *out-of-network benefit*.

Health savings accounts (HSAs) are fairly new. They combine high-deductible insurance plans with a tax-favored savings account used to pay the deductible and other self-pay medical expenses. If unused, the money continues to grow on a tax-deferred basis.

THE DIFFERENCES BETWEEN MEDICAL AND VISION EXAMS

Since the latter part of the 1990s, there has been a growing trend for employer groups to offer optional vision insurance as a policy separate from medical insurance. In some cases, routine exams and glasses or contact lenses are covered by vision insurance carriers that are subcontracted by the medical plan.

Vision insurance, for the most part, is used for routine eye exams and may include reduced prices on eyeglasses and contact lenses. These policies may have no copayment component, or the patient's responsibility may be substantially less than the copayment attached to the medical insurance. The frequency of exams may vary based on the policy. Many offer annual benefits, while others limit subscribers to biannual exams.

Routine care equates to a healthy eye exam, the focus of which is refractive in nature. When a medical condition is discovered (eg, cataracts, diabetic retinopathy), the exam may be converted to a *medical exam*. Alternately, the doctor may ask the patient to return for additional testing and another exam specific to the findings. Each vision carrier has its own rules as to covering diagnostic tests with a routine exam, if the refraction can be submitted to vision and the exam to the medical carrier, or if the vision carrier will deny a medical claim.

This is an area of confusion for the patient and often for the clinic as well. The best practices have a process in place to explain their policies to the patient from the time the initial call is made through check-out on the day of the appointment.

CODING

When a practice submits a claim to an insurance carrier, it is done by justifying the procedural codes with the diagnosis code(s). The former identifies the level of service, diagnostic test, or surgical procedure that was performed; the latter indicates the reason (justification) for the service provided.

Procedure Codes

The *Current Procedural Terminology* (CPT) index was developed by the American Medical Association in 1966 and is updated annually.[2] CMS adopted CPT in 1983 for reporting physician services.[2] The CPT index lists every level of service in medicine and includes explicit descriptions of each one. Although inpatient services are included in the book, we will focus our efforts solely on those used in the outpatient setting.

Evaluation and Management Codes

The *Evaluation and Management Codes* (E/M) are used by all of medicine to describe the level of service provided during an examination. They are subdivided into new patients, established patients, and consultations.

Until recently, a *new patient* was considered to be one that has never been seen in your office, or who has returned after a minimum of 3 years. The definition now includes patients who have been examined by one of the group's providers in another location in that 3-year time period. What this means is that if Dr. Smith's practice was acquired by ABC Eye Care, and Mrs. Jones was a former patient of Dr. Smith's, she is now an established patient of ABC Eye Care even though the Tax ID numbers used for billing are different. The determination of "established" or "new" patients is now made with the National Provider Identification (NPI) number instead of the Tax ID number (TIN). Likewise, if Dr. Smith is a contracted provider with multiple practices (ie, subspecialty care), she is considered an established patient at *all* locations (except for the initial visit with Dr. Smith).

Logic then tells us that all other patients are considered *established patients* as long as the previous visit, with either the same doctor in any location or any doctor within one clinic specialty, was within 3 years.

Until 2010, Medicare had a series of consultation codes that were paid at a higher level than the new patient visits. Although commercial carriers usually follow Medicare guidelines, there are some private payers that still allow consult codes to be used. So, what defines a *consultation* for billing purposes? There are several criteria that must be met:

▶ The patient (whether new or established) must be referred by another doctor. This can be an optometrist, one ophthalmologist to another, a primary care doctor, or a specialist (eg, endocrinologist or rheumatologist).

▶ There must be a written request for the consultation that becomes part of the patient's record that includes the reason for the consultation.

▶ The consulting doctor must send written communication back to the referring doctor with his/her findings and plan of treatment. Once the condition is under control, the patient is to be returned to the referring doctor.

TABLE 43-1	
CLASSIFICATION OF EXAM CODES USED IN EYE CARE	
Eye Codes	**Evaluation/Management Codes**
New Patient 92004 Comprehensive 92002 Intermediate	*New Patient* 99201 99202 99203 99204 99205
Established Patient 92014 Comprehensive 92012 Intermediate	*Established Patient* 99211 99212 99213 99214 99215

When Medicare allowed consultation billing, the chief complaint was to be written as "Referred by Dr. So-and-so for evaluation of such-and-such." Although Medicare has abandoned this code set, it is still good practice to word the chief complaint in this manner. This cues the ophthalmologist that the patient is likely new and that follow-up documentation is expected by the referring doctor.

The Eye Codes

This group of exam codes is specific to eye care providers. There are two classifications of these codes. The Intermediate Eye Exam (92002, 92012) is often undilated and the Comprehensive Eye Exam (92004, 92014) includes mydriasis/cycloplegia. But that is not the only difference.

The history requirement for the eye codes is far less stringent than that for the E/M codes. However, the CPT states that the intermediate service for both new (92002) and established (92012) patients must include a medical examination and evaluation with initiation of diagnostic and treatment programs (Table 43-1). This is for a new or existing problem, not necessarily related to the presenting complaint that requires a new diagnostic or management problem. The intermediate exam may or may not include dilation.

The comprehensive exam (92004 for new patients, 92014 for established patients) is an examination of the entire ocular system. Like the intermediate codes, these include history, general medical observation, and external and ophthalmoscopic examination. Work-up elements that are not required for the intermediate series but necessary for the comprehensive codes are confrontation visual fields and evaluation of motility. These exams also always include the initiation of diagnostic and treatment programs.

While most examinations will qualify for the eye codes, many do not; in these cases, the proper E/M code must be submitted. For example, if a patient returns for a follow-up on glaucoma, and the ordered optical coherence tomography (OCT) of the optic nerve indicates progression and the doctor changes or adds to the patient's medication, an eye code could be billed because there was a new diagnostic test and a modification to the treatment plan. If, however, the exam indicated a stable optic nerve and pressure, and there was no change to the treatment plan, an E/M code would have to be billed.

Elements of the Eye Exam

Chart documentation is the key to determining what billing code is submitted to the carrier. It must reflect everything that was done during the patient's encounter, just as a snapshot of a memorable event captures the moment. There is a key adage that "if it wasn't documented, it wasn't done."

History taking is the main driver of the exam. There are many components to a comprehensive history. These are the chief complaint (CC), the history of present illness (HPI), the review of systems (ROS), the patient's past medical history (PMH), and the patient's personal, family, and social history (PFSH). We will review each of these, although they are explained in more depth in Chapter 7.

The *chief complaint*, simply stated, is the reason the patient is sitting in the exam chair. The chief complaint must be the first thing documented in the visit note. It could be a consult requested by another eye care provider, a primary care physician, or a provider of specialty care. Or, if the visit is for follow-up care, it should be reflected in the previous note and carried forward as if they were subsequent chapters in a book. It may be that the patient has returned for follow-up, but is more concerned about a new symptom. That, too, should be discussed, but only after the original reason for the visit.

The new problem, whether in a new or established patient, must be documented as such. This might be worded as "Red OD for 2 days." The patient's past ocular history may or may not have any bearing on the new complaint.

The chief complaint is augmented by the *history of present illness*. This is the "story behind the story," much like the first paragraph of a news story provides the overview of the headline. In journalism the key facts answer the questions of who, what, where, when, how, and why. Once the answers to these questions are provided for the reader, the article continues with background information and other details.

In patient care, the information is substantiated with various quantifiers (various references may use other names for these elements, but they all cover the same data):

- ▸ Location
- ▸ Duration
- ▸ Timing
- ▸ Context
- ▸ Severity
- ▸ Quality
- ▸ Associated signs and symptoms
- ▸ Modifying factors (relief)

Although there are eight of them, the highest level E/M codes require only a minimum of four. There is no extra revenue offered for more, although quality care often requires it. A knowledgeable technician will ask pointed questions of the patient; these are questions that relate directly to the condition or symptom. The provider determines which ocular structures are examined based on the chief complaint.

Another part of a comprehensive history is the *review of systems*. When doing a full exam, the patient must be asked about 10 systems (respiratory, digestive, circulatory, etc) to qualify for a high-level E/M code. This is an inventory of how the patient is feeling *today*. The proper way to accomplish this is to ask the patient specific symptoms: Do you have palpitations? (Cardiovascular.) Headache? (Neurological.) Difficulty breathing? (Respiratory.) A rash? (Dermatological.) It is not necessary to ask multiple questions from the same system.

The patient's *past medical history* should include any serious illnesses, hospitalizations, and surgeries. Conditions for which the patient is taking medications must be included. The family history is usually limited to diabetes, cardiovascular issues (including hypertension), and cancer. ("Relatives" include parents, grandparents, and siblings.) The social history deals with lifestyle issues such as smoking and alcohol, recreational drugs, marital status, and occupation. For the highest level codes, you must cover and document at least three of these areas.

During an interval visit, the components of the PFSH only need to be updated. The systemic and ophthalmic medications must be reconciled at every visit.

The exam itself can include up to 11 ocular elements plus mental status for a total of 12. The elements of the eye and adnexa are:

1. Visual acuity (VA)
2. Confrontation visual field (CVF)
3. Ocular motility (extraocular muscle or cover testing)
4. Adnexa and eyelids
5. Conjunctiva
6. Cornea
7. Anterior chamber
8. Pupils and iris
9. Lens

SIDEBAR 43-2

FREQUENTLY USED MODIFIERS

▶ -24: Used with an exam code to indicate services were provided during the surgical global period, but not related to the surgical procedure.

- Example: Glaucoma patient returns for scheduled pressure check during the 90-day global period for cataract surgery, modifier -24 is applied to the exam code; glaucoma would be the diagnosis code.

▶ -25: Used with an exam code to indicate a separately identifiable (unrelated) procedure was performed in addition to the exam.

- Example: Patient presents with a new bleed for wet AMD. Doctor decides to do an intravitreal injection during that visit. Modifier -25 is applied to the exam code, and the injection and HCPCS code for the drug are also billed.

▶ -54 and -55: Used for comanagement. Both the surgeon and comanaging provider must indicate the date of surgery on the claims submitted during the global period. The surgeon applies modifier -54 to the surgical procedure submitted at the postoperative appointment and indicates the date that service was relinquished to the comanaging provider who appends -55 to the claims submitted during the global period.

- Example: At the 1-day postoperative visit following cataract surgery, the surgeon releases the patient to the referring optometrist. The claim is submitted with the surgical code and modifier -54. That date is included on the claim. At the subsequent follow-ups, the optometrist submits the claims with modifier -55.

▶ -57: Indicates the surgical procedure will be performed within 24 hours of the exam.

- Example: Patient is examined and the determination is made that a YAG capsulotomy will be performed the following day. Modifier -57 is appended to the exam code.

▶ -78: Relates to a surgical procedure. This is the indicator that the patient was returned to the operating room for a related or staged procedure.

- Example: A scleral buckle was performed to repair a retinal detachment. At the 1-week postoperative appointment, it was found to be incomplete. The patient was returned to the operating room. The second surgery will be billed with modifier -78.

▶ -79: Also relates to a surgical procedure. This indicates that the patient was returned to the operating room for a procedure that is unrelated to the original surgery.

- Example: The capsule broke during cataract surgery, sinking the nucleus. The patient is referred to a retinal surgeon in the same practice who performs a vitrectomy. That CPT code would be billed using modifier -79.

---

10. Intraocular pressure (IOP)

11. Fundus (discs, posterior segment)

12. The mental status element is referred to as "oriented to time, place, and person" (see Sidebars 9-3 and 9-4)

Medical decision-making is perhaps the most complex and difficult component of the examination to establish. There are several factors that go into this determination:

▶ The number of diagnoses and the number of management options that must be considered

▶ The amount and complexity of the data

▶ The table of risk, which includes complications, morbidity, and/or mortality

There are several reference tables in the CPT book (previously referred to as "The Index") designed to assist in appropriately assigning evaluation and management codes. These will indicate the number of elements needed in each area. The tally of elements designates the appropriate code.

Current Procedural Terminology Codes for the Eye and Adnexa

There are other CPT codes used in addition to the E/M and exam codes. These are the *procedural codes* that include diagnostic tests, in-office procedures, and surgical procedures performed in an ambulatory surgery center or hospital.

Modifiers

Modifiers are added to CPT codes to indicate that there were special circumstances surrounding the service provided to the patient. These might be used as a suffix on either the exam code or the code for the test itself (Sidebar 43-2). These are important to include because without them, the claims are likely to be denied.

SIDEBAR 43-3
MODIFIERS INDICATING SITE OF SERVICE

▶ -RT: Right side

▶ -LT: Left side

▶ E1: Left upper lid

▶ E2: Left lower lid

▶ E3: Right upper lid

▶ E4: Right lower lid

There are also codes used to indicate which eye had a unilateral test (eg, fluorescein angiography, extended ophthalmoscopy) or procedure (Sidebar 43-3).

Diagnostic Testing

Many of our diagnostic tests have their own procedure code, which means they can be billed as long as there is medical necessity and an order in the chart for them. For instance, an OCT is necessary to follow the progression of macular degeneration. But an OCT performed to rule out retinal pathology prior to cataract surgery is going to be denied by the insurance carrier. The published list of acceptable diagnoses for each diagnostic procedure is referred to as the *local carrier determination* (LCD). When multiple diagnoses are submitted with the exam code on a claim, it is critical that only the diagnosis code that justifies the test be submitted with it. Otherwise, it is likely that the test will be denied by the carrier.

There are two components that comprise the CPT code for a diagnostic test: technical and professional. The *technical* portion is the performance of the test. The *professional* component is the doctor's interpretation of the results. A practice indicates that the service was separated into two by adding the suffix -TC for the technical component and -26 for the professional component to the CPT code. The total payment of the two components is equal to the payment for the full CPT code, so these are most often billed as a single entity. There are several situations, however, that require breaking them down.

Occasionally, an outside doctor may request that your office perform a specific test because his/her practice does not have the equipment needed. With a written request to your office and the creation of a medical record for that patient, your office may perform the test, bill the technical portion, and send the results to the requesting doctor who will interpret them. He/She, in turn, will bill the professional component to the patient's insurance carrier.

Another such instance is when the requesting doctor in your practice has the patient return for testing during his/her extended absence, with the intention of reviewing the results after returning to the office.

There must be an order/request in the chart for every test that is going to be billed as a separately identifiable procedure. This includes the medical necessity for an A-Scan or optical biometry once the decision has been made for cataract surgery. In some cases, a patient may have the axial length measured using both technologies, but only one can be billed.

Most diagnostic tests are considered to be bilateral, whether one or both eyes are tested. The only test that is unilateral is extended ophthalmoscopy. This means that even if the service is provided on both eyes, each must be billed separately, with the indicator of -RT or -LT.

There are three categories of supervision as they apply to diagnostic tests. These indicate which tests can be performed when a doctor is out of the office, or how involved he/she must be during the test.

According to CMS, *general supervision* requires that the doctor order and interpret a specific test, but does not need to be physically present when it is performed. Tests that fall under general supervision include visual field testing, A-scans, optical biometry, and OCT. *Direct supervision* requires the physician to be present in the office and available to provide assistance and direction during the test if needed. Fluorescein angiograms fall into this group. The last category is *personal supervision*, indicating the provider must be in attendance in the room during the performance of the procedure. (To date, the only test that has this designation is oculoelectromyography.)

Surgical Coding

There are two groups of surgical procedures as they pertain to coding. Regardless of whether they are performed in the office or in a facility, they are considered major or minor procedures based on the *global period*. This refers to the number of days during which related care is bundled into the surgical fee. It begins with the day prior (major surgeries) or day of the procedure (minor procedures) through the postoperative period.

There are several 0-day (zero-day) global procedures, including the insertion of punctal plugs and intravitreal injections. The proper lid or eye modifiers must be added to the procedure code.

Minor procedures have a 10-day global period and are generally those that are performed in the office. Examples include the excision of a chalazion or hordeolum. In addition, these may be done during the same session as an exam, if time allows. If the procedure itself is the purpose of the exam, then the procedure is billed without inclusion of the exam.

The *major* procedures have a 90-day global period. These are usually performed in a hospital or ambulatory surgery center. Cataract surgery, glaucoma procedures, blepharoplasty, and scleral buckling are a few examples. All procedures performed in medicine are included in the CPT book.

In all these examples, it is necessary to append the correct modifier(s) to the procedure codes. These always include the eye or lid, but might also include other modifiers. Modifier -50 indicates to the payer that the same service was performed bilaterally during the same operative session by the same surgeon. Modifier -51 pertains to multiple, different procedures that are performed by the same surgeon during the same operative sessions. These, however, are paid so the highest reimbursing procedure is paid in full and all others are paid at 50% of the normal allowable amount.

It is important to note that laser procedures are considered major surgeries. However, the global period for peripheral iridotomy, argon or selective laser trabeculoplasty, and panretinal photocoagulation is 10 days; capsulotomy has a 90-day global period.

In order to eliminate billing individual components of minor or surgical procedures, the National Correct Coding Initiative (NCCI) was created and is reviewed regularly. Often included in a procedure are steps that could be billed separately, but are really an integral part of the procedure being reported. One example is the dilation and irrigation of a punctum; they were once billed separately, but because it is necessary to dilate the punctum prior to irrigation, they were combined into one CPT code. This term is often referred to as *bundling*.

Rules apply to surgical procedures with a 90-day global period also. For instance, CPT code 66984 is described as cataract extraction with the insertion of an intraocular lens (IOL) implant. Yet there are some factors that qualify the procedure as complex cataract surgery (CPT code 66982). These qualifiers include a miotic pupil, weak zonules, pediatric surgery, or intraoperative floppy iris syndrome. The operative report must reflect the condition and how it impacted the surgery.

Noncovered Services

Most services provided are billable to the insurance carrier. However, as diagnostic and therapeutic technologies advance, there are an increasing number of instances where patients must pay out-of-pocket for services that are not covered by insurance. These are cases when it is necessary to have patients sign a document indicating they have been informed that they may be responsible to pay for a specific service.

An *advanced beneficiary notice* (ABN) is used when the health care provider suspects or knows that Medicare may not pay for a service. The patient must be told why Medicare is likely not to pay, and provided with an estimate of costs. The patient then has several options:

▶ To pay for services out of pocket and have the provider bill Medicare. The practice will issue a refund if the claim is paid. The patient has the option to appeal any denial.

▶ To pay for services and *not* have the provider bill Medicare. The patient does not have the option to appeal any denial if Medicare is billed.

▶ To refuse services. With this choice the patient is not responsible for payment, and cannot appeal to see if Medicare would pay.

An ABN is not necessary when the service or product is stated as noncovered in the Medicare contract. Patients may be expected to pay for services when they are rendered. The most common situation of this type is the refraction/refractometry. Medicare doesn't cover routine eye exams (sometimes called "eye refractions") for eyeglasses or contact lenses.

The insertion of presbyopia-correcting and/or toric IOL at the time of cataract surgery was precedent-setting in May 2005.[3] This was the first instance where Medicare ruled that the patient is responsible for all charges related to the IOL (beyond the reimbursement for the monofocal [single vision] lens) because the costs related to the new technology exceed that for a conventional IOL. These have been ruled as pertaining to refractive error, and no ABN is required.

Cosmetic procedures are fully elective. In today's practice, these include injections of botulinum toxin or fillers. A blepharoplasty may be medically necessary if the patient's field of vision is obstructed, but when performed for cosmetic reasons, payment is the patient's responsibility. An ABN is required for services rendered.

When the diagnosis submitted does not meet Medicare's Local Medical Review Policy (LMRP) for the test or procedure, the claim may be denied as "not medically necessary." An example of this could be a topography performed prior to cataract surgery; topography is done for corneal pathology and is not considered necessary with a diagnosis of cataract.

Other denials may be received during the investigational stage of a new device or test. Until CMS has deemed that a procedure is medically necessary for a specific condition, claims are likely to be rejected. Another reason for denials is that the frequency of the CPT code that has been submitted exceeds the recommendations established by CMS. For example, many Medicare carriers allow up to two comprehensive (92004 or 92014) exams each year. More than that will cause a claim to be denied.

International Classification of Diseases Codes

As of October 1, 2015, the library of diagnostic codes changed radically from a five-digit code to an alphanumeric one that contains up to seven places.[4] With more specificity, the Centers for Disease Control and Prevention (CDC) is better able to track public health trends and causes of mortality.

The *International Classification of Diseases, 10th Edition* (ICD-10), code book has 22 chapters, each dedicated to a different bodily system. In some cases, the systemic condition is listed before the ocular manifestation, so eye care practices cannot limit themselves to the ocular chapter.

New to ICD-10 is the inclusion of laterality. For every diagnosis that can affect one or both eyes, the code must indicate the side(s) of the body affected by adding the number 1 for right, 2 for left, or 3 for both eyes.

Also new for ICD-10 is the designation of a stage for most types of glaucoma and of severity for diabetes. The American Glaucoma Society has classified the damage as mild, moderate, or severe. The additional classification "indeterminate" is used when testing (ie, visual fields) has not yet been performed.[5] Where diabetic coding in ICD-9 may have required multiple diagnoses, one code in ICD-10 now explains the ocular condition. Intrinsic to the diagnostic code are type (I or II), severity, eye(s), and whether or not diabetic macular edema is present.

In cases of injury or trauma, the seventh place of the code will indicate whether this is the first visit to this practice (by using the letter A), a follow-up to the trauma (letter D), or a sequela visit (letter S) related to the original injury. (*Sequelae* are disorders that occur due to some previous condition and are thus related to it.) The submission of an ICD-10 code for the first visit of an ocular injury must include CPT codes that indicate how and where the injury occurred. Subsequent related visits must indicate the original diagnosis in the second position, but not the cause of the injury. An example of this would be recurrent corneal erosion (-S) as the first diagnosis followed by corneal abrasion.

CHAPTER QUIZ

1. What is the difference between CPT and ICD codes?

2. What are the three parts of Medicare coverage?

3. What percentage of the contracted amount is paid by Medicare after the patient satisfies his/her deductible?

4. Who is considered a "new patient" for billing purposes?

5. List the quantifiers used to define the history of present illness.

6. The CPT codes that begin with "92" are examples of ____ .

7. Define a routine eye exam.

8. What two components comprise the CPT code for diagnostic tests?

9. What are the three categories of supervision for diagnostic tests and provide an example of each.

10. What is the purpose of a modifier?

11. What is an advanced beneficiary notice? When is it used?

Answers

1. The CPT code is a numerical description of services performed, whether it is an exam, minor office procedure, diagnostic test, or major surgery. The ICD code is used to describe the diagnosis or diagnoses pertinent to the visit that are used to substantiate the procedural codes.

2. Part A covers inpatient hospital stays, Part B is used for outpatient coverage, and Part D is used for prescription drugs.

3. 80%. The patient is responsible for paying the remaining 20% or having a secondary insurance policy that covers the remainder.

4. One that has never been seen in your office, or who has returned after a minimum of 3 years, as well as patients that have been examined by one of the group's providers in another location in that 3-year time period.

5. Quantifiers used to define the history of present illness:
   - Location
   - Duration
   - Timing
   - Context
   - Severity
   - Quality
   - Associated signs and symptoms
   - Modifying factors

6. Eye codes

7. Routine care equates to a healthy eye exam, the focus of which is refractive in nature.

8. Technical component and professional component

9. General supervision—Visual field test, A-scan, optical biometry, OCT; Direct supervision—Fluorescein angiography; Personal supervision—Oculoelectromyography.

10. Modifiers are added to CPT codes to indicate that there were special circumstances surrounding the service provided to the patient.

11. An advanced beneficiary notice (ABN) is used when the health care provider suspects or knows that Medicare may not pay for a service. The patient is notified that Medicare might not pay, and the estimated cost.

REFERENCES

1. Medicaid and CHIP coverage. Centers for Medicare & Medicaid Services HealthCare.gov website. www.healthcare.gov/do-i-qualify-for-medicaid/#howmed. Accessed July 4, 2016.

2. CPT process: how a code becomes a code. American Medical Association website. www.ama-assn.org/ama/pub/physician-resources/solutions-managing-your-practice/coding-billing-insurance/cpt/cpt-process-faq/code-becomes-cpt.page. Accessed July 4, 2016.

3. CMS Rulings. Centers for Medicare & Medicaid Services website. www.cms.gov/Regulations-and-Guidance/Guidance/Rulings/downloads/cmsr0501.pdf. Accessed July 4, 2016.

4. Deadline for ICD-10 allows health care industry ample time to prepare for change. Centers for Medicare & Medicaid Services website. www.cms.gov/Newsroom/MediaReleaseDatabase/Press-releases/2014-Press-releases-items/2014-07-31.html. Posted July 17, 2014. Accessed July 4, 2016.

5. Fellman RL, Mattox CG, Ross KM, Viccherelli S. Know the new glaucoma staging codes. American Academy of Ophthalmology's EyeNet magazine website. www.aao.org/eyenet/article/know-new-glaucoma-staging-codes?october-2011. Accessed July 4, 2016.

44

HEALTH CARE COMPLIANCE AND REGULATORY ISSUES

Gloria Garcia-Garza, COA, CMC
Cheryl Pelham

Health care compliance to rules and regulations has become a very prominent topic in the medical industry. For years, the US government did not have guidelines for pricing procedures, categorizing visits, and billing frequency, or for determining the legitimacy of charges. Monitoring and ensuring that procedures and fees were medically necessary was not scrutinized. Thus, health care compliance and other regulatory issues arose. Simply defined, *health care compliance* means to run a health care practice ethically, operating within the laws and directives provided by the government.

Note: Throughout this book we have attempted to keep in-text references to websites to a minimum. This chapter must be the exception, due in large part to the changeable nature of laws and regulations. The reader is invited to take advantage of the many online sources mentioned, making sure to access the most current versions available.

PREVENTING FRAUD AND ABUSE OF THE HEALTH CARE SYSTEM

What Is Fraud?

Medicare/Medicaid fraud involves several areas: knowingly submitting false statements and/or making misrepresentations to obtain health care payments when no such payments exist; soliciting, paying, and/or accepting payments to reward referrals for items or services reimbursed by health care programs; making prohibited referrals for health services; billing for services never provided; falsifying records in order to receive supplies; billing for services never provided; and falsely billing for services at a higher level than what was actually provided. Consult the website https://www.cms.gov/Outreach-and-Education/Medicare-Learning-Network-MLN/MLNProducts/Downloads/Fraud-Abuse-Products.pdf for additional information.

The Governing Bodies in Compliance

Office of Inspector General

In 1976, the *Office of Inspector General* (OIG) was directed to create guidelines to help ensure fair and legitimate charges, thus setting rules and regulations for individuals and companies participating in federal programs. Procedures to conduct reviews, audits, evaluations, and inspections of practices and medical facilities were developed, and acts were passed to address these concerns. The OIG employs lawyers, auditors, and law enforcement personnel to assist in these endeavors. A brief description outlining the numerous departments within the OIG is provided at oig.hhs.gov/about-oig/about-us/.

Ledford JK, Lens A, eds.
Principles and Practice in Ophthalmic Assisting: A Comprehensive Textbook (pp 705-714).
© 2018 Taylor & Francis Group.

When individuals or organizations are convicted of fraud and abuse of the health care system, the OIG issues what is referred to as exclusions. *Exclusions* are entities (be they individual or organizational) that are found to have participated in and have been convicted of Medicare/Medicaid fraud and/or abuse. Penalties for such activity can reach tens of thousands of dollars per violation, in addition to the possibility of imprisonment and/or permanent blocking of further participation in Medicare/Medicaid programs. Consult https://www.cms.gov/Outreach-and-Education/Medicare-Learning-Network-MLN/MLNProducts/Downloads/Fraud-Abuse-Products.pdf for further discussion.

Department of Health and Human Services

The *Department of Health and Human Services* (DHHS) is the government's principal agency for protecting the health of all Americans and providing essential human services such as health care. More information can be found at the DHHS website, https://www.dhhs.gov/.

Centers for Medicare & Medicaid Services

The *Centers for Medicare & Medicaid Services* (CMS) is a federal agency within DHHS. The Medicare and Medicaid programs were signed into law in 1965, providing health care insurance for those who qualify, specifically older adults, persons who are retired, people with disabilities, and those living below the poverty line. Visit www.cms.gov for additional links concerning this agency.

Occupational Safety and Health Administration

With the Occupational Safety and Health Act of 1970, Congress created the *Occupational Safety and Health Administration* (OSHA). OSHA's purpose is to ensure safe and healthy conditions for the US workforce by setting and enforcing standards, as well as providing training, outreach, education, and assistance in clarifying rules and regulations. The website www.oig.hhs.gov provides a review of the reports and publications on fraud, compliance, the Recovery Act Oversight, and exclusion.

REGULATORY ACTS AND LAWS IN HEALTH CARE

The *Federal Registry* is a collection of US codes (rules/regulations) containing not only regulations, but proposed rules, public notices, executive orders, proclamations, and other presidential documents. These regulations have been codified in what is referred to as the *Code of Federal Regulations* (CFRs). A wealth of information on how to locate specific codes can be found at www.archives.gov/federal-register/tutorial/online-html.html#CFR.

Health Insurance Portability and Accountability Act

The *Health Insurance Portability and Accountability Act* (HIPAA), overseen by DHHS, was passed in 1996 to establish a national framework for security standards and protection of confidentiality with regard to health care data and information. All those who participate in health care, such as health insurance companies, health care clearinghouses (for-profit billing services), and health care providers, *must* comply with HIPAA regulations. HIPAA regulations are based on three areas:

1. Administrative: Standards for the electronic transmission of health information.

2. Security: Entities maintaining *protected health information* (PHI) must preserve the security and integrity of PHI and *personal identifiable information* (PII). PII is information that identifies an individual, enabling that person to be contacted.

3. Privacy: General rules for the use and disclosure of PHI utilized by providers, business associates, and others (Sidebar 44-1).

HIPAA is designed to protect the privacy of all patients, providing the right of patients to have their information kept private and secure. There are both federal and state laws, with monetary and criminal penalties for violations. HIPAA gives state and federal authorities the power to enforce the Act and penalize violators.

This Act permits health care staff members to use and share PHI to perform their jobs for three reasons without patient permission: for health care administrative processes, for treatment, and for payment. Only staff members who "need to know" may have access to PHI. HIPAA requires health care providers to obtain permission from a patient before sharing PHI with family or friends.

Helpful Definitions

HIPAA's privacy and security rules apply to all *covered entities* (CEs). Covered entities include health plans, health care clearinghouses, and most provider organizations, such as physician practices, therapists, dentists, hospitals, ambulatory facilities, nursing homes, home health agencies, and pharmacies.

Under HIPAA regulations, there are transaction standards for *electronic data interchange* (EDI) of health care data. *Transactions* are electronic exchanges involving the transfer of information between two parties for specific purposes, such as a care provider sending a claim to a health plan showing code sets and requesting payment for medical services rendered. Covered entities must adhere to established content and format requirements of each transaction.

Codes and Identifiers

Code sets are specific alphanumeric codes created to identify diagnoses and procedures (see Chapter 43). There are four code sets: the *Healthcare Common Procedure Coding System* (HCPCS; for ancillary services and procedures); *Current Procedural Terminology* (CPT-4; these are procedures performed by the physician); the *International Classification of Diseases* (ICD-10; diagnosis codes and codes for hospital inpatient procedures); and the *National Drug Codes* (NDC; 10-digit codes assigned to each drug used in the United States and compiled for use by professionals who need to know specific information regarding any given drug).

Finally, DHHS adopted standards for unique identifiers for providers and employers that must be used in all exchanges. The first of these unique numbers is issued by the Internal Revenue Service (IRS) and is referred to as the *Employer Identification Number* (EIN), initiated on July 30, 2002.

The second unique number is the *National Provider Identifier* (NPI), a standard established under HIPAA. These numbers are free of information revealing who the provider is, where the provider is located, or what type of health care is conducted. All providers who must comply with HIPAA will ultimately need to share these numbers with health plans, clearinghouses, and other entities in order to process billing. These numbers are linked to the billing process and to the IRS, which not only allows billing to take place but also supplies information to the federal government in terms of statistics and payment information for each practice.

General HIPAA Definitions

A *business associate* is a person or company that has access to the clinic's network, electronic health records (EHRs), server rooms, and/or reports that contain PHI. Examples might include a certified public accountant, a malpractice insurance company, a retained lawyer, or a billing clearinghouse. HIPAA requires that a contract be made between the covered entity and the business associate, stipulating that health information is used and disclosed according to regulations and that it is protected at all times. A list of your clinic's business associates and their current, signed business agreements should always be available.

HIPAA requires providers to make a good faith effort to obtain each patient's written acknowledgment that he/she had access to or received a copy of the practice's *Privacy Notice*. A privacy notice is a document explaining what is done and not done by the practice with a patient's personal/health information. It also outlines steps that can be taken by the patient in the event of a complaint, and who the patient can contact to report such concerns. This acknowledgment must be signed by the patient at the first encounter, or as soon as possible. It only needs to be signed once in the lifetime of the patient unless there are

---

SIDEBAR 44-1
PRIVACY DO'S AND DON'TS

▶ Do not discuss PHI in public areas such as a cafeteria, elevator, lounge, or hallway.

▶ Keep records secure, allowing access only on a need-to-know basis for payment, health care operations, or other authorized purposes.

▶ Use and maintain secure usernames and passwords.

▶ Log off computer while away from the desk.

▶ Turn computer screens away from public view or use privacy screens.

▶ Do not leave papers containing PHI in plain sight; after using, return to the secured location or destroy by shredding.

▶ Don't discuss a patient's condition or treatment with patient's family members or visitors.

▶ Do not post pictures taken in a clinic (or any other information about patients) on social media sites.

▶ Never take PHI outside a facility unless it is part of your job description and a policy is implemented to ensure PHI protection in transporting from and to a secured site.

▶ An employee may not view the medical records of family members, friends, or celebrities unless there is an actual "need to know" to perform his/her job.

---

significant changes to the notice itself. Patients also have a right to request and receive a copy of the notice, so have a few available for this purpose.

There are times when release of PHI may be permitted or required by other laws and regulations. These exceptions must be listed on the privacy notice. Examples of when your organization may be permitted or required to release patient information include responding to court orders, reporting certain information to public health agencies, reporting certain information about medical devices to the Food and Drug Administration, and reporting suspected child abuse or domestic violence to the police or state child welfare agency.

HIPAA Violation Tiers Structure

Violating HIPAA privacy or security rules can result in civil and/or criminal penalties. The civil penalties for violations are based on a four-item tier system.

▶ Tier A: The offender did not know he/she violated the law.

- Fines: No less than $100, no more than $50,000 for each violation, or up to $1,500,000 for identical violations during a calendar year
▸ Tier B: Violation due to *reasonable cause* (defined as when a covered entity performs an act of omission or commission knowingly [or would have known if reasonable diligence had been used]) but did not commit the act as willful neglect.
- Fines: No less than $1,000, no more than $50,000 for each violation, or up to $1,500,000 for identical violations during a calendar year
▸ Tier C: Violation due to willful neglect, but corrected within a required time period. The correction period is generally 30 days. However, it depends on the nature of the damage done. The Office for Civil Rights (OCR), under the DHHS, has the authority to make such determinations based on the facts collected concerning the exposure of the information.
- Fines: No less than $10,000, no more than $50,000 for each violation, or up to $1,500,000 for identical violations during a calendar year
▸ Tier D: Violation due to willful neglect, and was not corrected.
- Fines: No less than $50,000 for each violation or no more than $1,500,000 for identical violations during a calendar year

Criminal penalties for wrongful disclosure of PHI can include not only large fines, but incarceration as well. The criminal penalties increase as the severity of the offense increases. Consult the website www.hipaa.com/hipaa-final-rule-enforcement-four-penalty-tiers/ for further information.

A confidentiality agreement should be signed by all visitors who may have incidental access to PHI. Examples might include drug reps who will be in the clinic or in any area that contains PHI, as well as contracted cleaning personnel and all regular employees. A *confidentiality agreement* states that the signer will abide by all rules under HIPAA protecting PHI, as well as all rules established in the practice or facility regarding PHI.

Health Information Technology for Economic and Clinical Health Act

The *Health Information Technology for Economic and Clinical Health Act* (HITECH) was passed in 2009. HITECH protects patient information created, stored, and transmitted electronically. It also regulates the requirements for incorporating meaningful use for EHRs and sharing patient information through health information technology systems.

Meaningful use is defined as an organization using computer equipment and software technology that has been EHR certified by the CMS in order to ensure the technology being used is secure. Review further information on meaningful use at www.cms.gov. The HITECH website is www.hhs.gov/hipaa/for-professionals/special-topics/HITECH-act-enforcement-interim-final-rule/index.html.

Affordable Care Act

The *Affordable Care Act* (ACA), also known as the *Patient Protection and Affordable Care Act* (PPACA), was signed into law in 2010. The intent of this act is to allow patients to have more control over their health care by being able to make more informed decisions about their care and coverage. This act also stipulates monetary penalties for those who do not obtain health insurance. The federal website, https://www.healthcare.gov, can be used, if desired, to obtain the required coverage depending on individual eligibility requirements. More information can be found at www.hhs.gov/healthcare/rights/index.html.

Emergency Medical Treatment and Labor Act

The *Emergency Medical Treatment and Labor Act* (EMTALA) was passed in 1986 to ensure patient access to emergency medical care and to prevent the practice of *patient dumping* (where noninsured patients are not treated because they did not have a way to pay for needed treatments). Such patients might be transferred to a public hospital solely for financial reasons without consideration of the patient's medical condition or stability. Further reading on this topic can be found at www.cms.gov/Regulations-and-Guidance/Legislation/EMTALA/.

False Claims Act

The *False Claims Act*, also known as the "Lincoln Law," is a primary act used to combat fraud and was enacted during the Civil War in 1863. This bill was passed because when the government had to purchase supplies for the Army, it was sold cheap or defective supplies at exaggerated prices. Now companies that defraud the government in this manner are liable for damages and monetary penalties from $5,000 to $10,000 for each false claim. This act also pertains to submitting *any* false claim. The False Claims Act website is located at https://oig.hhs.gov.

American Recovery and Reinvestment Act

The *American Recovery and Reinvestment Act* (ARRA) of 2009 is a federal law that includes provisions for making improvements in the privacy and security standards for health information. One tenet of ARRA concerns business associates being held accountable for any compliance failures of HIPAA or applicable regulations by others in the practice. The Act also provides guidance in determining the minimum of necessary private data that is sufficient for a person to perform his/her job.

Stark Laws I, II, and III

The Stark law is related to the federal anti-kickback law, which is discussed later in this section. *Stark Laws I, II, and III* (also known as the Physician Self-Referral Law) were named after US Congressman Pete Stark, who sponsored the initial bill in 1989. This law prohibits a physician from making referrals to an entity in which he/she (or immediate family) has a financial relationship, unless the financial relationship fits into an exception set forth in the statute.

A recent exception permits referral source physicians who are members of a group practice to refer a patient for imaging or other health services within their practice. This exception basically permits group practices to own, operate, and receive compensation for imaging and other health-related services provided within the group. This is generally meant for imaging services such as magnetic resonance imaging, positron emission tomography scans, and computed tomography scans. Because ophthalmology is such a specialized field and requires very specific diagnostics not provided in any other setting, imaging such as optical coherence tomography and fluorescein angiography does not fall under the Stark law. A more detailed explanation can be found at https://www.cms.gov/Medicare/Fraud-and-Abuse/PhysicianSelfReferral/index.html.

Civil Monetary Penalties Law

The *Civil Monetary Penalties* (CMP) law stipulates fines for engaging in:
► Submitting false claims for work not provided
► Violating the anti-kickback statute (discussed next)
► Submitting claims knowing that the claim being submitted is already stipulated as an unlawful payment

The above are but a few on this list. The actual code can be found at www.law.cornell.edu/uscode/text/42/1320a-7a.

Anti-Kickback Statute

The *Anti-Kickback Statute* (AKS) was originally passed in 1972 in order to protect patients as well as health care programs from the influence money can exert when it comes to decisions of patient care. It stipulates that payments cannot be offered, paid, or received, willfully or knowingly, to any federally funded program in order to obtain referrals or services by Medicare or Medicaid.

There is also a condition in the AKS that is referred to as *safe harbors*. Since the AKS is somewhat ambiguous in some circumstances, the OIG has outlined 13 regulatory safe harbors or situations where the AKS does not apply. Consultation with a health law professional is recommended. Refer to www.oig.hhs.gov/fraud/docs/safeharborregulations/safefs.htm for more details.

Criminal Health Care Fraud Statute

The *Criminal Health Care Fraud Statute* specifies penalties for committing the following:
► Knowingly or willfully planning or trying to plan and pursue the defrauding of any health care program
► Knowingly or willfully planning or trying to plan by fraud in any manner, the obtaining of monies or property under the care of any health care program, in connection with the receiving of payment for such property or services

This statute states that the penalties for knowingly and willfully committing any of the above infractions can be prison and/or fines. A more detailed discussion can be reviewed at www.cms.gov.

Breach Notification Rule

Health care workers must be very cognizant of how PHI is treated. Yet at times, due to the rush of the moment or carelessness, violations can occur. The *Breach Notification Rule* addresses situations where PHI and/or PII has been viewed or stolen by an unauthorized party.

Since every unauthorized PHI exposure situation is different, it is incumbent upon each practice to establish risk assessment analysis procedures and notification policies. These must be fully outlined and explained, ensuring continuous compliance and remedy.

Investigative steps must be provided and followed, if the occasion arises. During the specific risk assessment of a PHI exposure, a determination must be made as to whether the probability is low that PHI has in fact been improperly disclosed or viewed. Such determination is referred to as the *low-probability standard* and can be determined by following these guidelines:
► Has the disclosed PHI revealed types of identifiers disclosing patient identity?
► Was the PHI actually viewed or acquired?
► Who was the person using the unauthorized PHI?
► How was the PHI exposure corrected?

The outcome of the investigation will determine steps followed, as to who is notified and when. Time is of the essence during these investigations. It is highly recommended that this topic be further explored at www.hhs.gov, which provides the rule in detail. This site also gives instructions on how to submit breach reports online.

Informed Consent

Informed consent means that the patient has been notified of the condition he/she may have, the treatment involved, the risks of that treatment, alternatives to that treatment, and the problems that may arise if treatment is not performed or completed.

This discussion can take several forms and includes various media. For example, in eye care practices it is common for a patient considering cataract surgery to watch a video about the procedure. However, there must be some direct communication between the patient and the doctor (or his/her designated representative) that includes an opportunity for the patient to ask questions. Reading the consent form does not take the place of the actual discussion between the medical designee and the patient.

Once this discussion has taken place, the patient must indicate consent to proceed with treatment by signing a *consent form*. This form is placed in the patient's medical record. If English is not the primary language used during this discussion, it must be so noted in the record, showing who the interpreter was and his/her relationship to the patient. Review www.omic.com/informed-consent-obtaining-and-verifying for additional information regarding this topic. More information on informed consent is found elsewhere in this book; please consult the Index.

Failure to establish informed consent can result in unwanted legal issues. Such failure is ethically unacceptable.

Trade Regulation Rules for Ophthalmic Practices

In July 2004, Congress enacted the *Fairness to Contact Lens Consumers Act*, which allows consumers more leeway when purchasing contacts. The *Contact Lens Rule* was then issued as a guide for prescribers and sellers of contact lenses, imposing prescription release and verification requirements.

The Act states that eye care providers are required to release contact lens prescriptions to patients, and that purchase of contact lenses can be made at any outlet and not just the shop belonging to the prescriber. The Act also covers rules regarding fees that cannot be levied under certain conditions, record-keeping, prescription verification processes, rules regarding the expiration of prescriptions, what prescribers can and cannot do, what are considered deceptive and unfair business practices, advertising rules and regulations, and how to file complaints. Visit www.ftc.gov to research further, or contact the Federal Trade Commission's Division of Advertising Practices, the Bureau of Consumer Protection.

In the event a website is maintained by your practice or facility, go to https://www.ftc.gov/tips-advice/business-center/guidance/advertising-faqs-guide-small-business. This site provides guidelines, requirements, and regulations as to what can be placed on your website regarding information pertaining to the sale of contact lenses.

Red Flags Rule

The *Red Flags Rule* stipulates that certain businesses and organizations must develop and implement policies and procedures to enable the thorough identification of patients. This is done to protect clients from those who steal medical information (medical identity theft). In order to accomplish this level of protection, such policies might include taking photographs of patients, comparing insurance card information with patient identification information (from an ID card, driver's license, or passport), and contacting insurance companies in order to verify patient information.

To determine whether your practice must comply with this rule, go to https://www.ftc.gov/tips-advice/business-center/guidance/fighting-identity-theft-red-flags-rule-how-guide-business.

NON-GOVERNMENTAL COMPLIANCE ORGANIZATIONS

The Joint Commission (TJC; formerly the Joint Commission on Accreditation of Healthcare Organizations, or JCAHO) is an accreditation and certification organization that is known nationwide. Its mission is "to continuously improve health care for the public, in collaboration with other stakeholders, by evaluating health care organizations and inspiring them to excel in providing safe and effective care of the highest quality and value."[1]

American National Standards Institute

The *American National Standards Institute* (ANSI) is a private, nonprofit organization that oversees the development of voluntary standards for products, services, processes, systems, and personnel in the United States. Voluntary consensus pertains to non-governmental organizations coming to an agreement to create criteria for such items, entities, and persons.

Everything from ophthalmic implants to contact lenses and all tools and products associated with them fall under ANSI standards (Table 44-1). Procedures, such as visual acuity testing and ophthalmic data processing, also appear under ANSI Ophthalmic. ANSI standards are published by Standards Developing Organizations (SDOs). These SDOs solicit input from interested parties desiring to produce specifications that are fair, promote

TABLE 44-1

ANSI STANDARDS RELATED TO EYE CARE AND OCULAR PRODUCTS

ANSI Z80.31-2012	Optics—Specifications for Single-Vision Ready-to-Wear Near-Vision Spectacles
ANSI Z80.5-2010	Requirements for Ophthalmic Frames
ANSI Z80.1-2010	Prescription Ophthalmic Lenses
ANSI Z80.3-2009	Nonprescription Sunglasses and Fashion Eyewear Requirements
ANSI Z80.20-2010	Contact Lenses—Standard Terminology, Tolerances, Measurements, and Physicochemical Properties
ANSI Z80.18-2010	Contact Lens Care Products—Vocabulary, Performance Specifications, and Test Methodology
ANSI Z80.9-2010	Devices for Low Vision
ANSI Z80.7-2013	Optics—Intraocular Lenses
ANSI Z80.30-2010	Toric Intraocular Lenses
ANSI Z80.12-2007 (R2012)	Multifocal Intraocular Lenses
ANSI Z80.13-2007 (R2012)	Phakic Intraocular Lenses
ANSI Z80.27-2001 (R2011)	Aqueous Shunts for Glaucoma Application
ANSI Z80.11-2012	Laser Systems for Corneal Reshaping
ANSI Z80.10-2009	Tonometers
ANSI Z80.17-2013	Focimeters
ANSI Z80.21-1992 (R2004)	General-Purpose Clinical Visual Acuity Charts
ANSI Z80.23-2008 (R2013)	Corneal Topography Systems—Standard Terminology, Requirements
ANSI Z80.25-1996 (R2002)	Ophthalmic Instruments—Fundamental Requirements and Test Methods

standardization, and generate advancement while not placing the industry, workers, or patients in jeopardy due to unsafe exposures. Go to ansidotorg.blogspot.com/2012/02/ophthalmic-standards.html#ixzz3rhXizhe3 for more information.

INDIVIDUAL AND SMALL GROUP PHYSICIAN PRACTICES COMPLIANCE PROGRAMS

In small group or individual practices, compliance programs must still be established and maintained. Although an actual *compliance officer* (CO) may not be hired solely for this position, such duties can be delegated to one or more individuals within the practice.

While there currently may not be an official requirement to maintain a CO, it is a wise decision to do so. Eventually, it may become mandatory. By already having such a program in place, the practice will be kept up-to-date. It will also be an advantage to have a compliance program in place in the event a complaint is made to state or federal authorities for any reason. You can study the Federal Registry concerning your practice's compliance program by visiting oig.hhs.gov/compliance/compliance-guidance/index.asp.

Security—Physical, Administrative, and Technical Policies

Securing information through technology is possible by employing measures that protect computers from online viruses and malicious software. The following is a breakdown of measures that can be exercised in order to safeguard all information available on company computers.

Passwords and Personal User IDs

Login information policies must be created and implemented for user IDs and passwords, holding staff accountable for their assigned login details. Although procedures and disciplinary actions will differ from practice to practice, they must be both clear and enforced. It is recommended that such policies be read and signed by each employee, and the document placed in respective personnel files. Key features are that unique login codes are never shared, login information must not be written down and posted by computers, and each password must be strong and changed on a regular basis. Suggestions as to how to create strong passwords is easily available on the Internet.

Protecting Against Computer Viruses and Malware

Malware is malicious software that can destroy information stored on company computers, as well as copy passwords or PHI that has been stored or sent.

Computer *viruses* are independent programs designed to inflict damage or steal information. They are often transmitted by email attachments or by visiting innocent-looking but malevolent websites. Once policies and procedures are established in the practice, zero tolerance should be exercised regarding accessing sites or emails outside of work requirements.

Unauthorized Software

Unauthorized software is software that is not standard to the practice and must not be placed on company computers unless expressly permitted. Such software might include music, remote-access software, and games. These can threaten the network by allowing malicious software access to the entire computerized structure of the practice or facility. In addition, such programs may tie up an inordinate amount of computer space. Employees must be trained not to install or open such files without permission from technical support.

Unauthorized Hardware

External devices such as thumb drives, DVDs, CDs, or USB (universal serial bus) connected devices can potentially infect the company's protected network, allowing unauthorized downloads of PHI to an unknown receiver. The company's technical support department should have a way to monitor the system and know when a USB or external device has been plugged into the company's network. In addition, employees should not be allowed to plug in personal equipment or recharge personal items using office computers.

Securing Authorized Hardware

Any external devices such as laptops, tablets, or smart phones used by the practice must be passcode protected. Information stored on a laptop or mobile device should also be encrypted. *Encryption* means that information is coded or scrambled so that it cannot be read by anyone who doesn't have the software key to read it. In the event that such a device is lost or stolen, these safeguards can help reduce PHI exposure. PHI should not be stored on portable devices unless it has been encrypted.

When mobile devices are not in use, they should be individually locked and placed in secured drawers or a briefcase. If a device is stolen or lost, policy must require that an incident report be filed as soon as possible. All portable devices should be equipped with a way to remotely erase all information from the device.

Email Security

Email is usually not secure (that is, any email can be retrieved with little trouble by a third and unintended party). For that reason, your organization should adopt strict policies regarding how it transmits PHI. Some companies ban the inclusion of PHI in any email unless it is secured. There are several companies that provide this service for a monthly or yearly fee.

Faxing

HIPAA does not address faxing PHI specifically, but it does protect faxed information. A fax cover sheet should include a confidentiality statement and should not include any PHI. Sidebar 44-2 identifies more tips.

Reporting Violations

If an employee has a concern or witnesses a HIPAA or HITECH violation, he/she is to be encouraged to report it to the compliance officer. The reporting person has the choice to remain anonymous, and if the identity is revealed, he/she must be protected from any retaliation. Individuals reporting violations cannot be punished.

If there is suspicion that a patient is not the person he or she claims to be, immediately alert your supervisor so that he/she may alert the proper authorities. Identity theft is serious. Medical identity theft can have financial and life-threatening consequences.

CONSTRUCTING A COMPLIANCE PROGRAM

A compliance program is a voluntary aspect of the OIG designed to help prevent erroneous claims and fraudulent activity, as well as to ensure PHI is protected. This guideline addresses the need to have policies and protocols in place providing direction and procedures to inhibit fraud and wrongdoing within a practice. The guidelines recommend that each facility provide anonymity while encouraging staff and physicians to report concerns. This document is available on the OIG website at https://oig.hhs.gov/compliance/compliance-guidance/index.asp (in the "Electronic Reading Room") or by calling the OIG Public Affairs Office at (202) 619-1343.

While a compliance program is not hard to design and implement, there is some initial time-consuming training involved, and the larger the practice the slower the process. Policy and procedure development provides a way to communicate and ensures that the clinic's policies and procedures are followed. The website located at oig.hhs.gov/compliance/compliance-guidance/index.asp has compliance program advice geared to many types of operations including hospitals, small group and individual practices, nursing homes, pharmaceutical manufacturers, hospice programs, and third-party medical billing companies.

The OIG suggests a seven-part compliance program, which can serve as a starting point to put your own program together. Sidebar 44-3 shows a simplified listing.

DISASTER PREPAREDNESS PLANS

Disaster preparedness is something most businesses do not give ample thought to when it comes to planning ahead. Disasters can take the form of floods, tornadoes, hurricanes, severe storms causing electrical outages, etc. Or, it can be something less imposing such as your Internet provider suffering down time due to any number of problems. Regardless of the reason, the fact still remains that all digital records become vulnerable, as well as physical files.

Policies and procedures should be set in place to address these vital needs. Are back-ups of all information made on a consistent basis? Are copies of these back-ups kept in secure locations where they can be obtained so the practice can continue seeing patients? What processes will need to be established to ensure ongoing patient care? These are some questions that arise. Many more will undoubtedly come up as these policies and procedures are outlined during planning sessions.

Help can be obtained from your clinic's technical support team to address the hardware and software questions. Other help can be obtained by contacting the Centers for Disease Control and Prevention (www.emergency.cdc.gov), and an actual checklist can be printed from www.cms.gov that will help tremendously in preparing any plan.

Additional information can be found at www.cdc.gov/phpr/healthcare/planning.htm.

SIDEBAR 44-3
OFFICE OF INSPECTOR GENERAL SEVEN-POINT COMPLIANCE PROGRAM

1. Assign a compliance specialist
2. Written policies and procedures
3. Training
4. Effective lines of communication
5. Internal monitoring and auditing should be random and ongoing
6. Immediate response to detected violations
7. Disciplinary mechanisms

CHAPTER QUIZ

1. Fraud involves six areas. Briefly list each.

2. Why was the Office of Inspector General instructed to create guidelines regarding federal programs?

3. Why was the Occupational Safety and Health Administration created?

4. The acronym HIPAA stands for what? What is its purpose?

5. Name a criminal penalty for wrongfully disclosing protected health information.

6. Define informed consent.

7. What are the stipulations of the Red Flags Rule?

8. What is the American National Standards Institute? What is its acronym?

9. What is a compliance program?

10. Name some advantages of establishing a compliance program within your organization.

Answers

1. Fraud involves:
   a. Submitting and/or making false statements and/or misrepresentations in order to obtain health care payments

    b. Rewarding with payments in obtaining referrals for items or services

    c. Providing referrals to receive health services

    d. Billing for services never provided

    e. Falsifying records in order to receive supplies

    f. Billing for a service or services at a higher level than what was actually provided

2. The OIG guidelines were developed in order to ensure fair and legitimate charges.

3. OSHA was created to ensure safe and healthy working conditions.

4. HIPAA stands for Health Insurance Portability and Accountability Act. Its purpose is to establish a framework for security and protection standards regarding health care data and information.

5. Wrongfully disclosing PHI can result in large fines and/or incarceration.

6. Informed consent means that a patient has been informed of a condition he/she may have, the treatment and risks of such treatment, as well as possible risks if treatment is not performed or delayed.

7. The Red Flags Rule states that some businesses and organizations should develop and implement policies and procedures regarding the thorough identification of patients, so as to inhibit identity theft.

8. The American National Standards Institute is a private, nonprofit organization overseeing the development of standards for products, services, processes, systems, and personnel in the United States with the voluntary consensus of non-governmental organizations from various industries. The acronym is ANSI.

9. A compliance program is a set of policies and procedures designed for any given practice, detailing measures protecting every facet of patient and worker actions and information, per governmental and/or non-governmental standards.

10. Some advantages of establishing a compliance program within your organization is to ensure your practice is up to date in rules and regulations that may affect your workers and your patients. In the event your practice is visited by an inspecting entity, having such a plan in place will show you are concerned and serious about maintaining patient and worker protection in all aspects of your practice.

Reference

1. The Joint Commission mission statement. The Joint Commission website www.jointcommission.org/the_joint_commission_mission_statement/. Accessed July 4, 2016.

APPENDICES

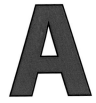

REVIEW OF SCIENCES AND APPLICATIONS

Jan Ledford, COMT

MATHEMATICS

The Number Line

You probably remember the number line from grade school math. It is a line with zero ("0") in the middle and numbers descending to the negative to the left and ascending to the positive to the right (Figure A-1). There are an indefinite number of points between the numbers on the line, but in optics we usually work in nothing smaller than 0.25.

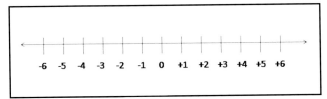

Figure A-1. The number line.

If you start at 0 and move two full steps to the right, you land on +2 (positive two). If you start at 0 and move two full steps to the left, you land on -2 (negative two). The confusion can begin when you don't start at 0, but at some other point. For example, suppose you start at +3 and move three steps to the right. You land on +6. If you start at +2 and move left five steps, you land on -3.

But try this (Figure A-2). Start at +3.00 (Point A). Move to the right to 5.50 (Point B). The question is this: how many "steps" did you move to get from Point A to Point B? And was this in a plus (positive) or minus (negative) direction?

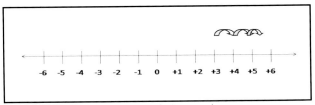

Figure A-2. Number line example (see text).

With the number line, moving left is always toward the negative and moving right is always toward the positive, no matter where you start. In the example above, we moved to the right, so we are adding. This is equivalent to the mathematical formula: $3.00 + X = 5.50$. When you look at it that way, the answer is a pretty obvious 2.50.

Try another one (Figure A-3). Point A is -1.00. Point B is -3.00. In moving from A to B, you moved left, so this is subtraction. The problem is translated as: $-1.00 - X = -3.00$. Again, it's easy to see that the answer is 2.00 (remember, subtracting a positive from a negative results in another negative: $-1.00 - 2.00 = -3.00$).

Ledford JK, Lens A, eds.
Principles and Practice in Ophthalmic Assisting:
A Comprehensive Textbook (pp 717-731).
© 2018 Taylor & Francis Group.

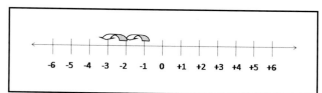

Figure A-3. Number line example (-1.00 -2.00; see text).

Many optical instruments we use every day are based on the number line, the lensometer being the most obvious. If you look at the power drum on a manual lensometer, you'll see what I mean. (Lensometry is covered in detail in Chapter 19.) From point 0, if you turn the wheel toward yourself, you move the number line in a plus direction (numbers usually inked in black or white). If you turn the wheel away from yourself, you are moving in the direction of minus numbers (usually inked in red).

If the patient has spherical lenses, then the mires (target lines) clear together at the same point, and the reading on the number line is the power of the lens. However, if the patient has astigmatism, the lensometer mires clear in two separate places. You must clear the first set of thin lines and note (write down) the number on the power wheel/number line (Point A). Then you must clear the second set of broad lines and again see the number on the power wheel (Point B)…but this is NOT the second number you're going to write down (which is where people get into trouble). The question is "How many steps did I have to go to get from the first reading to the second?" *That* is the second number you will record.

For example (Figure A-4), the thin lines clear at +2.00. In order to clear the wide lines, you find that you must turn the wheel away from you; these lines clear at 0.

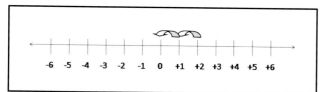

Figure A-4. Lensometry example (+2.00 -2.00; see text).

Step one: Are we moving in a plus or minus direction? Minus.

Step two: Where did we start, and what is the spherical power of this lens? +2.00.

Step three: Where did we end up? Plano (0). Caution: Don't write down "0" as the cylinder power. This is a common mistake.

Step four: How many "steps" did it take to get from +2.00 to 0? Written out, the equation is +2.00 + X = 0. Solving for X, the answer is -2.00. *This* is the cylindrical power of the lens.

Answer: The power of this lens is +2.00 -2.00. Of course, if this were a real-life example, the cylinder axis would also be noted.

Other instruments that work on a number line-type system include the Prince rule (as a measuring device, this is simply a positive/plus number line), the keratometer (another positive number line), and the Geneva lens measure (has a positive, black scale and a negative, red scale).

On the number line, if you were going to straddle the number 5 by one full step on either side (Figure A-5), the steps would correspond to the numbers 4 (going one step toward the minus) and 6 (going one step toward the plus), with 5 perfectly in the middle. The concept of *straddling* is important in refractometry. As the term implies, straddling is when an object is halfway between, or resting equally between two points.

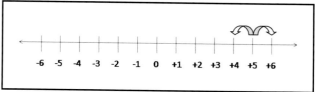

Figure A-5. Straddling.

We use straddling most often when refining the cylinder axis and power. The Jackson cross cylinder actually shows the patient one step toward the minus on one side (the red dot) and one step toward plus on the other side (the white dot). In between is the actual setting that you are evaluating.

Suppose you are refining the cylinder axis. The cylinder is currently set at 90 degrees (°). The cross cylinder shows the patient an equal distance clockwise and counterclockwise, pivoting on the 90° mark. Once the patient tells you which choice seems clearest, you move a little farther in the indicated direction. *When both choices seem the same, it means you are straddling the correct setting.* The same applies when refining the cylinder power.

You can also use this technique with spheres if the patient seems to have trouble discerning between choices. Suppose the patient says that +1.25, +1.50, and +1.75 all look the same. Use straddling and show the patient first the +1.25 and then the +1.75 (straddling the +1.50). If both choices look about the same, then +1.50 is the better endpoint.

Basic Math

The concepts of basic math are used daily in the eye clinic. For example, one might "count the clicks" during refractometry, then multiply by 0.25 to find lens power. (I like to use this when measuring the reading add; that way I don't have to do the subtraction!) Removing the working distance after retinoscopy might mean reducing the sphere power in the refractor by six clicks.

A "math problem" might also be called an *equation*. The prefix *equa-* denotes things that are the same (ie, equal), so an equation tells us that two (or more) items (mathematical expressions) on either side of the = sign are the same. The "math" in the equation (ie, +, −, X, and ÷) are called *operations*.

In basic math, a plain, unadorned equation is solved left to right, if only addition and subtraction OR only multiplication and division are involved. (Note: The colors in the equations show how the numbers flow through the resolution.) For example:

4 − 2 + 10 − 3
is worked 4 − 2 = 2
then 2 + 10 = 12
then 12 − 3 = **9**

After that, you get into something called the order of operations. This is a set of rules regarding equations that contain addition/subtraction AND multiplication/division. The order of operations says that multiplication/division must be solved first, from left to right, then addition and subtraction, from left to right, in equations that contain a mix of these operations.[1] For example:

49 − 7 X 6 + 8 ÷ 2
is worked as 7 X 6 = 42 and 8 ÷ 2 = 4
then 49 − 42 + 4 = **11**

In math, brackets are used to group things together. Parentheses are a type of bracket, as are "square" or "box" brackets [ ] and "curly" brackets { }. Anything in brackets of any kind is solved first. For example, if there is an equation within an equation, set off by parenthesis ( ), then the equation in the parentheses is calculated first:

49 − (7 + 6) + (8 ÷ 2)
is worked as 49 − (13) + (4)
then left to right 49 − 13 + 4 = **40**

Different kinds of brackets can even be used together, in the same equation. In such a case, start with the equation that is innermost.

100 − (7 X [2 + 3])
is worked as innermost set of brackets first: [2 + 3] = 5
then outer set of brackets: (7 X 5) = 35
then 100 − 35 = **65**

The same problem without the extra brackets would be:

100 − (7 X 2 + 3)
worked as multiplication first: 7 X 2 = 14
then the addition: 14 + 3 = 17
and finally 100 − 17 = **83**

Just move the brackets around and you get a whole different answer, even though the numbers and operations stay the same. So pay attention!

Here is the mathematical order of life:

1. In an equation with ONLY addition/subtraction or ONLY multiplication/division, solve LEFT to RIGHT. (This applies to equations in brackets, as well.)

2. In an equation MIXING addition/subtraction AND multiplication/division, solve the multiplication/division FIRST, then the addition/subtraction. (This applies to equations in brackets, as well.)

3. If the equation has brackets, solve inside the brackets FIRST, following Rules 1 and 2. If there are more than one kind of bracket in an equation, start with the innermost first, following Rules 1 and 2.

4. Exponents are thrown in there as well (eg, 7922^2), but you don't want to go there, do you? Me neither. (But if you *must* know, they are solved between brackets and multiplication/division.)

Algebra

Sometimes matters optical turn algebraic on us. In *algebra*, letters or symbols (called *variables*) are used to represent values that are unknown. Still, the basic tenets of math apply. One difference is that if two variables are written next to each other, this means to multiply them together (eg, *ab* means that you will multiply the two values *a* and *b*).

Variables are "stand-ins" for an unknown number in the equation. In eye care, these are most often found in formulas that tell you how to figure something out. Examples include calculating the dioptric power of a lens and the amount of induced prism.

Solving for Variables

Solving math problems is much easier if you remember that you can do anything you like to an equation (add, subtract, multiply, divide) and it won't change the result IF you do the SAME THING to BOTH sides of the equation.

For example, 2 + 2 = 3 + 1

If you add 5 to each side of the equation, the result on one side is still equal to the result on the other side:

2 + 2 + 5 = 3 + 1 + 5
becomes 9 = 9

Remember, you must do the SAME THING to both sides of the equation. (If you forgot to add the 4 to the left side, for example, you'd have 2 + 2 = 3 + 1 + 4, and 4 does not equal 8!)

Similarly, when using variables, you could have something like

a + b = c + d

You could divide each side by 3, and one side of the equation will still equal the other:

$$\frac{a+b}{3} = \frac{c+d}{3}$$

You could also multiply each side by 17, and one side will equal the other. Or subtract 2/17 from each side...you get the idea.

Plugging Into Formulas

Solving mathematical formulas is not difficult as long as you plug the *right* numbers into the *right* places. If the formula uses variables, there must be a notation that tells you what each variable stands for, and (if applicable) what type measurement must be used. For example, the most basic of optical formulae is probably the one that expresses the relationship between focal distance and diopters:

F = 1/D

where F = focal distance in meters

and D = power of lens in diopters

Here you are given the formula itself, plus a note that tells you what each variable stands for, as well as the specific measurement used. Using the correct form of measurement is key, because if you use the wrong one (eg, inches instead of meters, centimeters instead of millimeters), then the formula won't work and your answer will be incorrect.

You must also put the correct variable in its place. For example, if you enter diopters as F, then you won't be able to get the right answer either. That's what I mean by plugging in the right number(s) in the right place(s).

Suppose you want to figure out the focal length of an 8 diopter lens.

Plug in:

F = 1/8 diopters

F = 0.125 meters

Or suppose you've used the Allen cards to measure a child's vision. The Allen cards are based on a testing distance of 30 feet (see Chapter 8), and the child's vision was 15/30. But you want to convert the acuity to the 20 foot system. The equation would look like this:

$$\frac{15}{30} = \frac{20}{x}$$

Breaking it down, we start with the first fraction: 15/30 = 0.5

Now we can multiply both sides by x/1: 0.5

x = 20

Now we can divide both sides by 0.5:

x = 40

The conversion is 20/40.

Alternately, you can cross-multiply. This makes the equation 15x = (20 X 30). 15x = 600. Then divide both sides by 15 and you get the same answer: x = 40.

Metric System Basics

The metric system is used in most countries except the United States. The metric system is easy to use because it's based on increments of 10. Most optical formulas are designated in the metric system, so it's important to know.

These are the basic metric units most commonly used in ophthalmology:

► Weight/mass: Grams

► Length: Meters

► Volume/capacity: Liters

The size of a unit can be divided into units of 10, and are designated by a prefix (in eye care, we are usually using the three smaller units) as follows:

► micro- (μ) 1/1 million (0.000001, or 10^{-6})

► milli- (m) 1/1000 (0.001, or 10^{-3})

► centi- (c) 1/100 (0.01, or 10^{-2})

► 1 basic unit (eg, gram, liter, meter)

► kilo- (K) 1000 (10^3)

So if you have 2.5 cm and need to convert it to millimeters, you know there are 10 mm in every centimeter. So you can just move the decimal one space to the right for an answer of 25.0 mm. (Note: Be careful moving the decimal right and left! Before solving an equation involving metric units, stop and think.)

Sometimes it is necessary to convert US units into metric units (Table A-1). Focal length, for example, is calculated in meters. But suppose you're given the focal length in inches and asked for the dioptric power of the lens? You'll first need to convert the inches to meters, then plug into the formula.

TABLE A-1
METRIC CONVERSIONS
meters X 39.37 = inches
meters X 3.28 = feet
feet X 3.04 = meters
inches X 25.40 = millimeters
inches X 2.54 = centimeters
centimeters X 0.393 = inches
pounds X 453.6 = grams
kilograms X 2.205 = pounds
pounds X 0.453 = kilograms
ounces X 28.35 = grams
pints X .473 = liters
liters X 2.114 = pints

Suppose your focal length is 18 inches. There are 2.54 cm in 1 inch. The formula is:

F = 1/D

where F = focal distance in meters

and D = power of lens in diopters

There are 2.54 cm in an inch (*Think*: The answer should be more than 18…), so you can multiply 18 by 2.54 = 45.72 cm. But the formula calls for *meters* (*Think*: Since a meter is a larger unit, the answer will be tiny…). There are 100 cm in a meter, so move the decimal two places to the left, and the answer is 0.4572 meters. Now you can properly plug into the formula and solve from there:

0.4572 m = 1/D

Divide both sides by 0.4572:

1 = 1/0.4572 D

D = 2.187226596 diopters

Rounding Off

Sometimes we don't want or need to deal with all the integers in a number. Take, for example, the calculation we just did for the dioptric power of a lens with a focal length of 18 inches. We really only need accuracy to the 1/100, because diopters are not calculated any smaller than that. So we could round off the meters to the nearest 100th, to the second place to the right of the decimal. By and large, if the number you are rounding off is 5 or more, you would round *up*. If the number you are rounding off is 4 or less, you would round *down*. So we'd round off the answer above, which would be 2.19 D because the number in the third decimal place (7) is 5 or more.

Another example would be calculating the spherical equivalent (SE) of a lens. Suppose you had:

-7.25 + 1.75 X 80

You remember (from Chapter 4) that to find the SE you take half of the cylinder and add it to the sphere. Half of 1.75 = 0.875.

Add that to the sphere: -7.25 + 0.875 = -6.375. Round that off to two decimal places and you'd have -6.38 because the number in the third decimal place (5) is 5 or more. (Take it a step farther, because we only talk about lenses in 0.25 increments. So your choices are -6.25 or -6.50. In this case, -6.38 is closer to -6.50 [think number line], so -6.50 would be chosen.)

Geometry

Plane geometry deals with points, lines, and two-dimensional shapes, and is commonly used to demonstrate optical principles. A *point* is simply a dot; it has a location but nothing else (such as width, height, or direction) so it is one dimensional. You can extend one or more lines from (or to) any single point. In optics, we use lines to represent light rays and points to represent where these light rays either come from (source) and spread out (diverge) or else come together and meet (converge to a

focal point). Thus, lines and points are used to describe refraction and reflection as detailed in Chapter 4.

Two lines that run in the same direction and never touch are said to be *parallel* (Figure A-6). In optics we often talk about parallel light rays because they are considered to be from infinity and do not stimulate accommodation.

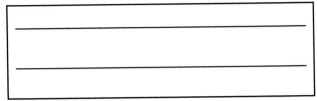

Figure A-6. Parallel lines never meet (intersect or converge).

When two lines meet at the same point (called the *vertex*), an *angle* is formed between the two lines. In optics, when we talk about an angle, it is something that can be measured (in degrees). If you stood in the middle of a circle and turned all the way around, you would have rotated 360°. If you are in the middle and turn from east to west, this would be a 180° turn. Or if you turned from south to east, this would be 90°. Two lines that are 90° from each other are said to be *perpendicular* (Figure A-7).

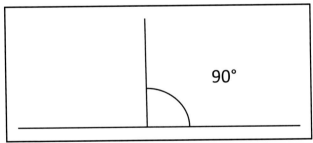

Figure A-7. If two lines are perpendicular, they are 90° apart.

You probably remember using a protractor in school to measure angles (Figure A-8). The cylinder axis dial on the refractor is a protractor of sorts, indicating the orientation (from 001° to 180°) of the cylindrical lens you are using to correct astigmatism. (Although in reality we generally think of axis in terms of direction, rather than angle.)

One degree can be further divided into 60 *minutes* (60') and is usually denoted specifically as *minutes of arc*. Each minute of arc can be subdivided into 60 seconds (60") of arc. These designations apply to visual acuity testing (where a Snellen letter is made up of five parts, each of which subtends [extends to the eye] 1' of arc), as well as to stereo vision testing (where the finest is 20" of arc). If the

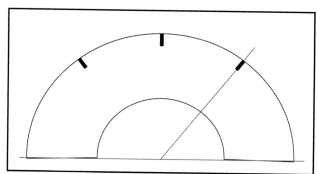

Figure A-8. Using a protractor to measure a 45° angle.

width of your thumb is 2° when held at arm's length, you begin to understand just how subtle visual discrimination can be.

A circle is an example of a two-dimensional shape (Figure A-9). The *circumference* is the distance around the circle itself. By definition, a circle is all of the points that are the same distance from the central point. The *radius* is the distance from the center of the circle to the edge. The *diameter* is the distance from one side of the circle to the other through the center (or, 2 X the radius).

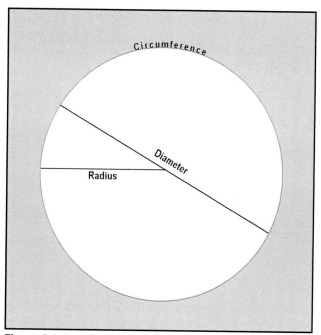

Figure A-9. A circle and its parameters.

Diameter is an important feature of contact lenses, measured in millimeters. A common soft contact lens diameter is 14.0, meaning that the lens is 14 mm across. We also use corneal diameter when calculating intraocular lens implant parameters as well as fitting contact lenses and prior to refractive surgery.

Dividing a circle into four equal parts with perpendicular lines at 90° and 180° yields four quadrants. We often speak of quadrants in visual field testing (eg, an

inferior left quadrantanopsia). If we want to indicate half of the circle (ie, two consecutive quadrants), then we use the prefix *hemi-* (eg, a temporal or nasal hemianopsia if the defect is the left or right half, or a superior or inferior altitudinal hemianopsia if the defect is the upper half or lower half, respectively).

Solid geometry involves three-dimensional objects such as spheres, prisms, and cylinders. However, these objects are often represented by drawings vs actual physical items. So for us, solid geometry is also more useful as illustrations. One important exception is contact lenses.

A contact lens is like a slice of a (hollow) sphere. The dimensions of the contact, or its parameters, depend on several things, such as the size of the sphere itself and just where you decide to slice it (Figure A-10). Thus, increasing lens diameter makes the lens tighter and increases the *vault*. (If you put a contact lens on a surface with curve-side up, the vault is the distance from that surface to the height of the lens's curve measured in millimeters.)

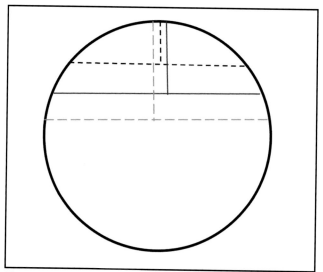

Figure A-10. As the diameter of a contact lens increases, the vault increases as well.

A contact's parameters also depend on the *base curve*; that is, how large is the "sphere" from which you slice it. A steeper base curve comes from a smaller sphere (Figure A-11).

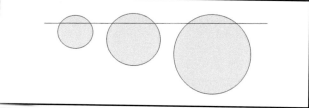

Figure A-11. A smaller circle has a steeper base curve, even when the vault is the same.

The concept of a sphere is also used in visual field testing. The fovea is considered the central point of the field. *Meridians* are lines that emanate from the center of the field. The most important are the 180° (horizontal) and 90° (vertical), but field testing involves other meridians as well, usually at regular intervals. (The tangent screen, for example, has a meridian stitched into it every 22.5°.)

The cornea is not a perfect sphere, but we routinely analyze its curves. Keratometry measures the curvature of 3 mm of the corneal cap (the central 4 to 6 mm of the anterior surface of the cornea). Corneal topography can be used to map out the curves of the entire tissue surface.

Basic Statistics

The purpose of this section is not to teach you how to "do" statistics, but rather to provide enough basic terminology for understanding test and research results. It will be easier to understand the definitions if we make up a study and follow it through the steps.

Example: You are studying the intraocular pressure (IOP) of women with glaucoma, ages 55 to 60, who are using Eyedrop X. The IOPs after using the drop for 3 months are: 10, 11, 11, 12, 14, 14, 15, 16, 16, 16, 18, 22, 24, 27. (Note: In reality a test group of 14 subjects would be way too small. But in this case we need manageable numbers we can handle.)

The *mean* is the same thing as the *average*. All the scores in a group are added together and divided by the number of participants. In our study the total is 226. Divide by 14, and the mean is 16.14.

However, the mean is not actually a very useful piece of information in this case. Look at the list. Only three persons in the study actually have an IOP of 16. A value called the *standard deviation* tells us how spread out the data are. If 16.14 is the middle of our data set, the standard deviation tells us if the other values in the data set are clustered close to 16.14 or spread out all over the place. If the standard deviation is 0, this indicates that every measurement is the same; there is no variation (deviation) from the mean. Thus, the closer the standard deviation is to 0, the more reliable the information because each measurement is pretty close to the mean. In our study, the standard deviation is 5.08. (I ran our numbers through a calculator at calculator.net.) The higher the standard deviation, the less representative the mean is of the actual data set. In other words, the standard deviation tells us the "average distance each data point is from the mean."[2]

Another indicator of the reliability of the mean is the *range*. The range is simply the difference between the highest and lowest values in a set. In our example the lowest IOP was 10, the highest was 27. So the range is 27 – 10, or 17. The smaller the range, the more closely the data points are to each other.

There are a few more terms you might run into as you peruse medical studies.

The *median* looks at the data and says what value is in the middle of the list. The formula is (N + 1)/2 = the *location* of the median, where N is the number of participants. In our case, (14 + 1)/2 = 15/2 = 7.5. *This is not the median itself*; it tells you the *position* of the median in a given series, so that half the scores are above and half are below this point. In our results list above, the median will be located at position 7.5, or halfway between the seventh (15) and eighth IOP (16) in the list. This corresponds to a median IOP of 15.5. The median is used to identify trends. (In our study, we would need to follow our patients over a long period of time in order to have a meaningful median.)

Mode is the most frequently appearing number in a set. In our example there are three 16's, two 14's, and two 11's. The mode is 16. This statistic helps identify repeated occurrences.

The concept of *reliability* is important in eye care. Suppose a patient who is a glaucoma suspect has his/her first visual field test and the results show an enlarged blind spot. You may be asked to repeat the field again to see if you get the same result twice. Thus reliability is another way of talking about consistency. In other words, if the conditions under which the visual field was performed is consistent (ie, room lighting, test strategy, correct trial lens used), and we get the same (or very similar) results as before, we consider the tests to be reliable.

In field testing, reliability is actually calculated. This is done by documenting false negatives, false positives, and fixation losses. In a false positive, the patient responds when there is no stimulus, is trigger happy, and pushes the button faster than the machine is presenting, or is just guessing. With a false negative, the patient does not respond to a stimulus that the machine has already determined should be seen (ie, a brighter-than-ever light in a spot where the patient has responded before). These two factors, in addition to fixation losses, are called *catch trials*. I think of this as the instrument "trying to catch" the patient being inconsistent. The catch trial results are then used to determine how reliable the test results are.

Many automated optical instruments employ statistical calculations besides the Humphrey Field Analyzer. The Tono-pen, optical coherence tomographer, pachymeter, A-scan, etc, all use statistics to average data and give you an idea of whether or not the results are reliable.

Statistical significance is a way of indicating whether or not a result is just a fluke, a chance occurrence, or is really due to the effects of something. In other words, what is the probability that the result is just luck (good or bad)? For example, if you tossed a coin 20 times and it came up heads 12 times and tails 8 times, you would not think this an unlikely result; the difference would not be significant. But if you flip the coin 20 times and it comes up heads every time but one, you don't need to do the math to realize that this is improbable. Your results are significant. There are formulas to use to calculate statistical significance, but you don't really want to go there, do you? Me neither.

UNDERSTANDING RESEARCH

While most of us will not be directly involved in research, we want to be current in our field. This includes finding the information we need to care for our patients, taking continuing education courses for certification, and looking things up just because we're curious.

Research is vital to any branch of medicine (or science, for that matter). It has a language all its own. There are some key terms you need to understand when you read an article that refers to a specific study, or when you read the study itself. This section is necessarily simplified, but is intended to help you look at a study, ask the right questions about its validity, and judge the results for yourself.

The study is identified in the title of the paper. It tells you the purpose of the research by identifying the specific problem or topic that the study was designed to evaluate. This might be to evaluate a treatment or to better understand how something works. For example, clinical trials are studies required when evaluating new medications.

The *study group* is the identified group of interest in the study. This could be a specific group of people (eg, persons with retinitis pigmentosa), a specific finding (eg, the relationship between sleep apnea and glaucoma), etc.

The *experimental group* consists of those in the study who receive or do the factor you are testing for. This may also be referred to as the *treatment group*.

A *control group* is the part of the study that does not experience whatever factor the research is evaluating. For example, if the study is about the effectiveness of a treatment, you must compare the subjects in the treatment group to another group that did not receive the treatment. The control group must be the same as the study group in every other way, however. For example, if the study is about a glaucoma treatment, you would compare the persons with glaucoma receiving the treatment with other persons with glaucoma not receiving the treatment. You wouldn't compare them to persons who don't have glaucoma at all.

The idea that the control and experimental groups must be similar in every way except for the one variable being studied may seem to be extreme. In our glaucoma treatment example, both groups have glaucoma and one group is going to receive a specific treatment. But the rules of research are strict. The study must be able to prove that any difference between the groups *must* be due to the medication itself (ie, cause and effect), and not due to anything else (eg, the fact that a drop of some kind was instilled into the eye).

So both groups will receive eye drops. The study group will take an eye drop with the new medication in it, and the control group will use a benign eye drop with no medication in it. The control group is getting a *placebo*, or the eye drop equivalent of "sugar pills." In this way the study can later prove that the medication is what made any difference in the study's tests.

Interestingly enough, using a placebo can backfire in some studies. Suppose you were testing the efficacy of a new tear drop and part of the evaluation was a survey filled out by the participants regarding how they *feel*. A person taking a placebo doesn't know if he/she is receiving the medicated version or not. Just the fact that he/she is being given *something* might produce, in his/her mind, some type of result. This is called the *placebo effect*, where the results are obtained from a person in the control group. This contaminates the results of the overall study.

So how is the selection made to put a person in one group or the other? Who knows which patients get the medication and which ones get the placebo?

If all things are equal between the study and control groups, the usual selection method is *randomized*. This amounts to the toss of the dice. Randomization is important because it removes the possibility of *selection bias*; that is, that the researchers could later be accused of selecting the persons to receive the treatment because those persons had some kind of propensity to respond positively to it. There are computer programs that make the assignment, removing the human factor altogether.

In studies that do not involve human subjects, placebos are not generally required unless there is the possibility that the researchers themselves might need to prove that they do not have some sort of bias. This brings up the question of who knows what, or who is "blind" to what's going on.

A *single-blind study* means that the subjects (humans) do not know who is receiving treatment and who is receiving a placebo. The experimenters, however, are aware of who is getting what, injecting the possibility of bias. In a *double-blind study*, neither the subjects nor the evaluators know which is which.

Quantitative data are derived from measuring something, like IOP. *Categorical data* are derived from putting things in a group with commonalities (women, ages 55 to 60 years, have glaucoma, use Eyedrop X).

Most medical research papers (*primary* or *original* research articles) follow a standard format. In simple terms, the research design involves asking a question, formulating a possible answer (the hypothesis), then designing a way to test the hypothesis. The arrangement of such a report will vary depending on the type of study as well as the publication, but this format is common:

▶ Abstract—This is the "short version" in 250 words or less.

▶ Introduction
  • Presentation of the problem
  • Purpose of the study
  • Statement of authors' position

▶ Review of literature

- ▶ Methods and materials
  - • Study design
  - • Participants
  - • Materials and instrumentation
- ▶ Results
- ▶ Discussion
- ▶ Conclusion
- ▶ References

Clinical trials involve research to determine if a drug, device, or treatment is safe and effective. The well-known Age Related Eye Disease Study (AREDS), while it involved other data as well, included clinical trials to find out what supplements (and at what dose) were of most benefit to patients with age-related macular degeneration as well as cataracts. The Food and Drug Administration (FDA) has strict requirements for clinical trials prior to approving any type of treatment.

The Early Treatment Diabetic Retinopathy Study (ETDRS) and the AREDS and AREDS2 are examples of *prospective* studies (Sidebar A-1). These multicenter studies gathered and evaluated data about the progression and occurrence of the diabetic eye disease, age-related macular degeneration, and cataracts. In other words, they monitored the progress of these disorders over a period of time, looking for outcomes and evaluating treatments. Each study was multi-faceted, and some segments of AREDS2 are ongoing.

A *retrospective* study is done after the fact. Suppose a large clinic wants to know how well their potential acuity meter (PAM) readings match up to best-corrected vision (BCV) in their patients who have had cataract surgery in the past year. They would look back at the records of all patients having cataract surgery in the past 12 months and see who had preoperative PAM readings and what their postoperative BCV turned out to be. In this case, the question is answered with data that had already been gathered (although not for the purpose of a study).

A *case study* is a report of an interesting or unusual occurrence. It is not research in that the subject is not being tested in any way. An example would be reporting on an incident where a patient had an angle-closure glaucoma attack within 24 hours of blepharoplasty surgery.

A *review of literature* does not involve research and experimentation. Rather, it means that the author has looked through literature regarding a specific topic and has prepared a report. There is so much information out there that such a review needs to be pretty specific to be useful. For example, suppose the topic is methods of measuring IOP. The authors would have to decide from the beginning whether they would look at materials by juried medical journals (where the paper is judged by experts in the field before being accepted for publication), by service organizations (for the public? for medical professionals?), or by patients who remark on their experiences in having

their IOP checked. Specific publication dates might be stipulated as well. If the interest is in a historical perspective, then the review would include writings from antiquity up to the development of the Schiötz tonometer, for example. If the topic is a recent development, then only more current materials would be reviewed. Most research papers include a short section on literature review.

SCIENCE

The purpose of this section is to go over just a few of the most basic elements of science not covered elsewhere in this text. While I have broken the information down into divisions, some items here might cross over into several scientific disciplines.

Physics

Physics is the study of matter, energy, and interactions between the two. This includes the study of movement, light, radiation, and optics. Basic optics is covered in Chapter 4.

Motion

Kinetic refers to movement. *Static* means that an object is still. In eye care, these terms are generally used in visual field testing where we are referring to the movement or nonmovement of a test object. In kinetic testing the target is moved, usually from a point where it is not seen to a point where it is. The question is "When do you first see the target?" In static testing, the question is merely "Do you see this when I hold it here?"

Surface Tension and the Meniscus

The molecules of the surface of a liquid have an elastic quality where the surface area is minimized, or more tightly drawn together. This is called *surface tension*, and it is what allows "water skimmer" bugs to skate across the surface of a pond. In the eye, this phenomenon plays a role in the tear film.

Surface tension is part of what keeps tears on the eye. But when the amount of tears overcomes the surface tension of the fluid, the surface tension "breaks" and tears flow out of the eyes.

If you put some water in a narrow test tube, you can see that the surface of the water "dips" down a little bit. This is called a *meniscus* (plural, *menisci*), which occurs because surface tension is pulling the surface molecules in tighter than the fluid below. In the eye, the *tear meniscus* is the dip in the surface of the tear film where it is pooled at the lid margins. (Note that this is not the same as the precorneal tear film.) It is probably most easily seen at the lower lid margin, although there is one at the upper lid margin as well. One study suggests that 75% to 90% of

---

SIDEBAR A-1

TWO BENCHMARK STUDIES IN OPHTHALMOLOGY[3,4]

Early Treatment Diabetic Retinopathy Study (ETDRS)
Study size: 3711 patients
Length of study: Began December 1979, concluded July 1985
Comment: In spite of the fact that this is an "old" study, it remains a benchmark analysis of diabetic retinopathy (DR) with numerous side benefits, such as the development of the ETDRS eye chart for visual acuity, definitions of specific stages of DR, and a system of grading DR.
Questions:

▶ Can argon laser photocoagulation delay or prevent progression of early DR? (Yes.)

▶ Can aspirin therapy delay or prevent progression of early DR? (No.)

▶ When is the best time to use photocoagulation to treat DR? (At the nonproliferative stage.)

▶ How does diabetes affect visual function?

▶ How does photocoagulation affect visual function?

▶ What can we learn that will help identify risk factors for DR?

▶ What can we learn that will help us better understand diabetes and DR?

Age Related Eye Disease Study (AREDS)
Original study
Study size: 4757 patients
Length of study: Began 1992, concluded 2001
Questions:

▶ Can certain vitamins and minerals reduce the risk of advanced age-related macular degeneration (AMD) when taken daily? (Yes.)
  • Vitamin E
  • Vitamin C
  • Beta-carotene
  • Zinc

▶ Can certain vitamins and minerals reduce the risk of cataracts when taken daily? (No.)

Follow-up study: AREDS2
Study size: 4203 patients
Length of study: Began 2006, results released in 2013; portions of the study are ongoing
Questions:

▶ Can omega-3 fatty acids reduce the risk of advanced AMD? (No.)

▶ Can lutein and zeaxanthin reduce the risk of advanced AMD? (Not really, unless the diet is low in these nutrients.)

▶ What levels of beta-carotene and zinc are needed to affect the risk of advanced AMD? (Beta-carotene was removed and the level of zinc lowered as a result of the study.)

---

the total volume of tears on the eye are contained within the menisci; the rest would be the precorneal tear film.[5]

Biochemistry

Osmolarity is a measure of the concentration of particles in a solution expressed as total particles per liter. This term might be seen in discussions of dry eye, because studies suggest that increased tear osmolarity is associated with dry eye disease. This hyperosmolarity occurs as the water in the tears evaporates off the eye's surface, instigating an inflammatory response that damages the corneal epithelium and renders the tear film unstable.[6] Ocular medications can affect the osmolarity of the tear film.[7]

Dilution refers to weakening the concentration of something. In the case of a chemical splash to the eye, we irrigate the eye with water in order to decrease or dilute the concentration of the substance on the eye.

Tonicity describes the amount of solute (dissolved substances). If a solution applied to tissue is *isotonic*, it has the same tonicity as the cells, and there is no movement of water either way across the cell membranes. Ideally, eye medications should be isotonic with tears (0.9% sodium chloride). If the tonicity of the solution outside the membrane is *hypertonic* (ie, higher tonicity), it has a higher amount of solute. This triggers osmosis (covered momentarily).

The *pH* of a solution or substance tells us how alkaline (basic) or acidic (acid) it is. It is measured on a scale of 0 to 14. The middle of the scale (7) is neutral, being neither an acid nor a base. But once you edge down from 7, the closer you get to 0, the more acidic a substance is. (For example, battery acid has a pH of about 1. This is also about the pH in the human stomach.) From 7 up, the closer you get to 14, the stronger an alkali (base) you have. (Common bases are baking soda [about 8] and lye [11.5].)

The pH of human tears is about 6.5 to 7.6 (7.4 is often the number given). Eye medications are most comfortable if the pH is 7.4. Eye drops with an alkaline pH are the ones that sting. In contrast, the pH of normal saline is 5.5. While this is slightly acidic, it does not sting.

The pH of a solution that is accidentally splashed into the eye is important. While an acid will burn surface tissue, it does not penetrate. A base will burn the surface as well as bind with lipid (fat), so it penetrates, destroying tissue from the outside in. Common bases include many cleaning solutions (eg, bleach, lye) and lime-containing construction materials (eg, cement/concrete, mortar).

Biology

A *barrier* is anything (in biology usually a membrane) that blocks movement of something from one location to another. For example, the corneal epithelium is a barrier against injury to the deeper layers of the tissue. The conjunctiva is a barrier against anything becoming "lost" behind the eye.

Some barriers are *selectively (semi-) permeable*, allowing certain things in or out. In the eye, there is the blood-retinal barrier and the blood-aqueous barrier, where there is an exchange of materials back and forth but not of blood itself. Barriers also represent a challenge to the delivery of medication to the ocular tissues. Permeability may also be named specifically, such as *oxygen permeability*.

Diffusion is the process by which a high concentration of particles (most often in a gaseous form) move to an area of lower concentration until the concentration of particles is equal throughout. Note that the particles do the moving. An example is air freshener diffusing through a room.

Osmosis is a specific type of diffusion, where *water* moves through a barrier in order to equalize the concentration of particles on either side. When we apply sodium chloride drops to an eye with corneal edema, osmosis occurs (Figure A-12). Water is drawn out of the cornea in an attempt to dilute the sodium chloride content on the other side of the tissue. Thus, the sodium chloride is acting as an *osmotic*, and the cornea clears as the excess fluid is moved out of the tissue.

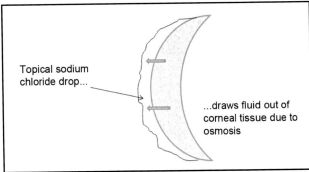

Topical sodium chloride drop...

...draws fluid out of corneal tissue due to osmosis

Figure A-12. Applying an osmotic (sodium chloride in this case) draws fluid out of the tissue.

Anatomy

Cells

Cells are the building blocks of living things. Each cell is its own little microcosm with inner structures that perform specific functions.

Animal cells are surrounded by a *cell membrane*. (Plants have a cell wall.) The cell membrane selectively allows nutrients in and wastes out. The nucleus (roughly in the cell's center) is the "brain" of the cell, controlling the activities of the cell and its parts and containing the cell's genetic information. It is separated from the rest of the cell by a membrane. The cytoplasm is the fluid inside the cell (ie, between the cell membrane and the nuclear membrane), and it contains the cell structures (called *organelles*).

One of the organelles is the *mitochondria*. These are the "power house of the cell" and function in energy production and use. The *endoplasmic reticulum* (ER) is a series of membranes that runs throughout the cytoplasm, linking the cell membrane and the nuclear membrane. It provides a transportation system for material moving through the cell. *Ribosomes* are tiny particles (sometimes attached to the ER) that produce protein. They are assisted by the *golgi bodies*, which manufacture and store hormones and enzymes. *Lysosomes*, little sacs that are part of the golgi bodies, contain digestive enzymes to help the cell process nutrients. If a lysosome bursts and releases these enzymes into the cell, the result may be cell death. *Vacuoles* are "storage pods" for nutrients and waste.

TABLE A-2 THE FOUR TISSUE TYPES IN THE EYE	
Tissue Type	**In the Eye**
Connective	Bones of orbit; blood supply of orbit, skin/lids, extraocular muscles, globe, uvea; orbital fat; orbital septa, sclera; vitreous humor, corneal stroma, canal of Schlemm
Epithelial	Epithelium of skin and conjunctiva, corneal epithelium, lens
Muscle	Extraocular muscles, muscles of lids and face, iris, ciliary muscle
Nerve	Optic nerve (sensory), retina (sensory), extraocular muscle supply (motor), lids/face (motor and sensory), iris/pupil (autonomic)

Tissues

A group of similar cells that perform the same function are called *tissues*. Understanding that a human being starts from a single cell really makes you appreciate how that one cell divides and differentiates. You've heard of *stem cells*? In the embryo, these are early cells that have the potential to morph into virtually any cell type the body needs; thus, they are thought of as being *plastic*. Stem cells are also found in certain nonembryonic tissues including bone marrow. There is great interest in stem cells, with the hope, for example, that one day we will be able to generate new retinal cells to replace those ravaged by macular degeneration or other problems.

The animal organism has four types of tissue. *Connective tissue* includes bones and blood. *Epithelial tissue* (epithelium) makes up coverings for organs and the body itself. *Muscle tissue* is obviously for movement, and *nerve tissue* provides for the transmission of impulses.

Within these four tissue types there is further specialization and adaptation. For example, the corneal epithelium is different from the epithelium of the skin, although both provide a covering.

Organs and Systems

When two or more types of tissue are grouped together to perform a specific function, this entity is known as an *organ*. The eye is a highly specialized organ that contains all four types of tissue (Table A-2).

A group of organs that work together to perform a function that meets a major need of the organism as a whole is called a *system*. (This is what's referred to in history taking when we perform a review of systems.) These systems are musculoskeletal, cardiovascular, gastrointestinal, endocrine, integumentary, psychiatric, genitourinary, hematologic/lymphatic, allergic/immunologic, respiratory, and neurological. (For billing and compliance, the American Academy of Ophthalmology additionally lists eyes; constitution; and ear, nose, mouth, and throat.[8]) Most of these are self-explanatory, but we'll look at several of them a little more closely.

The endocrine system is made up of organs (called *glands*) that produce *hormones*, which are chemicals that regulate metabolism and growth (among other things). Hormones are transported via the circulatory system.

We usually think of skin when we think about the integumentary system. But it also includes hair, nails, and brow/eyelashes.

The hematologic/lymphatic system is made up of the blood and lymph.

The allergic/immunologic system includes organs that are involved in protecting the body from foreign materials that can cause disease or otherwise harm the body.

The Nervous System

While each of the systems is part of or has an effect on the eye and vision, the nervous system is of key interest. It is also very complex. This section is simplified but covers the basics.

Note: Since some of the abbreviations overlap, I will only abbreviate those that we will be using frequently in this section.

The nervous system (Figure A-13) can be divided by where the nerves originate in the body.

The *central nervous system* (CNS) is the brain and spinal cord.

The *peripheral nervous system* (PNS) consists of nerves that branch off the spinal cord and extend to the muscles, organs, arms, legs, face, neck, torso, etc. These nerves are divided into *somatic* (also called *voluntary* nerves, involved in voluntary movement), *autonomic* ("automatic" activities such as breathing, heartbeat, pupil size), and *enteric* (controls digestion).

The 12 *cranial nerves* (CN) are part of the peripheral system. (Technically, however, the optic nerve is not a true peripheral nerve.) A cranial nerve might be motor (instigates movement), sensory, or both (mixed). Seven of the 12 cranial nerves are involved with the eye in some way.

The motor nerves of the somatic nervous system are of two types: afferent and efferent. The *afferent nerves* transmit impulses from the sense organs and muscles to the CNS. *Efferent nerves* transmit impulses from the CNS to the sense organs and muscles. Thus, an afferent

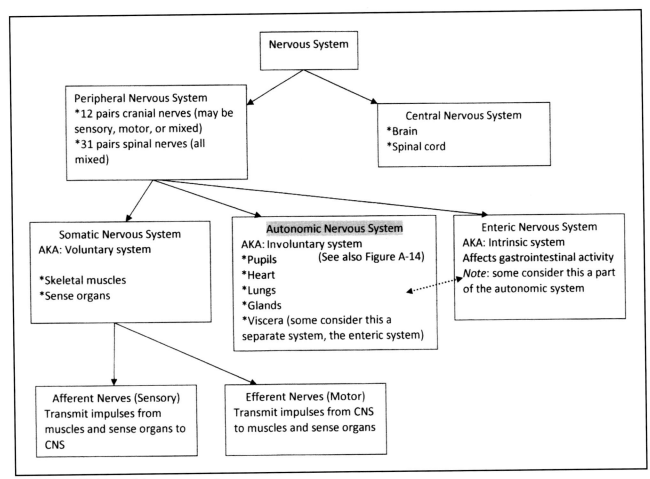

Figure A-13. Divisions of the nervous system.

pupillary defect (APD) is a problem in the transmission of impulses from the eye to the brain.

The *autonomic nervous system* (ANS; also called the *visceral* or *involuntary nervous system*) involves impulses to the internal organs and smooth muscle. It is divided into parasympathetic and sympathetic branches (Figure A-14). Understanding these two divisions and how they work is important in appreciating the actions of some ocular medications.

The parasympathetic nervous system (PSNS; also called the *cholinergic pathway*) operates when the body is in a relaxed state. Blood pressure, heart rate, and breathing rate are all steady and normal. The sympathetic nervous system (SNS; also called the *adrenergic pathway*), however, kicks in under stress. The pupils dilate, blood flow to the limbs increases (and blood flow to the viscera decreases), and breathing and heart rate become more rapid so that the body can respond to the threat. This is often called the "fight or flight" response. Once the threat

is neutralized, the parasympathetic system responds to calm the body down again ("digest and rest").

The biochemicals of the autonomic nervous system are the *neurotransmitters*. These transmit impulses across the *synapses* (spaces between nerve cells and other cells). Neurotransmitters activate receptor cites on other cells, rather like specialized keys that only fit into specific locks.

Acetylcholine (ACh) is the main neurotransmitter of the parasympathetic nervous system; *adrenaline* (epinephrine) and *noradrenaline* (norepinephrine) are transmitters of the sympathetic nervous system. An *agonist* is a substance that gives neurotransmitters an assist. They bind to a receptor and cause the neurotransmitter's response. An *antagonist* is a substance that blocks the action of a neurotransmitter.

Follow the flowchart in Figure A-14 for a basic understanding of how adrenergic drugs affect the sympathetic and parasympathetic systems, and how they are used in eye care.

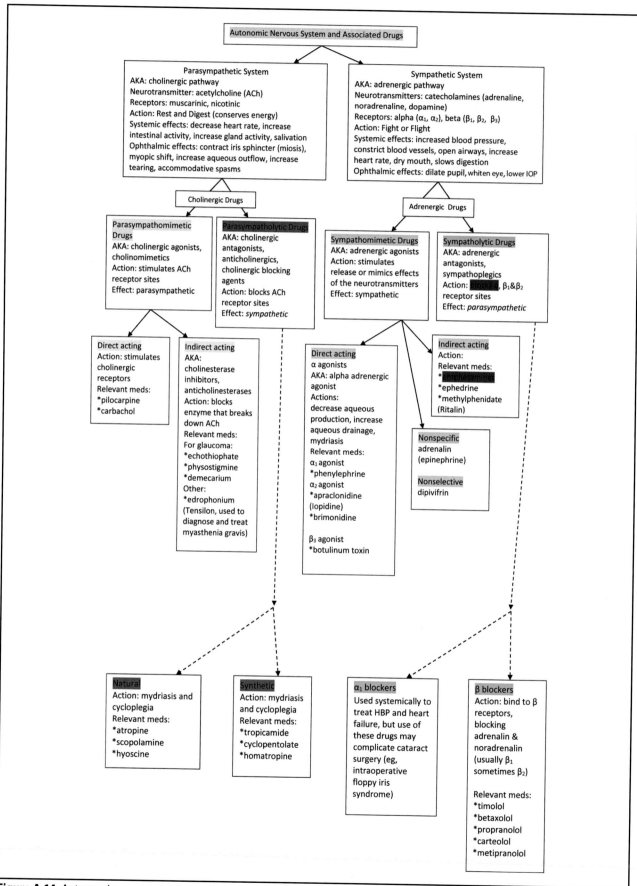

Figure A-14. Autonomic nervous system and associated drugs.

ACKNOWLEDGMENTS

The author would like to thank Al Lens, Aaron V. Shukla, Ken Woodworth, and Jennifer Cahill for their assistance with this appendix.

REFERENCES

1. The order of operations. Houghton Mifflin Harcourt's Education Place® website. https://www.eduplace.com/math/mathsteps/4/a/index.html. Accessed September 23, 2017.

2. Understanding standard deviation. Bacon Bits [Blog] of DataPig Technologies. http://datapigtechnologies.com/blog/index.php/understanding-standard-deviation-2/. Posted March 26, 2014. Accessed July 7, 2016.

3. Royle P. National Centers for Biotechnology Information. Early Treatment Diabetic Retinopathy Study (ETDRS). www.mrcophth.com/importanttrialsinophthalmology/etdrs.html. Accessed July 13, 2016.

4. Browne J. A summary of AREDS 1 and AREDS 2. www.optometrystudents.com/a-summary-of-areds-1-and-areds-2/. Posted May 21, 2013. Accessed July 13, 2016.

5. Holly FJ. Physical chemistry of the normal and disordered tear film. *Trans Ophthalmol Soc UK.* 1985:104(Pt 4):374-380. Cited by: Park DI, Lew H, Lee SY. Tear meniscus measurement in nasolacrimal duct obstruction patients with Fourier-domain optical coherence tomography: novel three-point capture method. *Acta Ophthalmologica.* 2011;90(3). doi:10.1111/j.1755-3768.2011.02183.x/pdf.

6. Lemp MA, Foulks GN. The definition & classification of dry eye disease. Guidelines from the 2007 International Dry Eye Workshop. Ophthalmology Management website. www.ophmanagement.com/archive.aspx?searchOptions=rbIssue&tm=4/1/2008. Accessed April 17, 2016.

7. Dutescue RM, Panfil C, Schrage N. Osmolarity of prevalent eye drops, side effects, and therapeutic approaches. *Cornea.* 2015;34(5)560-566. doi:10.1097/ICO.0000000000000368.

8. Vicchrilli SJ. E&M documentation requirements: a look at "review of systems." AAO Young Ophthalmologists website. www.aao.org/young-ophthalmologists/yo-info/article/em-documentation-requirements-look-at-review-of-sy. Posted May 20, 2014. Accessed July 7, 2016.

BIBLIOGRAPHY

Agents which influence the autonomic nervous system. Carteret Community College website. www.carteret.edu/keoughp/lfreshwater/pharm/Blackboard/PNS/Agents%20Which%20Influence%20the%20Autonomic%20Nervous%20System.htm. Accessed July 17, 2016.

Math is fun website. www.mathisfun.com. Accessed June 15, 2016.

The figures in this appendix were contributed by the following, who are associated with this book as authors:
Jan Ledford: Figures A-1 through A-8, A-10, A-11, A-13, A-14
Al Lens: Figures A-9, A-12

B

In-Office Training

Savory Turman, COMT, OCS

The career of an ophthalmic/optometric technician seems to be relatively unknown in the medical field. In general medical practice, thousands of medical assistants graduate every year. The dental field does not suffer from a lack of hygienists, either. However, with only slightly more than a dozen technical schools offering ophthalmic technician programs, eye clinics must often train their own assistants. Thus, it's imperative for a practice to develop its own training program.

NOTES ON HIRING

Sometimes the hardest decision of a training program can be who to bring into it. Making the right hiring decisions is a crucial part of what drives your program. Obviously, we'd all love to hire only amazing, experienced technicians, but the opportunity to do that is rare. For untrained talent, look at personality, likability, and desire to learn. Find people who have a track record of learning quickly, being reliable, getting along well with others, and tackling challenges.

Incorporating several interactions with prospective team members by formulating an interviewing system that has several steps can give you more exposure to the candidate. More exposure to the candidate can often prevent "buyer's remorse" by giving you more opportunities to observe his/her interactions with yourself and your teammates. You can also draw conclusions as to the desire that the candidates have to join your company. Do they do their research into your business in between your communications?

Below is an example of how your interviewing structure may work:

- Step 1: Résumé review—Here you can weed out those whose résumés are unprofessional or perhaps indicate an inability of keeping a position for more than a few months.

- Step 2: Phone interviews—Often you can tell within 5 minutes of speaking with an interviewee whether or not you'd like to spend 30 minutes with him/her in a face-to-face interview. Listen for pleasantness in the voice, a friendliness that translates through the phone, and an easy ability to communicate well. Senior techs could be asked to participate in this process. This not only helps with administrative tasks, it allows staff to feel that they are part of the hiring process.

- Step 3: Face-to-face interview—Consider conducting your face-to-face interviews with your next-in-command participating. Having a member of your staff interview with you can give another perspective of both the interview and the candidate. Observe the way the potential employee speaks to you and about others. Find out what his/her long- and short-term

Ledford JK, Lens A, eds.
*Principles and Practice in Ophthalmic Assisting:
A Comprehensive Textbook* (pp 733-772).
© 2018 Taylor & Francis Group.

SIDEBAR B-1
SAMPLE CONFIDENTIALITY STATEMENT

I, _____, understand that in the performance of my duties as an Employee/Intern/Observer of Clinic and its related entities and practices, I will have access to confidential information.

Confidential information is defined as any information found in a patient's medical and/or demographic and billing records, and personal and work-related information in an employee's personnel record. Information pertaining to all phases of operation of Clinic is considered property of Clinic and is subject to all rules of confidentiality. All information relating to a patient's care, treatment, or condition constitutes confidential information. Employees/Interns/Observers shall never discuss a patient's medical condition with other personnel, friends, or family. Confidential matters should not be topics for conversation at coffee breaks or in areas where they might be overheard. A patient's presence in the Clinic could also indicate the nature of the patient's illness and therefore should not be disclosed without proper authorization. Any unauthorized disclosure by Employees/Interns/Observers could render the Clinic liable for damages on grounds of defamation or invasion of privacy.

Any Employee/Intern/Observer who violates the confidentiality of medical, employee-related information, or Clinic business operations is subject to serious disciplinary action, up to and including immediate termination from employment/internship or right to observe. I further understand that I could be subject to legal action. I am also obligated to report to the human resource manager any violations of this policy of which I am aware.

I certify by my signature that I have read and agree to comply with this confidentiality statement as well as Clinic Notice of Privacy practices.

Date: _____

Signature: _____

Original to be placed in employee's permanent personnel file, Copy to be placed in orientation and training session file.

---

goals are and ask yourself if your company may be able to help meet those goals. Ask for examples of when he/she provided great customer service, as well as times when his/her ideas conflicted with those of his/her teammates or supervisors. Solicit in-depth answers from the candidate. Don't allow yes/no answers for questions that require more detailed responses. Ask follow-up questions that may solicit the actual information that you are seeking. Pay attention to the candidate's grammar, tone, and overall communication skills. The way you perceive him/her at this first meeting will probably be the way your patients perceive him/her. Make sure this perception will reflect well on your practice.

▶ Step 4: Clinical shadowing—After signing a confidentiality agreement (Sidebar B-1), have the candidate shadow in the clinic to give him/her an idea of the day-to-day life of a technician. The shadowing experience can last for an hour or two, just to expose the potential hire to clinic flow and function, and how a technician is expected to interact with patients. Encourage candidates to ask questions of your staff. You'll also want to make sure that you have the interviewee shadow a more experienced technician who is skilled, knowledgeable, and very comfortable in the exam room. You want your candidate to have a great experience without jeopardizing the quality of the patients' experience during the shadowing process. A senior tech who is part of your training team will be able to handle this process better than someone who is relatively new to the clinic.

▶ Step 5: Post-shadowing interview—In person or over the phone, asking the candidate about the experience while observing in the clinic can give you an idea of whether or not he/she may enjoy the patient interaction and the clinic. This should also give you an idea of the level of enthusiasm present in the potential hire.

This process may sound time-consuming and intensive, even overkill. But when weighed against the possibility of hiring someone who will not make it through a few weeks or months at your company, you can see that reducing turnover in the "pre-hiring" stages is the wisest and least time-consuming option.

Overall, you want to hire someone who will treat every patient as if he/she is the only patient of the day. You want someone who will reflect the goals and values of your company and will be a shining example of customer service and patient care. Notice this in your day-to-day life. You can see these qualities in the barista at your local coffee shop, in the waitress who serves your lunch, or in your child care provider. Your goal should be to employ people who not only want to work, but who will bring enthusiasm and energy to their day. That energy and enthusiasm will translate to patients and boost customer service.

THE TRAINING PLAN

There are a multitude of deterrents that clinics and staff experience during a training program. One of the biggest mistakes is to "wing it." When you do not have a guideline for training, things tend to slip through the cracks, and oftentimes, adequate training is not provided. A new technician cannot be successful without appropriate training, both in skills and ophthalmic/optometric knowledge. You may teach technicians to perform refractometry, but until they understand basic optics, it will continue to be an exercise in moving a dial. (*"So what if the refraction is -1.00 more than Mr. Jones walked in here with? He sees 20/20, either way."*)

In designing a plan for your program, first outline your goals for the training (Sidebar B-2). As Dr. Stephen Covey, author and motivational speaker often stated, you should "begin with the end in mind."[1] What is your desired outcome when a tech "graduates" from training? For most clinics, the need for a skilled technician is what drives the program, and this goal molds the direction of training. For example, a desired outcome could be a technician who has knowledge of anatomy, physiology, ocular and systemic diseases, pharmacology, optics, eye examinations, specialty testing, scribing, coding, and basic surgical assisting. In addition, the student will need to learn skills, clinical protocols and expectations, and basic professional office behavior.

For a training program to be fruitful, you cannot shortchange it. It is unrealistic to shove everything you need to teach new techs into 2 weeks. Depending on how much time will be devoted to straight training, you should allow several weeks. Some clinics may stretch that a bit, but again, the time frame can be adjusted as desired/needed. Just beware of shortening it too much. You'll cheat and discourage your new techs, and ultimately yourself and the practice, if you do. Make sure to reevaluate your timeline after each "class" of new techs to see what, if any, adjustments should be made.

A reasonable time frame for this venture should be between 6 to 10 weeks, depending on your training format. If you can spare 8 hours a day, 5 days a week, a new tech can be knowledgeable and adequately skilled in 8 weeks or less. Many clinics do not have the luxury of giving all day, every day, to train new staff, so longer training programs will suit the practice better. Find a workable option for your company by outlining your plans and then learn from those outlines. Your first "class" will teach you like no other! You'll know if your notions are achievable or if you are overshooting reality.

To avoid potential pitfalls, be sure to outline your training program. Have a list of goals to be met by the end of the week. For example:

SIDEBAR B-2
A PRO'S PERSPECTIVE

"My first goal when entering into a training period with new techs is to spark a love of ophthalmology in them. To watch the face of a trainee hearing how we detected a brain tumor by a visual field test or an aneurysm by finding a third nerve palsy is exciting. Amid the wonder that they display, you can often see the future of ophthalmology and the possibilities of where their careers will take them."

Week 1:

▶ Day 1: Orientation, tour of clinic, and shadow trainer

▶ Day 2: Computer orientation, electronic health record training, visual acuity training

▶ Day 3: Begin chief complaint training, follow trainer throughout examinations

▶ Day 4: Textbook: Start covering basic ophthalmic technician skills, anatomy and physiology; use computer-based learning to reinforce topics of anatomy, physiology, and eye examination

▶ Day 5: Perform chief complaints with trainer observation, perform visual acuities with trainer observing

In order to stay on track, consider using checklists for your training program. (Sample skill evaluation sheets can be found at the end of this appendix.) These checklists could be given to the trainee for the trainer to complete. Every skill that is mastered should be verified by the trainer and possibly the manager. Checklists will also help trainees realize exactly how far they've come and what they've accomplished in a short period of time.

Templates can also be useful. From learning about surgical procedures (Table B-1) to mastering terminology, you can design your own that will be customized to your trainees.

A combined approach of book study and clinical skills training is the best format. While the bulk of the training will be teaching clinical skills, teaching only skills is a mistake. Physicians want technicians who can process the information they gather and make informed decisions on how to proceed with the eye examination. If you simply teach skills, you lose that critical thinking portion of the examination. You can train skills quickly and efficiently, but staff will not learn anatomy, physiology, etc. They will not be able to complete a thorough work-up with a patient or answer many of the patient's questions.

In addition to a great textbook, you should gather other teaching materials for your students. A packet of patient educational materials, a list of clinical abbreviations, a history of your company, and any outside articles

TABLE B-1
TEMPLATE FOR LEARNING ABOUT OPHTHALMIC SURGICAL PROCEDURES

Procedure:
Indication(s):
Risks:
Benefits:
Preoperative tests and measurements:
Notes on surgery (special instruments, anesthesia, etc):
Postoperative patient education
     Eye care:
     Ocular medications:
     Restrictions:
     Warnings:
Postoperative evaluation
     What normal looks like:
     Tests and measurements:

or other resources pertinent to training will be helpful tools. A model eye, preferably with parts that are removable, is key. Many people are visual learners so being able to point out anatomical structures will be helpful.

Make sure you have a quiet area for teaching/study, ideally outside of the clinical area, if possible. You will want to schedule this time as well. Most likely you will allocate more resources to clinical skills training, so you will need to utilize the "out of clinic" hours to their fullest advantage. Consider writing quizzes for the new techs. This will show you how much information is being retained throughout the training period and process. In addition, testing will encourage staff to take time for self-study and to pay attention to what they are being taught.

Be open to new ideas. After each cycle of training, you will probably find that your training program has evolved from its original format. The beauty of creating a training program is that you can allow this development and progression. Each group of new students will show you gaps and strengths in the program and will allow for a more complete course for the next set of trainees. For example, maybe you find that you should switch the order of learning and teach the basics of comprehensive eye exams before optics training, if trainees are quickly learning the components of an eye exam before they fully understand refractometry.

TRAINING AND THE REST OF THE STAFF

You must have overall staff and doctor buy-in for training to be successful. One of the best things about staff being on board with training is that experienced techs can assist, answer questions, and doublecheck results for newer techs when needed.

Selection of trainers is very important to the overall process. Ask experienced techs if they have a desire to help with training and building the training program. You will want to find technicians who are not only skilled, but who are enthusiastic about eye care, your company, and being a technician. Solicit input from those on the floor everyday who will be working alongside the new techs. They should be more than willing to help further the efficiency and education of the team. In addition, new technicians usually look to their trainers as career-long mentors. Make sure that they have great examples to look up to!

Doctors who are brought into the training process are doctors who can envision the desired outcome. The technician they are teaching today is the tech who will sustain their practice in the future, one that they will be able to rely on, and one whose test results they trust. Present the training program and request that the doctors give feedback to new staff. Technicians appreciate hearing from the physicians. It also boosts the techs' confidence to have the doctors take time to invest in them and their careers.

CLOSING REMARKS

As you dive into training new staff, don't overlook the continuing education and training of long-term technicians. A refresher of basics, as well as growing the current knowledge base of experienced techs, will keep your team engaged and strong. Review the fundamentals of checking anterior chamber angles, have a class on refractometry troubleshooting, or discuss the building of a good chief complaint. Review new technology at a staff meeting. Discuss more complete charting in electronic medical records. Ask the physician to talk about emergency protocols. Anything to further training and evolve the team will be beneficial to your staff and your patients. There will be days in a busy practice when it seems easier to let training fall by the wayside, but you must be diligent to pursue time to train new staff. New techs will one day be your "pillar techs," so you have to give them the foundation they need. True, some days may seem monotonous, but if you foster a sense of excitement for their careers, new techs retain the "what if" of the exam: "What if today I find an APD that helps diagnose a tumor?" "What if today I do a visual field that confirms a stroke?" "What if today I see a postop corneal transplant patient who can now read 20/30 instead of 20/200?" Every day in eye care, we have that potential. Amid all the in-depth learning about our fascinating optical system, the core of the training program should be to keep techs engaged in their jobs and to cultivate a spirit of learning and growth.

With an increased need for trained eye care personnel, you will likely have a harder time finding certified (or even well-trained!) techs. Make sure you work hard to develop a training program that will continue to flourish and supply your office with new team members for years to come.

REFERENCE

1. Covey S. *The Seven Habits of Highly Effective People: Powerful Lessons in Personal Change.* London, England: Simon and Schuster; 1989.

HISTORY		
Task: History Taking	**Satisfactory**	**Unsatisfactory**
States purpose/scope of task ▸ To answer the question "Why are you here? How can we help you today?" ▸ To provide practitioner with necessary information about the reason(s) for patient's visit		
Cites situations indicating need for task ▸ Required for every visit		
Patient preparation/education ▸ Establish rapport ▸ Assurance of confidentiality		
Self-preparation ▸ Eye contact ▸ Body language ▸ Speaks clearly		

Performs steps of procedure
▸ Chief complaint
▸ History of present illness
  • Frequency
  • Onset
  • Location
  • Duration
  • Associated signs and symptoms
  • Relief
  • Severity
▸ Past ophthalmic history (diseases, disorders, injuries, surgeries, treatments, refractive correction)
▸ General medical history
  • Review of systems (including systemic diseases/disorders)
  • Past surgical history
  • Current medications
  • Allergies
▸ Social history
▸ Family history		

Documentation ▸ Accurately records patient's responses to questions ▸ Provides record of reason for patient's visit ▸ Helps establish exam level		
NOTES:		

VISUAL ASSESSMENT		
Task: Distant Visual Acuity Testing	**Satisfactory**	**Unsatisfactory**
States purpose/scope of distant visual acuity testing ▶ To determine patient's vision in each eye at a 20 foot/6 meter distance		
Cites situations indicating need for test ▶ Every exam/appointment ▶ Prior to any procedures		
Patient preparation/education ▶ Explanation of procedure ▶ With and/or without correction		
Identifies/prepares proper equipment ▶ Disinfected occluder ▶ Distant vision chart		
Performs steps of procedure ▶ Selects appropriate optotype ▶ Proper test distance ▶ Proper occlusion ▶ Appropriate encouragement to identify smallest optotype possible ▶ Uses pinhole as appropriate		
Performs appropriate disposal/processing/cleaning ▶ Disinfects occluder		
Documentation ▶ Records accurately ▶ Includes appropriate notations (eg, test used, alterations in test distance, patient cooperation)		
NOTES:		

VISUAL ASSESSMENT		
Task: Pinhole Test	**Satisfactory**	**Unsatisfactory**
States purpose/scope of the pinhole test ▶ To determine if subnormal vision is due to refractive error or possibly to pathology		
Cites situations indicating need for the pinhole test ▶ Situations where patient's vision is not as good as expected ▶ Establish baseline acuity that can be expected with refractometry ▶ Per clinic protocol		
Patient preparation/education ▶ Explanation/instruction of procedure		
Identifies/prepares proper equipment ▶ Disinfected occluder ▶ Disinfected pinhole		
Performs steps of procedure ▶ Proper occlusion of fellow eye ▶ Appropriate encouragement to identify smallest optotype possible		
Performs appropriate disposal/processing/cleaning ▶ Disinfects pinhole/occluder		
Documentation ▶ Records accurately ▶ Includes appropriate notations (eg, that pinhole was used, patient cooperation)		
NOTES:		

VISUAL ASSESSMENT		
Task: Near Acuity Testing	**Satisfactory**	**Unsatisfactory**
States purpose/scope of near acuity testing ► To determine patient's vision for near tasks		
Cites situations indicating need for near acuity testing ► Complete eye exams ► When patient is having near vision problems ► Per clinic protocol		
Patient preparation/education ► Explanation of procedure ► Uses any existing near vision correction (eg, bifocals, reading glasses, over-the-counter readers)		
Identifies/prepares proper equipment ► Disinfected occluder ► Appropriate near card ► Tape measure		
Performs steps of procedure ► Selects appropriate optotype ► Occludes properly ► Maintains proper distance ► Makes sure patient is using proper part of multifocal, if worn		
Performs appropriate disposal/processing/cleaning ► Disinfects occluder		
Documentation ► Records accurately ► Includes appropriate notations (eg, test used, alterations in test distance, patient cooperation)		
NOTES:		

VISUAL ASSESSMENT		
Task: Vision Testing With Allen Cards	**Satisfactory**	**Unsatisfactory**
States purpose/scope of test		
▶ Method of distance acuity testing that uses pictures of common objects		
Cites situations indicating need for test		
▶ Patients who are unable to identify numbers or letters but who can identify common objects/pictures		
Patient preparation/education		
▶ Explanation of procedure		
▶ Verify patient's identification of each picture		
Identifies/prepares proper equipment		
▶ Allen cards		
▶ Disinfected occluder		
▶ Measure/estimation of patient's distance from target		
Performs steps of procedure		
▶ Proper room lighting		
▶ Identification of correct eye to test first		
• Right eye, by convention		
• An amblyopic eye		
▶ Maintains proper occlusion (parent to assist, if appropriate)		
▶ Appropriate patient encouragement		
Performs appropriate disposal/processing/cleaning		
▶ Disinfects occluder		
Documentation		
▶ Accurately records testing distance		
▶ Records farthest distance where pictures are identified accurately		
NOTES:		

PUPILLARY ASSESSMENT		
Task: Pupil Evaluation, Reaction to Light	**Satisfactory**	**Unsatisfactory**
States purpose/scope of pupil evaluation ▶ To evaluate the neurological connections between the eye and brain		
Cites situations indicating need for pupil evaluation ▶ Complete eye exams ▶ Prior to any dilation ▶ Neurological work-up		
Patient preparation/education ▶ Explanation of procedure		
Identifies/prepares proper equipment ▶ Pen/muscle light		

Performs steps of procedure
▶ Dims lights appropriately
▶ Provides distant fixation point
▶ Performs direct pupil evaluation of each eye
  • Notes pupil reaction
  • Notes pupil size
  • Notes pupil shape
▶ Performs consensual pupil evaluation/swinging flashlight test
  • Swings flashlight from one eye directly to the other (ie, without a pause in between)		

Documentation
▶ Documents pupil sizes
▶ Documents any anomalies in pupil shape
▶ Documents pupillary anomalies
  • Marcus Gunn/afferent pupillary defect
    ▪ By direct observation of affected pupil
    ▪ By reverse (observation of unaffected pupil)
  • Horner's syndrome
  • Tonic pupil		

NOTES:		

PUPILLARY ASSESSMENT		
Task: Pupillary Accommodative Response	**Satisfactory**	**Unsatisfactory**
States purpose/scope of test		
▶ To evaluate pupils for light-near disparity		
Cites situations indicating need for test		
▶ To differentiate tonic pupils		
Patient preparation/education		
▶ Explanation of procedure		
Identifies/prepares proper equipment		
▶ Distant target		
▶ Accommodative target		
Performs steps of procedure		
▶ Uniform room lighting		
▶ Observes pupils as patient looks at distant target		
▶ Observes pupils as patient switches to look at near target		
▶ Repeat as necessary for evaluation		
· Does each pupil contract at near and expand at distance?		
· Do pupils contract and expand at same rate/to same size?		
▶ Compare near response to light response		
Documentation		
▶ Accurate notations regarding findings		
NOTES:		

OCULAR MOTILITY		
Task: Cover/Uncover Test	**Satisfactory**	**Unsatisfactory**
States purpose/scope of test ▸ To determine the presence of a strabismus and its direction		
Cites situations indicating need for test ▸ Complete eye exams ▸ Pediatric work-ups ▸ Patients complaining of diplopia		
Patient preparation/education ▸ Explanation of procedure ▸ Full correction, if worn, for both near and/or distance		
Identifies/prepares proper equipment ▸ Distant and near acuity charts ▸ Disinfected occluder		

Performs steps of procedure
▸ Selection of appropriate target
▸ Properly covers then uncovers one eye
▸ Monitors patient fixation
▸ Accurately identifies direction of deviation
▸ Accurately differentiates between
  • Tropia
  • Phoria
▸ Accurately identifies
  • Any fixation preference
  • Intermittent vs constant
▸ Selects and performs additional tests as indicated by results		

Performs appropriate disposal/processing/cleaning ▸ Disinfects occluder		
Documentation ▸ Accurately records test results		
NOTES:		

Ocular Motility		
Task: Cross/Cover Test	**Satisfactory**	**Unsatisfactory**
States purpose/scope of cross/cover test		
► To identify presence and direction of deviation		
Cites situations indicating need for cross-cover test		
► Complete eye exams		
► Pediatric work-ups		
► Patients complaining of diplopia		
Patient preparation/education		
► Explanation of procedure		
► Full correction, if worn, for both near and/or distance		
Identifies/prepares proper equipment		
► Distant and near acuity charts		
► Disinfected occluder		
Performs steps of procedure		
► Selection of appropriate target		
► Properly covers one eye then rapidly shifts cover to the other eye, not allowing binocular fixation in between		
► Monitors patient fixation		
► Accurately identifies presence of:		
• Ortho-		
• Eso-		
• Exo-		
• Hyper-		
• Hypo-		
► Appropriately initiates further testing to discern between tropia and phoria		
Performs appropriate disposal/processing/cleaning		
► Disinfects occluder		
Documentation		
► Accurately documents presence and direction of deviation		
NOTES:		

OCULAR MOTILITY		
Task: Krimsky Measurement	**Satisfactory**	**Unsatisfactory**
States purpose/scope of test ▶ Provides a measurement of the amount of strabismic deviation		
Cites situations indicating need for test ▶ Situations where measuring with prism and cover is not feasible		
Patient preparation/education ▶ Explanation of procedure		
Identifies/prepares proper equipment ▶ Fixation/muscle light ▶ Prisms		
Performs steps of procedure ▶ Monitors patient's fixation on muscle light ▶ Performs initial evaluation of reflex position, accurately identifying presence of: 　• Ortho- 　• Eso- 　• Exo- 　• Hyper- 　• Hypo- ▶ Selects prism 　• Prism base placed appropriately 　• Adjusts prism power until reflexes are positioned equally		
Documentation ▶ Documents type of measurement done ▶ Documents prism diopter of estimate ▶ Documents direction of deviation		
NOTES:		

OCULAR MOTILITY		
Task: Hirschberg Measurement	**Satisfactory**	**Unsatisfactory**
States purpose/scope of test		
▶ Provides estimate of the amount of a strabismic deviation		
Cites situations indicating need for test		
▶ Situations where measuring with prisms is not possible or feasible		
Patient preparation/education		
▶ Explanation of procedure		
Identifies/prepares proper equipment		
▶ Muscle light		
Performs steps of procedure		
▶ Monitors patient's fixation on muscle light		
▶ Performs initial evaluation of reflex position, accurately identifying presence of:		
• Ortho-		
• Eso-		
• Exo-		
• Hyper-		
• Hypo-		
▶ Appropriately estimates the magnitude of the deviation		
Documentation		
▶ Documents type of measurement done		
▶ Documents direction of deviation		
▶ Calculates approximate prism diopter of estimate		
NOTES:		

OCULAR MOTILITY		
Task: Measuring Strabismus With Prism	**Satisfactory**	**Unsatisfactory**
States purpose/scope of test		
▶ To measure/quantify strabismic deviations		
Cites situations indicating need for test		
▶ Strabismus detected on cover testing for extraocular muscle evaluation		
▶ Pre-and postoperative strabismus surgery measurements		
Patient preparation/education		
▶ Explanation of procedure		
Identifies/prepares proper equipment		
▶ Disinfected occluder		
▶ Appropriate distant/near target(s)		
▶ Prisms (loose, bar, Risley)		
Performs steps of procedure		
▶ Determines direction of prism base		
▶ Utilizes appropriate target		
▶ Properly employs cross/cover		
▶ Adds/subtracts prism until null point achieved		
Performs appropriate disposal/processing/cleaning		
▶ Disinfects occluder		
Documentation		
▶ Accurately records prism power		
▶ Accurately records direction of base		
NOTES:		

OCULAR MOTILITY		
Task: Amblyopia Therapy: Parent/Patient Education	**Satisfactory**	**Unsatisfactory**
States purpose/scope of task		
▶ To educate parents (and patient, if appropriate) regarding the purpose and method of amblyopia therapy		
Cites situations indicating need for task		
▶ When initiating and during amblyopia treatment		
Identifies/prepares proper equipment		
▶ Handouts		
▶ Samples (patch, occluder, drops, etc) for demonstration/dispensing		
▶ Optotype samples for at-home practice as appropriate		
Performs steps of procedure		
▶ Explains amblyopia and importance of therapy		
▶ Explains goals of therapy		
▶ Explains and demonstrates method of therapy		
▶ Answers parent questions		
▶ Offers encouragement and clinic's support		
Documentation		
▶ Records in chart		
· Type of education		
· Who was present		
· Materials given		
NOTES:		

OCULAR MOTILITY		
Task: Range of Motion Test	**Satisfactory**	**Unsatisfactory**
States purpose/scope of test ▶ To evaluate the movement of the extraocular muscles		
Cites situations indicating need for test ▶ Complete eye exams ▶ Extraocular muscle evaluations ▶ Pediatric exams ▶ Facial trauma ▶ Patient complaints of diplopia ▶ Patient complaints of pain when moving eyes		

Patient preparation/education
▶ Explain procedure
   • Keep head still
   • Follow light with eyes		

Identifies/prepares proper equipment ▶ Appropriate target/muscle light		
Performs steps of procedure ▶ Observes light reflexes in primary gaze ▶ Moves light to diagnostic positions of gaze ▶ Monitors patient head position ▶ Initiates further testing as appropriate		
Documentation ▶ Records that test was done ▶ Accurately records any irregularities in position ▶ Accurately records any pattern ▶ Records any irregularities in movement ▶ Notes any patient complaints of pain		
NOTES:		

OCULAR MOTILITY		
Task: Stereo Testing	**Satisfactory**	**Unsatisfactory**
States purpose/scope of stereo testing		
▶ To evaluate/quantify fusion		
Cites situations indicating need for stereo testing		
▶ Extraocular muscle evaluations		
▶ Pediatric exams		
▶ Patient complaints about "depth perception"		
▶ Aid in differentiating between small phoria and tropia		
Patient preparation/education		
▶ Habitual correction worn, if any		
▶ Polarized glasses worn over habitual correction		
▶ Keep both eyes opened		
Identifies/prepares proper equipment		
▶ Polarized glasses (disinfected at areas of patient contact)		
▶ Testing plates/booklet		
Performs steps of procedure		
▶ Stereo testing done prior to any other tests that would break fusion		
▶ Glasses properly placed		
▶ Target(s) properly introduced		
▶ Appropriate encouragement to "guess" next level		
Performs appropriate disposal/processing/cleaning		
▶ Polarized glasses disinfected on points of patient contact		
Documentation		
▶ Accurately records seconds of arc		
▶ Makes any pertinent notes (eg, "patient won't touch fly")		
NOTES:		

OCULAR MOTILITY		
Task: Near Point of Convergence	**Satisfactory**	**Unsatisfactory**
States purpose/scope of test ▶ To screen for convergence insufficiency		
Cites situations indicating need for test ▶ Pediatric eye exams ▶ Patient symptoms • Trouble concentrating when reading • Slow reading • Avoidance of near tasks • Asthenopia • Eyes tire with near tasks		
Patient preparation/education ▶ Explanation of procedure ("Try to keep the target from going double")		
Identifies/prepares proper equipment ▶ Appropriate near target		
Performs steps of procedure ▶ Gradually brings target closer • Objective: Observes when one eye finally looses fixation and drifts • Subjective: Patient states when target has doubled ▶ Accurately estimates or measures distance where binocular fixation is lost		
Documentation ▶ Properly documents findings in patient record		
NOTES:		

OPTOMETRIC/SPECTACLE SKILLS		
Task: Manual Lensometry	**Satisfactory**	**Unsatisfactory**
States purpose/scope of task		
▶ To evaluate and ascertain the prescription/prism in a pair of spectacles		
Cites situations indicating need for task		
▶ Full exams		
▶ Refractive exams		
▶ Refractive problems		
▶ Glasses problems		
Identifies/prepares proper equipment		
▶ Lensometer		
Performs steps of procedure		
▶ Adjusts/focuses eyepiece		
▶ Identifies multifocal		
▶ Properly places spectacles on stage		
▶ Identifies presence of cylinder; properly reads in + or − cylinder as per clinic protocol		
▶ Accurately notes sphere, cylinder, and axis readings		
▶ Identifies presence of prism		
• Direction of base		
• Strength of prism		
• Ground-in or decentered		
▶ Repositions properly to read add		
▶ Accurately notes power of add		
Performs appropriate disposal/processing/cleaning		
▶ Cleans patient's glasses		
Documentation		
▶ Accurately records findings		
• Cylinder power and axis if present		
• Multifocal power and type if present		
• Prism base and power if present		
NOTES:		

OPTOMETRIC/SPECTACLE SKILLS		
Task: Finding/Marking Lens Centers	**Satisfactory**	**Unsatisfactory**
States purpose/scope of task ▶ To locate and identify the optical center(s) of prescription lens(es)		
Cites situations indicating need for task ▶ To aid in proper alignment of lenses/frames ▶ To aid in proper alignment of prescribed induced prism ▶ Troubleshooting spectacle problems involving diplopia and/or asthenopia		
Identifies/prepares proper equipment ▶ Lensometer		
Performs steps of procedure ▶ Adjusts instrument eyepiece ▶ Places spectacles properly on stage ▶ Properly centers mires ▶ Lenses dotted by using marking device on instrument ▶ In case of progessive addition lenses, uses proper template to mark lens landmarks prior to reading and marking with lensometer ▶ Uses millimeter rule to measure distance between optical centers		
Performs appropriate disposal/processing/cleaning ▶ Cleans patient's glasses		
Documentation ▶ Properly documents distance between optical centers ▶ Accurately calculates induced prism, if required		
NOTES:		

OPTOMETRIC/SPECTACLE SKILLS		
Task: Pupillary Distance (Manual)	**Satisfactory**	**Unsatisfactory**
States purpose/scope of test		
▶ To provide measurement necessary to properly align spectacle lenses		
Cites situations indicating need for test		
▶ Patients receiving a spectacle prescription as per clinic protocol		
▶ Patients having glasses problems		
• Diplopia (decentration)		
• "Pulling" (decentration)		
Patient preparation/education		
▶ Explanation of procedure		
Identifies/prepares proper equipment		
▶ Penlight (if needed)		
▶ Millimeter rule		
Performs steps of procedure		
▶ Proper distance from patient (about 16 inches)		
▶ Properly positions millimeter rule		
▶ Monitors patient fixation		
▶ Takes reading at center of pupils or outside to inside limbus		
Documentation		
▶ Accurately documents reading in millimeters		
NOTES:		

OPTOMETRIC/SPECTACLE SKILLS

Task: Vertex Distance	Satisfactory	Unsatisfactory
States purpose/scope of test ▶ To measure distance between the surface of the eye and the back surface of spectacle lens		
Cites situations indicating need for measuring vertex distance ▶ A change in vertex distance that changes the effective power of the lens ▶ High-powered spectacle lenses (±4.00 or higher; some references say ±3.00 or higher) ▶ Contact lens power conversions ▶ Situations where patient wears spectacles farther from the eye than usual		

Patient preparation/education
▶ Explanation of procedure
  • Must keep eyes shut
  • Will feel instrument foot gently touch upper lid		

Identifies/prepares proper equipment ▶ Distometer • Disinfected points of patient contact		
Performs steps of procedure ▶ Spectacles worn in habitual position ▶ Patient's eyes are gently closed • In cases of dermatochalasis, extra fold of skin is lifted up out of the way ▶ Properly places instrument foot gently on lid ▶ Depresses plunger, takes reading on gauge ▶ Repeats for other eye		
Performs appropriate disposal/processing/cleaning ▶ Properly disinfects points of patient contact on distometer		
Documentation ▶ Properly records measurement for each eye		
NOTES:		

OPTOMETRIC/SPECTACLE SKILLS

Task: Writing Glasses Prescriptions	Satisfactory	Unsatisfactory
States purpose/scope of task		
▶ To provide patient with a prescription for spectacle lenses		
Cites situations indicating need of task		
▶ Only as directed by practitioner		
Patient preparation/education		
▶ Prescription expiration date		
▶ Not for contact lenses		
▶ Verify address if Rx to be mailed		
Identifies/prepares proper equipment		
▶ Office prescription form		
Performs steps of procedure		
▶ Identifies standard form used by clinic		
▶ Properly transcribes sphere, cylinder power, and axis		
▶ Properly transcribes add(s) for multifocal, if appropriate		
▶ Properly transcribes prism power and direction, if appropriate		
▶ Makes appropriate notations on Rx (eg, for reading only, postoperative glasses, increase by +0.25 if progressive addition lenses)		
▶ Obtains practitioner's signature		
▶ Appropriately releases Rx to patient/optician		
Documentation		
▶ Accurately records in chart that Rx was given/released and to whom		
NOTES:		

OPTOMETRIC/SPECTACLE SKILLS		
Task: Near Point of Accommodation and Accommodative Amplitude	**Satisfactory**	**Unsatisfactory**
States purpose/scope of test ▶ To quantify the amount of accommodation a patient has		
Cites situations indicating need for test ▶ Patients in pre-presbyopic and early presbyopic ages		
Patient preparation/education ▶ Patient instructed to report when letters *first* begin to blur (will still be able to read them)		

Identifies/prepares proper equipment
▶ Refractor
   • Disinfected points of patient contact
   • Best distance correction in place
   • Both apertures open
▶ Prince rule
▶ Rotating near chart		

Performs steps of procedure ▶ Reading card is gradually brought closer until patient reports blurring ▶ Asks if patient can "force your eyes to focus?" ▶ Accurately interprets endpoint		
Performs appropriate disposal/processing/cleaning ▶ Disinfects points of patient contact on refractor		
Documentation ▶ Accurately records near point of accommodation in inches or centimeters and/or ▶ Records accommodative amplitude in diopters		
NOTES:		

VISUAL FIELD ASSESSMENT		
Task: Confrontation Visual Fields	**Satisfactory**	**Unsatisfactory**
States purpose/scope of test ▶ Rough screening of peripheral vision 　• General idea of whether or not the external limitations are grossly normal 　• General idea of where any defects may be located ▶ Does not quantify, generally does not identify scotomas ▶ Not adequate for glaucoma diagnosis/management		
Cites situations indicating need for test ▶ Part of a routine eye exam ▶ Required for driving and other licenses/certifications/applications ▶ Patient complaints of field loss ▶ On testing visual acuity, patient consistently eliminates optotypes in certain areas of the chart (eg, patient does not report seeing first several optotypes on the left of each acuity line) ▶ As indicated by medical diagnoses (eg, pituitary tumor, stroke) ▶ As indicated by patient complaints (eg, light flashes, floaters, other retinal detachment symptoms)		
Patient preparation/education ▶ Explanation of procedure ▶ Proper occlusion ▶ Proper fixation ▶ Primary gaze ▶ Proper head position		
Performs steps of procedure ▶ Recognize possible physical restrictions (nose, brows) ▶ Selects appropriate target ▶ If kinetic: 　• Moves from nonseeing to seeing 　• Moves target at uniform speed ▶ If static: 　• Holds hand/target stationary at appropriate distance from patient ▶ Checks all four quadrants of each eye ▶ Further testing as appropriate		
Documentation ▶ Properly diagrams defects in written chart ▶ Properly describes defects in electronic health record		
NOTES:		

VISUAL FIELD ASSESSMENT

Task: Amsler Grid	Satisfactory	Unsatisfactory
States purpose/scope of test ▶ Evaluation of the central 10 degrees of peripheral vision		

Cites situations indicating need for test
▶ Patients with macular degeneration
▶ Patient complaints/symptoms
  • Missing letters when reading
  • Straight lines appear wavy
  • Areas of missing vision near center
  • Changes on patient's home-testing Amsler grid		

Patient preparation/education ▶ Explanation of procedure • Look at center dot and hold fixation there		
Identifies/prepares proper equipment ▶ Disinfected occluder/patch ▶ Amsler grid chart ▶ Pen/pencil ▶ Patient's habitual correction for near		

Performs steps of procedure
▶ Proper use of optical correction for near
▶ Proper distance for use of grid
▶ Proper occlusion
▶ Monitor patient fixation
▶ Asks patient relevant questions
  • Can you see the center dot?
  • As you look at the dot, are you aware of all four corners?
  • Are all the lines straight and square?
  • Is any area of the grid blocked out or missing?
▶ Has patient sketch any anomalies on grid		

Performs appropriate disposal/processing/cleaning ▶ Disinfects occluder/patch		
Documentation ▶ Patient demographics, date, eye tested ▶ Grid added to paper chart ▶ Description of results if electronic record		
NOTES:		

VISUAL FIELD ASSESSMENT		
Task: Automated Perimetry	**Satisfactory**	**Unsatisfactory**
States purpose/scope of test		
▶ To quantify and qualify patient's peripheral vision		
Cites situations indicating need for test		
▶ Glaucoma diagnosis		
▶ Glaucoma follow-up		
▶ Evaluate field defects identified on confrontation testing		
▶ Patient complaint of field loss		
▶ Neurological testing		
▶ Patient taking medication that can affect the retina/optic nerve		
▶ Patient with pituitary tumors and brain disorders		
▶ Patient with certain systemic diseases (multiple sclerosis, etc)		
Patient preparation/education		
▶ Explanation of procedure		
▶ Appropriately selects which eye to test first		
▶ Eye patch applied properly		
▶ Properly positions patient		
▶ Properly positions trial lens(es), if used		
▶ Eyelid taped, if necessary or appropriate		
▶ Appropriate fixation target selected		
Identifies/prepares proper equipment		
▶ Perimeter		
• Points of patient contact properly disinfected		
• Printer paper, storage media/discs		
• Instrument calibrated (self-calibration cycle)		
• Patient information entered properly		
• Appropriate test selected		
▶ Disinfected eye patch		
▶ Disinfected signaling device		
▶ Trial lens set (thin-rimmed, clean)		
▶ Appropriate trial lens(es) inserted		
▶ Appropriate patient seating		
Performs steps of procedure		
▶ Runs demo test as appropriate		
▶ Monitors fixation/alignment		
▶ Appropriately encourages patient periodically		
▶ Changes/removes trial lens(es) as appropriate		
▶ Troubleshoots common problems		
• Repeated fixation loss		
• Instrument cannot find blind spot		
• Head movement		
• Upper lid obstructing field		
• Excessive false positives/false negatives		
• Slow patient reaction time		
▶ Changes testing strategy as appropriate		

(continued)

VISUAL FIELD ASSESSMENT		
Task: Automated Perimetry (continued)	**Satisfactory**	**Unsatisfactory**
Performs appropriate disposal/processing/cleaning ▶ Points of patient contact properly disinfected ▶ Trial lenses cleaned as appropriate ▶ Eye patch properly disinfected ▶ Signaling device properly disinfected ▶ Test properly saved on instrument and disc		
Documentation ▶ Appropriate printout selected ▶ Appropriate notations made concerning patient (cooperation, excessive movement, etc)		
NOTES:		

TONOMETRY		
Task: Goldmann Applanation Tonometry	**Satisfactory**	**Unsatisfactory**
States purpose/scope of test		
▶ To quantify intraocular pressure (IOP)		
▶ To aid in diagnosing and following glaucoma		
Cites situations indicating need for test		
▶ Routine eye exams		
▶ Glaucoma follow-up exams		
▶ Patients taking topical steroids		
▶ Per clinic protocol		
Patient preparation/education		
▶ Explanation of procedure		
▶ Instillation of fluorescein/topical anesthetic		
▶ Positioned in slit lamp		
▶ Patient relaxed, breathing gently		
Self-preparation		
▶ Proper hand hygiene or gloving		
Identifies/prepares proper equipment		
▶ Calibration at regular intervals		
▶ Disinfected points of patient contact on slit lamp		
▶ Disinfected tonometer tip		
▶ Tonometer tip turned appropriately if greater than 3 diopters of astigmatism		
Performs steps of procedure		
▶ Topical anesthetic and dye instilled		
▶ Properly positions patient at slit lamp		
▶ Sets instrument to correct magnification, beam height and width, and cobalt blue filter		
▶ Properly positions instrument		
▶ Holds eyelids properly, as appropriate		
▶ Applanates properly		
▶ Monitors patient fixation and breathing		
▶ Turns drum on instrument to obtain reading		
▶ Obtains proper endpoint of mires		
▶ Reads measurement correctly from drum		
▶ Patient reminded not to rub eyes while they are numb		
Performs appropriate disposal/processing/cleaning		
▶ Proper disposal of gloves, if used		
▶ Performs hand hygiene		
▶ Disinfects points of patient contact on slit lamp		
▶ Disinfects tonometer prism as per clinic protocol		
▶ Instrument calibrated regularly		
Documentation		
▶ Accurately records pressure in patient chart		
▶ Notes method of IOP check (ie, "AT" for applanation tonometry)		
▶ Notes time of IOP check		
▶ Other notes as appropriate (eg, patient cooperation, appearance of mires)		
NOTES:		

TONOMETRY		
Task: Tono-Pen Tonometry	**Satisfactory**	**Unsatisfactory**
States purpose/scope of test ▶ To measure intraocular pressure ▶ To screen for glaucoma		
Cites situations indicating need for test ▶ On routine exams as per clinic protocol ▶ Patients who cannot be positioned at slit lamp		
Patient preparation/education ▶ Explanation of procedure ▶ Instills topical anesthetic		
Self-preparation ▶ Proper hand hygiene or gloving		
Identifies/prepares proper equipment ▶ Tono-pen ▶ Tono cover ▶ Topical anesthetic		
Performs steps of procedure ▶ Instrument calibrated regularly ▶ Tono cover properly placed ▶ Instills topical anesthetic ▶ Patient fixating steadily ▶ Proper applanation until reading is obtained ▶ Interprets reliability rating and repeats measurement as needed		
Performs appropriate disposal/processing/cleaning ▶ Proper disposal of gloves, if worn ▶ Proper hand cleansing ▶ Disposal of Tono cover		
Documentation ▶ Enters reading accurately in chart ▶ Notes method of measurement (eg, Tono-pen) ▶ Notes time of measurement		
NOTES:		

ANGLE EVALUATION		
Task: Angle Evaluation (Muscle Light)	**Satisfactory**	**Unsatisfactory**
States purpose/scope of test		
► To ascertain if the angles are open enough to safely dilate pupils		
Cites situations indicating need for test		
► Prior to dilation, if slit lamp is not available		
Patient preparation/education		
► Patient instructed to look at fixation light/target		
Self-preparation (in the event of touching patient)		
► Proper hand hygiene or gloving		
Identifies/prepares proper equipment		
► Muscle light		
Performs steps of procedure		
► Patient fixation in primary gaze		
► Muscle light directed from side: Temporally then nasally		
► Evaluates shadow on iris		
► Properly estimates angle status		
► Identifies narrow, at-risk angles		
► Performs/requests slit lamp evaluation as necessary		
Performs appropriate disposal/processing/cleaning (in the event of touching patient)		
► Proper disposal of gloves, if used		
► Proper cleansing of hands, if patient was touched		
Documentation		
► Notation of test done		
► Notation of technique used		
► Notation of estimate for each eye		
► Notation of further evaluation as necessary		
NOTES:		

ANGLE EVALUATION		
Task: Angle Evaluation (Slit Lamp/Van Herick Method)	**Satisfactory**	**Unsatisfactory**
States purpose/scope of test ▶ To ascertain if the angles are open • To safely dilate patient • To assist in diagnosis of narrow angles • To assist in diagnosis of angle-closure glaucoma		
Cites situations indicating need for test ▶ Prior to instilling dilating drops ▶ In evaluation of painful red eye		
Patient preparation/education ▶ Patient properly and comfortably positioned at slit lamp		
Self-preparation (in the event of touching patient) ▶ Proper hand hygiene or gloving		
Identifies/prepares proper equipment ▶ Slit lamp microscope • Disinfected points of contact on slit lamp		
Performs steps of procedure ▶ Patient fixation in primary gaze ▶ Light directed from 60° temporally, then nasally ▶ Evaluates light/dark interval ▶ Properly identifies angle status ▶ Identifies narrow, at-risk angles ▶ Requests further evaluation as necessary		
Performs appropriate disposal/processing/cleaning ▶ Disinfects points of contact on slit lamp ▶ Proper disposal of gloves, if used ▶ Proper cleansing of hands, if patient was touched		
Documentation ▶ Notation of test done ▶ Notation of technique used ▶ Notation of estimate for each eye ▶ Notation of further evaluation as necessary		
NOTES:		

COLOR VISION TESTING		
Task: Ishihara Color Plate Testing	**Satisfactory**	**Unsatisfactory**
States purpose/scope of test ▶ To determine if a red/green color defect is present ▶ Does not quantify degree of defect		
Cites situations indicating need for test ▶ Pediatric exams according to protocol ▶ Patients who complain of color vision problems ▶ Patients taking medications that can affect color vision ▶ Patients requiring the test for licensing, etc ▶ Per clinic protocol		
Patient preparation/education ▶ Explanation of procedure		
Identifies/prepares proper equipment ▶ Ishihara color plates ▶ Answer key ▶ Disinfected occluder/patch (if appropriate) ▶ Patient wears routine near vision correction		

Performs steps of procedure
▶ Proper room lighting
▶ Selects occlusion appropriately
   • Monocular testing if suspected acquired anomaly
   • Binocular testing if suspected genetic anomaly
▶ Guides patient through viewing plates
▶ Records responses		

Performs appropriate disposal/processing/cleaning ▶ Disinfects occluder/patch (if used)		
Documentation ▶ Notation of test done ▶ Properly documents results (OD and OS, or OU)		
NOTES:		

TEAR TESTING		
Task: Schirmer's Tear Test	**Satisfactory**	**Unsatisfactory**
States purpose/scope of various types of Schirmer's tear tests ▶ Evaluation of tear production 　• Schirmer's Tear Test I: Does not use topical anesthetic, and evaluates reflex tear production (< 10 mm of wetting in 5 minutes is abnormal) 　• Schirmer's Tear Test II: Uses topical anesthetic, and evaluates baseline tear production (< 5 mm of wetting in 5 minutes is abnormal; some consider this test unreliable)		
Cites situations indicating need for test ▶ Diagnosis of dry eye ▶ Before contact lens fitting ▶ Preoperative work-up for plastic surgery ▶ Patient complaints/symptoms		
Patient preparation/education ▶ Explanation of procedure		
Self-preparation ▶ Proper hand hygiene or gloving		
Identifies/prepares proper equipment ▶ Tear strips ▶ Topical anesthetic for Schirmer's Tear Test II ▶ Timer ▶ Millimeter rule		
Performs steps of procedure ▶ Instills topical anesthetic for Schirmer's Tear Test II ▶ Opens strip packet, maintaining sanitation ▶ Folds strip at notch ▶ Inserts strips properly into lower cul-de-sac ▶ Correctly times test ▶ Removes strips at end of testing time ▶ Accurately measures strip wetting using millimeter rule ▶ Identifies test results indicating tearing disorder		
Performs appropriate disposal/processing/cleaning ▶ Proper disposal of gloves, if used ▶ Proper cleansing of hands ▶ Proper disposal of used strips		
Documentation ▶ Records type of test used ▶ Records anesthetic, if used ▶ Accurately records wetting measurements		
NOTES:		

TEAR TESTING

Task: Tear Break-Up Time	Satisfactory	Unsatisfactory
States purpose/scope of test ▶ Evaluation of tear film stability (normal is > 15 seconds)		
Cites situations indicating need for test ▶ Patient complaints suggesting dry eye ▶ Preoperative documentation ▶ Pre-fit evaluation for contact lenses		
Patient preparation/education ▶ Explanation of procedure		
Self-preparation ▶ Proper hand hygiene or gloving		
Identifies/prepares proper equipment ▶ Slit lamp microscope with cobalt filter • Properly disinfected points of patient contact ▶ Fluorescein dye (drops or strips)		
Performs steps of procedure ▶ Properly instills fluorescein ▶ Patient instructed first to blink, then to stare without blinking ▶ Properly times the seconds from last blink to appearance of first dry spots on cornea		
Performs appropriate disposal/processing/cleaning ▶ Proper disposal of gloves, if used ▶ Proper cleansing of hands ▶ Properly disinfected points of patient contact on slit lamp		
Documentation ▶ Accurately records test results		
NOTES:		

SURFACE TISSUE EVALUATION		
Task: Topical Rose Bengal Evaluation	**Satisfactory**	**Unsatisfactory**
States purpose/scope of test ▶ To evaluate for damaged surface tissue (cornea and conjunctiva)		
Cites situations indicating need for test ▶ Diagnosis of dry eye		
Patient preparation/education ▶ Explanation of procedure		
Self-preparation ▶ Proper hand hygiene or gloving		
Identifies/prepares proper equipment ▶ Topical anesthetic (proparacaine 0.5%) ▶ Rose bengal strips or drops ▶ Irrigation fluid ▶ Paper towels/tissues ▶ Slit lamp microscope • Disinfected points of patient contact		
Performs steps of procedure ▶ Properly anesthetizes the eye ▶ Properly introduces rose bengal via drop or strip ▶ Gently irrigates eye after 30 seconds ▶ Observes eye with slit lamp, looking for staining patterns		
Performs appropriate disposal/processing/cleaning ▶ Proper disposal of gloves, if used ▶ Proper cleansing of hands ▶ Proper disposal of used strips and tissues ▶ Disinfected points of patient contact on slit lamp		
Documentation ▶ Accurately describes any staining pattern		
NOTES:		

MEASURING CORNEAL CURVATURE		
Task: Manual Keratometry	**Satisfactory**	**Unsatisfactory**
States purpose/scope of test		
▸ To measure corneal curvature		
Cites situations indicating need for test		
▸ Contact lens fitting		
▸ Intraocular lens calculations		
▸ Evaluate astigmatism		
Patient preparation/education		
▸ Explanation of procedure		
▸ Instillation of artificial tears, if appropriate		
▸ Positions patient at instrument		
▸ Instructs patient to look straight ahead		
Identifies/prepares proper equipment		
▸ Keratometer		
▸ Disinfected points of patient contact		
Performs steps of procedure		
▸ Adjusts/focuses eyepiece		
▸ Patient properly positioned at instrument		
▸ Adjusts patient alignment		
▸ Focuses mires		
▸ Accurately identifies axis		
▸ Properly positions drum and mires		
▸ Monitors patient fixation		
▸ Accurately reads measurement on instrument		
Performs appropriate disposal/processing/cleaning		
▸ Disinfects points of patient contact		
Documentation		
▸ Accurately records readings		
▸ Makes note of any additional findings (eg, blurred mires, patient head movement)		
NOTES:		

C

MEDICAL TERMINOLOGY

John P. Rowan, COMT

The difference between the right word and almost the right word is like the difference between lightning and a lightning bug.
—Mark Twain

Don't be afraid of medical terminology. Just hold on to your hat; here we go.

"Conjunctivitis"—Inflammation of the conjunctiva

"Lensectomy"—Removal of the lens

See? You can do this!

As documentation and coding become more precise and more important, ophthalmic medical personnel need to be well-versed in medical terminology.

You will encounter and use countless medical terms while reviewing or taking a patient's medical history. Similarly, if you scribe for the physician(s) in your office (see Chapter 6), you should know the meanings of the terms that you are asked to write. Or, perhaps you've listened to your boss speaking on the phone with another eye doctor about a patient, and thought, "I've heard these terms he's throwing around, but I'm not really sure what they all mean."

Note: This appendix is not intended to provide every term you might run across; there are books larger than this one devoted to nothing but medical terminology. Rather, we hope that with a good grounding in the fundamentals of how medical terms are constructed, you will be able to understand and use these words correctly and confidently in your work.

WORD PARTS

Note: For the purposes of this appendix and this approach to terminology, we present word parts in different categories. At the end of this appendix there is a chart of common word parts used in eye care.

Think about a couple of medical words you may have known since you were young: "appendectomy" ... "hepatitis" ... You'll notice that these terms are constructed from different parts. Getting a feel for these parts—what they are, what they do, and how they fit together—is the key to becoming comfortable with medical terminology. You will often find that parts of any given term look familiar (Table C-1). That's because many of our words are compound words. In medical terminology, these word parts are often borrowed from other languages (notably Latin and Greek).

The most common parts of a medical term are a *root word*, a *prefix* and/or a *suffix*, and a *combining form*. This is true not just for ophthalmic terminology, but for medical terms of all kinds. From ophthalmology, let's try

Ledford JK, Lens A, eds.
Principles and Practice in Ophthalmic Assisting:
A Comprehensive Textbook (pp 773-778).
© 2018 Taylor & Francis Group.

Word Part	Definition	Think Of	Example(s) in Eye Care
cry-	cold	cryogenics	cryopexy: applying a cryotherapy instrument to the sclera in order to repair or reattach a detached section of the retina by freezing
cyst-	bladder, bag	(having a) cyst	conjunctival cyst: fluid-filled, blister-like lesion on the conjunctiva
extra-	outside of	extracurricular	extraocular: outside the eye … the six extraocular muscles are on the outside surface of the eye
hem-	half	hemisphere	hemianopsia: absence of vision in one-half of the visual field … word parts are "hemi" (half), "an" (absence), "opsia" (seeing)
infra-	beneath, below	infrastructure	infrared: the portion of the electromagnetic spectrum below the visible red part
intra-	within	intramural (sports)	intraocular: within the eye, as in intraocular pressure
neo-	new	neonatal	neovascularization: formation of new blood vessels, such as beneath the retina (wet age-related macular degeneration) or around the edge of the cornea
pan-	all	Pan-American Games	panretinal photocoagulation: laser treatment over a large area of the retina
retr-	behind	retroactive	retrobulbar: behind the eyeball … retrobulbar injections of anesthesia are given to prevent eye movement during ocular surgery
trans-	across	transcontinental	transscleral: across the sclera (as an injection into the eye)
ultra-	beyond, excessive	ultramodern	ultraviolet: just beyond the violet end of the visible portion of the electromagnetic spectrum (ie, higher frequency, shorter wavelength); ultraviolet rays from the sun cause eye damage and skin damage
xer-	dry	Xerox copier	xerophthalmia: dryness (usually extreme) of the ocular surface

Table C-1: Medical Terminology

"cryoretinopexy." As with most terms, the root is in the center: "retin-." The prefix is "cry-," which means "cold" or "freezing." The suffix "-pexy" is "fixation" or "sticking." The term as a whole refers to the use of extreme cold to reattach a loose or detached part of the retina to its original place.

Notice that the combining form "o" appears between "retin-" and "-pexy." The combining form of a medical term is almost always a vowel (in fact, you'll notice that it is usually the letter "o"); it is used mainly to make the overall term pronounceable.

So much for dissection. Now let's go back and look at each term part in detail.

Prefixes

The first part of a multipart term is the *prefix*. Prefixes usually (but not always) indicate some quality of the root word to follow such as location, time, number, color, etc.

For example, think of the prefixes "pre-," "peri-," and "post-." "Pre-" means "before" or "in front of" and is used frequently in everyday speech: "Pre-theater menu," "premature," etc. This prefix can also refer both to time and to location: "Prenatal" refers to the time *before* childbirth; the "precorneal tear film" is *in front of* the cornea. "Peri-" means around: A "periocular" rash is *around* the eye. And finally, "post-" means after: "Postoperative" swelling occurs *after* surgery.

Prefixes Denoting Location or Position

ab-	away from
ad-	toward
amphi-	around, on both sides (of)
ante-	before
apo-	away from

cata-	down, against, back
circum-	around
contra-	against, opposite, counter
dia-	through
ecto-	outside, out
end-, endo-	in, within, inside
ento-	within
epi-	above, on, upon
eso-	inward
ex-, exo-	outside, away from, out of
extra-	on the outside, outside of, beyond
fore-	before, in front of
hyp-, hyph-, hypo-	under
infra-	beneath
inter-	between
intra-	within, inside
later-	side, on the side
meta-	beyond
pan-	entire, all
para-	beside, to the side of
per-	throughout
peri-	about, around
pro-	in front of, before
proxim-	near, nearest to
super-	over, over and above
supra-	above, over
ultra-	beyond, excessive(ly)

Prefixes Denoting Color

albin-	white
chlor-	green
cyan-	blue
erythro-	red
leuk-	white
melan-	black
xanth-	yellow

Prefixes Denoting Conditions or Qualities

aniso-	unequal
emmetr-	in proper measure
erythema-	redness, flushing
hyper-	increased, excessive
hypo-	decreased, deficient
macro-	large
mal-	bad
micro-	small, very small
mio-, meio-	less, smaller
necr-	dead
orth-	straight
pachy-	thick, thickness
poly-	many, much
steno-	narrow, constricted
syn-	together
xer-	dry

Prefixes Denoting Procedures

cente-	puncture
excis-	cutting out
incis-	cut into
sect-	cutting, dividing

Prefixes Denoting Organs/Tissues or Areas of the Body

angi-	blood or lymph vessels
cardio-	heart
cephal-	the head (but not the skull or brain)
cerebr-	the brain
cervic-	neck
chondr-	cartilage
crani-	the skull (not the brain)
cutane-	the skin
dent-	the teeth
encephal-	the brain
gastr-	stomach
gloss-	the tongue
hepat-	the liver
hist-	tissue
hemat-	blood
mast-	the breast(s)
mening-	membrane (especially those covering the brain and spinal cord)
my-	muscle(s)
nas-	the nose
nephr-	the kidney(s)
neur-	nerve(s)
oculo-	the eye
ophthal-	the eye
or-	the mouth
ost-	bone(s)
phleb-	vein (specifically; not just "blood vessel")
pneum-	the lung(s), air
psych-	the mind (not the brain)
pulm, pulmon-	the lung(s)
rhin-	the nose
sarc-	flesh
vas-	vessel

General "All-Purpose" Prefixes

alg-	pain
algesi-	pain
algesia-	pain
algesic-	pain
anis-	unequal
anomal-	irregular
attenuat-	diluted, weakened
auto-	self
bi-	two

brady-	slow
cau-	burn
chrom(at)-	color
cry-	cold
crypt-	hidden
cyst-	bag, bladder, sac containing fluid
dipl-	double
gran-	particle, grain
hemi-	half
heter-	other, different
hiat-	opening
homo-	the same
hydr-	water
mono-	one, single
morph-	form
multi-	many, much
pseud-	false
radi-	beam, ray, spoke
tachy-	fast, rapid
therm-	heat
tri-	three

Prefixes to Watch Out For

There are some similar-sounding, but opposite-meaning prefixes to watch out for.

ab- vs ad-	out or away vs in or toward (Sidebar C-1)
dys- vs eu-	abnormal or difficult vs normal or good
hyper- vs hypo-	above or excessive vs below or deficient
sub- vs supra-	below or under vs above

SIDEBAR C-1
AB- AND AD-

They look almost the same, they sound almost the same … but they have opposite meanings. "Ab" is the Latin word for "from" or "away from" (think of "abnormal"—literally, "away from normal"); "ad" is the Latin word for "toward" (think of "ad infinitum"). This is why, in verbally describing the action of extra-ocular muscles, practitioners often spell out the first two letters to avoid confusion or misunderstanding: "AD-duct" or "AB-duct."

It is also important to understand the difference and distinction between certain prefixes that sound similar and mean *almost* the same, but are NOT interchangeable.

intra-	within
inter-	between
para-	beyond, beside
per-	through
peri-	around, surrounding

Suffixes

A suffix appears at the end of a multipart term. Suffixes usually indicate a condition or quality, appearance, a disease or disorder, a specialty or specialist, or a procedure. The suffix makes the overall term specific and precise. Practice recognizing and using precise terms—remember, an "-otomy" is not the same as an "-ectomy"!

Suffixes Denoting Conditions or Qualities

-desis	binding
-dynia	pain
-ectasis, -ectasia	expansion, stretching
-emia	blood
-iasis	condition, pathology
-ism	condition (caused by)
-itis	inflammation (of)
-oma	tumor
-pathy	disease (of)
-penia	decrease, lessening
-plasia	development or growth
-plegia	paralysis
-rrhage, -rrhagia	bursting forth, abnormal excess discharge of fluid (usually blood)
-rrhea	abnormal flow or discharge
-rrhexis	rupture
-spasm	twitch
-trophy	development, growth

Suffixes Denoting Procedures

-centesis	surgical puncture to remove fluid
-cise	cut
-ectomy	surgical removal, excision
-lysis	disintegrate
-ostomy	surgical creation of a (new) opening
-otomy	incision, cutting
-pexy	fixation (as in to restore something to its original place)
-plasty	surgical repair (of)
-rrhaphy	to suture or stitch
-sect	cutting, dividing

General "All-Purpose" Suffixes

-algia	pain
-cide	causing death
-cidal	killing, pertaining to killing

-esthesia	feeling, sensation
-gen	original, beginning
-genesis	leading to the production of
-genous	producing
-gram	record, write
-graph	record created by an instrument
-meter, -metry	measure
-scope	instrument used to examine
-scopy	to view with a scope

Root Word Parts

In a medical term that includes a prefix and a suffix, the root word part is the center—literally and figuratively. Most medical terms, and therefore most root word parts, have to do with a part of the body. If you think of a sentence in which there is a subject (a noun) modified by adjectives, you can think of the root word in a medical term as the "subject" and the prefix and suffix as "modifiers." The root word part (to put it another way) is what the full medical term is "about." When confronted with a long and seemingly complex medical term, train yourself to focus first on the center, then look at the prefix and the suffix to zero in on exactly what the full term means.

WORD PARTS SPECIFIC TO OPHTHALMOLOGY

Table C-2 is a selection of word parts you are likely to see and hear in your work.

CHAPTER QUIZ

Match the definition to the word.
1. condition of unequal pupil diameters ____
2. incomplete development ____
3. on the opposite side of ____
4. inflammation of the eyelid ____
5. measurement of thickness ____
6. incision into junction of the upper/lower eyelids ____
7. softening of the cornea ____
8. study of the ears and throat ____
9. fungal infection involving or affecting the skin ____
10. overdevelopment or overgrowth ____
11. behind the globe (eyeball) ____
12. extreme or excessive sensitivity to light ____
13. surrounding the (optic) nerve ____
14. abnormal smallness of the head ____
15. under the tongue ____

TABLE C-2
WORD PARTS SPECIFIC TO OPHTHALMOLOGY/OPTOMETRY

Word Part	Pertains To
blephar-	eyelids
bulb-	globe, eyeball
canth-	angle(s) where upper and lower lids meet
cili-	eyelash
corne-	cornea
cycl-	ciliary body
dacry-	tear(s)
fund-	back of the eye (retina, optic disc, vessels)
ir-, irid-	iris
kerat-	cornea
lacrim-	tear(s)
ocul-, ophthalm-	eye
-opia, -opsia, -opsis	vision
opt-, optic	vision
palpebr-	eyelid
phac-, phak-	lens
phor-	to move, to carry
photo-	light
presby-	aging ("old man")
retin-	retina
scler-	sclera
tars-	tarsal plate (in eyelid)
trich-	hair (lash)
trop-	turn
uve-	uvea

a. hypertrophy
b. blepharitis
c. pachymetry
d. contralateral
e. photophobia
f. sublingual
g. anisocoria
h. microcephaly
i. hypoplasia
j. keratomalacia
k. otolaryngology
l. dermatomycosis
m. canthotomy
n. retrobulbar
o. peripapillary

Answers

1. g, anisocoria
2. i, hypoplasia
3. d, contralateral
4. b, blepharitis
5. c, pachymetry
6. m, canthotomy
7. j, keratomalacia

8. k, otolaryngology
9. l, dermatomycosis
10. a, hypertrophy
11. n, retrobulbar
12. e, photophobia
13. o, peripapillary
14. h, microcephaly
15. f, sublingual

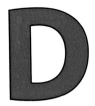

COMMONLY USED
OPHTHALMIC MEDICATIONS*†

Jan Ledford, COMT

Trade Name	Generic Name	Use	Manufacturer
Acular LS	ketorolac	NSAID	AGN, generic
Acuvail	bromfenac	NSAID	AGN
Akorn Artificial Tears	PVA	Artificial tears, PVA-based	Akorn
Akwa Tears Ointment	mineral oil, white petrolatum	Artificial tear gel/ointment	Akorn
Alamast	pemirolast	Allergy	Vistakon
Alaway (OTC)	ketotifen	Allergy, acute	B+L
Alocril	nedocromil	Allergy, chronic	AGN, generic
Alomide	lodoxamide	Allergy, chronic	ALC
Alphagan P	brimonidine	Glaucoma, alpha agonist	AGN
Alrex	loteprednol	Allergy, acute Corticosteroid, moderate strength	B+L
AzaSite	azithromycin	Antibiotic, other	Akorn
Azopt	brinzolamide	Glaucoma, carbonic anhydrase inhibitors	ALC
Bacitracin	bacitracin	Antibiotic	Perrigo
Bepreve	bepotastine	Allergy, acute	B+L
Besivance	besifloxacin	Antibiotic, fluoroquinolone	B+L
Betagan	levobunolol	Glaucoma, beta blocker	AGN, generic

Ledford JK, Lens A, eds.
Principles and Practice in Ophthalmic Assisting:
A Comprehensive Textbook (pp 779-784).
© 2018 Taylor & Francis Group.

Trade Name	Generic Name	Use	Manufacturer
Betimol	timolol hemihydrate	Glaucoma, beta blocker	Akorn
Betoptic-S	betaxolol	Glaucoma, beta blocker	ALC
Bimatoprost	bimatoprost	Glaucoma, prostaglandin analogue	Generic
Blephamide	prednisolone/sulfacetamide	Steroid/antibiotic combination	AGN
Blink Gel Tears	polyethylene glycol, hyaluronic acid	Artificial tear, liquid polyol-based	Abbott Labs
Blink Tears	polyethylene glycol, hyaluronic acid	Artificial tear, liquid polyol-based	Abbott Labs
Brimonidine	brimonidine	Glaucoma, alpha agonist	Generic
BromSite	bromfenac	NSAID	Sun Pharma
Ciloxan	ciprofloxacin	Antibiotic, fluoroquinolone	ALC, generic
Clear Eyes	PVA/povidone	Artificial tears, PVA-based	Prestige Brands
Combigan	brimonidine/timolol	Glaucoma, combination	AGN
Cosopt	dorzolamide/timolol	Glaucoma, combination	Akorn, generic
Cosopt PF	dorzolamide/timolol	Glaucoma, combination	Akorn
Crolom	cromolyn	Allergy, chronic	B+L, generic
Durezol	difluprednate	Corticosteroid, maximum strength	ALC
Elestat	epinastine	Allergy, acute	AGN, generic
Emadine	emedastine	Allergy, acute	ALC
Flarex	fluorometholone	Corticosteroid, moderate strength	ALC
FML drops and ointment	fluorometholone	Corticosteroid, moderate strength	AGN, generic
Freshkote	PVA/povidone	Artificial tears, PVA-based	FOCUS Labs
Garamycin	gentamicin	Antibiotic, aminoglycoside	Perrigo, generic
GenTeal Gel	HPMC	Artificial tear gel/ointment	Novartis
GenTeal Mild	HPMC	Artificial tears, methylcellulose-based	Novartis
GenTeal Moderate to Severe	HPMC/CMC	Artificial tears, methylcellulose-based	Novartis
Hylo-Comod	hyaluronic acid	Artificial tear, combination	URSAPHARM
Hylo-Fresh	hyaluronic acid	Artificial tear, combination	URSAPHARM
Hypotears	dextran, PVA	Artificial tear, combination	Novartis
Ilevro	nepafenac	NSAID	ALC
Istalol	timolol maleate	Glaucoma, beta blocker	B+L
Just Tears	CMC	Artificial tears, methylcellulose-based	Blairex
Lacril	HPMC	Artificial tears, methylcellulose-based	AGN

Trade Name	Generic Name	Use	Manufacturer
Lastacaft	alcaftadine	Allergy, Acute	AGN, generic
Liquivisc	carbomer	Artificial tear gel/ointment	URSAPHARM
Lotemax gel and ointment	loteprednol 0.5%	Corticosteroid, maximum strength	B+L
Lubrifresh PM	mineral oil, white petrolatum	Artificial tear gel/ointment	Major Pharmaceuticals
Lumigan	bimatoprost	Glaucoma, prostaglandin analogue	AGN
Maxitrol	dexamthasone/neomycin/ polymyxin B	Steroid/antibiotic combination	ALC
MiniDrops	PVA/povidone	Artificial tears, PVA-based	Optics Lab, Inc
Moxeza	moxifloxacin	Antibiotic, fluoroquinolone	ALC
Murine	naphazoline	Ocular decongestant	Prestige Brands
Murine Tears	PVA/povidone	Artificial tears, PVA-based	Prestige Brands
Naphcon	naphazoline	Ocular decongestant	ALC
Naphcon-A	naphazoline, pheniramine	Ocular decongestant/ antihistamine	ALC
Natural Balance Tears	HPMC	Artificial tears, methylcellulose-based	Major
Nature's Tears	HPMC	Artificial tears, methylcellulose-based	Bio-Logic Aqua Technologies
Neo-Poly-Bac	bacitracin/hydrocortisone/ neomycin/polymyxin b	Steroid/antibiotic combination	B+L
Neo-Poly-Dex	dexmethasone/neomycin/ polymyxin b	Steroid/antibiotic combination	B+L
Neosporin (drops)	polymyxin b/neomycin/ gramicidin	Antibiotic, polymyxin b combination	Generic
Neosporin (ointment)	polymyxin b/neomycin/ bacitracin	Antibiotic, polymyxin b combination	Generic
Nevanac	nepafenac	NSAID	ALC
Nutratear	PVA	Artificial tears, PVA-based	Medco Lab
Oasis Tears	glycerin	Artificial tear, liquid polyol-based	Oasis Medical
Oasis Tears Plus	glycerin	Artificial tear, liquid polyol-based	Oasis Medical
Ocuflox	ofloxacin	Antibiotic, fluoroquinolone	AGN, generic
Opcon-A	nephazoline/pheniramine	Ocular decongestant/ antihistamine	B+L
Opti-Clear	tetrahydrozoline	Ocular decongestant	Major
Optivar	azelastine	Allergy, acute	Meda, generic
Pataday	olopatadine	Allergy, acute	ALC
Patanol	olopatadine	Allergy, acute	ALC, generic
Poly-Pred	neomycin/polymyxin b/ prednisolone	Steroid/antibiotic combination	AGN

Trade Name	Generic Name	Use	Manufacturer
Polysporin	polymyxin b/bacitracin	Antibiotic, polymyxin b combination	Generic
Polytrim	polymyxin b/trimethoprim	Antibiotic, polymyxin b combination	AGN, generic
Pred Forte	prednisolone 1%	Corticosteroid, maximum strength	AGN, generic
Pred Mild	prednisolone 0.12%	Corticosteroid, moderate strength	AGN
Pred-G	gentamicin/prednisolone	Steroid/antibiotic combination	AGN
Preferin	phenylephrine	Ocular decongestant	AGN
Prolensa	bromfenac	NSAID	B+L
Refresh Celluvisc	CMC	Artificial tears, methylcellulose-based	AGN
Refresh Classic	PVA/povidone	Artificial tears, PVA-based	AGN
Refresh Lacri-Lube	mineral oil, white petrolatum	Artificial tear gel/ointment	AGN
Refresh Liquigel	CMC	Artificial tears, methylcellulose-based	AGN
Refresh Optive	polysorbate, CMC	Artificial tear, combination	AGN
Refresh Optive Advanced	CMC, castor oil, glycerin	Lipid-based artificial tear, combination	AGN
Refresh Optive Advanced PF	castor oil	Lipid-based artificial tear	AGN
Refresh Optive Advanced Sensitive	glycerin, CMC	Artificial tear, combination	AGN
Refresh Plus	CMC	Artificial tears, methylcellulose-based	AGN
Refresh PM Ointment	mineral oil, white petrolatum	Artificial tear gel/ointment	AGN
Refresh Tears	CMC	Artificial tears, methylcellulose-based	AGN
Restasis	cyclosporine	Treatment of inflammatory dry eye disease/increases tear production	AGN
Retaine CMC	CMC	Artificial tears, methylcellulose-based	OCuSOFT
Retaine MGD	glycerol	Lipid-based artificial tear	OCuSOFT
Rohto Hydra	HPMC	Artificial tears, methylcellulose-based	Rohto Labs
Simbrinza	brinzolamide/brimonidine	Glaucoma, combination	ALC
Similasan Dry Eye Relief	belladonna, euphrasia, mercurius sublimatus	Artificial tear, combination	Similasan Corp
Similasan Irritated Eye Relief	belladonna, euphrasia, hepar sulfuris	Artificial tear, combination	Similasan Corp
Soothe	glycerin/propylene glycol	Artificial tear, liquid polyol-based	B+L
Soothe Lubricant Eye Ointment	mineral oil, white petrolatum	Artificial tear gel/ointment	B+L
Soothe XP	polyethylene glycol, mineral oil	Lipid-based artificial tear, combination	B+L

Trade Name	Generic Name	User	Manufacturer
Systane	polyethylene glycol/ propylene glycol	Artificial tear, liquid polyol-based	ALC
Systane Gel Drops	polyethylene glycol/ propylene glycol	Artificial tear, liquid polyol-based	ALC
Systane Nighttime Ointment	mineral oil, white petrolatum	Artificial tear gel/ointment	ALC
Systane Ultra	polyethylene glycol/ propylene glycol	Artificial tear, liquid polyol-based	ALC
Tearisol	HPMC	Artificial tears, methylcellulose-based	Novartis
Tears Again Night & Day Gel	CMC	Artificial tear gel/ointment	OcuSoft
Tears Naturale	dextran, HPMC	Artificial tear, combination	ALC
Tears Naturale Forte	dextran, HPMC	Artificial tear, combination	ALC
Tears Naturale Free	dextran, HPMC	Artificial tear, combination	ALC
Tears Naturale II	glycerin, HPMC	Artificial tear, combination	ALC
Tears Naturale PM	mineral oil, white petrolatum	Artificial tear gel/ointment	ALC
Tears Renewed	HPMC	Artificial tear, combination	Akorn
Thera Tears	CMC	Artificial tears, methylcellulose-based	Advanced Vision Research
Timoptic	timolol maleate	Glaucoma, beta blocker	Valeant Ophthalmics, generic
Timoptic, Preservative Free	timolol maleate	Glaucoma, beta blocker	Valeant Ophthalmics
Timoptic-XE Gel	timolol maleate	Glaucoma, beta blocker	Valeant Ophthalmics, generic
Tobradex	dexamthasone/tobramycin	Steroid/antibiotic combination	ALC
Tobrex	tobramycin	Antibiotic, aminoglycoside	ALC, generic
Travatan Z	travoprost	Glaucoma, prostaglandin analogue	ALC
Travoprost	travoprost	Glaucoma, prostaglandin analogue	Generic
Trusopt	dorzolamide	Glaucoma, carbonic anhydrase inhibitors	Merck
Ultra Tears	HPMC	Artificial tears, methylcellulose-based	ALC
Vasocidin	prednisolone/sulfacetamide	Steroid/antibiotic combination	Novartis
Vexol	rimexolone	Corticosteroid, maximum strength	ALC
Vigamox	moxifloxacin	Antibiotic, fluoroquinolone	ALC
Viroptic	trifluridine	Antiviral	Pfizer
ViscoTears Liquid Gel	carbomer	Artificial tear gel/ointment	Novartis
Visine	tetrahydrozoline	Ocular decongestant	Johnson & Johnson
Visine Totality	glycerin, tetrahydrozoline, zinc sulfate, hypromellose, polyethylene glycol	Lubricant/decongestant/ astringent	Johnson & Johnson

Trade Name	Generic Name	Use	Manufacturer
Viva Drops	polysorbate	Artificial tear, polysorbate	Dakota Labs
Voltaren	diclofenac	NSAID	Novartis, generic
Xalatan	latanoprost	Glaucoma, prostaglandin analogue	Pfizer, generic
Xiidra	lifitegrast	Treatment of dry eye signs and symptoms	Shire US Inc
Zaditor (OTC)	ketotifen	Allergy, acute	ALC, generic
Zincfrin	phenylephrine, zinc sulphate	Ocular decongestant/astringent	ALC
Zioptan	tafluprost	Glaucoma, prostaglandin analogue	Akorn
Zylet	loteprednol/tobramycin	Steroid/antibiotic combination	B+L
Zymaxid	gatifloxacin	Antibiotic, fluoroquinolone	AGN, generic
Zyrtec Itchy Eye Drops	ketotifen	Allergy, acute	McNeil Consumer Healthcare

ABBREVIATION KEY

AGN: Allergan
ALC: Alcon
B+L: Bausch + Lomb
CMC: carboxy methylcellulose
HPMC: hydroxypropyl methylcellulose
MGD: meibomian gland disease
NSAID: nonsteroidal anti-inflammatory drug
OTC: over-the-counter
PF: preservative-free
PVA: polyvinyl alcohol

BIBLIOGRAPHY

Melton R, Thomas R. *Clinical Guide to Ophthalmic Drugs.* 20th anniversary ed. A supplement to *Review of Optometry.* 2016;May 15.

Moshirfar M, Pierson K, Hanamaikai K, Santiago-Caban L, Muthappan V, Passi SF. Artificial tears potpourri: a literature review. *Clin Ophthalmol.* 2014;8:1419-1433. Published online July 31, 2014. doi:10.2147/OPTH.S65263.

*It is impossible to include every over-the-counter and prescription eye medication; those listed are in common use at the time of publication. For diagnostic medications used in the eye clinic, see Chapter 22, Pharmacology.

†Color-coded caps are often used to designate different ocular drugs. See Table 22-1 in Chapter 22, Pharmacology.

GLOSSARY

accommodation: Adjustment of focal power of the eye from distance to near vision achieved by contraction of the ciliary muscle, which causes a thickening of the crystalline lens and a slight forward shift in its position, both of which increase its refractive power.

Adie's tonic pupil (AE-deez): Uneven constriction of the pupils of each eye upon accommodation (in near vision) in which the affected pupil reacts poorly to light and slowly to near; also called myotonic pupil, pupillotonia, tonic pupil, Adie's pupil, Adie's syndrome.

adnexa (ad-NEX-uh): General anatomic term for the structures surrounding an organ; the ocular adnexa are usually considered to include the eyelids, lacrimal apparatus, orbits, and other tissues within the orbits.

afferent nerve (A-fair-rent or AFF-er-ent): Nerve that conducts a sensory impulse (ie, information) from the peripheral point of origin into the central nervous system; another term for sensory nerve.

amblyopia (am-blee-OH-pee-uh): Impaired vision in one or both eyes that cannot be remedied with corrective lenses and has no obvious organic cause; colloquially known as lazy eye.

ametropia (am-i-TROH-pee-uh): General term for conditions in which the eye does not focus properly but can be corrected with eyeglasses or other vision aids; another term for refractive error.

Amsler grid (AM-zler): Visual field testing grid consisting of evenly spaced horizontal and vertical lines with a central dot to mark the point of fixation; used as a simple test for detecting defects or distortions in the central 20 degrees of the visual field.

aniseikonia (an-i-suh-KOH-nee-uh): Unequal retinal image sizes, especially as seen in corrected anisometropia, resulting in distorted spatial perception.

anisocoria (an-i-suh-KOHR-ee-uh): Uneven size of pupils in the two eyes, usually reserved to describe more than a 1-mm difference in diameter.

anisometropia (an-i-sum-uh-TROH-pee-uh): A difference between the refractive power of the two eyes, usually defined as more than a 2-diopter difference.

anterior chamber (AC): Area within the eye consisting of the structures in front of the iris and behind the cornea; it is filled with aqueous humor.

anterior segment: General term usually describing structures of the eye, including the lens and all structures anterior to the lens (thus including the anterior and posterior chambers).

Ledford JK, Lens A, eds.
Principles and Practice in Ophthalmic Assisting:
A Comprehensive Textbook (pp 785-796).
© 2018 Taylor & Francis Group.

antimetropia (an-ti-mah-TROH-pee-uh): Condition in which one eye is hyperopic while the fellow eye is myopic.

aphakia (a-FAY-kee-uh): Absence of the lens of the eye.

aqueous humor: Clear, watery liquid that fills the anterior and posterior chambers of the eye; typically referred to simply as aqueous.

Argyll-Robertson pupil (ar-GILL RAH-bert-suhn): Condition in which a pupil constricts upon accommodation but does not react to varying direct or consensual light; usually associated with syphilis.

astigmatism (ah-STIG-mah-tiz-um): Refractive error attributable to the presence of an elliptical rather than spherical shape of the refracting surfaces of the eye (usually the cornea), resulting in more than one focal point.

axis: General term for the imaginary line passing through a solid body; any one of several standard reference lines used to describe the anatomy and optical system of the eye, specifically: *cylinder a.* the orientation of a cylindrical lens; *optical* or *principal a.* axis passing through the optical center of the eye and perpendicular to the plane of the crystalline lens; *pupillary a.* axis centered on and perpendicular to the plane of the pupil; *visual a.* axis along which light rays travel from an object to the macula, also called line of sight.

binocular: Visual properties or processes that involve both eyes working together.

binocular vision: A way of expressing the manner in which the two eyes work together; *grade 1 b.v.* vision in which there is simultaneous perception; *grade 2 b.v.* vision in which there is simultaneous perception as well as fusion; *grade 3 b.v.* highest quality of vision in which there is simultaneous perception, fusion, and stereopsis.

biometry (bye-AHM-uh-tree): In ophthalmology, usually referring to ultrasonic measurements, especially A-scan.

blepharitis (blef-uh-RI-tis): Inflammation of the eyelid, most often referring to the edge of the lid along which the eyelashes are located.

blepharoplasty (BLEF-uh-roh-plas-tee): General term for plastic surgery of the eyelid(s) that can be reconstructive or cosmetic.

blindness: Partial (as in the following terms) or total lack of the visual sense; *cortical/cerebral b.* visual loss caused by pathology in the visual cortex or an interruption to the blood flow in these areas; *hysterical b.* state of visual impairment that has an emotional rather than physical or physiological cause; *legal b.* state of visual impairment defined by public law or legal contract precluding certain activities, such as driving, and qualifying individuals for certain benefits; legal blindness is usually defined as best-corrected acuity of 20/200 or less in the better-seeing eye or visual field of 20 degrees or less (regardless of visual acuity).

Bowman's capsule, layer, or membrane: Layer of the cornea lying above the corneal stroma and beneath the corneal epithelium; also called anterior basement membrane.

Brown syndrome: Condition in which fibrous adhesions of the tendon sheath of the superior oblique muscle prevent the eye from looking upward in adduction; also called sheath syndrome, superior oblique tendon sheath syndrome.

candela (can DEE luh) (cd): Standard metric unit used in measurement of the intensity of light.

capsulotomy (kap-suh-LOT-uh-me): 1. Surgical procedure to make an opening in a capsule, usually the lens capsule, as the first step in cataract extraction; 2. the opening made in the capsule in this manner; *posterior c.* surgical procedure to open the posterior capsule, often referring to the procedure performed with laser to open an opacified posterior capsule after cataract extraction.

cataract: Opacification of the crystalline lens, most commonly referring to that which occurs as a natural consequence of aging.

chalazion (kuh-LAY-zee-uhn or shuh-LAY-zee-uhn): Chronic granuloma of the eyelid resulting from blockage and inflammation of a meibomian gland.

chemosis (kee-MOH-sis): Swelling of the conjunctiva.

choroid (KOHR-oyd): Highly vascular tissue layer lying under the retina.

ciliary body (SIL-ee-air-ee): Ring-shaped structure joining the iris to the choroid and containing the ciliary muscle and ciliary processes.

ciliary or ciliaris muscle: Ring-shaped muscle in the ciliary body; it contracts when stimulated by a near target.

ciliary process: Finger-shaped extensions of the ciliary body that produce aqueous humor and provide an attachment for the zonules that support the lens capsule.

color vision: Subjective perception of the varying wavelengths of light.

concave: Having a curved, indented surface, like the inside of a bowl; a concave lens has minus (diverging) power.

cone cells: One of two types of light-sensitive cells in the retina (often simply referred to as cones), they are concentrated in the macula and function in the discrimination of color and fine detail mainly in the central field of view under lighted conditions; also called retinal cones.

confrontation visual fields: Gross method for measuring the approximate extent of the visual field; the examiner sits facing the test subject and holds a target far to the subject's side, then brings it slowly into the field of view; the subject reports when the object becomes visible; eyes are tested individually.

congruous (KAHN-groo-us): Similar in form.

conjunctiva (kahn-junk-TY-vuh): Ocular tissue lining the inner surface of the eyelids (ie, *palpebral c.*), which folds in to join with the tissue covering the sclera (ie, *bulbar c.*); the "pocket" of the fold is called the cul de sac.

conjunctivitis (kahn-junk-ti-VY-tus): Inflammation/infection of the conjunctiva; causes can include allergy, bacteria, fungi, chemicals, and viruses.

conoid of Sturm: Geometric representation of light refracted through a lens that is spherical along one axis and cylindrical along another.

contralateral: Anatomic term meaning on opposite sides.

converge: General term meaning coming together; 1. in optics, the bending of light rays such that they come together; 2. in ophthalmic usage, the turning of both eyes inward.

convergence: 1. In optics, the gathering together of parallel light rays to a point of focus after passing through a plus lens; 2. in ophthalmic usage, coordinated action of ocular muscles that draws both eyes inward to fixate upon the same point in space; the processes of convergence and accommodation normally are linked.

convex: Having a rounded, protruding surface, like a globe; a concave lens has plus (converging) power.

cover testing: Series of tests used to evaluate strabismus that utilize a fixation target and where one eye, then the other, is covered and uncovered as the examiner watches for eye movement(s).

cranial nerve(s) (CN): Twelve pairs of nerves (motor, sensory, and mixed) that originate in the brain, designated both by Roman numerals (I to XII) and names; six of them affect vision either directly or indirectly; the optic nerve is CN II.

crystalline lens: Proper term for the natural lens of the eye, usually called simply the lens, consisting of a soft outer cortex and nucleus in the center.

cycloplegia (sy-kluh-PLEE-jee-uh): Paralysis of the ciliary muscle (usually by eye drops instilled in the eye clinic) such that the eye does not accommodate in response to the usual stimuli.

cylinder (cyl): 1. In optics, a lens that is flat along one axis and curved along the perpendicular axis, or the property of a lens that is relatively flat along one axis and more curved along the perpendicular axis; 2. in refraction, the component of refractive error that can be corrected with a cylindrical lens (roughly synonymous with astigmatism).

depth perception: The ability to perceive three dimensions; it is not the same as stereopsis, as it is possible with only one eye.

dermatochalasis (DER-muh-toh-kuh-LAY-sis): General term referring to loose, baggy skin; in ophthalmology, generally referring to loose skin of the eyelids.

Descemet's membrane (DES-uh-mayz): Inner tissue layer of the cornea to which the corneal endothelium adheres.

deuteranomaly (DOO-tur-uh-NAH-muh-lee): Partial impairment of the green color mechanism resulting in poor red/green discrimination, although red is normally vivid.

deuteranopia, -opsia (DOO-tur-uh-NOH-pee-uh): Severe or total lack of the green color mechanism; red and yellow-green both look orange; red-orange, orange, and yellow are all the same strong red-orange color; magenta and green are gray tones; blue-green to purple are various confusing shades of blue.

dichromatism (die-KROH-muh-tiz-um): Condition in which only two of the three retinal cone pigments are present.

diopter (D): 1. Measure of the focusing power of a lens, defined as the reciprocal of the focal length measured in meters; 2. by analogy, degrees of myopia (designated as minus diopters) or hyperopia (designated as plus diopters), as well as astigmatism (cylinder diopters) described by the dioptric power of the lens needed to correct the defect; 3. measure of the refracting power of a prism.

diplopia (dip-LOH-pee-uh): Perception of two images where there is only a single object; colloquially known as double vision.

diverge: General term meaning moving away; 1. in optics, the bending of light rays such that they move away from each other; 2. in ophthalmic usage, the turning of both eyes outward, away from the midline.

divergence: 1. In optics, the spreading outward of parallel light rays after passing through a minus lens; 2. in ophthalmic usage, outward turning of both eyes.

Dua's layer (DOO-ah's): A corneal layer identified in 2013 that lies between the stroma and Descemet's membrane; there is some question whether it is indeed a separate layer or just part of the stroma.

Duane syndrome: Inherited abnormal function of the rectus muscles wherein the eye retracts into the orbit and the upper eyelid drops when the eye is rotated in toward the nose; usually monocular; also called retraction syndrome.

duction: Movement of one eye by the extraocular muscles; the direction of this movement is identified with prefixes, most commonly abduction (moving away from midline) and adduction (moving toward midline).

duochrome test: Use of a projector slide or chart that is green on one half and red on the other (split vertically) to prevent overminusing; also called bichrome test, red/green test.

ectopic (ek-TAH-pik): A dislocated organ or part, as in an ectopic lens or pupil.

ectropion (ek-TROH-pee-un): In ophthalmic usage, referring to a condition in which the lid turns outward from the eye, exposing the conjunctiva.

edema: Swelling due to fluid collection/retention.

efferent nerve (EF-ayr-uhnt): Nerve that conducts a central nervous system response to a sensory impulse, causing a reaction; another term for motor nerve.

emmetropia (em-uh-TROH-pee-uh): Condition in which the unaided eye properly focuses light from a distant object onto the retina.

endothelium: In general, a thin cell layer that lines blood and lymph vessels as well as serous cavities; in ophthalmology, usually referring to the endothelium of the cornea.

entopic phenomena (en-TAHP-ik): Visual perceptions that originate from within the eyeball or visual cortex, resulting from pressure or other atypical stimulation; can include dark or light spots, flashes, and "seeing stars."

entropion (en-TROH-pee-un): In ophthalmic usage, a folding inward of the lid, resulting in the lashes rubbing against the globe.

episclera (ep-ee-SKLAYR-uh): Outermost layer of the sclera containing fine connective tissue and blood vessels.

epithelium: The avascular outer layer of a tissue; in ophthalmology, usually referring to the corneal endothelium.

esophoria (E) (ee-soh-FOR-ee-uh): Phoria in which one eye turns inward when deprived of fusion.

esotropia (ET) (ee-soh-TROH-pee-uh): Type of strabismus in which one eye turns in toward the nose; also called convergent deviation, convergent strabismus, internal strabismus.

exophoria (X) (eks-oh-FOR-ia): Phoria in which an eye turns outward when deprived of fusion.

exophthalmos (eks-off-THAL-mus): Protrusion of the eye(s); also called proptosis.

exotropia (XT) (eks-uh-TROH-pee-uh): Type of strabismus in which one eye is turned outward; also called divergent deviation, divergent strabismus, external strabismus.

extraocular muscles (EOMs): Rectus and oblique muscles that attach to the outside of the eye and the inside of the bony orbit, responsible for movements of the eyeball; there are six, usually designated by name as well as left or right.

fixation: Looking directly at an object so that its image falls on the macula; requires that the eyes be steady and have a measure of visual function; also called central fixation; *binocular* or *bifoveal f.* ability to bring both eyes to bear upon the same object; requires coordination of ocular muscles; *eccentric f.* image does not fall on the macula but rather some peripheral retinal point.

flashes: Perception of sudden bursts of light in the absence of external stimuli, usually a symptom of retinal traction; also called light/lightning flashes.

floaters: Dark specks or strands in the field of view caused by cells or other nontransparent material in the vitreous.

fogging: Purposely blurring vision by the addition of plus lenses either to eliminate accommodation (in refractometry) or to semi-occlude the fogged eye.

fovea (FOH-vee-uh): Small depression in the center of the macula in which cone cells are densely packed; the area of fine central vision.

fundus: General term for the base of an organ or area; in ophthalmic usage, the retina, macula, optic disc, and retinal blood vessels as seen through an ophthalmoscope.

fusion: Binocular process in which each eye exerts the effort to fixate on the same object; *central f.* situation in which the image of an object falls on the fovea of each eye; *motor f.* action of the oculomotor system to align the eyes to achieve sensory fusion; *sensory f.* action of the brain in combining the slightly disparate images from each eye into one perceived, three-dimensional image.

glaucoma: Group of ocular disorders in which damage to the optic nerve and visual field loss are usually associated with high intraocular pressure; a leading cause of blindness throughout the world, in its early stages glaucoma has no symptoms but eventually causes irreversible vision loss.

hemianopia, -opsia (hem-ee-uh-NOH-pee-uh): Partial or total loss of vision in half the visual field in one or both eyes; the upper or lower portions of the visual field, as well as the right and left sides, can be affected.

hippus: Rhythmic contraction and dilation of the pupils independent of any stimulus, often seen when shining a light into one eye in order to evaluate pupillary reflexes; not usually indicative of pathology.

Hirschberg test (HERSH-burg): Identification of a tropia by noting the position of the reflections of a fixation light on the patient's corneas; if both reflections are on the visual axis (slightly nasal in most eyes), the eyes are orthotropic, but if the reflection is on the axis in one eye but not the other, a tropia may be present.

homonymous (huh-MON-uh-mus): When speaking of peripheral vision, a visual field defect that is on the same side in each eye (eg, both left halves of each visual field).

hordeolum (hor-DEE-oh-luhm or hor-dee-OH-luhm): Infection of one of the glands on the edge of the eyelid (*external h.* or sty) or in the palpebral conjunctiva (*internal h.*).

Horner's syndrome: Disorder of the third cranial nerve causing miosis, ptosis, and anhidrosis (lack of sweating) on the affected side.

horopter (hohr-AHP-ter or HOHR-ahp-ter): An imaginary arc that allows correlation of points in space to points on the retina; images in front of or behind the horopter will be perceived as doubled.

hyperemia (hy-per-EE-mee-uh): General medical term denoting presence of excessive blood.

hyperopia (hy-per-OH-pee-uh): Refractive error in which the eye focuses rays of light so that the focal point is theoretically behind the retina without accommodation; also called hypermetropia, farsightedness.

hyperphoria (hy-per-FOR-ee-uh): Phoria in which one eye drifts upward when fusion is broken (generally by occluding the eye).

hypertropia (hy-per-TROH-pee-uh): Strabismus in which the nonfixating eye turns upward relative to the fixating eye.

hyphema (hy-FEE-muh): Bleeding into the anterior chamber of the eye.

hypopyon (hy-POH-pee-ahn): Collection of pus (white blood cells) in the anterior chamber of the eye.

hypotony (hy-POT-uh-nee): In ophthalmic usage, abnormally low intraocular pressure (usually < 5 mm Hg).

hypoxia (hy-POK-see-uh): Abnormal reduction in the amount of oxygen available to a tissue; in ophthalmic usage, most frequently referring to lack of oxygen to the cornea related to contact lens wear; also called anoxia, oxygen deprivation.

hysterical: General medical term for a disorder triggered by emotional struggles; in ophthalmic usage, visual disorders due to emotional rather than organic causes, usually manifest in abnormal visual acuity or visual fields.

idiopathic (id-ee-o-PATH-ik): Disorder without a known cause.

incongruous (in-KAHN-groo-us): General term indicating dissimilarity in form; in ophthalmology, often used to refer to visual fields where the pattern of loss in one eye is dissimilar to that of the other eye.

inferior oblique (IO) muscle: Extraocular muscle lying underneath the eye around the equator of the globe and supplied by CN III (oculomotor nerve); responsible for elevating, abducting, and extorting the eye.

inferior rectus (IR) muscle: Extraocular muscle lying underneath the eye and supplied by CN III (oculomotor nerve); responsible for depressing, extorting, and adducting the eye.

injection: Condition in which tissue is red, swollen, and engorged with dilated blood vessels; most often in ophthalmic usage referring to conjunctival injection.

intraocular (in-trah-AHK-yuh-ler): General anatomic term for structure, entity, or process appearing or occurring within the eye.

intraocular pressure (IOP) (in-trah-AHK-yuh-ler): Pressure within the eye caused by the dynamics of the formation and drainage of aqueous humor.

ipsilateral (ip-suh-LAT-er-ul): Anatomic term meaning on the same side.

iridotomy (ir-i-DOT-uh-mee): Surgical procedure to remove iris tissue to facilitate the flow of aqueous humor and thus lower, or prevent a rise in, intraocular pressure.

iris: Mobile, vascular, ring-shaped structure that lies behind the cornea and in front of the crystalline lens and responsible for the color of the eye; its movements control the size of the pupil and, thus, the amount of light passing through to the retina; plural: irides.

iritis (i-RY-tis): Inflammation of the iris characterized by pain, photophobia, and redness; also called anterior uveitis.

isopter (I-sop-ter): General term for line on a chart or map connecting similar numerical values; in ophthalmic usage, lines on a visual field test chart connecting the border of an area that responds to the same test object.

keratitis (kayr-uh-TY-tis): General term for inflammation of the cornea.

keratoconus (KC) (kayr-uh-toh-KOH-nus): Progressive malformation of the cornea such that it is thin and cone-like in shape rather than rounded; causes painless visual distortion and loss; also called ectatic corneal dystrophy.

keratometer (kayr-uh-TOM-eh-ter): Any of several types of instruments used to measure the curvature of the cornea; the term usually refers to an instrument that measures the central 3 mm of the cornea.

Krimsky measurement/test (KRIM-skee): Method of measuring a tropia in which the examiner uses prisms to move a light reflex in the patient's pupils until the reflexes are in the same position in both eyes.

lacrimal apparatus/system: Collective term for the system that produces tears and drains them from the eye.

lamina cribrosa (LAM-in-uh krib-ROH-suh): Mesh-like area of sclera at the back of the eye through which retinal ganglion cells and blood vessels pass; also called cribriform plate, scleral foramen.

LASER: Acronym for "light amplification by stimulated emission of radiation," a process invented in the early 1960s to produce coherent light; there are many types of lasers with diverse medical applications, all of which are based upon the fact that specific wavelengths of light are absorbed by specific tissues or compounds within tissues, with various consequent reactions.

latent: General term describing a condition that is not immediately evident, such as a phoria or latent hyperopia.

lateral geniculate body (juh-NIK-yuh-lit): Area of the midbrain that receives visual impulses from the nerve fibers of the optic tract.

lateral rectus (LR) muscle: Extraocular muscle lying along the side of the eye near the temple, supplied by CN VI (abducens nerve) and responsible for abducting the eye; also called external rectus muscle.

lazy eye: Colloquial term for amblyopia; laypeople sometimes misapply the term to strabismus (ie, an eye that is lazy and thus turns or drifts).

lensmeter/lensometer: Instrument used to measure (or neutralize) the various components of curvature, and thus the refractive properties (ie, the "prescription") of a corrective lens.

limbus (LIM-bus): General anatomic term for the line along which two structures meet; most commonly in ophthalmic usage, the circular border between the cornea and sclera; also called corneoscleral junction.

low vision (LV): Visual impairment that cannot be remedied with corrective lenses or surgical intervention, usually describing a condition that renders an individual unable to perform normal daily functions; low vision is not synonymous with legal blindness.

lumen (LOO-mun): 1. General term for the hollow area inside a duct or tube (eg, the lumen of the lacrimal duct); 2. in optics, the standard unit of the amount of light flowing through a solid angle (ie, a space shaped like a cone); 1 lumen (1 lm) is defined as the flux of light through 1 steradian emitted by a light source with 1 candela intensity.

macula (MAK-yu-luh): General anatomic term derived from the Latin for spot or stain; most commonly in ophthalmic usage, the small yellowish area of the retina where cone cells are most densely packed (more properly called the macula lutea); the center of the macula is slightly depressed and known as the fovea, which in turn has a pit at its center called the foveola.

macular degeneration (MD) (MAK-yu-lar): General term for conditions in which the macular tissue breaks down, resulting in a loss of central vision; the visual loss is generally irreversible, although vitamin therapy, medicinal and laser treatment, and surgical therapies are employed to slow its progression.

Maddox rod: A lens composed of a series of high-powered cylinders (red or white); a point source of light viewed through the Maddox rod appears as a streak of light; used in measuring muscle deviations, especially phorias.

malingering (muh-LING-ger-ing): Situation in which the patient purposely gives false information during subjective testing in order to gain something (financial reimbursement, a pair of glasses, sympathy, a driver's license, a job, etc).

manifest: 1. General term describing a condition that is evident, such as a tropia or manifest hyperopia; 2. in optical use, refractometry that is performed without dilation or cycloplegia.

Marcus Gunn pupil (MG): Impairment of the normal response of the affected pupil to bright light when stimulated by the light; also called afferent pupillary defect, Gunn's pupil, relative afferent pupillary defect.

medial rectus (MR) muscle: Extraocular muscle lying along the side of the eye near the nose, supplied by CN III (oculomotor nerve) and responsible for adducting the eye; also called internal rectus muscle.

meibomian glands (my-BOH-mee-uhn): Glands located within the eyelids that produce oil; their secretions form the outer layer of the tear film; also called tarsal glands.

miosis (my-OH-sis): Constriction of one or both pupils in response to stimulation by bright light, to accommodation, or to certain drugs or disease processes.

mires: General term for a reference line or image of standard shape on a measuring device (eg, lensometer, keratometer).

monochromatic (mon-oh-kroh-MAT-ik): Characterized by a single color, as in an image of only one hue or light of a single wavelength (eg, laser light).

monochromatism (mon-oh-KROH-muh-tiz-uhm): Very rare condition in which only one of the three visual pigments is present.

monocular: Literally, "one eyed"; used alone to describe a patient with one functional eye or combined with another term to describe an ocular condition involving only one eye, as in monocular diplopia (ie, double image in one eye), etc.

monovision: Situation in which one eye sees at near and the other at distance, usually artificially created for the presbyope using contact lenses, intraocular lens implants, or refractive surgery.

mydriasis (mi-DRY-uh-sis): Dilation of one or both pupils, usually as a response to reduced light but also to certain drugs (as in office dilation) or disease processes.

myopia: Refractive error in which the eye focuses rays of light so that the focal point is in front of the retina, with the result that distant objects are not clearly seen; also called nearsightedness.

near point of accommodation (NPA): Distance from the eye to the nearest point clearly visible when accommodation is at its maximum.

near point of convergence (NPC): Nearest point where the eyes can maintain binocular vision by pulling together; the greatest degree of convergence that the eyes can attain.

neovascularization (nee-oh-vas-cu-lar-eh-ZAY-shun): Abnormal growth of blood vessels caused by some disorder or disease state, these new vessels are generally weak and prone to leakage and bleeding; *corneal n.* abnormal blood vessel growth into the cornea, usually associated with contact lens wear; *iris n.* also called iris rubeosis; *retinal n.* abnormal blood vessel growth into the retina, usually associated with diabetes and hypertension.

nystagmus (ny-STAG-muhs): Rapid, rhythmic, involuntary eye movements; nystagmus is classified according to the direction of motion (horizontal is the most common) and the stimuli that cause it to occur.

occipital lobe (ok-SIP-i-tl): That area of the brain, specifically the cerebrum, that is responsible for vision; located at the back of the brain.

ophthalmic artery: Main vessel bringing blood into the eye and orbit, entering the optic foramen, and dividing into vessels that enter the retina, lacrimal apparatus, extraocular muscles, etc.

ophthalmoscope: Instrument for viewing the inside of the eye; *binocular o.* ophthalmoscope with a head set that allows the examiner to use both eyes when viewing a subject's eye, thereby obtaining a three-dimensional image, also called *indirect o.; direct o.* hand-held ophthalmoscope where the examiner views with only one eye.

optic chiasm (KY-az-um): Point at which the two optic nerves meet; the nasal nerve fibers from each eye cross here, while the temporal fibers continue on the same side; also called chiasm, optic nerve decussation.

optic disc: Roughly circular area at the back of the eye where nerve fibers converge to form the optic nerve, creating a "blind spot" where images are not perceived; also called optic nerve head, optic papilla.

optic nerve (ON): Cranial nerve number two (CN II); the bundle of retinal nerve fibers that exits each eye; the optic nerves meet at the optic chiasm.

optic neuritis (nurh-I-tis): Inflammatory disorder of the optic nerve, often accompanied by pain, decreased vision, and central field defect.

optic radiations: "Fan" of afferent neurons as they leave the lateral geniculate body and travel to the occipital lobe of the brain.

optic tract: Visual nerve fibers that run from the chiasm to the lateral geniculate body.

ora serrata (OHR-uh ser-RAT-uh): Irregular anterior border of the retina where it attaches to the choroid, located adjacent to the pars plana of the ciliary body and approximately 8 mm posterior to the corneoscleral limbus.

orbit: Either of two spherical hollows in the skull that protect and provide attachments for the eyes, extraocular muscles, and surrounding tissues, commonly known as the eye socket.

orthokeratology (ortho-K) (or-thoh-kayr-uh-TOL-uh-jee): Treatment of refractive error by prescribing rigid contact lenses designed to gradually reshape the cornea.

orthophoria (or-thoh-FOR-ee-uh): Normal state in which the eyes remain properly oriented even if one or the other is occluded.

orthoptics (ohr-THOP-tiks): System for nonsurgical correction of strabismus and other defects of ocular motility.

overminus: The situation where a patient has accommodated during refractometry for distance and the examiner unwittingly provides excessive minus power (or insufficient plus power for hyperopes) to overcome it when evaluating; a distance measurement should prevent any accommodation.

pachymetry/pachometry (pak-im-uh-tree): Measurement of the thickness of the cornea using light or ultrasound; the instrument used to make the measurement is a pachymeter/pachometer.

palpebral (pal-PEE-brahl): Referring to the eyelids.

Panum's fusional area or fusional space (PAN-umz): Area in front of and behind the horopter where fusion occurs, making stereopsis possible.

perimetry: Technique of visual field testing that determines the boundaries of the field of view by presenting test targets (most often points of light) to the test subject, who fixates upon the middle of a blank screen and reports when the target becomes visible in the periphery.

phakic (FAY-kik): An eye in which the natural crystalline lens is present.

phoria (FOHR-ee-uh): Misalignment of the eyes present only when fusion is disrupted (eg, by occluding one eye); it is a latent deviation, usually held in check by fusion; also called heterophoria.

phoropter (FOHR-op-ter): Instrument fitted with a number of different types of lenses that are rotated into place in front of a test subject's eyes to determine the amount of vision correction necessary; when spelled Phoroptor, it denotes a brand name of one such instrument; also called refractor.

photopsia (foh-TAHP-see-uh): Appearance of flashes of light in the field of view attributable to some defect of the retina or optic tract, or a migraine aura.

photoreceptors: The cells in the retina that transmit nerve impulses when stimulated by light (ie, rod cells and cone cells); also called sensory receptors.

phthisis (TY-sis): General term for gradual loss of the bulk and structure of a bodily organ; in ophthalmic usage, most commonly referring to phthisis bulbi, a condition in which a blind eye shrivels, sometimes necessitating surgical removal.

pinguecula (ping-GWEK-yuh-luh): Abnormal, benign growth of yellowish membrane at the junction of the sclera and cornea.

posterior chamber (PC): Portion of the eye behind the iris and in front of the crystalline lens-zonule apparatus and ciliary body; it is part of the anterior segment and aqueous is formed here; not to be confused with posterior segment.

posterior segment (of the eye): General term describing the structures of the eye lying behind the lens-zonule apparatus and ciliary body; ophthalmic surgery is roughly divided into the categories of anterior segment (cornea, glaucoma, and cataract procedures) and posterior segment (retina and vitreous procedures); not to be confused with posterior chamber.

presbyopia (prez-bee-OH-pee-uh): Naturally occurring process of aging whereby changes in ocular tissues result in loss of accommodation and thus near vision, usually first noticeable soon after age 40 years; these changes are generally considered to be due to increasing rigidity of the crystalline lens and decreasing tone of the ciliary muscle.

prism: 1. General term for a transparent object having at least two flat surfaces at an angle to each other (most commonly a triangle in cross section, the top of which is the apex and the bottom of which is the base) that bends light rays from their original trajectory but in parallel paths; a prism bends light toward its base, thus when viewed through a prism, an object appears to move toward the prism's apex; prisms are used to measure various types of strabismus and to relieve double vision; 2. any component of an optical system that functions as a prism; *induced p.* prismatic effect that occurs when the visual axis of the patient is not aligned with the optical center of a lens.

prosthesis (prahs-THEE-sus): General medical term referring to an artificial body part; in ophthalmology, referring to a cosmetic artificial eye.

protanomaly (proh-tuh-NAHM-uh-lee): Partial impairment of the red color mechanism, resulting in red/green confusion with red appearing duller than normal.

protanopia, -opsia (proh-tuh-NOH-pee-uh): Severe or total lack of the red color mechanism; reds appear black and gray, the orange-yellow-greens all look yellow, blue/green is grayish, and blue looks the same as purple.

pseudophakia (SOO-doh-FAY-kee-uh): State in which an intraocular lens implant is present in the eye.

pseudostrabismus: The eyes appear crossed to the observer but on testing are found to be straight.

pterygium (tuh-RIJ-ee-uhm): Fully attached triangular membrane of fleshy tissue extending from a base in the conjunctiva extending across the sclera and onto the cornea; usually found nasally, but can be present temporally.

ptosis (TOH-sis): In ophthalmic usage, a drooping of the upper eyelid (blepharoptosis) or brow.

pupil (P): Opening in the center of the iris, normally circular, that controls the amount of light passing through the eye to the retina by opening (dilating) in dim light in a process called mydriasis and closing (constricting) in bright light in a process called miosis; *fixed p.* pupil in which there is no reaction to light or near; *peaked p.* pupil drawn to a point instead of being totally round, usually as a result of surgery or injury.

pupillary distance (PD): The distance between the eyes' visual axes; also called interpupillary distance (IPD).

quadrantanopia, -opsia (kwah-dran-tuh-NOH-pee-uh or kwah-drah-tuh-NOHP-see-uh): Loss of one-quarter of the visual field in one or both eyes; also called quadrant hemianopia.

refraction: 1. Bending of light as it passes from one transparent media to the next such that light is bent from its normal straight-line course; 2. in ophthalmic practice, the act of determining what power lens is needed to correct a refractive error, including the generation of a prescription for corrective lenses (which may be done only by a licensed professional); 3. in ophthalmic speech and literature, the power of a lens needed to correct an ametropia is referred to as the refraction of a given individual.

refractive error: General term for conditions in which the eye does not focus properly, but can be corrected with eyeglasses or other vision aids; includes myopia, hyperopia, and astigmatism; also called ametropia.

refractometry: Process of measuring a refractive error using lenses, which may be performed by an unlicensed professional; prescribing lenses using the measurement is the purview of licensed medical professionals.

retina: Transparent, light-sensitive structure lining the inside of the eye; lies between the vitreous body and the choroid; composed in part of the light-sensitive rod and cone cells.

retinal detachment (RD): Condition in which the bacillary layer (rod and cone cells) of the retina is partially or completely separated from the pigment epithelial layer, resulting in a loss of vision in the area that is detached.

retinal pigment epithelium (RPE): Dark, posterior-most layer of the retina providing attachment to the choroid as well as functioning in retinal nutrition; also called pigment epithelium.

retinitis (ret-in-I-tis): General term for inflammation of the retina, often associated with bacteria or fungi and characterized by loss of central vision and cells in the vitreous.

retinitis pigmentosa (RP) (ret-n-I-tis pig-men-TOH-sah): Inherited retinal dystrophy in which deposits of melanin pigment appear on the retina, accompanied by atrophy of retinal blood vessels and pallor of the optic disc, eventually leading to loss of vision.

retinopathy (ret-in-AH-path-ee): General term for any abnormal condition of the retina.

retinoscope (RET-in-uh-skohp): Hand-held instrument that projects a spot or streak of light that is reflected by the retina; the apparent motion and brightness of the reflected light when the instrument is moved allows the examiner to determine the refractive state of the eye; it is an objective test in that it does not require patient responses.

rod cells: One of two types of light-sensitive cells in the retina; often simply referred to as rods, they function primarily in peripheral and night vision.

saccades (suh-KAYDZ): Rapid refixation movements of the eyes from one point of fixation to another in a series of jerky steps, or as an effort to maintain prolonged fixation; also called saccadic movement.

Schlemm's canal (shlemz): Ring-shaped passage in the filtration angle through which aqueous humor drains into the bloodstream; also called canal of Schlemm, scleral canal.

sclera (SKLAYR-uh): Commonly called the "white" of the eye; the tough, fibrous tissue that makes up the major outer layer of the eye (lined inside by the choroid and retina); the optic nerve passes through it posteriorly at the lamina cribrosa, and anteriorly it joins with the clear cornea at the limbus.

scotoma (skuh-TOH-mah): Area within the borders of the visual field in which vision is impaired or absent; there is a natural scotoma where the optic nerve enters the eye, called the physiologic blind spot; plural: scotomata.

sign: Objective finding associated with a disorder that can be perceived or detected by the examiner.

sphere (sph): 1. In optics, a lens that refracts all incoming light to a single focal point; 2. in refraction, the component of refractive error that can be corrected with a spherical lens (myopia or hyperopia).

spherical equivalent (SE): 1. Representation of the average refractive power of a toric lens defined as the spherical power plus one-half the cylinder power; 2. similar calculation performed on the components of a spectacle prescription to describe the overall refractive error of an eye.

stereopsis (ster-ee-OP-sis): Three-dimensional vision possible only when binocular vision and fusion are present.

strabismus (struh-BIZ-muhs): Misalignment of the visual axes of the eyes (ie, the eyes are not straight); colloquially called cross-eyed or wall-eyed.

stroma: General anatomic term for the main structural element of a tissue or organ; *corneal s.* central layer of fibrous corneal tissue lying between Bowman's membrane and Dua's layer; *iris s.* connective tissue to which the sphincter muscles, nerves, and pigment of the iris adhere.

subconjunctival hemorrhage (SCH) (sub-kahn-junk-TY-vul): Bleeding between the conjunctiva and sclera, dramatic in appearance (initially a blood-red patch on the surface of the eye) but usually posing no threat and resolving without treatment.

superior oblique muscle (SO): Extraocular muscle lying across the top of the eye and supplied by CN IV (trochlear nerve) responsible for depressing, abducting, and intorting the eye.

superior rectus muscle (SR): Extraocular muscle lying across the top of the eye, supplied by CN III (oculomotor nerve), responsible for elevating, adducting, and intorting the eye.

suppression: Action of the brain to ignore the image from one eye during binocular vision as a result of anisometropia, deviation, or other visual disturbance.

symptom: Subjective indication or perception of a disorder as experienced and related by the patient; may or may not be objectively apparent to the examiner (eg, an examiner and patient can both see redness, but only the patient can feel pain).

tonometer (toh-NOM-eh-ter): Instrument that measures intraocular pressure; there are numerous types.

tonometry (toh-NOM-eh-tree): The act of measuring intraocular pressure using a tonometer.

trabecular meshwork (TM) (trah-BEK-yuh-ler): In ophthalmic usage, the porous tissues at the junction of the ciliary body and sclera through which aqueous humor drains from the anterior chamber of the eye; also called scleral trabeculae, trabeculum.

trabeculectomy (trah-BEK-yoo-LEK-tuh-mee): General term for a surgical procedure in which tissue is removed from the trabecular meshwork, most often to treat glaucoma by allowing aqueous humor to drain more easily from the eye.

transposition: Mathematical manipulation of a glasses or contact lens prescription in order to change from plus cylinder form to minus or vice versa; the procedure is as follows: algebraically add the spherical and cylindrical powers (this becomes the new spherical power), change the sign of the original cylinder (without changing its value), and rotate the axis by 90 degrees (if the original axis is 90 or less, add 90; if the original axis is over 90 degrees, subtract 90).

trichiasis (tri-KY-uh-sis): Condition in which individual lashes are turned inward toward the globe and irritate ocular surface tissues.

trichromatism (tri-KROH-muh-tiz-uhm): Condition in which all three visual pigments are present and color vision is normal; *anomalous t.* condition in which all three visual pigments are present but one is deficient, causing a defect in color vision, specifically deutanomaly, protanomaly, or tritanomaly.

tritanomaly (try-tuh-NAHM-uh-lee): Color vision defect in which the blue pigment is partially deficient, causing blue/green and yellow/green confusion; violets are perceived normally.

tritanopia, -opsia (try-tan-OP-see-uh): Severe or total lack of the blue color mechanism; reds and greens are normal, but yellow-green through purple (including blue) appear white and gray.

tropia (TROH-pee-uh): Constant (manifest) misalignment of the eyes in which they fail to fixate on the same object; commonly called crossed eyes; also called heterotropia, manifest strabismus; *horizontal t.* tropia in which the eyes deviate in or out (ie, left or right); *vertical t.* tropia in which the eyes deviate up or down.

ultrasound: Imaging technique that uses sound waves to produce an image; in ophthalmology, used to measure the axial length of the eye, thickness of the cornea, as well as to visualize the eye's inner structures.

uvea/uveal tract (YOO-vee-uh): The tissues of the eye that are heavily pigmented and consist primarily of blood vessels: the choroid, ciliary body, and iris (considered as a whole system).

uveitis (yoo-vee-I-tis): Inflammation of all or part of the uvea; *anterior u.* uveitis involving only the iris (iritis) and/or ciliary body (iridocyclitis); *intermediate/peripheral u.* inflammation of the ciliary body and vitreous; also called cyclitis, pars planitis, peripheral uveitis; *posterior u.* uveitis involving some part of the posterior uveal structures: the choroid (choroiditis), retina (retinitis), retinal blood vessels (retinal vasculitis), and/or optic nerve (papillitis, optic neuritis); often referred to simply as uveitis, creating confusion as to what is meant.

vergence: 1. In optics, the gathering together or spreading apart of parallel light rays, either naturally or as a result of passing through a lens; 2. in ophthalmic usage, motion of the eyes toward or away from one another; also called disjunctive movements.

version: Coordinated movement of both eyes in the same direction; also called conjugate movement.

vertex distance: Distance along the line of sight from the cornea to the back surface of a spectacle lens.

vision: Action of the eyes, nervous system, and brain in capturing reflected light from the environment and converting it to perceived images.

visual acuity (VA): Level of visual clarity; specifically, the ability to distinguish fine details, often expressed as a score on a vision test chart; *best-corrected v.a. (BCVA)* highest level of visual acuity that can be attained with corrective lenses in place; *corrected v.a. (VAcc)* visual acuity measured with current corrective lenses in place; *distance v.a.* acuity for far-off tasks, especially 20 feet or more; *near v.a.* acuity at close range, especially for reading; *uncorrected v.a. (UCVA or VAsc)* visual acuity measured without corrective lenses in place.

visual cortex: That part of the brain responsible for vision, primarily an area in the occipital lobe known as Brodmann area 17; also called striate cortex.

visual field (VF): 1. Area around the fixation point of each eye, generally circular in shape, in which objects are perceived; also called field of vision, peripheral vision, side vision; 2. in clinical usage, graphs representing the result of perimetry and other such tests are often simply referred to as visual fields.

visual pathway: The route of nerve fibers involved in vision; order is as follows: retina (rods, cones, nerve fiber layer), optic nerve, optic chiasm, optic tract, lateral geniculate body, optic radiations, occipital cortex.

visual purple: Light-sensitive retinal pigment found in the rod cells; it is synthesized in the dark, obliterated by light, and responsible for dark adaptation; also called rhodopsin.

vitrectomy (vih-TREK-tuh-mee): Surgical procedure involving partial or total removal of vitreous humor and any membranes, blood, or other tissue in the posterior segment.

vitreous, vitreous body/humor: Clear, fibrous, gel-like material filling the posterior segment of the eye, located behind the lens capsule and comprising about two-thirds of the total volume of the eye; typically referred to simply as the vitreous.

vitreous detachment: Condition in which the vitreous gel pulls away from the retina; symptoms often include floaters and flashes; also called posterior vitreous detachment (PVD).

xanthelasma/xanthoma (zan-thuh-LAZ-muh/zan-THOH-muh): Yellowish, raised, benign growth composed of fatty tissue, generally found on the upper lids but sometimes on the lower; may be associated with elevated cholesterol.

zonules: Fibers that attach the edge of the lens capsule to the ciliary body; also called ciliary zonules, zonules of Zinn.

Definitions taken from or adapted from Ledford JK, Hoffman J, Lens A. *Quick Reference Dictionary of Eyecare Terminology.* 5th ed. Thorofare, NJ: SLACK Incorporated; 2008.

FINANCIAL DISCLOSURES

Dr. Peter D. Anderson owns stock in Abbott Pharmaceuticals.

Dr. Eric Areiter has no financial or proprietary interest in the materials presented herein.

Sarah M. Armstrong has not disclosed any relevant financial relationships.

Jessica M. Barr has no financial or proprietary interest in the materials presented herein.

Laura Barry has no financial or proprietary interest in the materials presented herein.

Dr. Charles A. Beck has no financial or proprietary interest in the materials presented herein.

Ellie Bessarab has no financial or proprietary interest in the materials presented herein.

Dr. Gyula Bokor has not disclosed any relevant financial relationships.

Donna Bong has no financial or proprietary interest in the materials presented herein.

Dr. Adel Ebraheem has no financial or proprietary interest in the materials presented herein.

Sergina M. Flaherty has no financial or proprietary interest in the materials presented herein.

Wendy M. Ford has no financial or proprietary interest in the materials presented herein.

Gloria Garcia-Garza has not disclosed any relevant financial relationships.

Suzanne Hansen has no financial or proprietary interest in the materials presented herein.

Catherine Horan has not disclosed any relevant financial relationships.

Kesha Hyde has no financial or proprietary interest in the materials presented herein.

Dr. Sandra Johnson has not disclosed any relevant financial relationships.

Dr. Robert M. Kershner has no financial or proprietary interest in the materials presented herein.

Anna Kiss has no financial or proprietary interest in the materials presented herein.

Beth Koch has no financial or proprietary interest in the materials presented herein.

Paul M. Larson has no financial or proprietary interest in the materials presented herein.

Jan Ledford has no financial or proprietary interest in the materials presented herein.

Dr. Henry Lee has not disclosed any relevant financial relationships.

Al Lens has no financial or proprietary interest in the materials presented herein.

Dr. Sebastian Lesniak has not disclosed any relevant financial relationships.

Dr. Lisa Lystad has not disclosed any relevant financial relationships.

Roxanna Martin has not disclosed any relevant financial relationships.

Dr. Cynthia Matossian has no financial or proprietary interest in the materials presented herein.

Christine McDonald has no financial or proprietary interest in the materials presented herein.

Jacob P. McGinnis has not disclosed any relevant financial relationships.

Cheryl Pelham has not disclosed any relevant financial relationships.

Monique Rinke has not disclosed any relevant financial relationships.

Gayle Roberts has no financial or proprietary interest in the materials presented herein.

Sumáya "Sumi" Rodríguez has no financial or proprietary interest in the materials presented herein.

John P. Rowan has no financial or proprietary interest in the materials presented herein.

Colleen Schreiber has no financial or proprietary interest in the materials presented herein.

Dr. Aaron V. Shukla has no financial or proprietary interest in the materials presented herein.

Amanda J. Shuman has no financial or proprietary interest in the materials presented herein.

Jane T. Shuman occasionally trains scribes as part of her consulting services.

Adeline Stone has no financial or proprietary interest in the materials presented herein.

Savory Turman has no financial or proprietary interest in the materials presented herein.

Duanna VanCamp has not disclosed any relevant financial relationships.

Dr. James Walsh has no financial or proprietary interest in the materials presented herein.

Anne West-Ellmers has no financial or proprietary interest in the materials presented herein.

INDEX

A-scan, 7, 297, 483, 517
    basic sciences, 307–310
    procedures, 312–319, 325, 328
abbreviations, 70–71
abducens nerve, 13, 149, 479, 545
abnormal retinal correspondence, 142
Acanthamoeba, 407, 448, 454, 455, 495, 582
accommodation, 32, 47–48, 145
accommodative amplitude, 47, 201, 759
accommodative triad/reflex, 47
adenovirus, 553
administrative duties, 683–684
administrative personnel, 9–10
adrenaline, 13, 125, 474
Affordable Care Act, 69, 708
after-image test, 171
albinism, 504
alcohol use, 82, 87, 91, 126
Allen cards/pictures, 96, 98, 100, 103, 742
allergic conjunctivitis, 492–493
allergic reactions to medications, 424
allergies, medications for, 432
amblyopia, 137–177, 750
    management, 154–156
    types, 154
American National Standards Institute (ANSI), 368, 369, 372–373, 586, 710–711

Amsler grid, 128–129, 577, 761
anatomy, ocular, 11–26
    anterior segment, 17–20
    blood supply, 13–14, 549–550
    embryology, 23–26
    extraocular muscles, 15, 137–138
    eyelids, 15–16
    lacrimal system, 16–17
    lashes, 15–16
    nerve supply, 13, 15, 473–475, 549
    posterior segment, 20–23
        optic nerve, 22–23
        retina, 21–22
        vitreous body, 20–21
    skull, 11–13
        bony orbit, 11–13
    uveal tract, 20
anesthetics, 424–425
    general anesthesia, 425
    local anesthetics, 425
    topical anesthetics, 424–425
angle, of iris/cornea, 18, 31, 499, 523, 524, 525–526, 542, 576
    evaluation of, 127, 217, 230–231, 301, 329, 330, 531, 766–767
angle kappa, 166
angle of incidence, 41, 309

angle of reflection, 42, 309
anisocoria, 123, 124, 125, 479, 480, 545, 586
ankylosing spondylitis, 550
anterior chamber, 17–19, 230–231
anterior segment, 17–20
　　anterior chamber, 17–19
　　external globe, 17
　　posterior chamber, 19–20
anterior segment surgical procedures, 625–630
anti-infective agents, 428–431
　　antibacterials, 428–431
anti-inflammatory drugs, 431–432
　　corticosteroids, 431
　　nonsteroidal anti-inflammatory drugs, 431–432
antiglaucoma agents, 421, 427–428, 527–528, 534–535
aphakia 47, 230, 315, 627
apnea, 552
applanation tonometry
　　contact applanation tonometry, 237–244
　　noncontact applanation tonometry, 244–247
aqueous/anterior chamber, 499
　　cells, 499
　　flare, 499
　　hyphema, 499
　　hypopyon, 499
aqueous humor, 18, 31, 36, 45, 215, 224, 230–231, 450, 516,
　　523, 579, 627–628
arteriosclerosis, 550
arthritis, 552
artificial lubricants, 433–434
assistive personnel, 4–8
　　clinical specialties, 6–8
　　　　contact lenses, 6
　　　　corporate certified ophthalmic assistant, 8
　　　　eye bank technician, 8
　　　　imaging, 6
　　　　low vision, 6–7
　　　　orthoptics, 7–8
　　　　photography, 6
　　　　surgical assisting/surgical technologist, 7
　　　　ultrasound/sonography, 7
　　　　vision therapy, 7–8
　　licensed nursing staff, 5–6
　　medical assistant, 5
　　ophthalmic, 4–5
　　optometric, 5
asthma, 550
astigmatism 43, 46, 47, 52, 104, 154, 238, 240, 495, 578
　　contact lenses 382–383, 398–399, 400, 401, 402
　　correction 182, 183, 184, 185, 192, 194–196, 198–200,
　　　　515, 647–648, 650
　　irregular 46, 47, 181, 388, 519
atherosclerosis, 550
automated lensometry, 356
automated perimetry, 762–763
autorefractor, 58

autosomal dominant ophthalmic disease, 464–465
autosomal recessive ophthalmic disease, 465

B-scan, 7, 64
　　basic sciences, 307–310
　　procedures, 319–325
bacteria, 444–447
　　bacilli, 446
　　cocci, 445–446
　　spiral bacteria, 446–447
Bagolini test, 171
base-out test, 171
basic eye exam, 117–135
　　angle evaluation, 127
　　confrontation visual fields, 120–122
　　dilation, 127–128
　　extraocular muscle testing, 122
　　history taking, 119
　　lensometry, 120
　　muscle balance, 122
　　observation, 118–119
　　pupil assessment, 122–127
　　slit lamp, 127
　　tonometry, 127
　　visual acuity, 119
Bielschowsky head tilt test, 164, 165
binocular fixation preference, 108–109
binocular indirect ophthalmoscope, 62
binocular vision 48, 138, 140–143, 144, 150, 154, 155
　　testing 99, 118, 128, 157–158, 170–171, 172
biometer, 67–68
biometry procedures
　　contact biometry, 312–313
　　immersion biometry, 313–314
biomicroscopy, ultrasound, 328–330
blood-borne pathogens, 631–632
blowout fracture 150, 163–164, 561, 563–565, 629
blunt trauma, 558, 559, 560, 563, 567
botulinum, 174, 434
Brown syndrome, 151
brows/lids, 15–16, 27
　　disorders of, 485–488, 584, 585, 586
　　surgery of, 594, 623–624, 634, 637–639
　　trauma of, 560–561
Bruckner reflex test, 166
Burton lamp, 389

cataract, 19–20, 32, 154, 231, 511–522, 597–598
　　classification, 512–514
　　causes of, 513, 559, 560
　　surgery, 47, 514–517, 543, 627, 701
　　　　preoperative evaluation, 108, 109, 112, 311–314,
　　　　　　517–520
　　　　pre- and postoperative care, 520–521
　　symptoms of, 109, 511, 578
center thickness gauge, 394

central nervous system, drugs and, 422–424

chair-side assisting, 69–76

chemical eye injuries, 493, 559, 565

children, 48, 78–79, 88–89, 366, 374, 486, 490, 566–567, 605–607, 686–687
    strabismus, 146–147, 150–151, 153–157, 158, 172
    surgery, 425
    vision testing in, 93, 95, 96, 98, 99–100, 102–103, 106–108

circulator, 666–667

circulatory system, 549–550

clinical specimen, handling, 449–450

coding, 695–700
    evaluation codes, 697
    eye code, 697–698
    eye exam, elements of, 698–699
    International Classification of Diseases, 701–702
    management codes, 697
    procedure codes, 697–701

color vision, 34, 129–131

communication skills, 78–80

compliance programs, 711–713

complications of contact lens wear
    lens complications, 404–405
    ocular complications, 406–408
    solution reactions, 405–406

computer viruses, 712

cone cells, 22, 34, 93, 94, 112, 339, 612, 787

confocal microscope, 61

confocal scanning laser ophthalmoscopy, 303–304
    conducting scan, 304

confrontation visual fields, 120–122, 760

conjunctiva, 17, 228, 451, 490–493, 625
    conjunctivitis, 443, 446–447, 448–449, 454, 455, 491–493, 580
    growths, 490–491
    trauma, 561–562

conjunctival foreign body, 561–562

contact applanation tonometry, 237–244

contact lenses, 379–415
    complications with, 404–408
    contact lens fitting, 397, 399–402
    diopter/radius conversion, 380
    dispensing, 408–412
        insertion, 408
        removal, 408–411
        wearing schedules, 411–412
    fitting, 396–404
    follow-up care, 413–414
    instrumentation, 388–394
    lacrimal lens, 380–382
    lens care, 412–413
    optics, 379–383
    physical characteristics, 383–385
    pre-fit evaluation, 395–396
        slit lamp exam, 395–396
    presbyopic lenses, 402–404

residual astigmatism, 382–383

rigid contact lenses, 387
    manufacturing, 387
    materials, 387

soft contact lenses, 385–387
    manufacturing, 386–387
    materials, 385–386
    verifying, 394–395

specialty contact lenses, 387–388

vertex distance, 379–380

contact lenses clinical specialist, 6

cornea, 229–230, 493–498
    anatomy, 17
    corneal dystrophies, 496
        anterior basement membrane dystrophy, 496
        Fuchs' dystrophy, 496
    corneal ulcers, 494
    deposits, 496–498
    growths, 496–498
    keratitis, 495
    keratoconus, 495–496
    punctate epithelial erosions, 494
    recurrent corneal erosion, 494
    size, disorders of, 493–494
    superficial punctate keratitis, 494
    surface defects, 494–495

cornea evaluation, 60–61
    confocal microscope, 61
    corneal topographer, 61
    keratometer, 60
    pachymeter, 60–61
    slit lamp biomicroscope, 60
    specular microscope, 61

corneal diameter, 133

corneal procedures
    corneal inlay procedures, 648
    corneal relaxing incisions, 647–648
    laser-based surgery, 646–647
    limbal relaxing incisions, 647–648
    other corneal procedures, 648–649

corneal topographer, 61

corneal topography, 298–300, 390–392

corporate certified ophthalmic assistant, 8

cover testing, 160–162

cranial nerve palsies, 479–480
    disorders/palsies, 147–149, 479–480, 163
        CN II, 545. *See also* optic nerve
        CN III, 148, 151, 479, 480, 545
        CN IV, 149, 479, 545
        CN V, 564
        CN VI, 149, 479–480, 545
        CN VII, 488, 586

cranial nerves, 13, 15, 122, 123, 141, 151, 473–475, 728–730

crystalline lens, 19–20, 499–500
    luxation of lens, 500
    Mittendorf's dot, 500
    subluxation of lens, 500

culture, microbiological culture media, 452–453
curettes, 634
curtain over part of vision, 577
cutaneous sutures, removing, 636–642
cycloplegics, 425–426

dark adaptometry, 341–342
Department of Health and Human Services, 706
depth perception 29, 106, 128, 142, 172
    testing, 128
diabetes, 437–547, 550
    cataracts, 516
    diagnosing, 538–539
    effects on body, 539–540
    effects on eye, 541–545
    gestational diabetes, 538
    prediabetes, 538
    risk for diabetes, 538
    secondary diabetes, 538
    symptoms, 538
    treatment, 540–541
    type 1, 537–538
    type 2, 538
diabetic retinopathy, 504, 543–545
diagnostic imaging, 297–306
    confocal scanning laser ophthalmoscopy, 303–304
    corneal topography, 298–300
    laser interference biometry, 297–298
    optical coherence tomography, 300–303
    specular microscopy, 304–305
diameter gauge (V-gauge), 393–394
diffraction, 42–43
diffuse illumination, 221
dilation, 127–128
diplopia, 141, 578
direct focal illumination, 221
direct ophthalmoscope, 62
direct retroillumination, 221
disaster preparedness plans, 713–714
distance acuity systems, 97–98
distant visual acuity testing, 97–98, 739
double Maddox rod testing, 166–169
dry eye treatment, 433–434
    artificial lubricants, 433
    prescription treatments, 434
Duane syndrome, 151
ductions, 144
dyes, 228, 294–295, 426–427
    fluorescein, 114, 215, 228, 229, 230, 283–286, 388–389, 426, 561
    indocyanine green, 289–290, 427
    lissamine green, 228, 426–427
    methylene blue, 427
    rose bengal, 228, 229, 426

eczema, 550
electro-oculography, 340–341
electronic medical records, 692–694
    security, 692–693
    transferring information into, 693
electronystagmography, 342
electrophysical testing, 335–343
    dark adaptometry, 341–342
    electronystagmography, 342
    electro-oculography, 340–341
    electroretinography, 338–340
    visual evoked potential, 336–338
electroretinography, 338–340
    electroretinogram stimuli, 339
    electroretinogram waveforms, 339
    performing test, 339–340
    results, 340
    types of recording electrodes, 339
email security, 712
Emergency Medical Treatment and Labor Act, 708
endocrine system, 550
episclera/sclera, 493
eso deviations, 146–147
exo deviations, 147
exophthalmometry, 133
external photography, 291–293
extraocular muscles (EOMs) 15, 29–30, 137–175, 475
    accommodation 144–145, 146
    actions/movement 138, 143–145
    amblyopia 153–157, 172, 750
    binocular vision 138, 142, 143
    depth perception 142
    deviations 146–153
    exercises 173–174
    fixation 137–138, 153
    fusion 140–141, 157–160, 171–172
    innervation 13, 138, 143, 151, 475
        paralytic 147–149, 545, 546
    retinal correspondence 141–142, 153, 171–172
    stereopsis 128, 157–158, 752
    surgery 140, 174, 628
    testing 99, 122, 128, 139–140, 156–172, 475, 481, 745–753
eye bank technician, 8
eye exam, 117–135
    angle evaluation, 127
    confrontation visual fields, 120–122
    dilation, 127–128
    extraocular muscle testing, 122
    history taking, 119
    lensometry, 120
    muscle balance, 122
    observation, 118–119
    pupil assessment, 122–127

slit lamp, 127
tonometry, 127
visual acuity, 119
eyelid surgery, 623–625
reconstructive surgery, 624
eyelid trauma, 560–561
eyewear, 363–377

False Claims Act, 708
field of binocular single vision, 172
fixation 93, 108, 137–145, 146, 150–151, 156, 257
eccentric 93, 105, 153, 614
flashes, 21, 33, 502, 520, 577–578, 587
floaters, 20, 21, 33, 231, 502, 520, 577–578, 587
fluorescein angiography, 285–289
descriptive interpretation, 286–287
fundamentals, 285–286
perform, 288
prepare, 288
folliculitis, 493
forced ductions, 162–164
forceps, 633
frames, 363–369
dimensions, 368–369
fitting, 368
markings, 368
parts, 364–366
safety, 369
styles, 366–368
tilt, 375
fraud in health care, preventing, 705–706
Fuchs' dystrophy, 496
functional vision loss, 112–114, 611
fundus autofluorescence, 284–285
fundus photography, 275–284
mydriatic vs nonmydriatic systems, 276
parts of camera, 275–276
special techniques, 282–283
fungi, 447
fusion, 140–141, 157–160, 171–172

gene therapy, 468
genetic counseling, 467
genetics, 459–470
disease, 463–464
family history, 469–470
genetic inheritance, 460–463
genetic testing, 467–468
history of, 459–460
ophthalmic diseases, 464–467
sample collection, 469
Geneva lens clock/measure, 360–361
geometric optics, 41–45

glaucoma, 523–536, 600
central corneal thickness, 533
corneal hysteresis, 533
fundus examination, 531
fundus photography, 533
history taking, 529–531
imaging, 533
optic nerve, 526–527
optical coherence tomography, 533
patient education, 534–535
slit lamp evaluation, 531
tonometry, 531
treatment
medication, 421, 427–428, 527–528, 534–535
surgical treatment, 516, 528–529, 533–534, 542, 627–625
visual field testing, 531–533
gloving, 671
Goldmann applanation tonometry, 764
Goldmann visual fields, 253–267
calibration of Goldmann perimeter, 264
cleaning/maintenance of Goldmann perimeter, 267
performing Goldmann visual field test, 265–267
trial lens selection, 264–265
gonorrhea, 550
governing bodies in compliance, 705–706
gowning, 670–671

haloes around lights, 578
headaches, 480–481
migraine, 480–481
health care compliance, 705–714
compliance programs, 711–713
disaster preparedness plans, 713–714
Health Information Technology for Economic and Clinical Health Act, 708
Health Insurance Portability and Accountability Act, 706–709
hearing impaired patient, 686
Heidelberg Retina Tomograph, 63
helminths, 448
hemostats, 634
Hering's law of equal innervation, 143
Herpes viruses 430, 448–449, 454, 491, 553, 580, 582, 583, 585
Hess/Lees testing, 169–170
Hirschberg measurement, 164, 748
history taking, 77–92, 119, 156, 315–316, 397, 469–470, 481, 517, 529, 531, 545, 554–555, 565, 568–569, 587–588, 613, 650, 687, 738
AIDET model of patient satisfaction, 81, 90
communication skills, 78–81
documentation of, 70, 71, 319, 697

as guide for exam 87–89, 192
parts of, 82–87, 698, 728
types of questions, 81–82
home eye injuries, 568
horopter, 141
host defenses
immune system, 442–443
inflammatory response, 443
human immunodeficiency virus, 430, 501, 553, 631, 691
Humphrey field analyzer, 267–271
calibration of, 267–268
cleaning/maintenance for, 270–271
hyperopia, 43, 46, 104, 184, 186, 204–206, 543
hyperosmotics, 428
hypertension, 550–551
hypertensive retinopathy, 505
hysterical field/vision loss, 66, 112, 113, 263, 611

ice test, 172
imaging clinical specialist, 6
immune system, 442–443
in-office surgical procedures, 631–644
hand washing, 635
patient/site prep, 635
post-surgical patient education, 643
preoperative patient education, 643
surgical supplies, instruments, 632–635
tray set-up, 636
in-office training, 733–772
indentation tonometry
checking calibration, 236
disinfection, 236
technique, 236
indirect retroillumination, 221–222
indocyanine green angiography, 289–291
infants, vision testing in, 106–108
infectious conjunctivitis, 491–492
infectious disease transmission, 443–444
inflammatory response, 443
informed consent 520, 643, 661, 665, 690, 710
injuries related to abuse, 566–567
instrument care
cleaning, 673–674
disinfection, 675–676
inspection, 674
sterilization, 674–675
International Classification of Diseases, codes, 701–702
interpupillary distance. *See* pupillary distance
intracranial visual pathway
disorders of, 475–479
ischemic optic neuropathy, 478–479
multiple sclerosis, 477
ocular sarcoid, 477
optic nerve drusen, 478
pseudotumor cerebri, 478
stroke, 475–477

thyroid eye disease, 477–478
tumors, 477
intraocular pressure
anatomy/physiology of, 18, 31, 233, 523
factors affecting, 84, 234–235, 248
in glaucoma, 125, 523–527, 576
medications to lower, 427–428, 527–528
testing of. *See* tonometry
iris, 230
anatomy, 18–19
ischemic optic neuropathy, 478–479
Ishihara color plate testing, 768

keratoconus, 60, 300, 387, 388, 391, 465, 495–496, 648
keratometer, 60, 389–390
Krimsky measurement, 164, 166, 747

lacrimal kit, 634–635
lacrimal system, 488–490
abnormalities of tear production, dry eye syndrome, 489
infectious, 489
nasolacrimal duct obstruction, 489–490
tear production abnormalities, 488–489
lacrimal/tear system, 13, 16–17, 28–29, 131–132, 488–490, 625, 769–770
laser interference biometry, 297–298
laser surgery, 655–663
laser principles, 655–656
lasers, history of, 655
types of laser surgery, 658–661
laws in health care, 706–710
laws of ocular motility, 142–143
Leber congenital amaurosis, 504
lens centers, finding/marking, 755
lens forms, 369–374
index of refraction, 370
lens tints, coatings, 373–374
lens types, designs, 370–371
materials, 370
prism, 371–372
safety lenses, 372–373
lens power, 48, 347
lensometer/lensometry, 65–66, 348–356, 393
leukemia, 551
licensed practitioners, 3–14
doctor of osteopathy, 4
mid-level practitioners, 4
physician assistant, 4
ophthalmologist, 3
optometrist, 4
light reflex tests, 164–166
listening skills, 79–80
low vision, 611–619
aids, 614–615
disorders associated with, 611–612

history taking, 613
  resources, 617
  terminology, 611
  vision testing, 613–614
low vision aids
  nonoptical low vision aids, 614–615
  optical low vision aids, 614
low vision clinical specialist, 6–7
low vision patient, 686
lupus erythematosus, 552
Lyme disease, 551

macula/macular, 21-23, 34-35, 46, 71, 72, 93, 109, 112,
  253–261, 278, 301–303, 310, 318, 504, 506–507, 543–
  546, 603, 612, 628, 659, 790
macular degeneration, 287, 290, 336, 373, 433, 467, 506–
  507, 517, 603, 612, 658, 659, 725, 791
Maddox rod testing, 166–169
malingering, 66, 112–114, 158, 263, 272, 608
malware, risks, 712
manual keratometry, 772
manual lensometry, 348–356, 754
  manual lensometer use, 351–356
  parts of manual lensometer, 348–351
Marfan syndrome, 551
margin reflex distance, 132–133
Mayo stand set-up, 671
measuring AC/A ratio, 164
measuring strabismus with prism, 749
Medicaid, 706
medical record, 691–692
  access to, 691–692
  charges for, 692
  retention of, 692
medical terminology, 773–778
Medicare, 706
medications, ophthalmic, 779–784
mentally challenged patients, 687
metric system, 720–721
microbes, 441
  binomial nomenclature, 440
  host-microbe relationship, 441
  infectious disease, 441–442
  metric system, 439–440
  microscopy, 440–441
    electron microscopy, 441
    light microscopy, 440–441
  pathogens, 441
microbiology, 439–456
  bacteria, 444–447
  clinical laboratory communication, 455
  clinical specimen, handling, 449–450
  culture, 451–453
  fungi, 447
  helminths, 448
  host defenses

immune system, 442–443
  inflammatory response, 443
infectious disease, 441
laboratory testing, ocular infectious disease, 454
microbes, 441
  binomial nomenclature, 440
  metric system, 439–440
  microscopy, 440–441
microscopy, 450–451
nucleic acid-based tests, 453
prions, 449
protozoa, 448
serologic methods, 453
staining, 450–451
transmission, infectious disease, 443–444
viruses, 448–449
mid-level practitioners, physician assistant, 4
migraine headaches, 480–481
mitochondrial inheritance ophthalmic disease, 465–466
monofixation syndrome, 150–151
motor fusion, defined, 141
motor vehicle-related eye injuries, 567–568
multigenetic ophthalmic disease, 466–467
multiple sclerosis, 477
mydriatics, 425–426
myopia, 46, 48, 104, 184, 185–186, 315–316, 512, 513, 527,
  543, 646

nasolacrimal system. See lacrimal system
near acuity systems, 98–99
near acuity testing, 98–99, 103, 741
near point of accommodation, 759
near point of convergence, 160, 753
nerve palsies
  III N, 148, 479
  IV N, 148, 479
  VI N, 149, 479
nerve palsies, prism treatment, 174–175
neuro-ophthalmic disorders, 152
neuro-ophthalmology, 473–482
  headaches, 480–481
  history, 481
  imaging, 482–483
  intracranial visual pathway, disorders of, 475–479
  motility disorders, 479–480
  optic nerve, visual pathways, 475
  trauma, 479
  vision assessment, 481
  visual field testing, 482
night blindness, 504
non-English-speaking patients, 686
noncontact applanation tonometry, 244–247
normal retinal correspondence, 141–142
nucleic acid-based tests, 453
nystagmus, 152–153, 480

observation, 118–119
occupational injuries, 568
Occupational Safety and Health Administration, 706
ocular anatomy, 11–26
    anterior segment, 17–20
        anterior chamber, 17–19
        external globe, 17
        posterior chamber, 19–20
    blood supply, 13–14
    embryology, 23–26
    extraocular muscles, 15
    eyelids, 15–16
    lacrimal system, 16–17
    lashes, 15–16
    nerve supply, 13
        cranial nerves affecting eye, 13
    posterior segment, 20–23
        optic nerve, 22–23
        retina, 21–22
        vitreous body, 20–21
    skull, 11–13
        bony orbit, 11–13
    uveal tract, 20
ocular histoplasmosis syndrome, 505
ocular immunology specialty, 596–597
ocular motility, 137–177
ocular physiology, 27–37
    aqueous humor, 31
    blinking, 27–28
    blood, 36
    blood cells, 36
    bony orbit, 29
    conjunctiva, 30
    cornea, 30–31
    crystalline lens, 32
    dry eye, 28–29
    extraocular muscles, 29–30
    light, visual pathways, 35–36
    response to insult, 36–37
        allergy, 37
        infection, 36
        injury/inflammation, 36
    retina, 33–35
        macula, 34–35
        optic nerve head, 35
        photoreceptor layer, 33–34
    tear film, 28–29
        dry eye, 28–29
    uveal tract, 31–32
    vitreous, 32–33
ocular sarcoid, 477
ocular trauma, 557–572
    basic eye examination, 569
    classification, 557–558
    epidemiology, 557
    history taking, 568–569
    irrigation, 570

patient education, 570–571
precautions, 569
tissue reactions to injury, 558–559
triage, 569–570
types of injuries, 559–560
Office of Inspector General, 705–706
operating room personnel
    anesthesiologist, 666
    anesthetist, 666
    circulator, 666–667
    surgeon, 666
    surgical assistant, 666
operating room set-up
    back table, 667–668
    instrument stand, 668–669
    ophthalmic instruments, 669
    preparation table, 667
ophthalmic drug identification, 420
ophthalmic equipment, 57–68
    cornea evaluation, 60–61
        confocal microscope, 61
        corneal topographer, 61
        keratometer, 60
        pachymeter, 60–61
        slit lamp biomicroscope, 60
        specular microscope, 61
    imaging eye, 62–64
        anterior segment, 62–63
        diagnostic ultrasound, 64
        digital retinal camera, 63
        Heidelberg Retina Tomograph, 63
        optical coherence tomography, 64
    refractive error evaluation, 57–60
        autorefractor, 58
        phoropter, 57
        retinoscope, 58–60
        semiautomatic refractor/phoropter, 57–58
        trial lenses/frames, 58
ophthalmic medications, 779–784
ophthalmic photography, 275–296
    external photography, 291–293
    fluorescein angiography, 285–289
    fundus autofluorescence, 284–285
    fundus photography, 275–284
    indocyanine green angiography, 289–291
    patient services, 285
    slip lamp photography, 293–295
ophthalmic surgery, 623–630
    anterior segment procedures, 625–630
        anterior chamber reconstructive surgery, 627
        anterior vitrectomy, 627
        cataract procedures, 627
        conjunctiva, 625
        glaucoma surgery, 627–628
        intraocular lens implant, 627
        nonrefractive corneal surgery, 625–626
        orbital surgery, 629

retinal surgery, 628
strabismus surgery, 628
vitreous surgery, 628
brow surgery, 623–625
eyelid surgery, 623–625
reconstructive surgery, 624
lacrimal surgery, 625
ophthalmic ultrasound, 307–334
A-scan biometry, 310–311
biometry procedures, 312–314
contact biometry, 312–313
immersion biometry, 313–314
biometry results, 314–315
equipment, 312
exam, 315–320
maintenance, 330–333
physical principles, 307–309
standardized A-scan, 325–328
standardized B-scan, 319–325
ultrasound in ophthalmology, 309–310
optic nerve, 13, 22–23, 35, 502–504
coloboma, 503–504
cupping, 502–503
physiologic cupping, 502–503
drusen, 478, 503
optic neuritis, 503
pallor, 503
papilledema, 503
pseudopapilledema, 503
visual pathway, 22–23
visual pathways, 475
optical center of lens, 347–348
optical coherence tomography, 64, 300–303, 392
common abnormalities, 301–303
normal findings, 301
optical cross, 48–49
optical equipment
instruments, 65–68
biometer, 67–68
pupillometer, 67
transilluminator, 67
intraocular pressure evaluation, 64–65
lensometer, 65–66
peripheral vision evaluation, 66
perimeters, 66
tangent screen, 66
pupillometer, 65
radiuscope, 66
retina evaluation, 62
binocular indirect ophthalmoscope, 62
direct ophthalmoscope, 62
testing vision, 57
optical personnel, 8–9
ocularist, 8–9
ophthalmic laboratory technician, 9
optician, 8

prosthetist, 8–9
optical procedures, 347–361
automated lensometry, 356
frame measurement, 357–359
Geneva lens clock, 360–361
Geneva lens measure, 361
lens measurement, 357–359
lens power, 347
manual lensometry, 348–356
optical center of lens, 347–348
pupillary distance, 356
spectacle prescription format, 348
transposition, 348
vertex distance, 359–360
optics, 39–53
geometric optics, 41–45
lens power, 48
optical cross, 48–49
physical optics, 39–41
physiologic optics, 45–48
Prentice's rule, 50–51
prism power, calculating, 50
retinal image size, 48
spherical equivalent, 52
transposition, 51–52
vertex distance, 49–50
orbital disorders, 490
orbital injury, 563–565
orthoptics, 7–8

pachymeter, 60–61
painful eye, 580–583
painless red eye, 585
paralytic strabismus, 147–149
passwords, use of, 711
patterns of genetic inheritance, 460–463
pencil push-ups, 173
penetrating eye injuries, 562–563
penetrating trauma, 559
perimeters, 66
periorbital skin, 485–486
cancerous lesions, 485
nonmalignant lesions, 485–486
skin conditions affecting, 486
personal protective equipment, 671
pharmacology, 419–434
allergic reactions, 424
allergies, medications for, 432
anesthetics, 424–425
anti-infective agents, 428–431
anti-inflammatory drugs, 431–432
antiglaucoma agents, 427–428
botulinum, 434
central nervous system, drugs and, 422–424
cycloplegics, 425–426
dry eye treatment, 433–434

dyes, 426–427
hyperosmotics, 428
immunosuppressives, 432
medication characteristics, 420–422
mydriatics, 425–426
ophthalmic drug identification, 420
retinal disease, drugs for, 433
sealants, 434
side effects, 424
systemic drugs, ocular effects of, 434
phlyctenulosis, 493
phoropter, 57–58, 188, 190–192
photography, ophthalmic, 275–296. *See also* ophthalmic photography
photography clinical specialist, 6
photophobia, 583–584
physical optics, 39–41
physician assistant, 4
physiologic optics, 45–48
physiology, ocular, 27–37
    aqueous humor, 31
    blinking, 27–28
    blood, 36
    bony orbit, 29
    conjunctiva, 30
    cornea, 30–31
    crystalline lens, 32
    extraocular muscles, 29–30
    light, visual pathways, 35–36
    response to insult, 36–37
        allergy, 37
        infection, 36
        injury/inflammation, 36
    retina, 33–35
        macula, 34–35
        optic nerve head, 35
        photoreceptor layer, 33–34
    tear film, 28–29
        dry eye, 28–29
    uveal tract, 31–32
    vitreous, 32–33
pinhole test, 105, 111, 192, 588, 740
pinpoint illumination, 224–226
plus cylinder refractometry
    binocular balancing, 197
    duochrome test, 196–197
    initial sphere power, 193–194
    plus cylinder axis, 194–195
    plus cylinder power, 195–196
    sphere power, 196
posterior chamber, lens, 231–232
pregnant patients, 687
prematurity, retinopathy of, 505
Prentice's rule, 50–51
presbyopia, 19, 33, 46–47, 104, 179, 192, 369, 385, 387, 402–404, 543, 598, 599, 625, 645, 648, 650, 701, 793
prions, 449

prism power, calculating, 50
prism vergences, 159–160
prisms, 44–45
procedure codes, 697–701
protozoa, 448
proximal illumination, 222–224
pseudostrabismus, 147
pseudotumor cerebri, 478
psoriasis, 551
ptosis, 586
pupillary distance, 51, 65, 66, 348, 356–357, 369, 756
pupillometer, 65, 67, 356
pupil(s),
    abnormalities, 123, 124–125, 148, 388, 479, 480, 525, 542, 545, 581, 586, 627
        afferent pupillary defect (Marcus Gunn pupil), 113, 123, 125, 126, 558
    anatomy, 13, 18–19, 31–32, 112, 148
    dilation of, 127–128, 231, 421, 425–426. *See also* dilation
    evaluation/testing, 67, 122–127, 157, 403, 482, 531, 743–744
    physiology of, 31–32, 45, 47–48, 422–423, 474

quadrantanopia, 793

radiation injuries, 559–560, 565–566
radiuscope, 66, 392–393
range of motion test, 751
record keeping, 689–691
red filter test, 171–172
Red Flag Rule, 710
reflection, 41
refractive conditions
    aphakia 47, 230, 315, 627
    presbyopia 19, 32, 46–47, 100, 179
        correction 201–203, 204, 205, 402–404, 578, 649–650
        multifocal lenses 370–371
refractive errors
    astigmatism 43, 46, 47, 52, 104, 154, 238, 240, 495, 578
    hyperiopia 43, 46, 104, 184, 186, 204–206, 543
    myopia 46, 48, 104, 184, 185–186, 315–316, 512, 513, 527, 543, 646
refractive surgery, 645–654
    corneal procedures, 646–649
    history taking, 650–652
    intraoperative considerations, 652
    lens-based correction, 649–650
    measurements, 650–652
    postoperative considerations, 652–653
    pretesting, 650–652
refractometry, 188–206
    dynamic cross cylinder lens method, 201–202
    errors in refractometry, 206
    glasses check, 206
    instrumentation, 57–60, 188–191

minus cylinder refractometry, 197–201
plus cylinder refractometry, 193–197
power, 201–203, 204–205
range for add power, 202–203
set-up, 191–192
technique, 193
trial lenses method, 202
regulatory acts, 706–710
respiratory system, 549
reticle magnifier, 393
retina, 504–509
albinism, 504
congenital stationary night blindness, 504
detachments, 505
diabetic retinopathy, 504
fundus flavimaculatus, 504
hypertensive retinopathy, 505
Leber congenital amaurosis, 504
macula, 506–507
age-related macular degeneration, 507
central serous chorioretinopathy, 506
epiretinal membrane, 506–507
macular edema, 506
macular hole, 506
vitreomacular traction, 506
ocular histoplasmosis syndrome, 505
retinal artery, vein occlusions, 505–506
retinitis pigmentosa, 504
retinopathy of prematurity, 505
Stargardt's disease, 504
tears, 505
tumors, 507–508
lymphoma, 508
metastatic tumors, 508
retinoblastoma, 507–508
retinal correspondence, 141–142
tests, 171–172
retinal disease, drugs for, 433
retinal image size, 48
retinitis pigmentosa, 504
retinoscope, 58–60, 180–181
retinoscopy, 180–188
troubleshooting, 185
working distance, 183–184, 185–186
rheumatoid arthritis, 552
rod cells, 34, 339, 612, 794
rosacea, 552
rubella, 553–554
rubeola, 554

saccades, 143–144, 164
sarcoidosis, 554
Schirmer's tear test, 769
sclera, 17, 493
sclerotic scatter, 222
scribing, 69–76

documentation, 70–71
examination, 71–74
assessment, 72
findings, 71–72
plan, 72–74
scrubbing, 669–670
sealants, 434
sensorimotor unit, eyes as, 140–141
sensory fusion, defined, 140
set-up, operating room
back table, 667–668
instrument stand, 668–669
ophthalmic instruments, 669
preparation table, 667
Sherrington's law of reciprocal innervation, 143
sickle cell disease, 552
silicone oil, 315
single Maddox rod testing, 166–169
Sjögren's syndrome, 493
sleep apnea, 552
slip lamp photography, 293–295
slit lamp, 127
auxiliary items, 218
diopter lens, 217–218
goniolens, 217
Hruby lens, 217–218
parts of, 216–217
tonometer, 217
slit lamp biomicroscope, 60, 388–38
slit lamp microscopy, 213–232
anterior chamber, 230–231
auxiliary items, 217–219
conjunctiva, 228
cornea, 229–230
examination, 226–232
external, 228
focusing, 227–228
focusing oculars, 220
illumination, 220–226
diffuse illumination, 221
direct focal illumination, 221
direct retroillumination, 221
indirect retroillumination, 221–222
pinpoint illumination, 224–226
proximal illumination, 222–224
sclerotic scatter, 222
specular reflection, 226
tangential illumination, 221
transillumination of iris, 226
iris, 230
maintenance, 219–220
parts, 214–217
posterior chamber, lens, 231–232
troubleshooting, 219–220
smooth pursuit evaluation, 164
soft contact lenses, verifying, 394–395

sonography, clinical specialty, 7
special patient populations, 685–688
    aphasic, 686
    blind, 686
    deaf, 686
    hearing impaired, 686
    history taking, 89–91
    low vision, 686
    mentally challenged, 687
    non-English speaking, 686
    pregnant women, 687
    in wheelchair, 686
    young children, 686–687
specialties, 594–609
    cataract surgeons, 597–598
    cornea, 594–596
    electrophysiology, 607–608
    glaucoma, 600
    neuro-ophthalmology, 603–604
    ocular genetics, 604–605
    ocular oncology, 600–602
    oculoplastics, 594
    pediatrics, 607
    refractive surgery, 598–600
    research, 608
    strabismus, 605–607
    uveitis, 596–597
    vitreous, 602–603
specimen handling, 449–450
spectacle lenses, 369
spectacle prescription format, 348
spectacles, 363–377
specular microscope, 61
specular microscopy, 304–305
    conducting scan, 305
    image analysis, 305
specular reflection, 226
speculums, 634
spherical equivalent, 52, 196, 200, 203, 265
sports eye injuries, 566
standard (universal) precautions, 631–632
Stargardt's disease, 504
Stark Laws I, II, and III, 709
statistics, 723
stereo testing, 128, 157–158, 752
stereogram cards, 173–174
stereopsis assessment, 128
sterile fields, 672
Stevens-Johnson syndrome, 493, 552
strabismus. See also extraocular muscles
    accommodative, 145, 146–147, 172, 193, 198
    eso deviations, 146–147
    exo deviations, 146, 147
    paralytic, 147–149
    phoria, 122, 146, 161–162
    tropia, 122, 146–147, 161–162

stroke, 475–477
subspecialties, specialties, retina, 602–603
surgery, ophthalmic, 623–630
    anterior segment procedures, 625–630
        anterior chamber reconstructive surgery, 627
        anterior vitrectomy, 627
        cataract procedures, 627
        conjunctiva, 625
        glaucoma surgery, 627–628
        nonrefractive corneal surgery, 625–626
        orbital surgery, 629
        retinal surgery, 628
        strabismus surgery, 628
    eyelid surgery, 623–625
        reconstructive surgery, 624
    lacrimal surgery, 625
surgical assistant, 7, 666
surgical assisting, 665–679
    gloving, 671
    gowning, 670–671
    informed consent, 665
    instrument care, 673–676
    Mayo stand set-up, 671
    operating room personnel, 665–667
    operating room set-up, 667
    passing instruments, 672–673
    personal protective equipment, 671
    scrubbing, 669–670
    sterile fields, 672
surgical supplies, office, 633
surgical technologist, 7
sutures, 632
synoptophore, 170–170
syphilis, 552
systemic drugs, ocular effects of, 434
systemic lupus erythematosus, 552
systemic viral infections, 553–554

tangent screen, 66, 262–263
tangential illumination, 221
tear break-up time, 770
tear testing, 131–132
tears, retina, 505
temporal arteritis, 554
terminology, 684–685, 773–778
    charting, 684–685
    coding, 684–685
    federal incentives, 685
    insurance, 685
    medical, 773–778
    regulatory, 685
testing vision. See vision testing, visual acuity testing
thermal injuries, 560
thyroid eye disease, 151–152, 477–478, 554
tonometer, 45, 64–65, 217, 233–249

tonometry, 127, 233–251, 764–765. *See also* intraocular
  pressure, glaucoma
    applanation, 236–247
        contact applanation tonometry, 237–244
        noncontact applanation tonometry, 244–247
    cleaning, 247–248
    indentation, 235–236
        checking calibration, 236
        disinfection, 236
        technique, 236
    palpation, 235
    physics of, 234
    potential risks, 247
    sources of error, 247
total internal reflection, 41–42
trade regulation rules for ophthalmic practices, 710
training, in-office, 733–772
    hiring, 733–734
    history taking, 738
    training plan, 735–736
transient loss of vision, 577
transillumination of iris, 226
transilluminator, 67
transposition, 51–52, 348
trauma, ocular, 557–572
    basic eye examination, 569
    blunt trauma, 559
    chemical injuries, 559, 565
    classification, 557–558
    epidemiology, 557
    eyelid trauma, 560–561
    globe injury, 563–565
    history taking, 568–569
    home eye injuries, 568
    injuries related to abuse, 566–567
    irrigation, 570
    late complications, 558–559
    motor vehicle-related eye injuries, 567–568
    occupational injuries, 568
    orbital injury, 563–565
    patient education, 570–571
    penetrating eye injuries/trauma, 559, 562–563
    precautions, 569
    radiation injury, 559–560, 565–566
    sports eye injuries, 566
    thermal injury, 560, 565–566
    tissue reactions to injury, 558–559
    triage, 569–570
    types of injuries, 559–560

ulcers, corneal, 494
ultrasonography as clinical specialty, 7
ultrasound, ophthalmic, 307–334
    A-scan, 7, 297, 483, 517
        basic sciences, 307–310
        procedures, 312–319, 325, 328

    B-scan, 7, 64
        basic sciences, 307–310
        procedures, 319–325
    biomicroscopy, 328–330
    documentation, 319
    equipment, 309–310, 312–313, 319, 325, 328
    erroneous readings, 318
    gating, 317
    landmarking, 318
    maintenance, 330–333
    patient history, 315–316
    physical principles, 307–309
        frequency, 307–308
        gain, 309
        reflectivity, 309
        resolution, 308
        sound, 307–308
        velocity, 308–309
        wavelengths, 308
    quality checks, 317–318
    reproducibility, 317–318
    standardized A-scan, 325–330
    standardized B-scan, 319–325
        axial scans, 321–322
        longitudinal scan, 324
        screening technique, 325
        transverse scan, 322–323
universal/standard precautions, 631–632
uveal tract, 500–502
    choroid, 501
        melanoma, 501
        nevus, 501
    ciliary body, 501
        ciliary body melanoma, 501
    coloboma, 500
    iris, 500
        albinism, 500
        Lisch nodules, 500
        pigmentary dispersion syndrome, 500
    uveitis, 501–502
        anterior uveitis, 501
        causes of uveitis, 501–502
        intermediate uveitis, 501
        posterior uveitis, 501

vergence, 144–145
versions, 144
vertex distance, 49–50, 359–360, 374–375, 757
vertical deviation, 147
viral infections, 553–554
    adenovirus, 553
    herpes simplex, 553
    herpes zoster, 553
    human immunodeficiency virus, 553
    rubella, 553–554
    rubeola, 554

viruses, 448–449
vision testing. *See also* visual acuity testing
    contrast sensitivity, 108–109, 110
    glare testing, 109–111, 517
    macular photostress test, 112
    malingering, 112–114
    potential acuity, 111–112
visual acuity test types, 95–99, 105–106
visual acuity testing, 100–108, 119, 403, 613–614, 739–742
    documentation, 102–103, 105–106
    and fixation, 93
    infants/young children, 93, 95, 96, 99, 100, 103, 106–107, 742
    occlusion, 101
    optotypes, 94–97, 99–100, 108
    pinhole, 104, 740
    testing distance, 94
visual evoked potential, 336–338
visual fields, 253–274
    automated/Humphrey visual fields, 267–271
    confrontation, 120–122, 577, 613
    diagnostic use of, 271–273, 475–476, 613
    and glaucoma, 233, 262, 524, 530, 531–533
    Goldmann visual fields, 253–267
    instrumentation, 66, 262, 263–264, 267
    tangent screen, 262–263
    and visual pathway, 253, 255–256, 257–261, 475–476
vitreous, 11, 20–21, 32–33, 502
    asteroid hyalosis, 502
    posterior vitreous detachment, 502
    vitritis, 502

wheelchair-bound patients, 686
Wilson's disease, 554
word parts, 773–777
    prefixes, 774–776
    root word parts, 777
    suffixes, 776–777
Worth 4 dot test, 158–159

X-linked disease, 465
xanthelasma, 486, 542, 795

young children, 686–687
    vision testing in, 106
        central, steady, maintained, 107
        fix and follow, 106–107
        forced preferential looking, 107

zonules, 19, 32, 301, 329, 500, 511, 796